The Royal Marsden Manual of

Clinical Nursing Procedures

Student Edition

The Royal Marsden Manual of Clinical Nursing Procedures

Ninth Edition

Edited by

Lisa Dougherty

OBE, RN, MSc, DClinP

Nurse Consultant Intravenous Therapy

The Royal Marsden NHS Foundation Trust

Sara Lister

RN, PGDAE, BSc (Hons), MSc, MBACP

Head of Pastoral Care and Psychological Support

The Royal Marsden NHS Foundation Trust

Alexandra West-Oram

MSc, BSc (Hons), PG Dip (Ed), RN, RT

Programme Leader

The Royal Marsden School

The Royal Marsden NHS Foundation Trust

The ROYAL MARSDEN

NHS Foundation Trust

WILEY Blackwell

A John Wiley & Sons, Ltd., Publication

This edition first published 2015

Previous editions published 1992, 1996, 2000, 2004, 2008, 2011

Registered office:
John Wiley & Sons, Ltd, The Atrium, Southern Gate, Chichester, West Sussex, PO19 8SQ, UK

Editorial offices:
9600 Garsington Road, Oxford, OX4 2DQ, UK
The Atrium, Southern Gate, Chichester, West Sussex, PO19 8SQ, UK
111 River Street, Hoboken, NJ 07030-5774, USA

For details of our global editorial offices, for customer services and for information about how to apply for permission to reuse the copyright material in this book please see our website at www.wiley.com/wiley-blackwell

Library of Congress Cataloging-in-Publication Data is available for this title

A catalogue record for this book is available from the British Library.

Wiley also publishes its books in a variety of electronic formats. Some content that appears in print may not be available in electronic books.

Cover design by Design Deluxe

Set in 9/10 pt Lexia by Aptara, Inc., New Delhi, India
Printed and bound in Singapore by Markono Print Media Pte Ltd

1 2015

Brief table of contents

Detailed table of contents

6 Moving and positioning 201

7 Nutrition, fluid balance and blood transfusion 247

Part Four

Supporting the patient through treatment

Foreword to the ninth edition

As the Chief Nurse of The Royal Marsden NHS Foundation Trust, and a contributor and clinical user of the manual for many years, it is a special pleasure and honour to be asked to introduce the ninth Student edition of *The Royal Marsden Manual of Clinical Nursing Procedures*. The manual is internationally renowned and used by nurses across the world to ensure their practice is evidence based and effective. As information becomes ever more available to the consumers of healthcare, it is essential that the manual is updated frequently so that it reflects the most current evidence to inform our clinical practice.

More than ever in 2015, nurses need to be able to assure the public, patients and their families that care is based on the best available evidence. As nurses seeking to improve our care, it is essential that we are able to critically analyse our judgements in the light of current knowledge. For all of us working with patients and their families there is an imperative to question and renew our practice using the many sources of knowledge available to us. In the busy world of clinical practice in a ward, unit or in the community, it can be challenging to find time to search for the evidence and this is where the Student edition of *The Royal Marsden Manual of Clinical Nursing Procedures* is a real practical help.

As in the eighth edition, reviewing the evidence or sources of knowledge has been made more explicit with each level of evidence graded. This grading provides the reader with an understanding of whether the reference comes from a randomized controlled trial, national or international guidance, or from expert opinion. At its best, clinical nursing care is an amalgam of a sensitive therapeutic relationship coupled with effective care based on the best evidence that exists. Some areas of practice have attracted international research such as cardiopulmonary resuscitation and infection prevention and control; other areas of practice have not attracted such robust research and therefore it is more of a challenge to ensure evidence-based care. Each time a new edition of the manual is prepared, we reflect on the gaps in research and knowledge; this provides the impetus to develop new concept analyses and develop further research studies. In this new edition, the chapters have incorporated risk management, and legal and professional issues. In addition, the procedures were tried out by the student nurses from Kingston University and St Georges University of London to ensure they worked in practice. This new student edition incorporates a breadth of tools to support your learning including objectives at the beginning of each chapter, and a variety of learning activities that will either test your knowledge or prompt you to consider how you may apply what you are learning in practice.

As you look at the list of contributors to the manual you will see that this edition has continued to be written by nurses who are expert and active in clinical practice. This has the double advantage of ensuring that this manual reflects the reality of practice, but also ensures that nurses at The Royal Marsden NHS Foundation Trust are frequently reviewing the evidence and reflecting upon their care.

A textbook devoted to improving and enhancing clinical practice needs to be alive to the clinical practitioner. You will see that this edition has continued the improvement in format, including many more figures and photographs to make the manual more effective in clinical care.

As I commend this ninth Student edition of *The Royal Marsden Manual of Clinical Nursing Procedures* to you, I am aware that it will be used in many different countries and settings. Having had the privilege of visiting and meeting nurses across the world I know that there are more commonalities than differences between us. The common theme is, of course, the need to ensure that we as nurses provide care that is individually and sensitively planned and that it is based on the best available evidence. The Student edition of *The Royal Marsden Manual of Clinical Nursing Procedures* is a wonderful resource for such evidence and I hope it will be widely used in all clinical settings across the world.

Finally, I would like to pay a warm tribute to the excellent work undertaken by the three editors, Lisa Dougherty, Sara Lister and Alexandra West-Oram, and to all the nurses and allied health professionals at The Royal Marsden Hospital who have worked so hard on this ninth edition.

Dr Shelley Dolan
Chief Nurse
The Royal Marsden NHS Foundation Trust
Clinical Director
London Cancer Alliance

Acknowledgements

A book is a team effort and never more so than with this Student edition of *The Royal Marsden Manual of Clinical Nursing Procedures*.

Since the first edition of the manual was published in 1984, the range of procedures in nursing has grown in complexity, and the depth of the theoretical content underpinning them has increased considerably. Authors have, therefore, had to keep up-to-date with the ever-changing research evidence and write new, as well as update existing, material. This continues to be a collaborative task carried out by knowledgeable, expert nurses in partnership with members of the multidisciplinary team including pharmacists, physiotherapists, occupational therapists, dietitians, speech therapists, radiographers, anaesthetists, operating department practitioners and psychological care.

So, we must thank every member of the 'team' who has helped to produce this edition, for their time, effort and perseverance. An additional challenge has been to co-ordinate the increased number of contributors to each chapter. This responsibility has fallen to the lead chapter authors, so, for this, they deserve a special acknowledgement and thanks for their ability to integrate all the contributions and create comprehensive chapters.

We especially appreciate the work done by Anne Tibbles, Senior Lecturer Nursing, and the nursing students at Kingston University and St George's University of London, who reviewed all of the procedures used by students and gave us invaluable feedback on how they work in practice. We would also like to thank some other key people: Dale Russell and the library team of the David Adams Library at The Royal Marsden School of Cancer Nursing and Rehabilitation for their help and support in providing the references required by the authors and setting up the Endnote system; Stephen Millward and the medical photography team for all the new photographs; our families and friends who continue to encourage us, especially during the last two years – the time it takes to edit the manual; and, finally, our thanks go to Martin Davies, Magenta Styles, Karen Moore, Tom Bates and Helen Harvey at Wiley for their advice and support in all aspects of the publishing process.

Lisa Dougherty
Sara Lister
Alexandra West-Oram

List of contributors

Janice Barrett RN, BSc (Hons), PG Dip HE, MA
Sister, Critical Care Outreach
(Chapter 9: Respiratory care)

Helen Bass RGN, BSc (Hons) Nursing, MSc (Advancing Healthcare)
Lead Nurse, Clinical Education
(Chapter 8: Patient comfort and end-of-life care)

Helen Benson GPhC, MPharm (Hons), MSc
Associate Chief Pharmacist, Clinical Research and Development
(Chapter 12: Medicines management)

Louise Bisset Dip HE (Adult Nursing), BN (ICU)
Sister, Critical Care Outreach
(Chapter 9: Respiratory care)

Linda Bloomfield RGN, PG Cert, Dip HE (Nursing), DN Cert, OND
Discharge/Safeguarding Deputy
(Chapter 2: Assessment and discharge)

Grainne Brady BSc, Cert MRCSLT
Highly Specialist Speech and Language Therapist
(Chapter 7: Nutrition, fluid balance and blood transfusion)

Joanne Bull RN, MSc (Strategic Leadership and Expert Practice, Cancer), BN (Hons), Dip (Oncology)
Matron, Admissions and Preassessment, Clinical Assessment Unit, Outpatients and Rapid Diagnostic Assessment Centre
(Chapter 13: Perioperative care)

Nicholas Bultitude Registered ODP, BA (Hons), MSc (Healthcare Management)
Formerly, Divisional Operational Manager, Anaesthetics and Surgical Support
(Chapter 13: Perioperative care)

Maureen Carruthers RN, Dip (Oncology), BSc (Hons), MSc
Macmillan Matron, Palliative Care
(Chapter 8: Patient comfort and end-of-life care)

Suzanne Chapman MSc, BSc, RGN
Clinical Nurse Specialist, Pain Management
(Chapter 8: Patient comfort and end-of-life care)

Lydia Clark BA, BSc, Dip (Oncology)
Ward Sister
(Chapter 5: Elimination)

Michael Connolly MPhil, BSc, RGN
Consultant Nurse, Supportive and Palliative Care
South Manchester University Hospital
(Chapter 4: Communication)

Jill Cooper MSc, DMS, DipCOT
Head Occupational Therapist
(Chapter 6: Moving and positioning)

Michelle Davies BSc (Hons), RD
Home Enteral Feeding/Community Dietitian
(Chapter 7: Nutrition, fluid balance and blood transfusion)

Andrew Dimech RN, BN, MSc (ICU), Dip (Oncology)
Head, Clinical Technical Services
(Chapter 10: Interpreting diagnostic tests)

Laura Dopson BSc (Hons), RGN, NMP
Clinical Nurse Specialist, Pain Management
(Chapter 8: Patient comfort and end-of-life care)

Lisa Dougherty OBE, RN, MSc, DClinP
Nurse Consultant, Intravenous Therapy
(Chapter 12: Medicines management)

Andreia Fernandes RN, BSc, MSc
Clinical Nurse Specialist, Gynaecology Oncology
(Chapter 8: Patient comfort and end-of-life care; Chapter 10: Interpreting diagnostic tests)

Cathryn Forsythe RN, Dip HE, BSc (Hons)
Senior Staff Nurse, Critical Care
(Chapter 10: Interpreting diagnostic tests)

Sharon Giles BSc (Hons), MSc
MRI Research Radiographer
(Chapter 10: Interpreting diagnostic tests)

Rosie Goatley BSc (General Nursing, Intensive Care)
Sister, Critical Care Outreach
(Chapter 9: Respiratory care)

Amanda Gunning RGM
Lead Nurse, Stoma Care
(Chapter 5: Elimination)

Diz Hackman MSc, PG Dip (Physiotherapy)
Clinical Specialist Physiotherapist
(Chapter 6: Moving and positioning)

Ruth Hammond MSc (Advanced Cancer Practice) BSc (Adult Nursing)
Clinical Practice Educator
(Chapter 11: Observations)

Michael Hansford RMN, PG Dip (Counselling), MA (Counselling and Psychotherapy)
Staff Counsellor
(Chapter 4: Communication)

Zoe Hayman Registered Paramedic, Cert HE (Para Sci)
Resuscitation Lead
(Chapter 9: Respiratory care)

Nikki Hunter RN, BSc, MSc, MA
Complex Discharge Nurse
(Chapter 2: Assessment and discharge)

Kate Jones MCSP, HCPC, Dip (Physiotherapy), MSc
Clinical Specialist Physiotherapist
(Chapter 6: Moving and positioning)

Jon M. Knox RGN, Dip HE, BSc (Hons), PG Dip, RNIP, SCP
Advanced Nurse Practitioner, Plastics and Reconstructive Surgery
(Chapter 14: Wound management)

Sara Lister RN, PGDAE, BSc (Hons), MSc, MBACP
Head of Pastoral Care and Psychological Support
(Chapter 1: Introduction; Chapter 4: Communication)

Jennifer Mackenzie RN, BN, Cert (Intensive Care)
Sister, Critical Care
(Chapter 10: Interpreting diagnostic tests)

Katharine Malhotra MSc (Rehabilitation), PG Cert (Clinical Education), BSc (Hons) (Physiotherapy)
Allied Health Lecturer Practitioner
(Chapter 6: Moving and positioning)

Rebecca Martin RN, MSc, BSc (Hons), Independent Nurse Prescriber
Advanced Nurse Practitioner, Urology
(Chapter 5: Elimination; Chapter 13: Perioperative care)

Nuala McClaren BSc (General Nursing, Intensive Care)
Sister, Critical Care Outreach
(Chapter 9: Respiratory care)

Hayley McHugh BSc (Hons), RN, Cert (Intensive Care)
Senior Staff Nurse, Intensive Care
(Chapter 7: Nutrition, fluid balance and blood transfusion; Chapter 10: Interpreting diagnostic tests)

Wendy McSporran RGN, BSc (Hons), PG Dip
Transfusion Practitioner
(Chapter 7: Nutrition, fluid balance and blood transfusion)

Anita McWhirter GPhC, BSc (Hons), MSc
Pharmacy Clinical Services Manager
(Chapter 12: Medicines management)

Dee Mears DCR(R), DMS
CT Superintendent
(Chapter 10: Interpreting diagnostic tests)

Carolyn Moore MCSP, SRP
Superintendent Physiotherapist
(Chapter 6: Moving and positioning)

Philipa Nightingale BN, Nurse Practitioner
Senior Staff Nurse
(Chapter 2: Assessment and discharge)

Claire Nowell BSc (Hons), MSc
Senior Physiotherapist
(Chapter 6: Moving and positioning)

Luke Perrie BSc (General Nursing, Intensive Care), Independent Nurse Prescriber
Sister, Critical Care Outreach
(Chapter 9: Respiratory care)

Scott Pollock Dip (Social Work), BA (Hons), MSc
Discharge and Vulnerable Adult Lead
(Chapter 2: Assessment and discharge; Chapter 4: Communication)

Tessa Renouf RN, MSc (Advanced Cancer Practice), BSc (Hons), Dip (Oncology)
Lead Sister, Admissions and Preassessment Unit
(Chapter 13: Perioperative care)

Justin Roe BA (Hons), PG Dip, MSc, PhD, Cert MRCSLT
Joint Head, Speech and Language Therapy and Allied Health Professions Researcher, Project Lead
(Chapter 4: Communication; Chapter 7: Nutrition, fluid balance and blood transfusion)

Lara Roskelly RN, Dip (General, Community Psychiatric Nursing and Midwifery), Dip (ICU), Independent Nurse Prescriber
Matron, Critical Care Outreach and Resuscitation
(Chapter 9: Respiratory care; Chapter 10: Interpreting diagnostic tests)

Janet Schmitt BSc (Hons), PG Cert (Ed), MSc
Neuro-therapy Manager
(Chapter 6: Moving and positioning; Chapter 9: Respiratory care)

Richard Schorstein RN, BSc, PG Dip, Nurse Practitioner
Matron/Nurse Practitioner
(Chapter 2: Assessment and discharge)

Clare Shaw PhD (Nutrition), BSc (Hons) (Nutrition), PG Dip (Dietetics)
Consultant Dietitian
(Chapter 7: Nutrition, fluid balance and blood transfusion)

Louise Soanes RGN/RSCN, BSc, MSc
Teenage Cancer Trust Nurse Consultant, Adolescents and Young Adults
(Chapter 10: Interpreting diagnostic tests)

Heather Spurgeon RN, BSc (Critical Care Nursing), MSc (Adult Critical Care)
Matron, Critical Care and Theatres
(Chapter 11: Observations)

Anna-Marie Stevens MSc, BSc (Hons), RN
Macmillan Nurse Consultant, Palliative Care
(Chapter 8: Patient comfort and end-of-life care)

Nicola Tinne MSc (Advanced Cancer Practice), BSc (Cancer Nursing), Dip HE (Nursing Studies), RGN
Formerly, Clinical Nurse Specialist, Head and Neck Cancers
(Chapter 14: Wound management)

Richard Towers RGN, BSc (Hons), MSc, Professional Doctorate Nursing
Lead Nurse Counsellor/Lecturer Practitioner
(Chapter 4: Communication)

Simon Tuddenham RN, BN (Hons), BA (Hons)
Staff Nurse, Critical Care
(Chapter 10: Interpreting diagnostic tests)

Vanessa Franklin Urbina MSc (Nutrition and Dietetics), RD
Senior Specialist Dietitian
(Chapter 7: Nutrition, fluid balance and blood transfusion)

Susan Vyoral BSc (Hons), RD
Dietitian
(Chapter 7: Nutrition, fluid balance and blood transfusion)

Victoria Ward RN, BN (Hons), MSc
Matron/Nurse Practitioner
(Chapter 2: Assessment and discharge)

Paul Weaving BSc, RGN, MSc
Formerly, Associate Director, Infection Prevention and Control
(Chapter 3: Infection prevention and control)

Alexandra West-Oram MSc, BSc (Hons), PG Dip (Ed), RN, RT
Programme Leader, The Royal Marsden School
(Chapter 5: Elimination)

Catherine Wilson PhD, MSc, BSc (Hons), PG Dip (Ed), RN, Dip HE (Palliative Care), Cert Oncology Nursing
Head of School, The Royal Marsden School
(Chapter 4: Communication)

Barbara Witt RN
Nurse, Phlebotomist
(Chapter 10: Interpreting diagnostic tests)

Luv Wootton BSc (General Nursing, Intensive Care)
Sister, Critical Care Outreach
(Chapter 9: Respiratory care)

Lynn Worley RGN, RMN, BSc (Hons) (Cancer Practice)
Clinical Nurse Specialist, Plastic Surgery and Tissue Viability
(Chapter 14: Wound management)

The authors and Wiley are hugely grateful to the nursing staff and students at Kingston University and St George's University London for their help in the development of this edition.

Nursing staff

Cathy Chia RN, RM, RMN, Cert Ed, BSc (Hons), MSc
Senior Lecturer, Simulated Learning and Clinical Skills

Karen Elliott RN, BSC (Hons), PGCE
Senior Lecturer, Simulated Learning and Clinical Skills

Terry Firth RN, BA (Hons), RNT
Senior Lecturer, Simulated Learning and Clinical Skills.

Suchita Hathiramani MCSP, BSc, MSC, FHEA
Senior Lecturer, Simulated Learning and Clinical Skill

Francina Hyatt RN, Dip N, BSC (Hons)
Senior Lecturer, Simulated Learning and Clinical Skills

Jo Low
Clinical Skills Laboratory Manager

Tracey Marshall RN, BSc (Hons)
Nutrition Specialist Nurse, St George's Hospital

Barry Pearse RN, BA (Hons), PGCE
Senior Lecturer, Simulated Learning and Clinical Skills

Hazel Ridgers RN, DipHE, BA (Hons), MA
Senior Lecturer, Simulated Learning and Clinical Skills

Susan Rush RN, MSC, RNT
Associate Professor, Simulated Learning and Clinical Skills

Annie Spalton RN, Dip N, RNT
Senior Lecturer, Simulated Learning and Clinical Skills

Anne Tibbles TD, MSc, MA, PG Dip, PGCE, BSc (Hons), Dip N (Lond), RN
Senior Lecturer, Simulated Learning and Clinical Skills

Student cohorts

Diploma in Nursing students: September 2010 and February 2011

BSc Nursing students: September 2011 and September 2012

PG Dip Nursing students: February 2012 and September 2012

List of abbreviations

AAC	augmentive or alternative communication
AAGBI	Association of Anaesthetists of Great Britain and Ireland
ABG	arterial blood gas
ABPM	ambulatory blood pressure monitoring
AD	autonomic dysreflexia
ADH	antidiuretic hormone
ADR	adverse drug reaction
A&E	accident and emergency
AED	automated external defibrillator
AIDS	acquired immune deficiency syndrome
ALARP	as low as reasonably practicable
ALS	advanced life support
ALT	alanine aminotransferase
ANH	acute normovolaemic haemodilution
ANP	atrial natriuretic peptide
ANS	autonomic nervous system
ANTT	aseptic non-touch technique
AP	alkaline phosphatase/anteroposterior/alternating pressure
APTR	activated partial thromboplastin ratio
ARDS	adult respiratory distress syndrome
ART	assisted reproductive techniques
ASA	American Society of Anesthesiologists
AST	aspartate aminotransferase
AT	anaerobic threshold
AV	atrioventricular
AVPU	alert, verbal, pain, unresponsive
BAL	bronchoalveolar lavage
BIA	bio-electrical impedance analysis
BiPAP	bilevel positive airway pressure
BLS	basic life support
BME	black and minority ethnic
BMI	body mass index
BNF	British National Formulary
BP	blood pressure
BSE	bovine spongiform encephalopathy
CAUTI	catheter-associated urinary tract infection
CCU	coronary care unit
cfu	colony-forming unit
CHG	chlorhexidine gluconate
CJD	Creutzfeldt–Jakob disease
CLP	continuous low pressure
CMV	cytomegalovirus
CNCP	chronic non-cancer pain
CNS	central nervous system
CO	cardiac output
COAD	chronic obstructive airways disease
COPD	chronic obstructive pulmonary disease
CPAP	continuous positive airway pressure
CPET	cardiopulmonary exercise testing
CPNB	continuous peripheral nerve block
CPR	cardiopulmonary resuscitation
CRP	C-reactive protein
CSF	cerebrospinal fluid
CSP	Chartered Society of Physiotherapy
CSU	catheter specimen of urine
CT	computed tomography
CTZ	chemoreceptor trigger zone
CVA	cerebrovascular accident
CVAD	central venous access device
CVC	central venous catheter
CVP	central venous pressure
CXR	chest X-ray
DBE	deep breathing exercises
DIC	disseminated intravascular coagulation
DKA	diabetic ketoacidosis
DM	diabetes mellitus
DMSO	dimethylsulphoxide
DNA	did not attend
DNAR	do not attempt resuscitation
DPI	dry powder inhaler
DRE	digital rectal examination
DRF	digital removal of faeces
DVT	deep vein thrombosis
EBN	evidence-based nursing
EBP	evidence-based practice
ECF	extracellular fluid
ECG	electrocardiogram
ECM	extracellular matrix
EDTA	ethylenediamine tetra-acetic acid
ELISA	enzyme-linked immunosorbent assay
EMR	endoscopic mucosal resection
ENT	Ear, Nose and Throat
ESD	endoscopic submucosal dissection
ESR	erythrocyte sedimentation rate
ETT	endotracheal tube
EU	European Union
EWS	early warning scoring
FBC	full blood count
FEES	fibreoptic endoscopic evaluation of swallowing
FFP	fresh frozen plasma
FRC	functional residual capacity
FVC	forced vital capacity
FWB	fully weight bearing
GCS	Glasgow Coma Scale
GFR	glomerular filtration rate
GGT	gamma-glutamyl transpeptidase
GI	gastrointestinal
GMC	General Medical Council
GM-CSF	granulocyte macrophage-colony stimulating factor
GSL	general sales list medicine
GTN	glyceryl trinitrate
HBPM	home blood pressure monitoring
HBV	hepatitis B virus
HCA	healthcare assistant
HCAI	healthcare-associated infection
HCP	healthcare professional
HCV	hepatitis C virus
HDU	high-dependency unit
HEPA	high-efficiency particulate air
HFEA	Human Fertilisation and Embryology Authority
HFOT	high-flow oxygen therapy
HIV	human immunodeficiency virus
HLA	human leucocyte antigen
HME	heat and moisture exchanger

HOCF	Home Oxygen Consent Form
HOOF	Home Oxygen Ordering Form
HPA	Health Protection Agency
HPV	human papillomavirus
HR	heart rate
HSE	Health and Safety Executive
HTLV	human T cell leukaemia/lymphoma virus
IAD	incontinence-associated dermatitis
IASP	International Association for the Study of Pain
IBCT	incorrect blood component transfused
IC	inspiratory capacity
ICF	intracellular fluid
ICP	intracranial pressure
ICS	intraoperative cell salvage
ICSI	intracytoplasmic sperm injection
IM	intramuscular
INR	international normalized ratio
IO	intraosseous
IPCT	infection prevention and control team
ISC	intermittent self-catheterization
ITDD	intrathecal drug delivery
ITU	intensive therapy unit
IV	intravenous
JVP	jugular venous pressure
LA	local anaesthetic
LBC	liquid-based cytology
LCT	long-chain triglyceride
LMA	laryngeal mask airway
LMN	lower motor neurone
LOS	lower oesophageal sphincter
LPA	Lasting Power of Attorney
MAOI	monoamine oxidase inhibitor
MAP	mean arterial pressure
MAR	medicines administration record
MC&S	Microscopy, Culture and Sensitivity
MCT	medium-chain triglyceride
MDA	Medical Devices Agency
MDI	metered dose inhaler
MDT	multidisciplinary team
MESA	microepididymal sperm aspiration
MET	medical emergency team
MHRA	Medicines and Healthcare Products Regulatory Agency
MI	myocardial infarction
MIC	minimum inhibitory concentration
MMP	matrix metalloprotease
MPQ	McGill Pain Questionnaire
MRC	Medical Research Council
MRI	magnetic resonance imaging
MRSA	meticillin-resistant *Staphylococcus aureus*
MS	multiple sclerosis
MSCC	metastatic spinal cord compression
MSU	midstream urine
MUAC	mid upper arm circumference
MUST	Malnutrition Universal Screening Tool
NAT	nucleic acid testing
NBM	nil by mouth
NEWS	National Early Warning Score
NG	nasogastric
NHS	National Health Service
NHSCSP	NHS cervical screening programme
NIPEE	non-invasive positive end-expiration
NIV	non-invasive ventilation
NMC	Nursing and Midwifery Council
NMDA	N-methyl-D-aspartate
NPC	National Prescribing Centre
NPSA	National Patient Safety Agency
NPWT	negative pressure wound therapy
NRAT	Norgine Risk Assessment Tool
NRS	numerical rating scale
NSAID	non-steroidal anti-inflammatory drug
NWB	non-weight bearing
ODP	operating department practitioner
OGD	oesophagogastroduodenoscopy
OSCE	objective structured clinical examination
OT	occupational therapist
OTC	over the counter
P	pharmacy-only medicine
PACU	post-anaesthetic care unit
PAD	pre-operative autologous donation
PART	patient-at-risk team
PCA	patient-controlled analgesia
PCEA	patient-controlled epidural analgesia
PDPH	post-dural puncture headache
PE	pulmonary embolus
PEA	pulseless electrical activity
PEEP	positive end-expiratory pressure
PEF	peak expiratory flow
PEG	percutaneous endoscopically placed gastrostomy
PEP	post-exposure prophylaxis
PESA	percutaneous epididymal sperm aspiration
PGD	Patient Group Direction
PHCT	primary healthcare team
PHN	post-herpetic neuralgia
PICC	peripherally inserted central cannula
PN	parenteral nutrition
PNS	peripheral nervous system
POA	pre-operative assessment
POCT	point-of-care testing
POM	prescription-only medicine
PONV	post-operative nausea and vomiting
PPE	personal protective equipment
PRBC	packed red blood cell
PrP	prion protein
PSCC	primary/benign spinal cord compression
PT	physiotherapist
PTFE	polytetrafluoroethylene
PUO	pyrexia of unknown origin
PVC	polyvinyl chloride
PWB	partially weight bearing
PWO	partial withdrawal occlusion
RA	right atrium
RAS	reticular activating system
RBC	red blood cell
RCN	Royal College of Nursing
RCT	randomized controlled trial
RFID	radiofrequency identification tag
RIG	radiologically inserted gastrostomy
RNI	reference nutrient intake
RSV	respiratory syncytial virus
SA	sinoatrial
SaBTO	Safety of Blood, Tissues and Organs
SAP	Single Assessment Process
SARS	severe acute respiratory syndrome
SBAR	Situation, Background, Assessment, Recommendation
SC	subcutaneous
SCC	spinal cord compression
SCI	spinal cord injury
SGA	subjective global assessment
SHOT	Serious Hazards of Transfusion
SIMV	synchronized intermittent mandatory ventilation
SIRS	systemic inflammatory response syndrome
SIU	spinal injuries unit
SL	semi-lunar
SLT	speech and language therapist
SMBG	self-monitoring of blood glucose
SNRI	serotonin-norepinephrine reuptake inhibitor
SOP	Standard Operating Procedure
SPa	suprapubic aspirate

SSRI	selective serotonin reuptake inhibitor
SV	stroke volume
SVC	superior vena cava
swg	standard wire gauge
TACO	transfusion-associated cardiac overload
TA-GVHD	transfusion-associated graft-versus-host disease
TB	tuberculosis
TCA	tricyclic antidepressant
TED	thromboembolic deterrent
TENS	transcutaneous electrical nerve stimulation
TESE	testicular sperm extraction
TIVA	total intravenous anaesthesia
TPI	*Treponema pallidum* immobilization
TRALI	transfusion-related acute lung injury
TSE	transmissible spongiform encephalopathy
TSS	toxic shock syndrome
TTO	to take out
TURBT	transurethral resection of bladder tumour
TURP	transurethral resection of prostate
UMN	upper motor neurone
UTI	urinary tract infection
VAD	vascular access device
VAP	ventilator-associated pneumonia
VAT	Venous Assessment Tool
VBG	venous blood gas
vCJD	variant Creutzfeldt–Jakob disease
VDRL	Venereal Disease Research Laboratory
VEGF	vascular endothelial growth factor
VF	ventricular fibrillation
VPF	vascular permeability factor
V/Q	ventilation/perfusion
VT	ventricular tachycardia
VTE	venous thromboembolism
WBC	white blood cell
WBIT	wrong blood in tube
WHO	World Health Organization
WOB	work of breathing
WR	Wassermann reaction

Quick reference to the procedure guidelines

How to use your manual

Features contained within your textbook

The **overview page** gives a summary of the topics covered in each part.

Part One

Managing the patient journey

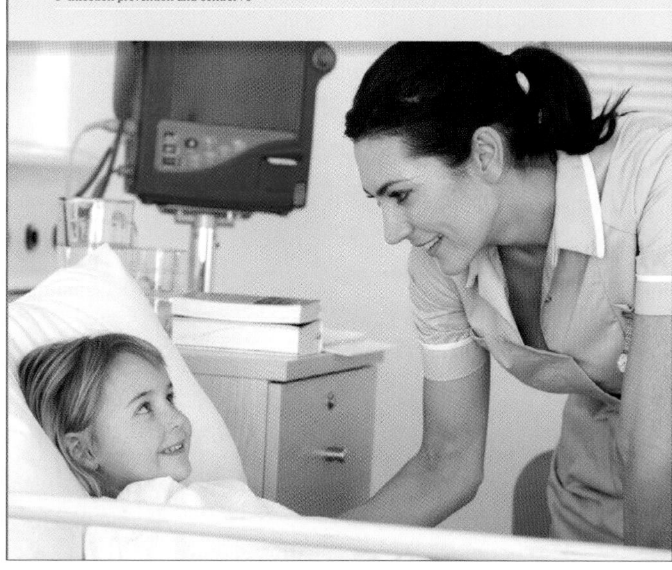

Learning outcomes give a summary of the topics covered in a chapter.

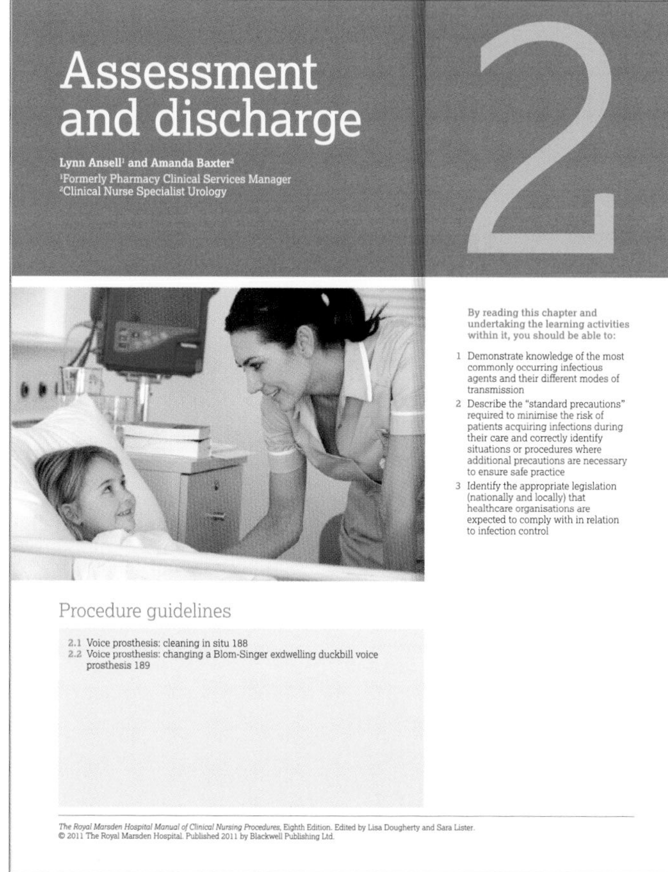

Assessment and discharge

2

Lynn Ansell[1] and Amanda Baxter[2]

[1]Formerly Pharmacy Clinical Services Manager

[2]Clinical Nurse Specialist Urology

By reading this chapter and undertaking the learning activities within it, you should be able to:

1 Demonstrate knowledge of the most commonly occurring infectious agents and their different modes of transmission
2 Describe the "standard precautions" required to minimise the risk of patients acquiring infections during their care and correctly identify situations or procedures where additional precautions are necessary to ensure safe practice
3 Identify the appropriate legislation (nationally and locally) that healthcare organisations are expected to comply with in relation to infection control

Procedure guidelines

2.1 Voice prosthesis: cleaning in situ 188
2.2 Voice prosthesis: changing a Blom-Singer exdwelling duckbill voice prosthesis 189

The Royal Marsden Hospital Manual of Clinical Nursing Procedures, Eighth Edition. Edited by Lisa Dougherty and Sara Lister.
© 2011 The Royal Marsden Hospital. Published 2011 by Blackwell Publishing Ltd.

Check your knowledge lets you check how much you think you know about the topic already.

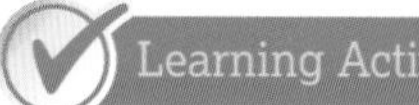

Learning Activity 3.1

Check your knowledge

Try this activity before you look at Box 3.1!

1 What do the following words mean?
- Pathogen.
- Colonization.

2 What is the difference between the following:
- Universal precautions and standard precautions?
- Source isolation and protective isolation?
- Barrier nursing and reverse barrier nursing?

Go to Box 3.1 to find the answers.

Learning in practice asks you to consider issues within your practice environment.

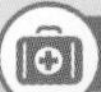

Learning Activity 2.5

Learning in practice: Complex discharge planning

Identify a patient who requires complex discharge planning. Review the discharge documentation for the patient and compare with the '**Guide to arranging a complex discharge home**' (see Box 2.8).

- Have all these steps been followed for your patient?
- Is there anything missing?
- What can you do to help?

Discuss this activity with a friend or your mentor to see if there is anything that could be done differently for this or future patients who have complex needs on discharge from hospital to home.

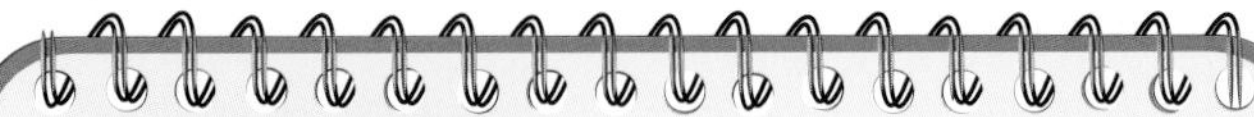

Case studies provide learning around a particular patient case.

Learning Activity 3.4 **Case study**

Mr Peters is a 74-year-old man who has a history of chronic obstructive pulmonary disease. He lives alone and became unwell 7 days ago, feeling fatigued with a productive cough and elevated temperature. He was diagnosed with a chest infection and admitted to hospital for intravenous antibiotics. Having completed his course of antibiotics yesterday, he has now had five episodes of diarrhoea in the last 12 hours. He is being cared for in a six-bedded bay on a male medical ward and is expecting his daughter to visit him later today with his two young grandchildren.

1 What precautions should be taken for this patient? For how long?
2 What information would you give to Mr Peters and why?
3 Would the precautions you take be any different if you were visiting Mr Peters in his own home? If so, how?

See the end of the chapter for the answers.

Scenarios challenge you to think how you would act in a given situation.

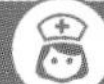

Learning Activity 5.2

Scenario: Urinary catheterization

You have been asked to catheterize a female patient (under supervision) who has been found to have urinary retention.

1 What factors should you consider prior to the procedure?
2 What steps can you take to minimize the risk of her developing a catheter-associated urinary tract infection?
3 What should you do after the procedure?

Hint: You should have come up with 4–5 points for each question.

See the end of the chapter for the answers.

Key point boxes at the end of each chapter highlight the essential points to remember.

Key points

- Many infections acquired by patients receiving healthcare are preventable through use of diligent hand hygiene and correct aseptic technique.
- The majority of healthcare-associated infections are endogenous (from organisms already present on an individual's body), highlighting the importance of effective skin cleansing prior to invasive procedures.
- Standard precautions must be taken with all patients at all times regardless of their infection status.
- Additional precautions may be required if patients are vulnerable to infection themselves or are colonized or infected with a micro-organism that may be a risk to others, or both.
- Infection prevention and control procedures must be followed at all times in order to minimize the risk of contamination and infection transmission.

Your textbook is full of **photographs**, **illustrations** and **tables**.

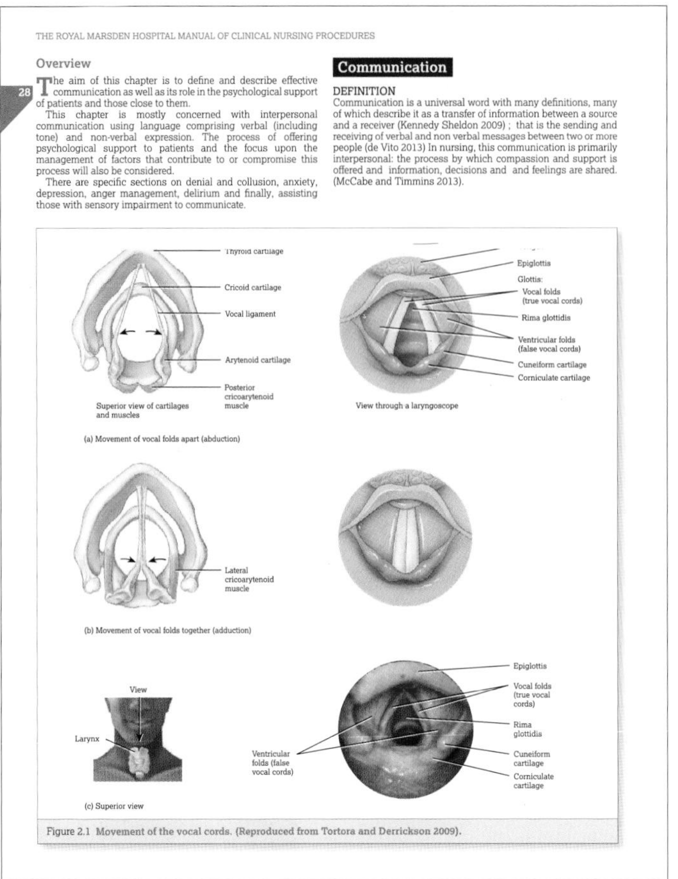

THE ROYAL MARSDEN HOSPITAL MANUAL OF CLINICAL NURSING PROCEDURES

28

Overview

The aim of this chapter is to define and describe effective communication as well as its role in the psychological support of patients and those close to them.

This chapter is mostly concerned with interpersonal communication using language comprising verbal (including tone) and non-verbal expression. The process of offering psychological support to patients and the focus upon the management of factors that contribute to or compromise this process will also be considered.

There are specific sections on denial and collusion, anxiety, depression, anger management, delirium and finally, assisting those with sensory impairment to communicate.

Communication

DEFINITION

Communication is a universal word with many definitions, many of which describe it as a transfer of information between a source and a receiver (Kennedy Sheldon 2009) ; that is the sending and receiving of verbal and non verbal messages between two or more people (de Vito 2013) In nursing, this communication is primarily interpersonal: the process by which compassion and support is offered and information, decisions and and feelings are shared. (McCabe and Timmins 2013).

Figure 2.1 Movement of the vocal cords. (Reproduced from Tortora and Derrickson 2009).

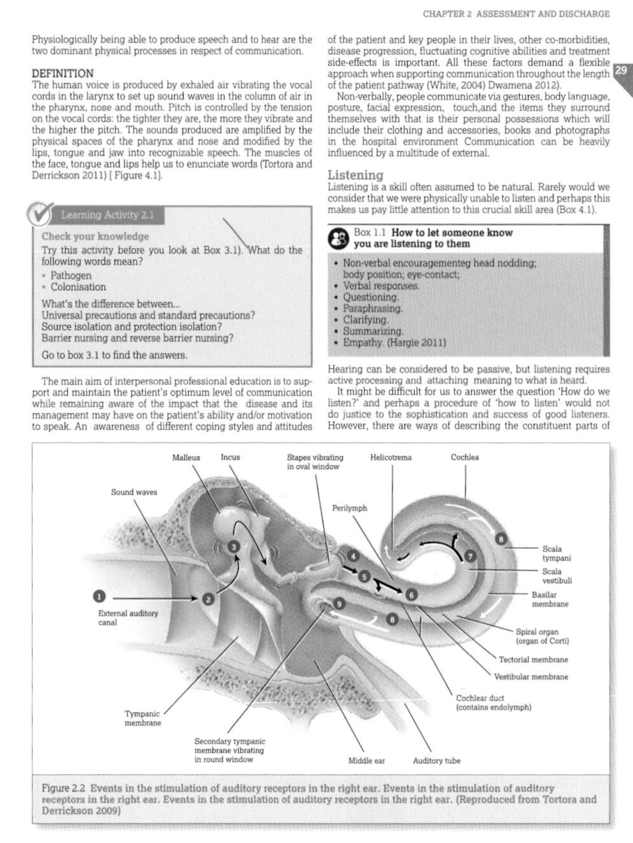

CHAPTER 2 ASSESSMENT AND DISCHARGE

29

Physiologically being able to produce speech and to hear are the two dominant physical processes in respect of communication.

DEFINITION

The human voice is produced by exhaled air vibrating the vocal cords in the larynx to set up sound waves in the column of air in the pharynx, nose and mouth. Pitch is controlled by the tension on the vocal cords: the tighter they are, the more they vibrate and the higher the pitch. The sounds produced are amplified by the physical spaces of the pharynx and nose and modified by the lips, tongue and jaw into recognizable speech. The muscles of the face, tongue and lips help us to enunciate words (Tortora and Derrickson 2011) [Figure 4.1].

Learning Activity 2.1

Check your knowledge

Try this activity before you look at Box 3.1). What do the following words mean?

- Pathogen
- Colonisation

What's the difference between...
Universal precautions and standard precautions?
Source isolation and protection isolation?
Barrier nursing and reverse barrier nursing?

Go to box 3.1 to find the answers.

The main aim of interpersonal professional education is to support and maintain the patient's optimum level of communication while remaining aware of the impact that the disease and its management may have on the patient's ability and/or motivation to speak. An awareness of different coping styles and attitudes of the patient and key people in their lives, other co-morbidities, disease progression, fluctuating cognitive abilities and treatment side-effects is important. All these factors demand a flexible approach when supporting communication throughout the length of the patient pathway (White, 2004) Dwamena 2012).

Non-verbally, people communicate via gestures, body language, posture, facial expression, touch,and the items they surround themselves with that is their personal possessions which will include their clothing and accessories, books and photographs in the hospital environment Communication can be heavily influenced by a multitude of external.

Listening

Listening is a skill often assumed to be natural. Rarely would we consider that we were physically unable to listen and perhaps this makes us pay little attention to this crucial skill area (Box 4.1).

Box 1.1 **How to let someone know you are listening to them**

- Non-verbal encouragementeg head nodding; body position; eye-contact;
- Verbal responses.
- Questioning.
- Paraphrasing.
- Clarifying.
- Summarizing.
- Empathy. (Hargie 2011)

Hearing can be considered to be passive, but listening requires active processing and attaching meaning to what is heard.

It might be difficult for us to answer the question 'How do we listen?' and perhaps a procedure of 'how to listen' would not do justice to the sophistication and success of good listeners. However, there are ways of describing the constituent parts of

Figure 2.2 Events in the stimulation of auditory receptors in the right ear. Events in the stimulation of auditory receptors in the right ear. Events in the stimulation of auditory receptors in the right ear. (Reproduced from Tortora and Derrickson 2009)

Learning exercises help you test yourself after each chapter.

Now Test Yourself

This section provides a range of exercises/activities to further test your learning. For additional exercises visit **www.royalmarsdenmanual.com/student**.

What have you learnt?

1 For which of the following modes of transmission is good hand hygiene a key preventative measure? (circle as many as are relevant)

A Airborne
B Direct contact
C Indirect contact
D Droplet
E All of the above

2 If you were told by a nurse at handover to take 'standard precautions' what would you expect to be doing?

A Taking precautions when handling blood and 'high risk' body fluids so as not to pass on any infection to the patient
B Wearing gloves, aprons and mask when caring for someone in protective isolation
C Asking relatives to wash their hands when visiting patients in the clinical setting
D Using appropriate hand hygiene, wearing gloves and aprons when necessary, disposing of used sharp instruments safely and providing care in a suitably clean environment to protect yourself and the patients.

3 *Hand hygiene:* when caring for a patient who has, or is suspected of having, *Clostridium difficile* why should you use soap and water rather than alcohol handrubs?

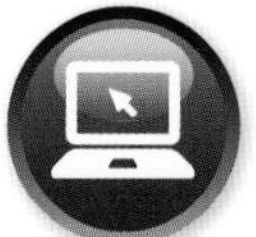

The **website icon** indicates that you can find more learning exercises on a topic by visiting the companion website.

About the companion website

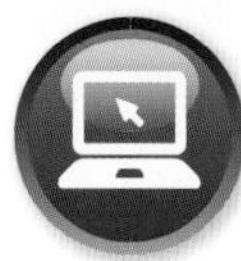

Don't forget to visit the companion website for this book:

www.royalmarsdenmanual.com/student

There you will find valuable material designed to enhance your learning, including:

- Interactive multiple choice questions
- Step-by-step: drag and drop the steps of Clinical procedures into the correct order. Check whether you have the right sequence and print out a copy for handy reference.
- Flashcards: view figures with labels off and labels on for self-testing
- References from the book

Scan this QR code to visit the companion website

Introduction

1

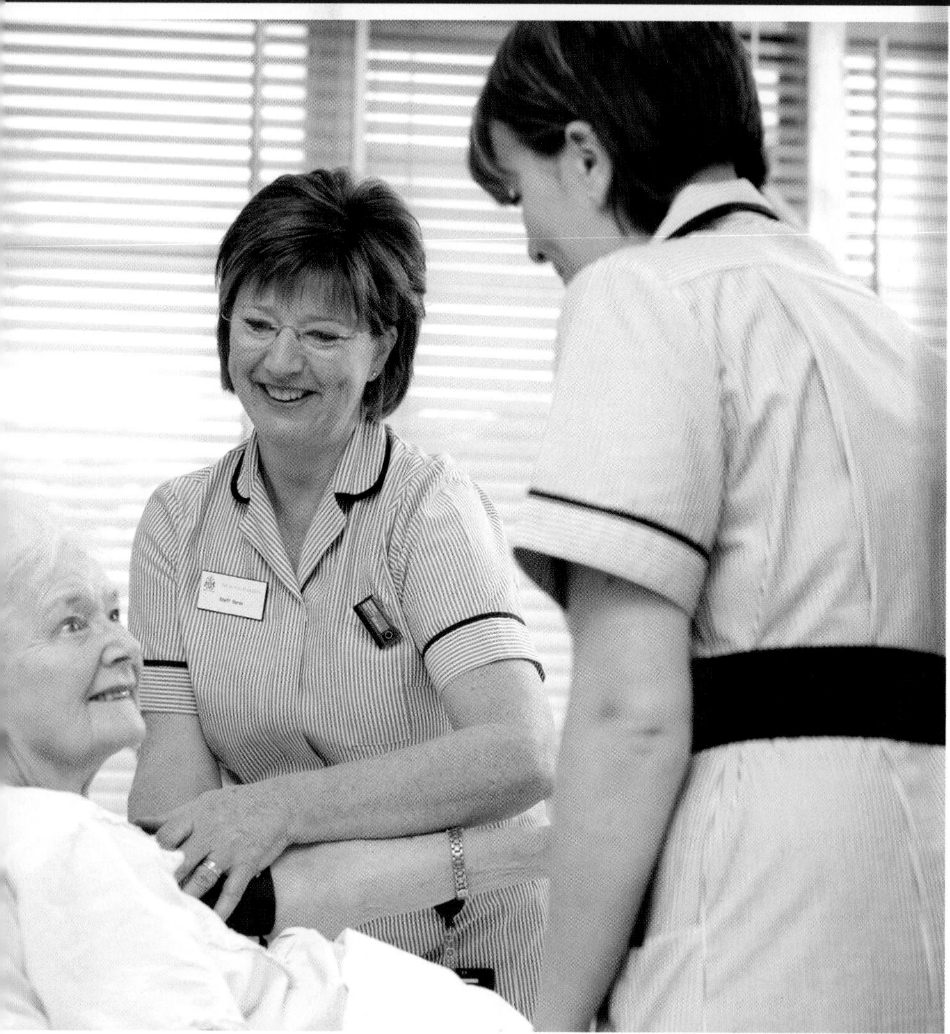

The Royal Marsden Manual of Clinical Nursing Procedures: Student Edition, Ninth Edition. Edited by Lisa Dougherty, Sara Lister and Alexandra West-Oram

Overview

The first edition of *The Royal Marsden Manual of Clinical Nursing Procedures* was produced in the early 1980s as a core procedure manual for safe nursing practice within The Royal Marsden Hospital, the first cancer hospital in the world. Implicit behind that first edition was the drive to ensure that patients received the very best care – expertise in carrying out clinical procedures combined with an attitude of respect and compassion.

Thirty years later these attitudes are still fundamental. The Chief Nurse Jane Cummings has 'committed to make sure all patients receive the very best care with compassion and clinical skill' (DH 2013). The values and behaviours of this compassionate practice are: *Care, Compassion, Competence, Communication, Courage and Commitment* – the 6Cs (DH 2013). This manual of clinical procedures focuses on bringing together current evidence, acting as an essential resource for practice and providing the theory underpinning *Competence*, one of the 6Cs.

This ninth student edition includes a range of new learning features throughout each chapter that have been designed to support student nurses as they use this manual to support learning in clinical practice. In line with the ninth professional edition, it focuses for the first time on procedures that are applicable in all areas of acute inpatient hospital care. (Procedures specific to the care of the cancer patient can be found in the new companion volume *The Royal Marsden Clinical Cancer Nursing Procedures*.) The Manual is informed by the day-to-day practice in the hospital and conversely is the corporate policy and procedure document for the adult inpatient service of the organization. It therefore does not cover all aspects of acute nursing practice or those relating to children's or community nursing. However, it does contain the procedures and changes in practice that reflect modern acute nursing care.

Core to nursing, wherever it takes place, is the commitment to care for individuals and to keep them safe so that when and wherever the procedures are used, they are to be carried out within the framework of the Nursing and Midwifery Code, Appendix 1 (NMC 2015). In respect of clinical competency, the NMC Code states that you must:

- have the knowledge and skills for safe and effective practice without direct supervision
- keep your knowledge and skills up to date throughout your working life
- recognize and work within the limits of your competence (NMC 2015).

The Manual has been structured to enable nurses to develop competency, recognizing that competence is not just about knowing how to do something but also about understanding the rationale for doing it and the impact it may have on the patient.

Some of the procedures in the Manual will be newer for nursing. Developing new roles and taking responsibility for new procedures have obvious risks attached, and although every individual nurse is accountable for their own actions, every healthcare organization has to take vicarious liability for the care, treatment and procedures that take place. An organization will have expectations of all its nurses in respect of keeping patients, themselves and the environment safe. There are obvious ethical and moral reasons for this: 'Nurses have a moral obligation to protect those we serve and to provide the best care we have available' (Wilson 2005, p.118). Risk management has therefore become an integral part of day-to-day nursing work. For this reason, the risk management implications of the areas of practice have been integrated into each chapter.

Evidence-based practice

The moral obligation described above extends to the evidence upon which we base our practice. Nursing now exists in a healthcare arena that routinely uses evidence to support decisions and nurses must justify their rationales for practice. Where historically, nursing and specifically clinical procedures were based on rituals rather than research (Ford and Walsh 1994, Walsh and Ford 1989), evidence-based practice (EBP) now forms an integral part of practice, education, management, strategy and policy. Nursing care must be appropriate, timely and based on the best available evidence.

What is evidence-based practice?

Evidence-based practice has been described by Sackett, a pioneer in introducing EBP in UK healthcare, as:

> 'the conscientious, explicit and judicious use of current best evidence in making decisions about the care of the individual patients. The practice of evidence-based medicine means integrating individual clinical expertise with the best available external clinical evidence from systematic research' (Sackett et al. 1996, p.72).

Despite the emphasis on research in EBP, it is important to note that where research is lacking, other forms of evidence can be equally informative when making decisions about practice. Evidence-based practice goes much wider than research-based practice and encompasses clinical expertise as well as other forms of knowing, such as those outlined in Carper's seminal work (1978) in nursing. These include:

- empirical evidence
- aesthetic evidence
- ethical evidence
- personal evidence.

This issue is evident throughout this Manual where clinical expertise and guidelines inform the actions and rationale of the procedures. Indeed, these other types of evidence are highly important as long as we can still apply scrutiny to their use.

Porter (2010) describes a wider empirical base upon which nurses make decisions and argues for nurses to take into account and be transparent about other forms of knowledge such as ethical, personal and aesthetic knowing, echoing Carper (1978). By doing this, and through acknowledging limitations to these less empirical forms of knowledge, nurses can justify their use of them to some extent. Furthermore, in response to Paley's (2006) critique of EBP as a failure to holistically assess a situation, nursing needs to guard against cherry-picking, ensure EBP is not brandished ubiquitously and indiscriminately and know when judicious use of, for example, experiential knowledge (as a form of personal knowing) might be more appropriate.

Evidence-based nursing (EBN) and EBP are differentiated by Scott and McSherry (2009) in that EBN involves additional elements in its implementation. Evidence-based nursing is regarded as an ongoing process by which evidence is integrated into practice and clinical expertise is critically evaluated against patient involvement and optimal care (Scott and McSherry 2009). For nurses to implement EBN, four key requirements are outlined (Scott and McSherry 2009).

1. To be aware of what EBN means.
2. To know what constitutes evidence.
3. To understand how EBN differs from evidence-based medicine and EBP.
4. To understand the process of engaging with and applying the evidence.

We contextualize our information and decisions to reach best practice for patients and the ability to use research evidence and clinical expertise together with the preferences and circumstances of the patient to arrive at the best possible decision for that patient is recognized (Guyatt et al. 2004).

Knowledge can be gained that is both propositional, that is from research and generalizable, and non-propositional, that is implicit knowledge derived from practice (Rycroft-Malone et al. 2004). In more tangible, practical terms, evidence bases can be drawn from a number of different sources, and this pluralistic approach needs to be set in the context of the complex clinical environment in which nurses work in today's NHS (Pearson et al. 2007, Rycroft-Malone et al. 2004). The evidence bases can be summarized under four main areas.

1 Research
2 Clinical experience/expertise/tradition
3 Patient, clients and carers
4 The local context and environment (Pearson et al. 2007, Rycroft-Malone et al. 2004)

Grading evidence in The Royal Marsden Manual of Clinical Nursing Procedures

The type of evidence that underpins procedures is made explicit by using a system to categorize the evidence which is broader than that generally used. It has been developed from the types of evidence described by Rycroft-Malone et al. (2004) in an attempt to acknowledge that 'in reality practitioners draw on multiple sources of knowledge in the course of their practice and interaction with patients' (Rycroft-Malone et al. 2004, p.88).

The sources of evidence, along with examples, are identified as follows.

1 *Clinical experience (E)*
- Encompasses expert practical know-how, gained through working with others and reflecting on best practice.
- *Example*: (Dougherty 2008: E). This is drawn from the following article that gives expert clinical opinion: Dougherty, L. (2008) Obtaining peripheral vascular access. In: Dougherty, L. & Lamb, J. (eds) *Intravenous Therapy in Nursing Practice*, 2nd edn. Oxford: Blackwell Publishing.

2 *Patient (P)*
- Gained through expert patient feedback and extensive experience of working with patients.
- *Example*: (Diamond 1998: P). This has been gained from a personal account of care written by a patient: Diamond, J. (1998) *C: Because Cowards Get Cancer Too*. London: Vermilion.

3 *Context (C)*
- Can include audit and performance data, social and professional networks, local and national policy, guidelines from professional bodies (e.g. Royal College of Nursing [RCN]) and manufacturer's recommendations.
- *Example*: (DH 2001: C). This document gives guidelines for good practice: DH (2001) *National Service Framework for Older People*. London: Department of Health.

4 *Research (R)*
- Evidence gained through research.
- *Example*: (Fellowes et al. 2004: R). This has been drawn from the following evidence: Fellowes, D., Wilkinson, S. & Moore, P. (2004) Communication skills training for healthcare professionals working with cancer patients, their families and/or carers. *Cochrane Database of Systematic Reviews*, 2, CD003751. DOI: 10.10002/14651858.CD003571.pub2.

The levels that have been chosen are adapted from Sackett et al. (2000) as follows.

1 a Systematic reviews of randomized controlled trials (RCTs)
  b Individual RCTs with narrow confidence limits
2 a Systematic reviews of cohort studies
  b Individual cohort studies and low-quality RCTs
3 a Systematic reviews of case–control studies
  b Case–control studies
4 Case series and poor-quality cohort and case–control studies
5 Expert opinion

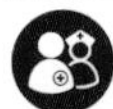
Box 1.1 **Levels of evidence**

1a Systematic reviews of RCTs
1b Individual RCTs with narrow confidence limits
2a Systematic reviews of cohort studies
2b Individual cohort studies and low-quality RCTs
3a Systematic reviews of case–control studies
3b Case–control studies
4 Case series and poor-quality cohort and case–control studies
5 Expert opinion

RCTs, randomized controlled trials.

Source: Adapted from Sackett et al. (2000). Reproduced with permission from Elsevier.

The evidence underpinning all the procedures has been reviewed and updated. To reflect the current trends in EBP, the evidence presented to support the procedures within the current edition of the Manual has been graded, with this grading made explicit to the reader. The rationale for the system adopted in this edition will now be outlined.

As we have seen, there are many sources of evidence and ways of grading evidence, and this has led us to a decision to consider both of these factors when referencing the procedures. You will therefore see that references identify if the source of the evidence was from:

- clinical experience and guidelines (Dougherty 2008: E)
- patient (Diamond 1998: P)
- context (DH 2001: C)
- research (Fellowes et al. 2004: R).

If there is no written evidence to support a clinical experience or guidelines as a justification for undertaking a procedure, the text will be referenced as an 'E' but will not be preceded by an author's name.

For the evidence that comes from research, this referencing system will be taken one step further and the research will be graded using a hierarchy of evidence. The levels that have been chosen are adapted from Sackett et al. (2000) and can be found in Box 1.1.

Taking the example above of Fellowes et al. (2004) 'Communication skills training for healthcare professionals working with cancer patients, their families and/or carers', this is a systematic review of RCTs from the Cochrane Centre and so would be identified in the references as: Fellowes et al. (2004: R 1a).

Through this process, we hope that the reader will be able to more clearly identify the nature of the evidence upon which the care of patients is based and that this will assist when using these procedures in practice. You may also like to consider the evidence base for other procedures and policies in use in your own organization.

Structure of the Manual

The chapters have been organized into four broad sections that represent as far as possible the needs of a patient along their care pathway. The first section, *Managing the patient journey*, presents the generic information that the nurse needs for every patient who enters the acute care environment. The second section of procedures, *Supporting the patient with human functioning*, relates to the support a patient may require with normal human functions such as elimination, nutrition and respiration. The third section, *Supporting the patient through the diagnostic process*, includes procedures that relate to any aspect of supporting a patient through the diagnostic process, from simple procedures such as taking a temperature to preparing a patient for complex procedures such as a liver biopsy. The final section, *Supporting the patient through treatment*, includes the procedures related to specific types of treatment or therapies the patient is receiving.

Structure of chapters in the student edition

The structure of each chapter is consistent throughout the book.

- *Learning outcomes*: each chapter starts by identifying what the reader can expect to have achieved after working through the chapter and completing the learning activities within it.
- *Overview*: as the chapters are larger and have considerably more content, each one has an overview to guide the reader, informing them of the scope and the sections included in the chapter
- *Learning activities*: each chapter includes a range of learning activities that encourage both reflection in, and on, practice. These include 'learning in practice' activities where students are asked to consider issues within their own practice environment, 'scenarios' that ask the student to consider what they would do in a given situation and 'case studies' where students work through questions to identify how a particular patient case may be managed. See Box 1.2.
- *Definition*: each section begins with a definition of the terms and explanation of the aspects of care, with any technical or difficult concepts explained.
- *Anatomy and physiology*: each section includes a discussion of the anatomy and physiology relating to the aspects of nursing care in the chapter. If appropriate, this is illustrated with diagrams so the context of the procedure can be fully understood by the reader.
- *Related theory*: if an understanding of theoretical principles is necessary to understand the procedure then this has been included.
- *Evidence-based approaches:* this provides background and presents the research and expert opinion in this area. If appropriate, the indications and contraindications are included as well as any principles of care.
- *Legal and professional issues:* this outlines any professional guidance, law or other national policy that may be relevant to the procedures. If necessary, this includes any professional competences or qualifications required in order to perform the procedures. Any risk management considerations are also included in this section.
- *Pre-procedural considerations:* when carrying out any procedure, there are certain actions that may need to be completed, equipment prepared or medication given before the procedure begins. These are made explicit under this heading.
- *Procedure:* each chapter includes the current procedures that are used in the acute hospital setting. They have been drawn from the daily nursing practice at The Royal Marsden NHS Foundation Trust. Only procedures about which the authors have knowledge and expertise have been included. Each procedure gives detailed step-by-step actions, supported by rationale, and where available the known evidence underpinning this rationale has been indicated.
- *Problem solving and resolution*: if relevant, each procedure will be followed by a table of potential problems that may be encountered while carrying out the procedure as well as suggestions as to the cause, prevention and any action that may help resolve the problem.
- *Post-procedural considerations*: care for the patient does not end with the procedure. This section details any documentation the nurse may need to complete, education/information that needs to be given to the patient, ongoing observations or referrals to other members of the multiprofessional team.
- *Complications*: any ongoing problems or potential complications are discussed in a final section which includes evidence-based suggestions for resolution.
- *Illustrations*: colour illustrations have been used to demonstrate the steps of some procedures. This will enable the nurse to see in greater detail, for example, the correct position of hands or the angle of a needle.
- *Summary of learning and reflection on practice:* at the end of each chapter there is a series of questions for students to work through. 'Learning for practice' then draws on students' individual learning from the chapter, asking them to identify five key points that they will be able to apply to their clinical practice.
- *Key points:* each chapter ends with a number of key points that draw together essential learning points from the chapter content.
- *References and reading list*: the chapter finishes with a combined reference and reading list. Only recent texts from the last 10 years have been included unless they are seminal texts. A list of websites has also been included.

Box 1.2 **Key to learning activities**

- *Learning in practice*: these activities enable students to consider issues within their own practice environment, encouraging exploration and discussion with mentors and colleagues.
- *Scenarios*: students are asked to consider what they would do in a given clinical situation.
- *Case studies*: students work through questions to identify how a particular patient case may be managed.
- *Summary of learning and reflection on practice:* at the end of each chapter there is a series of questions for students to work through. 'Learning for practice' then draws on students' individual learning from the chapter, asking them to identify five key points that they will be able to apply their clinical practice.
- *Key points:* each chapter ends with a number of key points that draw together essential learning points from the chapter content.

Where applicable, the answers to the questions are provided at the end of each chapter.

This book is intended as a reference and a resource, not as a replacement for practice-based education. None of the procedures in this book should be undertaken without prior instruction and subsequent supervision from an appropriately qualified and experienced professional. We hope that *The Royal Marsden Manual of Clinical Nursing Procedures* will continue to be a resource to deliver high-quality care that maximizes the well-being and improves the health outcomes of patients in acute hospital settings.

Conclusion

It is important to remember that even if a procedure is very familiar to us and we are very confident in carrying it out, it may be new to the patient, so time must be taken to explain it and gain consent, even if this is only verbal consent. The diverse range of technical procedures that patients may be subjected to should act as a reminder not to lose sight of the unique person undergoing such procedures and the importance of individualized patient assessment in achieving this.

When a nurse
Encounters another
What occurs is never a neutral event
A pulse taken
Words exchanged

A touch
A healing moment
Two persons
Are never the same
(Anon in Dossey et al. 2005)

Nurses have a central role to play in helping patients to manage the demands of the procedures described in this Manual. It must not be forgotten that for the patient, the clinical procedure is part of a larger picture, which encompasses an appreciation of the unique experience of illness. Alongside this, we need to be mindful of the evidence upon which we are basing the care we deliver. We hope that through increasing the clarity with which the evidence for the procedures in this edition is presented, you will be better able to underpin the care you deliver to your patients in your day-to-day practice.

REFERENCES

Carper, B. (1978) Fundamental patterns of knowing in nursing. *ANS Advances in Nursing Science*, 1(1), 13–23.

DH (2001) *National Service Framework for Older People*. London: Department of Health.

DH (2013) *Compassion in Practice*. NHS Commissioning Board. Leeds: Department of Health.

Diamond, J. (1998) *C: Because Cowards Get Cancer Too*. London: Vermilion.

Dossey, B.M., Keegan, L. & Guzzetta, C.E. (2005) *Holistic Nursing: A Handbook for Practice*, 4th edn. Sudbury, MA: Jones and Bartlett.

Dougherty, L. (2008) Obtaining peripheral vascular access. In: Dougherty, L. & Lamb, J. (eds) *Intravenous Therapy in Nursing Practice*, 2nd edn. Oxford: Blackwell Publishing.

Fellowes, D., Wilkinson, S. & Moore, P. (2004) Communication skills training for health care professionals working with cancer patients, their families and/or carers. *Cochrane Database of Systematic Reviews*, 2, CD003751.

Ford, P. & Walsh, M. (1994) *New Rituals for Old: Nursing Through the Looking Glass*. Oxford: Butterworth-Heinemann.

Guyatt, G., Cook, D. & Haynes, B. (2004) Evidence based medicine has come a long way. *BMJ*, 329 (7473), 990–991.

NMC (2015) *The Code: Standards of Conduct, Performance and Ethics for Nurses and Midwives*. London: Nursing and Midwifery Council.

Paley, J. (2006) Evidence and expertise. *Nursing Enquiry*, 13(2), 82–93.

Pearson, A., Field, J. & Jordan, Z. (2007) *Evidence-Based Clinical Practice in Nursing and Health Care: Assimilating Research, Experience, and Expertise*. Oxford: Blackwell Publishing.

Porter, S. (2010) Fundamental patterns of knowing in nursing: the challenge of evidence-based practice. *ANS Advances in Nursing Science*, 33(1), 3–14.

Rycroft-Malone, J., Seers, K., Titchen, A., Harvey, G., Kitson, A. & McCormack, B. (2004) What counts as evidence in evidence-based practice? *Journal of Advanced Nursing*, 47(1), 81–90.

Sackett, D.L., Rosenberg, W.M., Gray, J.A., Haynes, R.B. & Richardson, W.S. (1996) Evidence based medicine: what it is and what it isn't. *BMJ*, 312(7023), 71–72.

Sackett, D.L., Strauss, S.E. & Richardson, W.S. (2000) *Evidence-Based Medicine: How to Practice and Teach EBM*, 2nd edn. Edinburgh: Churchill Livingstone.

Scott, K. & McSherry, R. (2009) Evidence-based nursing: clarifying the concepts for nurses in practice. *Journal of Clinical Nursing*, 18(8), 1085–1095.

Walsh, M. & Ford, P. (1989) *Nursing Rituals, Research and Rational Actions*. Oxford: Heinemann Nursing.

Wilson, C. (2005) Said another way. My definition of nursing. *Nursing Forum*, 40(3), 116–118.

Part One
Managing the patient journey

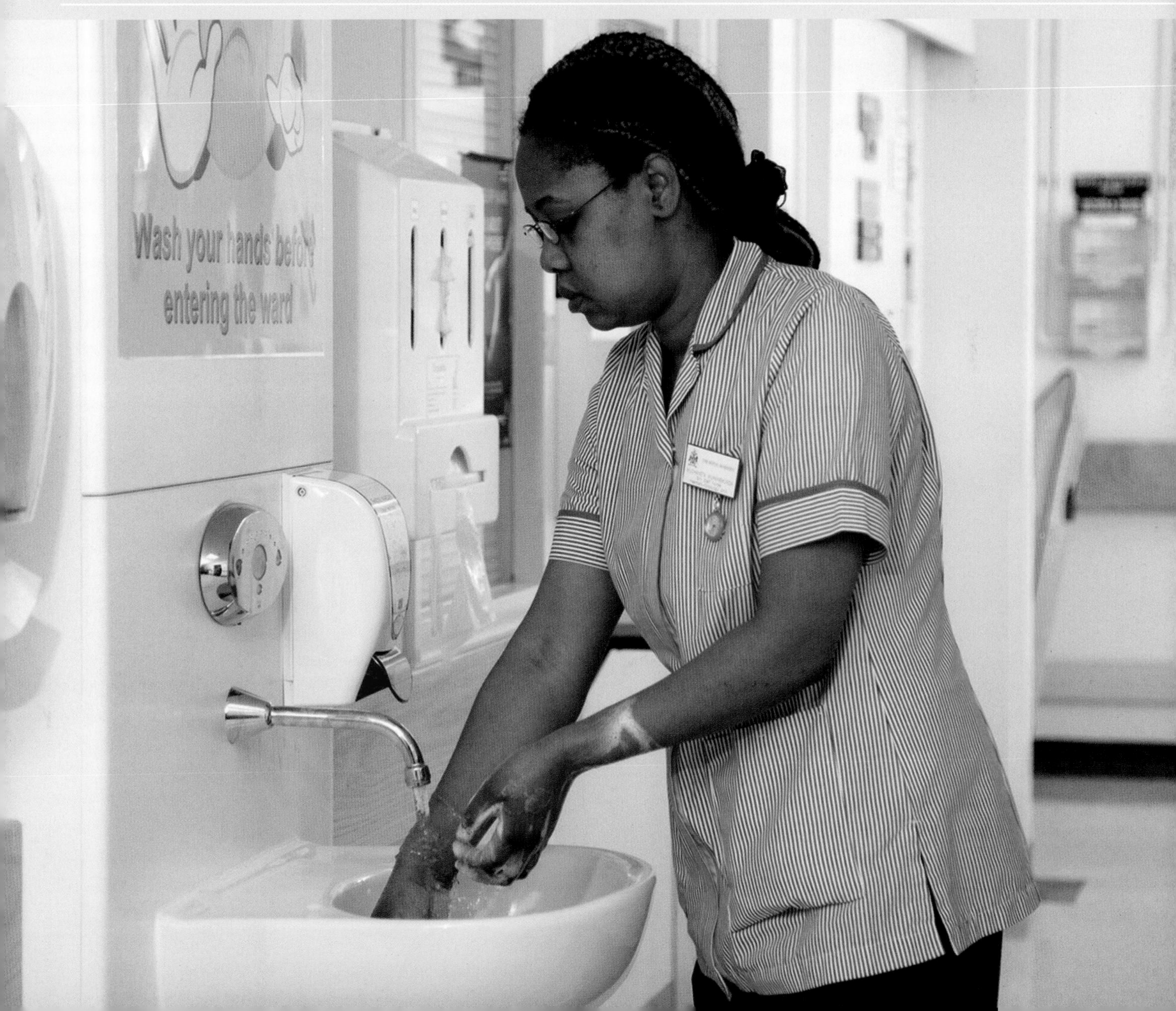

Assessment and discharge

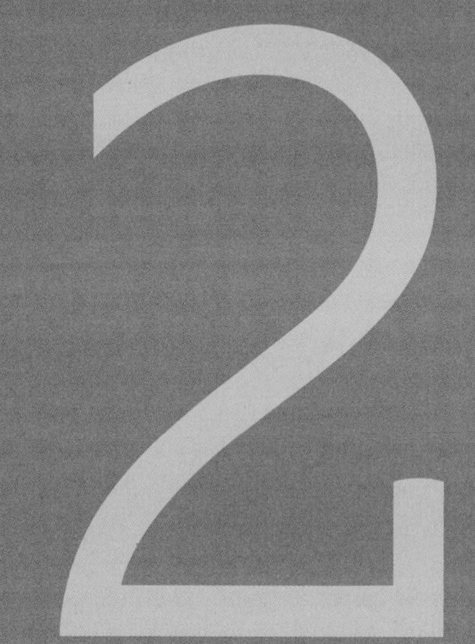

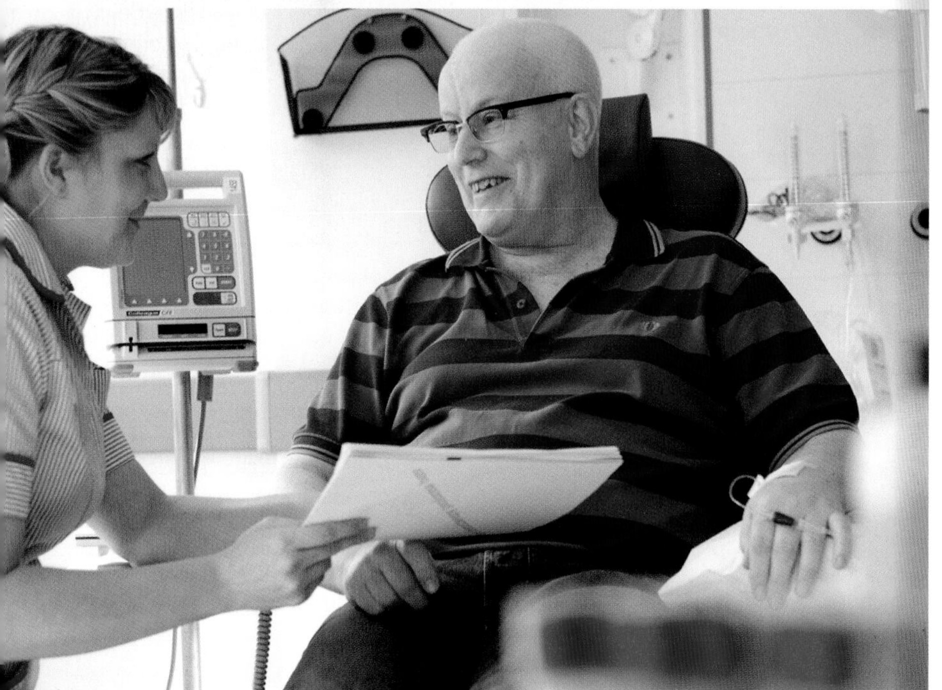

By reading this chapter and undertaking the learning activities within it, you should be able to:

1 Demonstrate a critical understanding of the principles and structure of nursing assessment, so that such frameworks and tools can be used to identify patient problems/ nursing diagnoses and monitor the effectiveness of care.

2 Construct a comprehensive nursing care plan for a patient that includes clear identification of the patient's problems, measurable outcomes and realistic nursing interventions.

3 Identify the key considerations when planning a discharge for a patient from hospital to the community to ensure the patient receives safe and effective ongoing care.

The Royal Marsden Manual of Clinical Nursing Procedures: Student Edition, Ninth Edition. Edited by Lisa Dougherty, Sara Lister and Alexandra West-Oram

Overview

This chapter will give an overview of a patient's care from assessment through to discharge.

Assessment forms an integral part of patient care and is considered to be the first step in the process of individualized nursing care. It provides information that is critical to the development of a plan of action that enhances personal health status.

Assessment decreases the potential for, or the severity of, chronic conditions and helps the individual to gain control over their health through self-care (RCN 2004). Early and continued assessments are vital to the success of the management of patient care. It is critical that nurses have the ability to assess patients and document their findings in a systematic way.

Discharge planning is key to ensuring that patients return to the community with the appropriate care to support them and their carers at home. The process can also reduce hospital length of stay and unplanned readmission to hospital, and improve the co-ordination of services following discharge from hospital (Shepperd et al. 2013).

The nurse's ability to assess the needs of the patient and carer (Atwal 2002) is central to a good discharge.

Inpatient assessment and the process of care

DEFINITION

Assessment is the systematic and continuous collection, organization, validation and documentation of information (Berman et al. 2010). It is a deliberate and interactive process that underpins every aspect of nursing care (Heaven and Maguire 1996). It is the process by which the nurse and patient together identify needs and concerns. It is seen as the cornerstone of individualized care, a way in which the uniqueness of each patient can be recognized and considered in the care process (Holt 1995).

RELATED THEORY

Principles of assessment

The purpose of the nursing assessment is to get a complete picture of the patient and how they can be helped. An effective assessment will provide the nurse with information on the patient's background, lifestyle, family history and the presence of illness or injury (Crouch and Meurier 2005). The nursing assessment should focus on the patient's response to a health need rather than disease process and pathology (Wilkinson 2007). The process of assessment requires nurses to make accurate and relevant observations, to gather, validate and organize data and to make judgements to determine care and treatment needs. It should have physical, psychological, spiritual, social and cultural dimensions, and it is vital that these are explored with the person being assessed. The patient's perspective of their level of daily activity functioning (Horton 2002) and their educational needs is essential to help maximize their understanding and self-care abilities (Alfaro-LeFevre 2014). It is only after making observations of the person and involving them in the process that the nurse can validate their perceptions and make appropriate clinical judgements.

Effective patient assessment is integral to the safety, continuity and quality of patient care, and fulfils the nurse's legal and professional obligations in practice. The main principles of assessment are outlined in Box 2.1.

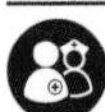

Box 2.1 **Principles of assessment**

1. Patient assessment is patient focused, being governed by the notion of an individual's actual, potential and perceived needs.
2. It provides baseline information on which to plan the interventions and outcomes of care to be achieved.
3. It facilitates evaluation of the care given and is a dimension of care that influences a patient's outcome and potential survival.
4. It is a dynamic process that starts when problems or symptoms develop, and continues throughout the care process, accommodating continual changes in the patient's condition and circumstances.
5. It is essentially an interactive process in which the patient actively participates.
6. Optimal functioning, quality of life and the promotion of independence should be primary concerns.
7. The process includes observation, data collection, clinical judgement and validation of perceptions.
8. Data used for the assessment process are collected from several sources by a variety of methods, depending on the healthcare setting.
9. To be effective, the process must be structured and clearly documented.

Source: Adapted from Alfaro-LeFevre (2014), NMC (2015), Teytelman (2002), White (2003).

Structure of assessment

Structuring patient assessment is vital to monitoring the success of care and detecting the emergence of new problems. There are many conceptual frameworks or nursing models, such as Roper's Activities of Daily Living (Roper et al. 2000), Orem's self-care model (Orem et al. 2001) or Gordon's Functional Health Patterns Framework (Gordon 1994). There remains, however, much debate about the effectiveness of such models for assessment in practice, some arguing that individualized care can be compromised by fitting patients into a rigid or complex structure (Kearney 2001, McCrae 2012). Nurses therefore need to take a pragmatic approach and utilize assessment frameworks that are appropriate to their particular area of practice. This is particularly relevant in today's rapidly changing healthcare climate where nurses are taking on increasingly advanced roles, working across boundaries and setting up new services to meet patients' needs (DH 2006a).

Nursing models can serve as a guide to the overall approach to care within a given healthcare environment and therefore provide a focus for the clinical judgements and decision-making processes that result from the process of assessment. During any patient assessment, nurses engage in a series of cognitive, behavioural and practical steps but do not always recognize them as discrete decision-making entities (Ford and McCormack 1999). Nursing models give novice practitioners a structure with which to identify these processes and to reflect on their practice in order to develop the analytical, problem-solving and judgement skills needed to provide an effective patient assessment.

Nursing models have been developed according to different ways of perceiving the main focus of nursing. These include adaptation models (e.g. Roy 1984), self-care models (e.g. Orem et al. 2001) and activities of daily living models (e.g. Murphy et al. 2000). Each model represents a different view of the relationship between four key elements of nursing: health, person, environment and nursing. It is important that the appropriate model is used to ensure that the focus of assessment data collected is effective for particular areas of practice (Alfaro-LeFevre 2014, Murphy et al. 2000). Nurses must also be aware of the rationale for implementing a particular model since the choice will determine the nature of patient care in their day-to-day work. The approach should be sensitive enough

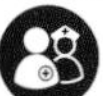

Box 2.2 **Gordon's functional health patterns**

- Health perception – health management
- Nutrition – metabolic
- Elimination
- Activity – exercise
- Sleep – rest
- Cognitive – perceptual
- Self-perception – self-concept
- Coping – stress tolerance
- Role – relationship
- Sexuality – reproductivity
- Value – belief

Source: Gordon (1994). Reproduced with permission from Elsevier.

to discriminate between different clinical needs and flexible enough to be updated on a regular basis (Allen 1998, Smith and Richardson 1996).

The framework of choice at the Royal Marsden Hospital is based on Gordon's Functional Health Patterns (Gordon 1994; Box 2.2). The framework facilitates an assessment that focuses on patients' and families' problems and functional status and applies clinical cues to interpret deviations from the patient's usual patterns (Johnson 2000). The model is applicable to all levels of care, allowing all problem areas to be identified. The information derived from the patient's initial functional health patterns is crucial for interpreting both the patient's and their family's pattern of response to the disease and treatment.

EVIDENCE-BASED APPROACHES

Collecting data

Data collection is the process of gathering information about the patient's health needs. This information is collected by means of interview, observation and physical examination and consists of both objective and subjective data. Objective data are measurable and can be detected by someone other than the patient. They include vital signs, physical signs and symptoms, and laboratory results. Subjective data, on the other hand, are based on what the patient perceives and may include descriptions of their concerns, support network, their awareness and knowledge of their abilities/disabilities, their understanding of their illness and their attitude to and readiness for learning (Wilkinson 2007). Nurses working in different settings rely on different observational and physical data. A variety of methods have been developed to facilitate nurses in eliciting both objective and subjective assessment data on the assumption that, if assessment is not accurate, all other nursing activity will also be inaccurate.

Studies of patient assessment by nurses are few but they indicate that discrepancies between the nurses' perceptions and those of their patients are common (Brown et al. 2001, Lauri et al. 1997, McDonald et al. 1999, Parsaie et al. 2000). Communication is therefore key for, as Suhonen et al. (2000) suggest, 'there are two actors in individual care, the patient and the nurse' (p.1254). Gaining insight into the patient's preferences and individualized needs is facilitated by meaningful interaction and depends both on the patient's willingness and capability in participating in the process and the nurse's interviewing skills. The initial assessment interview not only allows the nurse to obtain baseline information about the patient, but also facilitates the establishment of a therapeutic relationship (Crumbie 2006). Patients may find it difficult to disclose some problems and these may only be identified once the nurse–patient relationship develops and the patient trusts that the nurse's assessment reflects concern for their well-being.

While the patient is the primary source of information, data may be elicited from a variety of other secondary sources including family and friends, other healthcare professionals and the patient's medical records (Kozier 2012, Walsh et al. 2007).

Assessment interviews

An assessment interview needs structure to progress logically in order to facilitate the nurse's thinking (an example of such a structure can be found in Box 2.3) and to make the patient feel comfortable in telling their story. It can be perceived as being in three phases: the introductory, working and end phases (Crumbie 2006).

It is important at the beginning to build a rapport with the patient. It is vital that the nurse demonstrates interest and respect

Box 2.3 **Carrying out a patient assessment using functional health patterns**

Pattern	Assessment and data collection are focused on
Health perception – management	• The person's perceived level of health and well-being, and on the practices they use for maintaining health. • Habits that may be detrimental to health are also evaluated. • Actual or potential problems related to safety and health management may be identified as well as needs for modifications in the home or for continued care in the home.
Nutrition and metabolism	• The pattern of food and fluid consumption relative to metabolic need. • Actual or potential problems related to fluid balance, tissue integrity. • Problems with the gastrointestinal system.
Elimination	• Excretory patterns (bowel, bladder, skin). • Excretory problems such as incontinence, constipation, diarrhoea and urinary retention may be identified.
Activity and exercise	• The activities of daily living requiring energy expenditure, including self-care activities, exercise and leisure activities. • The status of major body systems involved with activity and exercise is evaluated, including the respiratory, cardiovascular and musculoskeletal systems.
Sleep and rest	• The person's sleep, rest and relaxation practices. • Dysfunctional sleep patterns, fatigue, and responses to sleep deprivation may be identified.

(continued)

Box 2.3 **Carrying out a patient assessment using functional health patterns *(continued)***

Pattern	Assessment and data collection are focused on
Cognitive and perceptual ability	• The ability to comprehend and use information. • The sensory and neurological functions.
Perception/concept of self	• The person's attitudes toward self, including identity, body image and sense of self-worth. • The person's level of self-esteem and response to threats to their self-concept may be identified.
Stress and coping	• The person's perception of stress and its effects on their coping strategies. • Support systems are evaluated, and symptoms of stress are noted. • The effectiveness of a person's coping strategies in terms of stress tolerance may be further evaluated.
Roles and relationships	• The person's roles in the world and relationships with others. • Satisfaction with roles, role strain or dysfunctional relationships may be further evaluated.
Sexuality and reproduction	• The person's satisfaction or dissatisfaction with sexuality patterns and reproductive functions. • Concerns with sexuality may be identified.
Values and belief	• The person's values, beliefs (including spiritual beliefs) and goals that guide their choices or decisions.

Source: Adapted from Gordon (1994). Reproduced with permission from Elsevier.

in the patient from the very start of the interview. Some of the questions asked are likely to be of a searching and intimate nature, which may be difficult for the patient to disclose. The nurse should emphasize the confidential nature of the discussion and take steps to reduce anxiety and ensure privacy since the patient may modify their words and behaviour depending on the environment. Taking steps to establish trust and develop the relationship early will set the scene for effective and accurate information exchange (Silverman et al. 2013).

In the middle working phase, various techniques can be employed to assist with the flow of information. Open questions are useful to identify broad information that can then be explored more specifically with focused questions to determine the nature and extent of the problem. Other helpful techniques include restating what has been said to clarify certain issues, using verbal and non-verbal cues to encourage the patient, verbalizing the implied meaning, using silence and summarizing (Kozier 2012, Silverman et al. 2013). It is important to recognize that there may be times when it is not possible to obtain vital information directly from the patient; they may be too distressed, unconscious or unable to speak clearly, if at all. In such situations, appropriate details should be taken from relatives or friends and recorded as such. Effort should equally be made to overcome language or cultural barriers by the use of interpreters.

The end phase involves a further summary of the important points and an explanation of any referrals made. In order to gain the patient's perspective on the priorities of care and to emphasise the continuing interest in their needs, a final question asking about their concerns can be used (Alfaro-LeFevre 2014). Examples include: 'Tell me the most important things I can help you with', 'Is there anything else you would like to tell me?', 'Is there anything that we haven't covered that still concerns you?' or 'If there are any changes or you have any questions, do let me know'. Box 2.4 provides a summary of the types of assessment.

LEGAL AND PROFESSIONAL ISSUES

The NHS *Knowledge and Skills Framework* (DH 2004a) states that the specific dimensions of 'assessment and care planning to meet people's health and wellbeing needs' and 'assessment and treatment planning related to the structure and function of physiological and psychological systems' are core to nursing posts in all settings. In undertaking this work, staff will need to be aware of their legal obligations and responsibilities, the rights of the different people involved, and the diversity of the people they are working with.

Nurses have an obligation to record details of any assessments and reviews undertaken, and provide clear evidence of the

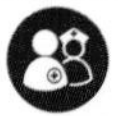

Box 2.4 **Types of patient assessment**

Mini assessment

A snapshot view of the patient based on a quick visual and physical assessment. Consider patient's ABC (airway, breathing and circulation), then assess mental status, overall appearance, level of consciousness and vital signs before focusing on the patient's main problem.

Comprehensive assessment

An in-depth assessment of the patient's health status, physical examination, risk factors, psychological and social aspects of the patient's health that usually takes place on admission or transfer to a hospital or healthcare agency. It will take into account the patient's previous health status prior to admission.

Focused assessment

An assessment of a specific condition, problem, identified risks or assessment of care; for example, continence assessment, nutritional assessment, neurological assessment following a head injury, assessment for day care, outpatient consultation for a specific condition.

Ongoing assessment

Continuous assessment of the patient's health status accompanied by monitoring and observation of specific problems identified in a mini, comprehensive or focused assessment.

Source: Ahern and Philpot (2002), Holmes (2003), White (2003).

arrangements that have been made for future and ongoing care (NMC 2010). This should also include details of information given about care and treatment.

PRE-PROCEDURAL CONSIDERATIONS

Assessment tools

The use of assessment tools enables a standardized approach to obtaining specific patient data. This can facilitate the documentation of change over time and the evaluation of clinical interventions and nursing care (O'Connor and Eggert 1994). Perhaps more importantly, assessment tools encourage patients to engage in their care and provide a vehicle for communication to allow nurses to follow patients' experiences more effectively.

Assessment tools in clinical practice can be used to assess the patient's general needs, for example the supportive care needs survey (Bonevski et al. 2000), or to assess a specific problem, for example the oral assessment guide (Eilers et al. 1988). The choice of tool depends on the clinical setting although in general, the aim of using an assessment tool is to link the assessment of clinical variables with measurement of clinical interventions (Frank-Stromborg and Olsen 2004). To be useful in clinical practice, an assessment tool must be simple, acceptable to patients, have a clear and interpretable scoring system and demonstrate reliability and validity (Brown et al. 2001).

More tools are used in practice to assess treatment-related symptoms than other aspects of care, possibly because these symptoms are predictable and of a physical nature and are therefore easier to measure. The most visible symptoms are not always those that cause most distress (Holmes and Eburn 1989); however, an acknowledgement of the patient's subjective experience is therefore an important element in the development of assessment tools (McClement et al. 1997, Rhodes et al. 2000).

The use of patient self-assessment tools appears to facilitate the process of assessment in a number of ways. It enables patients to indicate their subjective experience more easily, gives them an increased sense of participation (Kearney 2001) and prevents them from being distanced from the process by nurses rating their symptoms and concerns (Brown et al. 2001). Many authors have demonstrated the advantages of increasing patient participation in assessment by the use of patient self-assessment questionnaires (Rhodes et al. 2000).

The methods used to facilitate patient assessment are important adjuncts to assessing patients in clinical practice. There is a danger that too much focus can be placed on the framework, system or tool that prevents nurses thinking about the significance of the information that they are gathering from the patient (Harris et al. 1998). Rather than following assessment structures and prompts rigidly, it is essential that nurses utilize their critical thinking and clinical judgement throughout the process in order to continually develop their skills in eliciting information about patients' concerns and using this to inform care planning (Edwards and Miller 2001).

Learning Activity 2.1

Learning in practice: Patient assessment

- Make a list of all the different assessment tools you have observed being used in practice.
- Have a look at the types of patient assessment listed in Box 2.4 and classify each assessment as either a mini, comprehensive, focused or ongoing assessment.
- If there are any that you are not sure about, discuss with a colleague or your mentor.

Principles of an effective nursing assessment

The admitting nurse is responsible for ensuring that an initial assessment is completed when the patient is admitted. The patient's needs identified following this process then need to be documented in their care plan.

Box 2.5 discusses each area of assessment, indicating points for consideration and suggesting questions that may be helpful to ask the patient as part of the assessment process.

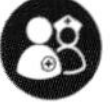

Box 2.5 **Points for consideration and suggested questions for use during the assessment process**

1 Cognitive and perceptual ability

Communication

The nurse needs to assess the level of sensory functioning with or without aids/support such as hearing aid(s), speech aid(s), glasses/contact lenses, and the patient's capacity to use and maintain aids/support correctly. Furthermore, it is important to assess whether there are or might be any potential language or cultural barriers during this part of the assessment. Knowing the norm within the culture will facilitate understanding and lessen miscommunication (Galanti 2000).

- How good are the patient's hearing and eyesight?
- Is the patient able to express their views and wishes using appropriate verbal and non-verbal methods of communication in a manner that is understandable by most people?
- Are there any potential language or cultural barriers to communicating with the patient?

Information

During this part of the assessment, the nurse will assess the patient's ability to comprehend the present environment without showing levels of distress. This will help to establish whether there are any barriers to the patient understanding their condition and treatment. It may help them to be in a position to give informed consent.

- Is the patient able and ready to understand any information about their forthcoming treatment and care? Are there any barriers to learning?
- Is the patient able to communicate an understanding of their condition, plan of care and potential outcomes/responses?
- Will he or she be able to give informed consent?

Neurological

It is important to assess the patient's ability to reason logically and decisively, and determine that he or she is able to communicate in a contextually coherent manner.

- Is the patient alert and orientated to time, place and person?

(continued)

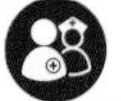

Box 2.5 **Points for consideration and suggested questions for use during the assessment process *(continued)***

Pain

To provide optimal patient care, the assessor needs to have appropriate knowledge of the patient's pain and an ability to identify the pain type and location. Assessment of a patient's experience of pain is a crucial component in providing effective pain management. Dimond (2002) asserts that it is unacceptable for patients to experience unmanaged pain or for nurses to have inadequate knowledge about pain. Pain should be measured using an assessment tool that identifies the quantity and/or quality of one or more of the dimensions of the patient's experience of pain.

Assessment should also observe for signs of neuropathic pain, including descriptions such as shooting, burning, stabbing, allodynia (pain associated with gentle touch) (Jensen et al. 2003, Rowbotham and Macintyre 2003).

- Is the patient pain free at rest and/or on movement?
- Is the pain a primary complaint or a secondary complaint associated with another condition?
- What is the location of the pain and does it radiate?
- When did it begin and what circumstances are associated with it?
- How intense is the pain, at rest and on movement?
- What makes the pain worse and what helps to relieve it?
- How long does the pain last, for example, continuous, intermittent?
- Ask the patient to describe the character of pain using quality/sensory descriptors, for example, sharp, throbbing, burning.

For further details regarding pain assessment, see Chapter 8: Patient comfort and end-of-life care.

2 Activity and exercise

Respiratory

Respiratory pattern monitoring addresses the patient's breathing pattern, rate and depth.

- Does the patient have any difficulty breathing?
- Is there any noise when they are breathing such as wheezing?
- Does breathing cause them pain?
- How deep or shallow is their breathing?
- Is their breathing symmetrical?
- Does the patient have any underlying respiratory problems such as chronic obstructive pulmonary disease, emphysema, tuberculosis, bronchitis, asthma or any other airway disease?

In this section it is also important to assess and monitor smoking habits. It is helpful to document the smoking habit in the format of pack-years. A *pack-year* is a term used to describe the number of cigarettes a person has smoked over time. One pack-year is defined as 20 manufactured cigarettes (one pack) smoked per day for 1 year. At this point in the assessment, it would be a good opportunity, if appropriate, to discuss smoking cessation. A recent meta-analysis indicates that if interventions are given by nurses to their patients with regard to smoking cessation the benefits are greater (Rice and Stead 2008). For further details see Chapter 9: Respiratory care.

Cardiovascular

A basic assessment is carried out and vital signs such as pulse (rhythm, rate and intensity) and blood pressure should be noted. Details of cardiac history should be taken for this part of the assessment. Medical conditions and previous surgery should be noted.

- Does the patient take any cardiac medication?
- Does he/she have a pacemaker?

Physical abilities, personal hygiene/mobility/toileting, independence with activities of daily living

The aim during this part of the nursing assessment is to establish the level of assistance required by the person to tackle activities of daily living such as walking and steps/stairs. An awareness of obstacles to safe mobility and dangers to personal safety is an important factor and part of the assessment.

- Is the patient able to stand, walk and go to the toilet?
- Is the patient able to move up and down, roll and turn in bed?
- Does the patient need any equipment to mobilize?
- Has the patient good motor power in their arms and legs?
- Does the patient have any history of falling?

The nurse should also evaluate the patient's ability to meet personal hygiene, including oral hygiene, needs. This should include the patient's ability to make arrangements to preserve standards of hygiene and the ability to dress appropriately for climate, environment and their own standards of self-identity.

- Can the patient take care of their own personal hygiene needs independently or do they need assistance?
- What type of assistance do they need: help with mobility or fine motor movements such as doing up buttons or shaving?

It might be necessary to complete a separate manual handling risk assessment – see Chapter 6: Moving and positioning.

3 Elimination

Gastrointestinal

During this part of the assessment it is important to determine a baseline with regard to independence.

- Is the patient able to attend to their elimination needs independently and is he/she continent?
- What are the patient's normal bowel habits? Are bowel movements within the patient's own normal pattern and consistency?
- Does the patient have any underlying medical conditions such as Crohn's disease or irritable bowel syndrome?

- Does the patient have diarrhoea or is he/she prone to or have constipation?
- How does this affect the patient?

For further discussion see Chapter 5: Elimination.

Genitourinary
The assessment is focused on the patient's baseline observations with regard to urinary continence/incontinence. It is also important to note whether there is any penile or vaginal discharge or bleeding.
- Does the patient have a urinary catheter *in situ*? If so, list the type and size. Furthermore, note the date the catheter was inserted and/or removed. Urinalysis results should also be noted here.
- How often does the patient need to urinate? (Frequency)
- How immediate is the need to urinate? (Urgency)
- Do they wake in the night to urinate? (Nocturia)
- Are they able to maintain control over their bladder at all times? (Incontinence – inability to hold urine)

For further discussion see Chapter 5: Elimination.

4 Nutrition

Oral care
As part of the inpatient admission assessment, the nurse should obtain an oral health history that includes oral hygiene beliefs, practices and current state of oral health. During this assessment it is important to be aware of treatments and medications that affect the oral health of the patient.
- If deemed appropriate, use an oral assessment tool to perform the initial and ongoing oral assessment.

During the admission it is important to note the condition of the patient's mouth.
- Lips – pink, moist, intact.
- Gums – pink, no signs of infection or bleeding.
- Teeth – dentures, bridge, crowns, caps.

For full oral assessment, see Chapter 8: Patient comfort and end-of-life care.

Hydration
An in-depth assessment of hydration and nutritional status will provide the information needed for nursing interventions aimed at maximizing wellness and identifying problems for treatment. The assessment should ascertain whether the patient has any difficulty eating or drinking. During the assessment the nurse should observe signs of dehydration, for example dry mouth, dry skin, thirst or whether the patient shows any signs of altered mental state.
- Is the patient able to drink adequately? If not, please explain why not.
- How much and what does the patient drink?
- Note the patient's alcohol intake in the format of units per week and the caffeine intake measured in number of cups per day.

Nutrition
A detailed diet history provides insight into a patient's baseline nutritional status. Assessment includes questions regarding chewing or swallowing problems, avoidance of eating related to abdominal pain, changes in appetite, taste or intake, as well as use of a special diet or nutritional supplements. A review of past medical history should identify any relevant conditions and highlight increased metabolic needs, altered gastrointestinal function and the patient's capacity to absorb nutrients.
- What is the patient's usual daily food intake?
- Do they have a good appetite?
- Are they able to swallow/chew the food – any dysphagia?
- Is there anything they don't or can't eat?
- Have they experienced any recent weight changes or taste changes?
- Are they able to eat independently?

(Arrowsmith 1999, BAPEN and Malnutrition Advisory Group 2000, DH 2005)
For further information, see Chapter 7: Nutrition, fluid balance and blood transfusion.

Nausea and vomiting
During this part of the assessment you want to ascertain whether the patient has any history of nausea and/or vomiting. Nausea and vomiting can cause dehydration, electrolyte imbalance and nutritional deficiencies (Marek 2003), and can also affect a patient's psychosocial well-being. They may become withdrawn, isolated and unable to perform their usual activities of daily living.
Assessment should address questions such as:
- Does the patient feel nauseous?
- Is the patient vomiting? If so, what is the frequency, volume, content and timing?
- Does nausea precede vomiting?
- Does vomiting relieve nausea?
- When did the symptoms start? Did they coincide with changes in therapy or medication?
- Does anything make the symptoms better?
- Does anything make the symptoms worse?
- What is the effect of any current or past antiemetic therapy including dose, frequency, duration, effect, route of administration?
- What is the condition of the patient's oral cavity?

(Adapted from Perdue 2005). For further discussion see Chapter 5: Elimination.

(continued)

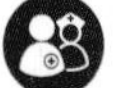

Box 2.5 **Points for consideration and suggested questions for use during the assessment process *(continued)***

5 Skin

A detailed assessment of a patient's skin may provide clues to diagnosis, management and nursing care of the existing problem. A careful skin assessment can alert the nurse to cutaneous problems as well as systemic diseases. In addition, a great deal can be observed in a person's face, which may give insight to his or her state of mind.

- Does the patient have any sore places on their skin?
- Does the patient have any dry or red areas?

Furthermore, it is necessary to assess whether the patient has any wounds and/or pressure sores. If so, you would need to complete a further wound assessment. For further information see Chapter 14: Wound management.

6 Controlling body temperature

This assessment is carried out to establish baseline temperature and determine if the temperature is within normal range, and whether there might be intrinsic or extrinsic factors for altered body temperature. It is important to note whether any changes in temperature are in response to specific therapies (e.g. antipyretic medication, immunosuppressive therapies, invasive procedures or infection (Bickley et al. 2013)). White blood count should be recorded to determine whether it is within normal limits. See Chapter 11: Observations.

- Is the patient feeling excessively hot or cold?
- Have they been shivering or sweating excessively?

7 Sleep and rest

This part of the assessment is performed to find out sleep and rest patterns and reasons for variation. Description of sleep patterns, routines and interventions applied to achieve a comfortable sleep should be documented. The nurse should also include the presence of emotional and/or physical problems that may interfere with sleep.

- Does the patient have enough energy for desired daily activities?
- Does the patient tire easily?
- Has he/she any difficulty falling asleep or staying asleep?
- Does he/she feel rested after sleep?
- Does he/she sleep during the day?
- Does he/she take any aids to help them sleep?
- What are the patient's normal hours for going to bed and waking?

8 Stress and coping

Assessment is focused on the patient's perception of stress and on his or her coping strategies. Support systems should be evaluated and symptoms of stress should be noted. It includes the individual's reserve or capacity to resist challenge to self-integrity, and modes of handling stress. The effectiveness of a person's coping strategies in terms of stress tolerances may be further evaluated (adapted from Gordon 1994).

- What are the things in the patient's life that are stressful?
- What do they do when they are stressed?
- How do they know they are stressed?
- Is there anything they do to help them cope when life gets stressful?
- Is there anybody who they go to for support?

9 Roles and relationships

The aim is to establish the patient's own perception of the roles and responsibilities in their current life situation. The patient's role in the world and their relationships with others are important to understand. Assessment in this area includes finding out about the patient's perception of the major roles and responsibilities they have in life, satisfaction or disturbances in family, work or social relationships. An assessment of home life should be undertaken which should include how they will cope at home post discharge from hospital and how those at home will cope while they are in hospital, for example dependants, children or animals, and if there are any financial worries.

- Who is at home?
- Are there any dependants (include children, pets, anybody else they care for)?
- What responsibilities does the patient have for the day-to-day running of the home?
- What will happen if they are not there?
- Do they have any concerns about home while they are in hospital?
- Are there any financial issues related to their hospital stay?
- Will there be any issues related to employment or study while they are in hospital?

10 Perception/concept of self

Body image/self-esteem

Body image is highly personal, abstract and difficult to describe. The rationale for this section is to assess the patient's level of understanding and general perception of self. This includes their attitudes about self, perception of abilities (cognitive, affective or physical), body image, identity, general sense of worth and general emotional pattern. An assessment of body posture and movement, eye contact, voice and speech patterns should also be included.

- How do you describe yourself?
- How do you feel about yourself most of the time?

- Has it changed since your diagnosis?
- Have there been changes in the way you feel about yourself or your body?

11 Sexuality and reproduction

Understanding sexuality as the patient's perceptions of their own body image, family roles and functions, relationships and sexual function can help the assessor to improve assessment and diagnosis of actual or potential alterations in sexual behaviour and activity.

Assessment in this area is vital and should include relevant feelings about the patient's own body, their need for touch, interest in sexual activity, how they communicate their sexual needs to a partner, if they have one, and the ability to engage in satisfying sexual activities.

This may also be an opportunity to explore with the patient issues related to future reproduction if this is relevant to the admission. Below are a few examples of questions that can be used.

- Are you currently in a relationship?
- Has your condition had an impact on the way you and your partner feel about each other?
- Has your condition had an impact on the physical expression of your feelings?
- Has your treatment or current problem had any effect on your interest in being intimate with your partner?

12 Values and beliefs

Religious, spiritual and cultural beliefs

The aim is to assess the patient's spiritual, religious and cultural needs to provide culturally and spiritually specific care while concurrently providing a forum to explore spiritual strengths that might be used to prevent problems or cope with difficulties. Assessment is focused on the patient's values and beliefs, including spiritual beliefs, or on the goals that guide his or her choices or decisions. A patient's experience of their stay in hospital may be influenced by their religious beliefs or other strongly held principles, cultural background or ethnic origin. It is important for nurses to have knowledge and understanding of the diverse cultures of their patients and take their different practices into account.

- Are there any spiritual/cultural beliefs that are important to you?
- Do you have any specific dietary needs related to your religious, spiritual or cultural beliefs?
- Do you have any specific personal care needs related to your religious, spiritual or cultural beliefs (i.e. washing rituals, dress)?

13 Health perception and management

Relevant medical conditions, side-effects/complications of treatment

Assessment of the patient's perceived pattern of health and well-being and how health is managed should be documented here. Any relevant history of previous health problems, including side-effects of medication, should be noted. Examples of other useful information that should be documented are compliance with medication regimen, use of health promotion activities such as regular exercise and if the patient has annual check-ups.

- What does the patient know about their condition and planned treatment?
- How would they describe their own current overall level of fitness?
- What do they do to keep well: exercise, diet, annual check-ups or screening?

POST-PROCEDURAL CONSIDERATIONS

Decision making and nursing diagnosis

The purpose of collecting information through the process of assessment is to enable the nurse to make a series of clinical judgements, which are known in some circumstances as nursing diagnoses, and subsequently decisions about the nursing care each individual needs. The decision-making process is based upon the clues observed, analysed and interpreted and it has been suggested that expert nurses assess the situation as a whole and make judgements and decisions intuitively (Hedberg and Satterlund Larsson 2003, King and Clark 2002, Peden-McAlpine and Clark 2002), reflecting Benner's (1984) renowned novice-to-expert theory. However, others argue that all nurses use a logical process of clinical reasoning in order to identify patients' needs for nursing care and that, while this becomes more automatic with experience, it should always be possible for a nurse to explain how they arrive at a decision about an individual within their care (Gordon 1994, Putzier and Padrick 1984, Rolfe 1999). A further notion is that of a continuum, where our ability to make clinical judgements about our patients lies on a spectrum, with intuition at one end and linear, logical decisions (based on clinical trials, for example) at the other (Cader et al. 2005, Thompson 1999). Factors that may influence the process of decision making include time, complexity of the judgement or decision to be made, as well as the knowledge, experience and attitude of the individual nurse.

Nursing diagnosis is a term which describes both a clinical judgement that is made about an individual's response to health or illness, and the process of decision making that leads to that judgement. The importance of thorough assessment within this process cannot be overestimated. The gathering of comprehensive and appropriate data from patients, including the meanings attributed to events by the patient, is associated with greater diagnostic accuracy and thus more timely and effective intervention (Alfaro-LeFevre 2014, Gordon 1994, Hunter 1998).

The concept of a 'nursing diagnosis' has historically generated much debate within the nursing literature. It is therefore important to clarify the difference between a nursing diagnosis and a patient problem or care need. 'Patient problems' or 'needs' are common terms used within nursing to facilitate communication about nursing care (Hogston 1997). As patient problems/needs may involve solutions or treatments from disciplines other than nursing, the concept of a 'patient problem' is similar to but broader than a nursing diagnosis. Nursing diagnoses describe problems that may be dealt with by nursing expertise (Leih and Salentijn 1994).

The term 'nursing diagnosis' also refers to a standardized nursing language, to describe patients' needs for nursing care, that originated in America over 30 years ago and has now been developed, adapted and translated for use in numerous other countries. The language of nursing diagnosis provides a classification of over 200 terms (NANDA-I 2008), representing judgements that are commonly made with patients/clients about phenomena of concern to nurses, enabling more consistent communication and documentation of nursing care.

Most significantly, the use of common language enables nurses to clearly and consistently express what they do for patients and why, making the contribution of different nursing roles clearly visible within the multidisciplinary care pathway (Delaney 2001, Elfrink et al. 2001, Grobe 1996, Moen et al. 1999). Secondly, an increasingly important reason for trying to structure nursing terms in a systematic way has been the need to create and analyse nursing information in a meaningful way for electronic care records (Clark 1999, Westbrook 2000). The term 'nursing diagnosis' is not commonly used within the UK as no definitive classifications or common languages are in general use; however, for the aforementioned reasons, the adaptation and implementation of standard nursing languages within clinical practice in the UK are being explored (Chambers 1998, Lyte and Jones 2001, Westbrook 2000).

Planning and implementing care

Nursing diagnoses provide a focus for planning and implementing effective and evidence-based care. This process consists of identifying nursing-sensitive patient outcomes and determining appropriate interventions (Alfaro-LeFevre 2014, Shaw 1998, White 2003).

- To determine the immediate priorities and recognize whether patient problems require nursing care or whether a referral should be made to someone else.
- To identify the anticipated outcome for the patient, noting what the patient will be able to do and within what time frame. The use of 'measurable' verbs that describe patient behaviour or what the patient says facilitates the evaluation of patient outcomes (Box 2.6).
- To determine the nursing interventions, that is, what nursing actions will prevent or manage the patient's problems so that the patient's outcomes may be achieved.
- To record the care plan for the patient which may be written or individualized from a standardized/core care plan or a computerized care plan.

Outcomes should be patient focused and realistic, stating how the outcomes or goals are to be achieved and when the outcomes should be evaluated. Patient-focused outcomes centre on the desired results of nursing care, that is, the impact of care on the patient, rather than on what the nurse does. Outcomes may be short, intermediate or long term, enabling the nurse to identify the patient's health status and progress (stability, improvement or deterioration) over time. Setting realistic outcomes and interventions requires the nurse to distinguish between nursing diagnoses that are life-threatening or an immediate risk to the patient's safety and those that may be dealt with at a later stage. Identifying which nursing diagnoses/problems contribute to other problems (for example, difficulty breathing will contribute to the patient's ability to mobilize) will make the problem a higher priority. By dealing with the breathing difficulties, the patient's ability to mobilize will be improved.

The formulation of nursing interventions is dependent on adequate information collection and accurate clinical judgement during patient assessment. As a result, specific patient outcomes may be derived and appropriate nursing interventions undertaken to assist the patient to achieve those outcomes (Hardwick 1998). Nursing interventions should be specific to help the patient achieve the outcome and should be evidence based. When determining what interventions may be appropriate in relation to a patient's problem, it may be helpful to clarify the potential benefit to the patient after an intervention has been performed, as this will help to ensure its appropriateness.

It is important to continue to assess the patient on an ongoing basis whilst implementing the care planned. Assessing the patient's current status prior to implementing care will enable the nurse to check whether the patient has developed any new problems that require immediate action. During and after providing any nursing action, the nurse should assess and reassess the patient's response to care. The nurse will then be able to determine whether changes to the patient's care plan should be made immediately or at a later stage. If there are any patient care needs that require immediate action, for example consultation or referral to a doctor, recording the actions taken is essential. Involving the patient and their family or friends will promote the patient's well-being and self-care abilities. The use of clinical documentation in nurse handover will help to ensure that the care plans are up to date and relevant (Alfaro-LeFevre 2014, White 2003).

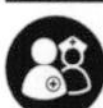
Box 2.6 **Examples of measurable and non-measurable verbs for use in outcome statements**

Measurable verbs (use these to be specific)

- State; verbalize; communicate; list; describe; identify
- Demonstrate; perform
- Will lose; will gain; has an absence of
- Walk; stand; sit

Non-measurable verbs (do not use)

- Know
- Understand
- Think
- Feel

Source: Alfaro-LeFevre (2014). Reproduced with permission from Lippincott Williams & Wilkins.

Learning Activity 2.2 **Case study: Developing an individualized care plan**

Core care plans and care pathways are being used increasingly to plan and deliver patient care. However, patients will inevitably have problems or health needs (nursing diagnoses) for which there is not a core care plan, so it is vitally important that nurses are able to develop comprehensive and individualized care plans for patients no matter what their condition.

Read the following case study:
Anna is a 27-year-old woman who was admitted to the ward with abdominal pain via the Emergency Department. She is currently nil by mouth and on intravenous fluids. She is very anxious about her mum, who is wheelchair bound and currently being looked after by a family friend; Anna is her main carer at home.

Develop a care plan for Anna to include the following:
- Nursing diagnoses (what are her problems or health needs?)
- Outcomes (what would you realistically hope to achieve for each of her nursing diagnoses?)
- Nursing interventions (what actions do the nursing team need to take to help achieve these outcomes?)

See the end of the chapter for the answers.

Evaluating care

Effective evaluation of care requires the nurse to critically analyse the patient's health status to determine whether the patient's condition is stable, has deteriorated or improved. Seeking the patient's and family's views in the evaluation process will facilitate decision making. By evaluating the patient's outcomes, the nurse is able to decide whether changes need to be made to the care planned. Evaluation of care should take place in a structured manner and on a regular basis by a Registered Nurse. The frequency of evaluation depends on the clinical environment within which the individual is being cared for as well as the nature of the nursing diagnosis (problem) to which the care relates.

- What are the patient's self-care abilities?
- Is the patient able to do what you expected?
- If not, why not?
- Has something changed?
- Are you missing something?
- Are there new care priorities?

These questions will help to clarify the patient's progress (Alfaro-LeFevre 2014, White 2003). It is helpful to consider what is observed and measurable to indicate that the patient has achieved the outcome.

Documenting

Nurses have a professional responsibility to ensure that healthcare records provide an accurate account of treatment, care planning and delivery, and are viewed as a tool of communication within the team. There should be 'clear evidence of the care planned, the decisions made, the care delivered and the information shared' (NMC 2010) (Box 2.7). The content and quality of record keeping are a measure of standards of practice relating to the skills and judgement of the nurse (NMC 2010).

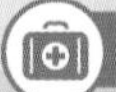

Learning Activity 2.3

Learning in practice: Record keeping

When you are in your clinical area, find out whether there are record keeping guidelines and how these are used and monitored.

Hint: Ask about a documentation audit. How is this done? How often?

Much of the record keeping that nurses do is mandatory for each patient on every admission to hospital.

- What would you do if you noticed a patient did not have a required assessment (for example, a pressure ulcer risk assessment) carried out as part of their admission?
- Who would you discuss this with?

For further information and guidance on record keeping, refer to NMC (2010) *Record Keeping: Guidance for Nurses and Midwives*.

Box 2.7 **The Royal Marsden Hospital Guidelines for Nursing Documentation (2011) (adopted in line with NMC (2010) Record keeping)**

General principles

1 Records should be written legibly in black ink in such a way that they cannot be erased and are readable when photocopied.
2 Entries should be factual, consistent, accurate and not contain jargon, abbreviations or meaningless phrases (e.g. 'observations fine').
3 Each entry must include the date and time (using the 24-hour clock).
4 Each entry must be followed by a signature and the name printed as well as:
  - the job role (e.g. staff nurse or clinical nurse specialist)
  - if a nurse is a temporary employee (i.e. an agency nurse), the name of the agency must be included under the signature.
5 If an error is made, this should be scored out with a single line and the correction written alongside with date, time and initials. Correction fluid should not be used at any time.
6 All assessments and entries made by student nurses must be countersigned by a Registered Nurse.
7 Healthcare assistants:
  - can write on fluid balance and food intake charts
  - must not write on prescription charts, assessment sheets or care plans.

Assessment and care planning

1 The first written assessment and the identification of the patient's immediate needs must begin within 4 hours of admission. This must include any allergies or infection risks of the patient and the contact details of the next of kin.
2 The following must be completed within 24 hours of admission and updated as appropriate:
  - completion of nutritional, oral, pressure sore and manual handling risk assessments
  - other relevant assessment tools, for example pain and wound assessment.
3 All sections of the nursing admission assessment must be completed at some point during the patient's hospital stay with the identification of the patient's care needs. If it is not relevant or if it is inappropriate to assess certain functional health patterns, for example the patient is unconscious, then indicate the reasons accordingly.
  The ongoing nursing assessment should identify whether the patient's condition is stable, has deteriorated or improved.
4 Care plans should be written wherever possible with the involvement of the patient, in terms that they can understand, and include:
  - patient-focused, measurable, realistic and achievable goals
  - nursing interventions reflecting best practice
  - relevant core care plans that are individualized, signed, dated and timed.
5 Update the care plan with altered or additional interventions as appropriate.
6 The nursing documentation must be referred to at shift handover so it needs to be kept up to date.

(continued)

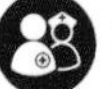

Box 2.7 **The Royal Marsden Hospital Guidelines for Nursing Documentation (2011) (adopted in line with NMC (2010) Record keeping)** ***(continued)***

Principles of assessment

Assessment should be a systematic, deliberate and interactive process that underpins every aspect of nursing care (Heaven and Maguire, 1996).

Assessment should be seen as a continuous process (Cancer Action Team 2007).

Structure of assessment

The structure of a patient assessment should take into consideration the specialty and care setting and also the purpose of the assessment.

When caring for individuals with cancer, assessment should be carried out at key points during the cancer pathway and dimensions of assessment should include background information and assessment preferences, physical needs, social and occupational needs, psychological well-being and spiritual well-being (Cancer Action Team 2007).

Functional health patterns provide a comprehensive framework for assessment, which can be adapted for use within a variety of clinical specialties and care settings (Gordon 1994).

Methods of assessment

Methods of assessment should elicit both subjective and objective assessment data.

An assessment interview must be well structured and progress logically in order to facilitate the nurse's thinking and to make the patient feel comfortable in telling their story.

Specific assessment tools should be used, where appropriate, to enable nurses to monitor particular aspects of care, such as symptom management (e.g. pain, fatigue), over time. This will help to evaluate the effectiveness of nursing interventions while often providing an opportunity for patients to become more involved in their care (O'Connor and Eggert 1994).

Decision making and nursing diagnosis

Nurses should be encouraged to provide a rationale for their clinical judgements and decision making within their clinical practice (NMC 2015).

The language of nursing diagnosis is a tool that can be used to make clinical judgements more explicit and enable more consistent communication and documentation of nursing care (Clark 1999, Westbrook 2000).

Planning and implementing care

When planning care, it is vital that nurses recognize whether patient problems require nursing care or whether a referral should be made to someone else.

When a nursing diagnosis has been made, the anticipated outcome for the patient must be identified in a manner which is specific, achievable and measurable (NMC 2015).

Nursing interventions should be determined in order to address the nursing diagnosis and achieve the desired outcomes (Gordon 1994).

Evaluating care

Nursing care should be evaluated using measurable outcomes on a regular basis and interventions adjusted accordingly (see Box 2.8).

Progress towards achieving outcomes should be recorded in a concise and precise manner. Using a method such as charting by exception can facilitate this (Murphy 2003).

Documenting and communicating care

The content and quality of record keeping are a measure of standards of practice relating to the skills and judgement of the nurse (NMC 2010).

In addition to the written record of care, the important role that the nursing shift report, or 'handover', plays in the communication and continuation of patient care should be considered, particularly when considering the role of electronic records.

Observation

DEFINITION

Observation is the conscious, deliberate use of the physical senses to gather data from the patient and the environment. It occurs whenever the nurse is in contact with the patient. At each patient contact, it is important to try and develop a sequence of observations. These might include the following.

1 As you enter the room, observe the patient for signs of distress, e.g. pallor, laboured breathing, and behaviours indicating pain or emotional distress.
2 Scan for safety hazards, e.g. are there spills on the floor?
3 Look at the equipment, e.g. urinary catheter, intravenous pumps, oxygen, monitors.
4 Scan the room – who is there and how do these people interact with the patient?
5 Observe the patient more closely for data such as skin temperature, breath sounds, drainage/dressing odours, condition of dressings, drains, need for repositioning (Wilkinson 2007).

Accurate measurements of your patient's vital signs provide crucial information about body functions (see Chapter 11: Observations).

Discharge planning

DEFINITION

Discharge planning is defined by Rorden and Taft (1990) as 'a process made up of several steps or phases whose immediate goal is to anticipate changes in patient care needs and whose long-term goal is to ensure continuity of health care'. Discharge planning should involve the development and implementation of a plan to facilitate the transfer of an individual from hospital to an appropriate setting and include the multidisciplinary team, the patient and their carers. Furthermore, it involves building on, or adding to, any assessments undertaken prior to admission (DH 2003).

INTRODUCTION

Discharge planning is a routine feature of health systems in many countries (Shepperd et al. 2013). The evidence suggests that a structured discharge plan tailored to the individual is best practice (Shepperd et al. 2013); therefore, effective, safe discharge planning needs to be patient and carer focused. There is consistent evidence to suggest that best practice in hospital discharge involves multidisciplinary teamwork throughout the process (Borrill et al. 2000). The multidisciplinary approach, where all staff have a clear understanding of their roles and responsibilities, will also help to prevent inappropriate readmissions and delayed discharges (Stewart 2000). This approach also promotes the highest possible level of independence for the patient, their partner and family by encouraging appropriate self-care activities.

Ineffective discharge planning has been shown to have detrimental effects on a patient's psychological and physical well-being and their illness experience (Cook 2001, Kissane and Zaider 2010, Lees 2013). Planning care, providing adequate information and involving patients, families and healthcare professionals will keep disruption to a minimum.

To achieve the best quality of life for patients and carers, there needs to be effective co-ordination in terms of care planning and delivery of that care over time (Day et al. 2009, NMC 2009, Øvretveit 1993). Discharge co-ordinators are, in general, health or social care professionals who have both hospital and community experience. Their role is to advise, help with planning, and assist the co-ordination of the differing care providers that the patient may need when leaving hospital, particularly when the nursing and care needs are complex. For complex discharges, it is helpful if a key worker, for example the discharge co-ordinator, is appointed to manage the discharge and, where appropriate, for family meetings/case conferences to take place and include the patient/carer, multidisciplinary team and primary healthcare team (PHCT) and representatives (Department of Evaluation in Healthcare Organisations 2001).

Patients with additional needs

There are groups of patients who may have additional needs on discharge and the approach taken may have to be tailored to meet these additional needs. If, for example, the patient has dementia or a learning disability, the approach to their discharge plan may need to be adjusted. If, for example, the patient has been assessed as lacking capacity to make a decision about where they live then the principles of the Mental Capacity Act (2005) must be employed to ensure the family and carers are involved. Where the patient is assessed as lacking capacity and has no relatives or friends and so is 'unbefriended' as defined by the Mental Capacity Act (2005), a referral should be made to the local Independent Mental Capacity Advocacy Service (Mental Capacity Act 2005). There is a concern that where a person has a degree of cognitive impairment, there will be an assumption that they cannot return home or that they need care. These assumptions should be challenged and decisions made on the basis of an assessment, including a mental capacity assessment. The assessment should evidence that the principles of the Mental Capacity Act (2005) have been applied.

For patients who may have additional needs on discharge, it is worth exploring what support services may be available and to identify what services were in place prior to admission. For example, if the person has a learning disability they may have a learning disability nurse in the community; involving them in the patient's discharge would ensure a safer transition for the patient and enable access to a professional who has knowledge and expertise in the field of learning disabilities but also in the needs of the patient.

Discharge processes (DH 2004b) endorse the value of co-ordination in a climate of shorter hospital stays and timely patient discharge. Poor discharge planning may result in patients remaining in hospital for longer than is necessary. Research has demonstrated that a high level of communication between the professionals planning the discharge and the providers of services outside the hospital setting is an effective mode of preventing readmission (Shepperd et al. 2013). McKenna et al. (2000) suggest that an indicator of poor discharge practice is poor communication amongst the multidisciplinary team (MDT), and between the hospital and community. For patients with complex needs, see Box 2.8 for additional support and guidance for decision making and planning. This should be used in conjunction with the discharge checklist (Figure 2.1).

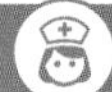 Learning Activity 2.4

Scenario: Discharge planning

You are caring for a patient who is known to have dementia.

1 What particular issues should you consider prior to discharge?
2 Does the patient lack capacity?
3 Does he/she have family/carers who should be involved in their care decisions?
4 Is it appropriate for him/her to return to their previous living arrangements?
5 If the patient lacks capacity and the answer to questions 3 and 4 is 'no', who should you get involved in their care?
6 What other support services might you want to get involved in his/her discharge?

See the end of the chapter for the answers.

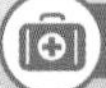 Learning Activity 2.5

Learning in practice: Complex discharge planning

Identify a patient who requires complex discharge planning. Review the discharge documentation for the patient and compare with the '**Guide to arranging a complex discharge home**' (see Box 2.8).

- Have all these steps been followed for your patient?
- Is there anything missing?
- What can you do to help?

Discuss this activity with a friend or your mentor to see if there is anything that could be done differently for this or future patients who have complex needs on discharge from hospital to home.

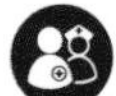

Box 2.8 **Guide to arranging a complex discharge home**

NB: This is not an exhaustive list and MUST BE DISCUSSED with the complex discharge co-ordinator/specialist sister, discharge planning, palliative care

Complex discharge definition

- A large package of care involving different agencies.
- The patient's needs have changed since admission, with different services requiring co-ordination.
- The family/carer requires intensive input into discharge planning considerations (e.g. psychological interventions):
  - patients who are entitled to NHS Continuing Healthcare and who require a package of care on discharge
  - patients for repatriation.

1 Comprehensive assessment by nurse on admission and document care accordingly

(a) Provisional discharge date set.	• This will only be an approximate date, depending on care needs, equipment, and so on. • It should be reviewed regularly with multidisciplinary team. • Discharge should not be arranged for a Friday or weekend.
(b) Referrals to relevant members of multidisciplinary team.	For example, occupational therapist, physiotherapist, social services.
(c) Referral to community health services (in liaison with multidisciplinary team).	For example, community nurse (who may be able to arrange for night sitters), community palliative care team.
(d) Request equipment from community nurse and discuss with family.	For example, hoist, hospital bed, pressure-relieving mattress/cushion, commode, nebulizer.
	If oxygen is required, medical team to complete Home Oxygen Ordering Form (HOOF) and Home Oxygen Consent Form (HOCF) for oxygen cylinders and concentrators at home. Fax to relevant oxygen supplier.

2 Discuss at ward multidisciplinary meeting, arrange family meeting/case conference as required, and invite all appropriate healthcare professionals, including community staff

(a) Appoint discharge co-ordinator at the multidisciplinary meeting.	• To act as co-ordinator for referrals and point of contact for any discharge concerns. • To plan and prepare the family meeting/case conference and to arrange a chairperson and minute-taker for the meeting. • Patient's named nurse to liaise with discharge co-ordinator.
(b) Formulate a discharge plan at meeting.	• At the meeting, formulate a discharge plan in conjunction with patient, carers, and all hospital and community personnel involved and agree a discharge date; an occupational therapist home visit may be required.
(c) Ascertain discharge address.	• Liaise with services accordingly. • It is important to agree who will care for patient/where the patient will be cared for, for example ground/first floor. • Ascertain type of accommodation patient lives in so that the equipment ordered will fit in appropriately. • **NB: If not returning to own home, a GP will be required to take patient on as a temporary resident.**
(d) Confirm PROVISIONAL discharge date.	• This will depend on when community services and equipment can be arranged. • This must be agreed with the patient and family/informal carer/s.

3 Ascertain whether community nurse is able to undertake any necessary clinical procedures in accordance with their local trust policy, for example care of skin-tunnelled catheters. Consider alternative arrangements if necessary

(a) Confirm equipment agreed and delivery date.	• **NB: Family must be informed of delivery date and also requested to contact ward to inform that this has been received.**
(b) Confirm start date for care.	• For example, social services/community nurse/community palliative care.

(c) Confirm with patient/family agreed discharge date.	• Liaise with complex discharge co-ordinator for Community Services Arrangements Form. • Check community services are able to enter patient's home as necessary.
4 Forty-eight hours prior to discharge, fax and telephone community nurse with Community Care Referral Form and discuss any special needs of patient, for example syringe driver, oxygen, wound care, intravenous therapy, methicillin-resistant *Staphylococcus aureus* or other infection status. Give written information and instructions	
a Arrange transport and assess need for escort/oxygen during transport. b Ongoing review. c If NO change within 24 hours of discharge, confirm that: – patient is medically fit for discharge – all community services are in place as agreed – patient has drugs to take out (TTO) and next appointment – access to home, heating and food are checked.	• Should be in place for any change in patient's condition/treatment plan. • If there is a change, notify/liaise with multidisciplinary team and community services. • Ensure patient has drugs TTO with written and verbal instructions. • Next in/outpatient appointment as required. • Check arrangements for patient to get into home (front door key), heating, food and someone there to welcome them home, as appropriate.
5 Hospital equipment, for example syringe drivers: ensure clearly marked and arrangements made for return	
6 After discharge, follow-up phone call to patient by ward nurse/complex discharge co-ordinator as agreed to ensure all is well	

The ten steps to discharge planning

The DH has identified ten steps to discharge planning to assist with the planning of discharge and transfer from hospital and intermediate care (DH 2010).

1. Start planning for discharge or transfer before or on admission.
2. Identify whether the patient has simple or complex discharge and transfer needs, involving the patient or carer in your decision.
3. Develop a clinical management plan for every patient within 24 hours of admission.
4. Co-ordinate the discharge or transfer of care process through effective leadership and handover of responsibilities at ward level.
5. Set an expected date of discharge or transfer within 24–48 hours of admission and discuss with the patient and carer.
6. Review the clinical management plan with the patient each day, take necessary action and update progress towards the discharge or transfer date.
7. Involve patients and carers so that they can make informed decisions and choices that deliver a personalized care pathway and maximize their independence.
8. Plan discharges and transfers to take place over 7 days to deliver continuity of care for the patients.
9. Use a discharge checklist 24–48 hours before transfer.
10. Make decisions to discharge and transfer patients each day.

EVIDENCE-BASED APPROACHES

Single Assessment Process

The Single Assessment Process (SAP) is a key part of the *National Service Framework for Older People* (DH 2001), but is not used comprehensively in the UK. The SAP is designed to replace fragmented assessments carried out by different agencies with one seamless procedure (Hunter 1998). It is based on the recognition that many older people have wide-ranging welfare needs and that agencies need to work together to ensure that assessment and subsequent care planning are effective and co-ordinated, and that care is holistic and centres on the whole person (Lymbery 2005). This standard aims to ensure that the NHS and social care services treat older people as individuals and enable them to make choices about their own care, by producing a comprehensive 'individualized care plan' that will set out their full needs and entitlements (Taylor 2012). The SAP aims to make sure older people's needs are assessed thoroughly and accurately, but without procedures being needlessly duplicated by different agencies, and that information is shared appropriately between health and social care agencies.

LEGAL AND PROFESSIONAL ISSUES

There is a requirement in discharge planning for nurses to share information about patients with health and social care providers in the community and, in doing so, there needs to be consideration regarding consent to share information and using safe procedures to ensure information is only shared with those who require it. Failing to apply good information governance processes could result in information being shared inappropriately and the breaching of a patient's right to confidentiality. Patients need to consent to their information being shared and, where the patient lacks capacity to share information, then sharing needs to be considered in the patient's 'best interest' based on a mental capacity best interest assessment (Mental Capacity Act 2005, p.3).

PRE-PROCEDURAL CONSIDERATIONS

It is essential that nurses are aware of their organization's discharge procedures, policies and protocols. If a patient is to be admitted for an elective procedure and has attended pre-assessment, discharge needs should be identified at this point to allow effective planning and potential services notified in advance of any admission. This is even more pertinent where patients are being admitted for a short length of stay. These discussions with patients and their families can also help them to determine what they may need on discharge and to plan accordingly.

The role of informal carers

Engaging and involving patients and informal carers, family member or friends who provide care in an unpaid capacity as

Patient's Name:... Hospital No.:..................

THE ROYAL MARSDEN

Complex Discharge Planning Sheet

Document the patient & carer involvement in discharge decisions and any change of discharge date or arrangements

SIGNATURE WHEN ACTIONED			COMMENTS
Discussed / agreed discharge date & arrangements e.g. Is heating organized? Is access sorted e.g. keys available / steps considered?	Patient informed	Sig Date/Time	**Provisional discharge date:............** **Agreed discharge date:.................**
	Carer informed	Sig Date/Time	
Equipment Access INTRANET for information about Discharge - Community Liaison • Discharge checklists for specific needs • Home equipment	Not applicable	Sig Date/Time	*Consider whether the patient needs: bed, hoist, mattress, commode, oxygen, nebulizer, syringe drivers at home*
	• Specify equipment & document in the discharge planning progress notes the arrangements as appropriate. • Obtain or print relevant discharge checklist(s) and complete as part of the patient's documentation		
Take home medication/ equipment	Medication ordered	Sig Date/Time	
	Nutritional supplements ordered	Sig Date/Time	
	Dressings ordered	Sig Date/Time	
	Appliances ordered e.g. stoma & continence aids	Sig Date/Time	
	Medication explained & given to patient	Sig Date/Time	
	Patient's own medication returned including controlled drugs	Sig Date/Time	
Ability to self medicate If **NOT ABLE**, name the person who will prompt or give medication post discharge	Able	Sig Date/Time	Is a dosette box required? Yes ❑ *Note arrangements in discharge planning progress notes* Named person: Self medication chart provided Yes ❑
	Not able	Sig Date/Time	
Follow up appointment Note Check if any investigations are required e.g. EDTA, X-ray or scans	Ordered	Sig Date/Time	Sick note given ❑ N/A ❑
	Given to patient	Sig Date/Time	
	No follow up	Sig Date/Time	
Transport - specify on transport form if : • Walker • Chair • Stretcher • Oxygen • Escort	Not required	Sig Date/Time	Date of transport booking: Booking reference no: 'Do not attempt resuscitation' letter completed by medical staff for ambulance staff provided Yes ❑
	Required	Sig Date/Time	
	Booked	Sig Date/Time	
Property / valuables (including key to access home)	Returned to patient	Sig Date/Time	
	Not applicable	Sig Date/Time	

Figure 2.1 **Complex discharge planning sheet.**

Communication & written information to: Community nurse; Community Palliative Care Team, Hospice Home Care Team

- Document in the discharge planning progress notes the nature of communication with others and action required or taken
- Note whether Community Referral form(s) or Hospice form faxed and/or given to the patient

Community nurse	Referral not required	Sig	**Comments**
		Date/Time	Copy of Referral form given to patient
	Referral required	Sig	Yes ❑
		Date/Time	
	Date of referral	Sig	
		Date/Time	
	Referral form faxed	Sig	
		Date/Time	
Date of first visit agreed with community staff		Sig	
Yes ❑ No ❑ Not specified ❑		Date/Time	
Community Palliative Care Team / Hospice Home Care Team	Referral not required	Sig	**Comments**
		Date/Time	Copy of Referral form given to patient
	Referral required	Sig	Yes ❑
		Date/Time	
	Date of referral	Sig	
		Date/Time	
	Referral form faxed	Sig	
		Date/Time	
Date of first visit agreed with community staff		Sig	
Yes ❑ No ❑ Not specified ❑		Date/Time	
Other e.g. Marie Curie Nurse, Stoma Nurse, Continence Advisor,			**Comments**
Specify:	Referral required	Sig	Copy of Referral form given to patient
		Date/Time	Yes ❑
	Date of referral	Sig	
		Date/Time	
	Referral form faxed	Sig	
		Date/Time	
Date of first visit agreed with community staff		Sig	
Yes ❑ No ❑ Not specified ❑		Date/Time	

Communication & written information to Community Social Services

- Clarify if section 2 and 5 notification forms required or whether the patient requires information, advice and/or carer's assessment by hospital social services (complete RMH Social Services Trigger Form)
- Be aware whether Community Care (Delayed Discharge) Act 2003 section 2 or section 5 notification sent to community social services. **If section 5 notification sent - ensure section 5 confirmation received from community social services prior to discharging the patient.**
- Document in the discharge planning progress notes the nature of communication with others and action required or taken

Community Social Services	Referral not required	Sig	**Comments**
		Date/Time	
	Required	Sig	
		Date/Time	

Figure 2.1 ***(Continued)***

equal partners is central to successful discharge planning (DH 2003, Holzhausen et al. 2001). The Picker Report, an independent patient survey, identified that 16% of patients questioned reported that they did not feel involved in their discharge (Garrett and Boyd 2008). The hospital discharge process is also a critical time for informal carers, placing an increasing burden of care on them (Bauer et al. 2009, Higginson and Costantini 2008), yet Holzhausen et al. (2001) suggest they do not feel involved in the discharge process. It may be the first time they have been confronted with the reality of their role, the effect it may have on their relationship with the person needing care, their family and their employment (Hill and MacGregor 2001). Research suggests that if carers are unsupported, this can result in early readmission of the patient (Holzhausen et al. 2001). It is therefore important to involve carers as partners in the discharge planning process.

The Carers (Equal Opportunities) Act 2004 was implemented to support carers in a practical way by providing information, helping carers to remain at work and to care for themselves. Under the Act, carers are entitled to their own assessment and many support services can be provided, including respite, at no charge. Carers are often unaware that they are entitled to an assessment and may be able to access care and support as a carer. It is important that carers are made aware of this and part of this might be as simple as letting them know that the role they play with their family member is that of a carer: many people would see themselves as a wife, husband or daughter rather than a carer.

It is important to recognize that in some families, children may take on a caring role and their needs may go unrecognized (Naked Flame Research 2004). Informing community health and social care providers that there are young carers involved, with prior consent from the parents, may enable the young carers to access additional support services (Carers UK 2012, Naked Flame Research 2004). Young carers may struggle with the responsibilities of providing care to parents and their function can frequently go unrecognized, making the young carer feel isolated and distressed.

Throughout discharge planning, carers' needs should be recognized and acknowledged. Carers may have different needs from patients and there may be conflicting opinions about how the patient's care needs can be met. It is not uncommon for patients to report that their informal carer is willing to provide all care but the carer is not in agreement with this. Healthcare professionals should allow carers sufficient time and provide appropriate information to enable them to make decisions. They should also provide written information on the discharge plan and ensure adequate support is in place before discharge takes place (DH 2010). This will promote a successful and seamless transfer from hospital to home.

The discharge planning process and the primary/secondary care interface

The discharge planning process can be initiated by any member of the PHCT or social services staff in the patient's home, prior to admission, in pre-admission clinics or on hospital admission (Huber and McClelland 2003). Importance is attached to developing a primary care-led NHS, reinforced by the government's White Paper *The New NHS: Modern, Dependable* (DH 1998). The focus on quality, patient-centred care and services closer to where people live will be dependent on primary, secondary and tertiary professionals working together (Davis 1998).

However, it is important to note that the Community Care (Delayed Discharges) Act (DH 2003) introduced a system of reimbursement to NHS bodies from social services departments for delays caused by the failure of social services departments to provide timely assessment and/or services for a patient being discharged from an acute hospital bed. An awareness of the process and required timescales is essential to ensure that a patient's discharge is not delayed because social services have had insufficient time to respond to a request for an assessment.

The discharge planning process takes into account a patient's physical, psychological, social, cultural, economic and environmental needs. It involves not only patients but also families, friends, informal carers, the hospital multidisciplinary team and the community health/social services teams (Maramba et al. 2004, Salantera et al. 2003), with the emphasis on health and social services departments working jointly. However, a new emphasis is being placed on personalized care in the community, with patients purchasing and managing their own care package (Darzi 2008). Giving patients greater control and choice over the services they need requires the professionals to ensure that they have provided information regarding all the possible alternatives for care open to the patient and their carers (Darzi 2008).

As well as patient experience, discharge planning is considered a factor in reducing the length of hospital stay, which has a financial impact for the NHS (DH 2004b, Bull and Roberts 2001, Mardis and Brownson 2003, Nazarko 1998). Given the huge cost of inpatient care, it is important to ensure that procedures are in place, and complied with, to facilitate patients being discharged at the earliest opportunity. However, the notion of a seamless service may be idealistic because of increasing time constraints and the complex care needs of high-dependency patients (Smith 1996).

A significant proportion of patients, 3–11%, return to hospital within 28 days because of complications that have arisen as a consequence of their health. Readmission rates can be reduced through the health assessments and planning that take place in hospital (NHS Institute for Innovation and Improvement 2014). This reinforces the fact that good discharge planning can not only support a better experience for the patient and their carers on discharge but could in fact prevent further unnecessary admissions to hospital.

Box 2.9 **Discharge against medical advice form**

Name:

Hospital No:

Address:

I wish to discharge myself against medical advice and accept full responsibility for my actions.

Signed:

Date:

Time:

Statement to be signed by the Doctor
I have discussed with the patient the medical reasons why he/she should remain in the hospital.

Signed:

This form should be filed with the patient's medical records
NB: If concerned about support in the community for the patient, contact social services, the complex discharge co-ordinator or the on-call sister in charge out of hours for advice.

Occasionally the discharge process may not proceed as planned; a discharge may be delayed for a number of reasons and a system should be in place to record this. Patients may take their own discharge against medical advice and this should be documented accordingly (Box 2.9). When patients are assessed as requiring care or equipment but decline these, this does not negate the nurse's duty to ensure a discharge is safe. A discussion should take place with the patient and carer to assess how they intend to manage without the required care/equipment in place. It is crucial that the community services are aware of assessed needs that are not being met through patient choice or lack of resources. It is critical that the community teams who will be supporting the patient when they return home are notified and where possible this should be in writing, such as sending them a copy of the 'Discharge against medical advice' form (see Box 2.9 and Box 2.10).

When patients are informed by their medical teams that there are no further treatment options and advised that their prognosis may be poor, they may decide they want to go home urgently and plans would need to be set up at short notice.

Voluntary services

In many areas voluntary sector providers have begun to forge ways to deliver efficient, high-quality, patient-centred care. Evidence suggests that partnerships between the NHS and voluntary sectors have the potential to address a number of priorities, including prevention and shifting treatment, care and support into the community (Addicott 2013). Therefore, it is worth exploring what voluntary services are available locally that could support patients in the return to the community, ranging from practical support such as small home improvements to befriending services.

Reablement and intermediate care

The provision of reablement or enablement and intermediate care packages constitutes what are known as 'supported discharges'. The aim is to support the patient in making the transfer from hospital to community, thereby avoiding lengthy

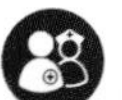
Box 2.10 **Patients taking discharge against medical advice**

Nursing staff responsibility

If a patient wishes to take their own discharge, the ward sister/co-ordinator should contact:

- a member of the medical team
- the manager on call
- the complex discharge co-ordinator.

The complex discharge co-ordinator will inform social services if appropriate. Out of hours, following a risk assessment, the manager on call will contact the local social services department, if appropriate, and inform the hospital social services department the following day.

Medical staff responsibility

The doctor, following consultation with the patient, should complete the appropriate form prior to the patient leaving the hospital. The form must be signed by the patient and the doctor and filed in the medical notes. The doctor must immediately contact the patient's GP.

stays for rehabilitation in an acute hospital bed (DH 2010). This may be a short stay in a residential rehabilitation unit or community hospital. This can also be provided in the patient's own home with additional services such as occupational therapy and physiotherapy being provided to support a personal care package. These services are normally short term and are likely to be reviewed within 6 weeks of discharge.

Reablement or enablement has been defined as 'services for people with poor physical or mental health to help them accommodate their illness by learning or re-learning the skills necessary for daily living. The focus is on restoring independent functioning rather than resolving health care issues, and on helping people to do things for themselves rather than the traditional home care approach of doing things for people that they cannot do for themselves' (DH 2010). Reablement or enablement focuses on dressing, using the stairs, washing and preparing meals. In some areas reablement or enablement may include social reintegration to support social activities. Although reablement overlaps with intermediate care, its focus on assisting people to regain their abilities is distinctive.

The *National Service Framework for Older People* (DH 2001) signalled the development of intermediate care as one of the major initiatives for services in the future. It is recognized that, if at all possible, older people are best cared for at home. To aid the transition period from hospital to home, intermediate care teams may provide a period of intensive care/rehabilitation following a hospital stay, which may take place in a care home or in the individual's own home. It is likely to be limited to a maximum of 6 weeks but there are local variations in practice. Intermediate care needs to have a person-centred approach, involving patients and carers in all aspects of assessment, goal setting and discharge planning. Its success depends on local knowledge of the service and interagency collaboration (Hancock 2003). There is growing evidence suggesting that intermediate care initiatives reduce admissions to acute hospitals and residential/nursing home placements (DH 2010, Foundation Trust Network 2012).

Social services care – Sections 2 and 5

If a patient does not meet the criteria for reablement, enablement or intermediate care, they may still receive assistance with personal care and domestic tasks through social services. However, it must be made clear to the patient and/or their family that they will be financially assessed and as a result may be charged for the service. In some local authorities, if the patient is assessed as 'self-funding', social services may only then offer a signposting services to private care providers. Where a patient is assessed as requiring care from social services to enable them to return home, then the trust should notify the local authority using the Community Care and Delayed Discharge Act processes.

The local authority will require a Section 2 no later than 72 hours prior to discharge but this should be done at the earliest opportunity. When the patient has been assessed and is ready for discharge, a Section 5 notification should be sent to the local authority at least 24 hours before discharge. How the local authority responds to the Section 2 may depend on what local arrangements are in place. Many local authorities have a social worker or social work department within the trust to facilitate the setting up of care packages for discharge. Other authorities may require additional assessments such as occupational therapy or medical reports to enable them to set up the care. It is not uncommon for local authorities to request an NHS Continuing Healthcare checklist to be completed as part of the process to assess if the patient might be entitled to NHS Continuing Healthcare funding.

NHS Continuing Healthcare

NHS Continuing Healthcare funding exists to support people with complex healthcare needs. It is provided to support the care that people need over an extended period of time as a result of disability, accident or illness, to address both physical and mental health needs. It may require services from the NHS and/or social care. It can be provided in a range of settings, for example, from a care home to care in people's own homes. NHS Continuing Healthcare is a package of care arranged and funded solely by the NHS. It should be awarded when it is established (through a comprehensive multidisciplinary assessment) that an individual's primary care need is a health need. There has been inconsistency in applying the criteria nationally (House of Commons Health Committee 2005), resulting in the Department of Health producing a *National Framework for NHS Continuing Healthcare* (DH 2009).

In November 2012 new national tools for NHS Continuing Healthcare were launched. These replace any previous tools, including the fast-track assessment for patients who have a rapidly deteriorating condition and a checklist to identify if a patient should be assessed using the full assessment. There is a legal obligation to inform patients of their right to be assessed for NHS Continuing Healthcare funding. There is an online resource booklet (www.gov.uk/government/publications/nhs-continuing-healthcare-and-nhs-funded-nursing-care-public-information-leaflet) informing patients of their rights and outlining the process (DH 2012). Patients who may be entitled to funding through this process could be paying unnecessarily for their care through social services as they will have been financially assessed or could be funding their own care. An important element of the new tools is the requirement for a signed consent rather than presumed consent (DH 2012).

Discharge to a care or nursing home

Discharging a patient to a care or nursing home requires careful thought as giving up their own home is one of the most traumatic events that a person has to consider. The impact on a patient and their carer may be significant, particularly where the person lives with a partner or family member and this would be a loss for both of them. A thorough multidisciplinary assessment is essential, taking into account the individual needs of the patient and their family or carer and exploring all the options before deciding on a care/nursing home. It is really important that carers are supported throughout this process. In most cases the family or carer will be the person who is looking for a care home placement. This can be quite a daunting process and it is worth providing a list of questions and things to look for when assessing a care or nursing home (Table 2.1).

Nursing and care home placements can be delayed while waiting for funding to be approved or waiting for a suitable bed to become available and it may therefore be necessary to consider an interim placement (DH 2003). It is important that the patient and carers are aware that there may be time limits on the stay in hospital so they will be required to find a suitable placement within an agreed timescale. Many hospitals have a policy to support staff where patients and their carers are delaying the process of arranging a nursing home placement.

Table 2.1 **Questions and things to look for when assessing a care or nursing home**

	Questions
First impressions	• Is the home easy for family and friends to visit, particularly those who have to rely on public transport? • Does the home have its own transport? • Is the main area accessible for disabilities, e.g. wheelchairs, poor sighted, hard of hearing? • Do the staff answer the door promptly? • Do the staff appear friendly and welcoming? • Does there appear to be a number of staff on duty? • Do the residents look well cared for and clean? • Is there an up-to-date registration certificate on display? It is usual to sign a visitors' book on arrival.
The accommodation	• Is the home/room clean and fresh? • Are the rooms single or shared? • Do the rooms have ensuite facilities? • Can you bring your own furniture and personal belongings? • Where are the nearest toilets, are they accessible? • Is there a telephone in the room and/or mobile phone reception? • Is there a wifi connection/is there a charge for this? • Are there quiet areas to sit in? • What are the meal times? • Is there a choice of meals/diets? • Is there a laundry service on site?
Personal needs	• How often do the hairdresser, dentist, chiropody, religious support, GP visit? • Does a resident change GP if they move from the local area? • Where are medications stored? • Can I get a newspaper? • What activities can I join in or hobbies to continue? • Does the home arrange outings? • Are there quiet areas for family/friends to visit? • Can they stay for meals? • Is there an overnight room where they can stay?
Finances and contracts	• What are the fees? • What services do the fees include, e.g. chiropody, hairdresser, etc.? • What are the terms and conditions? • Is there a reduction if the patient is admitted to hospital or goes on holiday? • What is the notice period/terminating contract? • When is the room available from?
Nursing needs	• How many qualified nursing staff are on duty day and night (in a nursing home)? • How often do qualified nursing staff review a resident (in a nursing home)? • How often does the community nursing team visit and review residents in the care home? • What is the daily care routine? • If the patient has very specific nursing needs, how will they be managed? Refer to the list given by the ward staff on the patient's specific health care needs. • How often do the community palliative care team visit the home? • How often is the GP or doctor in the home? • Although a difficult thing to consider, are they able to support patients to remain in the home for end-of-life care?

In 2007 there were important changes in the funding arrangements for adults requiring registered nursing care in nursing homes in England (DH 2013). All adults needing the skills and knowledge of a Registered Nurse to meet all or certain elements of their care needs have that care paid for by the NHS. The amount of funding, paid directly to the nursing home, is dependent on a comprehensive assessment of the patient's care needs by a Registered Nurse, who will usually be employed by the local Clinical Commissioning Group. NHS-funded nursing care was originally provided via payment 'bands', which relate to the level of nursing care required. However, the National Framework (DH 2006b), which came into effect in October 2007, replaced the banding system with a weekly rate for NHS-funded nursing care.

Equipment to facilitate a patient's discharge

Patients will frequently require equipment to enable them to return home. The equipment needs of each patient should be assessed at pre-admission and throughout their stay. From a nursing perspective, patients may require additional equipment such as oxygen, which should be prescribed using the appropriate national Home Oxygen Order Forms part A and B. However, in some hospitals this task is completed by a specialist respiratory nurse. It is useful to know how the local procedures work and how to access oxygen for patients at home. Consideration also needs to be given to the monitoring and reviewing of the patient on oxygen once at home.

Specialist ongoing care provisions for patients at home

Patients may require additional provisions to be put in place to facilitate a safe and timely discharge. Patients may be returning home having had interventions that mean they need specialist nursing input. There will be locally agreed policies and procedures in the community about what can be provided, therefore it is important to confirm that the individual patient's nursing needs can be met before discharge.

Nutritional needs on discharge

In some cases, patients may be receiving nutritional supplements via feeding tubes, known as enteral feeding. The common routes for enteral feeding in the community are:

- radiologically inserted gastrostomy (RIG)
- percutaneous endoscopically placed gastrostomy (PEG)
- jejunostomy
- nasogastric.

Community nurses and dieticians should be contacted in advance of a patient returning home with supportive feeding *in situ* to ascertain what information and support they need to facilitate the patient's safe and timely discharge.

Pumps and drains

For wound healing, in some cases patients may be discharged with drains or pumps *in situ*. It is important to confirm that the Clinical Commissioning Group will fund the equipment before discharge. The patient should be supplied with at least 1 week's supply of dressings, allowing the community nurse time to order additional supplies. This timescale may vary depending on local agreements between acute trust and community health providers.

Medication

Before a patient is discharged, the nurse needs to ensure that the patient and, where appropriate, the carer are competent to self-administer medication at home. In some areas tablet dispensers are provided, particularly for those who have difficulty opening containers. If carers/community nurses are involved, local policies need to be adhered to. A medicines administration record (MAR chart) should be given on discharge, clearly stating the name of the drug, dose and frequency and any other special instructions. Special considerations are required for medications prescribed for pumps and drivers, e.g. for patients who require end-of-life care of symptom management.

Patients with particular care needs on discharge

It is important to recognize that some patients may have additional needs that they have not considered themselves whilst in hospital (Box 2.11). If, for example, the patient lives alone or is very frail, simple tasks such as shopping for basic provisions may be very difficult. Consequently, some shopping may need to be done prior to discharge. The patient may have a family member, friend or neighbour who can do this but the patient may assume this task is going to be done when it has not been, thus leaving the patient at home with no basic provisions and no means of getting them. It is therefore really important to talk to the patient about how they might manage these tasks on discharge and consider other means of support such as Age UK or a local voluntary service.

For patients who are frail and at risk of falls, ensuring that they know that the community pendant alarm systems can be installed may provide the patient and family with some reassurance. Further information regarding these alarms and the local providers is usually held by the local authority.

Housing and impact on discharge

On discharge, consideration may need to be given to patient accommodation, such as the suitability of the accommodation and equipment needs, for example, if the patient's property is in a poor state or there are issues in relation to hoarding. A domiciliary visit may be required to ensure the property is habitable; this may need to be done by or with social services. It is also possible that prior to admission patients were homeless or they have become homeless during the admission. The patient may need to be supported to access accommodation through the local authority homelessness team. As part of the process, the patient will need to provide evidence of eligibility for social housing.

Issues of access to patient accommodation may impact on discharge plans. For example, the patient was mobile prior to admission and lives in third-floor accommodation with no lift, but is no longer mobile. However, the patient may still be discharged back to their property whilst the housing department reviews the accommodation and provides suitable alternative accommodation at a later date. Where the patient is a home owner, the housing department may be less likely to intervene and it may be down to the patient and their family to address this.

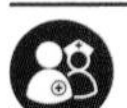

Box 2.11 **Patients with particular care needs on discharge**

- Live alone.
- Are frail and/or elderly.
- Have care needs which place a high demand on carers.
- Have a limited prognosis.
- Have serious illnesses and will be returning to hospital for further treatments.
- Have continuing disability.
- Have learning difficulties.
- Have mental illness or dementia.
- Have dependants.
- Have limited financial resources.
- Are homeless or live in poor housing.
- Do not have English as their first language.
- Have been in hospital for an 'extended stay'.
- Require aids/equipment at home.

Source: DH (2004b).

PRIOR TO DISCHARGE

It is important to continue to review the discharge needs of a patient up until the day of their discharge. There are certain issues that need to be addressed for all patients, such as transport to enable them to return home and that medications to take home have been ordered and are ready for discharge. For patients with more complex needs, it may be useful to use a discharge checklist; this can be commenced on the patient's admission and monitored throughout the patient's hospital stay (see Figure 2.1).

DISCHARGE AT THE END OF LIFE

The *End of Life Care Strategy* (DH 2008) requires that an assessment is made of the patient's preferred place of care and how and where they wish to be cared for at the end of life. Some patients may already have an advance care plan, within which will be recorded these wishes as well as any advance decision they have made about their end-of-life care. For some patients, these conversations may need to take place to ensure that they and their families are given the opportunity to make informed decisions about their wishes. It is important that these conversations are realistic and that patients and their families are aware of the services and potential gaps that might arise once the person is at home. For instance, if the patient believes that community nurses can be with them at any time day or night when a crisis occurs, this may set up the patient, family and community healthcare providers to fail.

The condition of a person nearing the end of life may change rapidly, so it is essential that choices are made and community services are accessed without delay. There may be occasions when a patient is reaching the end of life and the decision is made that their preferred place of care/death is home. Then every effort must be made to ensure that all practicable steps are taken to allow that to happen (Vaartio et al. 2006). Such discharges are often complex and multifactorial and require a multidisciplinary team to be flexible and responsive. It is important in the first instance to contact relevant community teams to highlight the need for a rapid response to any referrals being made. Community nursing, the community palliative care team and, where available, the community matron should be notified at the earliest opportunity. A fast-track NHS Continuing Healthcare funding application may need to be submitted to access funding for the care provision. The patient may also require essential equipment to enable them to return home, such as a profiling bed, commode or hoist; again, these should be ordered at the first opportunity.

Once care and equipment are in place and discharge is proceeding, ensure that a medical review takes place and that the GP, community nurses and community palliative care team are provided with a copy of the discharge summary (Figure 2.2). Telephone contact with the GP prior to discharge is essential to ensure they visit the patient at home.

The patient should be reviewed just prior to discharge by the medical team and any changes in their clinical condition or needs

Name: **Hospital No:**

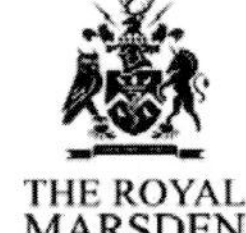

Patients Being Discharged Home for Urgent Palliative Care Checklist for Discharge

This form should be used to assist with planning an urgent discharge home for a patient with terminal care needs. It should be used in conjunction with the Discharge Policy.

Sign and date to confirm when arranged and equipment given. Document relevant information in the discharge planning section of the nursing documentation. Document if item or care is not applicable.

Appoint a designated discharge lead:

Name:.................................... Designation:.................................... Contact No:.................

	Date & Time	Signature, Print Name & Job Title
Patient / Family Issues		
Meeting with patient/family to discuss:- patient's condition and prognosis		
Plan agreed and discussed with patient and carers. Explain the level of care that will be provided in the community. Ensure an understanding that there will not be 24 hour nursing presence.		
Communication with Community Nurse and Community Palliative Care Team		
Discuss with patient/family: • Patient and family needs • The role of each service and the timing and frequency of visits • Community Service cover at night (to support family) e.g. Marie Curie or other local services • The need to complete the Continuing Care Application Form, if necessary. • Liaise with complex discharge co-ordinator if advice or fast tracking needed.		
Agreed planned date and time of community nurses first visit......................................		
Agreed planned date and time of community palliative care team first visit........................		
Night nursing service Start date.............................		
Communication with GP and Community Palliative Care Medical Team- Medical Responsibilities (Hospital medical team to organize – the nurse to confirm when arranged)		
Registrar to discuss patient's condition with GP and request home visit on day of discharge for death certification purposes. Agreed date and time of visit....................		
Oxygen: HOOF and HOCF completed and faxed to relevant company. Company to arrange delivery date and time with family. [Fax copies to GP for information only]		
Medical summary faxed to GP ❑ copy with patient ❑		
Registrar or Specialist Nurse to discuss with the Community Palliative Care team the patient's needs and proposed plan of care		
Adequate supply of drugs prescribed for discharge (TTOs) including crisis drugs e.g. s/c morphine, midazolam.		
Authorization for drugs to be administered by community nurses. Please refer to Subcutaneous Drugs policy and		

Figure 2.2 **Checklist for patients being discharged home for urgent palliative care.**

complete the discharge checklist for the McKinley T34 syringe pump.		
Prescription sheet of authorisation for drugs to be administered by community nurses. Faxed to Community Nurse and GP		
'Do Not Attempt Resuscitation' letter for Ambulance Crew		

Equipment - confirm delivery of equipment		
Electric, profiling hospital bed		
Pressure relieving equipment		
Commode/urinal/bed-pan		
Hoist/ slings/ sliding sheets		
Other, please state e.g. McKinley T34...		
Provide 4 days supply of:		
Dressings		
Sharps bin		
Continence aids		
Transport (confirm by ticking appropriate boxes) CHECK OTHER DISCHARGE DOCUMENTATION		
Escort (family/nurse)		
Family informed and aware that the patient may not survive the transfer journey and that the ambulance crew will not attempt resuscitation		
Written information and documentation		
Community Care Referral form completed and faxed for the attention of..		
Community Care Referral form and medical summary given to patient or relative (specify)		
Community Palliative Care Team form completed and faxed for the attention of...		
Patient/carer given list of contact numbers of community services **(including night service)**		
Medication list, stating reasons for drugs, given and explained to patient/ relative		
Confirm with the Hospital Consultant/Complex Discharge-Co-ordinator whether a bed should be held for this patient for 24hrs only (unless in exceptional circumstances following discussion with the Complex Discharge Co-ordinator)		

Signature/print name of designated ward based discharge lead:.................................

Date/Time..

File this form in the patient's records on discharge.

Figure 2.2 ***(Continued)***

should be shared with the community healthcare providers. It may even be necessary to review the decision and to have open and honest conversations with the patient and their family about what to expect in the coming hours, days or weeks.

POST-PROCEDURAL CONSIDERATIONS

A discharge delay is when a patient remains in hospital beyond the date agreed between the multidisciplinary team and beyond the time when they are medically fit to be discharged (DH 2003). For every patient who is 'delayed', NHS trusts are required to report the delay to their commissioners. It is the responsibility of the health authorities, in collaboration with local authorities, to monitor and address any issues that result in delays in the transfer of patients from an acute bed to their home or community bed, such as care home or rehabilitation bed. Trusts closely monitor bed activity and reporting varies from weekly to daily in winter months.

Learning for practice

After studying this chapter, list five key points you have learnt about assessment and discharge planning that you will be able to apply to your clinical practice.

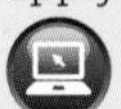

For further learning exercises visit **www.royalmarsdenmanual.com/student**.

Now Test Yourself

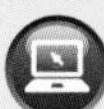

This section provides a range of exercises/activities to further test your learning. For additional exercises visit **www.royalmarsdenmanual.com/student**.

What have you learnt?

1 Within your clinical area, find the opportunity to either observe or carry out a patient admission assessment. Considering what you now know about that patient, go through the assessment questions in Box 2.5 and identify any 'gaps' in the patient assessment. What aspects of the assessment were not covered? Why?

2 If a patient has been assessed as lacking capacity to make their own decisions, what government legislation or 'act' should be referred to?
A Carers (Equal Opportunities) Act (2004)
B Mental Capacity Act (2005)
C Health and Social Care Act (2012)
D All of the above

3 How many steps to discharge planning were identified by the Department of Health (DH 2010)?
A 5 steps
B 8 steps
C 10 steps
D 12 steps

4 The single assessment process was introduced as part of the *National Service Framework for Older People* (DH 2001) in order to improve care for this group of patients
A True
B False

5 Under the Carers (Equal Opportunities) Act (2004) what are carers entitled to?
A Their own assessment
B Financial support
C Respite care
D All of the above

6 What is the main aim of the *End of Life Care Strategy* (DH 2008)?

See the end of the chapter for the answers.

Key points

- Assessment tools can be used to assess patients' general needs or to assess a specific problem.
- A comprehensive and systematic assessment is the key to planning and providing individualized patient care.
- Nurses have a professional responsibility to ensure that healthcare records provide an accurate account of the care process and are viewed as a tool of communication within the team.
- Effective discharge planning involving the multidisciplinary team helps to prevent inappropriate readmissions and delayed discharges while promoting the highest level of independence for the patient.
- When planning discharges, nurses are required to share information about patients with health and social care providers in the community. Principles of information governance must be adhered to, with care being taken to ensure that information is only shared as required and with the patient's consent.

REFERENCES

Addicott, R. (2013) *Working Together to Deliver the Mandate: Strengthening Partnerships Between the NHS and the Voluntary Sector.* London: King's Fund. Available at: www.kingsfund.org.uk/sites/files/kf/field/field_publication_file/working-together-to-deliver-the-mandate-jul13.pdf

Ahern, J. & Philpot, P. (2002) Assessing acutely ill patients on general wards. *Nursing Standard*, 16, 47–54.

Alfaro-LeFevre, R. (2014) *Applying Nursing Process: The Foundation for Clinical Reasoning.* Philadelphia: Lippincott Williams & Wilkins.

Allen, D. (1998) Record-keeping and routine nursing practice: the view from the wards. *Journal of Advanced Nursing*, 27, 1223–1230.

Arrowsmith, H. (1999) A critical evaluation of the use of nutrition screening tools by nurses. *British Journal of Nursing*, 8, 1483–1490.

Atwal, A. (2002) Nurses' perceptions of discharge planning in acute health care: a case study in one British teaching hospital. *Journal of Advanced Nursing*, 39, 450–458.

BAPEN & Malnutrition Advisory Group (2000) *Explanatory Notes for the Screening Tool for Adults at Risk of Malnutrition.* British Association for Parenteral and Enteral Nutrition, Malnutrition Advisory Group.

Bauer, M., Fitzgerald, L., Haesler, E. & Manfrin, M. (2009) Hospital discharge planning for frail older people and their family. Are we delivering best practice? A review of the evidence. *Journal of Clinical Nursing*, 18, 2539–2546.

Benner, P.E. (1984) *From Novice to Expert: Excellence and Power in Clinical Nursing Practice.* Menlo Park, CA: Addison-Wesley.

Berman, A., Kozier, B. & Erb, G.L. (2010) *Kozier and Erb's Fundamentals of Nursing.* Frenchs Forest, NSW: Pearson.

Bickley, L.S., Szilagyi, P.G. & Bates, B. (2013) *Bates' Guide to Physical Examination and History Taking.* Philadelphia: Lippincott Williams & Wilkins.

Bonevski, B., Sanson-Fisher, R., Girgis, A., Burton, L., Cook, P. & Boyes, A. (2000) Evaluation of an instrument to assess the needs of patients with cancer. *Cancer*, 88, 217–225.

Borrill, C., West, M., Shapiro, D. & Rees, A. (2000) Team working and effectiveness in healthcare. *British Journal of Healthcare Management*, 6, 364–371.

Brown, V., Sitzia, J., Richardson, A., Hughes, J., Hannon, H. & Oakley, C. (2001). The development of the Chemotherapy Symptom Assessment Scale (C-SAS): a scale for the routine clinical assessment of the symptom experiences of patients receiving cytotoxic chemotherapy. *International Journal of Nursing Studies*, 38, 497–510.

Bull, M.J. & Roberts, J. (2001) Components of a proper hospital discharge for elders. *Journal of Advanced Nursing*, 35, 571–581.

Cader, R., Campbell, S. & Watson, D. (2005) Cognitive Continuum Theory in nursing decision-making. *Journal of Advanced Nursing*, 49, 397–405.

Cancer Action Team (2007) Holistic Common Assessment of Supportive and Palliative Care Needs for Adults with Cancer: Assessment Guidance. London: Cancer Action Team.

Carers (Equal Opportunities) Act 2004; London: Stationery Office.

Carers UK (2012) Available at: www.carersuk.org

Chambers, S. (1998) Nursing diagnosis in learning disabilities nursing. *British Journal of Nursing*, 7, 1177–1181.

Clark, J. (1999) A language for nursing. *Nursing Standard*, 13, 42–47.

Cook, D. (2001) Patient autonomy versus parentalism. *Critical Care Medicine*, 29, N24–25.

Crouch, A.T. & Meurier, C. (eds) (2005) *Health Assessment.* Oxford: Blackwell Publishing.

Crumbie, A. (2006) Taking a history. In: Walsh, M. (ed) *Nurse Practitioners: Clinical Skills and Professional Issues*, 2nd edn. Edinburgh: Butterworth-Heinemann.

Darzi, L. (2008) *Our NHS, Our Future: NHS Next Stage Review: Leading Local Change.* London: Department of Health.

Davis, S. *Primary-Secondary care interface.* Conference proceedings, 25 March, 1998. NHS Executive.

Day, M.R., McCarthy, G. & Coffey, A. (2009) Discharge planning: the role of the discharge co-ordinator. *Nursing Older People*, 21, 26–31.

Delaney, C. (2001) Health informatics and oncology nursing. *Seminars in Oncology Nursing*, 17, 2–6.

Department of Evaluation in Healthcare Organisations (2001) *Evaluation of Professional Practice in Healthcare Organisations: Hospital Discharge Planning.* London: Department of Evaluation in Healthcare Organisations.

DH (1998) *The New NHS: Modern, Dependable.* London: Department of Health.

DH (2001) *National Service Framework for Older People.* London: Department of Health.

DH (2003) *Discharge from Hospital: Pathway, Process and Practice.* London: Department of Health.

DH (2004a) *The NHS Knowledge and Skills Framework (NHSKSF) and the Development Review Process.* London: Department of Health.

DH (2004b) *Achieving Timely 'Simple' Discharge from Hospital: A Toolkit for the Multi-Disciplinary Team.* London: Department of Health.

DH (2005) *Choosing a Better Diet: A Food and Health Action Plan.* London: Department of Health.

DH (2006a) *Modernising Nursing Careers: Setting the Direction.* London: Department of Health.

DH (2006b) *National Framework for NHS Continuing Healthcare and NHS-Funded Nursing Care in England. Consultation Document.* London: Department of Health.

DH (2008) *End of Life Care Strategy: Promoting High-Quality Care for all Adults at the End of Life.* London: Department of Health.

DH (2009) *The National Framework for NHS Continuing Healthcare and NHS-Funded Nursing Care*, July 2009 revised. London: Department of Health.

DH (2010) *Ready to Go? Planning the Discharge and the Transfer of Patients from Hospital and Intermediate Care.* London: Department of Health.

DH (2012) *The National Framework for NHS Continuing Healthcare and NHS-Funded Nursing Care*, November 2012 revised. London: Department of Health.

DH (2013) *NHS Continuing Healthcare and NHS-Funded Nursing Care: Public Information Leaflet.* London: Department of Health.

Dimond, B. (2002) *Legal Aspects of Pain Management.* Dinton, Wiltshire: Quay Books.

Edwards, M. & Miller, C. (2001) Improving psychosocial assessment in oncology. *Professional Nurse*, 16, 1223–1226.

Eilers, J., Berger, A.M. & Petersen, M.C. (1988) Development, testing, and application of the oral assessment guide. *Oncology Nursing Forum*, 15, 325–330.

Elfrink, V., Bakken, S., Coenen, A., McNeil, B. & Bickford, C. (2001) Standardized nursing vocabularies: a foundation for quality care. *Seminars in Oncology Nursing*, 17, 18–23.

Ford, P. & McCormack, B. (1999) Determining older people's need for registered nursing in continuing healthcare: the contribution of the Royal College of Nursing's Older People Assessment Tool. *Journal of Clinical Nursing*, 8, 731–742.

Foundation Trust Network (2012) *Briefing: FTN Benchmarking: Driving Improvement in Elderly Care Services.* London: Foundation Trust Network. Available at: www.foundationtrustnetwork.org

Frank-Stromborg, M. & Olsen, S.J. (eds) (2004) *Instruments for Clinical Healthcare Research.* Sudbury, MA: Jones and Bartlett Publishers.

Galanti, G.A. (2000) An introduction to cultural differences. *Western Journal of Medicine*, 172, 335–336.

Garrett, E. & Boyd, J. (2008) *Key Findings Report: Adult Inpatient Survey Results 2007.* Oxford: Picker Institute Europe. Available at: www.nhssurveys.org/survey/613

Gordon, M. (1994) *Nursing Diagnosis: Process and Application.* St Louis, MO: Mosby.

Grobe, S.J. (1996) The nursing intervention lexicon and taxonomy: implications for representing nursing care data in automated patient records. *Holistic Nursing Practice*, 11, 48–63.

Hancock, S. (2003) Intermediate care and older people. *Nursing Standard*, 17, 45–51.

Hardwick, S. (1998) Clarification of nursing diagnosis from a British perspective. *Assignment*, 4, 3–9.

Harris, R., Wilson-Barnett, J., Griffiths, P. & Evans, A. (1998) Patient assessment: validation of a nursing instrument. *International Journal of Nursing Studies*, 35, 303–313.

Health and Social Care Act 2012; London: Stationery Office.

Heaven, C.M. & Maguire, P. (1996) Training hospice nurses to elicit patient concerns. *Journal of Advanced Nursing*, 23, 280–286.

Hedberg, B. & Satterlund Larsson, U. (2003) Observations, confirmations and strategies – useful tools in decision-making process for nurses in practice? *Journal of Clinical Nursing*, 12, 215–222.

Higginson, I.J. & Costantini, M. (2008) Dying with cancer, living well with advanced cancer. *European Journal of Cancer*, 44, 1414–1424.

Hill, M. & MacGregor, G. (2001) *Health's Forgotten Partners? How Carers are Supported Through Hospital Discharge.* Manchester: Carers National Association.

Hogston, R. (1997) Nursing diagnosis and classification systems: a position paper. *Journal of Advanced Nursing*, 26, 496–500.

Holmes, H.N. (ed) (2003) *Three-Minute Assessmen.* Philadelphia: Lippincott Williams & Wilkins.

Holmes, S. & Eburn, E. (1989) Patients' and nurses' perceptions of symptom distress in cancer. *Journal of Advanced Nursing*, 14, 840–846.

Holt, P. (1995) Role of questioning skills in patient assessment. *British Journal of Nursing*, 4, 1145–1146, 1148.

Holzhausen, E., Clark, D. & Carers' National, A. (2001) *'You Can Take Him Home Now': Carers' Experiences of Hospital Discharge.* London: Carers National Association.

Horton, R. (2002) Differences in assessment of symptoms and quality of life between patients with advanced cancer and their specialist palliative care nurses in a home care setting. *Palliative Medicine*, 16, 488–494.

House of Commons Health Committee (2005). *NHS Continuing Care: Sixth Report of Session 2004-05, Vol 1. HC. 2004-05.* London: Stationery Office.

Huber, D.L. & McClelland, E. (2003) Patient preferences and discharge planning transitions. *Journal of Professional Nursing*, 19, 204–210.

Hunter, M. (1998) Rehabilitation in cancer care: a patient-focused approach. *European Journal of Cancer Care*, 7, 85–87.

Jensen, T.S., Wilson, P.R. & Rice, A.S. (2003) *Clinical Pain Management: Chronic Pain.* London: Arnold.

Johnson, T. (2000) Functional health pattern assessment on-line. Lessons learned. *Computers in Nursing*, 18, 248–254.

Kearney, N. (2001) Classifying nursing care to improve patient outcomes: the example of WISECARE. *Nursing Times Research*, 6, 747–756.

King, L. & Clark, J.M. (2002) Intuition and the development of expertise in surgical ward and intensive care nurses. *Journal of Advanced Nursing*, 37, 322–329.

Kissane, D.W. & Zaider, T. (2010) Bereavement. In: Hanks, G.W., Cherny, N.I., Christakis, N.A., Fallon, M., Kaasa, S., & Portenoy, R.K. *Oxford Textbook of Palliative Medicine.* 4th edn. Oxford: Oxford University Press.

Kozier, B. (2012) *Fundamentals of Nursing: Concepts, Process, and Practice.* Harlow, Essex: Pearson.

Lauri, S., Lepisto, M. & Kappeli, S. (1997) Patients' needs in hospital: nurses' and patients' views. *Journal of Advanced Nursing*, 25, 339–346.

Lees, L. (2013) The key principles of effective discharge planning. *Nursing Times*, 109, 18–19.

Leih, P. & Salentijn, C. (1994) Nursing diagnoses: a Dutch perspective. *Journal of Clinical Nursing*, 3, 313–320.

Lymbery, M. (2005) *Social Work with Older People: Context, Policy and Practice.* London: Sage.

Lyte, G. & Jones, K. (2001) Developing a unified language for children's nurses, children and their families in the United Kingdom. *Journal of Clinical Nursing*, 10, 79–85.

Maramba, P.J., Richards, S., Myers, A.L. & Larrabee, J.H. (2004) Discharge planning process: applying a model for evidence-based practice. *Journal of Nursing Care Quality*, 19, 123–129.

Mardis, R. & Brownson, K. (2003) Length of stay at an all-time low. *Health Care Manager*, 22, 122–127.

Marek, C. (2003) Antiemetic therapy in patients receiving cancer chemotherapy. *Oncology Nursing Forum*, 30, 259–271.

McClement, S.E., Woodgate, R.L. & Degner, L. (1997) Symptom distress in adult patients with cancer. *Cancer Nursing*, 20, 236–243.

McCrae, N. (2012) Whither nursing models? The value of nursing theory in the context of evidence-based practice and multidisciplinary health care. *Journal of Advanced Nursing*, 68, 222–229.

McDonald, M.V., Passik, S.D., Dugan, W., Rosenfeld, B., Theobald, D. E. & Edgerton, S. (1999) Nurses' recognition of depression in their patients with cancer. *Oncology Nursing Forum*, 26, 593–599.

McKenna, H., Keeney, S., Glenn, A. & Gordon, P. (2000) Discharge planning: an exploratory study. *Journal of Clinical Nursing*, 9, 594–601.

Mental Capacity Act 2005; London: Stationery Office.

Moen, A., Henry, S.B. & Warren, J.J. (1999) Representing nursing judgements in the electronic health record. *Journal of Advanced Nursing*, 30, 990–997.

Murphy, E.K. (2003) Charting by exception. *AORN Journal*, 78, 821–823.

Murphy, K., Cooney, A., Casey, D., Connor, M., O'Connor, J. & Dineen, B. (2000) The Roper, Logan and Tierney (1996) model: perceptions and operationalization of the model in psychiatric nursing within a health board in Ireland. *Journal of Advanced Nursing*, 31, 1333–1341.

Naked Flame Research (2004) *Understanding Sources of Help and Advice for Young People.* YouthNet. Available at: www.YouthNet.org

NANDA-I (2008) *Nursing Diagnoses: Definitions and Classifications, 2009-2011.* Oxford: John Wiley & Sons.

Nazarko, L. (1998) Improving discharge: the role of the discharge co-ordinator. *Nursing Standard*, 12, 35–37.

NHS Institute for Innovation and Improvement (2014) *Reduce Readmissions: Tool Generator.* Available at: www.institute.nhs.uk/scenariogenerator/tools/reduce_readmissions.html

NMC (2009). *Guidance for the Care of Older People.* London: Nursing and Midwifery Council. Available at: www.nmc-uk.org/documents/guidance/guidance-for-the-care-of-older-people.pdf

NMC (2010) *Record Keeping: Guidance for Nurses and Midwives.* London: Nursing and Midwifery Council. Available at: www.nmc-uk.org/Documents/NMC-Publications/NMC-Record-Keeping-Guidance.pdf

NMC (2015) *The Code: Standards of Conduct, Performance and Ethics for Nurses and Midwives.* London: Nursing and Midwifery Council. Available at: www.nmc-uk.org/Documents/Standards/The-code-A4-20100406.pdf

O'Connor, F.W. & Eggert, L.L. (1994) Psychosocial assessment for treatment planning and evaluation. *Journal of Psychosocial Nursing and Mental Health Services*, 32, 31–42.

Orem, D.E., Taylor, S.G. & Renpenning, K.M. (2001) *Nursing: Concepts of Practice.* St Louis, MO: Mosby.

Øvretveit, J. (1993) *Coordinating Community Care: Multidisciplinary Teams and Care Management.* Buckingham: Open University Press.

Parsaie, F.A., Golchin, M. & Asvadi, I. (2000) A comparison of nurse and patient perceptions of chemotherapy treatment stressors. *Cancer Nursing*, 23, 371–374.

Patton, K. & Thibodeau, G. (2010) *Anatomy and Physiology*, 7th edn. St Louis, MO: Mosby/Elsevier.

Peden-McAlpine, C. & Clark, N. (2002) Early recognition of client status changes: the importance of time. *Dimensions of Critical Care Nursing*, 21, 144–150.

Perdue, C. (2005) Understanding nausea and vomiting in advanced cancer. *Nursing Times*, 101, 32–35.

Putzier, D.J. & Padrick, K.P. (1984) Nursing diagnosis: a component of nursing process and decision making. *Topics in Clinical Nursing*, 5, 21–29.

RCN (2004) *Nursing Assessment and Older People: a Royal College of Nursing Toolkit.* London: Royal College of Nursing. Available at: www.rcn.org.uk/__data/assets/pdf_file/0010/78616/002310.pdf

Rhodes, V.A., Mcdaniel, R.W., Homan, S.S., Johnson, M. & Madsen, R. (2000) An instrument to measure symptom experience. Symptom occurrence and symptom distress. *Cancer Nuring*, 23, 49–54.

Rice, V.H. & Stead, L.F. (2008) *Nursing Interventions for Smoking Cessation.* Cochrane Database of Systematic Reviews. Available at: http://onlinelibrary.wiley.com/doi/10.1002/14651858.CD001188.pub4/pdf

Rolfe, G. (1999) Insufficient evidence: the problems of evidence-based nursing. *Nurse Education Today*, 19, 433–442.

Roper, N., Logan, W.W. & Tierney, A.J. (2000) *The Roper-Logan-Tierney Model of Nursing: Based on Activities of Living.* New York: Churchill Livingstone.

Rorden, J.W. & Taft, E. (1990) *Discharge Planning Guide for Nurses.* Philadelphia: W.B. Saunders.

Rowbotham, D.J. & MacIntyre, P.E. (2003) *Clinical Pain Management: Acute Pain.* London: Arnold.

Roy, C. (1984) *Introduction to Nursing: An Adaptation Model.* Englewood Cliffs, NJ: Prentice-Hall.

Salantera, S., Eriksson, E., Junnola, T., Salminen, E.K. & Lauri, S. (2003) Clinical judgement and information seeking by nurses and physicians working with cancer patients. *Psychooncology*, 12, 280–290.

Shaw, M. (1998) *Charting Made Incredibly Easy.* Springhouse, PA: Springhouse.

Shepperd, S., Lannin, N,A., Clemson, L.M., McCluskey, A., Cameron, I.D. & Barras, S.L. (2013) *Discharge Planning from Hospital to Home.* Available at: http://onlinelibrary.wiley.com/doi/10.1002/14651858.CD000313.pub4/pdf

Silverman, J., Kurtz, S.M. & Draper, J. (2013) *Skills for Communicating with Patients.* London: Radcliffe.

Smith, G.S. & Richardson, A. (1996) Development of nursing documentation for use in the outpatient oncology setting. *European Journal of Cancer Care*, 5, 225–232.

Smith, S. (1996) Discharge planning: the need for effective communication. *Nursing Standard*, 10, 39–41.

Stewart, W. (2000) Development of discharge skills: a project report. *Nursing Times*, 96, 37.

Suhonen, R., Valimaki, M. & Katajisto, J. (2000) Developing and testing an instrument for the measurement of individual care. *Journal of Advanced Nursing*, 32, 1253–1263.

Taylor, B.J. (2012) Developing an integrated assessment tool for the health and social care of older people. *British Journal of Social Work*, 42, 1293–1314.

Teytelman, Y. (2002) Effective nursing documentation and communication. *Seminars in Oncology Nursing*, 18, 121–127.

Thompson, C. (1999) A conceptual treadmill: the need for 'middle ground' in clinical decision making theory in nursing. *Journal of Advanced Nursing*, 30, 1222–1229.

Vaartio, H., Leino-Kilpi, H., Salantera, S. & Suominen, T. (2006) Nursing advocacy: how is it defined by patients and nurses, what does it involve and how is it experienced? *Scandinavian Journal of Caring Sciences*, 20, 282–292.
Walsh, M., Crumbie, A. & Watson, J.E. (2007) *Watson's Clinical Nursing and Related Sciences*. New York: Baillière Tindall/Elsevier.
Westbrook, A. (2000) Nursing language. *Nursing Times*, 96, 41.
White, L. (2003) *Documentation and the Nursing Process*. Clifton Park, NY: Thomson/Delmar Learning.
Wilkinson, J.M. (2007) *Nursing Process and Critical Thinking*, Upper Saddle River, NJ: Pearson Prentice Hall.

Answers

Learning Activity 2.2 Case study: Developing an individualized care plan

Core care plans and care pathways are being used increasingly to plan and deliver patient care. However, patients will inevitably have problems or health needs (nursing diagnoses) for which there is not a core care plan, so it is vitally important that nurses are able to develop comprehensive and individualized care plans for patients no matter what their condition.

Read the following case study:
Anna is a 27-year-old woman who was admitted to the ward with abdominal pain via the Emergency Department. She is currently nil by mouth and on intravenous fluids. She is very anxious about her mum, who is wheelchair bound and currently being looked after by a family friend; Anna is her main carer at home.

Develop a care plan for Anna to include the following:
- Nursing diagnoses (what are her problems or health needs?)
- Outcomes (what would you realistically hope to achieve for each of her nursing diagnoses?)
- Nursing interventions (what actions do the nursing team need to take to help achieve these outcomes?)

Example care plans
Anxiety related to being unable to care for her mother
For Anna to feel reassured that her mother is being looked after:

1 Allow time for Anna to discuss her home situation.
2 Support Anna to be able to speak with her mother over the phone.
3 Be flexible with visiting times to allow her mother to visit 'out of hours' if required.

Acute pain related to unknown cause
For Anna to state she is comfortable with pain score less than 3 (pain scale 0–10):

1 Assess pain hourly using a pain assessment chart.
2 Administer prescribed analgesia and monitor effect.
3 Provide Anna with information and support for any investigations she may have.

Risk for fluid deficit: nil by mouth
For Anna to state she does not feel dehydrated and to be in a slight positive fluid balance:

1 Administer prescribed IV fluids.
2 Maintain an accurate fluid balance chart.
3 Encourage Anna to rinse her mouth regularly.

Learning Activity 2.4 Scenario: Discharge planning

You are caring for a patient who is known to have dementia.
1 What particular issues should you consider prior to discharge?
2 Does the patient lack capacity?
3 Does he/she have family/carers who should be involved in their care decisions?
4 Is it appropriate for him/her to return to their previous living arrangements?
5 If the patient lacks capacity and the answer to questions 3 and 4 is 'no', who should you get involved in their care? Local Independent Mental Capacity Advocacy Service (Mental Capacity Act, 2005)
6 What other support services might you want to get involved in his/her discharge? For example: the hospital discharge team, social services, the mental health team?

Now Test Yourself What have you learnt?

1 Within your clinical area, find the opportunity to either observe or carry out a patient admission assessment. Considering what you now know about that patient, go through the assessment questions in Box 2.5 and identify any 'gaps' in the patient assessment. What aspects of the assessment were not covered? Why?

2 If a patient has been assessed as lacking capacity to make their own decisions, what government legislation or 'act' should be referred to?
A Carers (Equal Opportunities) Act (2004)
B Mental Capacity Act (2005)
C Health and Social Care Act (2012)
D All of the above

3 How many steps to discharge planning were identified by the Department of Health (DH 2010)?
A 5 steps
B 8 steps
C 10 steps
D 12 steps

4 The single assessment process was introduced as part of the *National Service Framework for Older People* (DH 2001) in order to improve care for this group of patients.
A True
B False

5 Under the Carers (Equal Opportunities) Act (2004) what are carers entitled to?
A Their own assessment
B Financial support
C Respite care
D All of the above

6 What is the main aim of the *End of Life Care Strategy* (DH 2008)?
A Identify a patient's preferred place of care.
B An assessment is used to identify how and where patients wish to be cared for at the end of life.

Infection prevention and control

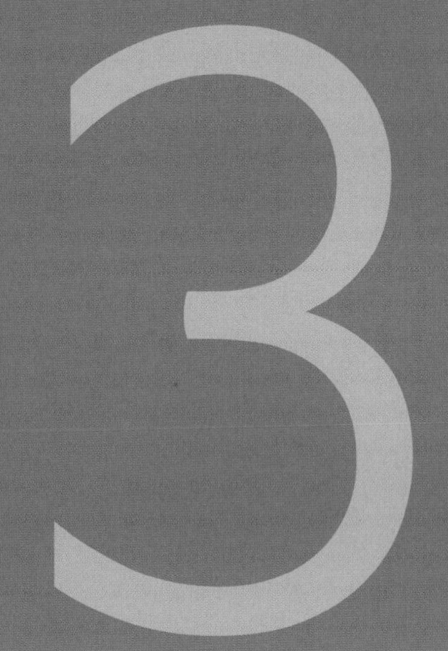

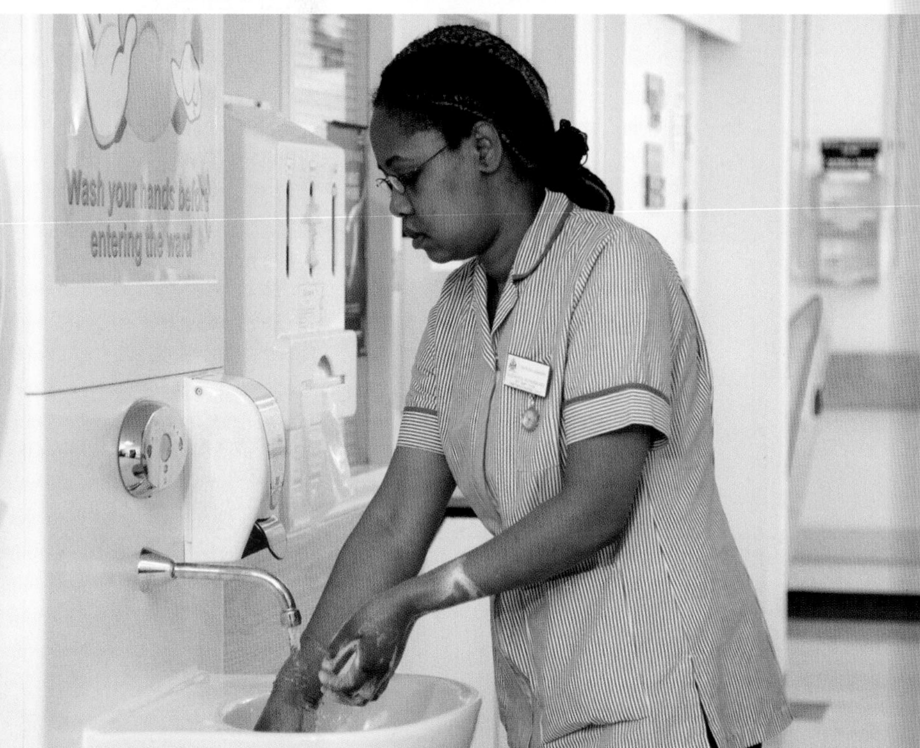

By reading this chapter and undertaking the learning activities within it, you should be able to:

1 Demonstrate knowledge of the most commonly occurring infectious agents and their different modes of transmission.
2 Describe the standard precautions required to minimize the risk of patients acquiring infections during their care, and correctly identify situations or procedures where additional precautions are necessary to ensure safe practice.
3 Identify the appropriate legislation (nationally and locally) that healthcare organizations are expected to comply with in relation to infection control.

Procedure guidelines

The Royal Marsden Manual of Clinical Nursing Procedures: Student Edition, Ninth Edition. Edited by Lisa Dougherty, Sara Lister and Alexandra West-Oram

Overview

This chapter describes the steps to be taken to minimize the risk of individuals acquiring infections during the course of care or treatment. Patients are most at risk but healthcare staff are also legally obliged to take reasonable and practicable precautions to protect themselves, other staff and anyone else who may be at risk in their workplace (Health and Safety at Work etc. Act 1974). The chapter describes the *standard precautions* that must be taken with all patients at all times regardless of their known infection status, and the additional precautions that need to be taken with some patients. Additional precautions can be required either:

- because the patient is colonized or infected with micro-organisms that may pose a particular risk to others, or
- because they are particularly vulnerable to infection themselves.

Note that it is quite possible for additional precautions to be required for both these reasons with one patient – someone who is more vulnerable to infection may well acquire an infection that poses a risk to others.

The chapter also describes the specific precautions that must be taken during invasive procedures, in particular aseptic technique. Related issues such as the safe management of healthcare waste are also considered briefly.

Learning Activity 3.1

Check your knowledge

Try this activity before you look at Box 3.1!

1 What do the following words mean?
  - Pathogen.
  - Colonization.

2 What is the difference between the following:
  - Universal precautions and standard precautions?
  - Source isolation and protective isolation?
  - Barrier nursing and reverse barrier nursing?

Go to Box 3.1 to find the answers.

Infection prevention and control

DEFINITIONS

'Infection prevention and control' has been defined as the clinical application of microbiology in practice (RCN 2010). More simply, it is a collective term for those activities intended to protect people from infections. Such activities are carried out as part of daily life by most individuals; for example, people wash their hands before eating to protect themselves from infection. The term is most often used in relation to healthcare, in particular with reference to preventing patients acquiring those infections most often associated with healthcare (such as wound infection) and preventing the transmission of micro-organisms from one patient to another (sometimes referred to as cross-infection).

Defined in Box 3.1 are some other terms used when discussing infection prevention and control. Confusion may sometimes arise because some of these terms are synonymous or have meanings which overlap, or are used in different ways by different people or organizations. This has been highlighted wherever possible.

RELATED THEORY

People who are receiving healthcare, whether in hospital or elsewhere, are at risk of infection (Loveday et al. 2014). There are many reasons for this; for example, people who are already ill may be less able to resist infection, and the invasive devices and procedures that are often used in healthcare often bypass some of the body's normal defences. If they are in hospital, this puts them in close proximity to other people who may also be more vulnerable to infection (Breathnach 2005, Gillespie and Bamford 2012). However, many infections acquired by patients receiving healthcare are preventable, as has been amply demonstrated by the 50% reduction in MRSA bacteraemia (bloodstream infections caused by meticillin-resistant *Staphylococcus aureus*) in English NHS hospitals between 2005 and 2008 (Health Protection Agency 2010a) and dramatic falls in the number of cases of *Clostridium difficile* infection in England (Health Protection Agency 2010b). These reductions were achieved by the systematic application and monitoring of established practices for the prevention and control of infection, including diligent hand hygiene and correct aseptic technique.

Box 3.1 **Terms used when discussing infection prevention and control**

Infectious agent

Anything that may be transmitted from one person to another, or from the environment to a person, and subsequently cause an infection or parasitic infestation. Infectious agents are most often micro-organisms such as bacteria or viruses.

Pathogen

A micro-organism that is capable of causing infection. Many micro-organisms are opportunistic pathogens; that is, they will cause infection in vulnerable individuals but not, normally, in healthy adults.

Colonization

When micro-organisms are present on or in a person but not currently causing any harm, that person is said to be colonized with those organisms. For example, human beings are normally colonized with huge numbers of several different species of bacteria.

Healthcare-associated infection (HCAI)

Any infection acquired as a result of a healthcare-related intervention or an infection acquired during the course of healthcare that the patient may reasonably expect to be protected from. For example, a person may acquire viral gastroenteritis in many circumstances but if they acquire it in hospital from another patient, it should be regarded as healthcare associated. This has replaced the term 'hospital-acquired infection'.

Cross-infection

Cross-infection is one term given to the transmission of infectious agents between patients within the healthcare setting. It may be direct transmission from one person to another, or indirect, for example via an incorrectly cleaned piece of equipment.

Universal precautions

Correctly called universal blood and body fluid precautions, these are the precautions that are taken with all blood and 'high-risk' body fluids. They are based on the principle that any individual may be infected with a bloodborne virus, such as HIV or hepatitis

B, and so pose a risk of infection; no individual can be regarded as completely 'risk free'. They are incorporated within standard precautions.

Standard precautions

The phrase 'standard precautions' is sometimes used interchangeably with 'universal precautions' (see above) but is used in this chapter and elsewhere (e.g. Health Protection Scotland 2009, Siegel et al. 2007) to describe the actions that should be taken in every care situation to protect patients and others from infection, regardless of what is known of the patient's status with respect to infection. Standard precautions include:

- hand hygiene at the '5 moments' described by the WHO (2009a), including before and after each patient contact
- care in the use and disposal of sharps
- the correct use of personal protective equipment for contact with all blood, body fluids, secretions and excretions (except sweat)
- providing care in a suitably clean environment with adequately decontaminated equipment
- the safe disposal of waste
- the safe management of used linen.

Transmission-based precautions

Additional infection control precautions taken with patients known or strongly suspected to be infected or colonized with organisms that pose a significant risk to other patients. The precautions will vary depending on the route by which the organism travels from one individual to another, but there will be common elements. Transmission-based precautions can be divided into:

- contact
- enteric
- droplet
- airborne.

Contact precautions

Additional infection control precautions to be taken with patients known or strongly suspected to be infected or colonized with pathogenic micro-organisms that are mainly transmitted through touch or physical contact. Contact precautions normally consist of isolation of the patient in a single room, where possible, and use of gloves and apron for any procedure involving contact with the patient or their immediate environment (Siegel et al. 2007).

Enteric precautions

Additional infection control precautions to be taken with patients suffering symptoms of infectious gastroenteritis, that is diarrhoea or vomiting that does not have an obvious mechanical or non-infectious cause. Enteric precautions should be taken from the first instance of diarrhoea or vomiting, regardless of whether a causative organism has been identified, until there is a definitive diagnosis that the symptoms do not have an infectious cause. Enteric precautions consist of prompt isolation of the patient in a single room with the door closed and use of gloves and apron for any procedure involving contact with the patient or their immediate environment (Chadwick et al. 2000, DH/HPA 2008).

Droplet precautions

Additional infection control precautions taken with patients known or strongly suspected to be infected or colonized with pathogenic micro-organisms that are mainly transmitted via droplets of body fluid expelled by an infected person. These are most often respiratory secretions expelled during coughing and sneezing but can include droplets from other sources such as projectile vomiting or explosive diarrhoea. The droplets are relatively large (>5 μm diameter) and do not remain suspended in the air for long so special ventilation is not normally required. Droplet precautions consist of isolation of the patient in a single room with the door closed and use of gloves and apron for any procedure involving contact with the patient or their immediate environment. Staff entering the room should wear a mask (Siegel et al. 2007).

Airborne precautions

Additional infection control precautions taken with patients known or strongly suspected to be infected or colonized with pathogenic micro-organisms that are mainly transmitted through the airborne route. These organisms are present in smaller droplets expelled by an infected person and so remain suspended in the air. Droplet precautions consist of prompt isolation of the patient in a single room, if possible with negative pressure ventilation or a positive pressure lobby, with the door closed, and use of gloves and apron for any procedure involving contact with the patient or their immediate environment. Staff entering the room should wear a fitted respirator (Siegel et al. 2007).

Some guidelines merge droplet and airborne precautions in order to provide a single set of instructions for staff caring for patients with any respiratory or airborne infection.

Isolation

Isolation is the practice of nursing a patient in a single-occupancy room to reduce the risk of spread of pathogens and to reinforce and facilitate additional infection control precautions.

Source isolation

The practice of isolating a patient for the main purpose of preventing the spread of organisms from that patient.

Protective isolation

The practice of isolating a patient for the main purpose of preventing the spread of organisms to that patient, normally used for patients with impaired immune systems.

Cohorting

When the number of patients with a particular infection or carrying a particular organism exceeds the single room capacity of a healthcare provider, they may be nursed together in a cohort. This is most often done for highly infectious conditions such as norovirus. Patients who require isolation but have different infections cannot be cohort nursed together because of the risk of cross-infection between them.

(continued)

Box 3.1 **Terms used when discussing infection prevention and control *(continued)***

Barrier nursing

The practice of nursing a patient who is carrying an infectious agent that may be a risk to others in such a way as to minimize the risk of transmission of that agent to others.

Reverse barrier nursing

The practice of nursing an individual who is regarded as being particularly vulnerable to infection in such a way as to minimize the transmission of potential pathogens to that person.

Common healthcare-associated infections

The 2011 national prevalence survey of patients in hospital in England with infections identified that 64 out of every 1000 patients in hospital at the time of the survey had an infection, a prevalence rate of 6.4%. Incidentally, this is another illustration of the fact that many healthcare-associated infections are preventable – the previous survey in 2006 showed a prevalence of 8.2% (Smythe et al. 2008). The most common types of infection were respiratory tract, urinary tract and surgical site infections (Health Protection Agency 2012). Less common types of infection, for example bacteraemia (bacteria infecting the bloodstream), may be more severe, so *all* procedures must be carried out in such a way as to minimize the risk of any infection.

Causes of infection

Infections are normally caused by micro-organisms. These are life forms too small to see with the naked eye. In some cases, for example prion diseases such as Creutzfeldt–Jakob disease (CJD), it can be unclear if the causative agent is actually living or not, while at the other extreme, infection control precautions will be applied to prevent the transmission of visible parasites such as scabies mites or enteric worms that may be metres in length (although their eggs are microscopic). The term 'infectious agent' is therefore often used to describe anything that may be transmitted from one person to another, or from the environment to a person, and subsequently cause an infection or parasitic infestation.

The major groups of micro-organisms are described below. Which group an infectious agent belongs to will have significant implications for the treatment of an infected individual – for example, antibiotics target bacteria but have no effect on viral infections – but for infection prevention and control it is more important to understand the *route of transmission* as this will dictate if any additional, transmission-based, precautions need to be in place (Siegel et al. 2007).

Types and classification of micro-organisms

Historically, the classification of micro-organisms was based on physical characteristics such as their size, shape or ability to retain a particular stain to make them visible under the microscope. Some of these distinctions are still useful, but classification is increasingly based on genetic characteristics, as analysis reveals the actual relationships between organisms. This can lead to confusion as new discoveries lead to species being reclassified and renamed. It should be noted that there can also be a wide variety of characteristics within each species, leading to significant variations in the severity of infection caused by different strains of the same organism. A good example of this is *Escherichia coli*. Every human being carries millions of these bacteria with no ill effects but infection with the toxin-producing O157 strain can cause serious illness.

This section describes the different types of organisms that may be encountered in a healthcare environment as well as the differences between and within the different types (Gillespie and Bamford 2012, Goering et al. 2012).

Bacteria

Bacteria are probably the most important group of micro-organisms in terms of infection prevention and control because they are responsible for many opportunistic infections in healthcare. A healthy human being will typically be host to one *quadrillion* (1000 trillion or 10^{15}) bacteria – around ten times as many organisms as there are cells in the human body. In normal circumstances the relationship between these bacteria and their host is commensal (i.e. their presence does not cause the host any problems) and may be mutually beneficial. For example, *E. coli* present in the gut can be an aid to digestion. However, when circumstances change, these commensal organisms can cause infections. If the *E. coli* in the example above are transferred from the gut to the urinary tract, a urinary tract infection can result.

Whether or not any particular situation will result in an infection depends on a wide range of factors and is not always predictable. What is certain is that bacterial infections cannot occur when bacteria are not present, hence the importance of measures designed to minimize the risk of transmission. However, the presence of bacteria does not necessarily indicate an infection – as noted above, many millions of bacteria live on and in the human body without causing harm – so the diagnosis of a bacterial infection and any decision about treatment must be made by considering a combination of the patient's symptoms and laboratory results that may indicate the presence of any particular bacteria (Gillespie and Bamford 2012).

Bacteria are what are known as *prokaryotes*, as opposed to *eukaryotes*, the term used for more complex organisms such as humans. This means that bacterial cells are much smaller and simpler than human cells, typically about the size of some of the structures such as mitochondria that exist within a mammalian cell. This small size means that bacteria do not have separate structures (such as a nucleus) within their cells. What bacteria do have and mammalian cells do not is a cell wall that contains the rest of the cell and gives it a distinctive shape (Goering et al. 2012). Some of these shapes are illustrated in Table 3.1. In terms of healthcare-associated infections, the most important bacteria are generally rod shaped or spherical.

The structure of the cell wall determines another important distinction in medically significant bacteria: whether they are Gram positive or Gram negative. The 'Gram' in these terms refers to Gram staining, named after its Dutch inventor, Hans Christian Gram (1853–1938), who devised the stain in 1884. Put simply, the structure of the cell wall determines whether or not the bacteria are able to retain a particular stain in the presence of an organic solvent such as acetone. The structure of the cell wall determines other characteristics of the bacteria, including their susceptibility to particular antibiotics, so knowing whether the cause of a bacterial infection is Gram positive or negative can help to determine appropriate treatment (Goering et al. 2012). The structure of the two different types of cell wall is shown in Figure 3.1.

Other structures visible outside the cell wall may include pili, which are rigid tubes that help the bacteria attach to host cells (or, in some cases, other bacteria for the exchange of genetic material), flagellae, which are longer, mobile projections that can help bacteria to move around, and capsules, that can provide protection or help the bacteria to adhere to surfaces. These are illustrated in Figure 3.2. The presence or absence of different structures will play a part in determining an organism's pathogenicity – its ability to cause an infection and the severity of that infection (Goering et al. 2012).

A final bacterial structure to consider is the spore. Bacteria normally reproduce by a process called binary fission – they

Table 3.1 **Bacterial shapes and arrangements**

	Shape/arrangements	Notes/example
	Coccus (sphere)	Different species divide in one plane to make pairs and chains or in multiple planes to make clusters
	Chain	*Streptococcus*
	Pair (diplococci)	*Neisseria*
	Cluster	*Staphylococcus*
	Straight rod	*Escherichia coli*
	Spore-forming rod	*Clostridium difficile*
	Comma-shaped	*Vibrio cholerae*
	Spiral-shaped	*Treponema pallidum*, which causes syphilis

create a copy of their genetic material and split themselves in two, with each 'daughter' cell being an almost exact copy of the parent (there are mechanisms by which bacteria can transfer genetic material between cells and so acquire characteristics such as antibiotic resistance, but they are beyond the scope of this chapter). However, some bacteria, notably *Clostridium difficile*, have the capacity, in adverse conditions, to surround a copy of their genetic material with a tough coat. Because this structure is created within the bacterial cell, it is sometimes referred to as an endospore, but is more often simply called a *spore*. Once the spore is formed, the parent cell dies and disintegrates, leaving the

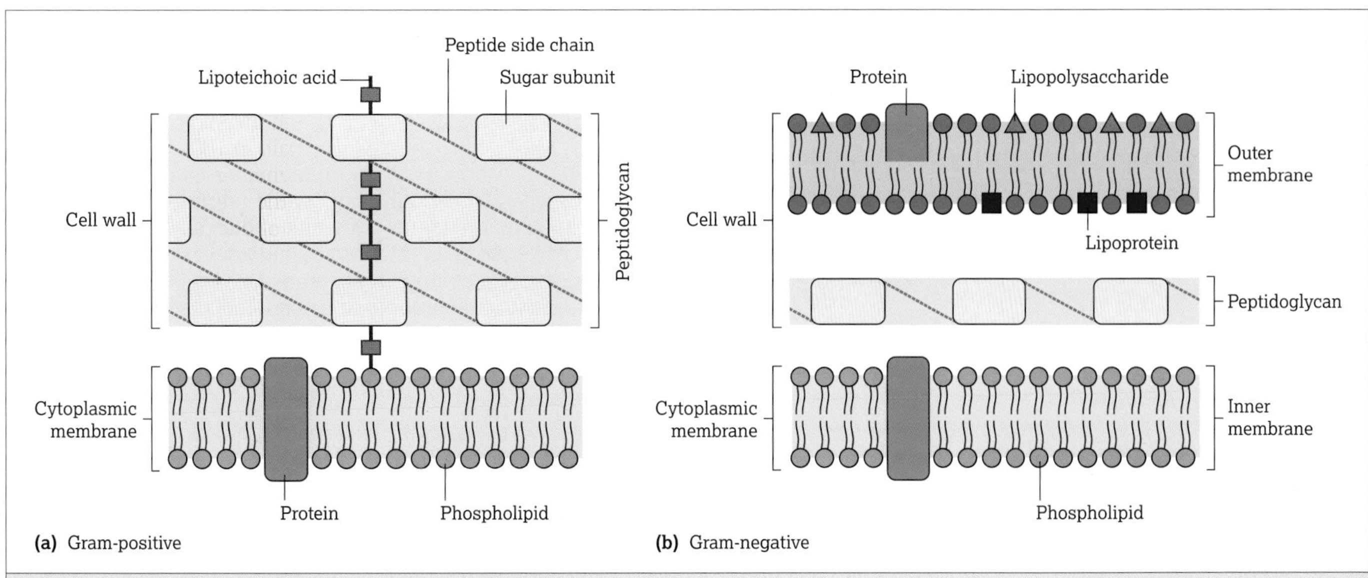

Figure 3.1 **Gram-positive (a) and Gram-negative (b) bacterial cell walls. Source: Adapted from Elliot et al. (2007). Reproduced with permission from John Wiley & Sons.**

Figure 3.2 **Bacterial structures.**

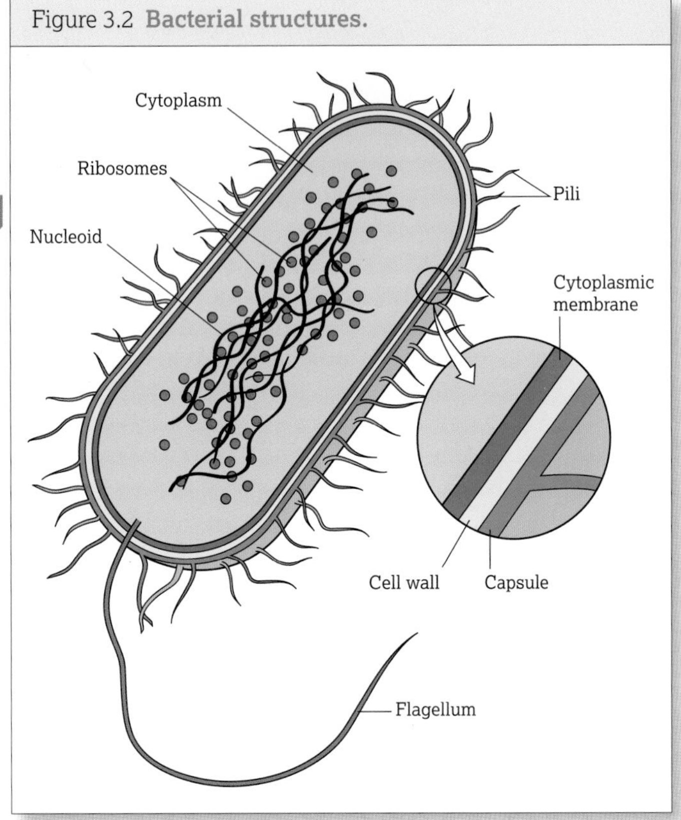

spore to survive until conditions are suitable for it to germinate into a normal, 'vegetative' bacterial cell that can then reproduce (Goering et al. 2012). Spores are extremely tough and durable. They are not destroyed by boiling (hence the need for high-temperature steam under pressure in sterilizing autoclaves) or by the alcohol handrubs widely used for hand hygiene – hence the need to physically remove them from the hands by washing with soap and water when caring for a patient with *Clostridium difficile* infection (DH/HPA 2008).

Some medically significant bacteria are listed in Table 3.2.

A few bacteria do not easily fit into the Gram-positive/negative dichotomy. The most medically significant of these are the Mycobacteria, which are responsible for diseases including tuberculosis and leprosy (Goering et al. 2012).

Viruses

Viruses are much smaller, and even simpler, than bacteria. They are often little more than a protein capsule containing some genetic material. They do not have cells, and some people do not even consider them to be alive. They have genes and will evolve through natural selection, but have no metabolism of their own.

Table 3.2 **Medically significant bacteria**

	Spherical	Rod-shaped
Gram positive	*Staphylococcus aureus* *Streptococcus* spp	*Clostridium difficile* *Clostridium tetanii* *Bacillus* spp
Gram negative	*Neisseria meningitides* *Neisseria gonorrhoeae*	*Pseudomonas aeruginosa* *Escherichia coli* *Legionella pneumophila* *Acinetobacter baumannii* *Salmonella*

The most significant characteristic of viruses is that they can only reproduce within a host cell, by using the cell's own mechanisms to reproduce the viral genetic material and to manufacture the other elements required to produce more virus particles. This often causes the death of the cell concerned (Goering et al. 2012).

The small size of viruses (poliovirus, for example, is only 30 nanometres (nm) across) means that most are smaller than the wavelengths of visible light. They can only be 'seen' with a specialist instrument such as an electron microscope, which will only be available in a very few hospital microbiology laboratories. Diagnosis of viral infections is normally by the patient's symptoms, with confirmation by laboratory tests designed to detect either the virus itself or antibodies produced by the patient's immune system as a response to infection (Goering et al. 2012).

There are viruses that specifically infect humans, or other animals, or plants, or even bacteria. This is one characteristic that can be used in classifying them. However, the main basis for classification is by the type of genetic material they contain. This can be DNA or RNA, and may be in a double strand, as seen in other organisms' DNA, or in a single strand. Other characteristics include the shape of the viral particle and the sort of disease caused by infection (Gillespie and Bamford 2012).

The life cycle of all viruses is similar and can be summarized as follows (Goering et al. 2012).

1 *Attachment*: a virus particle attaches to the outside of a host cell. Viruses are generally very limited in the types of cell that they can attach to, and normally infect only a single species or a limited range of related host organisms. Even a wide-ranging virus such as rabies is restricted to infecting mammals.
2 *Penetration*: the virus particle enters the host cell. The exact mechanism of this depends on the virus and the type of host.
3 *Uncoating*: the virus particle breaks down and exposes the viral genetic material.
4 *Replication*: the instructions contained in the viral genes cause the host cell mechanisms to create more viral particles.
5 *Release*: the new viral particles are released from the cell. Some viruses may 'bud' from the surface of the cell, acquiring their enclosing membranes in the process, but often release occurs due to cell rupture and destruction.

This process is illustrated in Figure 3.3.

A final point to consider in relation to viral structure and infection prevention and control is the presence or absence of a lipid envelope enclosing the viral particle. Those viruses that have a lipid envelope, such as herpes zoster virus (responsible for chickenpox and shingles), are much more susceptible to destruction by alcohol than those without, for example norovirus, which is a common cause of viral gastroenteritis (WHO 2009a).

Fungi

Like bacteria, fungi exist in many environments on Earth, including occasionally as commensal organisms on human beings. Unlike bacteria, they are eukaryotic, so their cells share some characteristics with other eukaryotes such as humans, but they are distinct from both animals and plants. Fungi are familiar to us as mushrooms and toadstools and the yeast that is used in brewing and baking. They also have many uses in the pharmaceutical industry, particularly in the production of antibiotics. Fungi produce spores, both for survival in adverse conditions, as bacteria do, and to provide a mechanism for dispersal in the same way as plants (Goering et al. 2012).

A few varieties of fungi are able to cause opportunistic infections in humans. These are usually found in one of two forms: either as single-celled yeast-like forms that reproduce in a similar fashion to bacteria, by dividing or budding, or as plant-like filaments called *hyphae*. A mass of hyphae together forms a *mycelium*. Some fungi may appear in either form, depending on environmental conditions. Fungal infections are referred to

Figure 3.3 **The viral life cycle. Source: Adapted from Perry (2007). Reproduced with permission from John Wiley & Sons.**

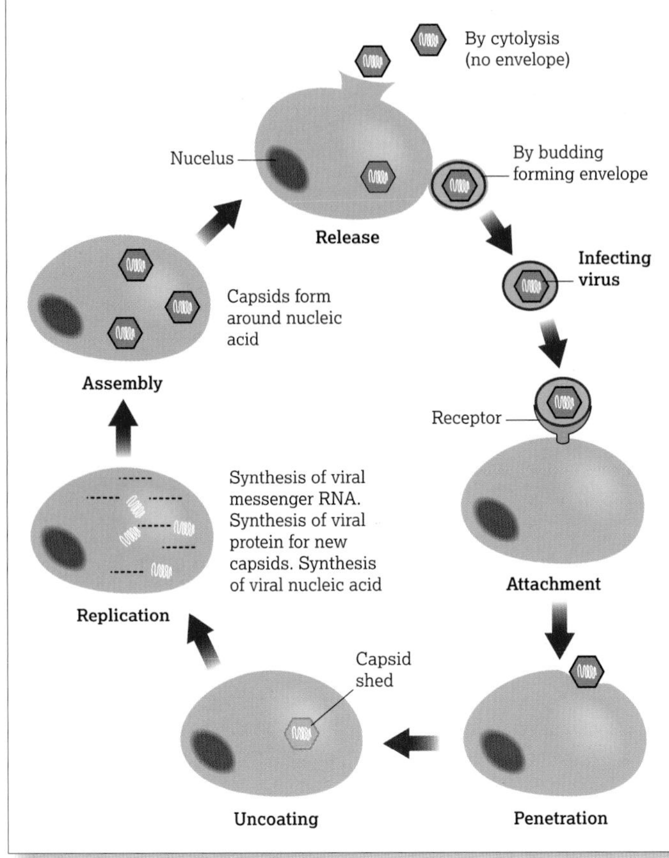

as *mycoses*. Superficial mycoses such as ringworm and thrush usually involve only the skin or mucous membranes and are normally mild, if unpleasant, but deeper mycoses involving major organs can be life threatening. These most frequently occur in patients who have severely impaired immune systems and may be an indicator of such impairment; for example, pneumonia caused by *Pneumocystis jirovecii* (previously *carinii*) is considered a clinical indication of AIDS. Superficial infections are generally transmitted by physical contact, whereas deeper infections can result, for example, from spores being inhaled. This is why it is important to ensure that patients with impaired immunity are protected from situations where the spores of potentially pathogenic fungi are likely to be released, for example during building work (Goering et al. 2012).

Protozoa

Protozoa are single-celled animals, some species of which are medically important parasites of human beings, particularly in tropical and subtropical parts of the world where diseases such as malaria are a major public health issue. Unlike bacteria, their relationship with humans is almost always parasitic – that is, their presence has an adverse effect on the host. The life cycles of protozoa can be complex, and may involve stages in different hosts.

Medically important protozoa include *Plasmodium*, the cause of malaria, *Giardia* and *Cryptosporidium*, which can cause gastroenteritis, and *Trichomonas*, which is a sexually transmitted cause of vaginitis (Gillespie and Bamford 2012).

The most common routes of infection with protozoa are by consuming them in food or water or via an insect vector such as a mosquito (Goering et al. 2012). Cross-infection in the course of healthcare is uncommon but not unknown.

Helminths

'Helminths' is a generic term for parasitic worms. A number of worms from three different groups affect humans: tapeworms, roundworms (nematodes) and flukes. Transmission is generally by ingestion of eggs or larvae, or of infected animals or fish, but some are transmitted via an insect vector and some, notably the nematode *Strongyloides*, have a larval stage that is capable of penetrating the skin (Gillespie and Bamford 2012).

Helminth infections can affect almost every part of the body, and the effects can be severe. For example, the *Ascaris* worm can cause bowel obstruction if there are large numbers present; *Brugia* and *Wuchereria* obstruct the lymphatic system and eventually cause elephantiasis as a result; and infection with *Toxocara* (often after contact with dog faeces) can result in epilepsy or blindness (Goering et al. 2012). However, cross-infection in healthcare is not normally considered a significant risk.

Arthropods

Arthropods (insects) are most significant in infectious disease in terms of their function as vectors of many viral, bacterial, protozoan and helminth-caused diseases. Some flies lay eggs in the skin of mammals, including humans, and the larvae feed and develop in the skin before pupating into the adult form, and some, such as lice and mites, are associated with humans for the whole of their life cycle. Such arthropod infestations can be uncomfortable, and there is often significant social stigma attached to them, possibly because the creatures are often visible to the naked eye. The activity of the insects and the presence of their saliva and faeces can result in quite severe skin conditions that are then vulnerable to secondary fungal or bacterial infection (Goering et al. 2012).

LICE

Species of *Pediculus* infest the hair and body of humans, feeding by sucking blood from their host. The adult animal is around 3 mm long and wingless, moving by means of claws. It cannot jump or fly, and dies within 24 hours if away from its host, so cross-infection is normally by direct contact or transfer of eggs or adults through sharing personal items (Wilson 2006).

SCABIES

Scabies is caused by the mite *Sarcoptes scabiei*, an insect less than 1 mm long, which burrows into the top layers of skin. Infestation usually starts around the wrists and in between the fingers because acquisition is normally by close contact with an infected individual. The female mites lay eggs in these burrows and the offspring can spread to other areas of skin elsewhere on the body. The burrows are visible as a characteristic rash in the areas affected. In immunocompromised hosts or in those unable to practise normal levels of personal hygiene, very high levels of infestation can occur, often with thickening of the skin and the formation of thick crusts. This is known as 'Norwegian scabies' and is associated with a much higher risk of cross-infection than the normal presentation. Scabies is most often associated with long-stay care settings, but there have been reported outbreaks associated with more acute healthcare facilities (Wilson 2006).

Prions

Prions are thought to be the causative agents of a group of diseases called transmissible spongiform encephalopathies (TSEs), the most well known of which are Creutzfeldt–Jakob disease (CJD) and its variant (vCJD). vCJD has been associated with the bovine spongiform encephalopathy (BSE) outbreak in Great Britain in the late 1980s and early 1990s. TSEs cause serious, irreversible damage to the central nervous system and are fatal. They are characterized by 'plaques' in the brain that are surrounded by holes that give the appearance of a sponge, hence the name. It used to be thought that this group of diseases was caused by so-called 'slow' viruses but they are now widely thought to be caused by prions, although this theory is not universally accepted. The theory is described below (Weaving 2007).

The prion protein (PrP) is a normally occurring protein found on the surface of some cells (PrPC). The disease-causing form of the protein (PrPCJD) appears to have an identical amino acid sequence but has a different three-dimensional shape. When the normal protein PrPC is exposed to the disease-causing form PrPCJD, it changes its conformation to that of PrPCJD. PrPCJD appears to progressively accumulate and be deposited in the brain, resulting in the characteristic 'plaques'. This process is slow compared to the replication of most micro-organisms and 'classic' CJD normally appears in older people.

One of the characteristics of vCJD is that it affects a much younger age group, although the incubation period still appears to be a number of years. There are currently no reliable tests to identify infection before the onset of symptoms, which has led to the worry that there could be a large pool of asymptomatic carriers of the vCJD infectious agent who may act as a reservoir for onward transmission via healthcare procedures. Routes of transmission already confirmed for CJD and vCJD include dura mater and corneal grafts, treatment with human-derived growth hormone, blood transfusion and surgical instruments. The infectious agent does not appear to be affected by decontamination processes such as autoclaving and chemical disinfection to the same extent as more familiar micro-organisms such as bacteria or viruses. This has led to extensive reviews of decontamination procedures in the UK and has resulted in an increased emphasis on effective washing to remove any residual organic material that may harbour the infectious agent, and on the tracking of instruments to individual patients to facilitate any look-back exercise should any patient be identified as suffering from CJD or vCJD at a later date (Weaving 2007).

Creutzfeldt–Jakob disease is a sporadic illness that affects around one person in every million and probably arises from a spontaneous genetic mutation. It should also be noted that only a very small number of people have developed vCJD. It appears that a combination of exposure to the infectious agent and genetic susceptibility is necessary for progression to the disease (related TSEs have a very strong genetic component), and there are numerous measures in place to prevent both the infectious agent entering the food chain and onward transmission through healthcare interventions. These appear to be the only routes of infection – there is no evidence of transmission via any other route. However, there is much that is unclear about the disease and the causative agent.

Mechanisms of infection

Whether or not a particular infectious agent will cause an infection in any given circumstance is dependent on many different factors, including how easily that agent can be transmitted, its *pathogenicity* (which is its ability to cause disease) and its *virulence* (which determines the severity of the infection produced) (Gillespie and Bamford 2012). It is generally accepted that for infection to occur, certain linked requirements need to be met; these links are often referred to as the *chain of infection* (Damani 2011). While the chain of infection will not be strictly accurate in every case – some 'links' may be missing or will overlap – it is an extremely useful model to use when considering how infection can be prevented, by breaking the 'links' in this chain. Some links are easier to break than others – for example, it is often easier to prevent an infectious agent entering a susceptible person than it is to prevent it leaving an infected one.

The chain of infection is illustrated in Figure 3.4 and the links are listed, with examples of how infection can be prevented at each link, in Table 3.3.

Modes of transmission

The mode of transmission is the method by which an infectious agent passes from one person or place to another. Considering the mode of transmission allows the practitioner to implement the measures required to prevent it.

Figure 3.4 **The chain of infection. A useful tool for seeing how to prevent transmission. How would you break each of the links in the chain?**

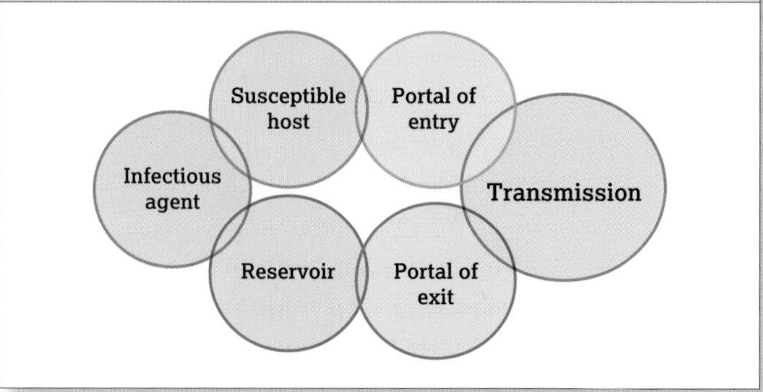

Direct contact

This is person-to-person spread of infectious agents through physical contact between people. It occurs through normal nursing activities and can happen during aseptic procedures if technique is poor. It can be prevented through good hand hygiene, the use of barriers such as aprons and gloves and non-touch technique for aseptic procedures (Loveday et al. 2014).

Indirect contact

This occurs when someone comes into contact with a contaminated object. Many items in the healthcare environment can become contaminated, but the most likely routes of spread are inadequately decontaminated items of equipment used for diagnosis or treatment. Transmission is prevented by effective cleaning, decontamination and good hand hygiene (DH/HPA 2008).

Droplet transmission

When people cough, sneeze or even talk, they expel droplets of respiratory secretions and saliva. These droplets will travel about a metre from the person expelling them, and may contain the agents responsible for respiratory infections such as influenza or tuberculosis. Transmission is prevented through isolating the affected patient and using masks, aprons and gloves to provide a barrier. Transmission of these infectious agents may also be reduced through good hand hygiene as transmission by indirect contact via contaminated surfaces is also possible (Crabtree and Henry 2011).

Airborne transmission

Airborne transmission also involves droplets or particles containing infectious agents, but on a small enough scale that the particles can remain suspended in the air for long periods of time. Infections spread via this route include measles and chickenpox. Prevention is as for droplet transmission.

Parenteral transmission

This is a form of contact transmission, where blood or body fluids containing infectious agents come into contact with mucous membranes or exposed tissue. In healthcare, this can occur through transplantation or infusion (which is why blood and organs for transplantation are screened for bloodborne viruses such as HIV) or through an inoculation injury where blood splashes into the eyes or a used item of sharp equipment penetrates the skin. This last type of incident is often referred to as a 'needlestick' injury. Transmission is prevented by good practice in handling and disposing of sharps and the appropriate use of protective equipment, including eye protection (UK Health Departments 1998). A European Union directive recently incorporated into UK legislation requires the use of 'safe' or needle-free devices wherever possible in order to reduce the risk of inoculation injury (Health and Safety Executive 2013).

Table 3.3 **Links in the chain of infection**

Link	Definition	Example	Examples of breaking the chain
Infectious agent	A potentially pathogenic micro-organism or other agent	Any potential pathogen	Removal of infectious agents through cleaning; destruction of micro-organisms through sterilization of equipment; treatment of patient with bacterial infection with antibiotics
Reservoir	Any location where micro-organisms or other agents may exist or reproduce	Human beings; the healthcare environment; stagnant water	Cleaning equipment and the environment; removing stagnant water by flushing low-use taps and showers and changing flower water regularly; minimizing the number of people present in high-risk situations such as surgery
Portal of exit	The route by which the infectious agent leaves the reservoir	Diarrhoea or vomit may carry norovirus; droplets expelled during coughing or sneezing may contain respiratory pathogens	Asking a patient with active tuberculosis infection to wear a mask in communal areas of the hospital
Mode of transmission	See 'Modes of transmission'		
Portal of entry	The route by which the infectious agent enters a new host	Organisms introduced into a normally sterile part of the body through use of an invasive device, for example urinary catheter; inhalation of airborne pathogens	Avoiding unnecessary invasive devices; using strict aseptic technique; staff members wearing masks when dealing with infectious agents that may be inhaled
Susceptible host	The person that the infectious agent enters has to be susceptible to infection	The very old and very young are more susceptible, as are people with underlying chronic illnesses	Ensuring adequate nutrition and personal hygiene; providing vaccination to healthcare workers

Faecal–oral transmission

This occurs when an infectious agent present in the faeces of an infected person is subsequently ingested by someone else and enters their gastrointestinal tract. It is the route of much gastrointestinal illness and water- and foodborne disease. There are often several steps involved. As an example, someone with infectious diarrhoea whose hand hygiene is poor is likely to contaminate any food they prepare; this exposes anyone who eats that food to infection. Transmission is prevented through isolating any patient with symptoms of gastroenteritis; effective hand hygiene by both staff and patients with soap and water (as many of these organisms are less susceptible to alcohol); appropriate use of gloves and aprons; and good food hygiene (DH/HPA 2008).

Vector transmission

Many diseases are spread through the action of a vector, most often an insect that travels from one person to another to feed. This route is not currently a concern in healthcare in England, but in some areas of the world, for example where malaria is endemic, protecting patients from vectors such as mosquitoes is an important element of nursing care.

These definitions are useful for considering the different routes by which infectious agents can spread but there is also overlap between the different categories: droplet and airborne spread, for example, or indirect contact and faecal–oral. Many agents will be spread by more than one route or there may be a combination of routes involved. In norovirus infection, for example, the overall mode of spread is faecal–oral but if someone is infected with norovirus, they may vomit and create an aerosol of droplets that contain the virus. Those droplets may be ingested directly from the atmosphere or they may settle on food, surfaces or equipment in the immediate vicinity. Anyone touching those surfaces will pick up the virus on their hands (indirect contact) and transmit it to their mouth either directly or via food.

Sources of infection

An individual may become infected with organisms already present on their body (endogenous infection) or introduced from elsewhere (exogenous infection). The majority of healthcare-associated infections (HCAIs) are endogenous, hence the importance of procedures such as effective skin decontamination prior to invasive procedures (Loveday et al. 2014).

Indicators and effects of infection

Generally, infection is said to have occurred when infectious agents enter a normally sterile area of the body and cause symptoms as a result. There are obvious exceptions to this (for example, the digestive tract is not sterile, being home to trillions of micro-organisms, but many types of infectious gastroenteritis are caused by particular organisms entering this area) but it is a useful working definition. The symptoms of infection are listed below. Not all symptoms will be present in all cases, and it should be noted that many symptoms are due to the body's response to infection and so may not be present in severely immunocompromised patients (Fishman 2011).

Symptoms of infection

- *Heat*: the site of the infection may feel warm to the touch, and the patient may have a raised temperature.
- *Pain*: at the site of the infection.
- *Swelling*: at the site of the infection.
- *Redness*: at the site of the infection.
- Pus.
- Feeling of general malaise.
- In *gastrointestinal infection*: abdominal pain and tenderness; nausea; diarrhoea and/or vomiting (Goering et al. 2012).
- In *urinary tract infection*: frequency of micturition; often confusion in the elderly; loin pain and/or abdominal discomfort (Goering et al. 2012).

EVIDENCE-BASED APPROACHES

Rationale

The principle of all infection prevention and control is preventing the transmission of infectious agents. However, the measures taken to reduce the risk of transmission must be reasonable, practicable and proportionate to the risk of transmission and the effects of infection with any particular agent. For example, while *Staphylococcus aureus* can cause severe infections, it is carried by around a third of the population and so isolating every patient carrying it would not be practicable. MRSA can cause equally serious infections, is resistant to many of the antibiotics that would normally be used to treat these infections and is carried by far fewer people, so it is both reasonable and practicable to take additional precautions to prevent its spread in healthcare. These may include isolation in an acute hospital but it would not be reasonable to segregate a colonized individual in a mental health unit where social interaction may form part of their care and the risk to other individuals is less.

The management of any individual who is infected or colonized with an organism that may pose a risk to other individuals must be based on a risk assessment that takes into account the following factors:

- how easily the infectious agent can be passed to other people
- the susceptibility to infection of other people being cared for in the same area and the likely consequences of their becoming infected
- the practicality of implementing particular infection prevention and control precautions within that area or institution (the number of single rooms available, for example)
- the individual's other nursing needs (Wilson 2006).

The infection prevention and control policies of health and social care providers are based on generic risk assessments of their usual client or patient group and should be adhered to unless there are strong reasons to alter procedures for a particular individual's care. In such circumstances, the advice of the infection prevention and control team (IPCT) should be sought first. Nurses working in organizations without an IPCT should identify the most appropriate source from which to seek advice, preferably before it is needed.

Indications

Infection prevention and control precautions must be taken with all patients, regardless of whether or not they are known to be carrying any particular infectious agent that may cause a hazard to others. This is because it is impossible to guarantee whether or not any given individual is free of any particular infectious agent and because many common micro-organisms may cause infections in some circumstances. Additional infection control precautions are indicated when:

- an individual is particularly vulnerable to infection because of some deficiency in their normal defence mechanisms; or
- they are known to be infected or colonized with an infectious agent that may pose a particular risk to others.

Contraindications

As mentioned previously, precautions to prevent the spread of infection must be based on a risk assessment that takes in all the relevant factors. In some cases precautions will need to be modified because of a patient's physical or psychological needs. Isolation, for example, has been demonstrated to have an adverse psychological effect on some individuals (Morgan et al. 2009).

Anticipated patient outcomes

The anticipated outcome is that no patient will acquire micro-organisms from any other individual during the course of healthcare or suffer an avoidable infection.

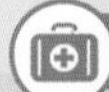
Learning Activity 3.2

Learning in practice

Find out what local guidance there is on the prevention and control of infections in your practice area.

- What measures are in place for meeting the 10 criteria of the hygiene code?
- Write down three steps you can take to help your clinical area meet the hygiene code.

LEGAL AND PROFESSIONAL ISSUES

In England, the Health and Safety at Work etc. Act 1974 is the primary piece of legislation relating to the safety of people in the workplace. It applies to all employees and employers, and requires them to do everything that is reasonable and practicable to prevent harm coming to anyone in the workplace. It requires employers to provide training and appropriate protective equipment and employees to follow the training that they have received, use the protective equipment provided, and report any situations where they believe inadequate precautions are putting anyone's health and safety at serious risk. This dovetails with the requirements of the Nursing and Midwifery Council (NMC 2015) for nurses to promote and protect the well-being of those in their care and to report their concerns in writing if problems in the environment of care are putting people at risk.

The requirement to protect individuals from healthcare-associated infections is further emphasized in England by the Health and Social Care Act 2008. This legislation is monitored and enforced by the Care Quality Commission, which assesses care providers against the requirements of the Code of Practice on the prevention and control of infections and related guidance (DH 2010a). Often referred to as the Hygiene Code, this has been applied to NHS hospitals in England, in one form or another, for some years and now applies to all providers of health or adult social care. Each provider must be registered with the Care Quality Commission and declare compliance with the ten criteria of the Hygiene Code. These criteria are summarized in Table 3.4. They also provide a useful guide for healthcare providers in other countries as to the elements an organization should have in place to facilitate effective infection prevention processes. For example, they could be used as the basis for a checklist for healthcare practitioners and organizations to assess the processes, policies and procedures that they have in place or may wish to have to help minimize the risk of infection to patients.

In England, nurses need to be aware of the measures that are in place in their workplace to ensure compliance with the Code of Practice. For example, many hospital trusts have a programme of regular visits to clinical areas by senior staff who will carry out an inspection against the criteria of the Code as if they were an external assessor. This programme ensures that senior staff are familiar with the Code and that everyone is familiar with the inspection process. In addition, nurses may need to carry out activities to promote compliance and provide evidence of assurance, such as audits of hand hygiene performance or compliance with aseptic technique. One such set of audits in place in many hospitals in England is the package produced by the Department of Health (2007a) and known collectively as *Saving Lives.* These are discussed in more detail later.

In addition to healthcare-specific requirements, items of legislation and regulation have also been devised with the objective of reducing the risk of infection in any situation that apply to healthcare as much as they do to any other business or workplace. These include legislation and regulation relating to food hygiene (Food Safety Act 1990), water quality (Health and Safety Commission 2001), waste management (Hazardous Waste Regulations 2005) and other issues that are peripheral

Table 3.4 **Criteria of the 2010 Hygiene Code of Practice**

Compliance criterion	What the registered provider will need to demonstrate
1	Systems to manage and monitor the prevention and control of infection. These systems use risk assessments and consider how susceptible service users are and any risks that their environment and other users may pose to them
2	Provide and maintain a clean and appropriate environment in managed premises that facilitates the prevention and control of infections
3	Provide suitable accurate information on infections to service users and their visitors
4	Provide suitable accurate information on infections to any person concerned with providing further support or nursing/medical care in a timely fashion
5	Ensure that people who have or develop an infection are identified promptly and receive the appropriate treatment and care to reduce the risk of passing on the infection to other people
6	Ensure that all staff and those employed to provide care in all settings are fully involved in the process of preventing and controlling infection
7	Provide or secure adequate isolation facilities
8	Secure adequate access to laboratory support as appropriate
9	Have and adhere to policies designed for the individual's care and provider organizations that will help to prevent and control infections
10	Ensure, so far as is reasonably practicable, that care workers are free of and are protected from exposure to infections that can be caught at work and that all staff are suitably educated in the prevention and control of infection associated with the provision of health and social care

Source: DH (2010a). © Crown copyright. Reproduced under the Open Government Licence v2.0.

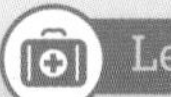 Learning Activity 3.3

Learning in practice

Have a look in your clinical area.

- Does the equipment for hand hygiene meet the criteria outlined in Table 3.4?
- Is the correct waste disposal equipment available?
- Do you have easy access to the essential PPE equipment (nonlatex disposable gloves, disposable aprons and eye protection)?

Make a note of any criteria that you think are not met.

- What can you do to help address this?
- In the clinical area, who might you discuss this with?

to healthcare but must be taken into account when developing policies and procedures for an NHS trust or other healthcare provider.

Competencies

The NMC Code (NMC 2015) states that all nurses must work within the limits of their competence. This means, for example, not carrying out aseptic procedures without being competent and confident that they can be carried out without increasing the risk of introducing infection through lack of knowledge or technique. However, there are some procedures for infection prevention and control that must be carried out as part of every care activity, and so all nurses must be competent in these if they are to provide any level of physical care at all. These are the *standard precautions* for infection prevention and control (Wilson 2006) and include:

- hand hygiene
- use of personal protective equipment such as gloves and aprons
- appropriate segregation and disposal of waste, in particular used sharps items and other equipment designated as single use
- appropriate decontamination of reusable equipment after use.

PRE-PROCEDURAL CONSIDERATIONS

Equipment

All infection prevention and control measures have the objective of preventing the transmission of infectious agents, whether by removing such agents from items that may be contaminated (hand hygiene and cleaning) or establishing a barrier (personal protective equipment and isolation). There are therefore some items that should be available for effective infection prevention and control in any situation where healthcare is provided. It is worth noting that it is a legal requirement in the UK for employers to provide suitable personal protective equipment when risks cannot be controlled in other ways, and for employees to use the equipment provided (Health and Safety Executive 2005).

Equipment for hand hygiene

It is essential that wherever care is provided, there are facilities for hand hygiene (WHO 2009a). Hand wash basins in clinical areas should have taps that can be turned on and off without using the hands; that is, they should be non-touch or lever operated (DH 2006). Basins used solely by clinical staff for hand hygiene should not have plugs (to encourage hand washing under running water) or overflows (because they are difficult to clean effectively and can be a reservoir for organisms such as *Pseudomonas* that may cause infection in vulnerable individuals) (DH 2013a). Basins that are also used by patients may require plugs, which will require careful management with some client groups to reduce the risk of flooding. In all cases, the taps should be positioned so that water does not fall directly into the outflow as this may lead to splashes containing organisms from within the drain. Taps should be of a mixer type that allows the temperature to be set before hand washing starts. Access to basins must be unobstructed by any furniture or equipment to ensure that they can easily be used whenever required (WHO 2009a).

Liquid soap dispensers should be positioned close to hand wash basins and care should be taken to ensure that soap cannot drip onto the floor from the dispenser and cause a slip hazard. Soap should be simple and unscented to minimize the risk of adverse reactions from frequent use. There is no advantage to using soap or detergents combined with or containing antimicrobial agents for routine hand washing. These preparations carry a higher risk of adverse reactions and should not be used routinely. Bar soap should not be used. For surgical scrub, the most commonly used preparations contain either chlorhexidine or povidone-iodine; both reduce bacterial counts significantly but chlorhexidine has a residual effect that prevents rapid regrowth. A paper towel dispenser should be fixed to the wall close to the hand wash basin. Hand towels should be of adequate quality to ensure that hands are completely dried by the proper use of one or two towels. To conveniently dispose of these towels, a suitable bin with a pedal-operated lid should be positioned close to the basin, but not so that it obstructs access to the basin (WHO 2009a).

Alcohol-based handrub should be available at the point of care in every clinical area for use immediately before care and between different care activities on the same patient (NPSA 2008). Dispensers may be attached to the patient's bed or bedside locker, and free-standing pump-top bottles can be used where appropriate, such as on the desk in a room used for outpatient clinics. Dispensers should not be sited close to sinks unless this is unavoidable because of the risk of confusion with soap, particularly if the dispensers are similar. Smaller sized personal issue bottles are appropriate where there is a risk that handrub may be accidentally or deliberately drunk, such as in paediatric areas or when caring for a patient with alcohol dependency (NPSA 2008). *Note*: Antiseptic handrubs based on non-alcoholic antiseptics are available but evidence suggests that alcohol is the most useful agent in terms of range and speed of antimicrobial activity (WHO 2009a).

Equipment for waste disposal

Also available should be disposal bags for domestic and clinical waste and a sharps bin if the procedure is to involve the use of any sharp single-use items (DH 2013b). The sharps bin should always be taken to the point of use (Loveday et al. 2014); do not transport used sharps in any other way or in any other container (UK Health Departments 1998). Bags and containers used for hazardous waste should be coloured according to their final disposal method (DH 2013b).

Personal protective equipment (PPE)

Other equipment required for infection prevention and control will depend on the activity being carried out, but basic PPE to provide a barrier to body fluids and micro-organisms – non-latex disposable gloves, disposable aprons and eye protection as a minimum – should be readily available in the clinical area (Loveday et al. 2014), and particularly where regular use is anticipated. For example, it is appropriate to have dispensers for gloves and aprons situated outside isolation rooms. All PPE sold in the UK must comply with the relevant regulations and standards, including being 'CE' marked to demonstrate that they meet these standards (Department of Trade and Industry 2002).

DISPOSABLE GLOVES

Gloves will be necessary in some circumstances but should be worn only when required (WHO 2009b). Non-sterile disposable gloves are most usefully available packaged in boxes of 100 ambidextrous gloves, in small, medium and large sizes. These boxes should be located close to the point of use, ideally in a fixed dispenser to make removing the gloves from the box as easy as possible. In the past, natural rubber latex was commonly used for these gloves but concerns about latex sensitivity mean that many healthcare organizations have adopted gloves made of alternative materials such as vinyl (RCN 2012). There is some evidence that vinyl may be a less effective barrier than latex (Kerr et al. 2004), but all gloves carry a risk of failure, often not visible to the naked eye (Kerr et al. 2004, Korniewicz et al. 2002), hence the need for hand hygiene regardless of whether or not gloves are worn. Whatever the material, these gloves are single use – they should be used for the task for which they are required and then removed and disposed of. They cannot be cleaned and reused for another task (Loveday et al. 2014, MHRA 2006).

DISPOSABLE APRONS

Single-use disposable aprons may be obtained either in a box or linked together on a roll. Presentation is not important as long as it is compatible with the dispensers in use and the product meets the requisite standards (i.e. is 'CE' marked). Aprons are normally made of thin polythene and are available in a range of colours. Different coloured aprons can be used to designate staff doing different tasks or working in different areas to give a visible reminder of the risk of cross-infection. As with disposable gloves, disposable aprons should be used for the task for which they are required and then removed and disposed of (Loveday et al. 2014, MHRA 2006).

STERILE GLOVES

Single-use sterile gloves, both latex and latex free, should be available in any area where their use is anticipated. Sterile gloves are packed as a left-and-right pair and are manufactured in a wide range of full and half sizes (similar to shoe sizes) so as to fit closely and provide the best possible compromise between acting as a barrier and allowing the wearer to work normally. Natural rubber latex is still one of the best materials for this, so sterile gloves are more often made of this than of alternative materials. Care must be taken to ensure alternatives are available for patients and staff with sensitivity to latex (RCN 2012).

STERILE GOWNS

To provide 'maximal barrier precautions' during surgery or other invasive procedures carrying a high risk of infection, or where infection would have serious consequences to the patient such as insertion of a central venous catheter, a sterile gown will be required in addition to sterile gloves. Modern sterile gowns are most often single-use disposable products made of water-repellent material as multiple-use fabric gowns may, over time, lose their effectiveness as a barrier (Leonas 1998).

EYE PROTECTION

Eye protection will be required in any situation where the mucous membranes of the eyes may be exposed to body fluid droplets created during aerosol-generating procedures or surgery with power tools. Both single-use and multiple-use options are available. Goggles are normally sufficient as long as they are worn in conjunction with a fluid-repellent mask. If greater protection is required, or a mask is not worn for any reason, a face shield should be used. Face shields may also be more appropriate for people who wear glasses. Prescription glasses will often not provide sufficient protection and should not be relied upon (UK Health Departments 1998).

MASKS AND RESPIRATORS

If dealing with organisms spread by the airborne or droplet route, a facemask or respirator will be required. When using a respirator (usually used to prevent the transmission of respiratory viruses), a good fit is essential to ensure that there is no leakage around the sides. Staff who are likely to need to use respirators should be 'fit tested' using a taste test to ensure that they have the correct size. A taste test consists of wearing the respirator while being exposed to a strong-tasting vapour (normally inside a hood to contain the vapour); if the subject can taste the vapour then the respirator is not properly fitted. Fit testing is normally carried out by the infection prevention and control team or occupational health department. Note that facial hair under the edge of the respirator will prevent a proper seal; staff with beards that prevent a proper seal will not be able to work safely if a respirator is required (Stobbe et al. 1988).

Single-use masks and respirators are normally the best option (and should be strictly single use). Multiple-use respirators are sometimes required for people whose face shape does not allow a good seal with disposable products (DH 2010b).

Assessment and recording tools

Assessment for infection prevention and control should take place at every level in an organization providing healthcare, from completing an assessment of infection risks (both to and from the patient) as part of the care planning process to the audit of compliance in a team, unit or hospital (DH 2010a). As mentioned previously, the Care Quality Commission assesses care providers in England against the requirements of the Hygiene Code. Other external assessors may also require evidence that procedures are in place to reduce the risk of healthcare-associated infection. Such evidence may include audits of compliance with hand hygiene against the WHO '5 moments' when hand hygiene should be performed at the point of care (WHO 2009a) or audits to demonstrate that all the elements of a procedure that carries a particular risk of infection have been carried out. Such procedures are sometimes referred to as 'high-impact interventions' because the risk of infection is such that improving adherence to good practice when they are carried out can have a significant impact on an organization's infection rates. The English Department of Health's *Saving Lives* toolkit (DH 2007a) is a collection of guidelines for high-impact interventions in the form of care bundles, and audits of those care bundles that can be used both for practice improvement and as evidence of good practice for internal and external assessment. All nurses should know which of these tools are being used in their workplace and actively participate in their completion.

At the level of individual patients, all additional precautions for infection prevention should be documented within the patient's individual plan of care. This should include regular reassessment and changes as necessary as the patient's condition alters. For example, a patient given antibiotics for a chest infection will be at increased risk of developing *Clostridium difficile* infection; if they develop diarrhoea, they must be isolated immediately. If the diarrhoea settles following treatment, they will no longer require isolation once they have been free of symptoms for 48 hours (DH/HPA 2008). When a procedure is carried out that requires additional precautions, for example aseptic technique, it should be documented in the record of that procedure that those precautions were adhered to or, if not, the reasons why they could not be implemented.

Specific patient preparation

Education

All patients should be informed about the risks of healthcare-associated infection and the measures that are known to reduce the risk of infection. In particular, patient education programmes that encourage the patient to ask healthcare workers 'Did you wash your hands?' have been demonstrated to increase compliance with hand hygiene (McGuckin et al. 2011). In addition, patients who are infected or colonized with infectious agents that require additional precautions to be implemented to reduce the risk of infection to other patients must be clearly told the nature of the infectious agent and its mode of spread, the risk to others, the details of the precautions required and the rationale behind them. Patients are likely to suffer anxiety if they are infected or colonized by such agents and this may be alleviated if they are provided with clear information. Similarly, there are adverse psychological effects of isolation and other precautions (Gammon 1998) and these are more likely to be mitigated if the patient has a clear understanding of why they are being implemented (Ward 2000).

Procedure guideline 3.1 **Hand washing**

Essential equipment

- Hand wash basin
- Liquid soap
- Paper towels
- Domestic waste bin

Pre-procedure

Action	Rationale
1 Remove any rings, bracelets and wristwatch still worn and roll up sleeves. (***Note***: It is good practice to remove all hand and wrist jewellery and roll up sleeves before entering any clinical area and the English Department of Health has instructed NHS trusts to implement a 'bare below the elbows' dress code.)	Jewellery inhibits good hand washing. Dirt and bacteria can remain beneath jewellery after hand washing. Long sleeves prevent washing of wrists and will easily become contaminated and so a route of transmission of micro-organisms (DH 2010c, **C**; WHO 2009a, **C**). Note that many organizations' dress codes allow staff to wear wedding rings while providing care. Although it can be argued that a smooth ring is less likely to retain dirt and bacteria than one with a stone or engraving, there is no evidence to suggest that wedding rings inhibit hand decontamination any less than other rings. **E**

(continued)

Procedure guideline 3.1 Hand washing *(continued)*

Action	Rationale
2 Cover cuts and abrasions on hands with waterproof dressing.	Cuts and abrasions can become contaminated with bacteria and cannot be easily cleaned. Repeated hand washing can worsen an injury (WHO 2009a, **C**). Breaks in the skin will allow the entry of potential pathogens. **E**
3 Remove nail varnish and artificial nails (most uniform policies and dress codes prohibit these). Nails must also be short and clean.	Long and false nails and imperfections in nail polish harbour dirt and bacteria that are not effectively removed by hand washing (WHO 2009a, **C**).
Procedure	
4 Turn on the taps and where possible direct the water flow away from the plughole. Run the water at a flow rate that prevents splashing.	Plugholes are often contaminated with micro-organisms that could be transferred to the environment or the user if splashing occurs (NHS Estates 2001, **C**).
5 Run the water until hand hot.	Warm water is more pleasant to wash with than cold so hand washing is more likely to be carried out effectively. **E** Water that is too hot could cause scalding. Soap is more effective in breaking down dirt and organic matter when used with hand-hot water (DH 2001, **C**).
6 Wet the surface of hands and wrists.	Soap applied directly onto dry hands may damage the skin. **E** The water will also quickly mix with the soap to speed up hand washing. **E**
7 Apply liquid soap and water to all surfaces of the hands.	Liquid soap is very effective in removing dirt, organic material and any loosely adherent transient flora. Tablets of soap can become contaminated, potentially transferring micro-organisms from one user to another, but may be used if liquid soap is unavailable (DH 2001, **C**). To ensure all surfaces of the hands are cleaned. **E**
8 Rub hands together for a minimum of 10–15 seconds, paying particular attention to between the fingers and the tips of fingers and thumbs (**Action figure 8a**). The areas that are most frequently missed through poor hand hygiene technique are shown in **Action figure 8b**.	To ensure all surfaces of the hands are cleaned. Areas that are missed can be a source of cross-infection (Fraise and Bradley 2009, **E**).
9 Rinse soap thoroughly off hands.	Soap residue can lead to irritation and damage to the skin. Damaged skin does not provide a barrier to infection for the healthcare worker and can become colonized with potentially pathogenic bacteria, leading to cross-infection (DH 2001, **C**).
10 Turn off the taps using your wrist or elbow. If the taps are not lever-type, turn them off using a paper hand towel to prevent contact.	To avoid recontaminating the hands. **E**
Post-procedure	
11 Dry hands thoroughly with a disposable paper towel from a towel dispenser.	Damp hands encourage the multiplication of bacteria and can potentially become sore (DH 2001, **C**).
12 Dispose of used paper towels in a black bag in a foot-operated waste bin.	Paper towels used to dry the hands are normally non-hazardous and can be disposed of via the domestic waste stream (DH 2013b, **C**). Using a foot-operated waste bin prevents contamination of the hands. **E**

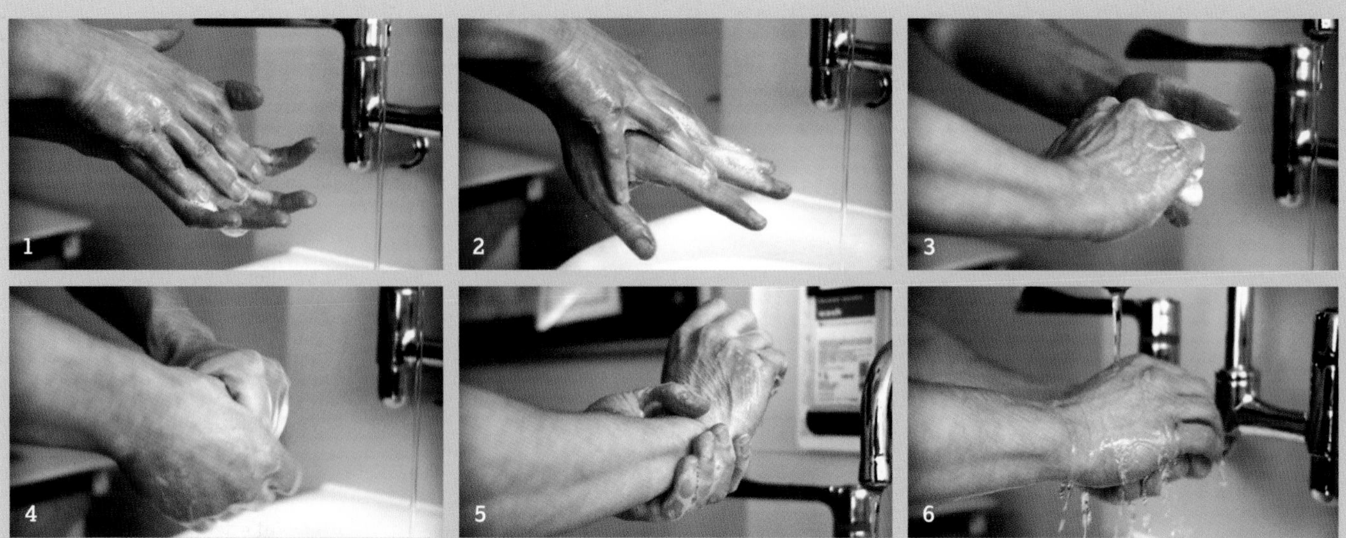

Action Figure 8a 1. Rub hands palm to palm. 2. Rub back of each hand with palm of other hand with fingers interlaced. 3. Rub palm to palm with fingers interlaced. Rub with back of fingers to opposing palms with fingers interlocked. Rub tips of fingers. Rub tips of fingers in opposite palm in a circular motion. 4. Rub each thumb clasped in opposite hand using a rotational movement. 5. Rub each wrist with opposite hand. 6. Rinse hands with water.

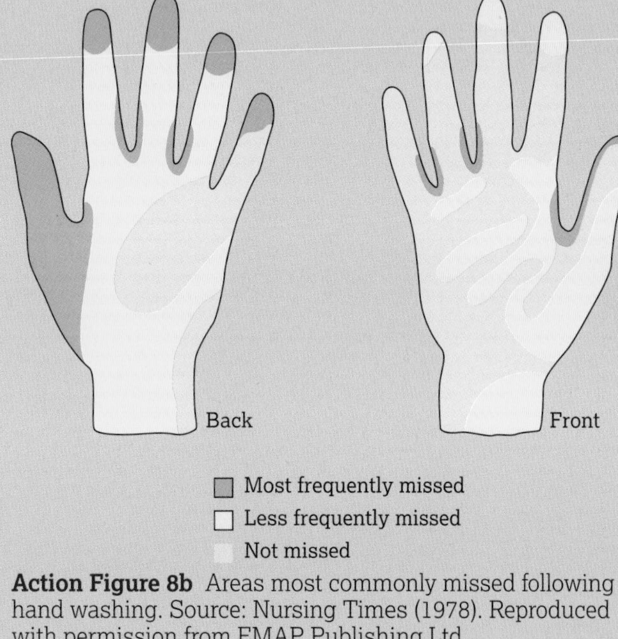

Action Figure 8b Areas most commonly missed following hand washing. Source: Nursing Times (1978). Reproduced with permission from EMAP Publishing Ltd.

Procedure guideline 3.2 Hand decontamination using alcohol handrub

Essential equipment

- Alcohol-based handrub

Procedure

Action	Rationale
1 Dispense the amount of handrub indicated in the manufacturer's instructions into the palm of one hand.	Too much handrub will take longer to dry and may consequently cause delays; too little will not decontaminate hands adequately. **E**

(continued)

Procedure guideline 3.2 Hand decontamination using alcohol handrub *(continued)*

Action	Rationale
2 Rub the alcohol handrub into all areas of the hands, until the hands are dry, using the illustrated actions in **Action figure 2**.	To ensure all areas of the hands are decontaminated. Alcohol is a rapid-acting disinfectant, with the added advantage that it evaporates, leaving the hands dry. This prevents contamination of equipment, whilst facilitating the application of gloves (WHO 2009a, **C**).

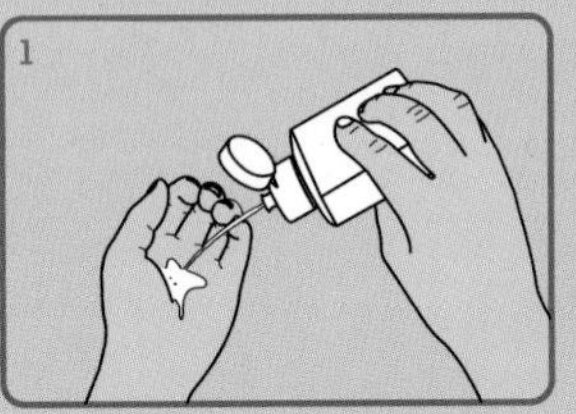

Apply a small amount (about 3 ml) of the product in a cupped hand

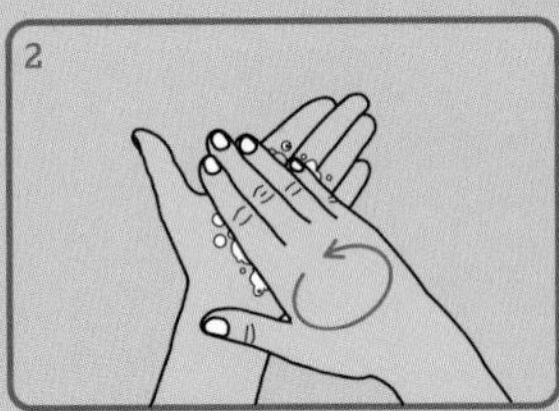

Rub hands together palm to palm, spreading the handrub over the hands

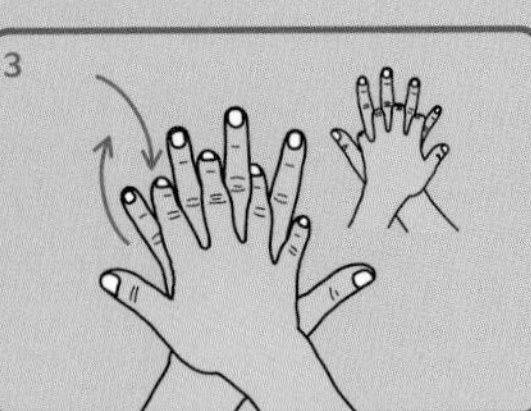

Rub back of each hand with palm of other hand with fingers interlaced

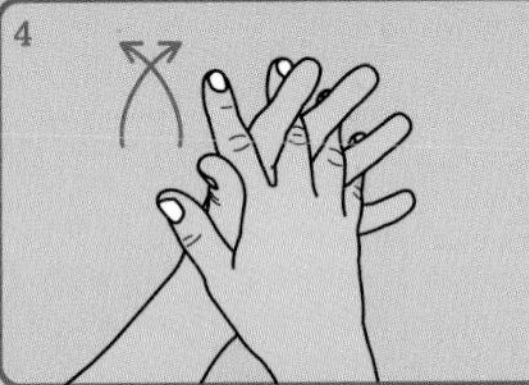

Rub palm to palm with fingers interlaced

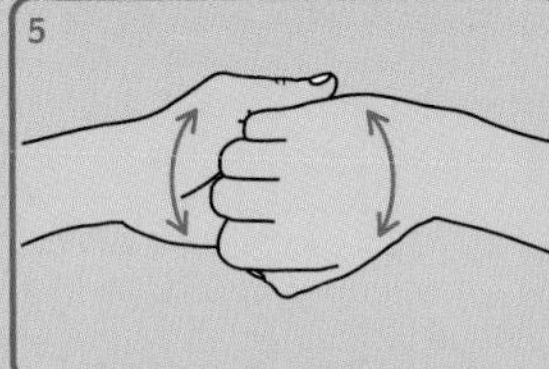

Rub back of fingers to opposing palms with fingers interlocked

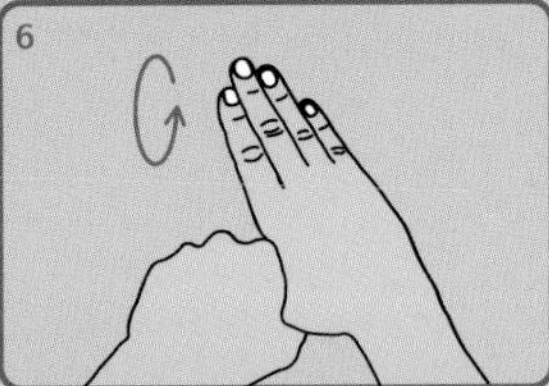

Rub each thumb clasped in opposite hand using a rotational movement

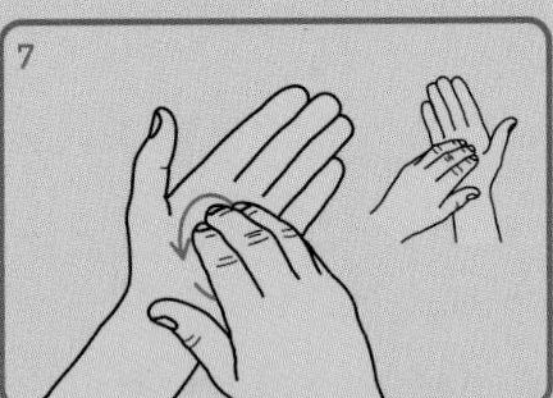

Rub tips of fingers in opposite palm in a circular motion

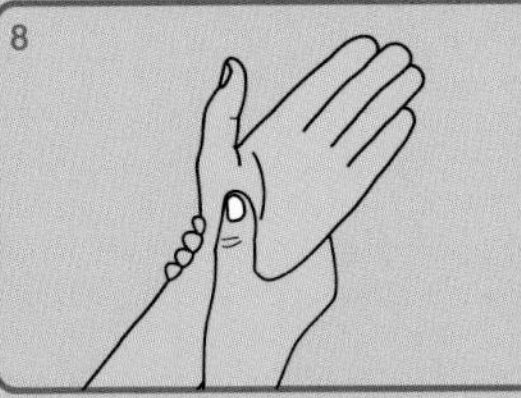

Rub each wrist with opposite hand

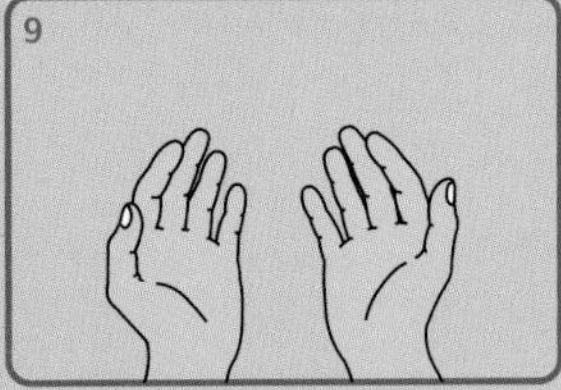

Wait until product has evaporated and hands are dry (do not use paper towels)

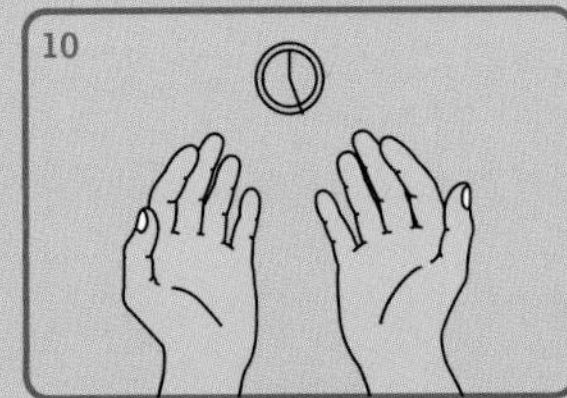

The process should take 15–30 seconds

cleanyourhands® campaign

NHS National Patient Safety Agency

Action Figure 2 Alcohol handrub hand hygiene technique – for visibly clean hands. Source: Adapted from WHO (2009a). © Crown copyright. Reproduced under the Open Government Licence v2.0.

Procedure guideline 3.3 Putting on and removing non-sterile gloves

Essential equipment

- Non-sterile gloves

Pre-procedure

Action	Rationale
1 Clean hands before putting on gloves.	Hands must be cleansed before and after every patient contact or contact with patient's equipment (Loveday et al. 2014, **C**).

Procedure	
2 Remove gloves from the box singly (**Action figure 2**), to prevent contamination of the gloves lower down. If it is likely that more than two gloves will be required (i.e. if the procedure requires gloves to be changed part-way through), consider removing all the gloves needed before starting the procedure.	To prevent cross-contamination. **E**
3 Holding the cuff of the glove, pull it into position, taking care not to contaminate the glove from the wearer's skin (**Action figure 3**). This is particularly important when the second glove is being put on, as the gloved hand of the first glove can touch the skin of the ungloved second hand if care is not taken.	To prevent cross-contamination (WHO 2009b, **C**).
4 During the procedure or when undertaking two procedures with the same patient, it may be necessary to change gloves. Gloves are single-use items and must not be cleansed and reused.	Disposable gloves are single-use items. They cannot be cleaned and reused for the same or another patient (MHRA 2006, **C**).
5 If gloves become damaged during use, they must be replaced.	Damaged gloves are not an effective barrier (WHO 2009b, **C**).
6 Remove the gloves when the procedure is completed, taking care not to contaminate the hands or the environment from the outside of the gloves.	The outside of the glove may be contaminated. **E**
7 Remove the first glove by firmly holding the outside of the glove wrist and pulling off the glove in such a way as to turn it inside out (**Action figure 7**).	Whilst removing the first glove, the second gloved hand continues to be protected. By turning the glove inside out during removal, any contamination is contained inside the glove. **E**
8 Remove the second glove by slipping the fingers of the ungloved hand inside the wrist of the glove and pulling it off whilst at the same time turning it inside out (**Action figure 8**).	By putting the fingers inside the glove, they will not be in contact with the potentially contaminated outer surface of the glove. **E**
Post-procedure	
9 Dispose of used gloves as 'hazardous infectious waste' (**Action figure 9**), that is, into an orange waste bag, unless instructed otherwise by the infection prevention and control team.	All waste contaminated with blood, body fluids, excretions, secretions and infectious agents thought to pose a particular risk should be disposed of as hazardous infectious waste. Orange is the recognized colour for hazardous infectious waste that does not require incineration and may be made safe by alternative treatment (DH 2013b, **C**).
10 After removing the gloves, decontaminate your hands.	Hands may have become contaminated (Loveday et al. 2014, **C**; WHO 2009b, **C**).

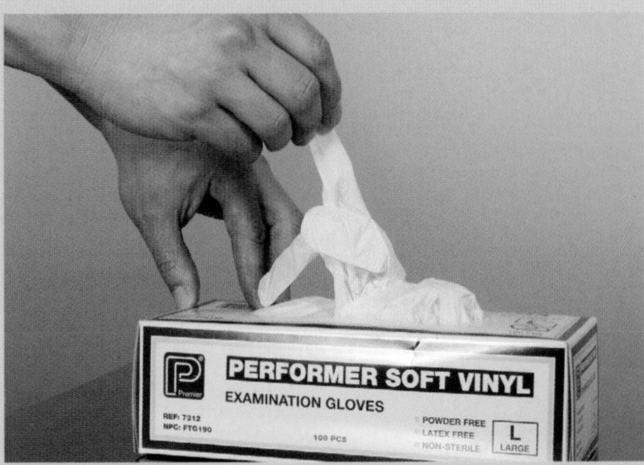

Action Figure 2 Remove gloves from the box.

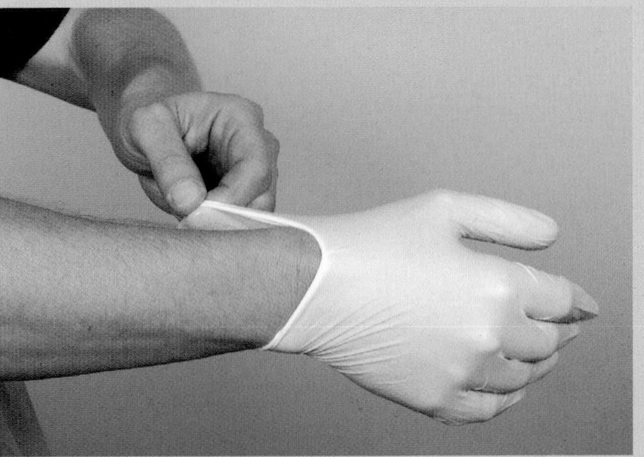

Action Figure 3 Holding the cuff of the glove, pull it into position.

(continued)

Procedure guideline 3.3 Putting on and removing non-sterile gloves *(continued)*

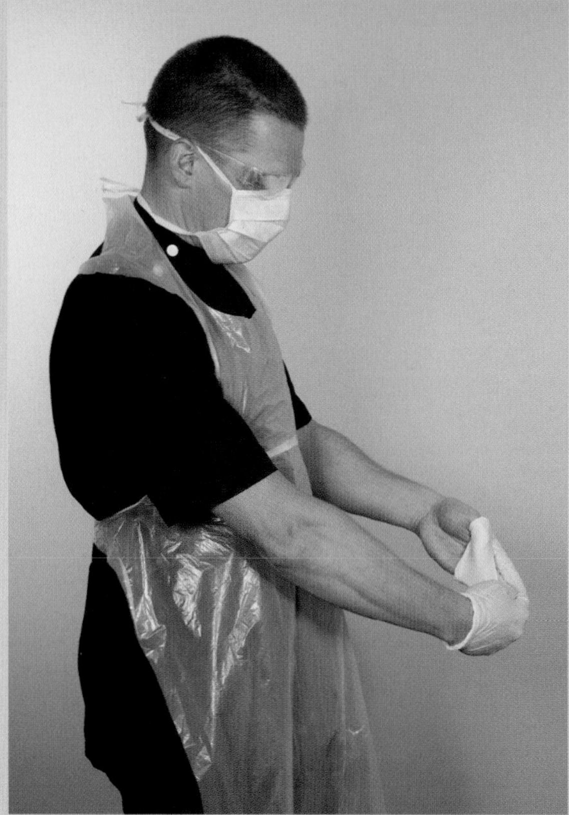

Action Figure 7 Remove the first glove by firmly holding the outside of the glove wrist, then pull off the glove in such a way as to turn it inside out.

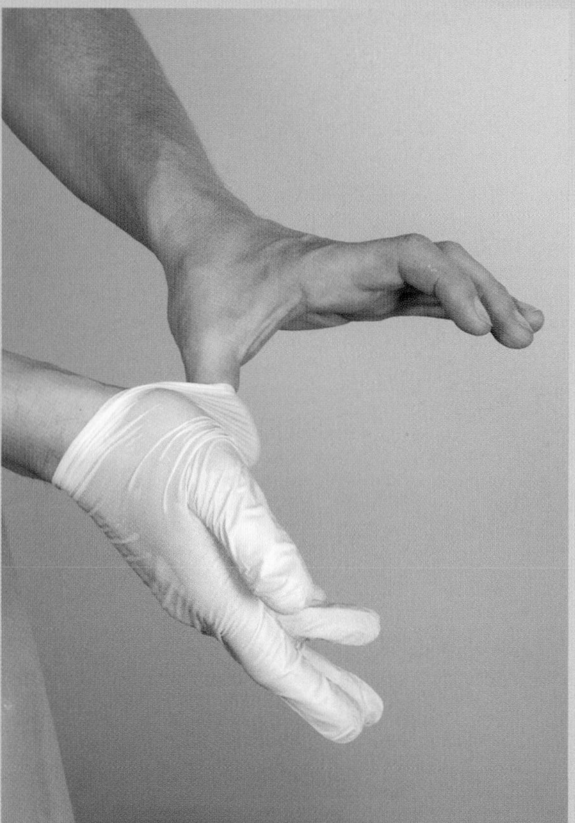

Action Figure 8 Remove the second glove by slipping the thumb of the ungloved hand inside the wrist of the glove and pulling it off while turning it inside out.

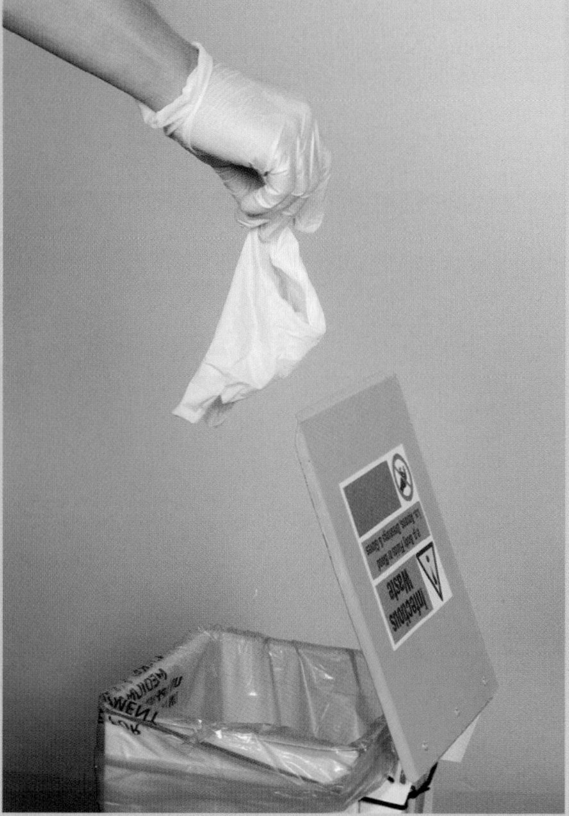

Action Figure 9 Dispose of used gloves into an orange waste bag.

Procedure guideline 3.4 Putting on and removing a disposable apron

Essential equipment

- Disposable apron

Pre-procedure

Action	Rationale
1 Remove an apron from the dispenser or roll using clean hands and open it out.	To make it easy to put on. **E**
Procedure	
2 Place the neck loop over your head and tie the ties together behind your back, positioning the apron so that as much of the front of your body is protected as possible (**Action figures 2a, 2b**).	To minimize the risk of contamination being transferred between your clothing and the patient, in either direction. **E**
3 If gloves are required, don them as described in Procedure guideline 3.3. At the end of the procedure, remove gloves first.	The gloves are more likely to be contaminated than the apron and therefore should be removed first to prevent cross-contamination (DH 2010b, **C**).
4 Remove the apron by breaking the ties and neck loop; grasp the inside of the apron and dispose of it (**Action figure 4**).	The inside of the apron should be clean. **E**
Post-procedure	
5 Dispose of used aprons as 'hazardous infectious waste', that is, into an orange waste bag, unless instructed otherwise by the infection prevention and control team.	All waste contaminated with blood, body fluids, excretions, secretions and infectious agents thought to pose a particular risk should be disposed of as hazardous infectious waste. Orange is the recognized colour for hazardous infectious waste that does not require incineration and may be made safe by alternative treatment (DH 2013b, **C**).
6 After removing the apron, decontaminate your hands.	Hands may have become contaminated (Loveday et al. 2014, **C**).

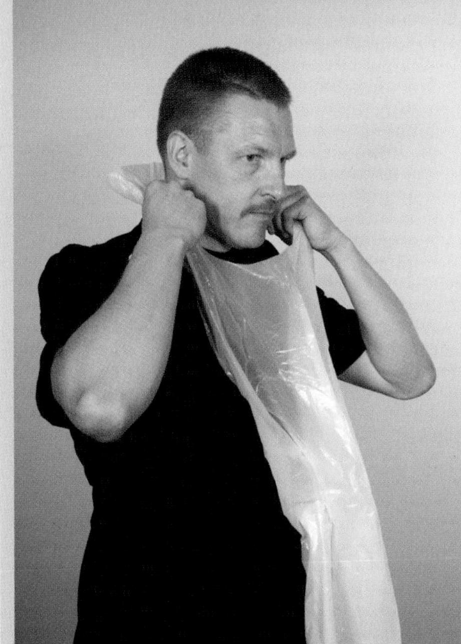

Action Figure 2a Place the neck loop of the apron over your head.

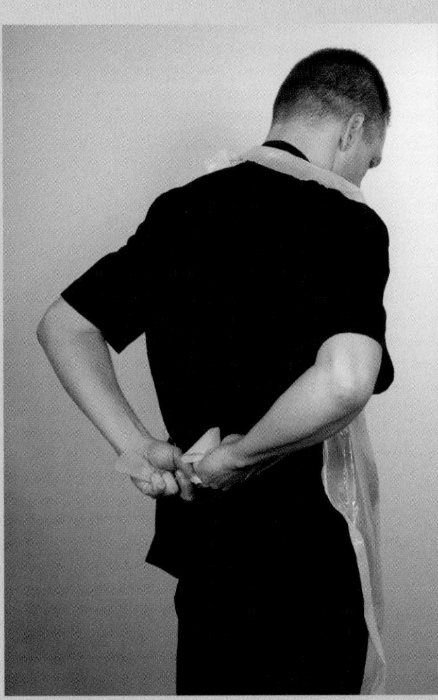

Action Figure 2b Tie the ties together behind your back, positioning the apron so that as much of the front of your body is protected as possible.

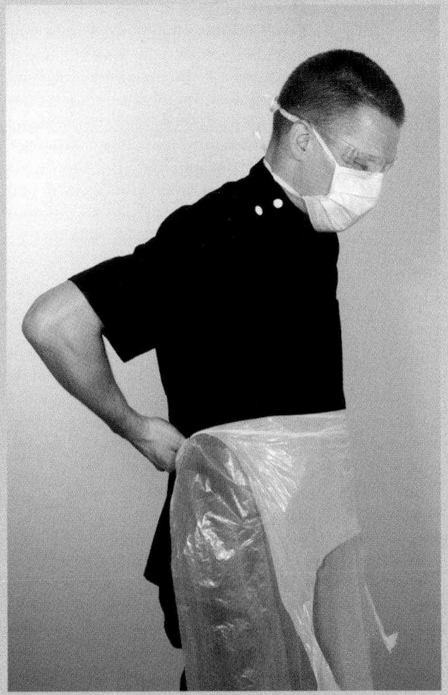

Action Figure 4 Remove the apron by breaking the neck loop and ties.

Procedure guideline 3.5 Putting on and removing a disposable mask or respirator

Essential equipment

- Disposable surgical mask or respirator

Pre-procedure

Action	Rationale
1 Remove surgical-type masks singly from the box, or remove individually wrapped items from their packaging, with clean hands.	To prevent contamination of the item or others in the box or dispenser. **E**
2 Remove glasses, if worn.	Glasses will obstruct the correct positioning of the mask or respirator and may be dislodged and damaged. **E**

Procedure

Action	Rationale
3 Place the mask/respirator over nose, mouth and chin (**Action figure 3**).	To ensure correct positioning. **E**
4 Fit the flexible nose piece over the bridge of your nose if wearing a respirator.	To ensure the best fit. **E**
5 Secure the mask or respirator at the back of the head with ties or fitted elastic straps and adjust to fit (**Action figure 5**).	To ensure the mask/respirator is comfortable to wear and remains in the correct position throughout the procedure. **E**
6 If wearing a respirator, perform a fit check. First, breathe in – respirator should collapse or be 'sucked in' to the face. Then breathe out – respirator should not leak around the edges.	To ensure that there is a good seal around the edge of the respirator so that there is no route for non-filtered air to pass in either direction. Note that this check should be carried out whenever a respirator is worn and is not a substitute for prior fit testing (DH 2010b, **C**).
7 Replace glasses, if worn.	To restore normal vision. **E**
8 At the end of the procedure, or after leaving the room in which the respirator is required, remove by grasping the ties or straps at the back of the head and either break them or pull them forward over the top of the head. Do not touch the front of the mask/respirator (**Action figures 8a, 8b**).	To avoid contaminating the hands with material from the outside of the mask/respirator (DH 2010b, **C**).
9 Dispose of used disposable items as 'hazardous infectious waste', that is, into an orange waste bag, unless instructed otherwise by the infection prevention and control team.	All waste contaminated with blood, body fluids, excretions, secretions and infectious agents thought to pose a particular risk should be disposed of as hazardous infectious waste. Orange is the recognized colour for hazardous infectious waste that does not require incineration and may be made safe by alternative treatment (DH 2013b, **C**).

Post-procedure

Action	Rationale
10 Clean reusable items according to the manufacturer's instructions, usually with detergent and water or a detergent wipe.	To avoid cross-contamination and ensure the item is suitable for further use (DH 2010b, **C**).

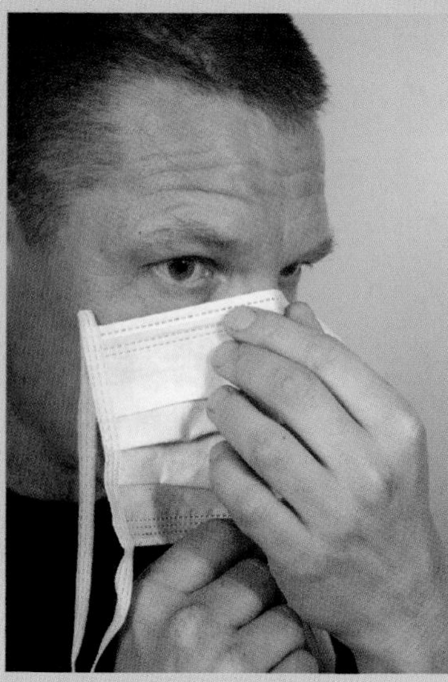

Action Figure 3 Place the mask over your nose, mouth and chin.

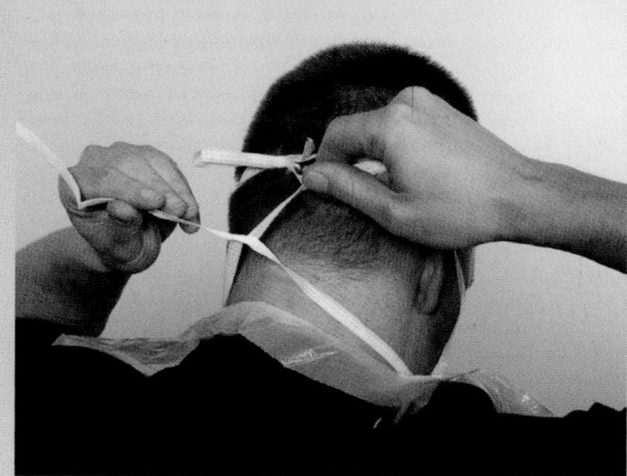

Action Figure 5 Secure the mask at the back of the head with ties.

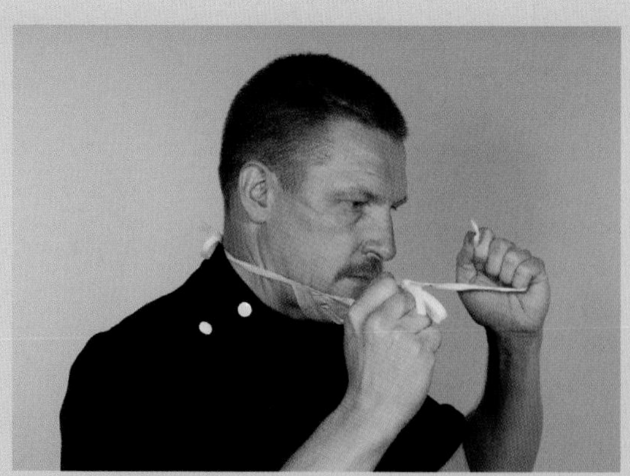

Action Figure 8a After use, remove the mask by untying or breaking the ties and pulling them forward.

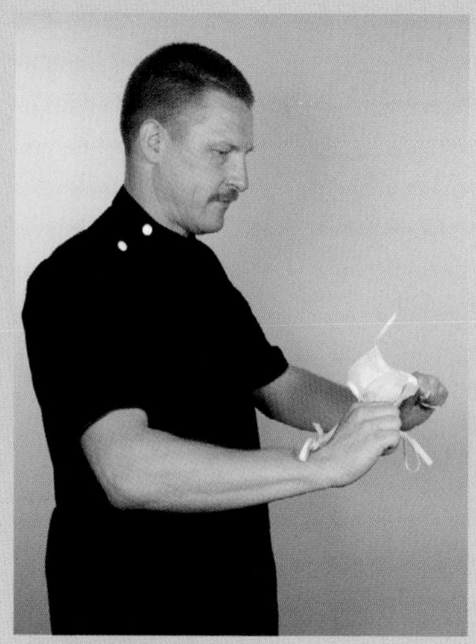

Action Figure 8b Do not touch the front of the mask.

Procedure guideline 3.6 Putting on or removing goggles or a face shield

Purpose

To protect the mucous membranes of the eyes, nose and mouth from body fluid droplets generated during aerosol-generating procedures or surgery with power tools.

Essential equipment

- Reusable or disposable goggles or face shield

Pre-procedure

Action	Rationale
1 Remove eye protection from any packaging with clean hands.	To prevent cross-contamination. **E**
2 Apply demister solution according to manufacturer's instructions, if required.	To ensure good visibility throughout the procedure. **E**
3 Position item over eyes/face and secure using ear pieces or headband; adjust to fit.	To ensure the item is comfortable to wear and remains in the correct position throughout the procedure. **E**
4 At the end of the procedure, remove by grasping the ear pieces or headband at the back or side of the head and lifting forward, away from the face. Do not touch the front of the goggles or face shield (**Action figure 4**).	To avoid contaminating the hands with material from the outside of the eye protection (DH 2010b, **C**).
Post-procedure	
5 Dispose of used disposable items as 'hazardous infectious waste', that is, into an orange waste bag, unless instructed otherwise by the infection prevention and control team.	All waste contaminated with blood, body fluids, excretions, secretions and infectious agents thought to pose a particular risk should be disposed of as hazardous infectious waste. Orange is the recognized colour for hazardous infectious waste that does not require incineration and may be made safe by alternative treatment (DH 2013b, **C**).
6 Clean reusable items according to the manufacturer's instructions, usually with detergent and water or a detergent wipe.	To avoid cross-contamination and ensure the item is suitable for further use. **E**

(continued)

Procedure guideline 3.6 Putting on or removing goggles or a face shield *(continued)*

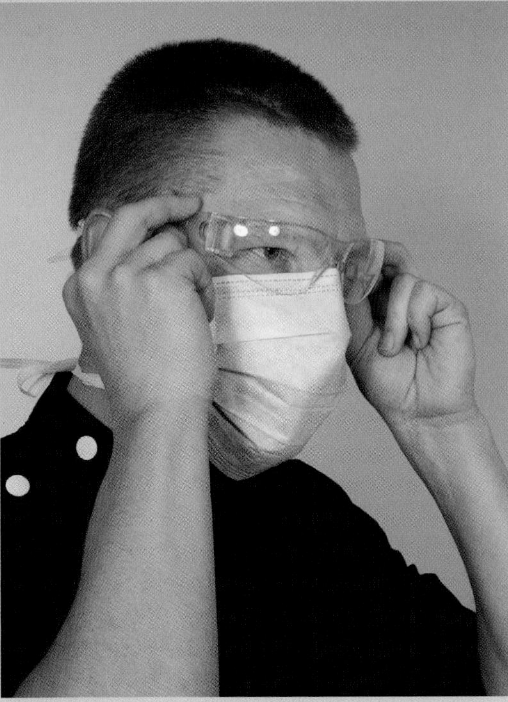

Action Figure 4 Don and remove eye protection by grasping the earpieces; do not touch the front.

Procedure guideline 3.7 Surgical scrub technique

Purpose

To reduce the release of bacteria from the hands while carrying out surgical or high-risk procedures. The difference from conventional hand washing is the reduction in the level of resident bacteria on the hands as well as removal of the majority of transient bacteria.

Essential equipment

- Hand wash basin or surgical scrub sink with sufficient space available under the outlet to allow easy rinsing of hands and forearms
- Liquid medicated soap
- Sterile towels
- Domestic waste bin

Optional equipment

Sterile scrubbing brush, nail file or other implement for cleaning beneath the nails. Note that WHO (2009a) guidelines recommend that scrubbing brushes should **not** be used as they may damage the skin and encourage the shedding of cells (including bacteria).

Pre-procedure

Action	Rationale
1 Remove any rings, bracelets and wristwatch still worn and roll up sleeves before entering the operating theatre or procedure area. (*Note*: Most organizations will require staff entering operating theatres to change into 'scrubs'.)	To ensure the ability of good hand washing as jewellery inhibits good hand washing. Dirt and bacteria can remain beneath jewellery after hand washing. Long sleeves prevent washing of wrists and will easily become contaminated and so a route of transmission of micro-organisms (DH 2010c, **C**; WHO 2009a, **C**).

Action	Rationale
2 Cover cuts and abrasions on hands with waterproof dressing.	Cuts and abrasions can become contaminated with bacteria and cannot be easily cleaned. Repeated hand washing can worsen an injury (WHO 2009a, **C**). Breaks in the skin will allow the entry of potential pathogens.
3 Remove nail varnish and artificial nails (most uniform policies and dress codes prohibit these). Nails must also be short and clean.	Long and false nails and imperfections in nail polish harbour dirt and bacteria that are not effectively removed by hand washing (WHO 2009a, **C**).
Procedure	
4 Turn on the taps and where possible direct the water flow away from the plughole. Run the water at a flow rate that prevents splashing.	Plugholes are often contaminated with micro-organisms that could be transferred to the environment or the user if splashing occurs (NHS Estates 2001, **C**).
5 Run the water until hand hot.	Warm water is more pleasant to wash with than cold so hand washing is more likely to be carried out effectively. **E** Water that is too hot could cause scalding. **E** Soap is more effective in breaking down dirt and organic matter when used with hand-hot water (DH 2001, **C**).
6 Wet the surface of hands, wrists and forearms.	Soap applied directly onto dry hands may damage the skin. **E** The water will also quickly mix with the soap to speed up hand washing. **E**
7 Apply medicated liquid soap and water to all surfaces of the hands.	Liquid soap is very effective in removing dirt, organic material and any loosely adherent transient flora. The bactericidal additive contributes to the reduction in numbers of bacteria. Chlorhexidine has a residual effect to prevent regrowth of bacteria for a period after hand decontamination (WHO 2009a, **C**).
8 Clean beneath the nails using a sterile implement (preferred) or soft scrubbing brush.	The area under the nails may harbour dirt and micro-organisms not easily removed by the other stages of the procedure (WHO 2009a, **C**). WHO guidelines suggest carrying out this stage before entering the operating theatre; experience indicates it is more easily incorporated into the surgical scrub procedure. **E**.
9 Start timing. Thoroughly wash the hands for 2 minutes, using the actions shown in Procedure guideline 3.1: Hand washing, **Action figure 3.13a**.	No advantage has been shown from scrub procedures lasting longer than 2 minutes (WHO 2009a, **C**).
10 Wash each arm from wrist to elbow for 1 minute, keeping the hand higher than the elbow at all times.	To avoid recontaminating the hands with water that has been used to clean the arms (WHO 2009a, **C**).
11 Rinse hands and arms thoroughly from fingertips to elbow, keeping the hands above the elbows at all times.	To avoid recontaminating the hands with water that has been used to clean the arms (WHO 2009a, **C**).
Post-procedure	
12 Dry hands thoroughly with a sterile paper or cloth towel. Dry in one direction only, from the fingertips to the elbow.	Damp hands encourage the multiplication of bacteria (DH 2001, **C**). Drying from hands to elbows only reduces the risk of contaminating hands with bacteria from parts of the arm that have not been washed. **E**.
13 Dispose of used paper towels in a black bag in an open or foot-operated waste bin.	Paper towels used to dry the hands are normally non-hazardous and can be disposed of via the domestic waste stream (DH 2013b, **C**). Using an open or foot-operated waste bin prevents contamination of the hands. **E**

WHO guidelines state that surgical procedures may be carried out one after the other without the need for further hand washing if hands are perfectly clean and dry, provided that the handrubbing technique for surgical hand preparation is followed (WHO 2009a). See Procedure guideline 3.2: Hand decontamination using alcohol handrub, **Action figure 2**.

Procedure guideline 3.8 Donning sterile gloves: open technique

Purpose

To have a barrier between the nurse's hands and the patient to prevent the transmission of infectious agents in either direction, and to prevent contamination of a vulnerable area or invasive device through contact with non-sterile gloves.

Note that in steps 4 and 5, below, either glove can be put on first. Simply exchange 'left' and 'right' in the description if you wish to put on the right-hand glove first.

Essential equipment

- Sterile disposable gloves
- All other equipment required for the procedure for which the gloves are required

Action	Rationale
Pre-procedure	
1 Clean hands using soap and water or alcohol-based handrub.	Hands must be cleansed before and after every patient contact or contact with patient's equipment (Loveday et al. 2014, **C**).
2 Prepare all the equipment required for the procedure, including setting up the sterile field and tipping sterile items on to it from packets if you do not have an assistant, but do not touch any sterile item before putting on gloves.	To avoid contaminating gloves with non-sterile packets. **E**
Procedure	
3 Open the packet containing the gloves and open out the inside packaging on a clean surface so that the fingers of the gloves are pointed away from you, taking care not to touch the gloves or allow them to come into contact with anything that is non-sterile (**Action figure 3**).	To prevent contamination of the gloves and to put them in the best position for putting them on. **E**
4 Clean hands using soap and water or alcohol-based handrub.	Hands must be cleansed before and after every patient contact or contact with patient's equipment (Loveday et al. 2014, **C**).
5 Hold the cuff of the left-hand glove with your right fingertips, at the uppermost edge where the cuff folds back on itself. Lift this edge away from the opposite edge to create an opening. Keeping them together, slide the fingers of the left hand into the glove, taking care not to contaminate the outside of the glove, while keeping hold of the folded edge in the other hand and pulling the glove onto the hand. Spread the fingers of the left hand slightly to help them enter the fingers of the glove (**Action figures 5a, 5b, 5c**).	To prevent contamination of the outside of the glove. **E**
6 Open up the right-hand glove with your left-hand fingertips by sliding them beneath the folded-back cuff. Taking care not to touch the left-hand glove or the outside of the right-hand glove, and keeping the fingers together, slide the fingers of the right hand into the right-hand glove. Again, spread your fingers slightly once inside the body of the glove to help them into the glove fingers (**Action figures 6a, 6b**).	To prevent contamination of the outside of the glove. **E**
7 When both gloves are on, adjust the fit by pulling on the body of the glove to get your fingers to the end of the glove fingers (**Action figures 7a, 7b**).	To ensure the gloves are comfortable to wear and do not interfere with the procedure. **E**
Post-procedure	
8 Remove the gloves when the procedure is completed, taking care not to contaminate the hands or the environment from the outside of the gloves.	The outside of the glove is likely to be contaminated. **E**
9 First, remove the first glove by firmly holding the outside of the glove wrist and pulling off the glove in such a way as to turn it inside out.	Whilst removing the first glove, the second gloved hand continues to be protected. By turning the glove inside out during removal, any contamination is contained inside the glove. **E**

Action	Rationale
10 Then remove the second glove by slipping the fingers of the ungloved hand inside the wrist of the glove and pulling it off whilst at the same time turning it inside out.	By putting the fingers inside the glove, the fingers will not be in contact with the potentially contaminated outer surface of the glove. **E**
11 Dispose of used gloves as 'hazardous infectious waste', that is, into an orange waste bag, unless instructed otherwise by the infection prevention and control team.	All waste contaminated with blood, body fluids, excretions, secretions and infectious agents thought to pose a particular risk should be disposed of as hazardous infectious waste. Orange is the recognized colour for hazardous infectious waste that does not require incineration and may be made safe by alternative treatment (DH 2013b, **C**).
12 After removing the gloves, decontaminate your hands.	Hands may have become contaminated (Loveday et al. 2014, **C**).

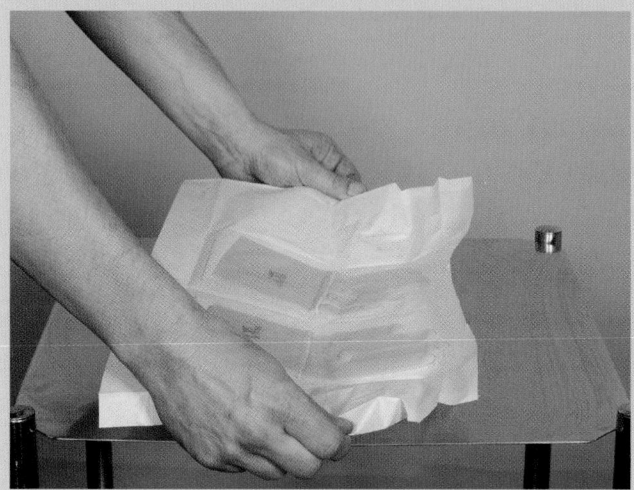

Action Figure 3 Open the packet containing the gloves onto a clean surface and open out the inside packaging so that the fingers of the gloves point away from you.

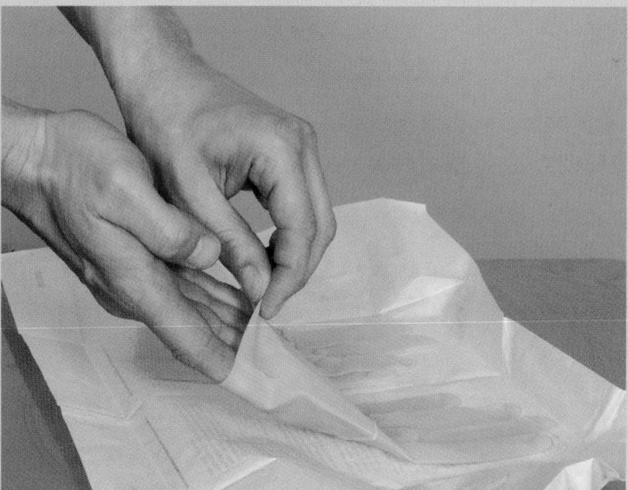

Action Figure 5a Hold the cuff of the first glove with the opposite hand and slide the fingertips of the other hand (that the glove is to go on) into the opening.

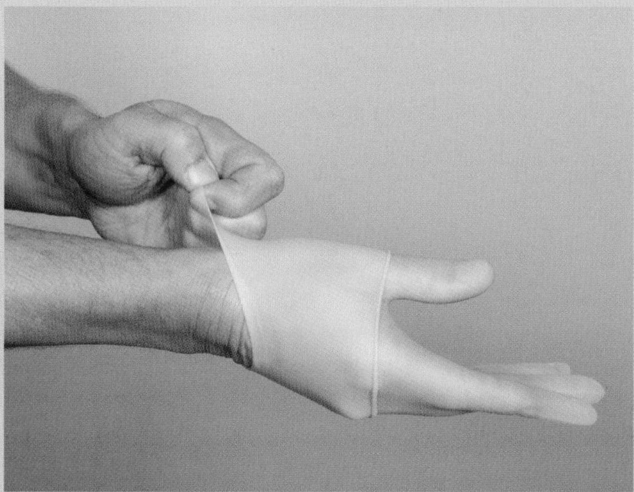

Action Figure 5b Keep hold of the folded edge and pull the glove onto your hand.

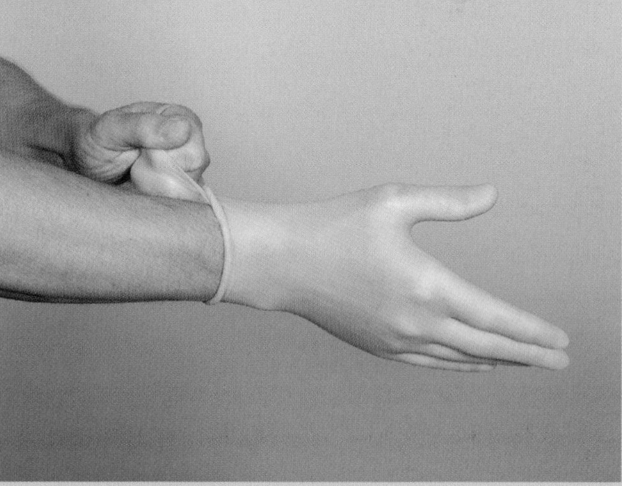

Action Figure 5c Spread your fingers slightly to help them enter the fingers of the glove.

(continued)

Procedure guideline 3.8 Donning sterile gloves: open technique *(continued)*

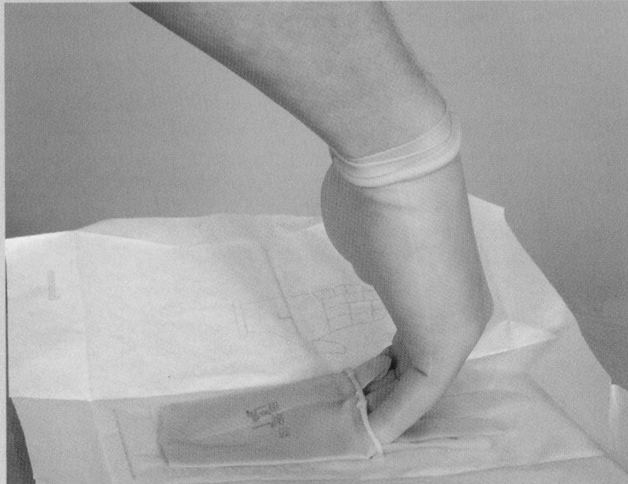

Action Figure 6a Slide the fingertips of your gloved hand beneath the folded cuff of the second glove.

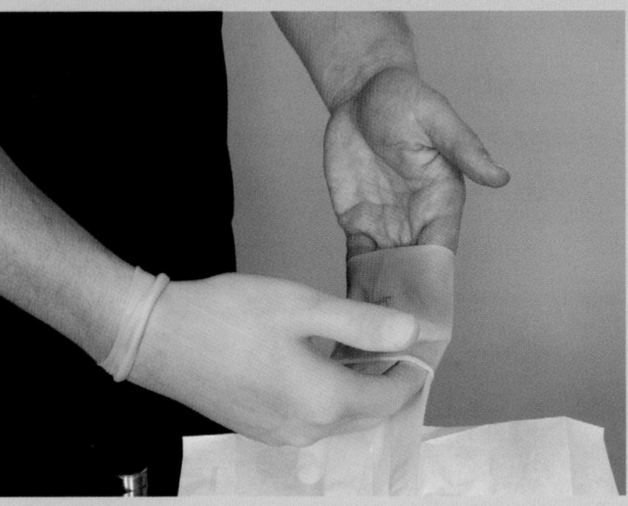

Action Figure 6b Slide the fingertips of your ungloved hand into the opening of the second glove.

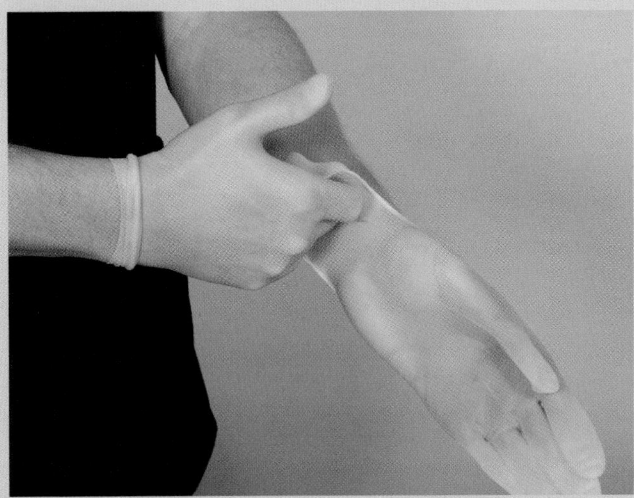

Action Figure 7a Pull the glove onto your hand, again spreading your fingers slightly to help them enter the fingers of the glove.

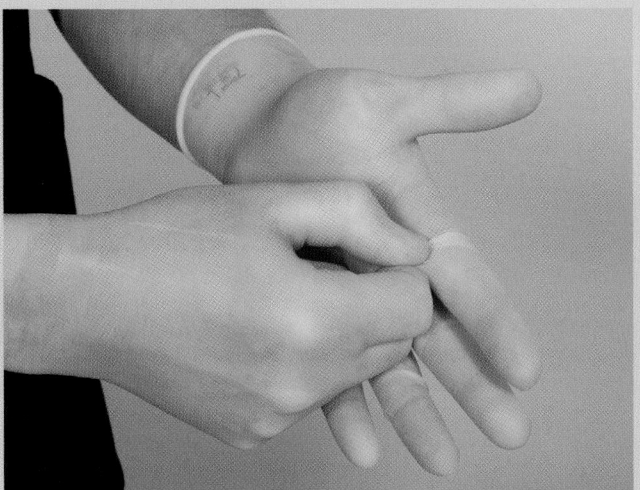

Action Figure 7b When both gloves are on, adjust the fit.

Procedure guideline 3.9 Donning a sterile gown and gloves: closed technique

Note 1: These procedures will normally require participants to also wear a mask and eye protection.
Note 2: An assistant is required to open sterile gloves and tie the back of the gown.

Essential equipment

- Sterile disposable gloves
- Sterile disposable or reusable gown

Pre-procedure

Action	Rationale
1 Prepare the area where gowning and gloving will take place. Open the gown pack with clean hands. Do not touch the inside of the package.	To ensure that there is adequate room to don gown and gloves and to avoid contaminating either. **E**

Action	Rationale
2 Wash your hands using a surgical scrub technique with either antiseptic hand wash solution or soap. Dry using a separate sterile paper towel for each hand and forearm. If hands have been washed with soap, apply an antiseptic handrub to the hands and forearms.	To both disinfect and physically remove matter and micro-organisms from the hands (WHO 2009a, **C**).
Procedure	
3 Open the inner layer of the gown pack, if present (**Action figures 3a, 3b**).	To allow the gown to be removed. **E**
4 Grasp the gown on its inside surface just below the neck opening (this should be uppermost if the gown pack has been opened correctly) and lift it up, holding it away from the body and any walls or furniture. The gown should fall open with the inside facing towards you (**Action figure 4**).	To open out the gown while keeping its outer surface sterile. **E**
5 Insert the free hand into the corresponding sleeve of the gown, pulling the gown towards you, until your fingers reach, but do not go beyond, the cuff of the sleeve (**Action figure 5**).	To pull on the gown while keeping its outer surface sterile. **E**
6 Release the inside surface of the gown and insert that hand into the corresponding sleeve, again until your fingers reach, but do not go beyond, the cuff of the sleeve. (**Action figure 6**). The assistant should help to pull the gown on and tie the ties, without touching any part of the gown other than the ties and rear edges.	To pull on the gown while keeping its outer surface sterile. **E**
7 The assistant opens a pair of sterile gloves and presents the inner packaging for you to take. Place this on the sterile area of the open gown package so that the fingers of the gloves point towards you (**Action figure 7**).	To prepare the gloves for donning while keeping them and the gown sterile. **E**
8 Open the inner packaging of the gloves. The fingers should be towards you, the thumbs uppermost and the cuffs folded over. Keeping your hands within the sleeves of the gown, slide the thumb of your right hand (still inside the sleeve) between the folded-over cuff and the body of the right glove. Pick up that glove. Grasp the cuff of that glove on the opposite side with the other hand (still inside its sleeve) and unfold it, pulling it over the cuff of the sleeve and the hand inside. Then push your right hand through the cuff of the sleeve into the glove. Repeat the process with the left hand. Once both hands are inside their respective gloves, there is no risk of contaminating the outside of the gloves or gown with your bare hands (**Action figures 8a, 8b, 8c, 8d, 8e, 8f, 8g**).	To don the gloves while keeping their outer surface sterile and ensuring that there is no risk of contaminating the outside of the gown. **E**
9 If you need to change a glove because it is damaged or contaminated, pull the sleeve cuff down over your hand as you do so and don the replacement glove using the technique above.	To minimize the risk of contaminating the gown or the sterile field. **E**
10 Dispose of used gloves and disposable gowns as 'hazardous infectious waste', that is, into an orange waste bag, unless instructed otherwise by the infection prevention and control team.	All waste contaminated with blood, body fluids, excretions, secretions and infectious agents thought to pose a particular risk should be disposed of as hazardous infectious waste. Orange is the recognized colour for hazardous infectious waste that does not require incineration and may be made safe by alternative treatment (DH 2013b, **C**).
Post-procedure	
11 At the end of the procedure, remove gown and gloves as a single unit by pulling the gown away from you so as to turn it and the gloves inside out (**Action figures 11a, 11b**).	To avoid cross-contamination of hands. **E**
12 Consign reusable gowns as infected linen according to local arrangements.	To minimize any risk to laundry workers from contaminated items (DH 2013c, **C**).
13 After removing the gloves and gown, decontaminate your hands.	Hands may have become contaminated (Loveday et al. 2014, **C**).

(continued)

Procedure guideline 3.9 Donning a sterile gown and gloves: closed technique *(continued)*

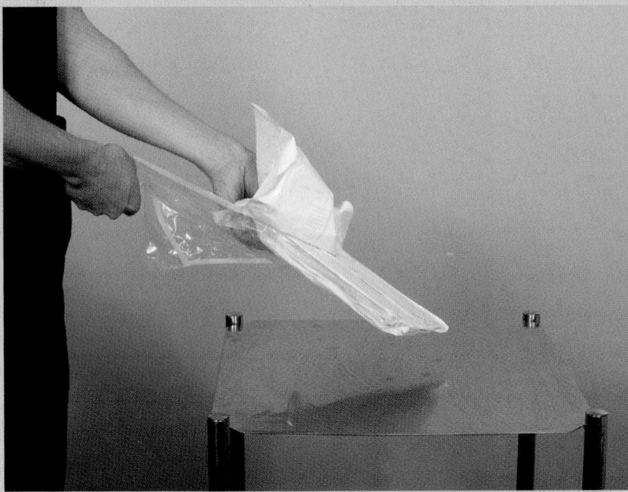

Action Figure 3a Open the gown pack with clean hands onto a clean surface. Do not touch the inner packet until after the surgical scrub.

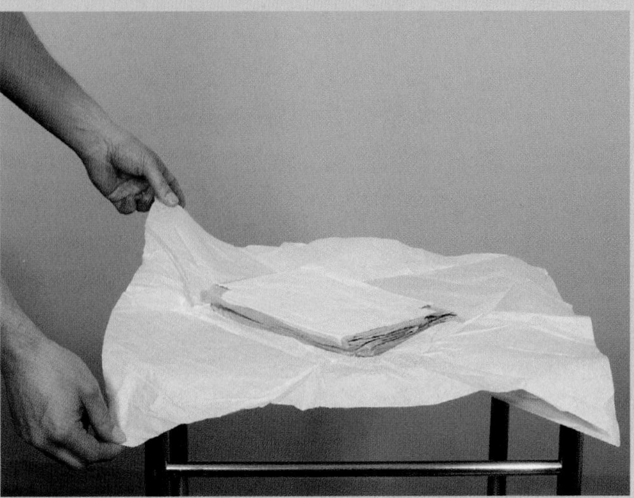

Action Figure 3b Open the inner layer of the pack; use sterile towels to dry hands and forearms if required.

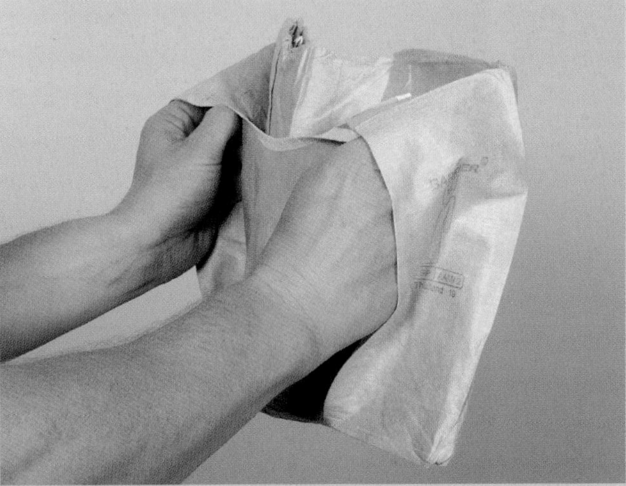

Action Figure 4 Lift up the gown by its inner surface and hold it away from the body.

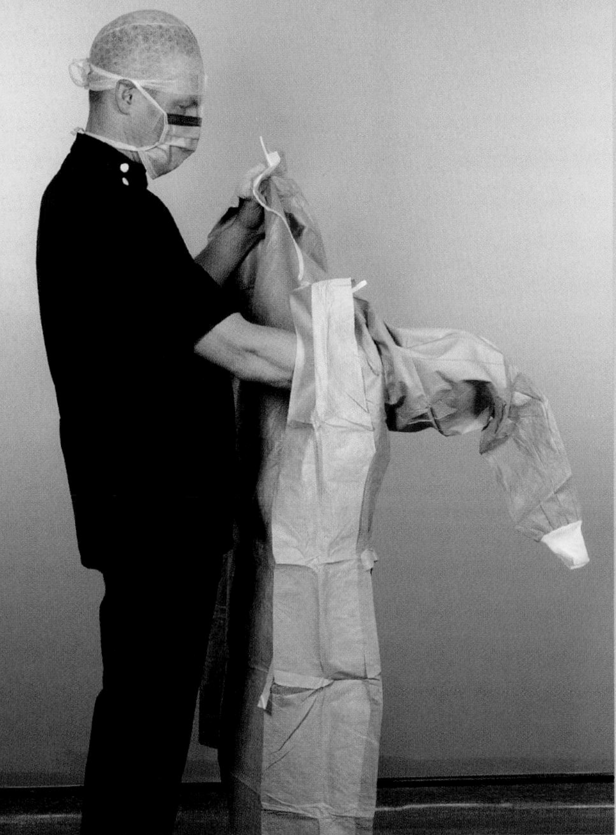

Action Figure 5 Put one hand into the corresponding sleeve and use the other hand to pull the gown towards you. Your hand should not go beyond the cuff.

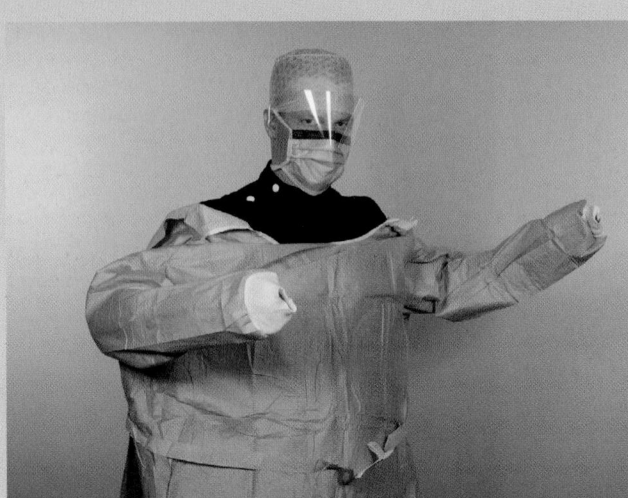

Action Figure 6 Put the other hand into the other sleeve. Again, your hand should not go beyond the cuff.

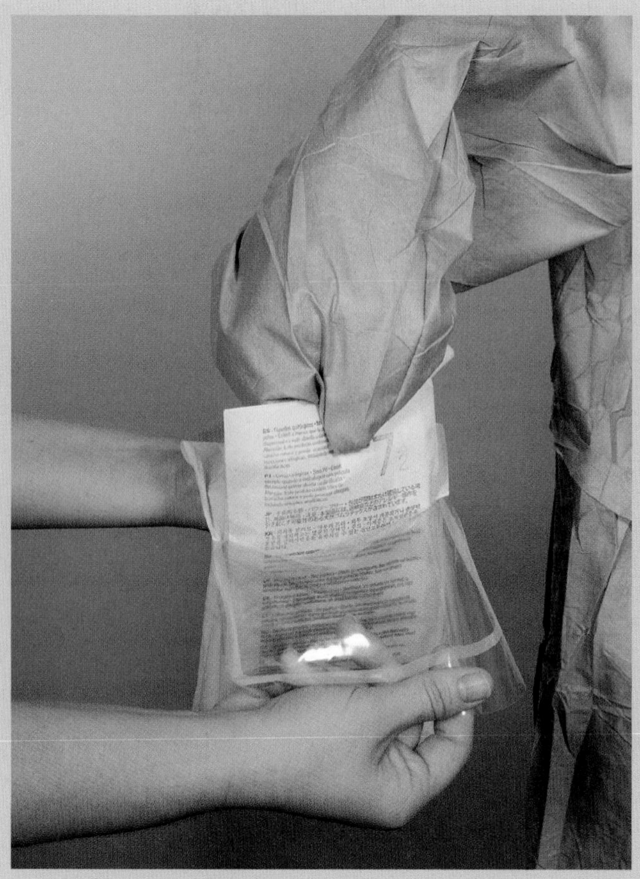

Action Figure 7 The assistant opens a pair of sterile gloves and presents the inner packaging for you to take.

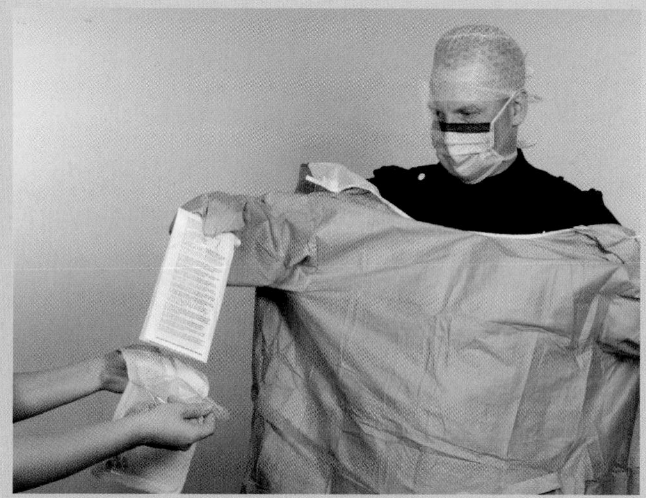

Action Figure 8a Take the gloves, keeping your hands inside your sleeves.

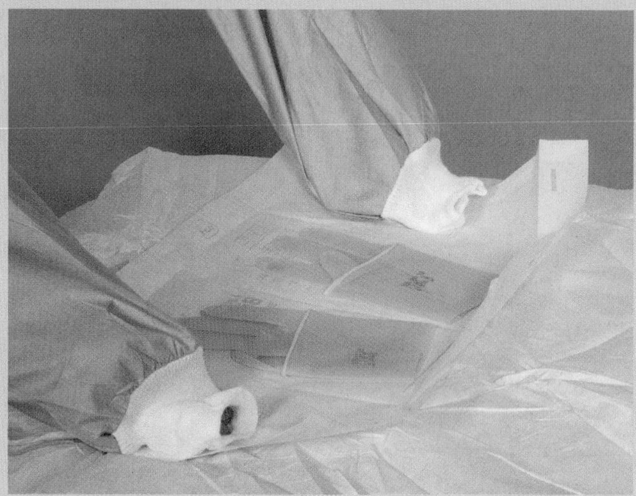

Action Figure 8b Open the inner glove packet on the sterile open gown package so that the glove fingers point towards you.

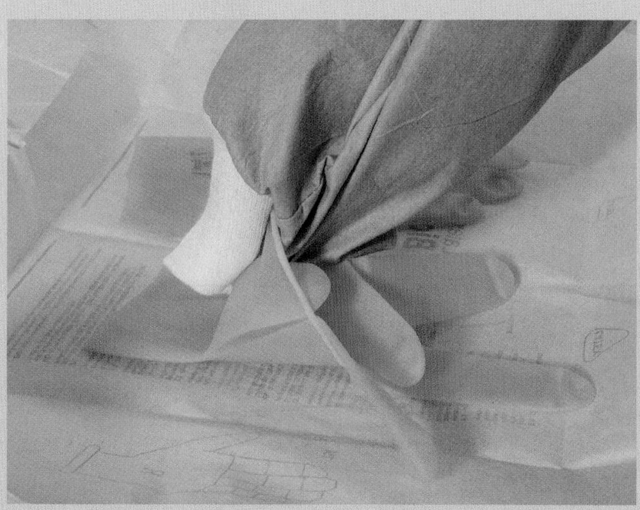

Action Figure 8c Slide the thumb of one hand (still inside the sleeve) under the folded-over cuff of the corresponding glove.

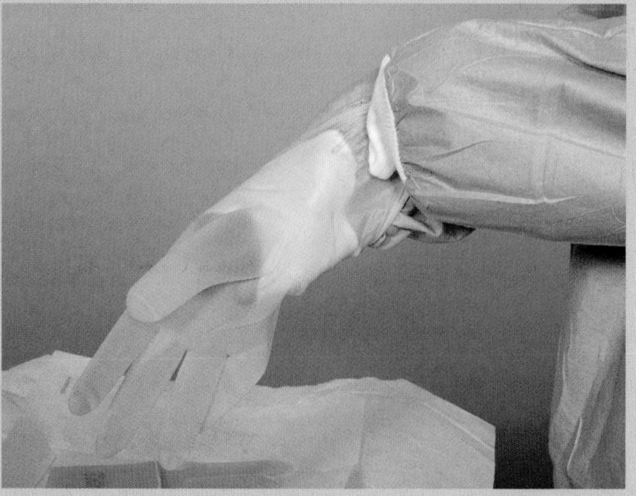

Action Figure 8d Push your hand through the cuff and into the glove.

(continued)

Procedure guideline 3.9 **Donning a sterile gown and gloves: closed technique *(continued)***

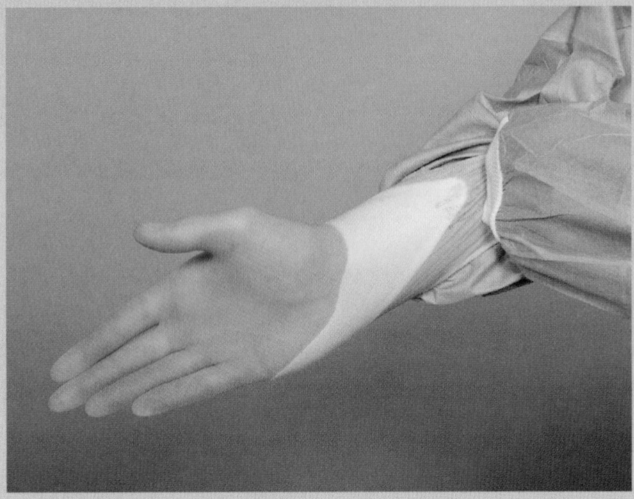

Action Figure 8e Pull the glove into position using the other hand (still inside its sleeve).

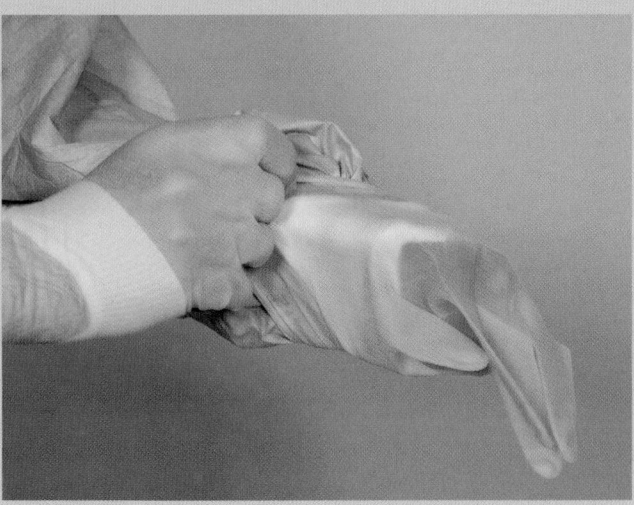

Action Figure 8f Repeat the process with the other glove.

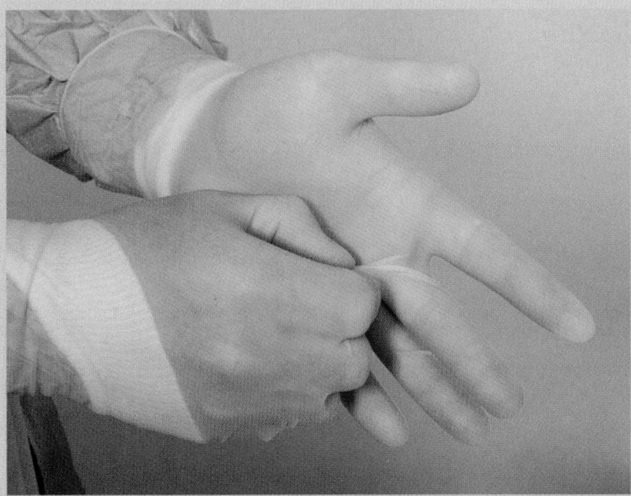

Action Figure 8g Adjust the fit when both gloves are on.

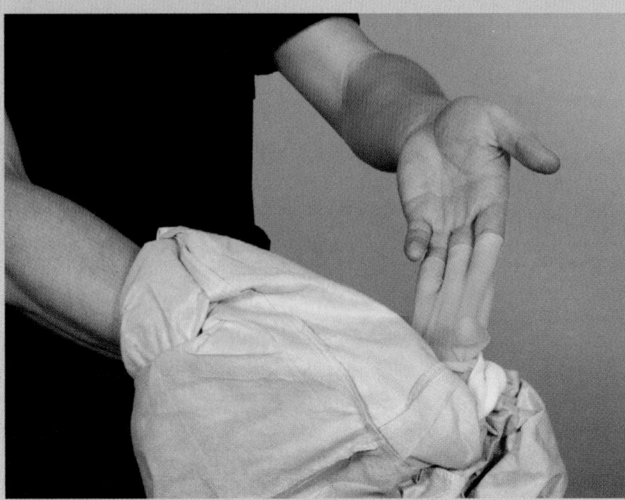

Action Figure 11b Turn it and the gloves inside out.

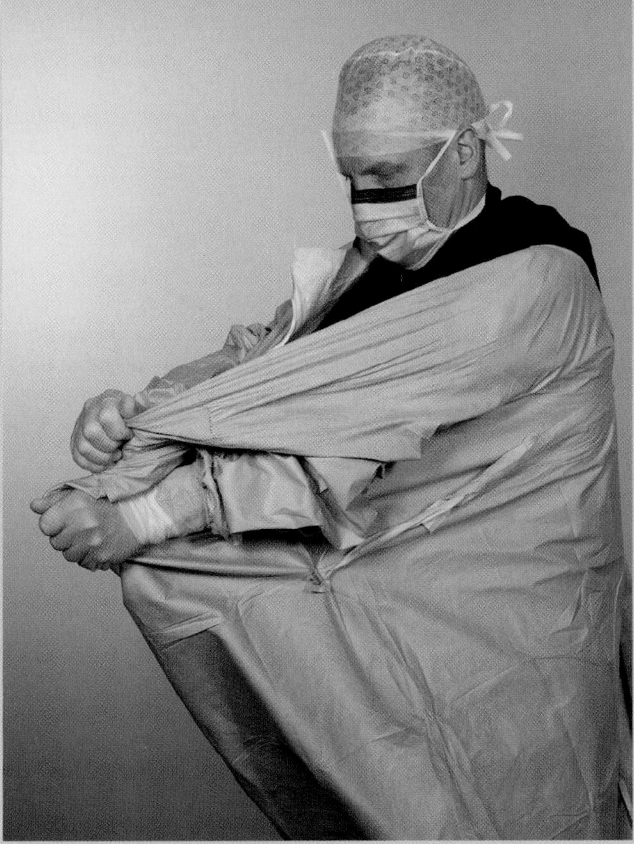

Action Figure 11a At the end of the procedure, remove gown and gloves as a single unit by pulling the gown away from you.

Aseptic technique

EVIDENCE-BASED APPROACHES

Rationale

Aseptic technique is the practice of carrying out a procedure in such a way that you minimize the risk of introducing contamination into a vulnerable area or contaminating an invasive device. Aseptic technique is required whenever you are carrying out a procedure that involves contact with a part of the body or an invasive device where introducing micro-organisms may increase the risk of infection. Note that the area or device on which you are working will not necessarily be sterile – wounds, for example, will be colonized with micro-organisms – but your aim must be to avoid introducing additional contamination.

Aseptic non-touch technique (ANTT) is the practice of avoiding contamination by not touching key elements such as the tip of a needle, the seal of an intravenous connector after it has been decontaminated, or the inside surface of a sterile dressing where it will be in contact with the wound (Rowley and Clare 2011). An example of non-touch technique is illustrated in Figure 3.5. Gloves are normally worn for ANTT but they are mainly for the practitioner's, rather than the patient's, protection. Non-sterile gloves are therefore perfectly acceptable.

As with other infection prevention and control measures, the actions taken to reduce the risk of contamination will depend on the procedure being undertaken and the potential consequences of contamination. Examples of different aseptic techniques and the measures required for them are given in Table 3.5. It is therefore difficult to provide a procedure guideline that will apply to the whole range of aseptic procedures. To provide a context, the following procedure contains steps for changing a wound dressing but is presented as a guide to aseptic technique in general. Local guidance and training should be sought before carrying out specific procedures. Some specific procedures are described in other chapters of this manual.

Figure 3.5 **Avoiding contamination by avoiding contact with the key elements. Source: Reproduced with permission from ICU Medical, Inc.**

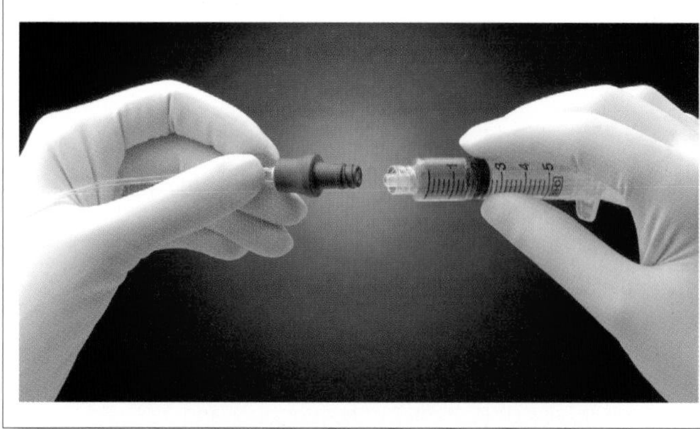

Table 3.5 **Examples of aseptic procedures**

Procedure	Precautions required
Surgical joint replacement	Must be carried out in an operating theatre with specialist ventilation by a team who will wear sterile gowns and gloves, or even full body suits with individual exhaust systems to eliminate airborne contamination
Urinary catheterization	Can be carried out in an open ward by a practitioner wearing an apron and sterile gloves
Peripheral intravenous cannulation	Can be performed wearing non-sterile gloves and using an appropriate non-touch technique

Procedure guideline 3.10 **Aseptic technique example: changing a wound dressing**

Essential equipment (will vary depending on procedure)

- Sterile dressing pack containing gallipots or an indented plastic tray, low-linting swabs and/or medical foam, disposable forceps, gloves, sterile field, disposal bag. Please note that in your organization there may be specific packs available for particular procedures, for example IV packs. Because the usage and availability of these vary between organizations, reference is generally made to 'sterile dressing pack'
- Fluids for cleaning and/or irrigation; 0.9% sodium chloride is normally appropriate
- Hypoallergenic tape (if required)
- Appropriate dressing (if required)
- Alcohol handrub (hand washing is an acceptable alternative but will take more time and may entail leaving the patient; alcohol handrub is the most appropriate method for hand hygiene during a procedure as long as hands are physically clean)
- Any extra equipment that may be needed during procedure, for example sterile scissors
- Traceability system for any reusable surgical instruments and patient record form
- Detergent wipe for cleaning trolley

Pre-procedure

Action	Rationale
1 Check that all the equipment required for the procedure is available and, where applicable, is sterile (i.e. that packaging is undamaged, intact and dry; that sterility indicators are present on any sterilized items and have changed colour where applicable).	To ensure that the patient is not disturbed unnecessarily if items are not available and to avoid unnecessary delays during the procedure. **E** To ensure that only sterile products are used (MHRA 2010, **C**).
2 Explain and discuss the procedure with the patient.	To ensure that the patient understands the procedure and gives their valid consent (NMC 2013, **C**).

(continued)

Procedure guideline 3.10 Aseptic technique example: changing a wound dressing *(continued)*

Procedure

Action	Rationale
3 Clean hands with alcohol handrub or wash with soap and water and dry with paper towels.	Hands must be cleaned before and after every patient contact and before commencing the preparations for aseptic technique, to prevent cross-infection (Loveday et al. 2014, **C**).
4 Clean trolley with detergent and water or detergent wipes and dry with a paper towel. If disinfection is also required (e.g. by local policy), use disposable wipes saturated with 70% isopropyl alcohol and leave to dry.	To provide a clean working surface (Fraise and Bradley 2009, **E**); alcohol is an effective and fast-acting disinfectant that will dry quickly (Fraise and Bradley 2009, **E**).
5 Place all the equipment required for the procedure on the bottom shelf of the clean dressing trolley.	To maintain the top shelf as a clean working surface. **E**
6 Take the patient to the treatment room or screen the bed. Ensure that any fans in the area are turned off and windows closed. Position the patient comfortably and so that the area to be dealt with is easily accessible without exposing the patient unduly.	To allow any airborne organisms to settle before the sterile field (and in this case, the wound) is exposed. Maintain the patient's dignity and comfort. **E**
7 Put on a disposable plastic apron.	To reduce the risk of contaminating clothing and of contaminating the wound or any sterile items from clothing. **E**
8 Take the trolley to the treatment room or patient's bedside, disturbing the curtains as little as possible.	To minimize airborne contamination. **E**
9 Loosen the adhesive or tape on the existing dressing.	To make it easier to remove the dressing. **E**
10 Clean hands with alcohol handrub.	Hands should be cleaned before any aseptic procedure (WHO 2009a, **C**). Using alcohol handrub avoids having to leave the patient to go to a sink. **E**
11 Open the outer cover of the sterile pack and, once you have verified that the pack is the correct way up, slide the contents, without touching them, onto the top shelf of the trolley.	To minimize contamination of the contents. **E**
12 Open the sterile field using only the corners of the paper.	So that areas of potential contamination are kept to a minimum. **E**
13 Open any other packs, tipping their contents gently onto the centre of the sterile field.	To prepare the equipment and, in the case of a wound dressing, reduce the amount of time that the wound is uncovered. **E**
14 Where appropriate, loosen the old dressing.	To minimize trauma when removing the old dressing. **E**
15 Clean hands with alcohol handrub.	Hands may have become contaminated by handling outer packets or the old dressing (Loveday et al. 2014, **C**).
16 Carefully lift the plastic disposal bag from the sterile field by its open end and, holding it by one edge of the open end, place your other hand in the bag. Using it as a sterile 'glove', arrange the contents of the dressing pack and any other sterile items on the sterile field.	To maintain the sterility of the items required for the procedure while arranging them so as to perform the procedure quickly and efficiently. **E**
17 With your hand still enclosed within the disposal bag, remove the old dressing from the wound. Invert the bag so that the dressing is contained within it and stick it to the trolley below the top shelf. This is now the disposal bag for the remainder of the procedure for any waste other than sharps.	To minimize risk of contamination by containing dressing in bag. **E** To ensure that any waste can be disposed of without contaminating the sterile field. **E**
18 Pour any solutions into gallipots or onto the indented plastic tray.	To minimize risk of contamination of solutions. **E**
19 Put on gloves, as described in Procedure guideline 3.3: Putting on and removing non-sterile gloves or Procedure guideline 3.8: Donning sterile gloves: open technique. The procedure will dictate whether gloves should be sterile or non-sterile.	Gloves should be worn whenever any contact with body fluids is anticipated (Loveday et al. 2014, **C**). Sterile gloves provide greater sensitivity than forceps for procedures that cannot be carried out with a non-touch technique and are less likely to cause trauma to the patient. **E**
20 Carry out the relevant procedure according to the guidelines.	

Post-procedure	
21 Make sure the patient is comfortable.	To minimize the risk of causing the patient distress or discomfort. **E**
22 Dispose of waste in orange plastic waste bags. Remove apron and gloves and discard into orange waste bag.	To prevent environmental contamination. Orange is the recognized colour for hazardous infectious waste (DH 2013b, **C**).
23 Draw back curtains or help the patient back to the bed area and ensure that they are comfortable.	To minimize the risk of causing the patient distress or discomfort. **E**
24 Check that the trolley remains dry and physically clean. If necessary, wash with liquid detergent and water or detergent wipe and dry thoroughly with a paper towel.	To remove any contamination on the trolley and so minimize the risk of transferring any contamination elsewhere in the ward (Loveday et al. 2014, **C**).
25 Clean hands with alcohol handrub or soap and water.	Hands should be cleaned after any contact with the patient or body fluids (WHO 2009a, **C**).
26 Document the procedure clearly, including details of who carried it out, any devices or dressings used, particularly any left *in situ*, and any deviation from prescribed procedure. Fix any record labels from the outside packaging of any items used during the procedure on the patient record form and add this to the patient's notes.	Provides a record of the procedure and evidence that any items used have undergone an appropriate sterilization process (DH 2007b, **C**; NMC 2010, **C**).

Source isolation

EVIDENCE-BASED APPROACHES

Rationale

Source isolation is used for patients who are infected with, or are colonized by, infectious agents that require additional precautions over and above the standard precautions used with every patient (Siegel et al. 2007). Source isolation is used to minimize the risk of transmission of that agent to other vulnerable persons, whether patients or staff. Common reasons for source isolation include infections that cause diarrhoea and vomiting, entailing the use of enteric precautions; infections that are spread through the air, entailing the use of airborne or droplet precautions; and infection or colonization with antibiotic-resistant bacteria, requiring contact precautions (Siegel et al. 2007). Note that the patient's other nursing and medical needs must always be taken into account and infection control precautions may need to be modified accordingly.

Patients requiring source isolation are normally cared for in a single room, although outbreaks of infection may require affected patients to be nursed in a cohort, that is, isolated as a group (Fraise and Bradley 2009). A single-occupancy room will physically separate patients who present a risk from others who may be at risk, and will act as a reminder to any staff dealing with that patient of the need for additional infection control precautions. Single-occupancy rooms used for source isolation should have en suite toilet and bathroom facilities wherever possible, and contain all items required to meet the patient's nursing needs during the period of isolation (e.g. instruments to assess vital signs); these should remain inside the room throughout the period of isolation. If this is not possible because insufficient equipment is available on the ward, any items taken from the room must be thoroughly cleaned and disinfected (normally with a chlorine solution) before being used with any other patient (Fraise and Bradley 2009).

The air pressure in the room should be negative or neutral in relation to the air pressure in the rest of the ward (note that some airborne infections will require a negative pressure room) (Siegel et al. 2007). A lobby will provide an additional degree of security and space for donning and removing personal protective equipment and performing hand hygiene. Some facilities have lobbies that are ventilated so as to have positive pressure with respect to both the rest of the ward and the single-occupancy room; this allows the room to be used for both source and protective isolation (DH 2013d). Where insufficient single rooms are available for source isolation, they should be allocated to those patients who pose the greatest risk to others, using a tool such as the one shown in Figure 3.6 (Jeanes et al. 2011). As a general rule, patients with enteric symptoms, that is diarrhoea and vomiting, or serious airborne infections, such as tuberculosis, have the highest priority for single-occupancy rooms. If this situation arises, it will mean that additional precautions will be required for some patients on the open ward; for example, gloves and aprons will still be required while caring for someone colonized with MRSA even if they are not isolated. Patients should receive a clear explanation of prioritization and thus why they may be isolated some times and not others; they may lose confidence in the care provided if it appears inconsistent without explanation.

Principles of care

Attending to the patient in isolation

MEALS

Meals should be served on normal crockery and the patient provided with normal cutlery. Cutlery and crockery should be washed in a dishwasher able to thermally disinfect items, that is, with a final rinse of 80°C for 1 minute or 71°C for 3 minutes. Disposable cutlery and crockery should only be used if specifically instructed by the infection prevention and control team. Disposables and uneaten food should be discarded in the appropriate bag.

Contaminated crockery is a potential vector for infectious agents, particularly those causing enteric disease, but thermal disinfection will minimize this risk (Fraise and Bradley 2009).

URINE AND FAECES

Wherever possible, a toilet should be kept solely for the patient's use. If this is not available, a commode should be left in the patient's room. Gloves and apron must be worn by staff when dealing with body fluids. Bedpans and urinals should be bagged in the isolation room and taken directly to the sluice for disposal. They should not be emptied before being placed in the bedpan washer or macerator unless the volume of the contents needs to be measured for a fluid balance or stool chart. Gloves and apron worn in the room should be kept on until the body waste is disposed of and then removed (gloves first) and discarded as infected waste.

This will minimize the risk of infection being spread from excreta, for example via a toilet seat or a bedpan (Loveday et al. 2014) and the risk of hands or clothing being contaminated by body waste.

(a)

Step 1	Identify infection or condition
Step 2	Use score card to: – record ACDP hazard group – record mode of transmission – record evidence for transmission – assess prevalence of infection in the hospital – determine antibiotic resistance – assess susceptibility of other patients – assess dispersal characteristics of patient
Step 3	Add all scores and compare total to chart to determine priority for isolation

(b)

Patient name: .... Date: .... Name and designation of person scoring: ....

Significant details, e.g. micro-organism(s): ....

Criteria	Classification	Score	Comments
ACDP	2	5	
	3	10	
	4	40	
Route	Airborne	15	
	Droplet	10	
	Contact/faecal–oral	5	
	Blood-borne	0	
Evidence of transmission	Strong (published)	10	
	Moderate (consensus)	5	
	Poor	0	
	Nil	–10	
Significant resistance	Yes	5	Such as MRSA, VRE, ESBL, Gent resistance
	No	0	
High susceptibility of other patients with serious consequences	Yes	10	Specific for various infections and patient populations
	No	0	
Prevalence in hospital	Sporadic	0	
	Endemic	–5	This reflects the burden of infection in the hospital and cohort measures may be more applicable
	Epidemic	–5	See above
Dispersal	High risk	10	This includes diarrhoea, projectile vomiting, coughing, confused wandering, infected patients, etc.
	Medium risk	5	
	Low risk	0	

TOTAL SCORE (document score in patient's notes):

Using the score to determine the priority for isolation:

Score	Priority for isolation
0–20	Low
25–35	Med
35+	High

(c)

Score	Priority for isolation
0–20	Low
25–35	Medium
35+	High

Figure 3.6 **Example of an isolation prioritization tool. (a) How to use the tool. (b) Score card. (c) Score. (d) Shortcut guide to priorities for isolation. (e) Infection identified (M-Z shown only). ACDP, Advisory Committee on Dangerous Pathogens; CJD, Creutzfeldt–Jakob disease; D&V, diarrhoea and vomiting; ESBL, extended-spectrum beta-lactamase producers; Gent, gentamicin; GRE, glycopeptide-resistant enterococci; ITU, intensive care unit; MDRTB, multidrug-resistant tuberculosis; MRSA, meticillin-resistant *Staphylococcus aureus;* NICU, neonatal intensive care unit; PVL, Panton-Valentine leukocidin; RSV, respiratory syncytial virus; SCBU, special care baby unit; TB, tuberculosis; TSE, transmissible spongiform encephalopathy; VHF, viral haemorrhagic fever; VRE, vancomycin-resistant enterococci. Source: Jeanes et al. (2011). Reproduced with permission from MA Healthcare Ltd.**

(d)

Clinical conditions	Score & priority for isolation	Mode of transmission	Specific guidance
Cellulitis	25	Contact	
Conjunctivitis	15	Contact	Several causes and can be problematic in babies
Diarrhoea with or without vomiting (D&V) (possible gastroenteritis or *Clostridium difficile*)	35–45	**Droplet**/faecal–oral	Isolate until a non-infectious cause is found or patient has been asymptomatic for at least 48 hours
Immunodeficiency	25		Score/criteria reflect susceptibility rather than organism. These patients are vulnerable to infection and should be placed in specialist ward. If they are particularly susceptible they need positive pressure isolation
Palliative care	20		Valid reason for side room use (see below)
Patients under close supervision or light sensitive	20		Valid reason for side room use and should be assessed on a case by case basis
Rash	>35	**Airborne**/ Droplet/contact	Isolate until a non-infectious cause is found or patient is no longer infectious
Wound oozing/infected	20 30	Contact	Susceptibility of other patients and dispersal potential is important. Medium risk is: open wound, copious secretions

(e)

Infection identified	Score & priority for isolation		Mode of transmission	Specific guidance
Measles	>35		Droplet	
Meningitis undiagnosed (viral or bacterial)	30–40		**Droplet**/faecal–oral	All meningitis cases should be isolated until cause is established. Meningococcal meningitis requires isolation until patient has received 48 hours of treatment
Meningococcal septicaemia	30–40		Droplet	Remain in isolation until 48 hours of treatment given
Meticillin-resistant *Staphylococcus aureus* (MRSA)	25	>35	Contact/ droplet	Risk assess for isolation. High risk includes: • major dispersers, i.e. dry or flaky skin, expectorating infected sputum • surgical, especially in orthopaedic, cardiac or neurosurgery areas • patients with multiple devices and interventions, e.g. ITU, NICU and SCBU • PVL MRSA Medium risk includes positive screening swab but otherwise well and not in areas identified above. These patients may be cohorted
Mumps	30–40		Droplet	
Norovirus/Small round structured virus (SRSV)	>45		**Faecal–oral**/ contact	
Respiratory syncytial virus (RSV)	25		Droplet	**A problem in newborn, children and immunodeficiency**
Rotavirus	25		**Droplet**/faecal–oral	**A problem in newborn, children and immunodeficiency**
Rubella	20	>30	Droplet	Susceptibility of non immune may be an issue Medium risk paediatrics and women's health
Salmonella or Shigella	20	>30	Faecal–oral	Dependent on potential for dispersal Medium risk for patients who are incontinent or have diarrhoea
Scabies (Confirmed)	20		Contact	
Scarlet fever	30		Droplet	
Severe acute respiratory syndrome (SARS)	40		**Droplet**/ contact	
Shingles (Herpes Zoster)	15	30	Contact	No isolation needed if lesions are covered or dried Medium risk is weeping lesions, non-immune women of childbearing age, babies and children and immunodeficient
Streptococcus pyogenes (Group A strep)	25		**Droplet**/ contact	Remain isolated for 24 hours following treatment
Tuberculosis (TB) non pulmonary	15		Contact	Dependent on site and stage of disease
Tuberculosis (TB) open pulmonary or exuding lesion	25	35	Contact/ airborne	Isolated for period of 10–14 days following commencement of treatment. **MDRTB patients should remain in isolation throughout hospital stay.** High risk: patients who have a cough, MDRTB
Typhoid fever	15	25	Faecal–oral	Dependant on potential for dispersal Medium risk for patients who are incontinent or have diarrhoea
Verotoxin producing strains of *Escherichia coli* (e.g. *E. coli* O157)	15	25	Faecal–oral	Dependant on potential for dispersal Medium risk for patients who are incontinent or have diarrhoea
Viral haemorrhagic fever (VHF) Lassa/Ebola/Marburg	>70		**Droplet**/ blood/contact	Blood and body fluids are highly infectious – **transfer to regional infectious diseases facility**

Figure 3.6 ***(continued)***

SPILLAGES

As elsewhere, any spillage must be mopped up immediately, using the appropriate method for the fluid spilt, and the area dried. This removes the risk of anyone slipping and removes and disinfects any contaminated fluid that may carry a risk of infection.

BATHING

If an en suite bathroom is not available, the patient must be bathed elsewhere on the ward. The patient does not need to use the bathroom last but the bathroom must be thoroughly cleaned after use so bathing them last will minimize any delays to other patients that this may cause. However, if the patient requires an early bath, for example because they are leaving the ward for an examination elsewhere, this must be catered for.

Thorough cleaning and disinfection of the bathroom will minimize the risk of cross-infection to other patients.

LINEN

Place infected linen in a red water-soluble alginate polythene bag, which must be secured tightly before it leaves the room. Just outside the room, place this bag into a red linen bag which must be secured tightly and not used for other patients. These bags should await the laundry collection in the area designated for this.

Placing infected linen in a red alginate polythene bag confines the organisms and allows laundry staff to recognize the potential hazard and avoid handling the linen (DH 2013c).

WASTE

Orange waste bags should be kept in the isolation room for disposal of all waste generated in the room. The top of the bag should be sealed and labelled with the name of the ward or department before it is removed from the room.

Cleaning the isolation room

1 Domestic staff must be instructed on the correct procedure to use when cleaning an isolation room, including an explanation as to why isolation is essential to reduce the risk of cross-infection, the materials and solutions used, and the correct colour coding for these materials. This will reduce the risk of mistakes and ensure that appropriate precautions are maintained (DH 2001).
2 Isolation rooms must be cleaned last, to reduce the risk of the transmission of contamination to 'clean' areas (NPSA 2009).
3 Separate cleaning equipment must be used for isolation rooms. Cross-infection may result from shared cleaning equipment (Wilson 2006).
4 Cleaners must wear gloves and plastic aprons while cleaning isolation rooms to minimize the risk of contaminating hands or clothing. Some PPE may also be required for the safe use of some cleaning solutions.
5 Floor (hard surface: carpeted rooms should not be used as isolation rooms). This must be washed daily with a disinfectant as appropriate. All excess water must be removed. Daily cleaning will reduce the number of bacteria in the environment. Organisms, especially Gram-negative bacteria, multiply quickly in the presence of moisture and on equipment (Wilson 2006).
6 Cleaning solutions must be freshly made up each day and the container emptied and cleaned daily. Disinfectants may lose activity over time; cleaning solutions can easily become contaminated (Dharan et al. 1999).
7 After use, the bucket must be cleaned and dried. Contaminated cleaning equipment and solutions will spread bacteria over surfaces being cleaned (Dharan et al. 1999).
8 Mop heads should be laundered in a hot wash daily as they become contaminated easily (Wilson 2006).
9 Furniture and fittings should be damp-dusted daily using a disposable cloth and a detergent or disinfectant solution by nursing or cleaning staff as dictated by local protocol, in order to remove dirt and a proportion of any organisms contaminating the environment (Wilson 2006).
10 The toilet, shower and bathroom areas must be cleaned at least once a day and if they become contaminated, using a non-abrasive hypochlorite powder, cream or solution. Non-abrasive powders or creams preserve the integrity of the surfaces.

Cleaning the room after a patient has been discharged

1 The room should be stripped. All bedlinen and other textiles must be changed and curtains changed (reusable curtains must be laundered and disposable curtains discarded as infectious waste). Dispose of any unused disposable items. Curtains and other fabrics readily become colonized with bacteria (Patel 2005); paper packets cannot be easily cleaned.
2 Impervious surfaces, for example locker, bedframe, mattress cover, chairs, floor, blinds, soap dispenser, should be washed with soap and water, or a combined detergent/chlorine disinfectant if sporicidal activity is required, and dried. Relatively inaccessible places, for example ceilings, may be omitted. Wiping of surfaces is the most effective way of removing contaminants. Spores from, for example, *Clostridium difficile* will persist indefinitely in the environment unless destroyed by an effective disinfectant; bacteria will thrive more readily in damp conditions; inaccessible areas are not generally relevant to any infection risk (Wilson 2006).
3 The room can be reused as soon as it has been thoroughly cleaned and restocked. Effective cleaning will have removed infectious agents that may pose a risk to the next patient.

Discharging the patient from isolation

If the patient no longer requires isolation but is still to be a patient on the ward, inform them of this and the reasons why isolation is no longer required before moving them out of the room. Also inform them if there is any reason why they may need to be returned to isolation, for example if enteric symptoms return.

If the patient is to be discharged home or to another health or social care setting, ensure that the discharge documentation includes details of their condition, the infection control precautions taken while in hospital and any precautions or other actions that will need to be taken following discharge. Suitable accurate information on infections must be supplied to any person concerned with providing further support or nursing/medical care in a timely fashion (DH 2010a).

Procedure guideline 3.11 **Source isolation: preparing an isolation room**

Essential equipment

- Single-occupancy room
- Patient equipment
- Personal protective equipment
- Hand hygiene facilities
- Patient information material

Pre-procedure

Action	Rationale
1 Identify the most suitable room available for source isolation, taking into account the risk to other patients and staff and the patient's other nursing needs.	To ensure the best balance between minimizing the risk of cross-infection and maintaining the safety and comfort of the isolated patient. **E**
Procedure	
2 Remove all non-essential furniture and equipment from the room. The remaining furniture should be easy to clean. Ensure that the room is stocked with any equipment required for patient care and sufficient but not excessive numbers of any disposable items that will be required.	To ensure the availability of everything required for patient care while minimizing the number of items that will require cleaning or disposal at the end of the isolation period and the amount of traffic of people and equipment into and out of the room. **E**
3 Ensure that a bin for clinical waste with an orange bag is present in the room. This will be used for all waste generated in the room. The bag must be sealed before it is removed from the room.	For containing contaminated rubbish within the room and minimizing further spread of infection. **E**
4 Place a container for sharps in the room.	To contain contaminated sharps within the infected area (DH 2013b, **C**).
5 Keep the patient's personal property to a minimum. All belongings taken into the room should be washable, cleanable or disposable. Contact the infection prevention and control team for advice as to how best to clean or wash specific items.	The patient's belongings may become contaminated and cannot be taken home unless they are washable or cleanable. **E**
6 Ensure that all PPE required is available outside the room. Wall-mounted dispensers offer the best use of space and ease of use but, if necessary, set up a trolley outside the door for PPE and alcohol handrub. Ensure that this does not cause an obstruction or other hazard.	To have PPE readily available when required. **E**
7 Explain the reason for isolation and the precise precautions required to the patient, their family and other visitors, providing relevant patient information material where available. Allow the patient to ask questions and ask for a member of the infection prevention and control team to visit the patient if ward staff cannot answer all questions to the patient's satisfaction.	Patients and their visitors may be more compliant if they understand the reasons for isolation, and the patient's anxiety may be reduced if they have as much information as possible about their condition. **E**
8 Fix a suitable notice outside the room where it will be seen by anyone attempting to enter the room. This should indicate the special precautions required while preserving the patient's confidentiality.	To ensure all staff and visitors are aware of the need for additional infection control precautions. **E**
9 Move the patient into the single-occupancy room.	To ensure isolation. **E**
10 Arrange for terminal cleaning of the bed space that the patient has been occupying.	To remove any infectious agents that may pose a risk to the next patient to occupy that bed (NPSA 2009, **C**).
Post-procedure	
11 Assess the patient daily to determine if source isolation is still required; for example, if enteric precautions have been required, has the patient been without symptoms for 48 hours?	There is often limited availability of isolation rooms (Wigglesworth and Wilcox 2006, **R1b**) so they must be used as effectively as possible. **E**

Procedure guideline 3.12 **Source isolation: entering the isolation room**

Essential equipment

- Personal protective equipment as dictated by the precautions required. Gloves and apron are the usual minimum; a respirator will be required for droplet precautions; eye protection if an aerosol-generating procedure is planned
- Any equipment required for any procedure you intend to carry out in the room

Pre-procedure

Action	Rationale
1 Collect all equipment needed.	To avoid entering and leaving the infected area unnecessarily. **E**

(continued)

Procedure guideline 3.12 Source isolation: entering the isolation room *(continued)*

Procedure

Action	Rationale
2 Ensure you are 'bare below the elbow' (see Procedure guideline 3.1: Hand washing).	To facilitate hand hygiene and avoid any contamination of long sleeves or cuffs that could be transferred to other patients. **E**
3 Put on a disposable plastic apron.	To protect the front of the uniform or clothing, which is the most likely area to come in contact with the patient. **E**
4 Put on a disposable well-fitting mask or respirator of the appropriate standard if droplet or airborne precautions are required, for example: (a) Meningococcal meningitis before completion of 24 hours of treatment (b) Pandemic influenza (c) Tuberculosis, if carrying out aerosol-generating procedure or the TB may be multiresistant.	To reduce the risk of inhaling organisms (DH 2010b, **C**; NICE 2006, **C**).
5 Don eye protection if instructed by infection prevention and control team (e.g. for pandemic influenza) or if conducting an aerosol-generating procedure (e.g. bronchoscopy or intubation) in a patient requiring airborne/droplet precautions.	To prevent infection via the conjunctiva (DH 2010b, **C**).
6 Clean hands with soap and water or alcohol handrub.	Hands must be cleaned before patient contact (WHO 2009a, **C**).
7 Don disposable gloves if you are intending to deal with blood, excreta or contaminated material, or if providing close personal care where contact precautions are required.	To reduce the risk of hand contamination (Loveday et al. 2014, **C**).
8 Enter the room, shutting the door behind you.	To reduce the risk of airborne organisms leaving the room (Kao and Yang 2006, **R1a**) and to preserve the patient's privacy and dignity. **E**

Procedure guideline 3.13 Source isolation: leaving the isolation room

Essential equipment

- Orange waste bag
- Hand hygiene facilities

Procedure

Action	Rationale
1 If wearing gloves, remove and discard them in the orange waste bag.	To avoid transferring any contamination on the gloves to other areas or items (Loveday et al. 2014, **C**).
2 Remove apron by holding the inside of the apron and breaking the ties at neck and waist. Discard it into the orange waste bag.	To avoid transferring any contamination on the apron to other areas or items (Loveday et al. 2014, **C**).
3 Clean hands with soap and water or alcohol handrub. Do not use alcohol handrub when patients require enteric precautions: wash with soap and water.	Hands must be cleaned after contact with the patient or their immediate environment (WHO 2009a, **C**); alcohol is less effective against *Clostridium difficile* spores and some enteric viruses and in the presence of organic material such as faeces (Fraise and Bradley 2009, **E**).
4 Leave the room, shutting the door behind you.	To reduce the risk of airborne spread of infection (Kao and Yang 2006, **R1a**).
5 Clean hands with soap and water or alcohol handrub. If the patient requires enteric precautions, hands should be cleaned with soap and water.	Hands must be cleaned after contact with the patient or their immediate environment (WHO 2009a, **C**). Alcohol is not effective on all organisms that cause enteric infections (Fraise and Bradley 2009, **E**).

Procedure guideline 3.14 Source isolation: transporting infected patients outside the source isolation area

Procedure

Action	Rationale
1 Inform the department concerned about the procedure required, the patient's diagnosis and the infection control precautions required at the earliest opportunity.	To allow the department time to make appropriate arrangements. **E**
2 If possible and appropriate, arrange for the patient to have the last appointment of the day.	The department concerned and any intervening areas will be less busy, so reducing the risk of contact with other vulnerable individuals, and additional cleaning required following any procedure will not disrupt subsequent appointments. **E**
3 Inform the portering service of the patient's diagnosis and the infection control precautions required; ensure that this information has been passed to any porters involved in transfer and reinforce the precautions required.	Explanation and reinforcement will minimize the risk of cross-infection through failure to comply with infection control precautions (Fraise and Bradley 2009, **E**).
4 Escort the patient if necessary.	To attend to the patient's nursing needs and to remind others of infection control precautions if required. **E**
5 If the patient has an infection requiring droplet or airborne precautions that may present a risk to people encountered in the other department or in transit, they will need to wear a mask or respirator of the appropriate standard. Provide the patient with the mask and explain why it is required and how and when it is to be worn (i.e. while outside their single-occupancy room) and assist them to don it if necessary.	To prevent airborne cross-infection. **E** Providing the patient with relevant information will reduce anxiety.

Learning Activity 3.4 Case study

Mr Peters is a 74-year-old man who has a history of chronic obstructive pulmonary disease. He lives alone and became unwell 7 days ago, feeling fatigued with a productive cough and elevated temperature. He was diagnosed with a chest infection and admitted to hospital for intravenous antibiotics. Having completed his course of antibiotics yesterday, he has now had five episodes of diarrhoea in the last 12 hours. He is being cared for in a six-bedded bay on a male medical ward and is expecting his daughter to visit him later today with his two young grandchildren.

1 What precautions should be taken for this patient? For how long?
2 What information would you give to Mr Peters and why?
3 Would the precautions you take be any different if you were visiting Mr Peters in his own home? If so, how?

See the end of the chapter for the answers.

Protective isolation

EVIDENCE-BASED APPROACHES

Rationale

Protective isolation is used to minimize the exposure to infectious agents of patients who are particularly at risk of infection. The evidence that protective isolation successfully reduces the incidence of infection is limited (Wigglesworth 2003), probably because many infections are endogenous (i.e. caused by the patient's own bacterial flora). However, it is used to reduce the risk of exogenous infection (cross-infection from other people or the environment) in groups who have greatly impaired immune systems (Fraise and Bradley 2009), such as autologous and allogenic bone marrow transplant patients. Patients who have compromised immune systems often have greatly reduced numbers of a type of white blood cell called a neutrophil; this condition is known as neutropenia and those people suffering from it are described as neutropenic. Neutropenia is graded from mild to severe according to how few neutrophils are in the circulation and hence how much the risk of infection is raised (Godwin et al. 2013).

Single-occupancy rooms used for protective isolation should have neutral or positive air pressure with respect to the surrounding area. High-efficiency particulate air (HEPA) filtration of the air in the room may reduce exposure to airborne pathogens, particularly fungal spores. A room with positive pressure ventilation must not be used for any patient infected or colonized with an organism that may be spread through an airborne route; in this circumstance, if an immunocompromised patient has such an organism, they should be nursed in a room with neutral air pressure or with a positive pressure lobby (DH 2013d).

Principles of care

Diet for the immunocompromised patient

- Educate the patient about the importance of good food hygiene in reducing their exposure to potential pathogens; they should choose only cooked food from the hospital menu and avoid raw fruit, salads and uncooked vegetables. Stress the importance of good hand hygiene before eating or drinking. Uncooked foods are often heavily colonized by micro-organisms, particularly Gram-negative bacteria (Moody et al. 2006); potential pathogens on the hands may be inadvertently consumed while eating or drinking.
- Educate the patient's family about the importance of good food hygiene, particularly good hand hygiene, and advise that any food brought in for the patient should be in undamaged, sealed tins and packets obtained from well-known, reliable firms and within the expiry date. Correctly processed and packaged foods are more likely to be of an acceptable food hygiene standard.

- Provide the patient with filtered water or sealed cartons of fruit juice (not fresh) to drink (Vonberg et al. 2005). Do not supply bottled water. Tap water may occasionally be contaminated with potential pathogens; long-life fruit juice has been pasteurized to remove micro-organisms; bottled water is not normally of any better quality than tap water and the bacterial count may increase after bottling (Rosenberg 2003).

Discharging the neutropenic patient

- Crowded areas, for example shops, cinemas, pubs and discos, should be avoided. Although the patient's white cell count is usually high enough for discharge, the patient remains immunocompromised for some time (Calandra 2000).
- Pets should not be allowed to lick the patient, and new pets should not be obtained. Pets are known carriers of infection (Lefebvre et al. 2006).
- Certain foods, for example take-away meals, soft cheese and pâté, should continue to be avoided. These foodstuffs are more likely to be contaminated with potential pathogens (Gillespie et al. 2005).
- Salads and fruit should be washed carefully, dried and, if possible, peeled, to remove as many pathogens as possible (Moody et al. 2006).
- Any signs or symptoms of infection should be reported immediately to the patient's general practitioner or to the discharging hospital. Any infection may have serious consequences if left untreated.

Procedure guideline 3.15 **Protective isolation: preparing the room**

Essential equipment

- Single-occupancy room
- Patient equipment
- Personal protective equipment
- Hand hygiene facilities inside and outside the room
- Patient information material detailing the other infection prevention precautions required
- Cleaning materials for the room

Pre-procedure

Action	Rationale
1 Identify the most suitable room available for protective isolation, taking into account the risk to the patient, the patient's other nursing needs and other demands on the available single rooms.	To ensure the best balance between minimizing the risk of infection, maintaining the safety and comfort of the isolated patient and the availability of single rooms for other purposes. **E**

Procedure

Action	Rationale
2 Remove all non-essential furniture and equipment from the room. The remaining furniture should be easy to clean. Ensure that the room is stocked with any equipment required for patient care and sufficient numbers of any disposable items that will be required.	To ensure the availability of everything required for patient care while minimizing the amount of cleaning required and the amount of traffic of people and equipment into and out of the room. **E**
3 Ensure that all PPE required is available outside the room. Wall-mounted dispensers offer the best use of space and ease of use but, if necessary, set up a trolley outside the door for PPE and alcohol handrub. Ensure that this does not cause an obstruction or other hazard.	To have PPE readily available when required. **E**
4 Ensure that the room is thoroughly cleaned before the patient is admitted.	Effective cleaning will remove infectious agents that may pose a risk to the patient (NPSA 2009, **C**).
5 Explain the reason for isolation and the precise precautions required to the patient, their family and other visitors, providing relevant patient information material where available. Allow the patient to ask questions and ask for a member of the infection prevention and control team to visit the patient if ward staff cannot answer all questions to the patient's satisfaction.	Compliance may be more likely if patients and their visitors understand the reasons for isolation; the patient's anxiety may be reduced if they have as much information as possible about their condition. **E**
6 Fix a suitable notice outside the room where it will be seen by anyone attempting to enter the room. This should indicate the special precautions required while preserving the patient's confidentiality.	To ensure all staff and visitors are aware of the need for additional infection control precautions. **E**
7 Move the patient into the single-occupancy room.	To minimize exposure to potentially harmful micro-organisms (Wigglesworth 2003, **E**).
8 Ensure that surfaces and furniture are damp-dusted daily using disposable cleaning cloths and detergent solution, and the floor is mopped daily using soap and water.	Damp-dusting and mopping remove micro-organisms without distributing them into the air. **E**

Procedure guideline 3.16 Protective isolation: entering the isolation room

Essential equipment

- Hand hygiene facilities
- Disposable plastic apron
- Additional equipment, including PPE, for any procedure to be undertaken

Pre-procedure

Action	Rationale
1 Collect all equipment needed.	To avoid entering and leaving the room unnecessarily. **E**
Procedure	
2 Ensure you are 'bare below the elbow' (see Procedure guideline 3.1: Hand washing).	To facilitate hand hygiene and to avoid transferring any contamination to the patient from long sleeves or cuffs. **E**
3 Put on a disposable plastic apron.	To provide a barrier between the front of the uniform or clothing, which is the most likely area to come in contact with the patient. **E**
4 Clean hands with soap and water or alcohol handrub.	To remove any contamination from the hands which could be transferred to the patient (WHO 2009a, **C**).
5 Close the room door after entering.	To reduce the risk of airborne transmission of infection from other areas of the ward and ensure that ventilation and air filtration systems work as efficiently as possible. **E**
Visitors	
1 Ask the patient to nominate close relatives and friends who may then, after instruction (see steps 1–5, above), visit freely. The patient or their representative should ask other acquaintances and non-essential visitors to avoid visiting during the period of vulnerability.	The risk of infection is likely to increase in proportion to the number of people visiting but unlimited visiting by close relatives and friends may diminish the sense of isolation that the patient may experience; however, large numbers of visitors may be difficult to screen and educate. **E**
2 Exclude any visitor who has had symptoms of infection or been in contact with a communicable disease in the previous 48 hours.	Individuals may be infectious both before and after developing symptoms of infection (Goering et al. 2012, **E**).
3 Educate all visitors to decontaminate their hands before entering the isolation room.	Hands carry large numbers of potentially pathogenic micro-organisms that can be easily removed (WHO 2009a, **C**).
4 Visiting by children, other than very close relatives, should be discouraged.	Children are more likely to have been in contact with infectious diseases but are less likely to be aware of this, and are more likely to develop infections because they have less acquired immunity. **E**

Prevention and management of inoculation injury

RELATED THEORY

Healthcare workers are at risk of acquiring bloodborne infections such as human immunodeficiency virus (HIV), the virus that causes acquired immune deficiency syndrome (AIDS), hepatitis B and hepatitis C. While the risk is small, five episodes of occupationally acquired HIV infection had nonetheless been documented in the UK up to 2002 (Health Protection Agency 2005). In 2006–7, 914 incidents of occupational exposure to bloodborne viruses were reported, of which between one-fifth and one-third could have been prevented through proper adherence to universal precautions and the safe disposal of hazardous waste (Health Protection Agency 2008). An understanding of the risk of infection and the preventive measures to be taken is essential in promoting a safer work environment (UK Health Departments 1998).

Bloodborne viruses are present in the blood and in other high-risk fluids that should be handled with the same precautions as blood. High-risk fluids include:

- cerebrospinal fluid
- peritoneal fluid
- pleural fluid
- pericardial fluid
- synovial fluid
- amniotic fluid
- semen
- vaginal secretions
- breast milk
- any other body fluid or unfixed tissue or organ containing visible blood (including saliva in dentistry).

Body fluids that do not need to be regarded as high risk, unless they are bloodstained, are:

- urine
- faeces
- saliva
- sweat
- vomit.

The most likely route of infection for healthcare workers is through the percutaneous inoculation of infected blood via a sharps injury (often called a needlestick injury) or by blood or other high-risk fluid splashing onto broken skin or a mucous membrane in the mouth, nose or eyes. These incidents are collectively known as inoculation injuries. A European Union directive recently incorporated into UK law requires healthcare organizations to use safe devices and systems of work to minimize the risk of inoculation injury (Health and Safety Executive 2013). Blood or another high-risk fluid coming into contact with intact skin is not regarded as an inoculation injury. It carries little or no risk due to the impervious nature of intact skin.

EVIDENCE-BASED APPROACHES

If the guidance in Box 3.2 is followed, it has been shown to reduce the risk of sharps injuries.

COMPLICATIONS

In the event of an inoculation injury occurring, prompt and appropriate action will reduce the risk of subsequent infection. These actions are described in Box 3.3 and should be taken regardless of what is thought to be known about the status of the patient whose blood has been inoculated. HIV, for example, has a 3-month 'window' following infection during which the patient has sufficient virus in their blood to be infectious but before their immune system is producing sufficient antibodies to be detected by the normal tests for HIV status.

Box 3.2 **Actions to reduce the risk of inoculation injury**

- Use safety devices as an alternative to sharp items wherever these are available (Health and Safety Executive 2013).
- Do not resheath used needles.
- Ensure that you are familiar with the local protocols for the use and disposal of sharps (e.g. location of sharps bins) and any other equipment before undertaking any procedure involving the use of a sharp item.
- Do not bend or break needles or disassemble them after use; discard needles and syringes into a sharps bin immediately after use.
- Handle sharps as little as possible.
- Do not pass sharps directly from hand to hand; use a receiver or similar receptacle.
- Discard all used sharps into a sharps container at the point of use; take a sharps container with you to the point of use if necessary. Do not dispose of sharps into anything other than a designated sharps container.
- Do not fill sharps bins above the mark that indicates that it is full.
- Sharps bins that are not full or in current (i.e. immediate) use should be kept out of reach of children and with any temporary closure in place.
- Sharps bins in use should be positioned at a height that enables safe disposal by all members of staff and secured to avoid spillage.
- Wear gloves in any situation where contact with blood is anticipated.
- Avoid wearing open footwear in any situation where blood may be spilt or where sharps are used.
- Always cover any cuts or abrasions, particularly on the hands, with a waterproof dressing while at work. Wear gloves if hands are particularly affected.
- Wear facial protection consisting of a mask and goggles or a face shield in any situation that may lead to a splash of blood or other high-risk fluid to the face. Do not rely on prescription glasses – they may not provide sufficient protection.
- Clear up any blood spillage promptly and disinfect the area. Use any materials or spillage management packs specifically provided for this purpose in accordance with the manufacturer's instructions.

Source: UK Health Departments (1998).

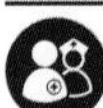

Box 3.3 **Actions to take in the event of inoculation injury**

- Encourage any wound to bleed to wash out any foreign material that has been introduced. Do not squeeze the wound, as this may force any virus present into the tissues.
- Wash any wound with soap and water. Wash out splashes to mucous membranes (eyes or mouth) with large amounts of clean water.
- Cover any wound with a waterproof dressing to prevent entry of any other foreign material.
- Ensure the patient is safe then report the injury as quickly as possible to your immediate line manager and occupational health department. This is because post-exposure prophylaxis (PEP), which is medication given after any incident thought to carry a high risk of HIV transmission, is more effective the sooner after the incident it is commenced (DH 2008).
- Follow any instructions given by the occupational health department.
- Co-operate with any action to test yourself or the patient for infection with a bloodborne virus but do not obtain blood or consent for testing from the patient yourself; this should be done by someone not involved in the incident.
- Complete a report of the incident according to local protocols.

Source: UK Health Departments (1998).

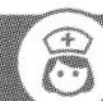

Learning Activity 3.5

Scenario: Inoculation injury

Once you have read through Boxes 3.2 and 3.3, consider the following scenario and write down your responses to each question.

A nurse was giving a patient a subcutaneous injection and sustained a needlestick injury after the injection had been administered.

- What should happen next?
- Who should be informed?
- What should be documented?
- Are there any additional precautions that should be taken?

Management of waste in the healthcare environment

DEFINITION

Waste is defined as 'any substance or object the holder discards, intends to discard or is required to discard' (European Parliament 2008).

EVIDENCE-BASED APPROACHES

Rationale

Waste material produced in the healthcare environment may carry a risk of infection to people who are not directly involved in providing healthcare but who are involved in the transport or disposal of that waste. All waste disposal is subject to regulation and hazardous waste is subject to further controls, depending on the nature of the hazard (DH 2013b). To ensure that everyone involved in waste management is aware of, and protected from, any hazard presented by the waste with which they are dealing, and that the waste is disposed of appropriately, a colour coding system is used. The colours in general use are shown in Table 3.6.

Waste receptacles are plastic bags or rigid plastic containers of the appropriate colour (Table 3.7).

Table 3.6 **Waste colours code**

Colour	Description
Yellow	**Waste which requires disposal by incineration** Indicative treatment/disposal required is incineration in a suitably permitted or licensed facility
Orange	**Waste which may be 'treated'** Indicative treatment/disposal required is to be 'rendered safe' in a suitably permitted or licensed facility, **usually alternative treatment plants (ATPs). However, this waste may also be disposed of by incineration**
Purple	**Cytotoxic and cytostatic waste** Indicative treatment/disposal required is **incineration** in a suitably permitted or licensed facility
Yellow/black	**Offensive/hygiene waste*** Indicative treatment/disposal required is **landfill** or municipal **incineration/energy from waste** at a suitably permitted or licensed facility
Red	**Anatomical waste for incineration†** Indicative treatment/disposal required is **incineration** in a suitably permitted facility
Black	**Domestic (municipal) waste** Minimum treatment/disposal required is **landfill**, municipal **incineration/energy from waste** or other municipal **waste treatment process** at a suitably permitted or licensed facility. Recyclable components should be removed through segregation. Clear/opaque receptacles may also be used for domestic waste
Blue	**Medicinal waste for incineration†** Indicative treatment/disposal required is **incineration** in a suitably permitted facility
	Amalgam waste For **recovery**

*The use of yellow/black for offensive/hygiene waste was chosen as these colours have historically been universally used for the sanitary/offensive/hygiene waste stream.
†The colours 'red' and 'blue' are new to the colour-coding system in this edition. Care should be taken when ordering red containers to ensure that they can be clearly differentiated from orange. The colour-coding should be agreed as part of a contract specification.
Source: DH (2013c). © Crown copyright. Reproduced under the Open Government Licence v2.0.

Table 3.7 **Waste containers**

Waste receptacle	Waste types	Example contents	Indicative treatment/disposal
'Over-stickers' with the radioactive waste symbol may be used on yellow packaging	Healthcare waste contaminated with radioactive material	Dressings, tubing, etc., from treatment involving low-level radioactive isotopes	Appropriately licensed incineration facility
	Infectious waste contaminated with cytotoxic and/or cytostatic medicinal products	Dressings/tubing from cytotoxic and/or cytostatic treatment	Incineration
SHARPS	Sharps contaminated with cytotoxic and cytostatic medicinal products*	Sharps used to administer cytotoxic products	Incineration
	Infectious and other waste requiring incineration including anatomical waste, diagnostic specimens, reagent or test vials, and kits containing chemicals	Anatomical waste from theatres	Incineration
SHARPS	Partially discharged sharps not contaminated with cytoproducts*	Syringe body with residue medicinal product	Incineration

(continued)

Table 3.7 **Waste containers *(continued)***

Waste receptacle	Waste types	Example contents	Indicative treatment/disposal
Solid / Liquid	Medicines in original packaging	Waste in original packaging with original closures	Incineration
Solid / Liquid	Medicines NOT in original packaging	Waste tablets not in foil pack or bottle	Hazardous waste incineration
	Infectious waste, potentially infectious waste and autoclaved laboratory waste	Soiled dressings	Licensed/permitted treatment facility
SHARPS	(i) Sharps not contaminated with medicinal products[†] *or* (ii) Fully discharged sharps contaminated with medicinal products other than cytotoxic and cytostatic medicines	Sharps from phlebotomy	Suitably authorized incineration or alternative treatment facility*
	Offensive/hygiene waste	Human hygiene waste and non-infectious disposable equipment, bedding and plaster casts	Deep landfill
	Domestic waste	General refuse,[‡] including confectionery products, flowers, etc.	Landfill
WHITE CONTAINER	Amalgam waste	Dental amalgam waste	Recovery

*The authorization type and content for alternative treatments in Northern Ireland, Scotland, England and Wales may differ. Not all facilities are authorized to process all types of waste.

Important: It is not acceptable practice to intentionally discharge syringes, etc., containing residual medicines in order to dispose of them in the fully discharged sharps receptacle. Partially discharged syringes contaminated with residual medicines should be disposed of in the yellow- or purple-lidded sharps receptacle shown above.

†The requirements for packaging are significantly affected by the presence of medicinal waste and the quantity of liquid present in the container.

‡General refuse is that waste remaining once recyclates (that is, paper, cardboard) have been removed.

Source: DH (2013c).

Learning Activity 3.6

Scenario: Waste disposal

You have just finished dressing a post-operative wound for a patient in which you have also removed some sutures. Identify which waste container(s) you would use to dispose of the following:

1 Soiled dressings and gauze swabs.
2 Plastic tray, plastic forceps.
3 10 mL plastic syringe containing some residual saline (used for irrigation).
4 Gloves and apron.
5 Stitch cutter.

See the end of the chapter for the answers..

LEGAL AND PROFESSIONAL ISSUES

The producer of hazardous waste is legally responsible for that waste, and remains responsible for it until its final disposal by incineration, alternative treatment or landfill (DH 2013b). In order to track waste to its point of origin, for example if it is necessary to identify where waste has been disposed of into the wrong waste stream, healthcare organizations should have a system of identifying waste according to the ward or department where it is produced. This may be through the use of labelling or dedicated waste carts for particular areas. When assembling sharps bins, always complete the label on the outside of the bin, including the date and the initials of the assembler. When sharps bins are closed and disposed of, they should be dated and initialled at each stage (DH 2013b).

Management of soiled linen in the healthcare environment

As with waste, soiled linen must be managed so as to minimize any risk to any person coming into contact with it. This is done by clearly identifying any soiled linen that may present a risk through the use of colour coding and limiting any contact with such linen through the use of water-soluble bags to contain the linen so that laundry staff do not have to handle it before it goes into the washer (DH 2013c).

Linen that may present a risk may be described as foul, infected or infested. The management of all hazardous linen is similar, so the following procedure applies to any linen that is wet with blood or other high-risk body fluids (see 'Prevention and management of inoculation injury') or faeces; has come from a patient in source isolation for any reason (that is, where enteric, contact or droplet/airborne precautions are in place); or is from a patient who is infested with lice, fleas, scabies or other ectoparasite. Note that this procedure can be much more easily carried out by two people working together.

Procedure guideline 3.17 **Safe disposal of foul, infected or infested linen**

Essential equipment

- Disposable gloves and apron
- Water-soluble laundry bag
- Red plastic or linen laundry bag in holder
- Orange waste bag

Pre-procedure

Action	Rationale
1 Assemble all the required equipment.	To avoid having to fetch anything else during the procedure and risk spreading contamination to other areas. **E**
2 Put on disposable gloves and apron.	To minimize contamination of your hands or clothing from the soiled linen. **E**
3 Separate the edges of the open end of the water-soluble laundry bag.	To make it easier to put the soiled linen in the bag. **E**
Procedure	
4 Gather up the foul, infected or infested linen in such a way that any gross contamination (e.g. blood, faeces) is contained within the linen.	To minimize any contamination of the surrounding area. **E**
5 If there are two people, one holds the water-soluble laundry bag open while the other puts the soiled linen into it. If one person, hold one edge of the open end of the water-soluble bag in one hand and place the soiled linen in the bag with the other. In either case, take care not to contaminate the outside of the bag.	So as to remove the need for laundry workers to handle foul, infected or infested linen before it is washed (DH 2013c, **C**).
6 Tie the water-soluble bag closed using the tie provided or by knotting together the edges of the open end.	To keep the soiled laundry inside the bag. **E**
7 Place the full water-soluble bag of soiled linen into the red outer laundry bag. Do not touch this bag.	To identify the linen as requiring special treatment. **E**
8 Remove gloves and apron and dispose of them into an orange waste bag.	To avoid transferring contamination to other areas (DH 2013b, **C**).
9 Wash hands and forearms with soap and water and dry hands thoroughly with a disposable paper towel.	To avoid transferring contamination to other areas (WHO 2009a, **C**).
10 Close the red outer laundry bag and transfer it to the designated collection area.	To ensure it does not cause an obstruction and is transferred to the laundry at the earliest opportunity. **E**

Learning for practice

After studying this chapter, list five key points you have learnt about infection prevention and control that you will be able to apply to your clinical practice.

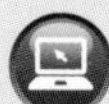 For further learning exercises visit **www.royalmarsdenmanual.com/student**.

Now Test Yourself

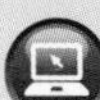

This section provides a range of exercises/activities to further test your learning. For additional exercises visit **www.royalmarsdenmanual.com/student**.

What have you learnt?

1 For which of the following modes of transmission is good hand hygiene a key preventative measure? (Circle as many as are relevant.)
  A Airborne
  B Direct contact
  C Indirect contact
  D Droplet
  E All of the above

2 If you were told by a nurse at handover to take 'standard precautions' what would you expect to be doing?
  A Taking precautions when handling blood and 'high risk' body fluids so as not to pass on any infection to the patient.
  B Wearing gloves, aprons and mask when caring for someone in protective isolation.
  C Asking relatives to wash their hands when visiting patients in the clinical setting.
  D Using appropriate hand hygiene, wearing gloves and aprons when necessary, disposing of used sharp instruments safely and providing care in a suitably clean environment to protect yourself and the patients.

3 Hand hygiene: when caring for a patient who has, or is suspected of having, *Clostridium difficile*, why should you use soap and water rather than alcohol handrubs?

4 What are the principles of caring for a patient in source isolation?
  - Can you think of an occasion where you have cared for such a patient?
  - Having studied this chapter and familiarized yourself with the principles of caring for this group of patients, is there anything that could/should have been done differently?

5 All individuals providing nursing care must be competent at the following procedures (circle all that are relevant):
  A Hand hygiene
  B Aseptic technique
  C Use of protective equipment
  D Disposal of waste
  E All of the above

See the end of the chapter for the answers.

Key points

- Many infections acquired by patients receiving healthcare are preventable through use of diligent hand hygiene and correct aseptic technique.
- The majority of healthcare-associated infections are endogenous (from organisms already present on an individual's body), highlighting the importance of effective skin cleansing prior to invasive procedures.
- Standard precautions must be taken with all patients at all times regardless of their infection status.
- Additional precautions may be required if patients are vulnerable to infection themselves or are colonized or infected with a micro-organism that may be a risk to others, or both.
- Infection prevention and control procedures must be followed at all times in order to minimize the risk of contamination and infection transmission.

REFERENCES

Breathnach, A. (2005) Nosocomial infections. *Medicine*, 33(3), 22–26.

Calandra, T. (2000) Practical guide to host defence mechanisms and the predominant infections encountered in immunocompromised patients. In: Glauser, M.P. & Pizzo, P.A. (eds) *Management of Infections in Immunocompromised Patients, Part I.* London: W.B. Saunders, pp. 3–16.

Chadwick, P.R., Beards, G., Brown, B., et al. (2000) Management of hospital outbreaks due to small round structured viruses. *Journal of Hospital Infection*, 45(1), 1–10. Available at: www.hpa.org.uk/web/HPAwebFile/HPAweb_C/1194947408355

Crabtree, A. & Henry, B. (2011) *Non-Pharmaceutical Measures to Prevent Influenza Transmission: The Evidence for Individual Protective Measures.* Winnipeg, Canada: National Collaborating Centre for Infectious Disease.

Damani, N.N. (2011) Basic concepts. In: Damani, N.N. *Manual of Infection Prevention and Control*, 3rd edn. Cambridge: Cambridge University Press.

Department of Trade and Industry (2002) *Product Standards: Personal Protective Equipment: Guidance Notes on the UK Personal Protective Equipment Regulations 2002 (S.I. 2002 No. 1144).* London: Department of Trade and Industry. Available at: www.bis.gov.uk/files/file11263.pdf (archived)

DH (2001) Standard principles for preventing hospital-acquired infection. *Journal of Hospital Infection*, 47(Supplement), S21–S37.

DH (2006) *Health Technical Memorandum 64: Sanitary Assemblies.* London: Stationery Office.

DH (2007a) *Saving Lives: Reducing Infection, Delivering Clean and Safe Care.* London: The Stationery Office. Available at: www.dh.gov.uk/en/Publicationsandstatistics/Publications/PublicationsPolicyAndGuidance/DH_078134 (archived)

DH (2007b) *Health Technical Memorandum 01-01: Decontamination of Reusable Medical Devices, Part A – Management and Environment (English edition).* London: Department of Health.

DH (2008) *HIV Post-Exposure Prophylaxis: Guidance from the UK Chief Medical Officers' Expert Advisory Group on AIDS.* London: Department of Health. Available at: www.dh.gov.uk/prod_consum_dh/groups/dh_digitalassets/@dh/@en/documents/digitalasset/dh_089997.pdf (archived)

DH (2010a) *The Health and Social Care Act 2008: Code of Practice on the Prevention and Control of Infections and Related Guidance.* London: Department of Health. Available at: www.dh.gov.uk/prod_consum_

dh/groups/dh_digitalassets/documents/digitalasset/dh_110435.pdf (archived)

DH (2010b) *Pandemic (H1N1) 2009 Influenza: A Summary of Guidance for Infection Control in Healthcare Settings.* London: Department of Health. Available at: www.dh.gov.uk/prod_consum_dh/groups/dh_digitalassets/@dh/@en/@ps/documents/digitalasset/dh_110899.pdf (archived)

DH (2010c) *Uniforms and Workwear: Guidance on Uniform and Workwear Policies for NHS Employers.* London: Department of Health. www.dh.gov.uk/prod_consum_dh/groups/dh_digitalassets/@dh/@en/@ps/documents/digitalasset/dh_114754.pdf (archived)

DH (2013a) *Health Technical Memorandum 04-01 Addendum: Pseudomonas Aeruginosa – Advice for Augmented Care Units.* London: Department of Health.

DH (2013b) *Health Technical Memorandum 07-01: Safe Management of Healthcare Waste.* London: Department of Health. Available at: www.gov.uk/government/uploads/system/uploads/attachment_data/file/167976/HTM_07-01_Final.pdf

DH (2013c) *Choice Framework for local Policy and Procedures 01-04 – Decontamination of linen for health and social care: Guidance for linen processors implementing BS EN 14065.* Department of Health, London. Available at: www.gov.uk/government/uploads/system/uploads/attachment_data/file/148539/CFPP_01-04_BS_EN_Final.pdf

DH (2013d) *Health Building Note 04-01 Supplement 1: Isolation Facilities for Infectious Patients in Acute Settings.* London: Department of Health. Available at: www.gov.uk/government/uploads/system/uploads/attachment_data/file/148503/HBN_04-01_Supp_1_Final.pdf

DH/HPA (2008) *Clostridium Difficile Infection: How to Deal with the Problem.* London: Department of Health/Health Protection Agency. Available at: www.hpa.org.uk/web/HPAwebFile/HPAweb_C/1232006607827

Dharan, S., Mourouga, P., Copin, P., et al. (1999) Routine disinfection of patients' environmental surfaces. Myth or reality? *Journal of Hospital Infection*, 42(2), 113–117.

Elliot, T., Worthington, A., Osman, H. & Gill, M. (2007) *Lecture Notes: Medical Microbiology and Infection*, 4th edn. Oxford: Blackwell Publishing.

European Parliament (2008) Directive 2008/98/EC of the European Parliament and of the Council of 19 November 2008 on waste and repealing certain Directives. *Official Journal of the European Union*, 22 November 2008. Available at: eur-lex.europa.eu/LexUriServ/LexUriServ.do?uri=OJ:L:2008:312:0003:0030:EN:PDF

Fishman, J.A. (2011) Infections in immunocompromised hosts and organ transplant recipients: essentials. *Liver Transplantation*, 17(Supplement 3), S34–S37.

Food Safety Act 1990. London: HMSO.

Fraise, A.P. & Bradley, T. (eds) (2009) *Ayliffe's Control of Healthcare-Associated Infection: A Practical Handbook*, 5th edn. London: Hodder Arnold.

Gammon, J. (1998) Analysis of the stressful effects of hospitalisation and source isolation on coping and psychological constructs. *International Journal of Nursing Practice*, 4(2), 84–96.

Gillespie, I.A., O'Brien, S.J., Adak, G.K., et al. (2005) Foodborne general outbreaks of *Salmonella enteritidis* phage type 4 infection, England and Wales, 1992–2002: where are the risks? *Epidemiology and Infection*, 133(5), 795–801.

Gillespie, S. & Bamford, K. (2012) *Medical Microbiology and Infection at a Glance*, 4th edn. Oxford: Blackwell Publishing.

Godwin, J.E., Braden, C.D. & Sachdever, K. (2013) Neutropenia. *Medscape Medical News,* 3 July 2013. Available at: http://emedicine.medscape.com/article/204821-overview

Goering, R., Dockrell, H., Zuckermann, M., et al. (2012) *Mims' Medical Microbiology*, 5th edn. London: Saunders.

Hazardous Waste (England and Wales) Regulations 2005 and the List of Wastes (England) Regulations 2005. London: HMSO.

Health and Safety at Work etc. Act 1974. London: HMSO.

Health and Safety Commission (2001) *Legionnaires' Disease: The Control of Legionella Bacteria in Water Systems. Approved Code of Practice and Guidance*, 3rd edn (L8). London: Health and Safety Executive.

Health and Safety Executive (2005) *Personal Protective Equipment at Work (2nd edn): Personal Protective Equipment at Work Regulations 1992 (as amended).* London: Health and Safety Executive.

Health and Safety Executive (2013) *Health and Safety (Sharp Instruments in Healthcare) Regulations 2013.* London: Health and Safety Executive.

Health Protection Agency (2005) *Occupational Transmission of HIV: Summary of Published Reports March 2005 Edition: Data to December 2002.* London: Health Protection Agency. Available at: http://www.hpa.org.uk/webc/hpawebfile/hpaweb_c/1194947320156]

Health Protection Agency (2008) *Eye of the Needle: United Kingdom Surveillance of Significant Occupational Exposures to Bloodborne Viruses in Healthcare Workers.* London: Health Protection Agency. Available at: www.hpa.org.uk/web/HPAwebFile/HPAweb_C/1227688128096

Health Protection Agency (2010a) *Results from the Mandatory Surveillance of MRSA Bacteraemia.* London: Health Protection Agency. Available at: www.hpa.org.uk/web/HPAweb&HPAwebStandard/HPAweb_C/1233906819629

Health Protection Agency (2010b) *Clostridium Difficile Mandatory Surveillance.* London: Health Protection Agency. Available at: www.hpa.org.uk/web/HPAweb&HPAwebStandard/HPAweb_C/1179746015058

Health Protection Agency (2012) *English National Point Prevalence Survey on Healthcare-associated Infections and Antimicrobial Use, 2011.* London: Health Protection Agency. Available at: www.hpa.org.uk/webc/HPAwebFile/HPAweb_C/1317134304594

Health Protection Scotland (2009) *Standard Infection Control Precautions.* Available at: www.hps.scot.nhs.uk/haiic/ic/standardinfectioncontrolprecautions-sicps.aspx

Jeanes, A, Macrae, B. & Ashby, J (2011) Isolation prioritisation tool: revision, adaptation and application. *British Journal of Nursing*, 20(9), 540–544.

Kao, P.H. & Yang, R.J. (2006) Virus diffusion in isolation rooms. *Journal of Hospital Infection*, 62(3), 338–345.

Kerr, L.N., Chaput, M.P., Cash, L.D., et al. (2004) Assessment of the durability of medical examination gloves. *Journal of Occupational and Environmental Hygiene*, 1(9), 607–612.

Korniewicz, D.M., El-Masri, M., Broyles, J.M., et al. (2002) Performance of latex and nonlatex medical examination gloves during simulated use. *American Journal of Infection Control*, 30(2), 133–138.

Lefebvre, S., Waltner-Toews, D., Peregrine, A., et al. (2006) Prevalence of zoonotic agents in dogs visiting hospitalized people in Ontario: implications for infection control. *Journal of Hospital Infection*, 62(3), 458–466.

Leonas, K.K. (1998) Effect of laundering on the barrier properties of reusable surgical gown fabrics. *American Journal of Infection Control*, 26(5), 495–501.

Loveday, H., Wilson, J.A., Pratt, R.J., et al. (2014) epic 3: National Evidence-Based Guidelines for Preventing Healthcare-Associated Infections in NHS Hospitals in England. *Journal of Hospital Infection* 86S1, S1-S70. Available at: http://www.his.org.uk/files/3113/8693/4808/epic3_National_Evidence-Based_Guidelines_for_Preventing_HCAI_in_NHSE.pdf

McGuckin, R., Storr, J., Longtin, Y., et al. (2011) Patient Empowerment and multimodal hand hygiene promotion: a win-win strategy. *American Journal of Medical Quality*, 26(1), 10–17.

MHRA (2006) *DB 2006(04) Single-use Medical Devices: Implications and Consequences of Reuse.* London: Medicines and Healthcare Products Regulatory Agency. Available at: www.mhra.gov.uk

MHRA (2010) Guidance notes on medical devices which require sterilization. In: MHRA *EC Medical Devices Directives: Guidance for Manufacturers on Clinical Investigations to be Carried Out in the UK,* Updated March 2010. London: MHRA, p. 40–41. Available at: www.mhra.gov.uk

Moody, K., Finlay, J., Mancuso, C., et al. (2006) Feasibility and safety of a pilot randomized trial of infection rate: neutropenic diet versus standard food safety guidelines. *Journal of Pediatric Hematology/Oncology*, 28(3), 126–133.

Morgan, D.J., Diekema, D.J., Sepkowitz, K. & Perencevich, E.N. (2009) Adverse outcomes associated with contact precautions: a review of the literature. *American Journal of Infection Control*, 37, 85–93.

NHS Estates (2001) *Infection Control in the Built Environment.* London: Stationery Office.

NICE (2006) *Tuberculosis, CG33.* London: National Institute for Health and Clinical Excellence. Available at: http://www.nice.org.uk/guidance/CG33

NMC (2010) *Record Keeping: Guidance for Nurses and Midwives.* London: Nursing and Midwifery Council. Available at: http://www.nmc-uk.org/Publications/Guidance/

NMC (2013) *Consent.* London: Nursing and Midwifery Council. Available at: http://www.nmc-uk.org/Nurses-and-midwives/Regulation-in-practice/Regulation-in-Practice-Topics/consent/

NMC (2015) *The Code: Standards of Conduct, Performance and Ethics for Nurses and Midwives.* London: Nursing and Midwifery Council. Available at: www.nmc-uk.org/Publications/Standards/The-code/Introduction/

NPSA (2008) *Patient Safety Alert, Second Edition, 2 September 2008: Clean Hands Save Lives.* London: National Patient Safety Agency. Available at: www.nrls.npsa.nhs.uk/resources/type/alerts/?entryid45=59848&q=0%C2%ACclean+hands%C2%AC%20

NPSA (2009) *Revised Healthcare Cleaning Manual.* London: National Patient Safety Agency. Available at: www.nrls.npsa.nhs.uk/EasySiteWeb/getresource.axd?AssetID=61814&type=full&servicetype=Attachment

Patel, S. (2005) Minimising cross-infection risks associated with beds and mattresses. *Nursing Times*, 101(8), 52–53.

Perry, C. (2007) *Infection Prevention and Control.* Oxford: Blackwell Publishing.

RCN (2010) *Infection Prevention and Control.* Available at: www.rcn.org.uk/development/practice/infection_control

RCN (2012) *Tools of the Trade: RCN Guidance for Health Care Staff on Glove Use and the Precention of Contact Dermatitis.* Available at: www.rcn.org.uk/__data/assets/pdf_file/0003/450507/RCNguidance_glovesdermatitis_WEB2.pdf

Rosenberg, F.A. (2003) The microbiology of bottled water. *Clinical Microbiology Newsletter*, 25(6), 41–44.

Rowley, S. & Clare, S. (2011) ANTT: a standard approach to aseptic technique. *Nursing Times*, 107(36), 12–14.

Siegel, J.D., Rhinehart, E., Jackson, M., Chiarello, L. & the Healthcare Infection Control Practices Advisory Committee (2007) *Guideline for Isolation Precautions: Preventing Transmission of Infectious Agents in Healthcare Settings.* Atlanta, GA: Centers for Disease Control. Available at: www.cdc.gov/ncidod/dhqp/pdf/isolation2007.pdf

Smythe, E.T., McIlvenny, G., Enstone, J.E., et al. (2008) Four Country Healthcare Associated Infection Prevalence Survey 2006: overview of the results. *Journal of Hospital Infection*, 69(3), 230–248.

Stobbe, T.J., daRoza, R.A. & Watkins, M.A. (1988) Facial hair and respirator fit: a review of the literature. *American Industrial Hygiene Association Journal*, 49(4), 199–204.

UK Health Departments (1998) *Guidance for Clinical Health Care Workers: Protection Against Infection with Blood-borne Viruses. Recommendations of the Expert Advisory Group on AIDS and the Advisory Group on Hepatitis.* London: Department of Health. Available at: www.dh.gov.uk/en/Publicationsandstatistics/Lettersandcirculars/Healthservicecirculars/DH_4003818 (archived)

Vonberg, R.P, Eckmanns, T., Bruderek, J. et al. (2005) Use of terminal tap water filter systems for prevention of nosocomial legionellosis. *Journal of Hospital Infection*, 60(2), 159–162.

Ward, D. (2000) Infection control: reducing the psychological effects of isolation. *British Journal of Nursing*, 9(3), 162–170.

Weaving, P. (2007) Creutzfeldt-Jakob disease. *British Journal of Infection Control*, 8(5), 26–29.

WHO (2009a) *WHO Guidelines on Hand Hygiene in Health Care: First Global Patient Safety Challenge: Clean Care is Safer Care.* Geneva: WHO. Available at: whqlibdoc.who.int/publications/2009/9789241597906_eng.pdf

WHO (2009b) *Glove Use Information Leaflet: Outline of the Evidence and Considerations on Medical Glove use to Prevent Germ Transmission.* Geneva: WHO. Available at: www.who.int/gpsc/5may/Glove_Use_Information_Leaflet.pdf

Wigglesworth, N. (2003) The use of protective isolation. *Nursing Times*, 99(7), 26.

Wigglesworth, N. & Wilcox, M.H. (2006) Prospective evaluation of hospital isolation room capacity. *Journal of Hospital Infection*, 63(2), 156–161.

Wilson, J. (2006) *Infection Control in Clinical Practice*, 3rd edn. London: Baillière Tindall.

Answers

Learning Activity 3.4 Case study

Mr Peters is a 74-year-old man who has a history of chronic obstructive pulmonary disease. He lives alone and became unwell 7 days ago, feeling fatigued with a productive cough and elevated temperature. He was diagnosed with a chest infection and admitted to hospital for intravenous antibiotics. Having completed his course of antibiotics yesterday, he has now had five episodes of diarrhoea in the last 12 hours. He is being cared for in a six-bedded bay on a male medical ward and is expecting his daughter to visit him later today with his two young grandchildren.

1 What precautions should be taken for this patient? For how long?
- Universal precautions (standard practice) and handwashing with soap and water.
- Source isolation (due to the risk of *Clostridium difficile* having been on antibiotics).
- Follow source isolation guidance for attending to the patient.
- Advise that young children do not visit in order to minimize the risk of infecting them.
- Remain isolated for 48 hours after the last episode of diarrhoea.

2 What information would you give to Mr Peters and why?
- What the suspected infectious agent is (*C. difficile*) and its modes of transmission.
- Why isolation is required and for how long.
- Precautions he should be taking, i.e. standard precautions.
- Precautions the nursing staff will be taking and advising his visitors to take.
- Advise that small children are potentially at increased risk of infection due to underdeveloped immunity so it is better for grandchildren not to visit at the present time.

3 Would the precautions you take be any different if you were visiting Mr Peters in his own home? If so, how?
- The same infection control procedures should be followed.
- Infectious waste bags should be provided if not within his home already.
- Advise to wash linen on a hot wash.
- Minimize visitors and advise them of procedures for effective hand hygiene.

Learning Activity 3.6 Scenario: Waste disposal

You have just finished dressing a post-operative wound for a patient in which you have also removed some sutures. Identify which waste container(s) you would use to dispose of the following:

1 Soiled dressings and gauze swabs. Orange bag

2 Plastic tray, plastic forceps. Orange bag

3 10 mL plastic syringe containing some residual saline (used for irrigation). Yellow sharps bin

4 Gloves and apron. Orange bag

5 Stitch cutter. Yellow sharps bin

Now Test Yourself **What have you learnt?**

1 For which of the following modes of transmission is good hand hygiene a key preventative measure? (Circle as many as are relevant.)

A Airborne
B Direct contact
C Indirect contact
D Droplet
E All of the above

2 If you were told by a nurse at handover to take 'standard precautions' what would you expect to be doing?

A Taking precautions when handling blood and 'high risk' body fluids so as not to pass on any infection to the patient
B Wearing gloves, aprons and mask when caring for someone in protective isolation
C Asking relatives to wash their hands when visiting patients in the clinical setting
D Using appropriate hand hygiene, wearing gloves and aprons when necessary, disposing of used sharp instruments safely and providing care in a suitably clean environment to protect yourself and the patients

3 Hand hygiene: when caring for a patient who has, or is suspected of having, *Clostridium difficile*, why should you use soap and water rather than alcohol handrubs?

'Spores are extremely tough and durable. They are not destroyed by boiling (hence the need for high temperature steam under pressure in sterilizing autoclaves) or by the alcohol handrubs widely used for hand hygiene – hence the need to physically remove them from the hands by washing with soap and water when caring for a patient with *Clostridium difficile* infection.' (DH/HPA 2008) – see section on 'Bacteria'.

4 What are the principles of caring for a patient in source isolation?

- Can you think of an occasion where you have cared for such a patient?
- Having studied this chapter and familiarized yourself with the principles of caring for this group of patients, is there anything that could/should have been done differently?

For the answers, see the section on "Source isolation: Principles of care, Attending to the patient in isolation".

5 All individuals providing nursing care must be competent at the following procedures (circle all that are relevant):

A Hand hygiene
B Aseptic technique
C Use of protective equipment
D Disposal of waste
E All of the above

Aseptic technique is an additional precaution that should only be performed by a nurse who is trained and competent to do so.

Part Two

Supporting the patient with human functioning

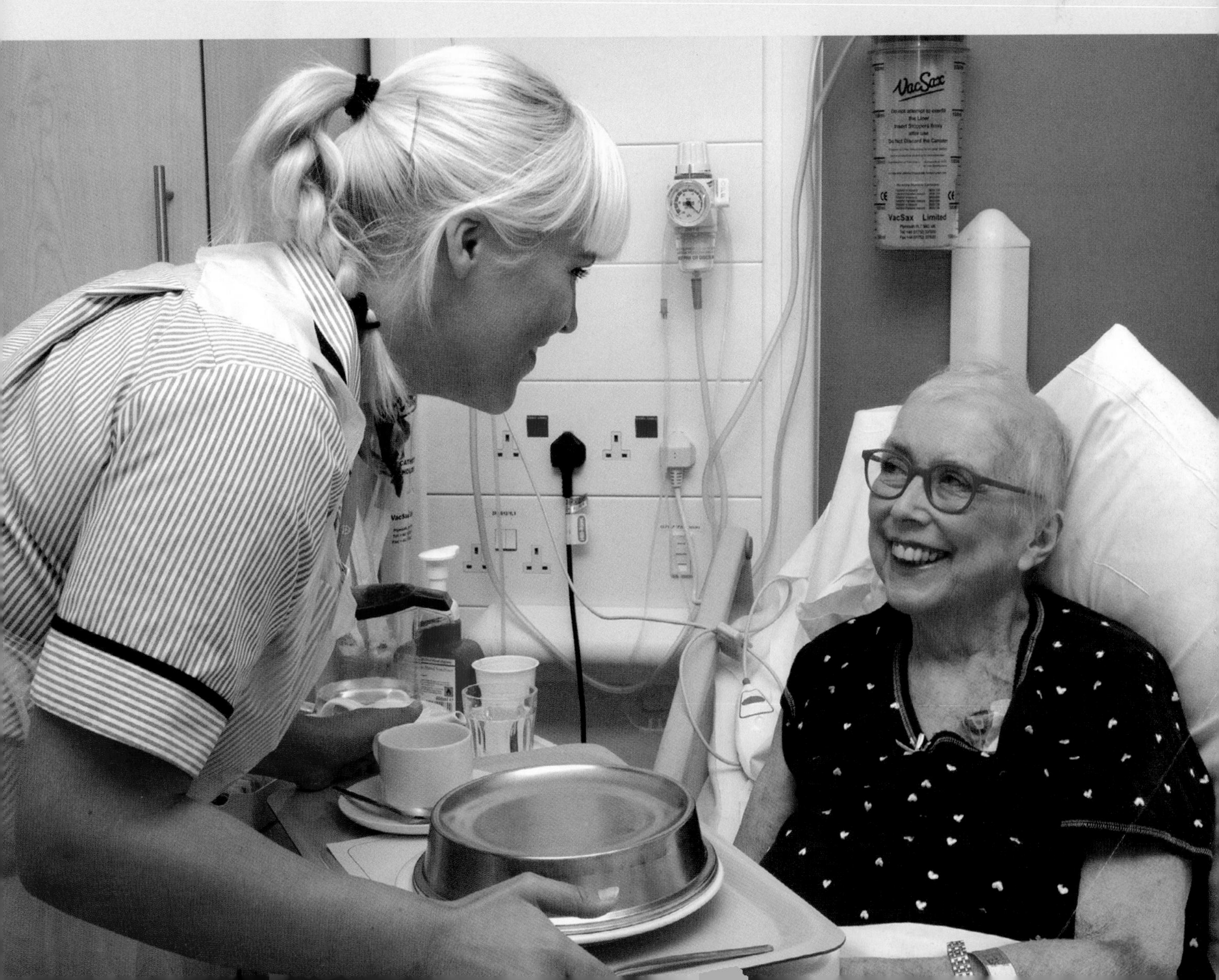

Communication

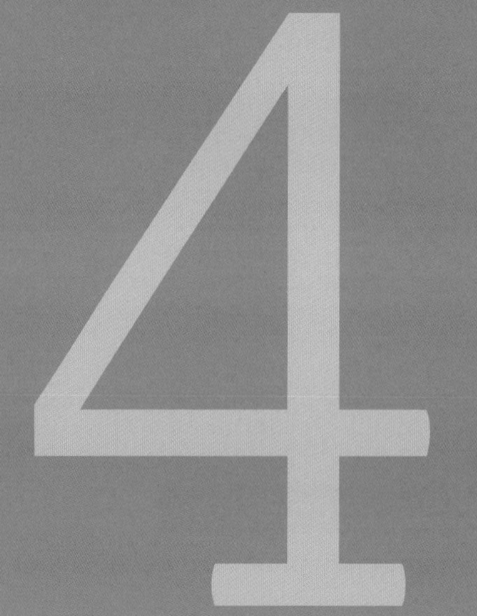

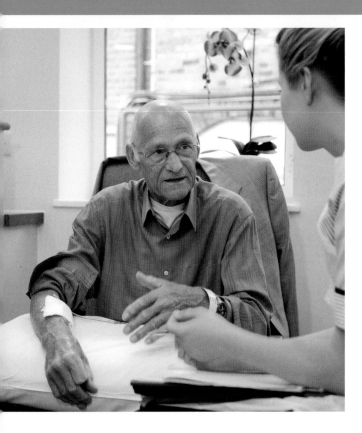

By reading this chapter and undertaking the learning activities within it, you should be able to:

1 Demonstrate an understanding of the important role communication plays in delivering safe, effective and individualized patient care.
2 Recognize the importance of non-verbal communication skills when communicating with patients, particularly for those patients whose verbal communication is impaired.
3 Develop an awareness of the importance of the nurse's role in giving information to patients.
4 Identify some strategies to help communicate with patients who have specific psychological needs.

Principles tables

The Royal Marsden Manual of Clinical Nursing Procedures: Student Edition, Ninth Edition. Edited by Lisa Dougherty, Sara Lister and Alexandra West-Oram

Overview

The aim of this chapter is to define and describe effective communication as well as its role in the psychological support of patients and those close to them. This chapter is mostly concerned with interpersonal communication using language comprising verbal (including tone) and non-verbal expression. The process of offering psychological support to patients and the management of factors that contribute to or compromise this process will also be considered.

There are specific sections on denial and collusion, anxiety, depression, anger management, delirium and finally, assisting those with sensory impairment to communicate.

Communication

DEFINITION

Communication is a universal word with many definitions, many of which describe it as a transfer of information between a source and a receiver (Kennedy Sheldon 2009); that is, the sending and receiving of verbal and non-verbal messages between two or more people (de Vito 2013). In nursing, this communication is primarily interpersonal: the process by which compassion and support are offered and information, decisions and feelings are shared (McCabe and Timmins 2013).

ANATOMY AND PHYSIOLOGY

Physiologically being able to produce speech and to hear are the two dominant physical processes involved in communication.

The human voice is produced by exhaled air vibrating the vocal cords in the larynx to set up sound waves in the column of air in the pharynx, nose and mouth. Pitch is controlled by the tension on the vocal cords: the tighter they are, the more they vibrate and the higher the pitch. The sounds produced are amplified by the physical spaces of the pharynx and nose and modified by the lips, tongue and jaw into recognizable speech. The muscles of the face, tongue and lips help to enunciate words (Tortora and Derrickson 2011) (Figure 4.1).

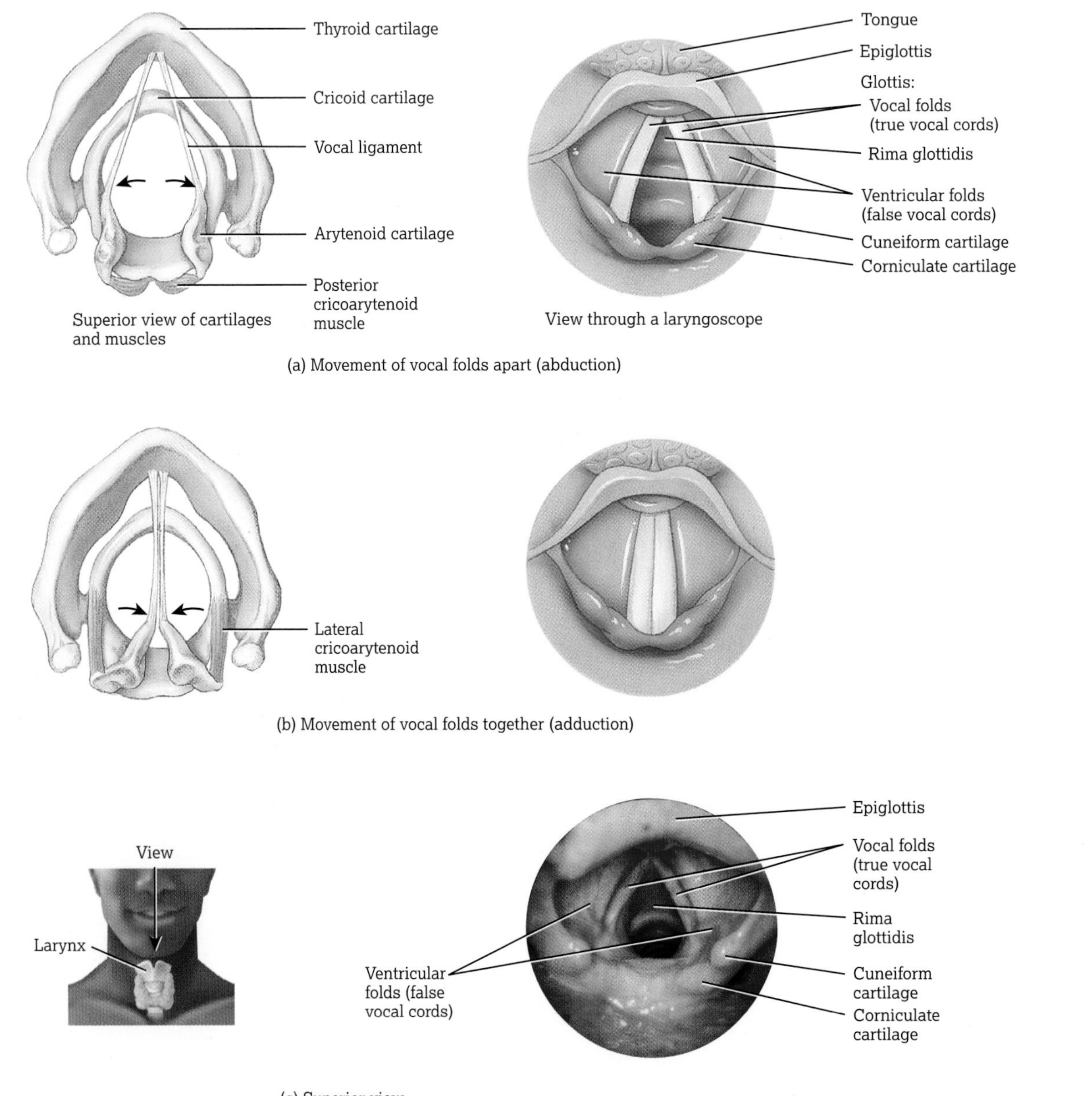

Figure 4.1 Movement of the vocal cords. *Source:* Tortora and Derrickson (2011). Reproduced with permission from John Wiley & Sons.

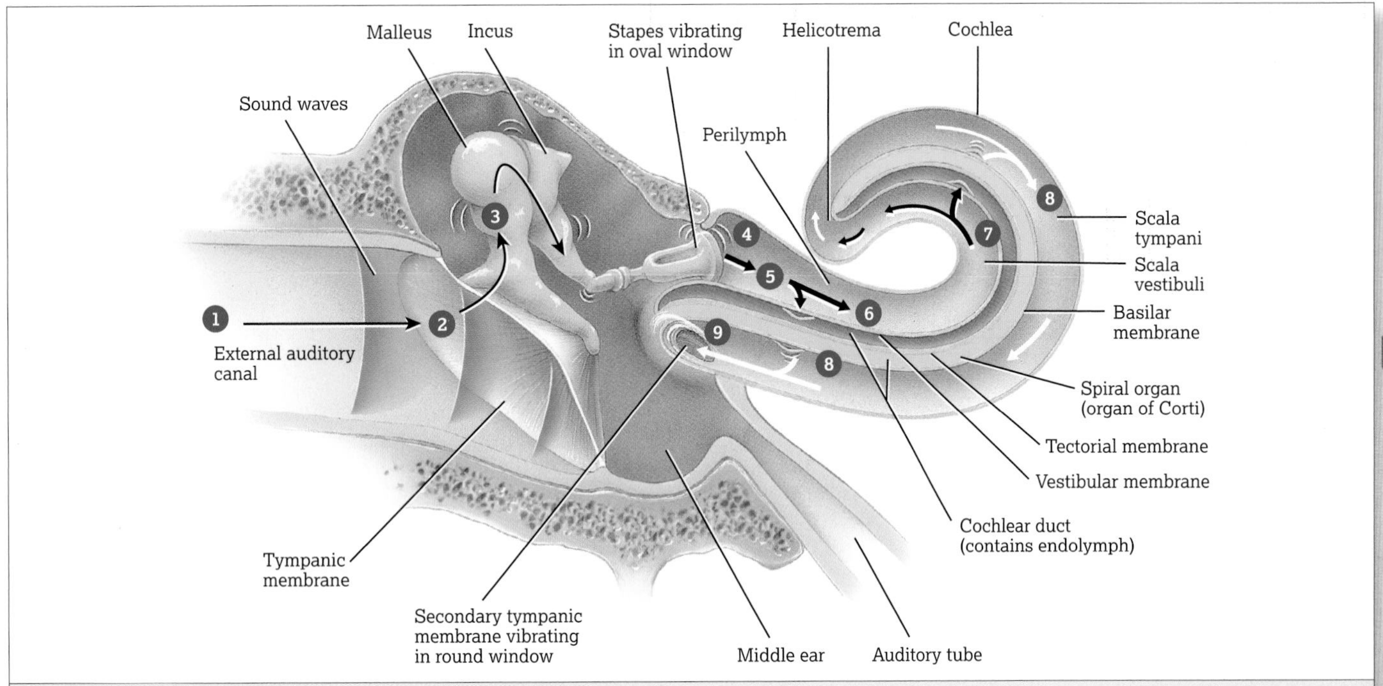

Figure 4.2 **Events in the stimulation of auditory receptors in the right ear.** ***Source:*** **Tortora and Derrickson (2011). Reproduced with permission from John Wiley & Sons.**

The ear contains receptors for sound waves and the external or outer ear is designed to collect them and direct them inward. As the waves strike the tympanic membrane, it vibrates due to the alternate compression and decompression of the air. This vibration is passed on through the malleus, incus and stapes of the middle ear. As the stapes vibrates, it pushes the oval window. The movement of the oval window sets up waves in the perilymph of the cochlea that ultimately lead to the generation of nerve impulses that travel to the auditory area of the cerebral cortex (Tortora and Derrickson 2011) (Figure 4.2).

The physiological process of communication is, however, much greater than just speech and hearing. The central nervous system is central to both verbal and non-verbal communication. Not only does it continually receive information but it also selects that which is important to respond to, so that overstimulation is avoided. Communication issues may arise if any of these processes are altered.

RELATED THEORY

There are many theories about interpersonal communication. One of the earliest theories is the idea that communication can be represented as a linear process (Miller and Nicholson 1976).

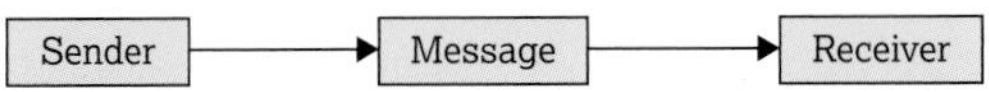

This Linear Model of Communication makes certain assumptions such as: that the receiver will be a willing participant in the process and open to receive the message; that all messages will be clear and the sender certain about their purpose (McCabe and Timmins 2013). However, such a model is unidirectional so more relevant for electronic media and not necessarily representative of the complexity of human communication.

The Transactional Model is more useful, recognizing that human communication is a simultaneous process, so each person involved is a communicator rather than just a sender or receiver (McCabe and Timmins 2013) (Figure 4.3). In addition, the model recognizes that the interpersonal context or environment affects the process significantly, as does the channel of communication (that is, visual, aural, gustatory, tangible or olfactory). This theory helps nurses to reflect on the multifaceted nature of communicating with patients and so recognize the many factors that can impact on an effective process.

Figure 4.3 **Transactional model of communication.** ***Source:*** **Adapted from Arnold and Underman Boggs (2011). Reproduced with permission from Elsevier.**

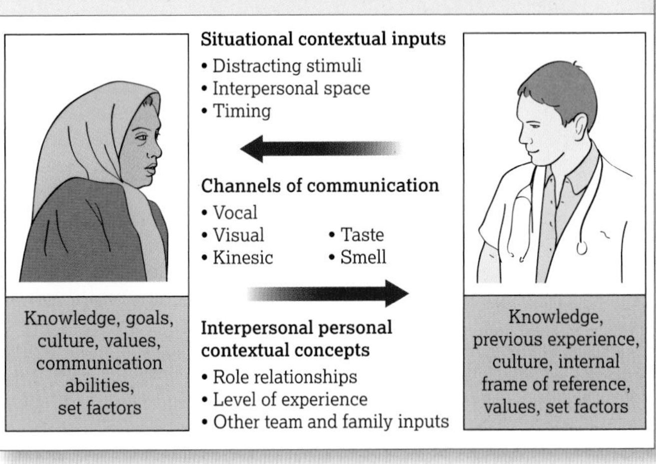

An aim of interpersonal professional communication trainingis to support and maintain the patient's optimum level of communication while remaining aware of the impact that the disease and its management may have on the patient's ability and/or motivation to speak. An awareness of different coping styles and attitudes of the patient and key people in their lives, other co-morbidities, disease progression, fluctuating cognitive abilities and treatment side-effects is important. All these factors demand a flexible approach when supporting communication throughout the length of the patient pathway (Dwamena et al. 2012, White 2004).

Non-verbally, people communicate via gestures, body language, posture, facial expression, touch, and the items they surround themselves with, such as their personal possessions which will include their clothing and accessories, books and photographs in the hospital environment. Communication can be heavily influenced by a multitude of external and internal factors, for example illness, culture, class, self-esteem, immediate environment, gender, status, mood and depression, and the influence of these factors needs to be carefully considered in each circumstance. All patients and relatives should be assessed for their psychological needs and tailored support offered to meet individual needs.

EVIDENCE-BASED APPROACHES

Effective communication is widely regarded to be a key determinant of patient satisfaction, compliance and recovery (Dwamena et al. 2012, Webster and Bryan 2009), yet poor communication is one of the most common causes of complaints in healthcare (DH 2013, Strachan 2004). Supportive communication is important to create an environment where the individual patient feels heard and understood and can be helped appropriately. Communication needs to be highly flexible, dependent upon cultural, social and environmental factors. Nurses need to communicate effectively with patients in order to deliver individualized safe care and treatment and to manage psychosocial concerns appropriately. People with illness want to be approached with a 'caring and humane attitude' that respects their privacy and dignity (Maben and Griffiths 2008, Webster and Bryan 2009). Patients want their personal values to be respected and to be treated as equals by health professionals. This can be achieved by taking the time to communicate, not controlling dialogue, listening and offering emotional support (Smith et al. 2005) and by striving for open, clear and honest communication (Heyland et al. 2006, Jenkins et al. 2001). The patient's dignity can be promoted by enabling the expression of concerns in a safe environment.

Patients want to be able to experience a meaningful connection and a sense of 'being known' by the staff they encounter (Thorne et al. 2005, Webster and Bryan 2009). Nurses need to be able to accurately assess how much patients want to share their thoughts and feelings without assuming that they either do or do not wish to.

Communication occurs in a time-pressured environment. Practical and technical tasks demand the nurse's time and tend to be prioritized above psychological support. The resulting communication may be limited and prevent effective exploration of psychological care issues. Without effective exploration, patients are not sufficiently encouraged to engage with and manage their own care. Nurses need to be aware of and consider other features of the environment that may contribute to the nature of the dialogue that takes place (Hargie 2011) – for example, the wearing of uniform. Patients may not expect to discuss psychosocial issues with nurses because of the communication bias toward physical and medical issues (Chant et al. 2004). The task-orientated short communication encounters that emerge do not encourage the disclosure of psychosocial concerns (Silverman et al. 2013).

Patient satisfaction is not necessarily related to the acquisition of specific communication skills (Dwamena et al. 2012, Thorne et al. 2005) but staff still need to be able to enquire about the nature and manner of support that patients want (so that satisfaction can be achieved wherever possible).

Listening and appropriate verbal responses that demonstrate empathy remain the key skills; if nothing else is achieved, adopting these qualities will be beneficial to patients and be a valuable use of time.

Listening

Listening is a skill often assumed to be natural. Rarely would we consider that we were physically unable to listen and perhaps this makes us pay little attention to this crucial skill area (Box 4.1).

The physical act of hearing is distinct from that of 'listening'. Hearing can be considered to be passive, but listening requires active processing and attaching meaning to what is heard.

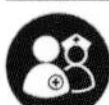

Box 4.1 **How to let someone know you are listening to them**

- Non-verbal encouragement, e.g. head nodding, body position, eye contact
- Verbal responses
- Questioning
- Paraphrasing
- Clarifying
- Summarizing
- Empathy

Source: Hargie (2011). Reproduced with permission from Taylor & Francis.

It might be difficult for us to answer the question 'How do we listen?' and perhaps a procedure of 'how to listen' would not do justice to the sophistication and success of good listeners. However, there are ways of describing the constituent parts of listening that, if followed, would make the person speaking appreciate that they were being listened to.

Problems can emerge as two people may interpret the meaning of the same dialogue differently. For example, if you ask the question 'How are you?' and the patient replies 'Getting by', do you assume they are doing well and coping or that this means they are struggling and 'putting on a brave face'?

Hopefully, you will be attending to numerous non-verbal cues to decipher what the patient actually means. If there is a suggestion of 'incongruence', where the patient says 'Getting by' in a low and sad-sounding voice coupled with a simultaneous lowering of the head, we might consider the latter assumption. Alternatively, if the patient sounds upbeat and looks you in the face with a smile, you might be reassured they mean the former.

There are strategies to promote successful listening, for example 'summarizing' and 'clarifying' (at suitable moments) what the patient is saying.

Non-verbal responses

Non-verbal communication generally indicates information transmitted without speaking. Included in this would be the way you sit or stand, facial expression, gestures and posture, whether you nod or smile and the clothes worn; all will have an impact on the total communication taking place (Hargie 2011). Argyle (1988) suggests that of communication that takes place between people, only 7% is verbal (cited in Jootun and McGhee 2011).

Egan (2013) usefully describes the acronym SOLER to summarize the constituent elements of non-verbal communication.

facing the patient **S**quarely
maintaining an **O**pen posture
Leaning slightly towards the patient to convey interest
having appropriate **E**ye contact, not staring nor avoiding (unless culturally appropriate)
being **R**elaxed

By learning an awareness of these factors and making this behaviour part of your normal demeanour, patients will be encouraged to talk more openly, facilitating emotional disclosure.

Saying nothing can also be interpreted as meaning something, so there is always communication however reluctant or silent you or the patient may be.

It can be argued that non-verbal information is more powerful than verbal information, for example in the case of 'incongruence' where the verbal message indicates one thing and the non-verbal suggests another. There is a tendency to believe the non-verbal message over the verbal in these instances. This highlights the need to communicate with genuine compassion. Without this, supportive communication can be severely reduced in its effectiveness.

Non-verbal communication becomes even more important in the case of people whose verbal communication is impaired, for example by stroke, trauma, learning disability, dementia or surgery. Patients need to be supported, ensuring, for example, that they have constant access to pen and paper; communication boards can be used to good effect and it is worth considering the use of information technology and communication software, if available. The experience of losing the ability to speak can be very isolating and frustrating and preparation of the patient and practice with communication aids is important to maximize the success of communication. It is essential that people with a speech deficit are given more time to communicate their needs, so patience and persistence are essential until interaction and understanding are gained at a satisfactory level.

Non-verbal behaviour to encourage patients to talk includes nodding/making affirming noises, for example 'Hmmm'. This 'affirming' is mostly done naturally, for example at points of eye contact, as specific points are made and during slight pauses in dialogue. It can be especially important to affirm when the patient is talking about psychological issues as they will need validation that this is an acceptable topic of conversation. Chambers (2003, p.878) suggests that for patients with 'limited verbal expression', nurses have a responsibility to build upon and recognize their non-verbal communication to support the development of a good working relationship with the patient.

Verbal responses

The way things are said makes a considerable difference, so attention needs to be paid to the tone, rate and depth of speech. This means sounding alert, interested and caring, but not patronizing. Speech should be delivered at an even rate, not too fast or too slow (unless presenting difficult or complex information).

Questioning

A skill that is used in close collaboration with listening is that of questioning. When specific information is required, for example in a crisis, closed questions are indicated, because they narrow the potential answer (Silverman et al. 2013) and allow the gathering of specific information for a purpose. Closed questions therefore are ones which are likely to generate a short 'yes or no' answer, for example 'Are you all right?'.

In care situations with significant life-changing implications, a broader assessment of the patient's perspective is required and there is also a need to show compassion and identify any underlying psychosocial issues. Open questions and listening are therefore required. Open questions do the opposite of closed questions; they broaden the potential answers (Silverman et al. 2013) giving the agenda and direction of the dialogue to the patient. So, for example, instead of asking 'Are you all right?', an open question would be 'How are you today?' or 'What has your experience of treatment been like?'.

A question that enquires about a patient's emotional experience indicates that this is also of interest to the nurse; for example, 'How did that make you feel?' or 'What are your main concerns?'.

Open questions cannot be used in isolation as the opportunity for open discussion can easily be blocked by failing to ensure that the rest of the fundamental communication elements are in place. Attention must therefore be paid to protecting sufficient time, verbal space (not interrupting) and encouragement (in the form of non-verbal cues, paraphrasing, clarifying and summarizing), so that the patient and/or relative can express their feelings and concerns.

Open questions may not be appropriate with people who have an acquired communication problem, such as changes to the oral cavity following head and neck surgery or if English is not their first language.

Asking one question at a time is important; it is easy to ask more than one question in a sentence and this can make it unclear where the focus is and lead the patient to answer only one part of the question.

Open questions can also be helpful to respond to cues that the patient may give about their underlying psychological state. Cues can be varied, numerous and difficult to define, but essentially these are either verbal or non-verbal hints of underlying unease or worry. Concerns may be easier to recognize where they are expressed verbally and unambiguously (del Piccolo et al. 2006).

Reflecting back

This is repeating the same words back to the patient, which signals that their focus is a legitimate topic for discussion (McCabe and Timmins 2013), but if this technique is overused it can sound unnatural (Silverman et al. 2013).

When it is used, it needs to be done with thought and include 'something of you in your response' (Egan 2013), meaning that you remain alert and caring.

Paraphrasing

This technique involves telling the patient what they have told you but using different words that retain the same meaning; for example:

> *Patient:* I need to talk to them but whenever they start to talk to me about the future, I just start to get wound up and shut down.
> *Nurse:* So when your family try to talk, you get tense and you stop talking …

Clarifying

The aim of this technique is to reduce ambiguity and help the patient define and explore the central or pivotal aspect of the issues raised. As nurses, we can be reluctant to explore emotional or psychological issues in too much depth, for fear that the issues raised are too emotional and hard to deal with (Perry and Burgess 2002). However, if the principles of good communication are applied and a focus on the patient's agenda is maintained, distressing and difficult situations can be heard and support offered to the patient.

The use of open questions is likely to raise certain issues that would benefit from further exploration. Clarification encourages the expression of detail and context to situations, helping to draw out pertinent matters, perhaps not previously considered by either the patient or the nurse. A mixture of open or closed questions can be used in clarification (Box 4.2).

It is sometimes necessary for the nurse to clarify their own position, perhaps acknowledging that they don't know something and cannot answer certain questions, for example 'I am not in a position to know if the treatment will work?'.

Sometimes not knowing can be a valuable position, as it prompts an enquiry about the patient's experience rather than making assumptions. The knowledge and experience gained through a nursing career may mean that the experience of the patient or relative is familiar; however, patients and relatives will benefit from the opportunity to share their experience in their own words and to feel 'heard' (Williams and Iruita 2004).

Box 4.2 **Open and closed questions**

- Are you feeling like that now? (closed)
- You seem to be down today, am I right? (closed)
- Can you describe how the experience made you feel? (closed)
- You say that you've not had enough information: can you tell me what you do know? (open)
- You mention that you are struggling: what kinds of things do you struggle with? (open)
- You say it's been hard getting this far: what has been the hardest thing to cope with? (open)

Summarizing

This intervention can be used as a way of opening or closing dialogue. An opening can be facilitated by recapping a previous discussion or outlining the understanding of the patient's position. Summarizing can be used to punctuate a longer conversation and highlight specific issues raised.

This serves several purposes.

- It informs the patient that they have been listened to and that their situation is understood.
- It allows the patient to correct any mistakes or misconceptions that may have arisen.
- It brings the conversation from the specific to the general (which can help to contextualize issues).
- It gives an opportunity for agreement to be reached about what may need to happen

An example of summarizing:

> 'It sounds like you are tired and are struggling to manage the treatment schedule. It also sounds like you don't have enough information and we could support you more with that …'

Summarizing can be a useful opportunity to plan and agree what actions are necessary, but if summarizing is used in this situation, it is important to avoid getting caught up with planning and solution finding; the patient will gain the greatest benefit from empathic attentive listening. In our nursing role, we are familiar with 'doing' and correcting problematic situations; and although interventions can be helpful in psychosocial issues, sometimes it is necessary not to act and to just 'be' with the patient, accepting their experience as it is, however difficult this may be.

Recognizing when to act and when to sit with distress can be difficult. However, it is important to develop this awareness and to accept that sometimes there are no solutions to difficult situations. The temptation to always correct problems might only serve to negate the patient's experience of being listened to (Connolly et al. 2010). Sometimes all the patient may want in that moment is to be listened to and heard.

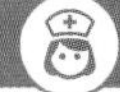 Learning Activity 4.1

Scenario: Listening and questioning

You are looking after a patient who has said they are worried about seeing the doctor.

- What open questions might you ask to start the conversation?
- How would you convey that you are listening to what they are saying?

You may want to role play this scenario with a friend or colleague.

Empathy

Sharing time and physical space with other people demands the development of a relationship. In nursing, the relationship with patients is defined by many factors, for example physical and medical care. In clinical roles, it is possible to be emotionally detached and to exist behind a 'professional mask' (Taylor 1998, p.74) but when working in a supportive role, a shared experience and bond are generated, inclusive of feelings.

Recognizing our own feelings is important to allow us to understand and to 'tolerate another person's pain' (McKenzie 2002, p.34). Nurses demonstrate empathy when there is a desire to understand the client (patient) as fully as possible and to communicate this understanding back to them (Egan 2013, p.97).

This means attempting to gain an appreciation of what the patient might be going through, taking into consideration their physical, social and psychological environment. This inferred information can be used to 'connect' with the patient, all the time checking that our interpretation of their experience is accurate. Even if the nurse has experienced similar events, it is important to determine the patient's thoughts and feelings as they can be very different.

Rogers (1975, p.2) seminally described the skill of empathy as: 'The ability to experience another person's world as if it were one's own, without losing the "as if" quality'. That means allowing ourselves to get into the patient's shoes and experience some of what they might be experiencing, without allowing ourselves to enter the experience wholly (it isn't our experience). Empathy allows for an opportunity to 'taste' and therefore attempt to understand the patient's perspective. Understanding emotions and behaviours in this way encourages an acceptance and positive negotiation of them. Maintaining the 'as if' quality protects us from adopting too great an emotional load. Having too much of a sense of loss or sorrow may prevent us from offering effective support, as we are drawn to focus on our own feelings more than is necessary or helpful for ourselves or the patient.

Empathy may not always come easily, especially if a patient is angry. What can be very useful in the development and use of empathy is the ability to step back from the situation and reflect upon what it is that you, as the nurse, feel and how this relates to what is happening for the patient.

Barriers to effective communication

Poor communication with patients can negatively affect decision making and quality of life (Dwamena et al. 2012, Fallowfield et al. 2001, Thorne et al. 2005).

The environmental conditions in which nurses work, with competing professional demands and time pressures, can reduce the capacity to form effective relationships with patients (Hemsley et al. 2012, Henderson et al. 2007).

There is a personal, emotional impact when providing a supportive role for patients with psychological and emotional issues (Botti et al. 2006, Dunne 2003, Turner et al. 2007) and it is therefore likely that blocking or avoidance of patients' emotional concerns relates to emotional self-preservation for the nurse. Young (2012) states that in caring for patients who have dementia, professional caregivers are likely to avoid communication which can result in further isolation and frustration in the patient which in turn could lead to anger.

When communicating and assessing patients' needs, nurses may be anxious about eliciting distress and managing expressed concerns. They may lack confidence in their ability to clarify patients' feelings without 'causing harm to the patient or getting into difficulty themselves' (Booth et al. 1996, p.526). As a consequence, nurses can make assumptions, rather than assessing concerns properly (Booth et al. 1996, Kelsey 2005, Schofield et al. 2008). To illustrate this point, Kruijver et al. (2001) demonstrated how nurses verbally focus upon physical issues, which accounted for 60% of communication with patients. Nurses often recognize this bias and suggest that they feel greater competence discussing physical rather than psychological issues and seek better skills to help them to manage challenging situations (McCaughan and Parahoo 2000). Being supported practically and emotionally by supervisors and/or senior staff can help to decrease blocking behaviours (Booth et al. 1996, Connolly et al. 2010). Clinical supervision can aid the transfer of communication skills into practice (Heaven et al. 2006).

Institutions, work environments and the nature of the senior staff within them can influence the nature of communication (Booth et al. 1996, Chant et al. 2004, McCabe 2004, Menzies-Lyth 1988, Wilkinson 1991). Nurses may improve their own practice by identifying where environmental barriers lie and attempting to mitigate the features of the clinical environment that inhibit psychological care. These barriers to communication may be even more significant for patients who have any cognitive or physical impairment, such as learning disability, dementia, hearing or sight impairment. Approaches to patients who have additional communication needs require consideration and planning.

Despite the difficulties outlined, it has been argued that nurses can communicate well when they are facilitated to provide individual patient-focused care (McCabe 2004).

 Learning Activity 4.2

Learning in practice: Barriers to effective communication

In your own clinical practice area, can you identify at least three environmental barriers to effective communication? How might you be able to overcome each of these?

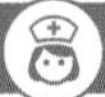 Learning Activity 4.3

Scenario: Blocking behaviours

You witness the following conversation between a nurse and a patient:

Nurse: Hello, I am looking after you this afternoon. Do you have any pain at the moment?
Patient: Yes I have a little bit of pain, but more importantly, my son hasn't visited for two days now, I want to tell him about the operation the doctors want me to have as I am getting rather worried about it.
Nurse: Right, well I will see if you can have some pain medication to help sort that out. That's a shame about your son not visiting, would you like me to call him?
Patient: Yes please.
Nurse: Ok, I will get your pain medication and call your son. Is there anything else that you want to talk about?

- Can you identify which of the nurse's responses are 'blocking' or avoiding the patient's emotional concerns?
- How might you respond differently in this situation?

LEGAL AND PROFESSIONAL ISSUES

There are a number of legal and professional concepts and issues that impact on effective communication and psychological support. These include:

- professional responsibility for effective communication
- confidentiality and appropriate disclosure of information about the patient
- consent communicating about a procedure and ensuring that a patient is fully cognisant of what it involves
- assessment of an individual's mental capacity to engage in care and treatment.

Professional responsibility for effective communication

The Francis Report (DH 2013) recommended that there should be an increased focus on a culture of caring, compassion and consideration in nursing. The steps to achieving this are set out in *Compassion in Practice* (DH 2012a). Underpinning this vision are six fundamental values: care, compassion, competence, communication, courage and commitment, and associated with these are six areas of action to support nursing staff in delivering excellent care.

Communication is one of the six fundamental values in the vision and is defined as:

> 'central to the caring relationships and to effective team working. Listening is as important as what we say and do and essential for 'no decision about me without me'. Communication is the key to a good workplace with benefits for those in our care and staff alike' (DH 2012a, p.13).

However, it is also important to note that 'Compassion: care given through relationships based on empathy, respect and dignity … also described as intelligent kindness' (DH 2012a, p.13) is also a fundamental professional responsibility.

This professional responsibility of every nurse to communicate effectively and compassionately is an explict standard of *The Code* (NMC 2015) (see Appendix: *The Code*):

> 'Make the care of people your first concern, treating them as individuals and respecting their dignity.
>
> - You must listen to the people in your care and respond to their concerns and preferences.
> - You must make arrangements to meet people's language and communication needs.
> - You must share with people, in a way they can understand, the information they want or need to know about their health.
> - You must uphold people's rights to be fully involved in their care'.

There are four essential features of maintaining dignity in communication.

1. *Attitude*. Being aware of the other person's experience, our attitudes towards them and how this affects the care provided.
2. *Behaviour*. Being respectful and kind, asking permission, giving your full attention and using understandable language.
3. *Compassion*. Being aware of and in touch with our own feelings and 'acknowledging the person beyond their illness' (Chochinov 2007, p.186).
4. *Dialogue*. Being able to demonstrate an appropriate knowledge of the patient's history, experience and family context (Webster and Bryan 2009). You might usefully make educated guesses about the likely experiences of the patient, for example 'It must have been difficult to have received the news at that point in your life'.

These qualities are recognized as so essential to nursing practice that the Francis Report (DH 2013) recommended that an aptitude test to explore an individual's qualities of caring and compassion should be included in the selection process of aspiring nurses.

Confidentiality

'Information provided in confidence should not be used or disclosed in a form that might identify a patient without his or her consent' (DH 2003, p.7). *The Code* (NMC 2015) states that every nurse must respect people's right to confidentiality, ensuring they are informed about how and why information is shared by those who provide their care. In addition, it is a legal obligation and should be part of the terms and conditions of employment of any healthcare professional (DH 2003).

However, if there is a concern that an individual may be at risk of harm, this must be appropriately disclosed following the guidance of the organization in which the nurse works.

Consent

One of the principles that guides the NHS in the Constitution is: 'NHS services must reflect the needs and preferences of patients, their families and carers. Patients, their families and carers where appropriate will be involved and consulted on all decisions about their care and treatment' (DH 2012b).

The NHS Constitution (DH 2012b) also states that a patient has the right to accept or refuse treatment that is offered and not be given any physical examination or treatment unless they have given valid consent.

The Code (NMC 2015) states that nurses have a responsibility to ensure they gain consent and that they must:

- gain consent before treatment or care starts
- respect and support people's rights to accept or decline treatment or care

- uphold people's rights to be fully involved in decisions about their care
- be aware of the legislation regarding mental capacity
- be able to demonstrate that they have acted in someone's best interests if emergency car has been provided.

For consent to be valid, it must be given voluntarily by a competent person who has been appropriately informed and who has the capacity to consent to the intervention in question (NMC 2013). This will be the patient or someone authorized to do so under a Lasting Power of Attorney (LPA) or someone who has the authority to make treatment decisions as a court-appointed deputy (DH 2009).

The validity of consent does not depend on a signature on a form. Written consent merely serves as evidence of consent. Although completion of a consent form is in most cases not a legal requirement, the use of such forms is good practice where an intervention such as surgery is to be undertaken (DH 2009).

If there is any doubt about the person's capacity to make a decision about consent, the nurse should determine whether or not the person has the capacity to consent to the intervention and secondly that they have sufficient information to be able to make an informed decision (DH 2009). This should be done before the person is asked to sign the form. Documentation is necessary and the nurse should record all discussions relating to consent, details of the assessment of capacity, and the conclusion reached, in the patient's notes (NMC 2013).

Obtaining consent is a process and not a one-off event (NMC 2013). Usually the person undertaking the procedure should be the person seeking to obtain consent. There may be situations when a nurse has been asked to seek consent on behalf of other staff. Providing the nurse has had training for that specific area, they may seek to obtain consent (NMC 2013).

As part of the nursing assessment, the nurse needs to establish if the person can understand the verbal communication, what they are being consented for and that they are able to read or write or communicate their decision in a reliable manner. If they are unable, they may be able to make their mark on the form to indicate consent by any reasonable means. If consent has been given validly, the lack of a completed form is no bar to treatment, but a form can be important evidence of such consent (DH 2009). If the patient is unable to consent because they do not understand the information or are unable to communicate their decision, the Mental Capacity Act 2005 allows decisions to be made in the patient's best interest. If the consent is about medical treatment then a best interest decision may be required; this will depend on the seriousness of the decision (Mental Capacity Act 2005).

Consent may be expressed by a person verbally, in writing or by implication (NMC 2013); an example of implied consent would be where a person, after receiving appropriate information, holds out an arm for their blood pressure to be taken. The nurse should ensure that the person has understood what examination or treatment is intended, and why, for such consent to be valid (DH 2009). It is good practice to obtain written consent for any significant procedure, such as a surgical operation or when the person participates in a research project or a video recording (NMC 2013).

A competent adult may refuse to consent to treatment or care and nurses must respect that refusal (NMC 2013). Where a patient declines an intervention, consideration must be given to the patient's capacity. If the patient is deemed to have capacity and refuses care, this needs to be recorded clearly in their notes.

Equality and diversity

An additional aspect of communication and psychological support from the legal persepctive is to ensure that it is as equitable as possible. The Equality Act (2010) reinforces the duty to ensure that everybody, irrespective of their disability, sex, gender, race, ethnic origin, age, relationship status, religion or faith, has equal access to information and is communicated with equitably. This means, for example, that provision is necessary to meet the information needs of blind and partially sighted people (Section 21 of the Disability Discrimination Act, October 1999).

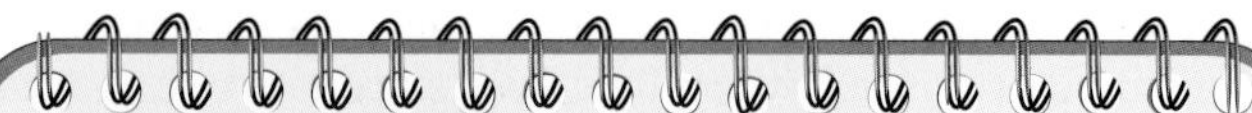

Learning Activity 4.4 Case study: Consent

Rose is a 79-year-old woman with dementia. She is having a pre-operative assessment prior to having a right hip replacement due to severe osteoarthritis. Rose has come to the department with her daughter, who lives with her and is her main carer. Her daughter informs you that Rose is capable of following simple instructions but she is struggling to understand why she is visiting the hospital today.

What steps do you need to take in order to gain consent for Rose to have her operation?

See the end of the chapter for the answers.

People from black and minority ethnic (BME) groups constitute 14% of the population in England and Wales (Jivraj 2012). Originating primarily from the Caribbean, Africa, South Asia and China, the majority of people falling into this group continue to maintain strong cultural links with their countries of origin even after being resident in the United Kingdom for several generations.

Communication needs are individual and information requirements are also culturally sensitive. People may hold different beliefs about why they have developed an illness, for instance thinking that they are being punished for something that they may or may not have done (Dein 2006, McEvoy et al. 2009).

Medical language is full of technical vocabulary and jargon which is often difficult to comprehend even for native English speakers. Macdonald (2004) suggests that people from BME groups may often come from communities where the opportunity for education is limited, thus making it difficult for them to comprehend the information that has been provided, particularly when their first language is not English. Macdonald (2004, p.131) states that 'sentences should be short, clear and precise'.

Patients from different ethnic backgrounds will often take a family member to health-related appointments. The family member is there to assist in the dialogue between the patient and the medical/nursing practitioner. Macdonald (2004) discusses the fact that communication is a two-way process and suggests that for it to be effective, the information provided needs to be patient focused. The process of translation and interpretation is never without potential problems, however, and it is important to try to find more effective ways of ensuring that the information provided is not misunderstood or misinterpreted (McEvoy et al. 2009).

In addition to the written word, there are also reputable telephone helplines that can facilitate the translation from one language to another. It is good practice that these services be utilized rather than relying on family or friends of the patient (Macdonald 2004). The reason for this is that the latter may not fully understand what they are being asked to translate, or might misconstrue or misrepresent what is being said (Macmillan Cancer Relief 2002).

Patients who are elderly may need additional support to be able to make informed decisions about care. Older patients are more likely to have hearing or sight loss although this should not be assumed. This needs to be considered when communicating as well as considering the patient's dignity. If a patient is hearing impaired there may be a temptation to shout, but in a busy clinical environment this might breach a patient's right to confidentiality and to be treated with dignity. Information provided in small print may be inappropriate and inaccessible for the patient, impacting on their ability to make an informed choice.

Patients with dementia may have additional communication needs, and there is a danger of assuming that because a person has dementia they will not be able to make decisions for themselves.

Daniel and Dewing (2012) suggest that this idea needs to be avoided as it fails to meet the requirements of the Mental Capacity Act (2005). The Mental Capacity Act (2005) makes it clear that consent must be decision specific and, as such, each significant decision needs to be assessed. If a patient with dementia has communication issues, it is important to work with them and their family to maximize their ability to be involved in decision making even when the person is assessed as lacking capacity. The Mental Capacity Act 'promotes the autonomy and rights of an individual who lacks decision-making capacity' (Griffith and Tengnah 2008, p.337).

In communication with people who have a learning disability, 50–90% experience communication difficulties, such as impaired speech, hearing or sight loss (Jones 2002, p.566). It is important to know what tools can be used to support this patient group to communicate their needs whilst receiving healthcare, the most important of which are the communication skills of the person providing the care (Chambers 2003). Many patients with learning disabilities will have a hospital or My Health passport which will include information on how best to communicate with the person. The person with a learning disability may have a communication book, which is full of symbols which they can use to communicate their needs.

With any patient who has additional communication needs, it is important to work with the people who know them well such as family, carers or other professionals. The family, carers and friends will be able to interpret the non-verbal communication more easily and so can support nurses in providing care; carers should be seen as partners in the caring process.

Mental Capacity Act (2005)

The Code also makes explicit the responsibility to be aware of the legislation regarding mental capacity, a factor that can have a significant impact on communication. The Mental Capacity Act (2005) sets out clear guidance and and has produced a code of practice to support professionals working with people who may have impairment in their capacity.

The first principle of the act is the presumption of capacity and so we must presume a person has mental capacity unless they:

- are unable to understand information given to them to make choices
- can understand but are unable to retain the information
- are unable to weigh up and relate the information accurately to their situation
- are unable to communicate their wishes or choices (by any means) (BMA 2007).

If any of these factors are in question, the Mental Capacity Act (2005) recommends that determining an individual's decision-making capacity is best achieved through multidisciplinary assessment. A separate assessment of capacity must take place for every decision involving the individual. It is important, however, to ensure that the person is involved as much as they can be in the decision making and that all reasonable steps have been made to support the patient to make the decision for themselves (Dimond 2008). Brady Wagner (2003) specifies four key areas that need to be fulfilled in order to have the capacity to make a decision.

1. Understanding the diagnosis and other information given regarding treatment and non-treatment options.
2. Manipulating those options and consequences in relation to one's personal values and goals.
3. Reasoning through a decision.
4. Communicating the preference/decision.

The mental capacity of an individual needs to be considered in any communication but particularly if it involves the patient making a decision about treatment or care options and in respect of consent. The assessment as to whether an individual has capacity or not can be a complex one and it is important to ensure that the principles of the Mental Capacity Act (2005) are applied in any decisions relating to a patient where there is a concern about impairment in the functioning of mind or brain and as such the person's capacity to communicate their consent is questioned (Daniel and Dewing 2012). At any time before making any referral or sharing patient information to enable access to further support, it is important that the patient fully understands and consents and where this is not possible, the decision may need to be made in the patient's best interests, ensuring the principles of the Mental Capacity Act (2005) are applied.

There are some patient groups in which the issue of commincation and consent may be more challenging, particularly when the person does not wish to engage in the care or treatment. If, for instance, a person with dementia was indicating by their non-verbal communication that they did not want to be treated but the treatment was required, in an adult with capacity this would be considered withdrawal of implied consent. In these situations where the adult has been assessed as lacking capacity and treatment is to be given, how the person is communicated with during this process is really important. The patient may feel threatened and anxious and so explaining what is happening, keeping calm and talking in a quiet voice may help facilitate the care without causing more distress to the patient.

Competencies

Communication is such an essential aspect of the role of anybody in healthcare that the NHS *Knowledge and Skills Framework* specifies four levels of skill in communication (Table 4.1). Nurses are expected to be competent as a minimum to level 3. This is a baseline and much work has been done in developing programmes to advance communication skills further.

The consistency of the success of training interventions has been widely discussed (Chant et al. 2004, Heaven et al. 2006, Schofield et al. 2008). The NHS Connected programme was developed initially to develop further the skills of key members of multidisciplinary teams in cancer care (Fellowes et al. 2004); this work has now been merged with the Health and Social Care Information Centre (http://systems.hscic.gov.uk/).

Ongoing development of communication skills should include learning how to negotiate barriers to good communication in the clinical environment, tailoring and individualizing communication approaches for different patients, conflict resolution and negotiation skills (Gysels et al. 2005, Roberts and Snowball 1999, Schofield et al. 2008, Wilkinson 1991).

Table 4.1 **NHS *Knowledge and Skills Framework*: four dimensions of communication competence**

1	2	3	4
Establish and maintain communication with other people on routine and operational matters	Establish and maintain communication with people about routine and daily activities, overcoming any differences in communication between the people involved	Establish and maintain communication with individuals and groups about difficult or complex matters, overcoming any problems in communication	Establish and maintain communication with various individuals and groups on complex potentially stressful topics in a range of situations

Source: Adapted from NHS Knowledge and Skills Framework and Development Review Guidance. Working draft, v6.0 (2003).

Courses with a behavioural component of communication training, that is, role-playing situations in the classroom, are preferable as this is indicated to influence effectiveness (Gysels et al. 2005).

If an issue appears to be beyond the scope of practice of the nurse, it is essential that further advice and help are sought to manage a patient's psychosocial needs. Self-care and supervision are key factors in maintaining the ability to support other people. This will mean having a balanced lifestyle, knowing self, and having relevant accessible support structures in place.

PRE-PROCEDURAL CONSIDERATIONS

Time

In an acute hospital environment time is always pressured. This has an impact on communication unless steps are taken to create time for effective, supportive communication to take place. From the patient's perspective, they need to know that they have the nurse's attention for a set period of time. It is therefore essential to be realistic and proactive with the patient to negotiate a specific conversation for a prescribed length of time at a prearranged point in the day. It is important to be realistic but also to keep to the arrangement, otherwise there is the potential for the patient to consider that their psychological needs are not important (Towers 2007).

Box 4.3 **Making the environment conducive to supportive communication**

- Can the patient safely and comfortably move to a more suitable area to talk with more privacy?
- Do they wish to move?
- Do they wish other people/members of the family to be there?
- Clear a space if necessary, respecting the patient's privacy and property.
- Check whether sitting on one side or another is preferable to them.
- Remove distractions, for example switch off a television, with the patient's permission.
- Is the patient able to sit comfortably?
- Will the patient be too hot or cold?
- As far as possible, choose a seat for yourself that is comfortable, and on the same level as the patient.
- Position your seat so you can have eye contact with each other easily without having to turn significantly.
- If you are in an open area on a ward, draw the curtains (with the patient's permission), to give you some privacy. Obviously, this does not prevent sound transfer and it is worth acknowledging the limitations of privacy.

Environment

Conversations in a hospital environment can be very difficult, especially if privacy is sought. However, there are actions that can be taken to make the environment as conducive as possible to enable supportive communication to take place (Towers 2007) (Box 4.3). This preliminary work might seem insignificant and time consuming but it underlines the importance of the communication to the patient and illustrates an interest in them.

Assessment

Nurses need to make careful assessments of the patient's communication and psychological needs. This will include an assessment of their communication style, skills and ability to relate (see Chapter 2: Assessment and discharge). In addition, nurses need to assess the psychological well-being of their patients. This will include observing their cognitive state, mood level, coping strategies and support networks. Patient needs and presentation are likely to vary at different points in the treatment journey. An ongoing professional relationship between a nurse and a patient can help identify alterations in mood and cognitive ability. Assessment and recording tools may be helpful in supporting discussions with patients as well as noting change over time.

Recording tools

The Distress Thermometer is a validated instrument for measuring distress (Gessler et al. 2008, Mitchell 2007, Ransom et al. 2006). It is similar to a pain analogue scale (0 = no distress, 10 = extreme distress) and is thus simple to use and understand (Mitchell et al. 2010) (Figure 4.4). The tool helps to establish which of the broad range of challenges that may face any unwell person is dominant at any given time. It provides a language to help patients talk about what is concerning them (Mitchell 2007). The patient marks where they feel they are at that moment or for an agreed period preceding the assessment. Trigger questions included with the Distress Thermometer can then be used to explore the nature of the distress, for example exploring family difficulties, financial worries, emotional or physical problems. A score of over 5 would warrant some supportive discussion and exploration of whether other support is necessary or desired. It may be that no further referral is necessary and the structured discussion this tool provides is sufficient in lowering the level of distress (NCCN 2010).

PRINCIPLES OF COMMUNICATION

Communication with a patient that is compassionate and supportive in a clinical environment cannot be described as a linear process but certain principles can increase its effectiveness.

Principles table 4.1 **Communication**

Principle	Rationale
Consider whether the patient is comfortable and doesn't need pain relief or to use the toilet before you begin.	Pain and the medication used to treat it and other distractions and discomforts may limit a patient's ability to reason and concentrate. E
Protect the time for psychosocial focus of conversation. This involves telling other staff that you don't wish to be disturbed for a prescribed period.	Patients may observe how busy nurses are and withhold worries and concerns unless given explicit permission to talk (McCabe 2004, R3b).
Set a realistic time boundary for your conversation at the beginning.	You may only have 10 minutes and therefore you need to articulate the scope of your available time; this will help you to avoid distraction and give your full attention during the time available. E

Principle	Rationale
Introduce yourself and your role and check what the patient wishes to be called.	This helps to establish initial rapport (Silverman et al. 2013, C).
Spend a short time developing a rapport and indicating your interest in the patient, for example comment on a picture by the bedside.	Patients want to feel known. P
Be ready to move the conversation on to issues that may be concerning the patient.	Be aware that some patients may stay with neutral topics as the central focus of the conversation and withhold disclosure of psychosocial concerns until later in a conversation (Silverman et al. 2013, C).
Suggest the focus of conversation, for example 'I would like to talk about how you have been feeling' or 'I wondered how you have been coping with everything'.	This indicates to the patient that you are interested in their psychological issues. E
Respond to and refer to cues.	Patients frequently offer cues – either verbal or non-verbal hints about underlying emotional concerns – and these need to be explored and clarified (Levinson et al. 2000, R3b; Oguchi et al. 2011, R3b).
Responding to cues: 'I noticed you seemed upset earlier. I have 10 minutes to spare in which we can talk about it if you wish' or 'You seem a little frustrated. Is now a good time to talk about how I can help you with this?'.	
If the patient does not wish to talk, respect this (it is still important that you have offered to talk and the patient may well wish to talk at another time).	The patient may not wish to talk at that moment or may prefer to talk to someone else. E
Ask open questions: prefix your question with 'what', 'how'.	Open questions encourage patients to talk (Hargie 2011, R5).
Use closed questions sparingly.	If patients have a complicated issue to discuss, closed questions can help them be specific and can be used for clarification as well as when closing dialogue (Hargie 2011, R5).
Add a psychological focus where you can, for example 'How have you felt about that?'.	This will help elicit information about psychological and emotional issues (Ryan et al. 2005, R3a).
Listen carefully and feed back your understanding of what is being said at opportune moments.	Listening is a key skill – it is an active process requiring concentration, verbal and non-verbal affirmations (Silverman et al. 2013; Wosket 2006, R5).
Be empathic (try to appreciate what the other person may be experiencing and recognize how difficult that is for them).	Empathy is about creating a human connection with your patient (DH 2012a, C; Egan 2013, R5).
Allow for silences.	This can give rise to further expression and allows useful thinking time for yourself and the patient (Silverman et al. 2013, C).
Initially avoid trying to 'fix' people's concerns and the problems that they express. It might be more powerful and important to simply sit, listen and show your understanding.	As an individual is listened to, they may feel comfort, relief and a sense of human connection essential for support (Egan 2013, R5).
Ask the patient how they think you may be able to help them.	The patient will know what they need better than you do. E
Avoid blocking (Box 4.4).	Blocking results in failing to elicit the full range of concerns a patient may have (Back et al. 2005, R3a).
When you are nearing the end of the time you have agreed to be with the patient, let the patient know; that is, mention that soon you will need to stop your discussion.	The patient can find this easier to accept if you have clearly expressed the time you had available in the first place (Towers 2007, R5).
Acknowledge that you may not have been able to cover all concerns and summarize what has been discussed, checking with the patient how accurate your understanding is.	The patient can correct any misinterpretations and this can lead to satisfactory agreement about the meeting. It also signifies closure of a meeting (Hargie 2011, R5).
If further concerns are raised at this point, you will need to make it clear that you cannot support them at the current time. Let the patient know when you or other staff may be available to talk again, or where else they may get further support.	Clarity and honesty are important, as is working within boundaries. Knowing the limits of your time and expertise will help to prevent confusion about where the patient can receive types of support. E

(continued)

Principles table 4.1 **Communication *(continued)***

Principle	Rationale
Agree any action points and follow up as necessary. If needs remain unmet, offer support from a clinical nurse specialist or a counselling service, if available. You must discuss what this means and be realistic with regard to waiting times. Consent from the patient for any further referral is essential (unless you consider the patient to be at risk).	Having made a suitable assessment, you can involve further support if appropriate. E
Document your conversation, having agreed with the patient what is appropriate to share with the rest of the team.	It is essential to document your conversation so other members of the team are informed and to meet your professional requirements (NMC 2010, C; NMC 2015, C).
Reflect upon your own practice.	You may have unintentionally controlled the communication or blocked expression of emotion. Reflection will increase your self-awareness and help develop your skills. E
Consider your own support needs. If you are affected by any discussions you have had, seek discussion with supportive senior members of staff or consider debriefing and/or supervision.	Clinical supervision supports practice, enabling registered nurses to maintain and improve standards of care (NMC 2008, C).

LONDON CANCER ALLIANCE West and South LCA — LONDON CANCER NORTH AND EAST

London Holistic Needs Assessment

For each item below, please select **yes** or **no** if they have been a concern for you during the last week, including today. Please also select **Discuss** if you wish to speak about it with your health professional.

Choose not to complete the assessment today by selecting this box ☐

Date:	Click here to enter text.
Name:	Click here to enter text.
Hospital/NHS number:	Click here to enter text.

Please **select the number** that best describes the overall level of distress you have been feeling during the last week, including today:

10 ☐ Extreme distress
9 ☐
8 ☐
7 ☐
6 ☐
5 ☐
4 ☐
3 ☐
2 ☐
1 ☐
0 ☐ No distress

For health professional use	
Date of diagnosis:	Click here to enter text.
Diagnosis:	Click here to enter text.
Pathway point:	Click here to enter text.

Practical concerns	**Yes**	**No**	**Discuss**
Caring responsibilities	☐	☐	☐
Housing or finances	☐	☐	☐
Transport or parking	☐	☐	☐
Work or education	☐	☐	☐
Information needs	☐	☐	☐
Difficulty making plans	☐	☐	☐
Grocery shopping	☐	☐	☐
Preparing food	☐	☐	☐
Bathing or dressing	☐	☐	☐
Laundry/housework	☐	☐	☐
Family concerns			
Relationship with children	☐	☐	☐
Relationship with partner	☐	☐	☐
Relationship with others	☐	☐	☐
Emotional concerns			
Loneliness or isolation	☐	☐	☐
Sadness or depression	☐	☐	☐
Worry, fear or anxiety	☐	☐	☐
Anger, frustration or guilt	☐	☐	☐
Memory or concentration	☐	☐	☐
Hopelessness	☐	☐	☐
Sexual concerns	☐	☐	☐
Spiritual concerns			
Regret about the past	☐	☐	☐
Loss of faith or other spiritual concern	☐	☐	☐
Loss of meaning or purpose in life	☐	☐	☐

Physical concerns	**Yes**	**No**	**Discuss**
High temperature	☐	☐	☐
Wound care	☐	☐	☐
Passing urine	☐	☐	☐
Constipation or diarrhoea	☐	☐	☐
Indigestion	☐	☐	☐
Nausea and/or vomiting	☐	☐	☐
Cough	☐	☐	☐
Changes in weight	☐	☐	☐
Eating or appetite	☐	☐	☐
Changes in taste	☐	☐	☐
Sore or dry mouth	☐	☐	☐
Feeling swollen	☐	☐	☐
Breathlessness	☐	☐	☐
Pain	☐	☐	☐
Dry, itchy or sore skin	☐	☐	☐
Tingling in hands or feet	☐	☐	☐
Hot flushes	☐	☐	☐
Moving around/walking	☐	☐	☐
Fatigue	☐	☐	☐
Sleep problems	☐	☐	☐
Communication	☐	☐	☐
Personal appearance	☐	☐	☐
Other medical condition	☐	☐	☐

Figure 4.4 **The London Holistic Needs Assessment tool.** ***Source:*** **Reproduced with permission from London Cancer Alliance (www.londoncanceralliance.nhs.uk/) and London Cancer (www.londoncancer.org/). Adapted with permission from the NCCN Clinical Practice Guidelines in Oncology (NCCN Guidelines®) for Distress Management V.2.2014.**

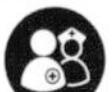 Box 4.4 **Characteristics of blocking behaviours**

Blocking can be defined as:

- failing to pick up on cues (ignoring emotional content)
- selectively focusing on the physical/medical aspects of care
- premature or false reassurance, for example telling people not to worry
- inappropriate encouragement or trivializing, for example telling someone they look fine when they have expressed altered body image
- passing the buck, for example suggesting it is another professional's responsibility to answer questions or sort out the problem (doctors or counsellors, for example)
- changing the subject, for example asking about something mundane or about other family members to deflect the conversation away from issues that may make the nurse feel uncomfortable
- jollying along, for example 'You'll feel better when you get home'
- using closed questions (any question that can be answered with a yes or a no is a closed question).

Source: Adapted from Faulkner and Maguire (1994).

Communicating with those who are worried or distressed

DEFINITION

Interpersonal communication is the process of discussion between healthcare professionals and patients and carers, which allows patients and carers to explore issues and arrive at decisions (NICE 2004).

RELATED THEORY

Patients will naturally have an emotional response to serious illness. At its most mild, this is seen as sadness and worry. At its most serious, however, patients experience severe psychological responses such as adjustment reactions, anxiety states or depression (NICE 2004). This is because illness changes lives, or at least threatens to. Nurses must know how to respond, therefore, to sad and worried patients. The ability to listen fully is perhaps the most frequently used skill or competence of a nurse. Noticing when a patient is worried, listening carefully to their concerns without interrupting, and responding helpfully are components of effective communication with an individual who is distressed. When health workers have such skills, patient outcomes are improved and staff feel more satisfied with their work (Fallowfield and Jenkins 1999, Fellowes et al. 2004, Ong et al. 2000, Razavi et al. 2000, Stewart 1996, Taylor et al. 2005).

Before learning how to listen and respond to patient worries, it is worth knowing about unhelpful communication habits. Health workers often focus on physical and practical concerns but ignore the emotional issues of patients (Booth et al. 1999, Maguire et al. 1996). This is despite the fact that patients hint at their worries (Uitterhoeve et al. 2010). It seems that health workers are eager to give advice, reassurance and information before hearing all the patient's concerns (Booth et al. 1999). This rush to fix problems may be one cause of incomplete listening.

EVIDENCE-BASED APPROACHES

Research evidence suggests that nurses and other health workers should listen to all of the concerns, even those that have no resolution (Booth et al. 1999, Pennebaker 1993). Nurses should enquire about the resources (help) that patients have around them and patients should be given an opportunity to describe for themselves what would help, before the health worker offers advice, information or reassurance (Booth et al. 1999, Tate 2010). It is also known to be helpful for health workers to use a structure in their own minds to organize their thoughts and questions (Silverman et al. 2013). Patients or their carers will often have disorganized thoughts because their thinking is clouded by emotions. A helpful health worker, on the other hand, needs to be calm, organized and sensitive. The SAGE & THYME model (Connolly et al. 2010) presented below is one way for nurses and other health workers to conduct a structured and evidence-based conversation. The model suggests a sequence of sensitive questions which allow the health worker to hear about strong emotions and remain calm themselves.

PRE-PROCEDURAL CONSIDERATIONS

Patients need privacy to discuss emotions and worries: they also need time. Nurses, therefore, should create the conditions for patients to describe their worries. Nurses are often busy because there are many competing demands for their time, yet proper listening requires time and privacy. Nurses create time and privacy to dress a wound. They dress wounds expertly, in a logical and sequential way which has been carefully learned and practised. Listening to the worries of the patient also needs uninterrupted time and a logical sequence. This skill must also be learned and mastered if the nurse is to become an expert listener.

Principles table 4.2 **SAGE & THYME**

Principle	Rationale
SETTING – think first about the setting. Can you respond to this hint from the patient now or should you return when you and they can protect ten minutes? Can you create some privacy? Would they like to talk?	Patients notice that nurses are busy and withhold worries unless given an explicit opportunity to describe their concerns (McCabe 2004, R3b). It is important to create the setting or environment within which patients or carers can disclose their concerns (Hase and Douglas 1986, R5).
ASK – ask the patient what is concerning or worrying them (don't worry yourself about problems that you cannot solve – just listen).	Patients frequently hint about their underlying concerns. These hints need to be noticed and responded to (Oguchi et al. 2010, R3b). Asking specifically about emotions encourages patients to describe psychological and emotional issues (Ryan et al. 2005, R3a). Specific questions about psychological concerns are important (Booth et al. 1999, R3b; Maguire et al. 1996, R3b).

(continued)

Principles table 4.2 **SAGE & THYME *(continued)***

Principle	Rationale
GATHER – gather all of the concerns, not just the first few (ask if there is something else). Repeat back to the patient what you have heard (this proves that you are listening) and make a list of all the concerns (actually write them down).	Listening is an active process, requiring concentration, silences and verbal affirmation that you hear what is being said (Silverman et al. 2013, R5; Wosket 2006, R5). It is important to hear all the patient's concerns, to summarize and check that you have understood correctly (Maguire et al. 1996, R3b; Pennebaker 1993, R3b).
EMPATHY – say something which suggests that you are aware of the burden of their worry, such as: 'I can see that you have a lot to be worried about at the moment'.	Empathy is about creating a human connection with your patient (Egan 2013, R5). Empathy shows that you have some sense of how the patient is feeling (Booth et al. 1999, R3b; Maguire and Pitceathley 2002, R3b).
TALK – ask who they have to talk to and what support they have. Make a list of all the people who would help. 'Who do you have that you can talk to about your concerns?'	Patients commonly rely on family and friends for support (Ell 1996, R5). Good social support is associated with enhanced coping skills for the patient (Chou et al. 2012, R3b). Supportive ties may enhance well-being by meeting basic human needs for companionship, intimacy and a sense of belonging (Berkman et al. 2000, R5). It is helpful to know what social support surrounds the patient (Stewart 1996, R5).
HELP – ask 'How do these people help?'	People's social networks may help them reinterpret events or problems in a more positive and constructive light (Thoits 1995, R5). The support from family and friends commonly involves reassurance, comfort and problem solving (Schroevers et al. 2010, R5).
YOU – ask the patient: 'What do you think would help?' or 'What would help?'	It is helpful to use a style of problem solving which seeks the patient's own solutions first (Booth et al. 1999, R3b; Tate 2010, R5).
ME – ask the patient: 'Is there something you would like me to do?'	It is helpful to use a negotiated style of communication which gives the patient control over what, if any, professional help they receive with their concerns or dilemmas (Fallowfield and Jenkins 1999, R3b).
END – summary and strategy. 'I now know what you are worried about and the support you have. I know what you think would help and what you want me to do. I'll get on with that and come back to you when I can. Is it OK to leave it there for now?'	It is important to know how to summarize and close an interaction (Bradley and Edinberg 1990, R5).

Problem-solving table 4.1 **Prevention and resolution (Principles table 4.2)**

Problem	Action
DIRECT REQUESTS Patients often have concerns at the same time as direct requests or direct questions. When listening for all the concerns, it is easy to be distracted by the direct request. The following is an example: 'I keep hearing different things and it makes me feel as though nobody really knows what is happening. That's scary for me. Am I having this scan or not?'	It is tempting to deal only with the direct request (about the scan) and to ignore the other cues and concerns (different messages, nobody knows what is happening, scary). However, the direct request cannot be ignored either. A clear-thinking nurse will notice both the direct question and the other cues and concerns. 'I hear that you are scared, that you feel that nobody knows what is going on, that you are getting different messages and that you want to know about the scan. I promise to find out about the scan; would you prefer me to do that straight away or can I come back to that once we've discussed you feeling scared and that nobody knows what is going on?' In this way, the direct question is addressed but the process of gathering concerns continues. You are back in SAGE because you have 'parked' the request about the scan. Alternatively, you find out immediately about the scan and then return to the other concerns.

Problem	Action
MISTAKING THE 'Y' OF THYME Some learners of the SAGE & THYME model mistake the You of THYME by wrongly interpreting this as a challenge to patients: 'What can you do for yourself?'	This is not recommended. It risks the unfair suggestion that the patient is not doing enough for themselves. Nurses should practise hearing themselves asking the correct questions as follows: 'What do you think would help?' and 'Is there something else that would help?' The questions relate to the patient's own ideas about what could be helpful: 'What do *you* think would help?' or 'What would help?'. These questions are important because research suggests that we should seek the patient's own ideas about what would help before we ask about what we can do to help.
NOBODY IN THE 'T' OF THYME Some patients will have no support. No people in their lives to help them think through or cope with the difficulties they face. This becomes obvious in the 'T' question in THYME ('Who do you have to talk to about your worries/concerns?').	In these circumstances, there is no purpose asking the 'H' question ('How do these people help?'). Move straight on to the next question: 'What do you think would help?'

Informing patients

Here we cover the principles of providing information to patients and discussing procedures to be carried out.

RELATED THEORY

Research conducted by the Picker Institute (Ellins and Coulter 2005) shows that 80% of people actively seek information about how to cope with health problems. Information is of prime importance in helping to support people in the decision-making process, particularly when they are vulnerable and feeling anxious. It is important that high-quality, reliable and evidence-based information should be accessible to patients, their relatives and carers at the right time, making it an integral part of their care (DH 2008a). This is reiterated in the White Paper *Our Health, Our Care, Our Say* (DH 2006), which states that 'people with a long-term condition and/or long-term need for support – and their carers – should routinely receive information about their condition' and the services available to them. Information prescriptions represent good practice for supporting the information needs of individuals (DH 2009). *High Quality Care for All* (DH 2008b) requires NHS organizations to provide accessible information to patients who have a learning disability.

EVIDENCE-BASED APPROACHES

With any procedure, it is essential that the patient (assuming consciousness and ability to make rational decisions) is psychologically prepared and consented. This requires careful explanation and discussion before a procedure is carried out.

As nurses, we can become so familiar with procedures that we expect them to be considered 'routine' by our patients. This can prevent us from providing thorough and necessary information and gaining acceptance and co-operation from our patients. We therefore need to avoid assuming that repetitive or frequent procedures do not require consent, explanation and potential discussion, for example taking a temperature.

It is important to consider giving information in small amounts and checking whether the patient understands what has been said after each part has been explained. Keep language simple and clarify common and complex medical terms, for example 'cannula', 'catheter'.

Check frequently whether the patient wishes you to continue to provide them with the same level of information. If confusion is arising, consider whether you are providing too much detail or using too many medical terms. Be aware whether the patient is paying attention or appears anxious (e.g. fidgety/non-attentive behaviour). Do not ignore these cues: name them. For example: 'I notice you seem a little anxious while I am describing this …' or 'You seem concerned about the procedure, what can I do to help?'. This recognition of behaviour will help to fully explore and support the patient's concerns.

Prior to starting, establish how the patient can communicate with you during the procedure; for example, confirm that they can ask questions, request more analgesia or ask for the procedure to stop (if this is realistic).

Information must be presented accurately and calmly and without 'false reassurance'; for example, do not say something 'will not hurt' or it 'will not go wrong', when it might. It is better to explain the risk and likely outcome. Explain that working with the nurse and co-operating with instructions are likely to improve the outcome and that every effort will be made to reduce risk and manage any problems efficiently.

Respect any refusal unconditionally; however, you may wish to explore the reasons for refusal and explain the potential (realistic) consequences. Document carefully and discuss with the multidisciplinary team. If a patient has had a procedure before, do not assume that they are fully aware of the potential experience or risks involved, which may well have changed.

Attention to good communication, honesty, confidence and calmness will help to reassure the patient, thus gaining their compliance and improving the potential outcome (Maguire and Pitceathly 2002).

Giving the right amount of information is important; for example, it has been shown that getting the level of information wrong (too much or too little) at diagnosis can significantly affect the subsequent level of coping (Fallowfield et al. 2002). Getting the level right can be achieved by simply asking how much people want to know and frequently checking if the level of information is satisfactory for the individual.

PRINCIPLES OF GIVING INFORMATION TO A PATIENT

The term 'giving information' implies that the healthcare professional's agenda is uppermost and results in a paternalistic model of care (Redsell and Buck 2009). Whilst this approach can at times be justified (e.g. in an emergency situation), wherever possible, it is important to allow patients the opportunity to be a partner in their care and to be involved in decision making (DH 2012b). In addition, the principles of 'facilitative' communication (Wilkinson 1991) remain relevant when giving information; this type of conversation is still a dialogue – therefore patients should be allowed time to speak, be listened to and to contribute.

There are many different theories and models for giving information to patients, but the following paragraphs are based on the principles of giving information taken from self-management and person-centred approaches to care.

Giving information implies that there is a message to be shared and someone who is to receive it. This means that the person receiving the information is able and willing to have information given to them. The first step to giving information is to assess the patient's readiness and ability to hear what is going to be said.

It is wise to ensure patients are comfortable and able to absorb information, so attend to analgesia, and allow them to visit the toilet if necessary. It is helpful to outline the purpose of the conversation at the beginning, before any information is shared – this will enable the patient to begin to actively listen, which requires concentration and is tiring. Therefore, make sure that the session is brief and that as much verbal information as possible is supplemented and reinforced with written and visual resources.

Patients should be asked their preferred role in the decision-making process before information is given, so that the style of delivery can be tailored to their preferences and wishes (Alexander et al. 2012, Redsell and Buck 2009). In addition, many patients will be well informed about their condition or have existing understanding or knowledge, so it is important to establish and assess patients' existing knowledge and ability/capacity to learn something new (Price 2013).

Information should be given in 'chunks' or small sections (Smets et al. 2013), pausing after a key point to allow the information to be absorbed and processed, and giving the patient the opportunity to respond, ask questions or make comments.

During the conversation, remember to use empathic statements (Egan 2013) and encourage the patient to express their worries and concerns. Giving information is more than a cognitive exercise – it also includes relational, affective aspects (Smets et al. 2013) and therefore, the principles of supportive communication apply, especially the need to notice, listen and respond to patients' cues and concerns.

Principles table 4.3 **Information giving**

Principle	Rationale
There are benefits if a patient is well informed.	Informed patients can better manage their health, illness, treatment and medication.
	Informed patients have lower rates of depression and anxiety.
	Informed patients have lower levels of pain, e.g. if they understand the causes of pain and the principles of pain management.
Be honest when giving information.	Patients value honesty from their healthcare professionals – it increases a sense of trust.
Patients can find it difficult to absorb information.	Anxiety, distressing symptoms, fear and denial can affect a person's ability or willingness to listen and retain information.
	Write down information so that there is a record of the conversation or instructions which can be followed. Keep the written information simple.
	Avoid using jargon or technical language or abbreviations when giving information to patients. If appropriate, use pictures, e.g. to explain anatomy. Colours can be used to colour code information if this would be helpful.
	Encourage a relative or friend to be present whilst information is being given – so that someone else is hearing what is being said and can support the patient later.
Information should be paced.	Giving too much information in one session can be overwhelming and prevent a patient from remembering what was said.
	Never rush information giving – patients will feel overwhelmed and exhausted. If you are short of time, give a small part of the information.
	Observe the patient closely – read their non-verbal cues and, if necessary, stop and allow them to process what they have been told.
Chunk and check.	Divide the information into small sections. Check that the patient has understood before moving on, e.g. ask 'Do you understand?', 'Is there something you would like to ask at this point?', 'Would you like to explain to me what I have just shared with you?'.
Encourage the patient to repeat back to you what you have explained.	You could ask the patient to explain what they are going to tell their family when they get home – this will help you to identify whether they have misunderstood anything you have told them.
Allow the patient to ask questions.	Listen carefully to the questions the patient asks you – these can indicate where misunderstandings have occurred.
Monitor the patient's response and non-verbal cues.	Receiving information is tiring. Be prepared to pause or stop the session and allow the patient time to absorb and process what has been explained.
Show empathy.	Remember that the information might have an emotional impact on the patient – acknowledge this and be supportive.

PRE-PROCEDURAL CONSIDERATIONS

Patient information

Patient information in this context refers to information about disease, its treatment, effects and side-effects, and the help and support available to people living with a chronic condition, their relatives and carers.

When writing information for patients and carers, consideration should be given to information already available on the chosen topic. The purpose of the information may be to:

- address frequently asked questions
- inform about a treatment or service
- reduce anxiety
- give reference material.

Ideas should be shared with other members of the team or clinical unit, and patients and carers involved, from the outset. The content of the material should be accurate and evidence based and meet the current Department of Health and NHS Litigation Authority requirements.

When writing the information, everyday language should be used as if speaking face to face and avoiding the use of jargon; 16% of adults in England do not have the literacy levels expected of an 11-year-old (DfES 2003). However, there is no need to be patronizing or use childish language. The Plain English campaign (www.plainenglish.co.uk) offers a downloadable guide entitled *How to Write Plain English*.

When producing written information for patients, it may be worth considering accessibility for patients who may be non-verbal or have a learning disability. An easy-to-read, information resource with pictures and images and few words can support people with learning disabilities to have a greater understanding of information and support their decision making.

Information should be dated and carry a planned review date. Sources of information should be acknowledged. This gives the reader confidence in the material.

The provision and production of information must take into account diversity in ethnicity, culture, religion, language, gender, age, disability, socio-economic status and literacy levels, as stated in the Department of Health publication *Better Information, Better Choice, Better Health* (2004). See Principles table 4.4: Giving information about a clinical procedure for the provision of information. Information should be ratified according to local trust policy. Where a trust does not produce patient information materials to meet specific patient needs, suitable alternative sources of information should be sought.

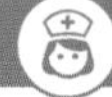

Learning Activity 4.5

Scenario: Patient information

You have been asked by the nurse in charge to explain to one of your patients about how to care for their surgical wound once they are discharged home. Using the principles of information giving (Principles table 4.3), how would you relay this information, ensuring they fully understand?

Other sources of information

Patients and their families may benefit from information and support available in the wider community, away from the environment of statutory health services. Sources of additional information include:

- *disease-specific national charities*, for example the Multiple Sclerosis Society or the British Heart Foundation: these organizations produce written material in booklet and fact sheet format, as well as having websites
- *the 'illness memoir' and internet blogs*: personal accounts are easily accessible online and through bookstores. It may help patients to hear other people's stories as this can reduce the sense of isolation and powerlessness and promote hope (Chelf et al. 2001). It must be borne in mind that not everyone will benefit from these sources of information
- *peer support*: the therapeutic benefits of groups are extensively documented (NICE 2004) and most of the support charities will have a directory of local and national groups available.

Principles table 4.4 Giving information about a clinical procedure

Principle	Rationale
Review the changing context of the patient's situation.	What may have been relevant before may now not be the same. People's circumstances and needs change. E
Prepare for discussion, ensuring you are familiar with the procedure, disease process, medication or other aspect of care to be discussed.	Accurate information giving is an essential part of nursing care. E
If possible, discuss the procedure some time before it is to be carried out for the first time. Provide the patient with leaflets, DVDs or videos, if available, so the patient has time to review the information at their own pace.	Give patients the opportunity to digest information in their own time (Lowry 1995, E). In certain groups it can be demonstrated to improve clinical outcomes, satisfaction, chances of meeting the targeted discharge date and quicker return to prior functional status (Lookinland and Pool 1998, R2b).
Introduce yourself.	Ensure the patient understands who you are and your role and specific aim. Promote patient satisfaction (Delvaux et al. 2004, R1b).
Maintain a warm and approachable demeanour. Do not rush.	Promote patient satisfaction (Delvaux et al. 2004, R1b).
Explain that you have a procedure to carry out, considering privacy in giving information.	Promote dignity/preserve confidentiality (NMC 2015, C).
Name the procedure. Elicit, clarify and check the information received by the patient.	Promote understanding and patient satisfaction. E

(continued)

Principles table 4.4 Giving information about a clinical procedure *(continued)*

Principle	Rationale
Explain the procedure, avoiding the use of medical jargon. Be prepared to repeat information or rephrase until the patient understands. (If the patient doesn't understand, they haven't consented.)	Establish mutual understanding. Gain compliance with procedure: minimize risk (NMC 2015, C). Improve outcome (Fellowes et al. 2004, R1a). Help patients manage side-effects and adhere to care and treatment Dwamena et al. 2012, R3a).
Confirm consent: ensure that the patient is happy for you to proceed. Allow the patient an opportunity to ask further questions or say no to the procedure. (If the patient fully understands what is involved, they may decide that they are not ready to proceed.)	Respecting the rights of the individual (NMC 2015, C). Obtaining consent correctly (NMC 2013, C).
Start the procedure, reiterating the main issues as you go along and keeping the patient updated on progress.	To maintain open dialogue and address issues and questions, as they arise. E
Make it clear when the procedure has finished and what has been achieved. Offer opportunity for discussion of implications, disclosing as much information as the patient wishes.	So that the patient is aware and has the information they need and want (Jenkins et al. 2001, R2b).

Communicating with those with specific psychological needs

Denial and collusion

DEFINITIONS

Denial is a complex phenomenon (Vos and Haes 2010) and can be considered a mechanism for slowing down and filtering the absorption of traumatic information, 'allowing for avoidance of painful or distressing information' (Goldbeck 1997, p.586).

Collusion is when two or more parties develop a shared, sometimes secret, understanding, that may involve withholding information from another person. It is important that health professionals resist invitations to collude with inaccurate patient understanding (Macdonald 2004). It can be argued that collusion is consistent with some patients' wishes (Helft 2005) and can be a necessary protection against unbearable facts and feelings (Vos and Haes 2010, p.227).

RELATED THEORY

Diagnosis of any potentially life-threatening illness is experienced in many different ways and can cause strong emotional responses. Patients are likely to feel a degree of distress and experience a wide range of emotions that may be lessened if healthcare professionals (HCPs) are truthful and open with patients about their diagnosis and prognosis.

People may use denial as a way of coping when faced with frightening situations. Denial can be conscious or unconscious and is commonly recognized in cancer settings (Vos and Haes 2010).

Literature on denial tends to be focused within the cancer field and prevalence rates are difficult to assess. Vos (2008) found that most lung cancer patients displayed some level of denial, which increased over the course of the illness. This was considered to be a normal phenomenon and not a sign of disturbed coping (Vos 2008). Denial may be conscious or unconscious (Vos and Haes 2011).

Nurses can be unsettled by the presentation of denial as it creates uncertainty about levels of understanding, coping and engagement with treatment. Family members and nurses can collude with patient denial, perhaps as a means of protecting the patient or themselves from facing the full impact and pain of the situation. Nurses need to be aware of the pitfalls of colluding with patient or family denial and consider how they may contribute to it.

As human beings, we live our lives in our own individual, unique ways and also deal with a life-threatening diagnosis in our own way. For some people, focusing on hope and cure is the priority, whilst for others it is first necessary to prepare themselves and their family for the possibility that their illness may be incurable. Denial is a complex, fluid process, as is living with a life-threatening diagnosis. Patients' understanding of what is happening to them can fluctuate from minute to minute.

Denial is not an 'all or nothing' phenomenon. A patient may accept his illness in the morning, but by evening deny that he has it (Dein 2005, p.251).

Medical and nursing staff, family members and patients may all be 'in denial' at some point – to protect either themselves or those they care about.

EVIDENCE-BASED APPROACHES

Assessment of denial

In order to try to understand as fully as possible the emotions that patients are experiencing and the resources they have for coping, a careful assessment of each patient's circumstances is important.

Nurses need to establish what information the patient has been given, before assuming that the patient is experiencing denial. We need to be sure that patients have been given adequate, digestible information, if necessary on several occasions.

It is helpful to view denial as a process (Vos and Haes 2011) and to see its expression along a continuum. This needs to be acknowledged in the assessment process.

Repeated assessments of denial may help us to understand how various factors might influence denial and to better understand its dynamic nature.

Complications

Balancing the reality of the illness with reasonable hope is often difficult for health professionals and caregivers (Kogan et al. 2013, Parker et al. 2010). When working with patients who we think are in denial, the challenge for healthcare professionals is not so much the confrontation of denial but rather the avoidance of collusion with it (Houldin 2000) as doing this offers the health professional the opportunity to avoid the distress.

Principles table 4.5 Supporting a person in denial

Principle	Rationale
Healthcare professionals should aim to provide honest information to patients with the use of good communication skills, to the depth and detail the patient requests.	This enables patients to have control over the rate at which they absorb and integrate news and information that may have life-threatening implications for them (Maguire 2000, R5).
Useful skills are those of listening, reflecting and summarizing.	This will establish a supportive relationship which in the future may provide the patient with the security to acknowledge the gravity of the information they have been given. E
If denial is affecting a treatment regime or decisions for the future, it may need to be gently challenged. This can be done by either questioning any inconsistencies in the patient's story or asking if at any point they have thought that their illness may be more serious.	These questions may help the patient get closer to knowledge they may already have about the seriousness of their illness. With the right support, they might be able to face their fears and be more fully involved in decisions about future care and treatment. E
If the patient remains in denial it shouldn't be challenged any further (Dein 2005).	'Confrontation, if pursued in an insensitive or dismissive way or in the absence of adequate trust and support mechanisms, may increase denial, may reduce treatment compliance, or may even precipitate a complete breakdown in the health care professional – patient relationship' (Goldbeck 1997, p.586).
The delivery of bad news and information giving needs to be recorded clearly. The degree to which the patient accepts the information is variable and needs to be respected and carefully documented.	Good communication can help prevent patients receiving mixed messages. E

Collusion can leave healthcare professionals, patients and relatives feeling confused. Recognizing collusion, challenging it and discussing our concerns with colleagues is important. Working with our multiprofessional team helps to improve communication and to ensure a collaborative approach to care. Drawing on the richness of experience of others can help.

Clinical supervision can provide a safe reflective space for healthcare professionals to explore their practice. It is an ideal place to explore the complex phenomenon of denial and collusion, and be supported with it.

Anxiety

DEFINITION

Anxiety is a feeling of fear and apprehension about a real or perceived threat and may cause excessive worry and heightened tension, affecting important areas of normal functioning (NICE 2011). The source of the feeling may or may not be known (Kennedy Sheldon 2009).

ANATOMY AND PHYSIOLOGY

Anxious feelings can result in physical symptoms related to the flight or fight response as the body responds to the threat, real or otherwise. The sympathetic nervous system releases adrenaline that is responsible for an increase in heart rate and therefore palpitations and raised blood pressure, faster, shallower breathing (hyperventilation), dizziness, dry mouth and difficulty swallowing, relaxation of sphincters leading to an increase in urinary and faecal elimination, reduction in blood supply to the intestines leading to feelings of 'butterflies', knotted stomach and nausea, increase in perspiration as the body seeks to cool down the tense muscles, and musculoskeletal pains (particularly in the back and neck) (Powell and Enright 1990). These are all unpleasant physical symptoms for the patient and can escalate further if not managed at an early stage.

RELATED THEORY

There are a number of theories about anxiety, its causes and how to manage it (Powell and Enright 1990). To be effective in supporting and communicating with a patient with anxiety, it is necessary to know that there are three aspects of feeling anxious.

- *Bodily sensations.*
- *Behaviour:* how the individual behaves when faced with the fear, especially if the behaviour involves avoiding it.
- *Thinking:* this is the ideas, beliefs and mental pictures about what might happen in the situation feared (Powell 2009).

Principles table 4.6 Supporting an anxious individual

Principle	Rationale
Listen to and incorporate individual needs and preferences to promote informed decison making about treatment and care.	If people feel in control they are likely to feel less worried (NICE 2011, C).
Be alert to the signs and symptoms of anxiety.	Early recognition and intervention may help to prevent worsening of symptoms. E
Encourage the patient to talk about the source of their anxiety if they can. Work openly to explore worries, information requirements and treatment options.	Patients may find some benefit from expressing their concerns and being heard. E

(continued)

Principles table 4.6 Supporting an anxious individual *(continued)*

Principle	Rationale
Listen and only when the patient has expressed all their concerns offer tailored information. Gentle challenging of misunderstanding about treatment, processes or outcomes may be beneficial if this is the source of the anxiety.	Information about a procedure, particularly an operation, can reduce anxiety and improve outcomes (Nordahl et al. 2003, R2b; Scott 2004, R3a).
If the patient doesn't know why they are feeling anxious, encourage them to describe what is happening in their body, when it started, what makes it worse, what makes it better.	Patient feels listened to and less alone, which may increase their sense of security and therefore reduce anxiety. E
Ask the patient if they have had the feelings before. What has helped previously (coping mechanisms) and what do they think may help this time?	The patient is encouraged to take control and apply their own coping mechanisms. E

Anxiety is a normal response to threatening events but can become a problem when it is frequent, exaggerated or experienced out of context (Blake and Ledger 2007). As levels of anxiety increase, awareness and interaction with the environment decrease, and recall and general function are also impaired (Kennedy Sheldon 2009). Anxiety can become a general and protracted problem, even when the immediate source of anxiety has abated.

EVIDENCE-BASED APPROACHES

Managing generalized anxiety is initially about early recognition and helping people understand the problem, providing them with appropriate information that might allay the source of anxiety. If this is not effective then people can choose between 'individual non-facilitated self-help, individual guided self-help or psychoeducational groups'. If these interventions are ineffective, individual high-intensity psychological interventions (involving cognitive behavioural therapy and relaxation) **or** drug treatments are advocated (NICE 2011).

Panic attacks (acute anxiety)

RELATED THEORY

The body has a normal response to fear and stress, but if this response is exaggerated, people might experience a sense of panic. A number of symptoms can be experienced including palpitations, nausea, trembling, weak legs and dizziness (Box 4.5). Panic attacks can have a sudden onset and may last 5–20 minutes (MIND 2013). The more these thoughts intrude, the more extreme the physiological response becomes (Powell 2009). An indication for many individuals that a panic attack is beginning is a feeling of tightness in the chest or being aware that their breathing is fast. If not managed, this progresses to hyperventilation (Powell 2009).

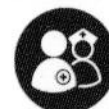

Box 4.5 **Criteria for defining a panic attack**

A discrete period of intense fear or discomfort in which four (or more) of the following symptoms develop abruptly and reach a peak within 10 minutes.

- Palpitations, pounding heart or accelerated heart rate
- Sweating
- Trembling or shaking
- Sensations of shortness of breath or smothering
- Feeling of choking
- Chest pain or discomfort
- Nausea or abdominal distress
- Feeling dizzy, unsteady, light-headed or faint
- Derealization or depersonalization
- Fear of losing control or going crazy
- Fear of dying
- Pins and needles in extremities
- Chills or hot flushes

Source: Adapted from Donohoe and Ricketts (2006). Reproduced with permission from Sage Publications Ltd.

EVIDENCE-BASED APPROACHES

Managing acute anxiety (including panic attacks) can help to avoid the development of a panic disorder and generalized anxiety disorder. Nurses can support patients to avoid anxiety attacks by taking time to talk issues through. If the anxiety has progressed further and the patient is experiencing the warning signs that they are on the verge of hyperventilation, it is helpful to:

- remind them that the symptoms they are feeling are not harmful
- help them to actively release tension in the upper body by encouraging them to sit up and drop their shoulders in a sideways widening direction. This makes hyperventilation more difficult since the chest and diaphragm muscles are stretched outwards
- breathe slowly … in to a count of 4 and out to a count of 4. (Slowing your own breathing down can help the patient)
- encourage them to concentrate on breathing out and trying to breathe through their nose (adapted from Powell 2009).

A panic or anxiety attack does not necessarily mean that the patient has a pathological disorder. Prompt treatment and management are important to prevent transient anxiety turning into a disorder (NICE 2011).

If the patient has a history of panic attacks and these become a prolonged problem for the individual, it is important to provide them with evidence-based information about treatment, including the use of medication (and its side-effects), self-help groups and individual intensive cognitive behavioural therapy (NICE 2011). It is important to include families and carers and support them to help.

PRE-PROCEDURAL CONSIDERATIONS

Pharmacological support

Panic disorder

Benzodiazepines, antipsychotics and sedating antihistamines are associated with a worse long-term outcome and pharmacological interventions should be either tricyclic or selective serotonin reuptake inhibitor (SSRI) antidepressant medication (NICE 2011).

Non-pharmacological support

The rebreathing technique

This involves the patient rebreathing the air they have just breathed out (Box 4.6, Figure 4.5). This air is high in carbon dioxide so has less oxygen. This means that there will be a lower amount of

Box 4.6 Rebreathing technique instructions for a patient

- Make a mask of your hands and put them over your nose and mouth and keep them there (see Figure 4.5).
- Breathe in and out through your nose once.
- Breathe in your own exhaled air through your nose.
- Breathe out hard through your mouth.

This should be done slowly without holding your breath. Repeat this four or five times but no more. Remain calm and relaxed while doing it.

Source: Adapted from Powell (2009). Reproduced with permission from Speechmark.

oxygen in the blood, thus activating the parasympathetic nervous system and promoting relaxation (Blake and Ledger 2007).

After the panic attack, it is important to reflect with the patient about what happened and try to identify any triggers. Explanation and education about physiological responses can help to show the patient the importance of slowing their breathing which will in turn give them a sense of control.

If these panic attacks continue or if the patient has a history of anxiety then the management of this will include a referral for psychological support (with consent). Medication may be indicated after assessment (NICE 2011).

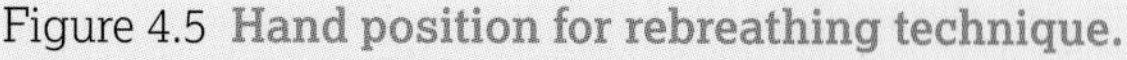

Figure 4.5 **Hand position for rebreathing technique.**

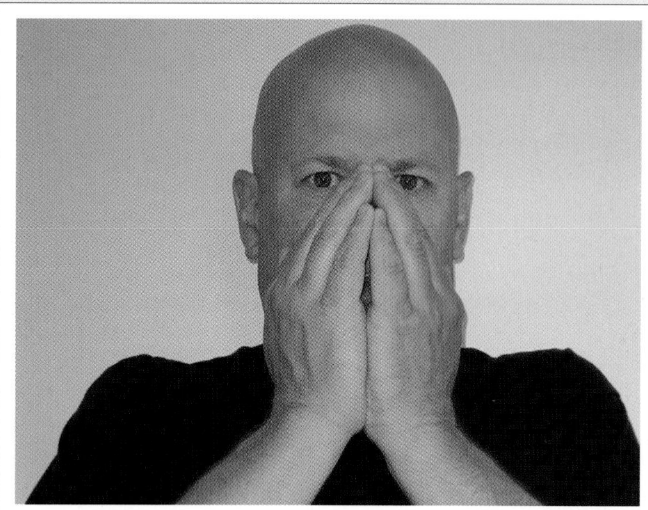

Principles table 4.7 **Supporting an individual having a panic attack**

Principle	Rationale
Firstly, exclude any physical reasons for the patient's distress such as an acute angina episode or asthma attack.	If the symptoms of a panic attack have a physical cause, management needs to be instigated as soon as possible. E
Remain calm and stay with the patient. Ask them about history of anxiety or panic attacks.	The patient will not be reassured by others reacting with tension or anxiety about the situation. E
Maintain eye contact with the patient. Consider holding the patient's hand.	This helps the patient to be connected to reality and engage with your attempts to support them. Some patients may be reassured by physical touch, but assess each individual for appropriateness. E
Guide the patient to breathe deeply and slowly, demonstrating where necessary.	This gives the patient an activity to concentrate on and may help normalize any carbon dioxide and oxygen blood imbalance. E

Depression

DEFINITION

Depression is a broad and heterogeneous diagnosis. Central to it is a depressed mood and/or loss of pleasure in most activities (NICE 2009b). Depression is often accompanied by symptoms of anxiety, and can be short-lived (sometimes dependent upon physical symptoms) or chronic.

RELATED THEORY

Depression is a common psychological response in patients with a chronic physical illness such as heart disease, diabetes and cancer. When this occurs, it is referred to as a 'co-morbid' depression. Co-morbid depression is difficult to detect as symptoms can be similar to the expected side-effects of the illness or treatment. For example, undetected depression rates in adult patients with cancer can be as high as 50% (Brown et al. 2009). Depression can be found in 20% of patients with a chronic physical illness (NICE 2009a), which is 2–3 times higher than individuals in good health. It is therefore essential that patients with a long-term physical illness are regularly assessed for anxiety and depression.

Box 4.7 sets out some of the symptoms of depression (NICE 2009a).

A normal low mood is differentiated from what is medically diagnosed as a depressive episode by the length of time the low mood is experienced. Low mood that persists for 2 weeks or more or rapid-onset/severe low mood are reasons for concern. The presence of other depressive symptoms contributes to a diagnosis as well as a consideration of how this low mood affects the individual's ability to interact socially. Depression frequently follows a pattern of relapse and remission and the key aim of intervention is to relieve symptoms (NICE 2009a).

EVIDENCE-BASED APPROACHES

Approaches to treatment of depression are influenced by the severity of the condition. Diagnosing depression has improved following the introduction of ICD-10 which lists ten depressive symptoms, dividing them into:

- subthreshold <4 symptoms
- mild 4 symptoms
- moderately depressed 5–6 symptoms, and

Box 4.7 **Symptoms that indicate a diagnosis of clinical depression**

Behavioural

- Tearfulness
- Irritability
- Socially withdrawn
- Changes to sleep patterns
- Lowered appetite
- Lack of libido
- Fatigue
- Diminished activity
- Attempts at self-harm or suicide

Physical

- Exacerbation of pre-existing pains
- Pains secondary to increased muscle tension
- Agitation and restlessness
- Changes in weight

Cognitive

- Poor concentration
- Reduced attention
- Pessimistic thoughts
- Recurring negative thoughts about oneself, past and future
- Mental slowing
- Rumination

Emotional

- Feelings of guilt
- Worthlessness
- Deserving of punishment
- Lowered self-esteem
- Loss of confidence
- Feelings of helplessness
- Suicidal ideation

- severe 7 or more symptoms with or without psychosis.
  - Symptoms need to be present for longer than 2 weeks.

Core management skills include risk assessment plus the following:

- good communication skills are required to enable the nurse to elicit information from the patient (Brown et al. 2009) and show understanding of the problem
- a sufficient understanding of the signs and symptoms of anxiety and depression and ability to make a preliminary assessment
- a sufficient understanding of antidepressant medication to enable an explanation of its actions to the patient
- an ability to 'refer on' when it is recognized that the issues are beyond the scope of experience. This must be done with the patient's consent
- awareness of the stigma attached to a diagnosis of depression, and protection of the patient's privacy and dignity
- sensitivity to diverse cultural ethnic and religious backgrounds considering variations in presentations of low mood
- awareness of any cognitive impairments or learning disabilities to ensure that specialist therapists are involved (where needed).

Use of available psychological support services can assist with the care and treatment of patients as well as providing a supervisory and support framework for staff. Working with psychological support services can enable nurses develop their assessment skills of anxiety and depression, helping them to identify the appropriate time for referral to a specialist service if required (Towers 2007).

PRE-PROCEDURAL CONSIDERATIONS

Pharmacological support

There are four main types of antidepressant: tricyclic, monoamine oxidase inhibitors (MAOI), selective serotonin reuptake inhibitors, (SSRI) and serotonin-norepinephrine reuptake inhibitors (SNRI) (RCPsych 2013). When a patient is prescribed antidepressants, the two main considerations are the presence of other physical health problems and the side-effects of the drugs which may affect the underlying physical disease.

There is little difference between the effectiveness of each type of antidepressant; however, there are clear differences in the side-effects of the different classes and types of antidepressants. Selective serotonin reuptake inhibitors are safer in overdose than tricyclic antidepressants (TCAs), which can be dangerous. There is, however, an increased risk of gastrointestinal bleeding with SSRIs so they should be avoided for patients who are taking non-steroidal anti-inflammatory drugs. Monoamine oxidase inhibitors can affect blood pressure, particularly when certain food types are eaten.

Serotonin-norepinephrine reuptake inhibitors are not appropriate for patients with heart conditions as they too increase blood pressure. Citalopram and sertraline (both SSRIs) are associated with fewer interactions and so are more likely to be prescribed if the patient has a long-term chronic condition (NICE 2009b).

Table 4.2 lists the most commonly prescribed antidepressants. The therapeutic effect of antidepressants may take some time to appear and treatment should continue for at least 6 months after a response to the treatment.

Nurses have an important role in exploring with the patient any concerns they may have about taking an antidepressant. The patient should be given all the necessary information regarding the optimum time to take the medication and the expected length of time before any therapeutic effect becomes apparent. Medication should be taken for at least 6 months following remission.

In general, treatment should not be stopped abruptly and discontinuation of treatment usually requires gradual reduction of dose over 4 weeks (NICE 2009b). Concerns regarding addiction require further information and reassurance confirming that this is unlikely to happen with modern antidepressant treatments. Further information on pharmacological intervention can be found in the NICE guidelines on depression (NICE 2009a).

Non-pharmacological support

Nurses can be involved in assessing depression in patients with physical illness. NICE guidance sets out a four-step model for managing a patient with depression. The first step (Box 4.8) could be managed by a nurse in an acute environment.

Assessment of how the patient's low mood has affected their usual daily activities such as eating, dressing and sleeping is important. The nurse can also encourage the patient to engage with activities that would be normal for them.

Table 4.2 Most commonly prescribed antidepressants

Medication	Trade name	Group
Amitriptyline	Tryptizol	Tricyclic
Clomipramine	Anafranil	Tricyclic
Citalopram	Cipramil	SSRI
Dosulepin	Prothiaden	Tricyclic
Doxepin	Sinequan	Tricyclic
Fluoxetine	Prozac	SSRI
Imipramine	Tofranil	Tricyclic
Lofepramine	Gamanil	Tricyclic
Mirtazapine	Zispin	NaSSA
Moclobemide	Manerix	MAOI
Nortriptyline	Allegron	Tricyclic
Paroxetine	Seroxat	SSRI
Phenelzine	Nardil	MAOI
Reboxetine	Edronax	SNRI
Sertraline	Lustral	SSRI
Tranylcypromine	Parnate	MAOI
Trazodone	Molipaxin	Tricyclic related
Venlafaxine	Efexor	SNRI

MAOI, monoamine oxidase inhibitor; NaSSA, noradrenergic and specific serotonergic antidepressant; SNRI, serotonin-norepinephrine reuptake inhibitor; SSRI, selective serotonin reuptake inhibitor.

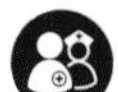

Box 4.8 Managing the patient with depression: NICE guidance, step 1

Key questions

1 During the last month, have you often been bothered by:
- feeling down, depressed or hopeless?
- having little interest or pleasure in doing things?

2 How long have you felt like this for?

If the patient answers 'yes' to question 1 and the time scale is longer than 2 weeks, it is important that a referral is made for further assessment by a healthcare professional with clinical competence in managing depression, such as a clinical psychologist or a registered mental health nurse, so they can determine if the patient has been bothered by 'feelings of worthlessness, poor concentration or thoughts of death' (NICE 2009a, p.4).

Other questions should assess for the following

- Other physical health problems that may be significantly affecting their mood such as uncontrolled pain, sleep disruption, excessive nausea and vomiting, physical limitations on their independence or body image disturbance.
- A history of psychological illness such as depression.
- A consideration of the medication the patient is taking, specifically medication for mental health problems. Have they been able to take it and absorb it or have they had any digestive issues?
- Social support for the patient: who else is around to support the person, are they isolated?

Source: Adapted from NICE (2009a).

Principles table 4.8 Communicating with a depressed person

Principle	Rationale
Initiate the conversation, develop rapport. Develop a person-centred communication style.	Good communication is essential to assess and individualize support (NICE 2009a, C).
Show understanding, caring and acceptance of behaviours, including tears or anger.	Accepting the patient as they are without attempting to block or contain their emotions helps them to express their feelings accurately. E
Encourage patient to identify their own abilities or strategies for coping with the situation.	Promote self-efficacy. E

Problem-solving table 4.2 Prevention and resolution (Principles table 4.8)

Problem	Cause	Prevention	Action
Patient expresses ideas of self-harm or taking their own life.	Low mood, depression.	Assess for risk: this can be as simple as remarking upon the person's low mood and asking them if they have ever thought of hurting themselves. Explore any expressions of suicidal ideas for intention to act. This can be achieved by asking if the patient has a plan. Crucially you will also need to explore what stops the patient from acting and what changes might cause them to act. If you consider the patient is at risk, explain to them that you need to refer them for further support.	If you have any concerns that the patient is at risk, follow the procedure of your organization. This may include contacting psychiatric liaison services or other psychological support.

Anger, aggression and violence management

DEFINITION

Anger is an emotional state experienced as the impulse to behave in order to protect, defend or attack in response to a threat or challenge. Of itself, anger is not classifed as an emotional disorder. This emotional state may range in intensity from mild irritation to intense fury and rage and becomes a problem when it is associated with poor impulse control.

RELATED THEORY

Nurses may be exposed to anger and aggression. Poor communication is frequently a precursor to aggressive behaviour (Duxbury and Whittington 2005). Aggression and abuse tend to be discussed synonymously in the literature and are reported to occur with some frequency in nursing (McLaughlin et al. 2009). Anger is felt or displayed when someone's annoyance or irritation has increased to a point where they feel or display extreme displeasure. Verbal aggression is the expression of anger via hostile language; this language causes offence and may result in physical assault. Verbal abuse may actually be experienced as worse than a minor physical assault (Adams and Whittington 1995).

Whatever the cause of anger or conflict, people can behave in a number of challenging ways and with varying degrees of resistance to social and hospital rules. People may simply refuse to comply with a request or may behave more aggressively, for example by pushing someone aside (without intent to harm) or by deliberately striking out at others. Mental capacity issues should be considered when assessing the causes of aggressive behaviours.

When patients do feel anger, they may feel too depleted by experiences of disease and treatment to express it (Bowes et al. 2002).

For some people, anger may be the least distressing emotion to display. Sometimes helplessness, sadness and loss are far harder to explore and show to others. Anger therefore can be a way of controlling intimacy and disclosure, but it can escalate to threatening, abusive or violent behaviour.

EVIDENCE-BASED APPROACHES

Prevention is the most effective method of managing anger; that is, diffusing stressful or difficult interactions before they become a crisis. Understanding why angry or challenging behaviour occurs can be helpful in establishing a comprehensive approach to prevention. NHS Protect (2013) proposes a framework for explaining challenging behaviour. This includes considering:

- *historical factors:* such as substance and alcohol abuse
- *current presentation:* diagnosis, physical factors such as pain
- *triggers or antecedents:* which include environmental factors such as other agitated individuals, busy or noisy areas and situational factors such as inconsistent staff attitude, time of day. Figure 4.6 presents this in more detail.

In some instances, challenging or difficult behaviour can be seen to be related to underlying stress and difficulty in a person's situation. Anger, aggression and violence may have 'biological, psychological, social and environmental roots' (Krug 2002, p.25). People frequently get angry when they feel they are not being heard or when their control of a situation and self-esteem are compromised. Institutional pressures can influence healthcare professionals to act in controlling ways and may contribute to patients' angry responses (Gudjonsson et al. 2004). Patients are often undergoing procedures that threaten them and they may consequently feel vulnerable and react aggressively as a result (NHS Protect 2013). Another source of anger can be when personal beliefs in the form of rules are broken by others. We therefore need to strive to be aware of individual and cultural values and work with them to avoid frustration and upset.

Figure 4.6 **Managing and assessing risk behaviours. A framework for explaining challenging behaviour.** ***Source:*** **NHS Protect (2013). Reproduced with permission from NHS Protect (www.nhsprotect.nhs.uk/reducingdistress).**

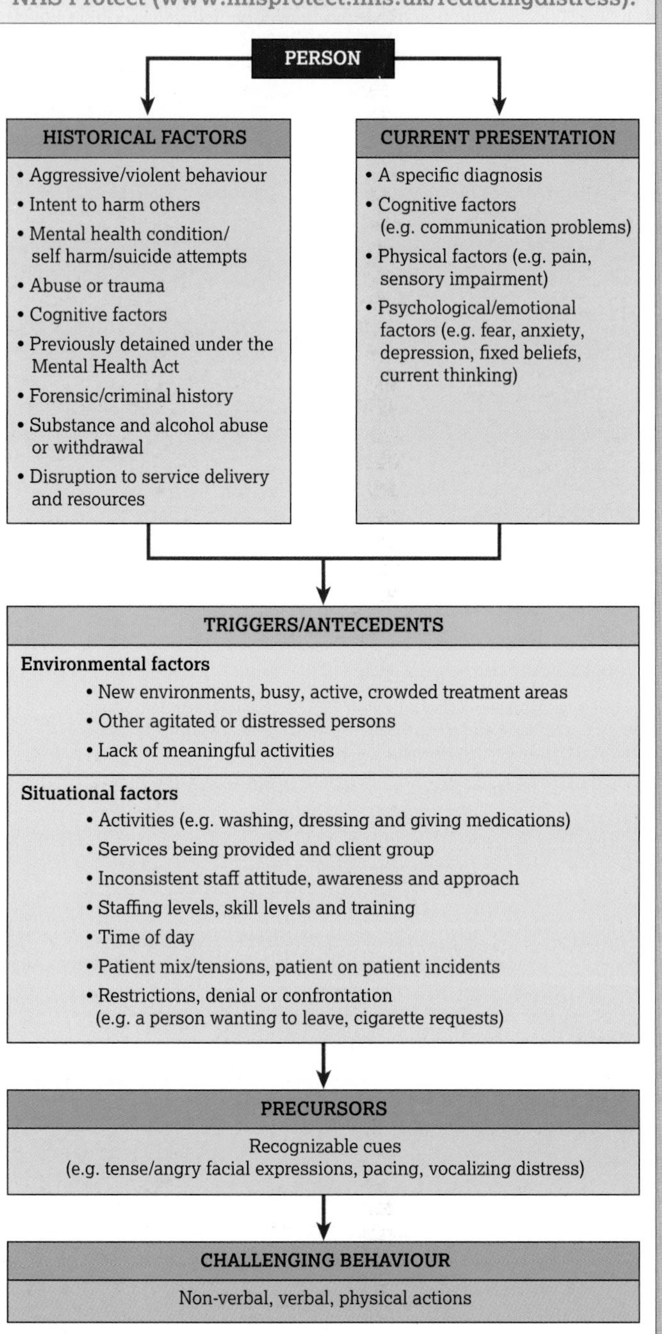

People also can become angry when they feel that they have not been communicated with honestly or are misled about treatments and their outcomes. To prevent people's frustration escalating into anger or worse, health professionals need to ensure that they are communicating openly, honestly and frequently (NHS Protect 2013).

Some patients may appear or sound aggressive when they are not intending to be and the nurse must therefore use good judgement to clarify their behaviour in these instances. Nurses need to be aware of their own boundaries and capabilities when dealing with challenging or abusive situations.

Threats, uncertainty and disempowerment may predispose people to anger, and living with and being treated for any serious

Box 4.9 **Warning signs that a patient is angry**

- Tense, angry facial signs, restlessness and increased volume of speech
- Prolonged eye contact and a refusal to communicate
- Unclear thought process, delusions or hallucinations
- Verbal threats and reporting angry feelings

condition can be sufficiently threatening and disempowering (NHS Protect 2013).

LEGAL AND PROFESSIONAL ISSUES

Nurses may be inclined to accept aggressive behaviour as part of the job (McLaughlin et al. 2009) due to being encouraged to be caring, compassionate and accepting of others. Despite this, nurses have the right to work without feeling intimidated or threatened and should not tolerate verbal or physical abuse, threats or assault. Personal comments, sarcasm and innuendo are all unacceptable.

Employers have a responsibility to adhere to Management of Health and Safety at Work Regulations (HM Government 2000, NHS Protect 2013). This involves providing a safe environment for people to work in and one that is free from threats and abuse. With any physical assault, the police should be involved.

PRE-PROCEDURAL CONSIDERATIONS

Assessment

Box 4.9 lists signs indicating that people may be angry. It is necessary to engage people sensitively and carefully to attempt to help them whilst maintaining a safe environment for all.

EVIDENCE-BASED APPROACHES

It is frequently possible to engage with and manage some of the underlying features without endangering anyone. People who are behaving aggressively probably do not normally act that way and may apologize when helped.

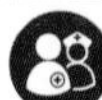

Box 4.10 **Phrases that might help when talking with an angry person**

- I can see that you are angry about this…
- I would like to help you try to sort this out, how can I do that?
- In order for me to help you, I need you to stop shouting.
- You are shouting at me and I can't help you until you stop.
- Please stop (unacceptable behaviour), you are making me and these other people quite frightened.
- Can you tell me what is making you so angry so that I might be able to help you sort it out?

Try to agree with the patient where possible (this can be a good way to defuse tensions).

- I can see how that would annoy you … let's see what we can do about it.
- What might I/we do, for you to … (comply with the rules/request)?

Talking down or de-escalation of situations where someone is being non-compliant can be achieved with careful assessment of the situation and skilful communication. NICE (2005) clinical guidelines on managing disturbed and violent behaviour recommend remaining calm when approaching someone and offering them choices. It is acknowledged, however, that there is little research indicating the correct procedure to follow. Box 4.10 suggestsphrases that might help when talking with an angry person.

Pharmacological support

Short-term use of a benzodiazepine, for example diazepam or lorazepam, may be indicated. Assess this carefully; that is, do not assume that it is necessary. Once a situation is more under control, you can ask if the person feels less angry and whether they feel that they need further support. Suggesting this at the wrong time or insensitively may inflame the situation.

A psychiatrist may prescribe an antipsychotic medication for short-term use, for example risperidone.

Principles table 4.9 **Communicating with a person who is angry**

Principle	Rationale
Remain calm.	
Verbally acknowledge the person's distress/anger and suggest you wish to help.	The person may respond positively and accept help (NHS Protect 2013, C).
Acknowledge issues that may be contributing, for example being kept waiting.	This helps the person feel that their concerns are understood. E
Consider what causes there may be, for example medication or disease (consider diabetes – hypo/hyperglycaemia), medical, circumstantial and so on.	Several factors might be influencing the behaviour. E
Consider safety – try to move to another area (ideally where you can sit down). If others might be intimidated or in danger, be clear about moving one of the parties away where practical, but do not endanger yourself in the process.	Maintain safety for all (NHS Protect 2013, C).
If a person's behaviour is hostile and intimidating, tell them you are finding their behaviour threatening and state clearly you wish them to stop/desist (see Box 4.10 for suggested phrases).	Some people may not be aware of the impact of their behaviour and will change it when it is pointed out that it is unacceptable (NHS Protect 2013, C).
Assess individual situations and make use of relatives or friends if they are present and can be of assistance in defusing the situation.	Sometimes people will listen more to a person who is close to them. E

(continued)

Principles table 4.9 **Communicating with a person who is angry *(continued)***

Principle	Rationale
Create some physical distance or summon assistance if the patient does not concur and continues to be threatening, abusive or passively non-compliant (e.g. refuses to move).	Maintaining safety for all. E
Warn the person that you will contact security staff/police if necessary – avoid threatening language. If possible, make a personal or practical appeal.	People need clear information about the consequences of their actions. E
Attempt to talk the individual down; that is, calm them down by remaining calm and professional yourself, keeping your voice at a steady pace and a moderate volume. Try to engage the person in conversation.	Your behaviour will have an impact on theirs (NHS Protect 2013, C).
Avoid personalizing the anger but do not accept unwarranted personal criticism.	If we personalize then we are likely to react in a way that exacerbates the situation but neither should you accept abuse. E
You may suggest walking with the patient to discuss issues but ensure you remain in a public/safe environment.	Changing the environment may help to recontextualize behaviour and movement channels agitation. E
The key communication skills discussed in the skills section will be helpful here but fundamentally you need to listen to what the grievance is, treat the person as an individual, preserve their dignity and attempt to help where you realistically can. Avoid passing the buck or blocking in another way.	People need to be heard and understood (NHS Protect 2013, C).
If a patient is no longer abusive or threatening but is struggling to reduce their anger, they may benefit from some further psychological support or medication to help them feel calmer.	The short-term use of some medication may be beneficial. C
In rare and extreme circumstances where patients are violent and do not respond to de-escalation attempts and where the safety of other people is compromised, you must take immediate action by involving security and the police. If they are an ambulant outpatient, you need to ask them to leave if their behaviour is not acceptable.	Maintaining safety for all. E
Restraint and sedation may be required in some cases. Follow individual hospital security/emergency procedures in these instances.	Maintain the safety of the patient and staff members (NHS Protect 2013, C).
Document the incident according to the hospital incident reporting process.	So such incidents can be investigated.

POST-PROCEDURAL CONSIDERATIONS

The ideal outcome for an encounter with an angry, aggressive or threatening person is that safety is not compromised and the healthcare professional is able to talk the person down, helping them to express the reason why they are angry. Follow-up support should be offered to help stop the person repeating the same behaviour. However, people should also be made aware of potential sanctions if they are unable to comply, for example withdrawal of treatment and involvement of the police.

It can be distressing to be exposed to threatening or abusive people and it is good practice to seek a debriefing interview. This can help you and the institution reflect upon the experience and procedures in place to manage such situations. Check with your occupational health or human resources department to establish where you can access support facilities.

Delirium

DEFINITION

Delirium is a distressing and underdiagnosed syndrome of acute alteration in mental state. The core clinical features that indicate a diagnosis of delirium are:

- impaired consciousness and attention
- disorientation, impaired recent memory, perceptual distortions, transient delusions
- psychomotor disturbances (hypo- or hyperactivity)
- disturbed sleep/wake cycle
- emotional disturbances (various) (ICD-10 1992).

Delirium can present in three forms.

- *Hypoactive delirium:* a subtype of delirium characterized by becoming withdrawn, quiet and sleepy.
- *Hyperactive delirium:* a subtype of delirium characterized by people who have heightened arousal and can be restless, agitated or aggressive.
- *Mixed:* with both hypoactive and hyperactive features.

RELATED THEORY

In most cases, delirium is caused by a general medical condition, intoxication or withdrawal of medication/substances which act upon the neurochemical balance of the brain (Ross 1991). Causative factors like infection, post-anaesthesia and medication (especially analgesics) need to be considered, particularly for sudden onset of delirium in the hospital environment.

The prevalence of delirium in hospital patients is between 20% and 50% (NICE 2010). Certain factors predispose to or are risk factors for developing delirium.

- Other serious illness such as uncontrollable cardiovascular or respiratory conditions, diabetes

- Multiple co-morbidities
- Older age
- Alcohol dependence syndrome
- Previous or existing other mental disorder, such as dementia
- Hypoalbuminaemia
- Infection
- Taking medications that affect the mind or behaviour
- Uncontrolled pain
- Taking high doses of analgesia (Irving et al. 2006)

Being an inpatient in a hospital environment can contribute to the development of delirium. The following factors can increase the risk.

- Patient not UK resident and/or English is not their first language.
- Changing clinical environment such as room or ward on a number of occasions.
- Absence of any means of gauging the time of day.
- Absence of family or other close friend.
- Catheterization.

The greater the number of risk factors present, the greater the likelihood of delirium developing (NICE 2010).

The disturbance can develop quickly and fluctuate during the course of a 24-hour period (DSM IV 1994). Environmental cues during the daytime act as stabilizing factors and this makes symptoms typically worse at night. The disturbance can resolve within hours/days or can last longer if co-existing with other problems like dementia. A patient's behaviour may change to indicate potential delirium before a full set of diagnostic symptoms is observable (Duppils and Wikblad 2004). There is considerable morbidity and mortality associated with delirium, delaying recovery and rehabilitation (Irving et al. 2006, NICE 2010). Recognizing and addressing delirium is important because of the distress it causes patients, families and staff (Lawlor et al. 2000). A marked feature of delirium is the variety and fluctuating nature of symptoms.

EVIDENCE-BASED APPROACHES

Nurses play a critical role in the prevention, early detection (Milisen et al. 2005) and management of delirium. Delirium is frequently iatrogenic (i.e. caused by medical intervention) and hence can often be corrected once the causative factor has been identified.

Addressing the causative factors as part of good nursing and medical care will help prevent the development of delirium. This means ensuring hydration and nutritional requirements are met and any electrolyte imbalances are monitored and corrected.

Nurses need to be aware that patients over the age of 65 (especially those having anaesthesia) will be highly prone to developing delirium so need to be monitored carefully over a period of time to pick up any early signs. The effect of analgesia (especially opiates) also needs to be considered.

The emergence of delirium can also be significant at the end of life and significantly complicate care (Delgado-Guay et al. 2008). Terminal restlessness is a term often used to describe this agitated delirium in end-of-life care, where the causes may require specific management different from that of other types of delirium (Travis et al. 2001). A progressive shutdown of body organs in the last 2–3 days of life (Lawlor et al. 2000) leads to irresolvable systemic imbalances. The management of delirium in end-of-life care therefore shifts from a focus on reversing the cause to alleviating the symptoms. Nurses should avoid medicating symptoms unless this is in the patient's best interests.

Principles of care

Initial screening for any cognitive issues on admission is important to identify predictive factors and establish a baseline of cognitive functioning. Involving the family can be crucial to an accurate assessment where there are existing changes.

If risk factors are identified, nursing care for an individual with delirium should focus on minimizing hyperarousal from the environment.

- Minimize the frequency of moving the patient from one ward/bed/room to another.
- Ensure that there is cognitive stimulation – television is working, patient is in an environment with other patients.
- Access to means of determining the time of day, e.g. clock/can see a window.
- Have access to hearing aids/glasses, etc.
- Encourage friends/relatives/spiritual advisors (if appropriate) to visit.

And in addition, nursing care should include optimizing physical health for the patient to maintain mobility (if appropriate), hydration and nutrition, and prevent constipation and incontinence. This will take place in parallel to the medical management which should focus intially on attempting to establish the potential reversible causes. These will include:

- newly started medications
- changes in dosage
- opioid toxicity, withdrawal from opioids or alcohol
- use of corticosteroids
- metabolic imbalances or organ failure affecting the processing and excretion of drugs
- infections
- hypercalcaemia
- constipation.

LEGAL AND PROFESSIONAL ISSUES

In the case of medium-term to longer-term delirium, another person may make decisions on the patient's behalf as long as this has been agreed as a part of a best interest assessment and the principles of the Mental Capacity Act have been applied. The best interest assessment must include the views of family or informal carers and the decision maker would generally be the lead clinician for the patient (Griffith and Tengnah 2008). However, if the patient has a Lasting Power of Attorney for welfare and this application has been registered with the Public Guardianship Office, then the relevant person will be able to make decisions on the patient's behalf.

The Mental Capacity Act sets out principles for protection of liberty when caring for someone with reduced capacity. This is reliant upon accurate and suitable assessment of capacity and best interests which are well documented and reviewed.

Physical restraint

Wherever possible, nurses must attempt to create an environment where restraint is not going to be necessary. It is a rare requirement and all feasible steps to avoid the use of restraint must be explored. Any action taken must be the 'least harmful' intervention in the circumstance. The aim is to balance the patient's right to independence with their and others' safety. However, if physical restraint is necessary to maintain the safety of the patient, then it requires careful ethical consideration.

Restraint takes many forms and must be meticulously judged for the potential to benefit or harm an individual. The delirium diagnosis prevention and management guidelines (NICE 2010) advise that the use of physical restraint should be a last resort, where the patient is putting themselves or others at risk of harm and all other means of management and deflection have been employed. When physical restraint is employed, this should be for the shortest period possible and with use of minimum force to ensure the patient is not harmed.

'Control and Restraint' is a formal term relating to a specific process for which training is required and clear procedures are to be followed. This is outside the remit of this book. The level of force applied must be justifiable, appropriate, reasonable and proportionate to a specific situation and should be applied for the minimum possible amount of time.

If restraint is required, nurses must explain to the patient why they are doing what they are doing (regardless of the patient's perceived capacity) and reduce the negative impact upon the patient's dignity as much as possible.

Documentation

Delirium is under-reported in nursing and medical note taking (Irving et al. 2006). Documentation outlining the onset of behaviours and symptoms is instrumental in assisting the medical team to identify the cause and likely solution to the problem. The documentation of the assessment and subsequent care must be detailed and accurate.

PRE-PROCEDURAL CONSIDERATIONS

Pharmacological support

Once diagnosed, symptoms that do not respond to non-pharmacological interventions can be treated with prescribed medication, including sedatives, for example haloperidol (NICE 2010). As far as possible, benzodiazepines are avoided as a side-effect of these can be delirium (BNF 2014). However, they may be used if delirium is caused by alcohol withdrawal.

Use of medication for sedation in the end-stages of life needs individual consideration and the family must be involved and communicated with regularly.

It is worth noting that health professionals and family members can mistake the agitation of delirium for symptoms of pain. If opioids are increased as a result, there will be a potential worsening of the delirium (Delgado-Guay et al. 2008).

Non-pharmacological support

Creating an environment conducive to orientation is important wherever possible, for example a quiet well-lit environment, where normal routines take place. Nurses must help patients to maximize their independence through activity as mobilization is seen to assist with orientation (Neville 2006). Nursing interventions include creating a well-lit room with familiar objects, limited staff changes (possibly requiring one-to-one nursing care), reduced noise stimulation and the presence of family or familiar friends.

Principles table 4.10 **Communicating with a patient with delirium**

Principle	Rationale
It is essential to ensure that aids for visual and hearing impairments are functional and are being used.	To maximize ability to communicate normally. E, C
Adjust environment to promote the patient's orientation, for example visible clock or calendar, photographs of family.	Maintain/promote orientation. E, C
Background noise should be kept to a minimum.	This can be very distracting for the patient. E, C
The healthcare professional should introduce themselves to the patient (do not assume they remember you). If possible, limit the number of individuals involved in care.	Promote consistency and reduce potential for confusion. E
Give simple information in short statements. Use closed questions.	Closed questions are less taxing and only require a yes or no answer. E
It is important to give explicit explanation of any procedures or activities carried out with the individual.	Maintain respect and dignity. E, C

POST-PROCEDURAL CONSIDERATIONS

Liaison with the patient's family is important so that they understand what is happening and what they can do to help. It must be recognized how distressing it can be to witness or spend time with a delirious member of the family. The family should therefore be given the opportunity to talk about their concerns and be updated with information about the cause and management.

Dementia

DEFINITION

'Dementia is an umbrella term describing a syndrome' (Westerby and Howard 2011, p.44). There are four common types of dementia and Elkins (2012) suggests that the percentages of people who have the different types of dementia are as follows: Alzheimer's (60%), vascular (15–30%), Lewy body (4–20%) and frontotemporal (2%). Weatherhead and Courtney (2012, p.114) state that 'dementia is not a normal part of the aging process, but almost all types of dementia are progressive and incurable. Dementia does not exclusively affect older people and so younger people can be affected and it is not uncommon for people with Down's syndrome to develop dementia at an earlier age'.

RELATED THEORY

Dementia can be caused by a number of illnesses and manifests as a decline in multiple areas of functioning, most notably mental and social function and ability to carry out activities of daily living (Westerby and Howard 2011). The number of people in the UK living with dementia is thought to be around 820,000 (Alzheimer's Research UK 2014) and it is thought that one quarter of inpatient beds are occupied by people who have dementia (Alzheimer's Society 2009). Older patients who have not had a formal diagnosis of dementia may not in fact have dementia but have depression which manifests in a similar way to dementia, demonstrating the importance of obtaining a diagnosis (Westerby and Howard 2011).

EVIDENCE-BASED APPROACHES

De Vries (2013) suggests that the 'decline in communication ability for older people with dementia is usually progressive and gradual, with the condition affecting expressive and receptive language abilities' (p.30). It is thought that those in the caring profession avoid communication with people who have dementia and this can have a negative impact on the person's experience and result in behaviour which can be challenging (Jootun and McGhee 2011). People who have dementia will frequently have word-finding difficulties so supporting communication can include finding suitable tools such as a communication book. The use of non-verbal skills such as simply allowing the person to point at what they want can help in the communication process. It is important to engage with the person with dementia and, although it may take more time, the results can be rewarding. Excluding or ignoring the patient can leave them feeling frustrated and angry (Tonkins 2011).

The use of family and carers is important as they may have a greater understanding of the verbal and non-verbal communication of the person with dementia. However, the involvement of family and carers should not exclude communication between the person with dementia and nurses; the person with dementia should be involved as much as possible in all communication relating to their care. As Jootun and McGhee (2011, p.41) suggest, it is important for the nurse to demonstrate sensitivity and to encourage the person to communicate in whichever way suits him or her the best.

Baillie et al. (2012) suggest that providing personal care to a person with dementia, if done sensitively, can help build on the relationship between them and the nurse. However, it is important to consider what the person with dementia might be experiencing. The person's reality may not be the same as the nurse's. The person with dementia may think they are at home and the nurse a family member.

LEGAL AND PROFESSIONAL ISSUES

The principles of the Mental Capacity Act apply to all patients and the first principle of the Act, the presumption of capacity, also applies to patients who have dementia. A person's capacity is decision specific and, as such, a person with dementia may be able to make decisions as long as they can show that they understand the decision they are making and the risk associated with the decision. If a patient with dementia declines care or treatment, they should be treated as an adult with capacity unless an assessment of capacity has indicated they lack capacity to make the decision. If this is the case, a best interest decision must be made in consultation with the patient's family. Where the person has no family and the decision relates to medical treatment or about where they will be living, a referral must be made to the Independent Mental Capacity Advocacy Service.

For people with dementia who are in hospital or a care setting, consideration needs to be given to the Deprivation of Liberty Act. If the patient is unable to consent to being in hospital and there are restictions on their liberty, they are not free to leave if they wish to, so they may be being deprived of their liberty.

PRE-PROCEDURAL CONSIDERATIONS

Equipment

People who have dementia may need no additional equipment other than the skills of the nurse communicating with them. However, tools such as communcation cards or books that allow patients to point to images may be very useful, such as images of the toilet, shower and food and drink.

Assessment

Assessing the pain of a person who has dementia and communication difficulties can also be challenging and so using non-verbal pain assessment tools should ensure that the patient's pain is appropriately assessed.

Principles table 4.11 Supporting communication for the person with dementia

Principle	Rationale
Be aware of what the patient's communication needs may be.	Knowing the patient's preferred style of communication or communication needs will enhance the patient's and nurse's experience.
Be aware of the patient's reality, orientating them and if necessary reinforcing this throughout the care intervention.	You may be speaking to a patient and they may not be able to understand the context.
Consider if the patient has other communication issues.	The patient may have a dementia but they may also have a hearing impairment and so they may understand what is being said but cannot hear what is being asked.
Consider the environment and the impact on the patient.	The patient may be distracted by the noise of a busy unit and finding a quieter space may help the communication process.
Avoid reinforcing a patient's reality when it is not real, and avoid telling them things that are not true.	Telling patient that a loved one, parent or husband has been dead for some years may be very distressing for the patient but so might telling them they are at home and they will see them later. Better to change the subject and orientate them to where they are.
Patients with dementia may need constant reorientation.	Due to anxiety and poor short-term memory, patients with dementia may forget what they have been told very quickly; for instance, when assisting with personal care or changing a dressing they may need to be reminded where they are.
Learn about the patient's past and occupation.	It is not uncommon for patients with dementia to behave as they did when they were in employment; for instance, a cleaner may want to go around the ward cleaning. These behaviours can give the patient a sense of value but can present risks.
Be aware of your body language and non-verbal communication; be open and approachable and be on the patient's level.	Patients with dementia may misinterpret non-verbal communication and this can cause them to become distressed or angry.
Use short simple sentences and avoid providing too many choices.	Patients with dementia may not recall everything that is being said, so shorter sentences will help; offering a choice of two at a time might be better than an entire list.

(continued)

Principles table 4.11 **Supporting communication for the person with dementia *(continued)***

Principle	Rationale
It is better to use closed rather than open-ended questions, such as 'Would you like a cup of tea?'.	Open questions can make it difficult for the person to respond, as they may struggle to remember the words they need.
If a person with dementia is struggling to find a word, help them find a way around it.	The person with dementia can become very frustrated when trying to find a word and may decide to withdraw from the conversation.
When giving instruction to the patient with dementia, give one instruction at a time.	To help maximize the person's independence; supporting them to do a task by helping them with the sequencing is enabling.
Avoid interruption when the person with dementia is speaking.	Interrupting the person whilst they are speaking may result in them losing what they wanted to say and can cause frustration.

Acquired communication disorders

DEFINITIONS

Aphasia/dysphasia (terms can be used interchangeably) is an acquired communication disorder that impairs a person's ability to process language. It does not affect intelligence but does affect how someone uses language. Any injury to the brain has the potential to change a person's ability to speak, read, write and understand others.

Aphasia may be temporary or permanent. Aphasia does *not* include speech impairments caused by damage to the muscles involved with speech; that is dysarthria.

Dysarthria is a motor speech disorder. Neurological and muscular changes may cause difficulty in producing or sustaining the range, force, speed and co-ordination of the movements needed to achieve appropriate breathing, phonation, resonance and articulation for speech (Royal College of Speech and Language Therapists 2006). Speech may sound flat, slurred, nasal or have a jerky rhythm; pitch, loudness and breath control can also be affected.

Dyspraxia of speech is different from dysarthria as it is not caused by muscle weakness or sensory loss but is a disorder of planning, initiating and sequencing purposeful/voluntary movement. Verbal expression may be hesitant with sound substitutions, for example saying 'tup of tea' for 'cup of tea'.

Dysphonia is a voice disorder and may be related to disordered laryngeal, respiratory and vocal tract function and reflect structural, neurological, psychological and behavioural problems as well as systemic conditions (Mathieson 2001).

RELATED THEORY

Language

It is now recognized that many areas of the brain are involved with language and cognitive processing and the complex relationship between structure and function is not fully understood. Impaired cognition is the most common deficit experienced by patients with primary brain tumours and has been reported to occur in up to 80% of cases (Mukand et al. 2001). Approximately 25% of patients with a primary brain tumour have a disturbance of language as part of their initial presentation (Recht et al. 1989).

The cause of cognitive and language impairment may be multifactorial and it may result from the location of the primary tumour, compression/oedema and/or as a consequence of treatment.

Cognitive and language impairments thus may not always have a direct relationship with the location of the primary brain tumour (Gaziano and Kumar 1999, Gehring et al. 2008, Scheibal et al. 1996).

Speech

Speech (dysarthria), voice (dysphonia) and swallowing (dysphagia) can be impaired by any brain tumours, involving the ventricular system, brainstem, cerebellum and cranial nerves (V, VII, IX, X, XI, XII), or by any tumour affecting the head and/or neck.

The brain is the organ of the body that is, above all others, linked with our sense of self. The importance of effective communication is considered at the beginning of this chapter and this need becomes more apparent with any communication disorder. Speech and language shape our thoughts, and language is necessary to make sense of or give meaning to our world. It is the currency of friendship (Parr et al. 1997) and is intrinsic and essential to our well-being. Its value and complexity may not become apparent until it is disrupted.

One of the key issues for patients with aphasia (disruption of language processing) is when we expect them to make sense of their disease, its treatment and management options. To do this, they need to use the very medium that is damaged – language. This may have an obvious or more subtle impact upon how the patient's psychological, emotional and social needs are met.

When patients have difficulty communicating, their sense of identity can become fragile and may be further undermined when they are in hospital. Understandably, in this environment, the focus is on their medical diagnosis, prognosis, treatments and side-effects. Facilitating their communication strengths allows us to help them understand, as well as supporting, acknowledging and respecting their individual needs.

Barriers to communication

- *Poor memory*: delayed language processing can further compromise short-term memory problems.
- *Reduced concentration and short attention span*: acute post-surgical; during and after radiotherapy treatment to the brain.
- *Distractibility*: increased sensitivity to background noise or visual distractions.
- *Generalized fatigue*: already using extra energy to process language, it becomes too effortful to chat.

EVIDENCE-BASED APPROACHES

Communication is a neurological function and the speech and language therapist has a key role in the specialist assessment and management of disorders/disruptions to this vital function (Giordana and Clara 2006). Patients with diseases affecting their central nervous system require input from a well co-ordinated multiprofessional team (NICE 2006), to support their complex changing care needs throughout the patient pathway (NICE 2006, NSF 2005, RCP, BSRM, NCPCS 2008).

PRE-PROCEDURAL CONSIDERATIONS

Equipment

Communication aids

Communication aids are referred to as augmentive or alternative communication (AAC). AAC may range from basic picture charts or books to electronic aids and computer programs and may support communication when the patient presents with a severe dysarthria or a severe expressive and/or receptive aphasia. Box 4.11 provides suggestions to facilitate realistic expectations and successful use of AAC.

Patients with various forms of communication difficulty

The person with aphasia

Principles table 4.12 **Supporting communication for the person with aphasia**

Principle	Rationale
Be aware of where the aphasic patient is within their disease trajectory.	
Be aware if the patient has impaired attention, concentration and/or memory.	This will affect what you say and how you check for understanding.
Minimize distractions, both visual and auditory.	Make it easier for both parties to concentrate.
Allow enough time, with a calm, friendly, encouraging approach.	Develop and maintain rapport.
Use a notebook to record key information.	This minimizes miscommunication particularly if the information is new or complex, the patient is anxious or their memory function is impaired.
Frequent signposting and checking of understanding.	To make sure the patient understands the purpose of the conversation.
Talk directly to the patient and ask them what is/isn't helpful.	So that communication is as effective as possible.
Have a pen and paper for both the patient and healthcare professional to use during the conversation.	Writing or drawing can support what is being said.
Speech should be clear, slightly slower and of normal volume.	To ensure the patient has time to process what is being said.
Use straightforward language, avoiding jargon.	Medical terminology is inevitably long and complex but can be clearly written in the notebook for future reference.
Say one thing at a time and pause between 'chunks' of information.	To allow time for understanding and for questions.
Structure questions carefully and make use of closed questions.	Limit the need for complex expression.
Regularly check the patient's understanding.	To ensure they continue to be involved in the conversation and are respected.
Declare a change of topic clearly.	It can be harder for some patients to recognize when the topic has changed.
Be prepared for their and your frustration. You might have to come back to a topic at another time.	Abilities may fluctuate, so what helps one moment might not work another time.

The person with impaired speech (dysarthria)

The dysarthria may range from mild, slightly slurred or imprecise speech to being unintelligible (this is different from aphasia where language is not affected).

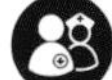

Box 4.11 **Suggestions to facilitate realistic expectations and successful use of augmentive or alternative communication**

- An early referral to the speech and language therapist to assess the appropriateness of the use of AAC.
- With the addition of any aid (no matter how simple or sophisticated), communication becomes more complex and difficult as it involves another step in the process; that is, it changes from a two-way to a three-way process.
- Patients need to be motivated to use aids.
- The use of aids requires planning, extra concentration and time, listening, watching and interpretation by both patient and conversation partner.

Principles table 4.13 Supporting communication for the person with dysarthria

Principle	Rationale
Be encouraging but honest and open if you are having difficulty understanding.	This allows the patient to repeat things or express things in another way that may be more understandable.
Ask if they use any strategies to help their speech.	Patients may well know what helps most.
Encourage a slower rate of speech and regular pauses.	Ensure adequate breathing between words and phrases.
Find a quiet environment to speak.	Reduce distractions and make it easier to concentrate.
Allow more time than usual.	So the person doesn't feel rushed while they are finding the words they wish to communicate.
Have pen and paper to hand, and encourage writing when necessary.	To provide another medium of communication.

The person with impaired voice (dysphonia)

The dysphonia may fluctuate from a mild hoarseness to not being able to voice at all. Early referral to a speech and language therapist for assessment and advice on vocal hygiene may be required.

Principles table 4.14 Supporting communication for the person with dysphonia

Principle	Rationale
Have pen and paper to hand, encourage writing when necessary.	Provide another medium of communication.
Encourage the patient to talk gently and avoid either shouting or whispering.	This can strain the voice.
Avoid having to talk where there is background noise.	To reduce the necessity for the individual to strain their voice unnecessarily.
Face-to-face communication is preferable. Keep telephone calls to a minimum.	The patient will then also be able to use non-verbal communication to transmit their message.
Encourage regular sips of water.	To maintain hydration and keep the throat area moist.
Use closed questions and discourage lengthy responses to questions.	So the individual doesn't need to make lengthy responses to questions.
Discourage frequent throat clearing. Instead, encourage a firm swallow if possible or gentle throat clearing.	To minimize straining of the throat.
Be aware if the room atmosphere is dry (placing a bowl of water beside the radiator will help humidify/moisten the air).	A humid atmosphere is preferable to reduce local irritation.

The person who is blind or partially sighted

Sight loss may vary from mild to complete. Any sight loss is a significant issue when caring for patients. They will rely more on other senses, especially their hearing. Good communication practice is essential and you may need to be the eyes for the patient and relay information they are not aware of; for example, the patient's visitor has arrived and is waiting. It is important to be open about the visual impairment and identify the preferred method(s) for each person. No single method will suit all. Even the same person might use different methods at different times and under different circumstances.

Blind and partially sighted people have the same information needs as everyone else and need accessible information in a suitable format such as large-print documents, Braille or audio information. Access to information facilitates informed decisions and promotes independence.

Principles table 4.15 Communication with a person who is blind or partially sighted

Principle	Rationale
Always say who you are when you arrive.	Visualcues are not available to the blind or partially sighted.
In situations where there might be confusion as to who is being spoken to, use the patient's name or a light touch when you are addressing them.	As above.
Explain precisely where you are.	So people can orientate towards you.

Principle	Rationale
Ensure glasses are clean and within reach.	
Clear and careful explanations and checking understanding verbally are essential.	We communicate a substantial essence of meaning non-verbally. Blind people therefore do not receive this information so it is harder to gain full understanding.
Indicate to a patient when you are leaving.	Normal cues are not available to the blind or partially sighted.

The person who is deaf or hard of hearing

As with blindness, the severity of the impairment will vary. If a hearing aid is used, make sure it is fitted and working. Remember that hearing aids amplify everything, even background noise. More severe hearing loss will not benefit from an aid and these patients might rely on lip reading and/or signing or writing.

Principles table 4.16 **Communicating with a person who is deaf or hard of hearing**

Principle	Rationale
Find a suitable place to talk, somewhere quiet with no noise or distractions, with good lighting. Make sure that the light is not behind you.	So the person can clearly see your face, and lip reading and expression can contribute to understanding.
Be patient and allow extra time for the consultation/conversation.	It is likely to take longer than normal.
Depending on the purpose of the consultation, writing down a summary of the key points might be helpful.	This will ensure the person has a record of what is said in case they have misunderstood or misheard what is said.
If the person is wearing a hearing aid, ask if it is on and if they still need to lip read.	This is because at times individuals may turn their hearing aids off because they aren't functioning or the interference from background noise is painful. They can then forget to switch the hearing aid on again.
If an interpreter is required, always remember to talk directly to the person you are communicating with, not the interpreter.	This is respectful and confirms that it is them you are addressing.
Make sure you have the listener's attention before you start to speak.	Otherwise they may miss crucial information.
Contextualize the discussion by giving the topic of conversation first.	Signposting helps people understand.
Talk clearly but not too slowly, and do not exaggerate your lip movements.	Lip reading is easier for people when you talk fairly normally.
Use natural facial expressions and gestures and try to keep your hands away from your face.	Blocking your face will make understanding more difficult.
Use plain language; avoid waffling, jargon and unfamiliar abbreviations.	Plain language will be more easily understood.
Check that the person understands you. Be prepared to repeat yourself as many times as necessary.	Many people need to have information repeated to understand it.

Learning for practice

After studying this chapter, list five key points you have learnt about communication that you will be able to apply to your clinical practice.

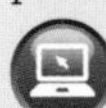 For further learning exercises visit **www.royalmarsdenmanual.com/student**.

Now Test Yourself

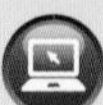

This section provides a range of exercises/activities to further test your learning. For additional exercises visit **www.royalmarsdenmanual.com/student**.

What have you learnt?

1 In non-verbal communication, what does 'SOLER' stand for?

2 Which of the following is NOT one of the six fundamental values for nursing, midwifery and care staff set out in *Compassion in Practice Nursing, Midwifery and Care Staff* (DH 2012a)?
A Care
B Compassion
C Communication
D Consideration

3 You inform a patient that you need to take his temperature, pulse and blood pressure. He agrees and puts out his arm. What type of consent does this demonstrate?
A Verbal
B Implied
C Written
D None of the above, consent is not required

4 What does 'SAGE' from the Sage and Thyme® model of communication stand for?
A Start, ask, gather, end
B Setting, ask, gather, empathy
C Setting, ask, gather, end
D Start, ask, gather, empathy

5 List three warning signs that indicate a patient may be angry.

See the end of the chapter for the answers.

Key points

- Communication can be heavily influenced by a range of external and internal factors, for example, illness, culture, class, self-esteem, immediate environment, gender, status, mood, depression.
- All patients and relatives should be assessed for their psychological needs and tailored support offered to meet individual needs.
- A range of verbal and non-verbal communication skills should be used when communicating with patients, with particular consideration given for those patients whose verbal communication is impaired.
- It is the professional responsibility of every nurse to communicate effectively and compassionately, respecting people's right to confidentiality, and involving patients in decisions about their care and treatment.
- Nurses have a responsibility to ensure that high quality, reliable and evidence-based information is available to patients and their families/carers in a timely manner.

Websites and useful addresses

Action for Blind People
Helpline: 0800 915 4666
Website: www.actionforblindpeople.org.uk

Depression Alliance
Telephone: 0845 123 23 20
Website: www.depressionalliance.org

Depression UK
Email: info@depressionuk.org
Website: www.depressionuk.org

NHS patient information toolkit, version 2.0 (2003)
Website: www.nhsidentity.nhs.uk/patientinformationtoolkit/patientinfotoolkit.pdf

Plain English Campaign
Telephone: 01663 744409
Website: www.plainenglish.co.uk

RNIB See It Right
Telephone: 020 7388 1266
Helpline: 0303 123 9999
Website: www.rnib.org.uk

Action on Hearing Loss
Information line : 0808 808 0123
Textphone: 0808 808 9000
Website: www.actiononhearingloss.org.uk

Royal College of Psychiatrists
Leaflet on delirium:
www.rcpsych.ac.uk/mentalhealthinfo/problems/physicalillness/delirium.aspx

Royal College of Speech and Language Therapists
Telephone: 020 7378 1200
Website: www.rcslt.org

Speakability
Helpline: 0808 808 9572
Website: www.speakability.org.uk

Stroke Association
Helpline: 0845 3033 100
Website: www.stroke.org.uk

REFERENCES

Adams, J. & Whittington, R. (1995) Verbal aggression to psychiatric staff: traumatic stressor or part of the job? *Psychiatric Care*, 2(5), 171–174.

Alexander, S.C., Sullivan, A.M., Back, A.L., et al. (2012) Information giving and receiving in haematological malignancy consultations *Psycho-Oncology*, 21, 297–306.

Alzheimer's Research UK (2014) *Defeating Dementia*. Available at: http://www.alzheimersresearchuk.org/dementia-statistics

Alzheimer's Society (2009) *Counting the Cost of Older People with Dementia in Hospital Wards*. London: Alzheimer's Society. Available at: www.alzheimers.org.uk/countingthecost

Argyle, M.(1988) *Bodily Communication*, 2nd edn. Abingdon: Routledge.

Arnold, E.C. & Underman Boggs, K. (2011) *Interpersonal Relationships – Professional Communication Skills for Nurses*, 6th edn. St Louis: Saunders.

Back, A.L., Arnold, R.M., Baile, W.F., et al. (2005) Approaching difficult communication tasks in oncology. *CA*, 55(3), 164.

Baillie, L., Cox, J. & Merritt, J. (2012) Caring for older people with dementia in hospital. Part one: challenges. *Nursing Older People*, 24(8), 33–37.

Berkman, L., Glass, T., Brissette, I. & Seeman, T. (2000) From social integration to health: Durkheim in the new millennium. *Social Science and Medicine*, 51(6), 843–857.

Blake, C. & Ledger, C. (2007) *Insight into Anxiety*. Waverley Abbey Insight Series. Farnham: CWR.

BMA (2007) *Mental Capacity Act. Guidance for Health Professionals*. London: BMA.

BNF (2014) *British National Formulary 67*. London: Pharmaceutical Press.

Booth, K., Maguire, P., Butterworth, T. & Hillier, V.F. (1996) Perceived professional support and the use of blocking behaviours by hospice nurses. *Journal of Advanced Nursing*, 24, 522–527.

Booth, K., Maguire, P. & Hillier, V.F. (1999) Measurement of communication skills in cancer care: myth or reality? *Journal of Advanced Nursing*, 30(5), 1073–1079.

Botti, M., Endacott, R., Watts, R., et al. (2006) Barriers in providing psychosocial support for patients with cancer. *Cancer Nursing*, 29(4), 309–316.

Bowes, D.E., Tamlyn, D. & Butler, L.J. (2002) Women living with ovarian cancer: dealing with an early death. *Health Care for Women International*, 23(2), 135–148.

Bradley, J.C. & Edinberg, M.A. (1990) *Communication in the Nursing Context*, 3rd edn. London: Prentice Hall International.

Brady Wagner, L.C. (2003) Clinical ethics in the context of language and cognitive impairment: rights and protections. *Seminars in Speech and Language*, 24(4), 275–284.

Brown, R.F., Byland, C.L., Kline, N., et al. (2009) Identifying and responding to depression in adult cancer patients. *Cancer Nursing*, 32(3), E1–E7.

Chambers, S. (2003) Use of non-verbal communication skills to improve nursing care. *British Journal of Nursing*, 12(14), 874–879.

Chant, S. Jenkinson, T., Randle, J. & Russell, G. (2004) Communication skills: some problems in nurse education and practice. *Journal of Clinical Nursing*, 11, 12–21.

Chelf, J.H., Agre, P., Axelrod, A., et al. (2001) Cancer-related patient education: an overview of the last decade of evaluation and research. *Oncology Nursing Forum*, 28(7), 1139–1147.

Chochinov, H.M. (2007) Dignity and the essence of medicine: the A, B, C, and D of dignity conserving care. *BMJ (Clinical Research Ed)*, 335(7612), 184–187.

Chou, A.F., Stewart, S.L., Wild, R.C., et al. (2012) Social support and survival in young women with breast carcinoma. *Psycho-Oncology*, 21(2), 125–133.

Connolly, M., Perryman, J., McKenna, Y., et al. (2010) SAGE & THYME™: a model for training health and social care professionals in patient-focussed support. *Patient Education and Counseling*, 79(1), 87–93.

Daniel, D. & Dewing, J. (2012) Practising the principles of the Mental Capacity Act. *Nursing and Residential Care*, 14(5), 243–245.

Dein, S. (2005) Working with the patient who is in denial. *European Journal of Palliative Care*, 12(6), 251–253.

Dein, S. (2006) *Culture and Cancer Care: Anthropological Insights in Oncology*. Maidenhead: Open University Press.

Delgado-Guay, M.O., Yennurajalingam, S. & Bruera, E. (2008) Delirium with severe symptom expression related to hypercalcemia in a patient with advanced cancer: an interdisciplinary approach to treatment. *Journal of Pain and Symptom Management*, 36(4), 442.

Del Piccolo, L., Goss, C. & Bergvik, S. (2006) The fourth meeting of the Verona Network on Sequence Analysis. 'Consensus finding on the appropriateness of provider responses to patient cues and concerns'. *Patient Education and Counseling*, 61, 473–475.

Delvaux, N., Razavi, D., Marchal, S., et al. (2004) Effects of a 105 hours psychological training program on attitudes, communication skills and occupational stress in oncology: a randomised study. *British Journal of Cancer*, 90, 106–114.

De Vito, J.A. (2013) *Essentials of Human Communication*, 8th edn. London: Pearson.

De Vries, K. (2013) Communicating with older people with dementia. *Nursing Older People*, 25(4), 30–38.

DfES (2003) *The Skills for Life Survey*. Norwich: Department for Education and Skills. Available at: www.dfes.gov.uk/research/data/uploadfiles/RB490.pdf

DH (2003) *Confidentiality: NHS Code of Practice*. Leeds: Department of Health.

DH (2004) *Better Information, Better Choice, Better Health*. London: Department of Health.

DH (2006) *Our Health, Our Care, Our Say: A New Direction for Community Services*. London: Department of Health.

DH (2008a) *Information Accreditation Scheme*. London: Department of Health. Available at: http://webarchive.nationalarchives.gov.uk/+/dh.gov.uk/en/Healthcare/PatientChoice/BetterInformationChoicesHealth/Informationstandard/index.htm

DH (2008b) *High Quality Care for All*. London: Department of Health.

DH (2009) *Information Prescriptions*. London: Department of Health.

DH (2012a) *Compassion in Practice Nursing, Midwifery and Care Staff: Our Vision and Strategy*. Leeds: Department of Health.

DH (2012b) *The Handbook to the NHS Constitution*. Leeds: Department of Health.

DH (2013) Report of the Mid-Staffordshire NHS Foundation Trust Public Inquiry. London: House of Commons.

Dimond, B. (2008) The Mental Capacity Act 2005 and the decision-making code of practice. *British Journal of Nursing*, 17, 110–112.

Donohoe, G. & Ricketts, T. (2006) Anxiety and panic. In: Feltham, C. & Horton, I. (eds) *The Sage Handbook of Counselling and Psychotherapy*. London: Sage.

DSM-IV (1994) *Diagnostic and Statistical Manual of Mental Disorders*, 4th edn. Washington, DC: American Psychiatric Association.

Dunne, K. (2003) The personal cost of caring. Guest editorial. *International Journal of Palliative Nursing*, 9(6), 232.

Duppils, G.S. & Wikblad, K. (2004) Delirium: behavioural changes before and during the prodromal phase. *Journal of Clinical Nursing*, 13 (5), 609–616.

Duxbury, J. & Whittington, R. (2005) Causes and management of patient aggression and violence: staff and patient perspectives. *Journal of Advanced Nursing*, 50 (5), 469–478.

Dwamena, F., Holmes-Rovner, M., Gaulden, C. M., et al. (2012) Interventions for providers to promote a patient-centred approach in clinical consultations. *Cochrane Database of Systematic Reviews*, 12, CD003267.

Egan, G. (2013) *The Skilled Helper. A Problem-Management and Opportunity-Development Approach to Helping*, 10th edn. Pacific Grove, CA: Brooks/Cole.

Elkins, Z. (2012) Optimising treatment and care for dementia patients. *Journal of Community Nursing*, 26(5), 9–14.

Ell, K. (1996) Social networks, social support and coping with serious illness: the family connection. *Social Science and Medicine*, 42(2), 173–183.

Ellins, J. & Coulter, A. (2005) *How Engaged are People in Their Healthcare? Findings of a National Telephone Survey*. Oxford: Picker Institute.

Equality Act (2010) Available at: www.equalities.gov.uk/equality_act_2010.aspx

Fallowfield, L. & Jenkins, V. (1999) Effective communication skills are the key to good cancer care. *European Journal of Cancer*, 35(11), 1592–1597.

Fallowfield, L., Ratcliffe, D., Jenkins, V. & Saul, J. (2001) Psychiatric morbidity and its recognition by doctors in patients with cancer. *British Journal of Cancer*, 84, 1011–1015.

Fallowfield, L., Jenkins, V.A. & Beveridge, H.A. (2002) Truth may hurt but deceit hurts more: communication in palliative care. *Palliative Medicine*, 16, 297–303.

Faulkner, A. & Maguire, P. (1994) *Talking to Cancer Patients and their Relatives*. Oxford: Oxford University Press.

Fellowes, D., Wilkinson, S. & Moore, P. (2004) Communication skills training for health care professionals working with cancer patients, their families and/or carers. *Cochrane Database of Systematic Reviews*, 2, CD003751.

Gaziano, J.E. & Kumar, R. (1999) Primary brain tumours. In: Sullivan, P. & Guilford, A.M. (eds) *Swallowing Intervention in Oncology*. San Diego: Singular Publishing Group, pp.65–76.

Gehring, K., Sitskoorn, M.M., Aaronson, N.K. & Taphoorn, J.B. (2008) Interventions for cognitive deficits in adults with brain tumours. *Lancet Neurology*, 7, 548–560.

Gessler, S., Low, J., Daniells, E., et al. (2008) Screening for distress in cancer patients: is the distress thermometer a valid measure in the UK and does it measure change over time? A prospective validation study. *Psycho-Oncology*, 17(6), 538.

Giordana, M.T. & Clara, E. (2006) Functional rehabilitation and brain tumours patients. A review of outcome. *Journal of Neurological Sciences*, 27, 240–244.

Goldbeck, R. (1997) Denial in physical illness. *Journal of Psychosomatic Research*, 43(6), 575–593

Griffith, R. & Tengnah, C. (2008) Mental capacity act: determining Best Interests. *British Journal of Community Nursing*, 13, 335–340.

Gudjonsson, G.H., Rabe-Hesketh, S. & Szmukler, G. (2004) Management of psychiatric in-patient violence: patient ethnicity and use of medication, restraint and seclusion. *British Journal of Psychiatry*, 184, 258–262.

Gysels, M., Richardson, R. & Higginson, I.J. (2005) Communication training for health professionals who care for patients with cancer: a systematic review of effectiveness. *Journal of Supportive Care in Cancer*, 13(6), 356–366.

Hargie, O. (2011) *Skilled Interpersonal Communication: Research, Theory and Practice*, 5th edn. Abingdon: Routledge.

Hase, S. & Douglas, A. J. (1986) *Human Dynamics and Nursing: Psychological Care in Nursing Practice.* Melbourne: Churchill Livingstone.

Heaven, C., Clegg, J. & Maguire, P. (2006) Transfer of communication skills training from workshop to workplace: the impact of clinical supervision. *Patient Education and Counseling*, 60, 313–325.

Helft, P.R. (2005) Necessary collusion: prognostic communication with advanced cancer patients. *Journal of Clinical Oncology*, 23(13), 3146–3150.

Hemsley, B., Balandin, S. & Worrall, L. (2012) Nursing the patient with complex communication needs: time as a barrier and a facilitator to successful communication in hospital. *Journal of Advanced Nursing*, 68(1), 116–126.

Henderson, A., van Eps, M.A., Pearson, K., et al. (2007) 'Caring for' behaviours that indicate to patients that nurses 'care about' them. *Journal of Advanced Nursing*, 60(2), 146.

Heyland, D.K., Dodek, P., Rocker, G., et al. (2006) What matters most in end-of-life care: perceptions of seriously ill patients and their family members. *Canadian Medical Association Journal*, 174(5), 627–633.

HM Government (2000) *Management of Health and Safety at Work: Management of Health and Safety at Work Regulations 1999 Approved Code of Practice and Guidance.* Sudbury: Health and Safety Executive.

Houldin, A. (2000) *Patients with Cancer. Understanding the Psychological Pain.* Philadelphia: Lippincott.

Irving, K., Fick, D. & Foreman, M. (2006) Practice development – delirium. Delirium: a new appraisal of an old problem. *International Journal of Older People Nursing*, 1(2), 106–112.

Jenkins, V., Fallowfield, L. & Saul, J. (2001) Information needs of patients with cancer: results from a large study in UK cancer centres. *British Journal of Cancer*, 84, 48–51.

Jivraj, S. (2012) How has ethnic diversity grown? 1991-2001-2011? *Dynamics of Diversity: Evidence from the 2011 Census.* Manchester: Joseph Rowntree Foundation, the University of Manchester. Available at: www.ethnicity.ac.uk

Jones, J. (2002) *Factsheet: Communication.* Worcester: British Institute of Learning Disabilities.

Jootun, D. & McGhee, D. (2011) Effective communication with people who have dementia. *Nursing Standard*, 25, 40–46.

Kelsey, S. (2005) Improving nurse communication skills with cancer patient. *Cancer Nursing Practice*, 4(2), 27–31.

Kennedy Sheldon, L. (2009) *Communication for Nurses.* Sudbury, MA: Jones and Bartlett.

Kogan, N.R., Dumas, M., & Cohen, S.R. (2013) The extra burdens patients in denial impose on their family caregivers. *Palliative and Supportive Care*, 11(2), 91–99.

Krug, E.G. (2002) *World Report on Violence and Health.* Geneva: World Health Organization.

Kruijver, I.P., Kerkstra, A., Bensing, J.M. & van de Weil, H.B. (2001) Communication skills of nurses during interactions with simulated cancer patients. *Journal of Advanced Nursing*, 34(6), 772–779.

Lawlor, P.G., Gagnon, B., Mancini, I.L., et al. (2000) Occurrence, causes, and outcome of delirium in patients with advanced cancer: a prospective study. *Archives of Internal Medicine*, 160(6), 786–794.

Levinson, W., Gorawara-Bhat, R. & Lamb, J. (2000) A study of patient clues and physician responses in primary care and surgical settings. *JAMA*, 284(8), 1021–1027.

Lookinland, S. & Pool, M. (1998) Study on effect of methods of pre-operative education in women. *AORN Journal*, 67(1), 203–213.

Lowry, M. (1995) Knowledge that reduces anxiety: creating patient information leaflets. *Professional Nurse*, 10(5), 318–320.

Maben, J. & Griffiths, P. (2008) *Nurses in Society: Starting the Debate.* London: King's College.

Macdonald, E. (2004) *Difficult Conversations in Medicine.* Oxford: Oxford University Press.

Macmillan Cancer Relief (2002) *Macmillan Black and Minority Ethnic Toolkit – Effective Communication with African-Caribbean and African Men Affected by Prostate Cancer.* London: Macmillan Cancer Relief.

Maguire, P. (2000) *Communication Skills for Doctors.* London: Arnold.

Maguire, P. & Pitceathly, C. (2002) Key communication skills and how to acquire them. *BMJ*, 325, 697–700.

Maguire, P., Booth, K., Elliott, C. & Jones, B. (1996) Helping health professionals involved in cancer care acquire key interviewing skills – the impact of workshops. *European Journal of Cancer*, 32A(9), 1486–1489.

Mathieson, L. (2001) *The Voice and Its Disorders*, 6th edn. London: Whurr.

McCabe, C. (2004) Nurse–patient communication: an exploration of patients' experiences. *Journal of Clinical Nursing*, 13, 41–49.

McCabe, C. & Timmins, F. (2013) *Communication Skills for Nursing Practice*, 2nd edn. Basingstoke: Palgrave Macmillan.

McCaughan, E. & Parahoo, K. (2000) Medical and surgical nurses' perceptions of their level of competence and educational needs in caring for patients with cancer. *Journal of Clinical Nursing*, 9, 420–428.

McEvoy, M., Santos, M.T., Marzan, M., Green, E.H. & Milan, F.B. (2009) Teaching medical students how to use interpreters: a three year experience. *Medical Education Online*, 14, 12.

McKenzie, R. (2002) The importance of philosophical congruence for therapeutic use of self in practice. In: Freshwater, D. (ed) *Therapeutic Nursing: Improving Patient Care Through Self-awareness and Reflection.* London: Sage Publications, p.22–38.

McLaughlin, S., Gorley, L. & Moseley, L. (2009) The prevalence of verbal aggression against nurses. *British Journal of Nursing*, 18(12), 25.

Mental Capacity Act (2005). Available at: www.opsi.gov.uk/acts/acts2005/ukpga_ 20050009_en_1

Menzies-Lyth, I. (1988) *Containing Anxiety in Institutions: Selected Essays.* London: Free Association Books.

Milisen, K., Lemiengre, J., Braes, T. & Foreman, M.D. (2005) Multicomponent intervention strategies for managing delirium in hospitalized older people: systematic review. *Journal of Advanced Nursing*, 52(1), 79–90.

Miller, G.R. & Nicholson, H.E. (1976) *Communication Inquiry: A Perspective on a Process.* Reading, MA: Addison-Wesley.

MIND (2013) *Anxiety and Panic Attacks.* Available at: www.mind.org.uk/information-support/types-of-mental-health-problems/anxiety-and-panic-attacks/

Mitchell, A.J. (2007) Pooled results from analysis of the accuracy of distress thermometer and other ultra short methods of detecting cancer related mood disorders. *Journal of Clinical Oncology*, 25, 4670–4681.

Mitchell, A.J., Baker-Glenn, E.A., Park, B., et al. (2010) Can the Distress Thermometer be improved by additional mood domains? Part II: What is the optimal combination of Emotion Thermometers? *Psycho-Oncology*, 19(2), 134–140.

Mukand, J.A., Blackinton, D.D., Crincoli, M.G., et al. (2001) Incidence of neurologic deficits and rehabilitation of patients with brain tumors. *American Journal of Physical Medicine and Rehabilitation*, 80(5), 346–350.

NCCN (2010) *Distress Management. Clinical Practice Guidelines in Oncology.* Fort Washington, PA: National Comprehensive Cancer Network. Available at: www.nccn.org

Neville, S. (2006) Practice development – delirium. Delirium and older people: repositioning nursing care. *International Journal of Older People Nursing*, 1(2), 113–120.

NHS Protect (2013) *Meeting Needs and Reducing Distress: Guidance on the Prevention and Management of Clinically Related Challenging Behaviour in NHS Settings.* London: NHS Protect. Available at: www.nhsprotect.nhs.uk/reducingdistress

NICE (2004) *Improving Supportive and Palliative Care for Adults with Cancer: The Manual.* London: National Institute for Health and Clinical Excellence.

NICE (2005) *The Short-Term Management of Disturbed/Violent Behaviour in In-Patient Psychiatric Settings and Emergency Departments Violence, CG25.* London: National Institute for Health and Clinical Excellence.

NICE (2006) *Guidance on Cancer Services: Improving Outcomes for People with Tumours of the Brain and Central Nervous System.* London: National Institute for Health and Clinical Excellence.

NICE (2009a) *Depression in Adults with a Chronic Physical Health Problem. Quick Reference Guide for Healthcare Professionals in General Hospital Settings.* London: National Institute for Health and Clinical Excellence.

NICE (2009b) *Depression with a Chronic Physical Health Problem: Quick Reference Guide: CG91.* London: National Institute for Health and Clinical Excellence. Available at: http://guidance.nice.org.uk/CG91/QuickRefGuide/pdf/English

NICE (2010) *Delirium: Diagnosis, Prevention and Managment, CG103.* London: National Institute for Health and Clinical Excellence.

NICE (2011) *Generalised Anxiety Disorder and Panic Disorder (With or Without Agoraphobia) in Adults: Management in Primary, Secondary and Community Care, CG113.* London: National Institute for Health and Clinical Excellence.

NMC (2008) *Clinical Supervision for Registered Nurses.* London: Nursing and Midwifery Council.

NMC (2010) *Record Keeping: Guidance for Nurses and Midwives.* London: Nursing and Midwifery Council.

NMC (2013) *Consent.* London: Nursing and Midwifery Council. Available at: www.nmc-uk.org/Nurses-and-midwives/Advice-by-topic/A/Advice/Consent

NMC (2015) *The Code: Standards of Conduct, Performance and Ethics for Nurses and Midwives.* London: Nursing and Midwifery Council.

Nordahl, G., Olofsson, N., Asplund, K. & Sjoling, M. (2003) The impact of preoperative information on state anxiety, postoperative pain and satisfaction with pain management. *Patient Education and Counseling*, 51(2), 169.

NSF (2005) *The National Service Framework for Long-Term Conditions.* London: Department of Health.

Oguchi, M., Jansen, J., Butow, P., et al. (2011) Measuring the impact of nurse cue-response behaviour on cancer patients' emotional cues. *Patient Education and Counseling*, 82(2), 163–168.

Ong, L.M., Visser, M.R., Lammes, F.B. & de Haes, J.C. (2000) Doctor–patient communication and cancer patients' quality of life and satisfaction. *Patient Education and Counseling*, 41(2), 145–156.

Parker, P.A., Ross, A.C., Polansky, M.N., et al. (2010) Communicating with cancer patients: what areas do physician assistants find most challenging? *Journal of Cancer Education*, 25(4), 524–529.

Parr, S., Byng, S., Gilpin, S. & Ireland, C. (1997) *Talking About Aphasia.* Buckingham: Open University Press.

Pennebaker, J.W. (1993) Putting stress into words: health, linguistic, and therapeutic implications. *Behaviour Research and Therapy*, 31(6), 539–548.

Perry, K.N. & Burgess, M. (2002) *Communication in Cancer Care.* Oxford: Blackwell Publishing.

Powell, T. (2009) *The Mental Health Handbook*, 3rd edn. Milton Keynes: Speechmark.

Powell, T. & Enright, S. (1990) *Anxiety and Stress Management.* London: Routledge.

Price, B. (2013) Six steps to teaching cancer patients. *Cancer Nursing Practice*, 12(6), 25–33.

Ransom, S., Jacobsen, P.B. & Booth-Jones, M. (2006) Validation of the Distress Thermometer with bone marrow transplant patients. *Psycho-Oncology*, 15(7), 604.

Razavi, D., Delvaux, N., Marchal, S., et al. (2000) Testing health care professionals' communication skills: the usefulness of highly emotional standardized role-playing sessions with simulators. *Psycho-Oncology*, 9(4), 293–302.

RCP, BSRM & NCPCS (2008) *Long-term Neurological Conditions: Management at the Interface Between Neurology, Rehabilitation and Palliative Care: Concise Guidance to Good Practice No 10.* London: Royal College of Physicians, British Society of Rehabilitation Medicine, National Council for Palliative Care Services.

RCPsych (2013) *Depression Leaflet.* London: Royal College of Psychiatrists, Public Education Editorial Board. Available at: www.rcpsych.ac.uk/healthadvice/problemsdisorders/depression.aspx

Recht, L.D., McCarthy, K., O'Donnell, B.F., et al. (1989) Tumor-associated aphasia in left hemisphere primary brain tumors: the importance of age and tumor grade. *Neurology*, 39(1), 48–48.

Redsell, S.A. & Buck, J. (2009) Health-related decision making: the use of information giving models in different care settings. *Quality in Primary Care*, 17(6), 377–379.

Roberts, D. & Snowball, J. (1999) Psychosocial care in oncology nursing: a study of social knowledge. *Journal of Clinical Nursing*, 8, 39–47.

Rogers, C.R. (1975) Empathic: an unappreciated way of being. *Counselling Psychologist*, 5, 2–10.

Ross, C.A. (1991) CNS arousal systems: possible role in delirium. *International Psychogeriatrics*, 3(2), 353–371.

Royal College of Speech and Language Therapists (2006) Therapists guidance on best practice in service organisation and provision. *Communicating Quality*, 3.

Ryan, H., Schofield, P., Cockburn, J., et al. (2005) Original article: How to recognize and manage psychological distress in cancer patients. *European Journal of Cancer Care*, 14(1), 7–15.

Scheibal, R.S., Meyer, C.A. & Levin, V.A. (1996) Cognitive dysfunction following surgery for intra-cerebral glioma. Influence of histopathology, lesion, location and treatment. *Journal of Neuro-Oncology*, 30, 61–69.

Schofield, P.E., Butow, P.N., Thompson, J.F. & Tattersall, M.H. (2008) Physician communication. *Journal of Clinical Oncology*, 26(2), 297–302.

Schroevers, M.J., Helgeson, V.S., Sanderman, R., et al. (2010) Type of social support matters for prediction of posttraumatic growth among cancer survivors. *Psycho-Oncology*, 19(1), 46–53.

Scott, A. (2004) Managing anxiety in ICU patients: the role of pre-operative information provision. *Nursing in Critical Care*, 9(2), 72–79.

Silverman, J.D., Kurtz, S.M. & Draper, J. (2013) *Skills for Communicating with Patients*, 3rd edn. London: Radcliffe.

Smets, E.M., Hillen, M.A., Douma, K.F., et al. (2013) Does being informed and feeling informed affect patients' trust in their radiation oncologist? *Patient Education and Counseling*, 90(3), 330–337.

Smith, C., Dickens, C. & Edwards, S. (2005) Provision of information for cancer patients: an appraisal and review. *European Journal of Cancer Care*, 14, 282–288.

Stewart, M.A. (1996) Effective physician-patient communication and health outcomes: a review. *Canadian Medical Association Journal*, 152, 1423–1433.

Strachan, H. (2004) Nursing information. *Communication. Research and Theory for Nursing Practice*, 18(1), 7–10.

Tate, P. (2010) *The Doctor's Communication Handbook.* London: Radcliffe Medical Press.

Taylor, B. (1998) Ordinariness in nursing as therapy. In: McMahon, R. & Pearson, A. (eds) *Nursing as Therapy.* Cheltenham: Stanley Thornes, pp. 64–75.

Taylor, C., Graham, J., Potts, H., Richards, M. and Ramirez, A. (2005) Changes in mental health of UK hospital consultants since the mid-1990s. *Lancet*, 366(9487), 742–744.

Thoits, P.A. (1995) Stress, coping, and social support processes: where are we? What next? *Journal of Health and Social Behavior,* Spec No, 53–79.

Thorne, S.E., Kuo, M., Armstrong, E.-A., et al. (2005) 'Being known': patients' perspectives of the dynamics of human connection in cancer care. *Psycho-Oncology*, 14(10), 887.

Tonkins, S. (2011) Dementia care. (Based on NS581 Jootun, D. & McGhee, G. (2011) Effective communication with people who have dementia. *Nursing Standard*, 25, 40–46.) *Nursing Standard,* 25(50), 59.

Tortora, G.J. & Derrickson, B.H. (2011) *Principles of Anatomy & Physiology*, 13th edn. Hoboken, NJ: John Wiley & Sons.

Towers, R. (2007) Providing psychological support for patients with cancer. *Nursing Standard*, 28(12), 50–58.

Travis, S., Conway, J., Daly, M. & Larsen, P. (2001) Terminal restlessness in the nursing facility: assessment, palliation, and symptom management. *Geriatric Nursing*, 22(6), 308–312.

Turner, J., Clavarino, A., Yates, P., et al. (2007) Oncology nurses' perceptions of their supportive care for patients with advanced cancer: challenges and educational needs. *Psycho-Oncology*, 16, 149–157.

Uitterhoeve, R.J., Bensing, J.M., Grol, R.P., et al. (2010) The effect of communication skills training on patient outcomes in cancer care: a systematic review of the literature. *European Journal of Cancer Care (English Language Edition)*, 19(4), 442–457.

Vos, M.S. (2008) Denial in lung cancer patients: a longitudinal study. *Psycho-Oncology*, 17, 1163–1171.

Vos, M.S. & de Haes, H.J. (2010) Complex rather than vague. *Lung Cancer*, 70(2), 227–228.

Vos, M.S. & de Haes, H.J. (2011) Denial indeed is a process. *Lung Cancer*, 72(1), 138.

Weatherhead, I. & Courtney, C. (2012) Assessing the signs of dementia. *Practice Nursing*, 23(3), 114–118.

Webster, C. & Bryan, K. (2009) Older people's views of dignity and how it can be promoted in a hospital environment. *Journal of Clinical Nursing*, 18(12), 1784–1792.

Westerby, R. & Howard, S. (2011) Early recognition and diagnosis. *Practice Nurse*, 42(16), 42–47.

White, H. (2004) Acquired communication and swallowing difficulties in patients with primary brain tumours. In: Booth, S. & Bruera, E. (eds) *Palliative Care Consultations Primary and Metastatic Brain Tumours.* Oxford: Oxford University Press, pp. 117–134.

Wilkinson, S. (1991) Factors which influence how nurses communicate with cancer patients. *Journal of Advanced Nursing*, 16, 677–688.

Williams, A.M & Iruita, V.F (2004) Therapeutic and non-therapeutic interpersonal interactions: the patient's persepctive. *Journal of Clinical Nursing*, 13(7) 806–815.

Wosket, V. (2006) *Egan's Skilled Helper Model: Developments and Applications in Counselling.* London: Routledge.

Young, T. (2012) Devising a dementia toolkit for effective communication. *Nursing & Residential Care*, 14(3), 149–151.

Answers

Learning Activity 4.4 Case study: Consent

Rose is a 79-year-old woman with dementia. She is having a pre-operative assessment prior to having a right hip replacement due to severe osteoarthritis. Rose has come to the department with her daughter, who lives with her and is her main carer. Her daughter informs you that Rose is capable of following simple instructions but she is struggling to understand why she is visiting the hospital today.

What steps do you need to take in order to gain consent for Rose to have her operation?

- Give a full explanation of the procedure to Rose and her daughter.
- Identify, with her daughter, the best way to communicate with Rose in order to help her understand the procedure, its consequences and potential complications (for example, short, simple sentences, closed questions).
- Establish whether Rose has the capacity to make a decision about consent (do not assume that Rose is unable to make such a decision).
- Refer to the multidisciplinary team to assess whether Rose is lacking capacity (in accordance with the Mental Capacity Act, 2005) and whether a best interest decision should be made in consultation with her daughter.

Now Test Yourself What have you learnt?

1 In non-verbal communication, what does 'SOLER' stand for?

Facing patient	**S**quarely
Maintaining	**O**pen posture
	Leaning slightly towards the patient
Having	**E**ye contact
Being	**R**elaxed

2 Which of the following is NOT one of the six fundamental values for nursing, midwifery and care staff set out in *Compassion in Practice Nursing, Midwifery and Care Staff* (DH 2012a)?
A Care
B Compassion
C Communication
D Consideration

3 You inform a patient that you need to take his temperature, pulse and blood pressure. He agrees and puts out his arm. What type of consent does this demonstrate?
A Verbal
B Implied
C Written
D None of the above, consent is not required

4 What does 'SAGE' from the Sage and Thyme® model of communication stand for?
A Start, ask, gather, end
B Setting, ask, gather, empathy
C Setting, ask, gather, end
D Start, ask, gather, empathy

5 List three warning signs that indicate a patient may be angry.
See Box 4.9 for the answers.

Elimination

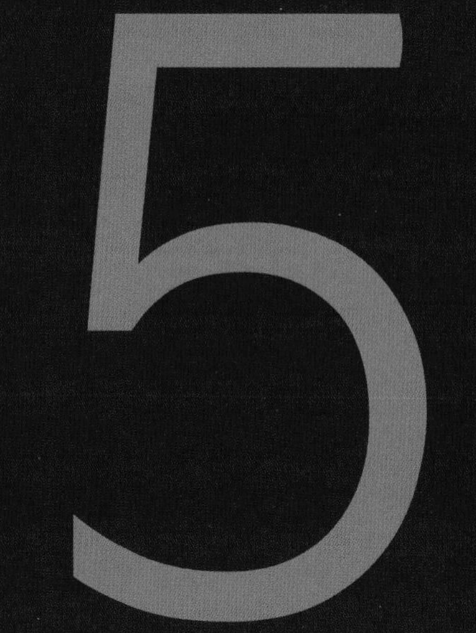

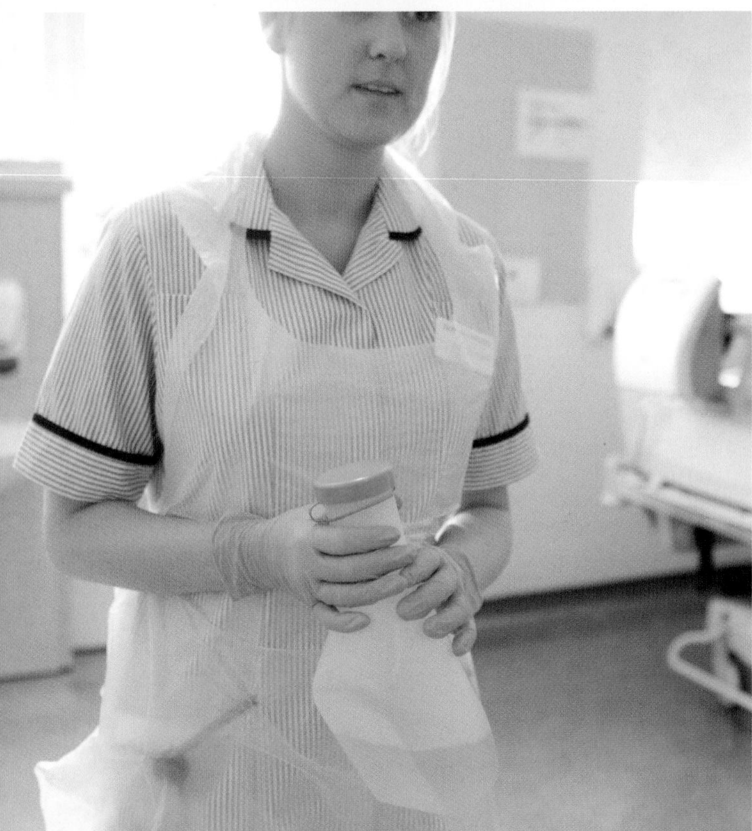

By reading this chapter and undertaking the learning activities within it, you should be able to:

1. Discuss the processes of normal elimination.
2. Identify different strategies to manage altered urinary elimination.
3. Demonstrate an ability to explore and discuss strategies to assess and support a patient with altered faecal elimination.
4. Demonstrate knowledge of the considerations prior to stoma formation and care of the patient with a newly formed stoma.

Procedure guidelines

The Royal Marsden Manual of Clinical Nursing Procedures: Student Edition, Ninth Edition. Edited by Lisa Dougherty, Sara Lister and Alexandra West-Oram

Overview

This chapter will provide an overview of elimination and is divided into four main sections. The first reviews normal elimination. The second examines altered urinary elimination, including penile sheaths, urinary catheterization, urinary diversions and bladder irrigation. The third section considers altered faecal elimination, including diarrhoea, constipation, enemas, suppositories, digital rectal examination and digital removal of faeces. The final section provides an overview of stoma care.

Normal elimination

This section reviews normal elimination processes including vomiting, urination and defaecation.

Vomiting

DEFINITION

Vomiting is a co-ordinated reflex whereby the diaphragm contracts, resulting in changes in intrathoracic pressure causing the forceful expulsion of gastric or intestinal contents through the oral cavity (Bennett 2009, Campos de Carvalho et al. 2007, Kelly and Ward 2013). Vomiting, and the associated sensation of nausea, are significant and distressing symptoms that patients may experience as a result of either disease or treatment (Bennett 2009). Post-operative nausea and vomiting affects up to 30% of surgical patients (Abraham 2008). Around 70–80% of cancer patients receiving chemotherapy experience nausea and vomiting associated with their treatment (Richardson et al. 2007) while approximately 60% of patients with advanced cancer report nausea and 30% report vomiting (Davis and Walsh 2000). Nausea and vomiting is experienced by 17–49% of patients with advanced non-malignant disease, including heart disease and kidney failure (Kelly and Ward 2013) and Twycross et al. (2009) report that nausea and vomiting is experienced by up to 70% of patients in their last week of life.

ANATOMY AND PHYSIOLOGY

The pathophysiology of nausea and vomiting is complex (Figure 5.1); two main centres within the brainstem are involved: the chemoreceptor trigger zone (CTZ) and the vomiting centre (Kelly and Ward 2013). Vomiting is ultimately controlled by the vomiting centre which receives input from a wide range of sources. Some of these inputs are directly connected to the vomiting centre but most are directed through the CTZ (Bennett 2009, Kelly and Ward 2013). The CTZ is an area of the brain that is not fully separated from the blood by the blood–brain barrier, allowing it to detect chemicals in the blood and cerebrospinal fluid and initiate vomiting where necessary. It is also stimulated by the vagus and vestibular nerves, which receive signals from the gut and inner ear respectively (Bennett 2009, Kelly and Ward 2013).

The causes of vomiting are often multifactorial and therefore thorough assessment of the risk factors, precipitating factors and alleviating factors is the key to identifying effective strategies for managing this symptom (Box 5.1).

Figure 5.1 **The emetic pathway.** ***Source:*** **Kelly and Ward (2013). Reproduced with permission from EMAP Publishing Ltd.**

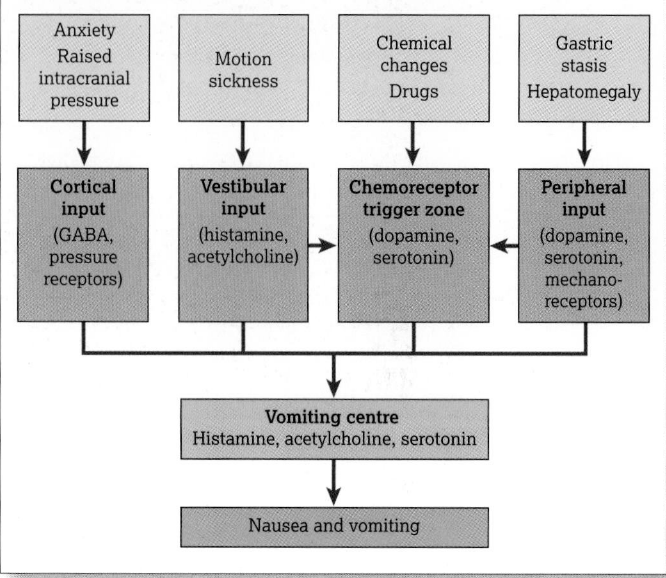

EVIDENCE-BASED APPROACHES

Assessment

Assessment may either focus on risk factors in the case of post-operative nausea and vomiting, in order to prevent or minimize the symptom occurring, or identifying causative factors where patients are already experiencing the symptoms. Risk assessment tools for post-operative nausea and vomiting consider a range of factors relating to the patient themselves (e.g. gender, age, history of motion sickness, smoker), the surgical procedure (e.g. duration, open versus laparoscopic, type of surgery) and the anaesthetic (e.g. type of agent, duration, premedication, use of opioids) (Hambridge 2013). In those patients who are already experiencing nausea and vomiting associated with other causes, a consistent and systematic approach should be used to determine the cause where possible and assess their symptoms (Kelly and Ward 2013).

Pharmacological and non-pharmacological approaches

Nausea and vomiting can be managed using pharmacological and non-pharmacological interventions. There are a range of non-pharmacological strategies available to manage nausea and vomiting. First, consideration needs to be given to any precipitating factors that can be controlled or removed, such as exposure to food

Box 5.1 **Common causes of vomiting**

- Direct irritation of the throat, oesophagus, stomach or intestine (e.g. food poisoning).
- Anticipatory vomiting: situations which have previously been associated with vomiting.
- Sensory stimuli: strong smells or tastes, seeing others vomiting.
- Toxins: presence of drugs or other toxins (e.g. alcohol) in the bloodstream.
- Disruption of the inner ear: motion sickness, middle ear infections, physical trauma.
- Organic disease or conditions: migraines, certain tumours.
- Recent surgery: either as a direct result of surgery to the gut or surrounding organs or from the drugs used perioperatively.
- Pregnancy.

Source: Adapted from Bennett (2009).

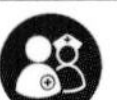

Box 5.2 **Classes of antiemetics**

Antihistamines

- Antihistamines block the histamine H1 receptor and are widely used. The main side-effects are the sedative potential and anticholinergic side-effects (e.g. dry mouth, constipation). Cyclizine tends to be less sedating than other antihistamines and is commonly used as a first-line treatment for post-operative nausea and vomiting or motion sickness.

Dopamine antagonists

Act by blocking the dopamine D2 receptors in the chemoreceptor trigger zone. Some antipsychotic drugs, such as the phenothiazines, have a strong affinity for these receptors but also block D2 receptors elsewhere, leading to side-effects such as restlessness and tremors, which may limit their use as an antiemetic, particularly in very young or older patients (Bennett 2009). Metoclopramide and domperidone act on D2 receptors in the chemoreceptor trigger zone (CTZ) but also act on receptors in the gastrointestinal tract which can reduce abdominal bloating. There is a particular risk of neurological side-effects with longer-term use and higher doses (BNF 2014). Levomepromazine is a 'broad-spectrum' antiemetic, acting on a range of receptors, that also has sedating and analgesic effects and so is often used in the palliative care setting.

5-HT3 antagonists

These are regarded as highly effective antiemetics which block 5-HT3 receptors in the CTZ and the gastrointestinal tract. They are commonly used to prevent chemotherapy-induced nausea and vomiting.

Steroids

Dexamethasone, a corticosteroid, is recognized for its antiemetic effect (Warren and King 2008), and is often used in conjunction with other antiemetics, although its mechanism of action is not clear.

Other antiemetics

Other categories of antiemetic include benzodiazepines, which work in the central nervous system to inhibit the GABA neurotransmitter; anticholinergics, such as hyoscine hydrobromide which acts directly on the vomiting centre and cannabinoids which inhibit nausea and vomiting caused by substances that irritate the CTZ, although the precise mechanism of action is not clearly understood. Neurokinin-1 antagonists are a relatively new category of antiemetic acting on NK1 receptors in the CTZ which have been found to be most effective in the treatment of chemotherapy-induced nausea and vomiting when used in conjunction with an HT3 antagonist and dexamethasone (BNF 2014, Dikken and Wildman 2013).

Source: Adapted from Bennett (2009), BNF (2014).

smells, large meals or malodour. Complementary therapies, such as acupressure and acupuncture, may be used but the evidence base for their effectiveness is relatively weak (Abraham 2008). Interventions including progressive muscle relaxation techniques (Campos de Carvalho et al. 2007) and hypnosis (Richardson et al. 2007) have been found to be effective in reducing nausea and vomiting associated with cancer chemotherapy but more research is required to establish the wider effectiveness of these approaches.

There is a wide variety of antiemetic drugs available, all of which act on one or more type of neuroreceptor, resulting in a central and/or peripheral effect. Bennett (2009) identifies nine categories of antiemetics, a summary of which can be found in Box 5.2. Table 5.1 summarizes the classification of drugs used to control nausea and vomiting.

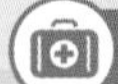

Learning Activity 5.1

Learning in practice: Nausea and vomiting

- List some of the different strategies you have seen being used in clinical practice to manage nausea and vomiting. Think of both the pharmacological and non-pharmacological approaches.
- Find out from the clinical team what complementary approaches to reduce nausea and vomiting are available to patients within the hospital and when, or to whom, these may be offered (you may need to ask a few different team members to find this out).

Procedure guideline 5.1 **Care of a patient who is vomiting**

Essential equipment

- Clean gloves and apron
- 2 × vomit bowls
- Tissues/wipes
- Bowl of warm water, wipes, towel

Pre-procedure

Action	Rationale
1 Ensure the patient is in a safe place and position to avoid any unnecessary injury or fall.	To maintain patient safety. **E**

(continued)

Procedure guideline 5.1 Care of a patient who is vomiting *(continued)*

Action	Rationale
2 Put on clean gloves and an apron.	To ensure procedure is as clean as possible (Fraise and Bradley 2009, **E**).
Procedure	
3 Close door/draw curtains around the patient's bed area.	To maintain privacy and dignity and avoid any unnecessary embarrassment for the patient (NMC 2015, **C**).
4 Provide the patient with a vomit bowl and tissues.	To reduce any risk of spillage and cross-infection (Fraise and Bradley 2009, **E**).
5 Remain with the patient.	To provide reassurance and maintain safety. **E**
6 Once the patient has stopped vomiting, remove used vomit bowl and offer warm water and towels for them to wash face and hands.	For infection prevention and control and patient comfort (Fraise and Bradley 2009, **E**).
7 Assist the patient to find a comfortable position and leave the second, clean vomit bowl with them.	To ensure comfort following the procedure. **E**
8 Take vomit bowl to the dirty utility (sluice) room and, where necessary, measure volume and note characteristics (colour, consistency and smell) of the vomit.	The characteristics of the vomit may help to determine the cause. **E**
Post-procedure	
9 Dispose of contents safely and place vomit bowl in the washer/disposal unit.	For infection prevention and control (Fraise and Bradley 2009, **E**).
10 Remove disposable apron and gloves. Wash hands using soap and water.	For infection prevention and control (Fraise and Bradley 2009, **E**).
11 Record volume and any notable characteristics of the vomit in the patient's notes.	To maintain accurate documentation (NMC 2010, **C**).
12 Return to the patient and assess nausea and vomiting at regular intervals.	To monitor and maintain patient's safety. **E**

Table 5.1 Classification of drugs used to control nausea and vomiting

Site/mode of action	Class	Example
Central nervous system		
Vomiting centre	Anticholinergic Antihistamine* 5-HT2 antagonist	Hyoscine hydrobromide, cyclizine, dimenhydrinate, phenothiazines, levomepromazine
Central nervous system	Neurokinin-1 antagonist	Aprepitant
Chemoreceptor trigger zone	Dopamine (D2) antagonist 5-HT3-antagonist	Haloperidol, phenothiazines, metoclopramide, domperidone, levomepromazine, granisetron, ondansetron, tropisetron
Cerebral cortex	Benzodiazepine Cannabinoid Corticosteroid	Lorazepam Nabilone Dexamethasone
Gastrointestinal tract		
Prokinetic	5-HT4 agonist Dopamine (D2) antagonist	Metoclopramide Metoclopramide, domperidone, levomepromazine

Site/mode of action	Class	Example
Antisecretory	Anticholinergic Somatostatin analogue	Hyoscine butylbromide Glycopyrronium Octreotide
Vagal 5-HT3 receptor blockade	5-HT3 antagonist	Granisetron, ondansetron, tropisetron
Anti-inflammatory	Corticosteroid	Dexamethasone

*Antihistamines and phenothiazines both have H1 receptor antagonistic and anticholinergic properties.
Vomiting is a significant yet complex symptom that requires a multifactorial approach to assess, prevent and manage it effectively.
Source: Adapted from Twycross and Back (2004).

Insertion of a nasogastric drainage tube

For patients who are vomiting large amounts, it may be appropriate to insert a nasogastric drainage tube in order to make the patient more comfortable, avoid any unnecessary trauma, such as to wounds, from the retching associated with vomiting and to more effectively monitor fluid output.

Anticipated patient outcomes

The patient has a nasogastric drainage tube inserted comfortably and safely. The position is checked and it is confirmed that the tube is placed in the stomach.

LEGAL AND PROFESSIONAL ISSUES

Those passing the nasogastric tube should have achieved competencies set by the local trust and be clear that the purpose of inserting the tube is for drainage of gastric contents only.

PRE-PROCEDURAL CONSIDERATIONS

Equipment

A wide-bore nasogastric drainage tube must be used for this procedure. This should not be confused with a fine-bore nasogastric tube that is used for the sole purpose of enteral feeding.

Specific patient preparation

The planned procedure should be discussed with the patient so they are aware of the rationale for insertion of a nasogastric tube. The decision to insert a nasogastric tube must be made by at least two healthcare professionals, including the senior doctor responsible for the patient's care. Verbal consent for the procedure must be obtained from the patient.

Contraindications

Prior to performing this procedure, the patient's medical and nursing notes should be consulted to check for potential complications. For example, anatomical alterations due to surgery, such as a flap repair, or the presence of a cancerous tumour can prevent a clear passage for the nasogastric tube, resulting in pain and discomfort for the patient and further complications. Patients who have recurrent retching or vomiting, swallowing dysfunction or are comatose have a high risk of placement error or migration of the tube so care must be taken when placing a nasogastric tube under these circumstances (NPSA 2011). The assessment of the patient, the risks and patient consent obtained should be clearly documented.

Procedure guideline 5.2 Insertion of a nasogastric (NG) drainage tube

Essential equipment

- Clean tray
- Receiver
- Nasogastric tube
- Drainage bag
- Tape
- Disposable gloves and apron
- Lubricating jelly
- Gauze squares
- 50 mL syringe

Pre-procedure

Action	Rationale
1 Explain and discuss the procedure with the patient.	To ensure that the patient understands the procedure and gives their valid consent (NMC 2013, **C**).
2 Arrange a signal by which the patient can communicate if they want the nurse to stop, for example by raising their hand.	To maintain communication and minimize discomfort and trauma to the patient during the procedure. **E**
3 Assist the patient to sit in a semi-upright position in the bed or chair. Place a pillow behind their head for support. Note: The head should not be tilted backwards or forwards.	To maintain a suitable position during the procedure to help correct insertion of the tube (Rollins 1997).

(continued)

Procedure guideline 5.2 Insertion of a nasogastric (NG) drainage tube *(continued)*

Action	Rationale
4 Using a small piece of tape, mark the distance to which the tube is to be passed by measuring the distance on the tube from the patient's earlobe to the bridge of the nose plus the distance from the earlobe to the bottom of the xiphisternum (the NEX measurement). See **Action figures 4a, 4b**.	To identify the length of tube that needs to be inserted to ensure it is in the correct position. **E**
5 Wash hands with bactericidal soap and water or bactericidal alcohol handrub, and assemble the equipment required. Put on disposable gloves and apron.	To ensure procedure is as clean as possible (Fraise and Bradley 2009, **E**).
Procedure	
6 Check the nostrils are patent by asking the patient to sniff with one nostril closed. Repeat with the other nostril.	To avoid any blockages or anatomical abnormalities. **E**
7 Lubricate about 15–20 cm of the tube with a thin coat of lubricating jelly that has been placed on a gauze swab.	To make insertion of the tube easier. **E**
8 Ensure receiver is placed beneath the end of the tube.	To prevent spillage and reduce risk of infection (Fraise and Bradley 2009, **E**).
9 Insert the proximal end of the tube into the clearer nostril and slide it backwards and inwards along the floor of the nose to the nasopharynx. If an obstruction is felt, withdraw the tube and try again in a slightly different direction or use the other nostril.	To avoid unnecessary trauma to the nose and nasopharynx.
10 As the tube passes down into the nasopharynx, ask the patient to start swallowing. Offer sips of water.	To help ensure that the tube passes easily into the oesophagus.
11 Advance the tube through the pharynx as the patient swallows until the tape-marked tube reaches the point of entry into the nostril (NEX measurement). If the patient shows signs of distress, for example gasping or cyanosis, remove the tube immediately.	Reaching the NEX measurement on the tube indicates that it should have advanced far enough down the oesophagus to be correctly positioned in the stomach. If there are signs of respiratory distress this may indicate the tube is incorrectly positioned in the bronchus. **E**
12 Secure the tube to the nostril with adherent dressing tape, for example Elastoplast, or an adhesive nasogastric stabilization/securing device. If this is contraindicated, a hypoallergenic tape should be used. An adhesive patch (if available) will secure the tube to the cheek.	To ensure the tube remains in the correct position. **E**
13 Use the syringe to gently aspirate any stomach contents and then attach the tube to a drainage bag.	Aspiration and/or drainage of stomach contents or bile will indicate that the tube is in the correct position in the stomach.
14 Assist the patient to find a comfortable position.	To ensure comfort following the procedure. **E**
Post-procedure	
15 If unsure of the tube's position, the following method can be used to test it.	
pH Test	
Aspirate 0.5–1 mL of stomach contents and test pH on indicator strips (NPSA 2011).	A pH level of between 1 and 5.5 reflects the acidity of the stomach and so is unlikely to be pulmonary aspirates (Metheny and Meert 2004; NPSA 2011, **C**). If a pH of 6 or above is obtained, then a second person should retest.
16 Remove gloves and apron and dispose of all equipment safely. Wash hands using soap and water.	For infection prevention and control (Fraise and Bradley 2009, **E**).
17 Record the procedure, NEX measurement, length of visible portion of the tube from tip of nose and tip position in the patient's notes.	To maintain accurate documentation (NMC 2010, **C**).

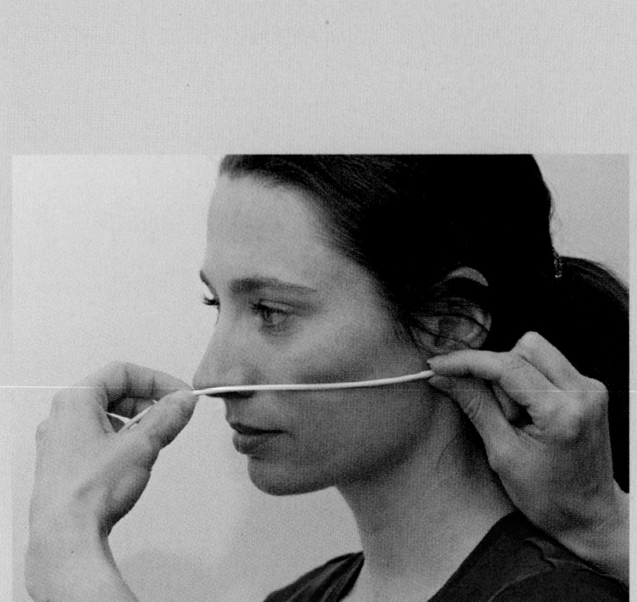

Action Figure 4a Measuring for a nasogastric tube: measure from the patient's ear lobe to the bridge of the nose.

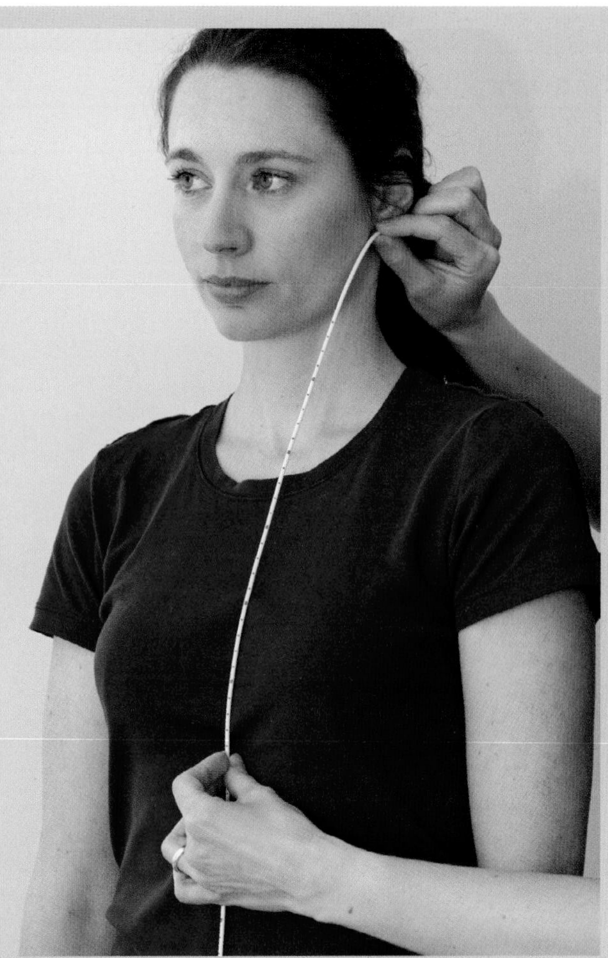

Action Figure 4b Measuring for a nasogastric tube: measure from the ear lobe to the bottom of the xiphisternum.

Removal of a nasogastric drainage tube

Prior to removal of a nasogastric drainage tube, the procedure should be explained to the patient and verbal consent obtained.

Procedure guideline 5.3 **Removal of a nasogastric tube**

Essential equipment

- Clean gloves and apron
- Contaminated waste disposal bag
- Bowl of warm water and wipes

Pre-proedure

Action	Rationale
1 Explain the procedure to the patient.	To ensure that the patient understands the procedure and gives their valid consent (NMC 2013, **C**).
2 Assist the patient to sit in a semi-upright position in the bed or chair. Support the patient's head with pillows.	To allow for easy removal of tube. **E**
3 Wash hands with bactericidal soap and water or bactericidal alcohol handrub, and assemble the equipment required. Apply apron and clean gloves.	Hands must be cleansed beforepatient contact to minimize cross-infections (Fraise and Bradley 2009, **E**).

(continued)

Procedure guideline 5.3 Removal of a nasogastric tube *(continued)*

Procedure

Action	Rationale
4 Remove any tape securing the nasogastric tube to the nose.	To assist in removal of nasogastric tube. **E**
5 Using a steady and constant motion, gently pull the tube until it has been completely removed.	To remove the nasogastric tube. **E**
6 Place the used nasogastric tube directly into the contaminated waste bag.	For infection prevention and control (Fraise and Bradley 2009, **E**).
7 Using warm water and wipes, clean the nose and face to remove any traces of tape.	To ensure patient comfort and dignity. **E**
8 Assist the patient to find a comfortable position.	To ensure comfort following the procedure. **E**
Post-procedure	
9 Remove gloves and apron and dispose of all equipment safely. Wash hands using soap and water.	For infection prevention and control (Fraise and Bradley 2009, **E**).
10 Document removal of nasogastric tube in care plan and patient's notes.	To ensure adequate records and to enable continued care of patient (NMC 2010, **C**).

Urinary elimination

DEFINITION

Urinary elimination is the excretion of urine from the body (Thibodeau and Patton 2010).

ANATOMY AND PHYSIOLOGY

The urinary tract (Figure 5.2) consists of the two kidneys, two ureters, the bladder and urethra. The urinary system produces, stores and eliminates urine. The kidneys are responsible for excreting wastes such as urea and ammonium and for the reabsorption of glucose and amino acids. They are involved with the production of hormones including calcitrol, renin and erythropoietin. The kidneys also have homeostatic functions, including the regulation of electrolytes, acid/base balance and blood pressure (Tortora and Derrickson 2011).

Each kidney excretes urine into a ureter, which arises from the renal pelvis on the medial aspect of each kidney. In adults, the ureters are approximately 25–30 cm long and 2–4 mm in diameter (Tortora and Derrickson 2011). The ureters are muscular tubes, which propel urine from the kidneys to the urinary bladder. They enter through the back of the bladder, running within the wall of the bladder for a few centimetres. Ureterovesical valves prevent the backflow of urine from the bladder to the kidneys.

The bladder sits on the pelvic floor and is a hollow, muscular, distensible organ which stores urine until it is convenient to expel it. Urine enters the bladder via the ureters and exits via the urethra. As the bladder fills, stretch receptors in the muscular wall signal the parasympathetic nervous system to contract the bladder, initiating the conscious desire to expel urine. In order for urine to be expelled, both the automatically controlled internal sphincter and the voluntary controlled external sphincter must be opened.

Urine leaves the bladder via the urethra. In females this lies in front of the anterior wall of the vagina and is approximately 3.8 cm long. In males it passes through the prostate and penis and is approximately 20 cm long (Tortora and Derrickson 2011).

Figure 5.2 **(a) Male and (b) female genitourinary tract.**

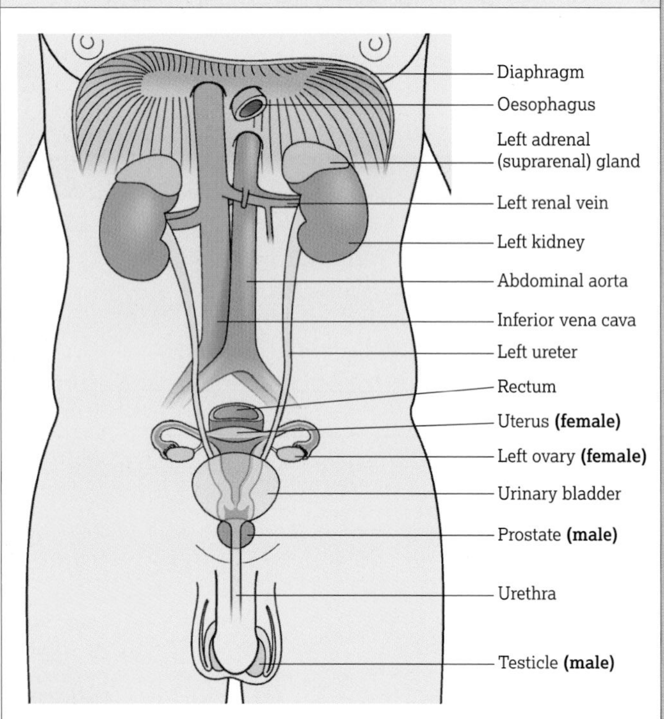

Faecal elimination

DEFINITION

Faecal elimination is the expulsion of the residues of digestion – faeces – from the digestive tract (Thibodeau and Patton 2010). The act of expelling faeces is called defaecation.

ANATOMY AND PHYSIOLOGY

This section will consider the normal structure and function of the bowel, which includes the small and large intestine (Figure 5.3). The small intestine begins at the pyloric sphincter of the stomach, coils through the abdomen and opens into the large intestine at the ileocaecal junction. It is approximately 6 m in length and is divided into three segments: the duodenum (25 cm), jejunum (2.5 m) and ileum (3.5 m) (Thibodeau and Patton 2010). The mucosal surface of the small intestine is covered with finger-like processes called villi, which increase the surface area available for absorption and digestion. A number of digestive enzymes are also secreted by the small intestine (Tortora and Derrickson 2011).

Figure 5.3 **The gastrointestinal tract.** ***Source:*** **Peate et al. (2014). Reproduced with permission from John Wiley & Sons.**

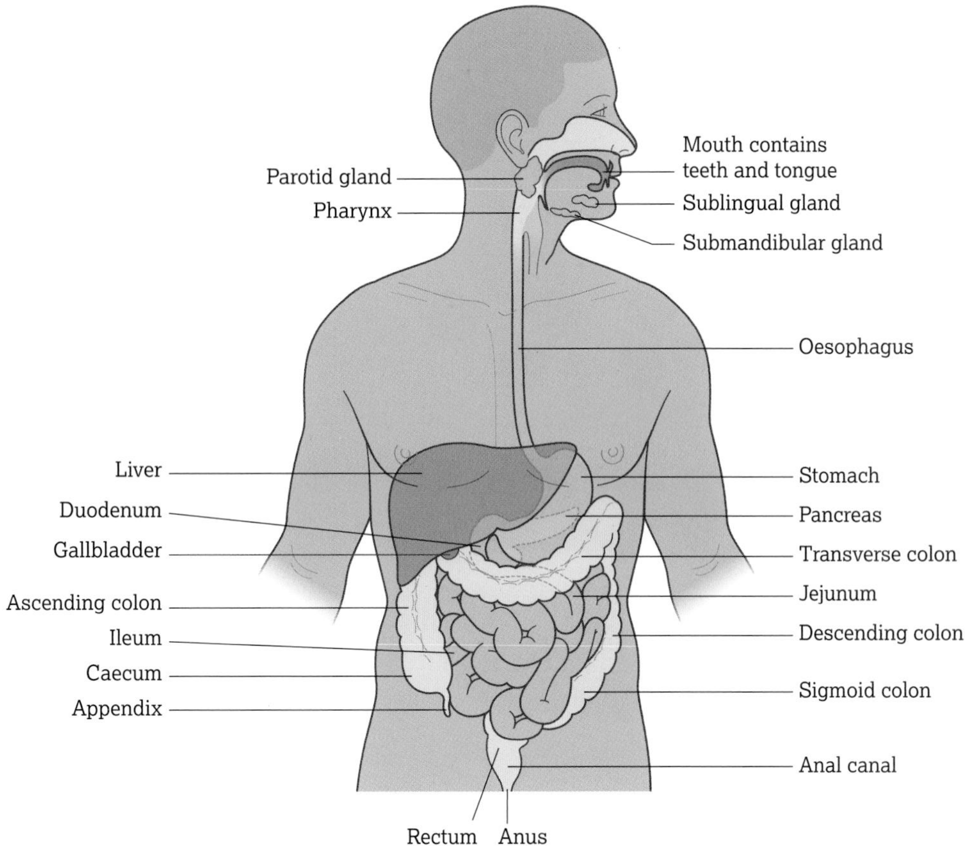

Movement through the small bowel is divided into two types, segmentation and peristalsis, and is controlled by the autonomic nervous system. Segmentation refers to the localized, concentric contraction of the intestine, aided by constant lengthening and shortening of the villi, mixing the intestinal contents and bringing particles of food into contact with the mucosa for absorption. Once the majority of a meal has been absorbed through this process, intestinal content is then pushed along the small intestine by repeated peristaltic wave-like actions. Intestinal content usually remains in the small bowel for 3–5 hours (Tortora and Derrickson 2011).

The total volume of fluid, including ingested liquids and gastrointestinal secretions, that enters the small intestine daily is about 9.3 litres. The small intestine is responsible for absorbing around 90% of the nutrients, electrolytes and water within this volume by diffusion, facilitated diffusion, osmosis and active transport (Tortora and Derrickson 2011). Water is able to move across the intestinal mucosa in both directions, but is influenced by the absorption of nutrients and electrolytes. As various electrolytes and nutrients are actively transported out of the lumen, they create a concentration gradient, promoting water absorption, via osmosis, in order to maintain an osmotic balance between intestinal fluid and blood. This ultimately leads to only about 1 litre of effluent passing through into the colon (Thibodeau and Patton 2010, Tortora and Derrickson 2011).

From the ileocaecal sphincter to the anus, the colon is approximately 1.5–1.8 m in length and 4–6 cm in diameter. Its main function is to eliminate the waste products of digestion by the propulsion of faeces towards the anus. In addition, it produces mucus to lubricate the faecal mass, thus aiding its expulsion. Other functions include the absorption of fluid and electrolytes, including sodium and potassium, the storage of faeces and the synthesis of vitamins B and K by bacterial flora (Thibodeau and Patton 2010, Tortora and Derrickson 2011).

Faeces consist of the unabsorbed end-products of digestion, bile pigments, cellulose, bacteria, epithelial cells, mucus and some inorganic material. They are normally semi-solid in consistency and contain about 70% water (Tortora and Derrickson 2011). The colon absorbs about 2 litres of water in 24 hours, so if faeces are not expelled they will gradually become hard due to dehydration and more difficult to expel. If there is insufficient roughage (fibre) in the faeces, colonic stasis occurs, which leads to continued water absorption and further hardening of the faeces. Faeces will, therefore, vary in consistency, as illustrated in the Bristol Stool Chart (Figure 5.4).

The movement of faeces through the colon towards the anus occurs by mass peristalsis, a gastrocolic reflex initiated by the presence of food in the stomach, which begins at the middle of the transverse colon and quickly drives the colonic contents into the rectum. This mass peristaltic movement generally occurs 3–5 times a day (Perdue 2005). In response to this stimulus, faeces move into the rectum (Norton 1996, Taylor 1997, Tortora and Derrickson 2011). This rectal distension triggers the desire to defaecate, also known as the 'call to stool'.

Assisting the patient with elimination

EVIDENCE-BASED APPROACHES

Principles of care

Elimination is a sensitive issue and providing effective care and management for problems associated with it can be problematic.

Figure 5.4 **Bristol Stool Chart.** ***Source:*** **Reproduced by kind permission of Dr KW Heaton, Reader in Medicine at the University of Bristol. © 2000–2014, Norgine group of companies.**

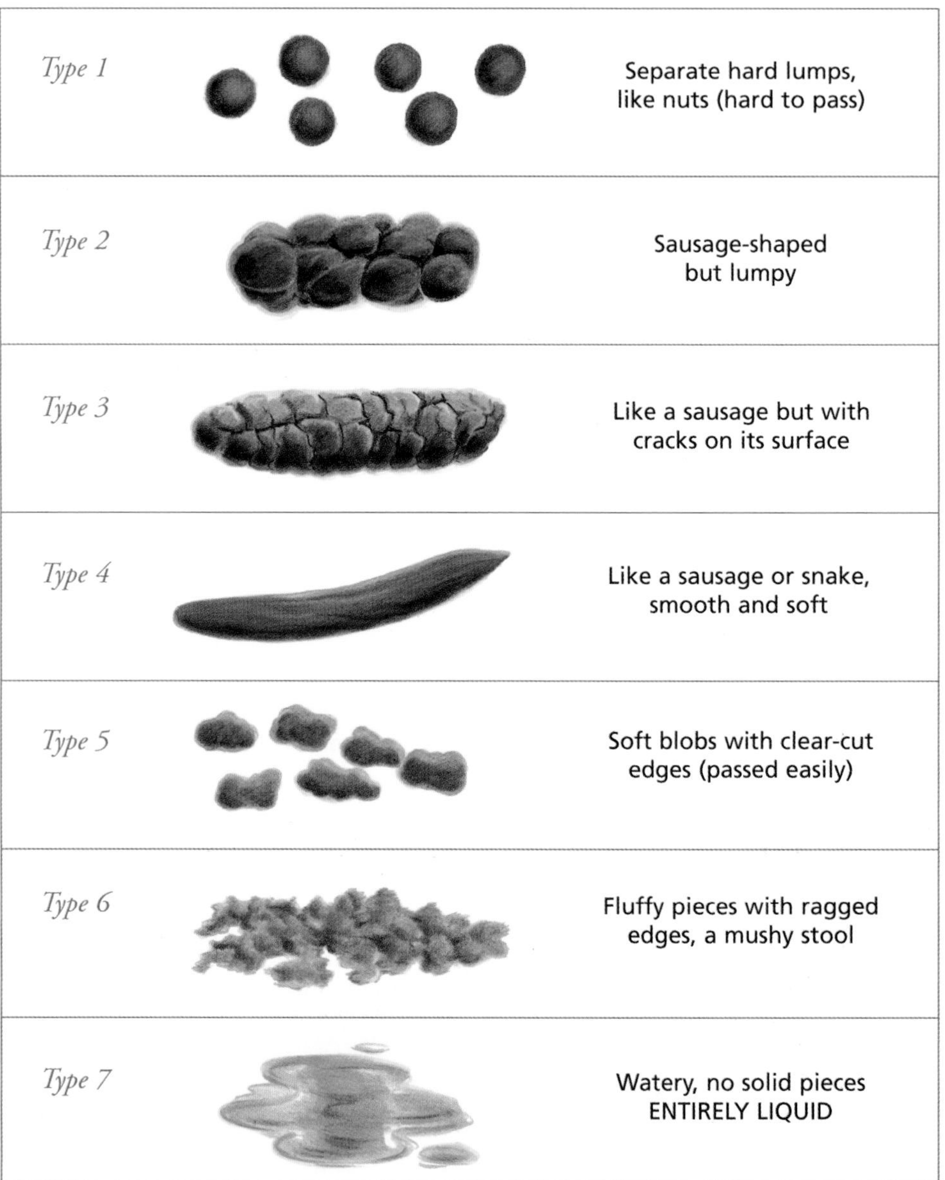

The difficulties associated with this can be minimized if the nurse seeks to respect the patient's dignity when carrying out procedures such as assisting them with using a bedpan or a commode.

LEGAL AND PROFESSIONAL ISSUES

The privacy and dignity of the patient must be respected at all times (NMC 2015). It is essential that the procedure is explained clearly to the patient to ensure consent is obtained and patient co-operation is agreed. A moving and handling assessment is vital in order to establish if additional equipment such as a hoist is required.

PRE-PROCEDURAL CONSIDERATIONS

Equipment

Before commencing the procedure, ensure that appropriate equipment and staff are available for safe moving and handling

Figure 5.5 **Slipper bed pan.**

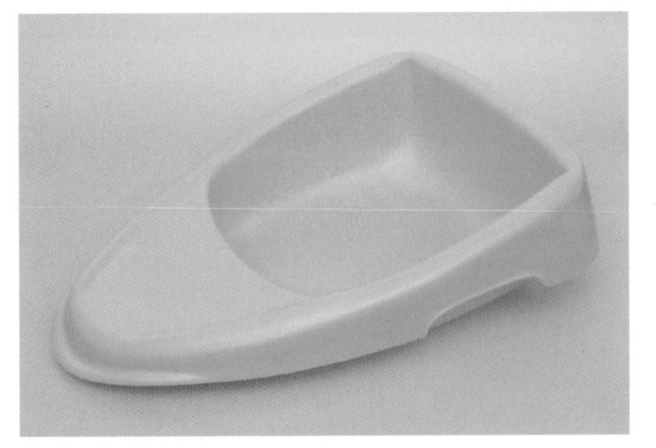

Figure 5.6 **Commode.**

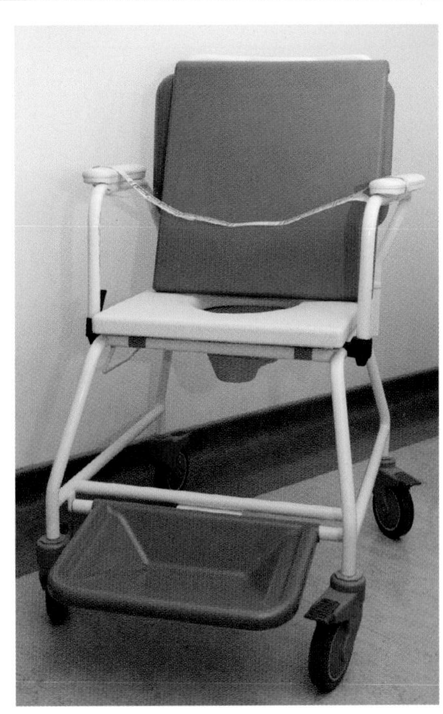

of the patient and, depending on the patient's mobility, that either a bedpan or commode is available for immediate use (Figure 5.5, Figure 5.6).

Pharmacological support

Incontinence-associated dermatitis (IAD) is a term used for skin breakdown resulting from exposure to urine or faeces and so is a common problem with either faecal and/or urinary incontinence (Doughty et al. 2012, Gray et al. 2007) and has been clearly differentiated from other forms of skin damage such as pressure ulcers or skin tears (Gray et al. 2012). Current nursing practice includes the use of a wide range of skin moisturizers and barrier creams with varying evidence about their efficacy or effectiveness (Gray et al. 2012). Ripley (2007) suggests that barrier products vary in both properties and uses but they can be effective in promoting skin integrity when selected appropriately. The same author recommends the development of protocols to support effective use of such products. A review suggests that the use of barrier creams with a pH near to that of normal skin can be useful in prevention of skin problems (Beeckman et al. 2009, Geraghty 2011). Recommendations from a recent international consensus conference advocate a consistently applied skin regime for the prevention and treatment of IAD which includes gentle perineal cleansing, moisturization and application of a skin protectant, but suggest that further research is required (Doughty et al. 2012, Gray et al. 2012).

Procedure guideline 5.4 **Slipper bedpan use: assisting a patient**

Essential equipment

- Disposable apron and gloves
- Manual handling equipment as appropriate
- Slipper bedpan and paper cover
- Additional nurse if required to assist with manual handling
- Toilet paper
- Wash bowl, warm water, disposable wipes and a towel

Pre-procedure

Action	Rationale
1 Carry out appropriate manual handling assessment prior to commencing procedure and establish whether an additional nurse or equipment such as a hoist is necessary.	To maintain a safe environment. **E**
Procedure	
2 Take the equipment to the bedside and explain the procedure to the patient.	To ensure that the patient understands the procedure and gives their valid consent (NMC 2013, **C**).
3 Wash hands, put on gloves and apron.	To ensure procedure is as clean as possible and minimize the risk of spreading infection (Fraise and Bradley 2009, **E**).
4 Close door/draw curtains around the patient's bed area.	To maintain privacy and dignity and avoid any unnecessary embarrassment for the patient (NMC 2015, **C**).

(continued)

Procedure guideline 5.4 Slipper bedpan use: assisting a patient *(continued)*

Action	Rationale
5 Remove the bedclothes and, providing there are no contraindications (e.g. if patient is on flat bedrest), assist the patient into an upright sitting position.	An upright, 'crouch-like' posture is considered anatomically correct for defaecation. Poor posture adopted while using a bedpan has been shown to cause extreme straining during defaecation. Patients should therefore be supported with pillows in order to achieve an upright position on the bedpan (Woodward 2012, **E**).
6 Ask the patient to raise their hips/buttocks and insert the bedpan beneath the patient's pelvis, ensuring that the wide end of the bedpan is between the legs, and the narrow end is beneath the buttocks.	A slipper bedpan provides more comfort for a patient who is unable to sit upright on a conventional bedpan (Nicol 2008, **E**).
7 Offer the patient the use of pillows and encourage them to lean forward slightly if possible.	To provide support and optimize positioning for defaecation (Woodward 2012, **E**). To ensure that the patient is in optimum position for eliminating. **E**
8 Once the patient is on the bedpan, encourage them to move their legs slightly apart and check to ensure that their positioning is correct.	To avoid any spillage onto the bedclothes and reduce risk of contamination and cross-infection. **E**
9 Cover the patient's legs with a sheet.	To maintain privacy and dignity (NMC 2015, **C**).
10 Ensure that toilet paper and call bell are within patient's reach and leave the patient, but remain nearby.	To maintain privacy and dignity (NMC 2015, **C**).
11 When the patient has finished using the bedpan, remove it, replace the paper cover and bring washing equipment to the bedside. Assist the patient to clean perianal area using warm water and soap. Apply a small amount of barrier cream to the perineal/buttock area if appropriate.	Talcum powder should not be used and barrier creams should be applied sparingly, gently layered on in the direction of the hair growth rather than rubbed into the skin (Le Lievre 2002, **E**).
12 Offer a bowl of water or moistened wipes for the patient to clean their hands.	For infection prevention and control and patient comfort (Fraise and Bradley 2009, **E**).
13 Ensure bedclothes are clean, straighten sheets and rearrange pillows, assisting patient to a comfortable position. Ensure call bell is within reach of the patient.	For patient comfort. **P**
14 Take bedpan to the dirty utility (sluice) room and, where necessary, measure urine output and note characteristics and amount of faeces using the Bristol Stool Chart (Figure 5.4).	To monitor and evaluate patient's elimination patterns. **E**
Post-procedure	
15 Dispose of contents safely and place bedpan in the washer/disposal unit.	For infection prevention and control (Fraise and Bradley 2009, **E**).
16 Remove disposable apron and gloves. Wash hands using soap and water.	For infection prevention and control (Fraise and Bradley 2009, **E**).
17 Record any urine output/bowel action in patient's documentation.	To maintain accurate documentation (NMC 2010, **C**).

Procedure guideline 5.5 Commode use: assisting a patient

Essential equipment

- Disposable apron and gloves
- Manual handling equipment as appropriate
- A clean commode with conventional bedpan inserted below seat
- Additional nurse if required
- Toilet paper
- Wash bowl, warm water, disposable wipes and a towel

Pre-procedure

Action	Rationale
1 Carry out appropriate manual handling assessment prior to commencing procedure and ensure that patient's weight does not exceed the maximum recommended for commode (see manufacturer's guidelines).	To maintain a safe environment. **E**

Action	Rationale
2 Wash hands, put on gloves and apron.	For infection prevention and control (Fraise and Bradley 2009, **E**).
3 Take the equipment to the bedside and explain the procedure to the patient.	To ensure that the patient understands the procedure and gives their valid consent (NMC 2013, **C**).
Procedure	
4 Close door/draw curtains around the patient's bed area.	To maintain privacy and dignity and avoid any unnecessary embarrassment for the patient (NMC 2015, **C**).
5 Remove the commode cover. Assist the patient out of the bed/chair and onto the commode.	
6 Once seated, ensure the patient's feet are positioned directly below their knees and flat on the floor. The use of a small footstool and/or pillows may help to achieve a comfortable position.	An upright, crouching posture is considered anatomically correct for defaecation. Pillows and a footstool can provide support and optimize positioning for defaecation (Woodward 2012, **E**).
7 Cover the patient's knees with a towel or sheet.	To maintain privacy and dignity (NMC 2015, **C**).
8 Ensure that toilet paper and call bell are within patient's reach and leave the patient, but remain nearby.	To maintain privacy and dignity (NMC 2015, **C**) and to prevent falls.
9 When the patient has finished using the commode, bring washing equipment to the bedside. Assist patient to clean perianal area using toilet paper and, where necessary, warm water and soap. Apply a small amount of barrier cream to the perineal/buttock area if appropriate.	Talcum powder should not be used and barrier creams should be applied sparingly, gently layered on in the direction of the hair growth rather than rubbed into the skin (Le Lievre 2002, **E**).
10 Offer a bowl of water for the patient to wash their hands.	For infection control and patient dignity (Fraise and Bradley 2009, **E**).
11 Assist the patient to stand and walk to bed/chair, ensuring that they are comfortably positioned. Ensure call bell is within reach of the patient.	For patient comfort. **P**
Post-procedure	
12 Replace cover on the commode and return to the dirty utility (sluice) room.	To reduce any risk of contamination or cross-infection (Fraise and Bradley 2009, **E**) and to avoid patient embarrassment (NMC 2015, **C**).
13 Remove pan from underneath the commode and, where necessary, measure urine output, and note characteristics and amount of faeces using the Bristol Stool Chart (see Figure 5.4).	To monitor and evaluate patient's elimination patterns. **E**
14 Dispose of contents safely and place pan in the washer/disposal unit.	For infection prevention and control (Fraise and Bradley 2009, **E**).
16 Clean commode using Actichlor Plus solution and label commode according to local guidelines to indicate it has been cleaned.	
17 Remove disposable apron and gloves. Wash hands using bactericidal soap and water.	For infection control purposes (Fraise and Bradley 2009, **E**).
18 Record any urine output/bowel action in patient's documentation.	To maintain accurate documentation (NMC 2010, **C**).

Altered urinary elimination

This section first examines urinary incontinence and then reviews different approaches to its management. Surgical interventions and supportive care for altered urinary elimination will be considered, including insertion of nephrostomy tubes and urinary diversions.

Urinary incontinence

RELATED THEORY

Urinary incontinence is a worldwide problem affecting 13% of men and 14% of women aged 65–74 years (Nethercliffe 2012). Nurses will encounter patients with incontinence in most care settings, so it is important that they are aware of the issues surrounding this sensitive subject (Lay 2012).

Risk factors include the following.

- Age (Devore et al. 2012).
- Neurological conditions (MS or MDN, spinal cord injury) (Nethercliffe 2012).
- Surgical procedures (hysterectomy, pelvic surgery) (Stothers and Friedman 2011).
- Diabetes (Stothers and Friedman 2011).
- Higher body mass index (Devore et al. 2012).

- Physical trauma (childbirth) (Nethercliffe 2012).
- Menopause.
- Cystitis and UTI (Getliffe and Dolman 2007).
- Enlargement of the prostate – benign prostatic hyperplasia.
- Prostate surgery.
- Prostate cancer.

EVIDENCE-BASED APPROACHES – PENILE SHEATHS

Rationale

Penile sheaths are external devices made from a soft and flexible latex or silicone tubing which are applied over the penis to direct urine into a urinary drainage bag from where it can be conveniently emptied (Figure 5.7). A penile sheath is a soft flexible sleeve that fits over the penis with an anti-reflux bulbous end, which is able to attach to any standard urinary drainage bag (Kyle 2011a). They are used by men to manage urinary incontinence.

Penile sheaths (also known as conveens) are only to be considered once other methods of promoting continence have failed, as the promotion and treatment of incontinence should be the primary concern of the nurse (Pomfret 2002). They should be considered as a preferable alternative to other methods of continence control, such as pads which can quickly become sodden (Pomfret 2002) and cause skin problems, and catheters, which have several potential complications (Jahn et al. 2012).

Indications

Penile sheaths may be used to relieve incontinence when no other means is practicable or when all other methods have failed. Penile sheaths are associated with many common problems which are identified by Woodward (2007) and Wells (2008); these include difficulty in fitting, leaking, kinking, falling off, allergies and urinary tract infections.

Contraindications

Penile sheaths are contraindicated for men with very small or retracted penises, sensitive skin and allergies (Booth 2009, Wells 2008).

PRE-PROCEDURAL CONSIDERATIONS

Equipment

Silicone types are now preferred due to concerns about latex allergies (Booth and Lee 2005).

Sizing and fitting

As modern sheaths come in a variety of sizes and the correct size can be determined by measuring the girth of the penile shaft, one of the most important considerations is to move away from the mentality that one size fits all. The penis should be measured in the flaccid state (Potter 2007). Most devices come with a manufacturer's sheath sizing guide with different diameters cut into it, so that the correct size can be easily determined. Sheaths are available in a variety of different sizes, which generally increase in increments of 5–10 mm, and in either standard or short lengths (Robinson 2006). Silicone sheaths are advantageous as they are transparent, allowing the patient's skin to be observed and to breathe by allowing the transmission of water vapour and oxygen (Booth and Lee 2005).

The main methods of fixation in current use follow two different approaches. First, the sheaths can be self-adhesive, so that the sheath itself has a section along its length with adhesive on the internal aspect that sticks to the penile shaft as it is applied. The second method is a double-sided strip of hypoallergenic or foam material applied in a spiral around the penis (which increases the surface area of the conveen adhered to the penis) and then the sheath is applied over the top. Newer devices have been developed which move away from the condom catheter-based system and employ a unique hydrocolloid 'petal' design which adheres only to a small area of the glans penis around the meatus, ensuring a comfortable and secure fit; these are ideal for men with a retracted penis (Wells 2008).

Figure 5.7 **Penile sheath.**

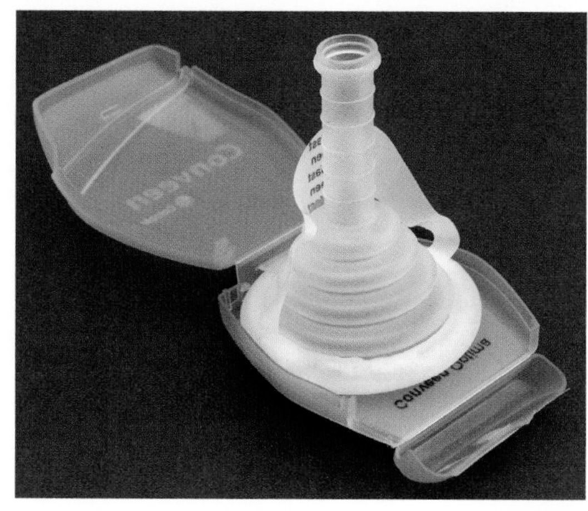

Procedure guideline 5.6 **Penile sheath application**

Essential equipment

- Bowl of warm water and soap
- Scissors or a disposable razor
- Clean disposable gloves and apron
- Drainage bag and stand or holder
- Selection of appropriate-sized penile sheaths
- Hypoallergenic tape or leg strap
- Bactericidal alcohol handrub
- Catheter leg bag

Pre-procedure

Action	Rationale
1 Explain and discuss the procedure with the patient.	To ensure that the patient understands the procedure and gives his valid consent (NMC 2013, **C**).

Action	Rationale
2 Screen the bed.	To ensure patient's privacy. To allow dust and airborne organisms to settle before the field is exposed (NMC 2015, **C**).
3 Prepare the trolley, placing all equipment required on the bottom shelf.	The top shelf acts as a clean working surface. **E**
4 Take the trolley to the patient's bedside, disturbing the screens as little as possible.	To minimize airborne contamination (Fraise and Bradley 2009, **E**).
5 Wash hands using bactericidal soap and water or bactericidal alcohol handrub.	To reduce risk of infection (Fraise and Bradley 2009, **E**).
6 Put on a disposable plastic apron.	To reduce risk of cross-infection from micro-organisms on the uniform (Fraise and Bradley 2009, **E**).
7 Assist the patient into a comfortable position. The patient can lie on the bed in the supine position or sit on the edge of the bed.	To ensure the appropriate area is easily accessible. **E**
Procedure	
8 Assist the patient to remove his underwear and ensure he has a sheet or disposable towels available and use to cover his thighs.	To maintain privacy and dignity (NMC 2015).
9 Position a disposable pad under the patient's buttocks and thighs.	To ensure urine does not leak onto bedclothes. **E**
10 Clean hands with a bactericidal alcohol handrub.	Hands may have become contaminated by handling the outer packs (Fraise and Bradley 2009, **E**).
11 Put on non-sterile gloves.	To reduce risk of cross-infection (Fraise and Bradley 2009, **E**).
12 With one hand retract the foreskin, if necessary, and with the other hand clean the penis with soap and water. Dry completely and reduce or reposition the foreskin.	To remove old adhesive and ensure sheath sticks to the skin. To prevent retraction and constriction of the foreskin behind the glans penis (paraphimosis) which may occur if this is not performed. **E**
13 Using the scissors or disposable razor, trim any excess pubic hair from around the base of the penis.	To prevent sheath from painfully pulling pubic hair when applied. **E**
14 Apply sheath following manufacturer's guidelines, ensuring that there is a space between the glans penis and the sheath. Squeeze the sheath gently around the penile shaft.	To prevent the sheath from rubbing the glans penis and causing discomfort and potential skin irritation and to ensure sheath has adhered to penis (Pomfret 2002, **C**).
15 Connect catheter bag and ensure tubing is not kinked.	To facilitate drainage of urine into catheter bag. **E**
16 Remove gloves and apron. Dispose of all waste and equipment in an orange plastic clinical waste bag and seal the bag.	Orange is the recognized colour for clinical waste (DEFRA 2005, **C**).
Post-procedure	
17 Provide any assistance the patient may need to dress, encouraging loose clothing where possible. Draw back the curtains once the patient is dressed.	To maintain the patient's dignity (NMC 2015, **C**) and to avoid any unnecessary kinking of the sheath or its tubing. **E**
18 Dispose of clinical waste bag in a larger bin.	To prevent environmental contamination (Fraise and Bradley 2009, **E**).
19 Record information in relevant documents; this should include: • reasons for applying penile sheath • date and time of application • sheath type • length and size • manufacturer • any problems negotiated during the procedure • a review date to assess the need for reapplication.	To provide a point of reference or comparison in the event of later queries (NMC 2010, **C**).

Problem-solving table 5.1 **Prevention and resolution (Procedure guideline 5.6)**

Problem	Cause	Action	Prevention
Leaking or backflow of urine under the sheath.	Penile sheath is the wrong size.	Remeasure penile shaft and select the correct size.	Measure penile shaft using the sizing tool.
Twisting or kinking of sheath.	Lack of care taken when applying, drainage tube unsecured.	Secure drainage bag to leg or stand.	Assess patient mobility before application and select suitable type and method of securing the drainage bag.
Difficulty fitting sheath to patient with retracted penis.	Anatomy of the patient.	Observe the penile length when the patient is sitting. If the length of the penis is less than 5 cm when sitting, use a hydrocolloid petal design sheath.	It may be that a penile sheath is not the most appropriate device in some cases.

Urinary catheterization

EVIDENCE-BASED APPROACHES

Rationale

Urinary catheterization is the insertion of a specially designed tube into the bladder using aseptic technique, for the purposes of draining urine, the removal of clots/debris and the instillation of medication. It is an invasive procedure and should not be undertaken without full consideration of the benefits and risks. The presence of a catheter can be a traumatic experience for patients and have huge implications for body image, mobility, pain and discomfort (Clifford 2000, RCN 2012a). Indwelling catheters are the primary source of urinary tract infections within acute care. It is essential that they are only used if clinically necessary (Murphy et al. 2014).

Indications

Urinary catheterization may be carried out for the following reasons.

- To empty the contents of the bladder, for example before or after abdominal, pelvic or rectal surgery, before certain investigations and before childbirth, if thought necessary.
- To determine residual urine.
- To allow irrigation of the bladder.
- To bypass an obstruction.
- To relieve retention of urine.
- To enable bladder function tests to be performed.
- To measure urinary output accurately, for example when a patient is in shock, undergoing bone marrow transplantation or receiving high-dose chemotherapy.
- To relieve incontinence when no other means is practicable.
- To avoid complications during the insertion of radioactive material (e.g. caesium into the cervix/uterus, brachytherapy for the prostate).

LEGAL AND PROFESSIONAL ISSUES

Competencies

Nurses performing female and/or male urinary catheterization must have demonstrated the appropriate level of competency to carry out this procedure and be sure it is within their scope of professional practice in accordance with *The Code* (NMC 2015).

PRE-PROCEDURAL CONSIDERATIONS

Patients should be assessed individually as to the ideal time to change their catheters. The use of a catheter diary will help to ascertain a pattern of catheter blockages so changes can be planned accordingly.

Equipment: catheter selection

A wide range of urinary catheters is available, made from a variety of materials and with different design features. Careful assessment of the most appropriate material, size and balloon capacity will ensure that the catheter selected is as effective as possible, that complications are minimized and that patient comfort and quality of life are promoted (Nazarko 2010, Pomfret 1996, Robinson 2001). Types of catheter are listed in Table 5.2 and illustrated in Figure 5.8, together with their suggested use. Catheters should be used in line with the manufacturer's recommendations, in order to avoid product liability (Fraise and Bradley 2009, NHS Supply Chain 2008).

Table 5.2 **Types of catheter**

Catheter type	Material	Uses
Balloon (Foley) two-way catheter: two channels, one for urine drainage and second, smaller channel for balloon inflation	Latex, PTFE-coated latex, silicone elastomer coated, 100% silicone, hydrogel coated	Most commonly used for patients who require bladder drainage (short, medium or long term)
Balloon (Foley) three-way irrigation catheter: three channels, one for urine, one for irrigation fluid, one for balloon inflation	Latex, PTFE-coated latex, silicone, plastic	To provide continuous irrigation (e.g. after prostatectomy). Potential for infection is reduced by minimizing the need to break the closed drainage system (Mulhall et al. 1993)
Non-balloon (Nelaton) or Scotts, or intermittent catheter (one channel only)	PVC and other plastics	To empty bladder or continent urinary reservoir intermittently; to instil solutions into bladder

PTFE, polytetrafluoroethylene; PVC, polyvinylchloride.

Figure 5.8 **Catheter types.**

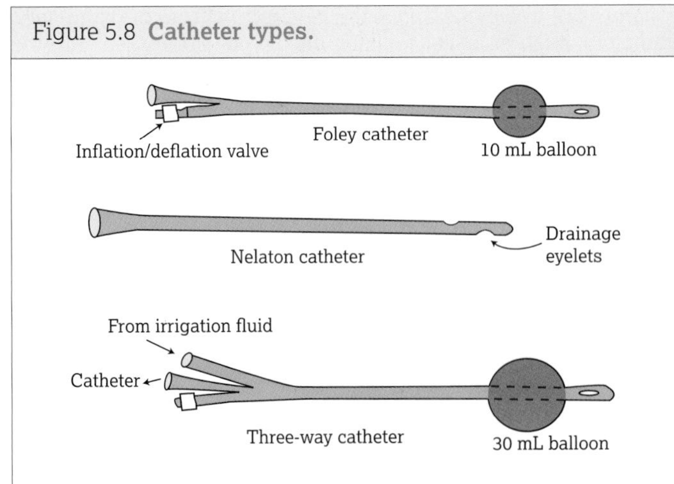

Balloon size

In the 1920s, Fredrick Foley designed a catheter with an inflatable balloon to keep it positioned inside the bladder. Balloon sizes vary from 2.5 mL for children to 30 mL. A 5–10 mL balloon is recommended for adults and a 3–5 mL balloon for children.

Care should be taken to use the correct amount of water to fill the balloon because too much or too little may cause distortion of the catheter tip. This may result in irritation and trauma to the bladder wall, consequently causing pain, spasm, bypassing and haematuria. If underinflated, one or more of the drainage eyes may become occluded or the catheter may become dislodged. Overinflation risks rupturing the balloon and leaving fragments of it inside the bladder (Robinson 2001). Catheter balloons should only be inflated once; deflation/reinflation or topping up is not recommended by the manufacturers as distortion of the balloon may occur (Nazarko 2009, Robinson 2004).

Catheter balloons must be filled only with sterile water (Hart 2008). Tap water and 0.9% sodium chloride should not be used as salt crystals and debris may block the inflation channel, causing difficulties with deflation (Head 2006). Any micro-organisms which may be present in tap water can pass through the balloon into the bladder (Stewart 1998).

Catheter size

Urethral catheters are measured in charrières (ch). The charrière is the outer circumference of the catheter in millimetres and is equivalent to three times the diameter. Thus a 12 ch catheter has a diameter of 4 mm. The bigger the catheter, the more the urethra is dilated. 12 ch is normally suitable for men and women (Nazarko 2012). The urethra is approximately 6 mm in diameter, this is equivalent to a size 16 ch catheter. This is useful to know as it has implications for patient comfort.

Potential side-effects of large-gauge catheters include:

- pain and discomfort
- pressure ulcers, which may lead to stricture formation
- blockage of paraurethral ducts
- abscess formation (Winn 1998)
- bypassing – urethral leakage.

The most important guiding principle is to choose the smallest size of catheter necessary to maintain adequate drainage (Robinson 2006). If the urine to be drained is likely to be clear, a 12 ch catheter should be considered. Larger gauge catheters may be necessary if debris or clots are present in the urine (Pomfret 1996, Winn 1998).

Length of catheter

There are three lengths of catheter currently available:

- female length: 23–26 cm
- paediatric: 30 cm
- standard length: 40–44 cm.

The shorter female length catheter is often more discreet and less likely to cause trauma or infections because movement in and out of the urethra is reduced. Infection may also be caused by the longer catheter looping or kinking (Pomfret 2002, Robinson 2001). In obese women or those in wheelchairs, however, the inflation valve of the shorter catheter may cause soreness by rubbing against the inside of the thigh, and the catheter is more likely to pull on the bladder neck; therefore, the standard length catheter should be used (Evans et al. 2001, Godfrey and Evans 2000, Pomfret 2004).

It is vital to stress that female catheters must not be used for male catheterization. This will cause trauma to the urethra as the balloon will be inflated inside it. It can cause haematuria, penile swelling, retention and impaired renal function. The NPSA have produced a rapid response report alerting clinical staff to the dangers of this (NPSA 2009).

Tip design

Several different types of catheter tip are available in addition to the standard round tip (Figure 5.9). Each tip is designed to overcome a particular problem.

- The *Tiemann-tipped catheter* has a curved tip with 1–3 drainage eyes to allow greater drainage. This catheter has been designed to negotiate the membranous and prostatic urethra in patients with prostatic hypertrophy. It is recomended that these catheters are only inserted by a urology specialist.
- The *whistle-tipped catheter* has a lateral eye in the tip and eyes above the balloon to provide a large drainage area. This design is intended to facilitate drainage of debris, for example blood clots.
- The *Roberts catheter* has an eye above and below the balloon to facilitate the drainage of residual urine.

Catheter material

A wide variety of materials is used to make catheters. The key criterion in selecting the appropriate material is the length of time the catheter is expected to remain in place. Three broad timescales have been identified.

- Short term (1–7 days), e.g. PVC and intermittent catheters.
- Short to medium term (up to 28 days), e.g. PTFE.
- Medium to long term (6–12 weeks), e.g. hydrogel and silicone coated.

The principal catheter materials are as follows.

Figure 5.9 **Catheter tips.**

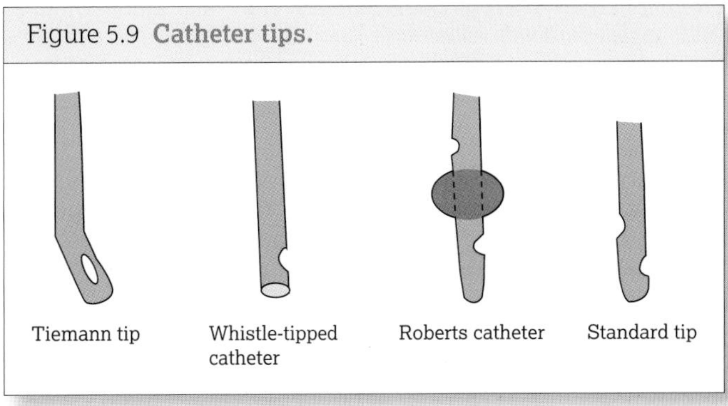

Polyvinyl chloride (PVC)
Catheters made from PVC or plastic are quite rigid. They have a wide lumen, which allows a rapid flow rate, but their rigidity may cause some patients discomfort. They are mainly used for intermittent catheterization or post-operatively. They are recommended for short-term use only (Pomfret 1996).

Latex
Latex is a purified form of rubber and is the softest of the catheter materials. It has a smooth surface, with a tendency to allow crust formation. Latex absorbs water and consequently the catheter may swell, reducing the diameter of the internal lumen and increasing its external diameter (Pomfret 2002, Robinson 2001). It has been shown to cause urethral irritation and therefore should only be considered when catheterization is likely to be short term.

Hypersensitivity to latex has been increasing in recent years (Woodward 1997) and latex catheters have been the cause of some cases of anaphylaxis (Young et al. 1994). Woodward (1997) suggests that patients should be asked whether they have ever had an adverse reaction to rubber products before catheters containing latex are utilized.

Teflon (polytetrafluoroethylene [PTFE]) or silicone elastomer coatings
A Teflon or silicone elastomer coating is applied to a latex catheter to render the latex inert and reduce urethral irritation (Bell 2010). Teflon is recommended for short-term use and silicone elastomer-coated catheters are used for long-term catheterization.

All silicone
Silicone is an inert material which is less likely to cause urethral irritation. Silicone catheters are not coated and therefore have a wider lumen. The lumen of these catheters, in cross-section, is crescent or D-shaped, which may induce formation of encrustation (Pomfret 1996). Because silicone permits gas diffusion, balloons may deflate and allow the catheter to fall out prematurely. These catheters may be more uncomfortable as they are more rigid than the latex-cored types. All-silicone catheters are suitable for patients with latex allergies. Silicone catheters are recommended for long-term use.

Hydrogel coatings
Catheters made of an inner core of latex encapsulated in a hydrophilic polymer coating are commonly used for long-term catheterization. The polymer coating is well tolerated by the urethral mucosa, causing little irritation. Hydrogel-coated catheters become smoother when rehydrated, reducing friction with the urethra. They are also inert and are reported to be resistant to bacterial colonization and encrustation (Woollons 1996). Hydrogel-coated catheters are recommended for long-term use.

Conformable catheter
Conformable catheters are designed to conform to the shape of the female urethra, and allow partial filling of the bladder. The natural movement of the urethra against the collapsible catheter is intended to prevent obstructions. They are made of latex and have a silicone elastomer coating. Conformable catheters are approximately 3 cm longer than conventional catheters for women.

Other materials
Research into new types of catheter materials is ongoing, particularly examining materials that resist the formation of biofilms (bacterial colonies that develop and adhere to the catheter surface and drainage bag) and consequently reduce the instances of urinary tract infections (Pratt et al. 2007).

Catheters coated with a silver alloy have been shown to prevent urinary tract infections (Schumm and Lam 2008). However, the studies that demonstrated this benefit were all small scale and a number of questions about the long-term effects of using such catheters, such as silver toxicity, need to be addressed. Argyria is a condition caused by the deposition of silver locally or systemically in the body, and can give rise to nausea, constipation and loss of night vision (Bardsley 2009, Pratt et al. 2007). There is some suggestion in the research that the use of silver alloy-coated catheters does reduce the onset of bacteriuria and may be beneficial when catheterization is in high-risk situations, for example diabetic and intensive care patients (Saint et al. 2000). However, research trials analysed by the Cochrane Collaboration (Schumm and Lam 2008) indicate that this asymptomatic bacteraemia was only seen in the first 5–7 days; after this, the catheter type made little difference (Plowman et al. 2001, Pratt et al. 2007).

Catheters coated with antibiotics such as gentamicin, rifampicin, nitrofurazone and nitrouroxone have been investigated in the search to find a product that will reduce instances of catheter-associated urinary tract infections (CAUTI). They may have a role to play in the management of trauma patients; nitrofurazone-impregnated catheters were shown to reduce urinary infections when compared with standard catheters in a trial by Stensballe et al. (2007). Whether this effect would be present in non-trauma patients and in the management of patients with long-term catheters is unknown. However, issues such as antibiotic sensitivity or resistance have not been fully investigated or assessed (Schumm and Lam 2008).

The cost implications for routine use of these impregnated catheters would be huge for the NHS (Johnson et al. 2006). However, a recent review of impregnated catheters found that silver alloy (antiseptic)-coated or nitrofurazone-impregnated (antibiotic) urinary catheters do reduce infections in hospitalized adults, and siliconized catheters may reduce adverse effects in men, but the evidence is weak (Schumm and Lam 2008). Trials with a specific catheter may be appropriate on an individual patient basis when other types of catheter management of recurrent infections have failed.

Drainage bags

A wide variety of drainage systems is available. When selecting a system, consideration should be given to the reasons for catheterization, intended duration, the patient's wishes, and infection control issues.

Urine drainage bags should only be changed according to clinical need; that is, when that catheter is changed or if the bag is leaking, or at times dictated by the manufacturer's instructions, for example every 5–7 days (Pratt et al. 2007). Urine drainage bags positioned above the level of the bladder and full bags cause urine to reflux, which is associated with infection. Therefore bags should always be positioned below the level of the bladder to maintain an unobstructed flow and be emptied appropriately. Urine drainage bags should be hung on suitable stands to avoid contact with the floor. In situations when dependent drainage is not possible, the system should be clamped until dependent drainage can be resumed (Kunin 1997). When emptying drainage bags, clean separate containers should be used for each patient and care should be taken to avoid contact between the drainage tap and the container (Pratt et al. 2007).

Urine drainage bags are available in a wide selection of sizes ranging from the large 2 litre bag, which is used more commonly in non-ambulatory patients and overnight, to 350–750 mL leg bags (Figure 5.10, Figure 5.11). There are also large drainage bags that incorporate urine-measuring devices, which are used when very close monitoring of urine output is required (Figure 5.12).

There are a number of different styles of drainage bags, from the body-worn 'belly bags' (Pomfret 2007) to the standard leg-worn bags. They allow patients greater mobility and can be worn under the patient's own clothes and therefore are much more discreet, helping to preserve the patient's privacy and dignity. Shapes vary from oblong to oval and some have cloth backing for greater comfort when in contact with the skin. Others are

Figure 5.10 **Urinary catheter bag, standard.**

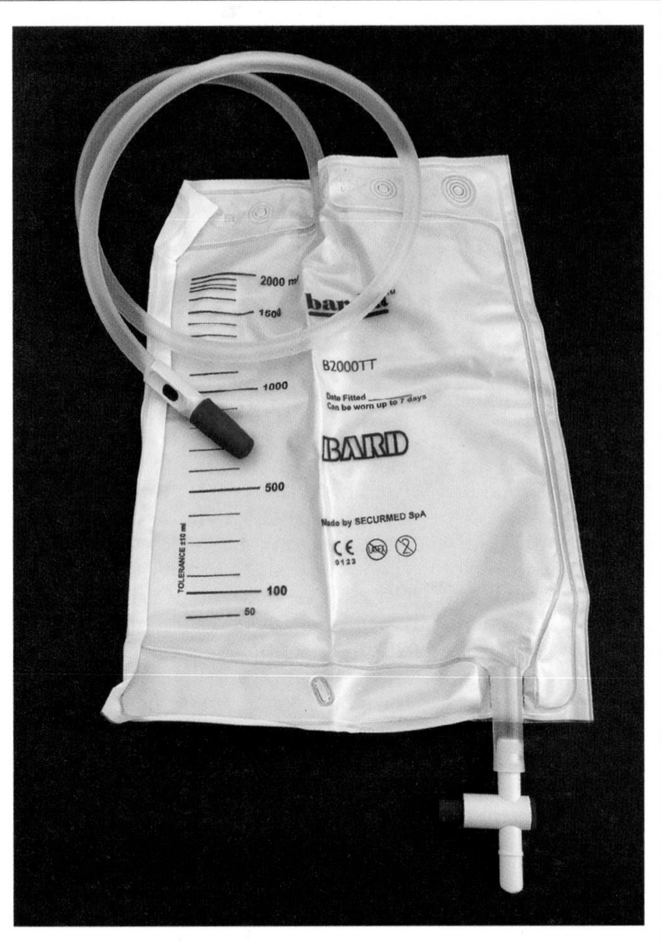

Figure 5.11 **Urinary catheter leg bag.**

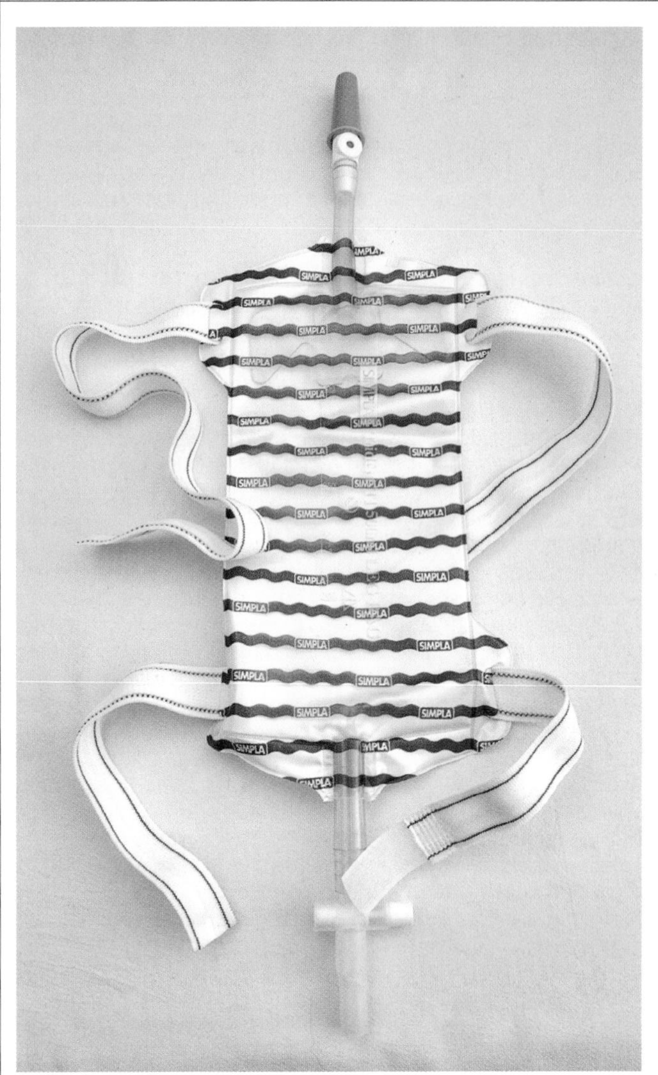

ridged to encourage an even distribution of urine through the bag, resulting in better conformity to the leg. The length of the inlet tube also varies (direct, short, long and adjustable length) and the intended position on the leg, that is thigh, knee or lower leg, determines which length is used (Robinson 2006, 2008). The patient should be asked to identify the most comfortable position for the bag (Pomfret 2007). The majority of drainage bags are fitted with an antireflux valve to prevent the backflow of urine into the bladder (Madeo and Roodhouse 2009). Several different tap designs exist and patients must have the manual dexterity to operate the mechanism (Robinson 2008). Most leg bags allow for larger 1–2 litre bags to be connected via the outlet tap, to increase capacity for night-time use.

It is advised to maintain a closed system of drainage to limit infection, but long-term catheter users may opt to wear a urinary drainage bag attached to their leg bag for larger capacity. Such changes disrupt the closed system but are essential to improve quality of life (Ostaszkiewicz and Paterson 2012).

A variety of supports is available for use with these bags, including sporran waist belts, leg holsters, knickers/pants and leg straps (Doherty 2006).

Leg straps

The use of thigh straps (e.g. Simpla G-Strap) and other fixation devices (e.g. Bard StatLock, Comfasure, Clinimed CliniFix) helps to immobilize the catheter and thus reduce the trauma potential to the bladder neck and urethra (Eastwood 2009). It is particularly appropriate for men, due to the longer length and weight of the

Figure 5.12 **Urinary catheter bag with urometer.**

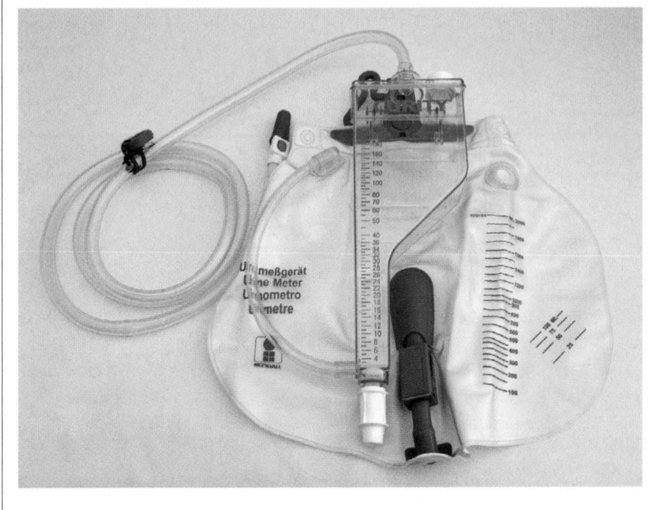

tube being used; however, some women may also find the extra support more comfortable. Guidance from the Royal College of Nursing (RCN 2012a) and NHS Scotland (NHSQIS 2004) reiterates the importance of catheter tetherage to promote patient comfort and to limit the potential complications of catheter migration and subsequent need for recatheterization. The application of these devices is not without potential complications; for example, restriction of the circulation to the limb may give rise to deep vein thrombosis while tension and traction to the urethra can cause trauma and necrosis, especially in men (Bierman and Carigan 2003).

Catheter valves

Catheter valves, which eliminate the need for drainage bags, are also available. The valve allows the bladder to be emptied intermittently and is particularly appropriate for patients who require long-term catheterization, as they do not require a drainage bag.

Catheter valves are only suitable for patients who have good cognitive function, sufficient manual dexterity to manipulate the valve and an adequate bladder capacity. It is important that catheter valves are released at regular intervals to ensure that the bladder does not become overdistended. These valves must not be used on patients following surgical procedures to the prostate or bladder, as pressure caused by the distending bladder may cause perforation or rupture; in most of these instances the urethral catheter is only required for a short period of time and free drainage is the preferred method. As catheter valves preclude free drainage, they are unlikely to be appropriate for patients with uncontrolled detrusor overactivity, ureteric reflux or renal impairment (Fader et al. 1997). Catheter valves are designed to fit with linked systems so it is possible for patients to connect to a drainage bag. This may be necessary when access to toilets may be limited, for example overnight or on long journeys.

Catheter valves are recommended to remain *in situ* for 5–7 days, which corresponds with most manufacturers' recommendations (Woodward 2013). More research is needed into the advantages and disadvantages of catheter valves.

Pharmacological support

Anaesthetic lubricating gel

The use of anaesthetic lubricating gels is well recognized for male catheterization, but there is some controversy over their use for female catheterization. In male patients the gel is instilled directly into the urethra and then external massage is used to move the gel down its length, unless a conforming gel such as Instillagel is used and then this is not necessary. In female patients, the anaesthetic lubricating gel or plain lubricating gel is applied to the tip of the catheter only, if it is used at all.

These differences in practice imply that catheterization is a painful procedure for men but is not so for women. This assumption is not based on any empirical or biological evidence. Other than the differences in length and route, the male and female urethra are very similar except for the presence of lubricating glands in the male urethra (Tortora and Derrickson 2011).

A study by Chung et al. (2007) showed that women who had lubricating gel prior to catheterization reported lower pain scores than those who did not. The use of anaesthetic gel also dilates the urethral folds, making insertion easier for the professional.There is a need for caution with the use of lidocaine in the elderly, those with cardiac dysrhythmias and those with sensitivity to the drug, as there is a danger of injury to the urothelial lining of the urethra during the procedure, allowing systemic absorption of the drug (BNF 2014).

Trauma can occur during catheterization, which in turn can increase the risk of infection. Using single-use lubrication gels with antiseptic properties can reduce these risks (BNF 2014, Pratt et al. 2007). Since there is a lack of research to clarify the efficacy of lubricating gels, practice must be based on the research evidence that is available and the physiology and anatomy of the urethra.

Procedure guideline 5.7 **Urinary catheterization: male**

Essential equipment

- Sterile pack containing gallipots, receiver, gauze swabs, disposable towels
- Disposable pad
- 0.9% sodium chloride
- Bactericidal alcohol handrub
- Hypoallergenic tape or leg strap for tethering
- Sterile gloves
- Sterile water
- Selection of appropriate catheters
- Syringe and needle (as required to obtain a urine sample)
- Sterile anaesthetic lubricating jelly
- Disposable plastic apron
- Universal specimen container
- Drainage bag and stand or holder
- Clean towel or similar

Pre-procedure

Action	Rationale
1 Explain and discuss the procedure with the patient.	To ensure that the patient understands the procedure and gives his valid consent (NMC 2013, **C**).
2 Screen the bed.	To ensure patient's privacy. To allow dust and airborne organisms to settle before the sterile field is exposed (Fraise and Bradley 2009, **E**).
3 Prepare the trolley, placing all equipment required on the bottom shelf.	The top shelf acts as a clean working surface. **E**
4 Take the trolley to the patient's bedside, disturbing the screens as little as possible.	To minimize airborne contamination (Fraise and Bradley 2009, **E**).

Action	Rationale
5 Assist the patient to get into the supine position with the legs extended on the bed.	To ensure the appropriate area is easily accessible. **E**
6 Remove underpants or pyjama trousers and use a towel to cover the patient's thighs and genital area.	To maintain patient's dignity and comfort (NMC 2015, **C**).
7 Wash hands using bactericidal soap and water or bactericidal alcohol handrub.	To reduce risk of infection (Fraise and Bradley 2009, **E**).
8 Put on a disposable plastic apron.	To reduce risk of cross-infection from micro-organisms on uniform (Fraise and Bradley 2009, **E**).
Procedure	
9 Open the outer cover of the catheterization pack and slide the pack onto the top shelf of the trolley.	To prepare equipment. **E**
10 Using an aseptic technique, open the sterile/catheter pack. Pour 0.9% sodium chloride into gallipot. Open an appropriately sized catheter onto the sterile field.	To reduce the risk of introducing infection into the bladder (NICE 2012, **C**).
11 Remove cover from the patient's genital area, maintaining the patient's privacy, and position a disposable pad under the patient's buttocks and thighs.	To ensure urine does not leak onto bedclothes. **E**
12 Clean hands with a bactericidal alcohol handrub.	Hands may have become contaminated by handling the outer packs (Fraise and Bradley 2009, **C**).
13 Put on sterile gloves.	To reduce risk of cross-infection (NICE 2012, **C**).
14 On the sterile field, place the catheter into the sterile receiver.	
15 Place a sterile towel across the patient's thighs.	To create a sterile field. **E**
16 With one hand, wrap a sterile topical swab around the penis. Use this to retract the foreskin, if necessary, and with the other hand clean the glans penis with 0.9% sodium chloride or sterile water.	To reduce the risk of introducing infection to the urinary tract during catheterization. **E**
17 Insert the nozzle of the lubricating jelly into the urethra. Squeeze the gel into the urethra, remove the nozzle and discard the tube. Massage the gel along the urethra using the barrel of the syringe.	Adequate lubrication helps to prevent urethral trauma. Use of a local anaesthetic minimizes the discomfort experienced by the patient (Bardsley 2005, **P**).
18 Squeeze the penis and wait approximately 5 minutes.	To prevent anaesthetic gel from escaping. To allow the anaesthetic gel to take effect. **E**
19 With one hand hold the penis firmly behind the glans, raising it until it is almost totally extended. Maintain this hold of the penis until the catheter is inserted and urine flowing.	This manoeuvre straightens the penile urethra and facilitates catheterization (Stoller 2004, **P**). Maintaining a grasp of the penis prevents contamination and retraction of the penis.
20 With the free hand, place the receiver containing the catheter between the patient's legs. Take the catheter and insert it into the penis for 15–25 cm until urine flows.	The male urethra is approximately 18 cm long (Bardsley 2005, **P**).
21 If resistance is felt at the external sphincter, increase the traction on the penis slightly and apply steady, gentle pressure on the catheter. Ask the patient to cough gently.	Some resistance may be due to spasm of the external sphincter. Coughing gently helps to relax the external sphincter. **E**
22 When urine begins to flow, advance the catheter almost to its bifurcation.	Advancing the catheter ensures that it is correctly positioned in the bladder. **E**
23 Gently inflate the balloon according to the manufacturer's direction, having ensured that the catheter is draining properly beforehand.	Inadvertent inflation of the balloon in the urethra causes pain and urethral trauma (Getliffe and Dolman 2007, **E**).
24 Withdraw the catheter slightly and attach it to the drainage system.	To ensure that the balloon is inflated and the catheter is secure. **E**

(continued)

Procedure guideline 5.7 Urinary catheterization: male *(continued)*

Action	Rationale
25 Support the catheter, if the patient desires, either by using a specially designed support, for example Simpla G-Strap, or by taping the catheter to the patient's leg. Ensure that the catheter does not become taut when patient is mobilizing or when the penis becomes erect. Ensure that the catheter lumen is not occluded by the fixation device or tape.	To maintain patient comfort and to reduce the risk of urethral and bladder neck trauma. Care must be taken in using adhesive tapes as they may interact with the catheter material (Fillingham and Douglas 2004, **E**; Pomfret 1996, **P**).
26 Ensure that the glans penis is clean and dry and then extend the foreskin.	Retraction and constriction of the foreskin behind the glans penis (paraphimosis) may occur if this is not done (Pomfret 2002, **E**).
Post-procedure	
27 Assist the patient to replace underwear and pyjamas and replace bed cover. Ensure that the area is dry.	If the area is left wet or moist, secondary infection and skin irritation may occur (Pomfret 2002, **E**).
28 Measure the amount of urine.	To be aware of bladder capacity for patients who have presented with urinary retention. To monitor renal function and fluid balance. It is not necessary to measure the amount of urine if the patient is having the urinary catheter routinely changed (Pomfret 2002, **E**).
29 If required, take a urine specimen for laboratory examination (see Chapter 11: Observations).	For further information, see Chapter 11, Procedure guideline 11.7 Urinalysis: reagent strip procedure.
30 Dispose of equipment including apron and gloves in an orange plastic clinical waste bag and seal the bag before moving the trolley.	To prevent environmental contamination. Orange is the recognized colour for clinical waste (DH 2005, **C**).
31 Draw back the curtains.	
32 Dispose of clinical waste bag in a larger bin.	To prevent environmental contamination (Fraise and Bradley 2009, **E**).
33 Wash hands thoroughly with bactericidal soap and water.	To reduce risk of infection (Fraise and Bradley 2009, **E**).
34 Record information in relevant documents; this should include: • reasons for catheterization • date and time of catheterization • catheter type, length and size • amount of water instilled into the balloon • batch number • manufacturer • any problems negotiated during the procedure • a review date to assess the need for continued catheterization or date of change of catheter.	To provide a point of reference or comparison in the event of later queries (NMC 2010, **C**).

Procedure guideline 5.8 Urinary catheterization: female

Essential equipment

- Sterile catheterization pack containing gallipots, receiver, gauze swabs, disposable towels
- Bactericidal alcohol handrub
- Hypoallergenic tape or leg strap for tethering
- Sterile water
- Syringe and needle
- Disposable plastic apron
- Drainage bag and stand or holder
- Clean towel or similar cover
- Disposable pad
- Sterile gloves
- Selection of appropriate catheters
- Sterile anaesthetic lubricating jelly
- Universal specimen container

Pre-procedure

Action	Rationale
1 Explain and discuss the procedure with the patient.	To ensure that the patient understands the procedure and gives her valid consent (NMC 2013, **C**).

2 Screen the bed.	To ensure patient's privacy. To allow dust and airborne organisms to settle before the sterile field is exposed (Fraise and Bradley 2009, **E**).
3 Prepare the trolley, placing all equipment required on the bottom shelf. (See also 'Equipment: catheter selection'.)	To reserve top shelf for clean working surface. **E**
4 Take the trolley to the patient's bedside, disturbing screens as little as possible.	To minimize airborne contamination (Fraise and Bradley 2009, **C**).
5 Remove patient's underwear. Assist patient to get into the supine position with knees bent, hips flexed and feet resting about 60 cm apart.	To enable genital area to be seen. **E**
6 Place a towel over the patient's thighs and genital area.	To maintain the patient's dignity and comfort (NMC 2013, **C**).
7 Ensure that a good light source is available.	To enable genital area to be seen clearly. **E**
8 Wash hands using bactericidal soap and water or bactericidal alcohol handrub.	To reduce risk of cross-infection (Fraise and Bradley 2009, **E**).
9 Put on a disposable apron.	To reduce risk of cross-infection from micro-organisms on uniform (Bardsley and Kyle 2008, **E**; Fraise and Bradley 2009, **E**).

Procedure

10 Open the outer cover of the catheterization pack and slide the pack on the top shelf of the trolley.	To prepare equipment. **E**
11 Using an aseptic technique, open sterile pack. Then open appropriately-sized catheter and place on sterile field.	To reduce risk of introducing infection into the urinary tract. **E**
12 Remove towel, maintaining the patient's privacy, and position a disposable pad under the patient's buttocks.	To ensure urine does not leak onto bedclothes. **E**
13 Clean hands with a bactericidal alcohol handrub.	Hands may have become contaminated by handling of outer packs, and so on (Fraise and Bradley 2009, **C**).
14 Put on sterile gloves.	To reduce risk of cross-infection (NICE 2012, **C**).
15 Place sterile towels under the patient's buttocks.	To create a sterile field. **E**
16 Using gauze swabs, separate the labia minora so that the urethral meatus is seen. One hand should be used to maintain labial separation until catheter is inserted and urine flowing.	This manoeuvre provides better access to the urethral orifice and helps to prevent labial contamination of the catheter. **E**
17 Clean around the urethral orifice with 0.9% sodium chloride using single downward strokes.	Inadequate preparation of the urethral orifice is a major cause of infection following catheterization. To reduce the risk of cross-infection (Fraise and Bradley 2009, **E**).
18 Place a small amount of the lubricating jelly/anaesthetic gel onto the tip of the catheter.	Adequate lubrication helps to prevent urethral trauma. Use of a local anaesthetic minimizes the patient's discomfort (Woodward 2005, **P**).
19 Place the catheter, in the sterile receiver, between the patient's legs.	To provide a temporary container for urine as it drains. **E**
20 Introduce the tip of the catheter into the urethral orifice in an upward and backward direction. Advance the catheter until 5–6 cm has been inserted.	The direction of insertion and the length of catheter inserted should relate to the anatomical structure of the area. **E**
21 If there is no urine present, remove the catheter gently and start procedure again. If urine is present, advance the catheter 6–8 cm.	This prevents the balloon from becoming trapped in the urethra.
22 Inflate the balloon according to the manufacturer's directions, having ensured that the catheter is draining adequately.	Inadvertent inflation of the balloon within the urethra is painful and causes urethral trauma (Getliffe and Dolman 2007, **P**).
23 Withdraw the catheter slightly and connect it to the drainage system.	To ensure that the balloon is inflated and the catheter is secure. **E**

(continued)

Procedure guideline 5.8 Urinary catheterization: female *(continued)*

Action	Rationale
24 Support the catheter, if the patient desires, either by using a specially designed support, for example Simpla G-Strap, or by taping the catheter to the patient's leg. Ensure that the catheter does not become taut when patient is mobilizing. Ensure that the catheter lumen is not occluded by the fixation device or tape.	To maintain patient comfort and to reduce the risk of urethral and bladder neck trauma. Care must be taken in using adhesive tapes as they may interact with the catheter material (Pomfret 1996, **P**).
Post-procedure	
25 Assist the patient to replace underwear and pyjamas and replace bed cover. Ensure that the area is dry.	If the area is left wet or moist, secondary infection and skin irritation may occur (Pomfret 2002, **E**).
26 Measure the amount of urine.	To be aware of bladder capacity for patients who have presented with urinary retention. To monitor renal function and fluid balance. It is not necessary to measure the amount of urine if the patient is having the urinary catheter routinely changed (Pomfret 2002, **E**).
27 If required, take a urine specimen for laboratory examination (see Chapter 11: Observations).	For further information, see Chapter 11, Procedure guideline 11.7 Urinalysis: reagent strip procedure.
28 Dispose of equipment including apron and gloves in an orange plastic clinical waste bag and seal the bag before moving the trolley.	To prevent environmental contamination. Orange is the recognized colour for clinical waste (DH 2005, **C**).
29 Draw back the curtains.	
30 Dispose of clinical waste bag in a larger bin.	To prevent environmental contamination (Fraise and Bradley 2009, **E**).
31 Wash hands thoroughly with bactericidal soap and water.	To reduce risk of infection (Fraise and Bradley 2009, **E**).
32 Record information in relevant documents; this should include: • reasons for catheterization • date and time of catheterization • catheter type, length and size • amount of water instilled into the balloon • batch number and manufacturer • any problems negotiated during the procedure • a review date to assess the need for continued catheterization or date of change of catheter.	To provide a point of reference or comparison in the event of later queries (NMC 2010, **C**).

Problem-solving table 5.2 Prevention and resolution (Procedure guidelines 5.7, 5.8)

Problem	Cause	Prevention	Action
Urethral mucosal trauma.	Incorrect size of catheter. Procedure not carried out correctly or skilfully. Movement of the catheter in the urethra.		Recatheterize the patient using the correct size of catheter. Check the catheter support and apply or reapply as necessary.
	Trauma to the urethral tissue due to rapid insertion of catheter.		Nurse may need to remove the catheter and wait for the urethral mucosa to heal.
Patient has a vasovagal attack.	This is caused by the vagal nerve being stimulated so that the heart slows down, leading to a syncope faint.		Lie the patient down in the recovery position (see Chapter 9: Respiratory care, Figure 9.32 Recovery position). Inform doctors.

Male			
Paraphimosis	Failure to extend the foreskin after catheterization or catheter toilet.		Always retract the foreskin. Clean and dry around the foreskin.
Female			
No drainage of urine.	Incorrect identification of external urinary meatus.	Ensure sufficient light to observe the area. Review the female anatomy prior to the procedure.	Check that catheter has been sited correctly. If catheter has been wrongly inserted in the vagina, leave it in position to act as a guide, reidentify the urethra and catheterize the patient. Remove the inappropriately sited catheter.
Difficulty in visualizing the urethral orifice.	This can be due to vaginal atrophy and retraction of the urethral orifice.		The index finger of the 'dirty' hand may be inserted in the vagina, and the urethral orifice can be palpated on the anterior wall of the vagina. The index finger is then positioned just behind the urethral orifice. This then acts as a guide, so the catheter can be correctly positioned (Jenkins 1998).

Suprapubic catheterization

EVIDENCE-BASED APPROACHES

Rationale

Suprapubic catheterization is the insertion of a catheter through the anterior abdominal wall into the dome of the bladder. The procedure is performed under general or local anaesthesia, using a percutaneous system (Robinson 2008). The National Patient Safety Agency (NPSA 2009) published a rapid response report stating that the insertion of a suprapubic catheter should be undertaken by experienced urology staff using ultrasound imaging. Pre-procedural considerations are those indicated when preparing a patient for a radiological intervention.

Indications

Suprapubic catheterization does offer some advantages over urethral catheterization (Rigby 2009). The risk of patients developing urinary tract infection is reduced, as the bacterial count on the abdominal skin is less than around the perineal and perianal areas, although bacteriuria and encrustation still occur in susceptible patients (Simpson 2001). Urethral integrity is retained and it allows for the resumption of normal voiding after surgery. Clamping the suprapubic catheter allows urethral voiding to occur, and the clamp can be released if voiding is incomplete. Pain and catheter-associated discomfort are reduced. Patient satisfaction is increased as, for some, their level of independence is increased and sexual intercourse can occur with fewer impediments (Fillingham and Douglas 2004).

Indications for the use of suprapubic catheters over indwelling catheters include the following.

- Post-operative drainage of urine after lower urinary tract and bowel surgery.
- Management of neuropathic bladders.
- Long-term conditions, for example multiple sclerosis (MS) or spinal cord injuries.
- People with long-term catheters – to minimize the risk of urethral infections or urethral damage (NPSA 2009).

However, there are a number of risks and disadvantages associated with suprapubic catheterization.

- Bowel perforation and haemorrhage at the time of insertion.
- Infection, swelling, encrustation and granulation at insertion site.
- Pain, discomfort or irritation for some patients.
- Bladder stone formation and possible long-term risk of squamous cell carcinoma.
- Urethral leakage (Addison and Mould 2000).

POST-PROCEDURAL CONSIDERATIONS

Care of a suprapubic catheter is the same as for a urethral catheter. Immediately following insertion of a suprapubic catheter, aseptic technique should be employed to clean the insertion site (Robinson 2008). Keyhole dressings around the insertion site may be required if secretions soil clothing, but they are not essential. Once the insertion site has healed (7–10 days), the site and catheter can be cleaned during bathing using soap, water and a clean cloth (Fillingham and Douglas 2004).

Procedure guideline 5.9 Urinary catheter bag: emptying

Essential equipment

- Alcohol wipe
- Disposable gloves
- Container (jug or urine bottle)
- Paper towel to cover the jug

Pre-procedure

Action	Rationale
1 Explain and discuss the procedure with the patient.	To ensure that the patient understands the procedure and gives their valid consent (NMC 2013, **C**).
2 Wash hands using bactericidal soap and water or bactericidal alcohol handrub, and put on disposable gloves.	To reduce risk of cross-infection (Fraise and Bradley 2009, **E**).
Procedure	
3 Open the cathether valve. Allow the urine to drain into the jug.	To empty drainage bag and accurately measure volume of contents. **E**
4 Close the outlet valve and clean it with an alcohol wipe.	To reduce risk of cross-infection (Fraise and Bradley 2009, **E**).
5 Cover the jug and dispose of contents in the sluice, having noted the amount of urine if this is requested for fluid balance records.	To reduce risk of environmental contamination (DEFRA 2005, **C**).
6 Wash hands with bactericidal soap and water.	To reduce risk of infection (Fraise and Bradley 2009, **E**).

Procedure guideline 5.10 Urinary catheter removal

Essential equipment

- Dressing pack containing sterile towel, gallipot, swab or non-linting gauze
- Needle and syringe for urine specimen, specimen container
- Disposable gloves and apron
- Syringe for deflating balloon

Pre-procedure

Action	Rationale
1 Catheters are usually removed early in the morning.	So that any retention problems can be dealt with during the day. **E**
2 Explain procedure to the patient and inform them of potential post-catheter symptoms, such as urgency, frequency and discomfort, which are often caused by irritation of the urethra by the catheter.	So that patient knows what to expect, and can plan daily activity.
3 Wash hands using bactericidal soap and water or bactericidal alcohol handrub, and put on disposable gloves.	To reduce risk of cross-infection (Fraise and Bradley 2009, **E**).
Procedure	
4 If a specimen is required, clamp below the sampling port until sufficient urine collects. Take a catheter specimen of urine using the sampling port.	To obtain an adequate urine sample and to assess whether postcatheter antibiotic therapy is needed (Fraise and Bradley 2009, **E**).
5 Wearing gloves, use saline-soaked gauze to clean the meatus and catheter, always swabbing away from the urethral opening.	To reduce risk of infection (Fraise and Bradley 2009, **E**).
Note: in women, never clean from the perineum/vagina towards the urethra.	To help reduce the risk of bacteria from the vagina and perineum contaminating the urethra. **E**
6 Release leg support.	For easier removal of catheter. **E**

7 Having checked volume of water in balloon (see patient documentation), use syringe to deflate balloon.	To confirm how much water is in the balloon. To ensure balloon is completely deflated before removing catheter. **E**
8 Ask patient to breathe in and then out; as patient exhales, gently (but firmly with continuous traction) remove catheter. Male patients should be warned of discomfort as the deflated balloon passes through the prostate gland.	To relax pelvic floor muscles. **E** It is advisable to extend the penis as per the process for insertion to aid removal. **E**
Post-procedure	
9 *Male*: clean meatus and make the patient comfortable. *Female*: clean area around the genitalia and make the patient comfortable.	To maintain patient comfort and dignity. **E**
10 Encourage patient to exercise and to drink 2–3 litres of fluid per day.	To prevent urinary tract infections. **E**
11 Dispose of equipment including apron and gloves in an orange plastic clinical waste bag.	To prevent environmental contamination. Orange is the recognized colour for clinical waste (DEFRA 2005, **C**).
12 Wash hands thoroughly with bactericidal soap and water.	To reduce risk of infection (Fraise and Bradley 2009, **E**).
13 Record information in relevant documents; this should include: • reasons for catheterization • date and time of catheterization • catheter type, length and size • amount of water instilled into the balloon • batch number and manufacturer • any problems negotiated during the procedure • a review date to assess the need for continued catheterization or date of change of catheter.	To provide a point of reference or comparison in the event of later queries (NMC 2010, **C**).

COMPLICATIONS

Infections

Catheterization carries an infection risk. Catheter-associated infections are the most common hospital-acquired infection, accounting for 40% of all hospital infections (Andreessen et al. 2012).

Key areas have been identified as having a direct link with the development of urinary tract infection.

- Assessing the need for catheterization and the length of time the catheter is *in situ* (Nazarko 2007). The risk of developing a catheter-associated infection increases with the length of time that a catheter is *in situ* (Bernard et al. 2012).
- Selection of the most appropriate type of catheter and drainage system to be used.
- The aseptic conditions and process by which the catheter is inserted and maintained as a closed drainage system.
- Training and competence of the person performing the procedure and those undertaking the aftercare, that is, patients, relatives and health professionals. Patient education is essential in preventing catheter-associated infections. Adequate information and teaching for patients may help to reduce infection if they can care for their catheters with good hygiene.

The maintenance of a closed drainage system is central in reducing the risk of catheter-associated infection. It is thought that micro-organisms reach the bladder by two possible routes: from the urine in the drainage bag or via the space between the catheter and the urethral mucosa (Ostaszkiewicz and Paterson 2012). To reduce the risk of infection, it is important to keep manipulation of the closed system to a minimum; this includes unnecessary emptying, changing the drainage bags or taking samples (Ostaszkiewicz and Paterson 2012). There is now an intregal catheter and drainage bag available to reduce the number of potential disconnection sites and infection risk. Before handling catheter drainage systems, hands must be decontaminated and a pair of clean non-sterile gloves should be worn (Pratt et al. 2007). All urine samples should only be obtained via the specially designed sampling ports using an aseptic technique.

Urinary tract infections (male): meatal cleaning

Cleaning the urethral meatus, where the catheter enters the body, is a nursing procedure intended to minimize infection of the urinary tract for men (DH 2003, Magnall and Watterson 2006). Studies examining the use of a variety of antiseptic, antimicrobial agents or soap and water found that there was no reduction in bacteriuria when using any of these preparations for meatal cleaning compared to routine bathing or showering (Pratt et al. 2007). Further studies support the view that vigorous meatal cleaning is unnecessary and may compromise the integrity of the skin, thus increasing the risk of infection (Leaver 2007, Saint and Lipsky 1999). Therefore it is recommended that routine daily personal hygiene with soap and water (NICE 2012) is all that is needed to maintain meatal hygiene (Pomfret 2004, Pratt et al. 2007). Nursing intervention is necessary if there is a poor standard of hygiene or a risk of contamination (Gilbert 2006); removal of a smegma ring, where the catheter meets the meatus, is important to prevent ascending infections and meatal trauma (Wilson 2005).

A urinary tract infection (UTI) may be introduced during catheterization because of faulty aseptic technique, inadequate urethral cleaning or contamination of catheter tip. UTI may be introduced via the drainage system because of faulty handling of equipment, breaking the closed system or raising the drainage bag above bladder level, causing urine reflux.

If a UTI is suspected, a catheter specimen of urine must be sent for analysis. The patient should be encouraged to have a fluid intake of 2–3 litres a day. Medical staff should be informed if the problem persists so that antibiotics can be prescribed.

Table 5.3 details other complications that may arise if a patient is catheterized.

Table 5.3 **Complications of catheterization**

Problem	Cause	Suggested action
Inability to tolerate indwelling catheter	Urethral mucosal irritation Psychological trauma Unstable bladder Radiation cystitis	Nurse may need to remove the catheter and seek an alternative means of urine drainage Explain the need for and the functioning of the catheter
Inadequate drainage of urine	Incorrect placement of a catheter Kinked drainage tubing Blocked tubing, for example pus, urates, phosphates, blood clots	Resite the catheter Inspect the system and straighten any kinks If a three-way catheter, such as a Foley, is in place, irrigate it. If an ordinary catheter is in use, milk the tubing in an attempt to dislodge the debris, then attempt a gentle bladder washout. Failing this, the catheter will need to be replaced; a three-way catheter should be used if the obstruction is being caused by clots and associated haematuria
Fistula formation	Pressure on the penoscrotal angle	Ensure that correct strapping is used
Penile pain on erection	Not allowing enough length of catheter to accommodate penile erection	Ensure that an adequate length is available to accommodate penile erection
Formation of crusts around the urethral meatus	Increased urethral secretions collect at the meatus and form crusts, due to irritation of urothelium by the catheter (Fillingham and Douglas 2004)	Correct catheter toilet
Leakage of urine around catheter	Incorrect size of catheter Incorrect balloon size Bladder hyperirritability	Replace with the correct size, usually 2 ch smaller Select catheter with 10 mL balloon Use Roberts tipped catheter As a last resort, bladder hyperirritability can be reduced by giving diazepam or anticholinergic drugs (Nazarko 2009)
Unable to deflate balloon	Valve expansion or displacement Channel obstruction	Check the non-return valve on the inflation/deflation channel. If jammed, use a syringe and needle to aspirate by means of the inflation arm above the valve Obstruction by a foreign body can sometimes be relieved by the introduction of a guidewire through the inflation channel Inject 3.5 mL of dilute ether solution (diluted 50/50 with sterile water or 0.9% sodium chloride) into the inflation arm Alternatively, the balloon can be punctured suprapubically using a needle under ultrasound visualization Following catheter removal, the balloon should be inspected to ensure it has not disintegrated, leaving fragments in the bladder *Note:* steps above should be attempted by or under the directions of a urologist. The patient may require cystoscopy following balloon deflation to remove any balloon fragments and to wash the bladder out
Dysuria	Inflammation of the urethral mucosa	Ensure a fluid intake of 2–3 litres per day. Advise the patient that dysuria is common but will usually be resolved once micturition has occurred at least three times. Inform medical staff if the problem persists
Retention of urine	May be psychological	Encourage the patient to increase fluid intake. Offer the patient a warm bath. Inform medical staff if the problem persists

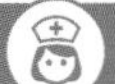 Learning Activity 5.2

Scenario: Urinary catheterization

You have been asked to catheterize a female patient (under supervision) who has been found to have urinary retention.

1 What factors should you consider prior to the procedure?
2 What steps can you take to minimize the risk of her developing a catheter-associated urinary tract infection?
3 What should you do after the procedure?

Hint: You should have come up with 4–5 points for each question.

See the end of the chapter for the answers.

Bladder irrigation

DEFINITION

Bladder irrigation is the continuous washing out of the bladder with sterile fluid, usually 0.9% normal saline (Ng 2001). Three-way catheters are used to wash out the bladder (Moslemi and Rajaei 2010).

EVIDENCE-BASED APPROACHES

Rationale

Indications

Bladder irrigation is performed to prevent the formation and retention of blood clots, for example following prostatic surgery such as transurethral resection of bladder tumour (TURBT) or transurethral resection of prostate (TURP). Other indications include irrigation for the delivery of pharmacological agents, irrigation for candida cystitis, prevention of haematuria following chemotherapy or surgical procedures (Moslemi and Rajaei 2010). On rare occasions bladder irrigation is performed to remove heavily contaminated material from a diseased urinary bladder (Cutts 2005, Fillingham and Douglas 2004, Scholtes 2002).

Principles of care

There are a number of risks associated with bladder irrigation (including introducing infection) and the procedure should not be undertaken lightly (McCarthy and Hunter 2001, NICE 2012). Prior to taking a decision to use bladder maintenance solutions, patients should be assessed. The guiding principle for effective catheter management always involves addressing the individual needs of the patient (Godfrey and Evans 2000). Assessment of all aspects of catheter care and irrigation should be undertaken, including:

- patient activity and mobility (catheter positioning, catheter kinking)
- diet and fluid intake
- standards of patient hygiene
- patient's and/or carer's ability to care for the catheter (Ng 2001, Rew 2005).

An important aspect of management for patients in whom a clear pattern of catheter history can be established is the scheduling of catheter changes prior to likely blockages (Yates 2004). In patients in whom no clear pattern emerges, or for whom frequent catheter changes are traumatic, acidic bladder washouts can be beneficial in reducing catheter encrustations (McCarthy and Hunter 2001, Yates 2004). The administration of catheter maintenance solutions to eliminate catheter encrustation can also be timed to coincide with catheter bag changes (every 5–7 days) so that the catheter system is not opened more than necessary (Yates 2004).

PRE-PROCEDURAL CONSIDERATIONS

Equipment

Catheters used for irrigation

A three-way urinary catheter must be used for irrigation in order that fluid may simultaneously be run into, and drained out from, the bladder (Cutts 2005, Ng 2001). A large-gauge catheter (16–24) is often used to accommodate any clot and debris which may be present. This catheter is commonly passed in theatre when irrigation is required, for example after prostatectomy (Forristal and Maxfield 2004). Occasionally, if a patient is admitted with a heavily contaminated bladder, for example blood clots, bladder irrigation may be started on the ward. If the patient has a two-way catheter, this must be replaced with a three-way type (Scholtes 2002).

It is recommended that a three-way catheter is passed if frequent intravesical instillations of drugs or antiseptic solutions are prescribed and the risk of catheter obstruction is not considered to be very great. In such cases, the most important factor is minimizing the risk of introducing infection and maintaining a closed urinary drainage system, for which the three-way catheter allows (Figure 5.13).

Pharmacological support

The agent most commonly recommended for irrigation is 0.9% sodium chloride which should be used in every case unless an alternative solution is prescribed. 0.9% sodium chloride is isotonic so it does not affect the body's fluid or electrolyte levels, enabling large volumes of the solution to be used as necessary (Cutts 2005). In particular, 2-litre bags of 0.9% sodium chloride are available for irrigation purposes. It has been proposed that sterile water should never be used to irrigate the bladder as it can be readily absorbed by osmosis (Addison 2000). However, a study has demonstrated that sterile water is a safe irrigating fluid for TURP (Moharari et al. 2008).

Although not a common complication, absorption of irrigation fluid can occur during bladder irrigation. This can produce a potentially critical situation, as absorption leads to electrolyte imbalance and circulatory overload. Absorption is most likely to occur in theatre where glycine irrigation fluid, devoid of sodium or potassium, is forced under pressure into the prostatic veins (Forristal and Maxfield 2004). The 0.9% sodium chloride cannot be used during surgery as it contains electrolytes which interfere with diathermy (Forristal and Maxfield 2004). However, the risk of absorption still remains while irrigation continues post-operatively. For this reason, it is important that fluid balance is monitored carefully during irrigation (Scholtes 2002).

Figure 5.13 Closed urinary drainage system with provision for intermittent or continuous irrigation.

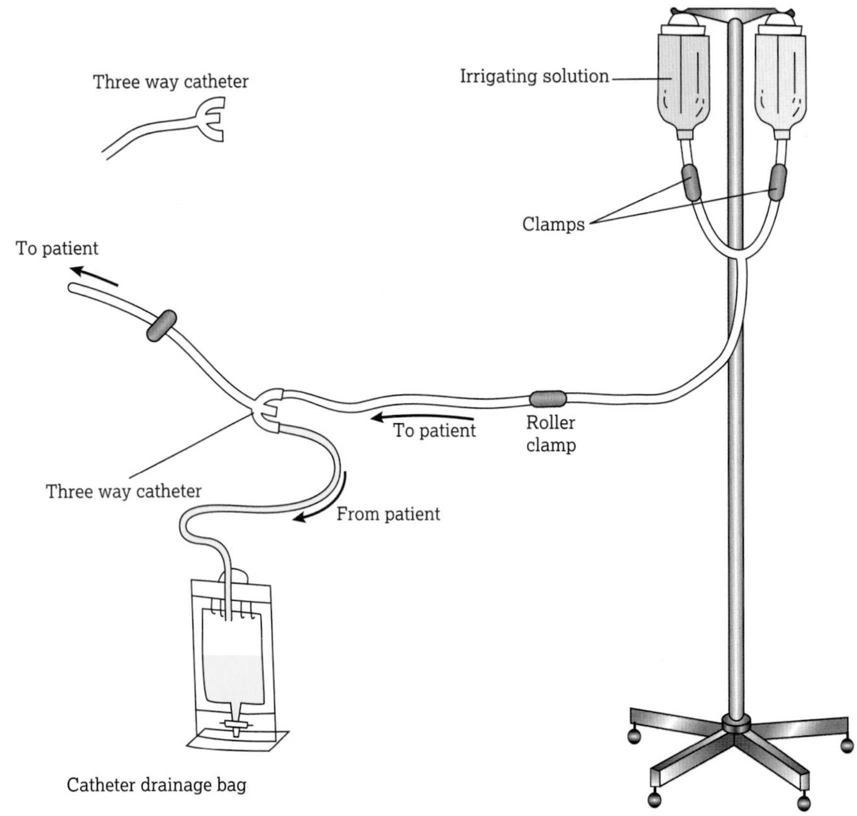

Procedure guideline 5.11 Commencing bladder irrigation

Essential equipment

- Sterile dressing pack and sterile gloves
- Chlorhexidine antiseptic solution
- Bactericidal alcohol handrub
- Clamp
- Disposable irrigation set
- Infusion stand
- Sterile jug
- Absorbent sheet
- Clean gloves and apron

Medicinal products

- Sterile irrigation fluid

Pre-procedure

Action	Rationale
1 Explain and discuss the procedure with the patient.	To ensure that the patient understands the procedure and gives their valid consent (NMC 2013, **C**).
2 Screen the bed. Ensure that the patient is in a comfortable position, allowing the nurse access to the catheter.	For the patient's privacy and to reduce the risk of cross-infection (Fraise and Bradley 2009, **E**).

Procedure	
3 Perform the procedure using an aseptic technique.	To minimize the risk of infection (Fraise and Bradley 2009, **E**).
4 Open the outer wrappings of the pack and put it on the top shelf of the trolley.	To prepare equipment. **E**
5 Insert the end of the irrigation giving set into the fluid bag and hang the bag on the infusion stand. Allow fluid to run through the tubing so that air is expelled.	To prime the irrigation set so that it is ready for use. Air is expelled in order to prevent discomfort from air in the patient's bladder. **E**
6 Clamp the catheter and place absorbent sheet under the catheter junction.	To prevent leakage of urine through the irrigation arm when the spigot is removed. **E** To contain any spillages.
7 Clean hands with a bactericidal alcohol handrub. Put on clean gloves.	To minimize the risk of cross-infection (Fraise and Bradley 2009, **E**).
8 Place a sterile paper towel under the irrigation inlet of the catheter and remove the spigot.	To create a sterile field. To prepare catheter for connection to irrigation set (Scholtes 2002, **E**).
9 Discard the spigot and gloves.	To prevent reuse and reduce risk of cross-infection (Fraise and Bradley 2009, **E**).
10 Put on sterile gloves. Clean around the end of the irrigation arm with sterile low-linting gauze and an antiseptic solution.	To remove surface organisms from gloves and catheter and to reduce the risk of introducing infection into the catheter (Fraise and Bradley 2009, **E**).
11 Attach the irrigation giving set to the irrigation arm of the catheter. Keep the clamp of the irrigation giving set closed.	To prevent overdistension of the bladder, which can occur if fluid is run into the bladder before the drainage tube has been unclamped (Scholtes 2002, **E**).
12 Release the clamp on the catheter tube and allow any accumulated urine to drain into the catheter bag. Empty the urine from the catheter bag into a sterile jug.	Urine drainage should be measured before commencing irrigation so that the fluid balance may be monitored more accurately (Scholtes 2002, **E**).
13 Discard the gloves.	These will be contaminated, having handled the cathether bag (Fraise and Bradley 2009, **E**).
14 Set irrigation at the required rate and ensure that fluid is draining into the catheter bag.	To check that the drainage system is patent and to prevent fluid accumulating in the bladder. **C**
Post-procedure	
15 Make the patient comfortable, remove unnecessary equipment and clean the trolley.	To reduce the risk of cross-infection (Fraise and Bradley 2009, **E**).
16 Wash hands.	To reduce the risk of cross-infection (Fraise and Bradley 2009, **E**).
17 Check blood results 8–12 hours after irrigation has been commenced.	To ensure reabsorption has not occurred.
18 Record information in relevant documents; this should include: • reason for irrigation • date and time irrigation commenced • volume, colour and characteristics of urine output.	To provide a point of reference or comparison in the event of later queries (NMC 2010, **C**).
19 Ensure an accurate fluid balance is commenced and maintained throughout irrigation (Figure 5.14 provides an example of a bladder irrigation chart).	

Figure 5.14 **Bladder irrigation chart.**

Patient name:			**Hospital no:**		
(A) Date and time	**(B) Volume put up**	**(C) Volume run in**	**(D) Total volume out**	**(E) Urine**	**(F) Urine running total**
10/7/14					
10.00	2000				
10.30			700		
11.10			850		
11.40		2000	600		
			2150	150	150
11.45	2000				
12.30			500		
13.15			700		
14.20		2000	800		
			2400	400	550
14.25	2000				
15.30			850		
17.00	Irrigation stopped	1200	800		
			1650	450	1000

Problem-solving table 5.3 **Prevention and resolution (Procedure guideline 5.11)**

Problem	Possible cause	Prevention	Suggested action
Fluid retained in the bladder when the catheter is in position.	Fault in drainage apparatus, for example: kinked tubing blocked catheter. Overfull drainage bag. Catheter clamped off.	Empty the drainage bag every 4 hours.	Straighten the tubing. 'Milk' the tubing. Wash out the bladder with 0.9% sodium chloride using an aseptic technique.

Problem	Possible cause	Prevention	Suggested action
Distended abdomen related to an overfull bladder during the irrigation procedure.	Irrigation fluid is infused at too rapid a rate. Fault in drainage apparatus.	Monitor fluid drainage rate every 15 minutes.	Slow down the infusion rate. Check the patency of the drainage apparatus.
Leakage of fluid from around the catheter.	Catheter slipping out of the bladder. Catheter too large or unsuitable for the patient's anatomy.		Insert the catheter further in. Decompress balloon fully to assess the amount of water necessary. Refill balloon until it remains *in situ*, taking care not to overfill beyond safe level (see manufacturer's instructions). If leakage is profuse or catheter is uncomfortable for the patient, replace with one of smaller size.
Patient experiences pain during the lavage or irrigation procedure.	Volume of fluid in the bladder is too great for comfort. Solution is painful to raw areas in the bladder.		Reduce the fluid volume within the bladder. Inform the doctor. Administer analgesia as prescribed.
Retention of fluid with or without distended abdomen, with or without pain.	Perforated bladder.		Stop irrigation. Maintain in recovery position. Call medical assistance. Monitor vital signs. Monitor patient for pain, tense abdomen.

Procedure guideline 5.12 Care of the patient during bladder irrigation

Essential equipment

- Gloves and apron
- Bactericidal alcohol handrub
- Clean jug

Medicinal products

- Sterile irrigation fluid

Procedure

Action	Rationale
1 Adjust the rate of infusion according to the degree of haematuria. This will be greatest in the first 12 hours following surgery (average fluid input is 6–9 litres during the first 12 hours, falling to 3–6 litres during the next 12 hours). The aim is to obtain a drainage fluid which is rosé in colour. Check the bags of irrigation fluid regularly and renew as required.	To remove blood from the bladder before it clots and to minimize the risk of catheter obstruction and clot retention (Scholtes 2002, **E**).
2 Check the volume in the drainage bag frequently when infusion is in progress, and empty bags before they reach their capacity, for example half-hourly or hourly, or more frequently as required.	To ensure that fluid is draining from the bladder and to detect blockages as soon as possible; also to prevent overdistension of the bladder and patient discomfort.
3 Annotate the fluid balance chart accurately. The fluid balance of all patients having bladder irrigation must be closely monitored.	So that urine output is known and any related problems, for example renal dysfunction, may be detected quickly and easily. **E**

POST-PROCEDURAL CONSIDERATIONS

Documentation

Bladder irrigation recording chart

The bladder irrigation recording chart (see Figure 5.14) is designed to provide an accurate record of the patient's urinary output during the period of irrigation. Record the time (column A) and the fluid volume in each bag of irrigating solution (column B) as it is put up.

When the irrigating fluid has all run from the first bag into the bladder, record the original volume in the bag in column C. Record the corresponding time in column A. Do not attempt to estimate the fluid volume run-in while a bag is in progress as this will be inaccurate. If, however, a bag is discontinued, the volume run-in can be calculated by measuring the volume left in the bag and deducting this from the original volume. This should be recorded in column C (Scholtes 2002).

The catheter bag should be emptied as often as is necessary, the volume being recorded in column D and the corresponding time in column A. The catheter bag must also be emptied whenever the bag of irrigating fluid is empty, and the volume recorded in column D.

When each bag of fluid has run through, add up the total volume drained by the catheter in column D, and write this in red. Subtract from this the total volume run-in (column C) to find the urine output (D – C = E). Write this in column E. Draw a line across the page to indicate that this calculation is complete and continue underneath for the next bag.

Nephrostomy tubes

RELATED THEORY

The nephrostomy tube is a pigtail drain inserted under fluoroscopic, ultrasonographic or computed tomography (CT) guidance, with a local anaesthetic, usually by an interventional radiologist. The procedure involves the passing of a needle and guidewire, followed by a pigtail drain, through the skin, subcutaneous tissue, muscle layers and the renal parenchyma into the renal pelvis (Grasso and Taylor 1996). The drain is attached to a drainage bag and the system is secured to the skin with a suture and a drain fixation dressing (Figure 5.15).

The percutaneous nephrostomy diverts urine away from the ureter and bladder into an externalized drainage bag (Hohenfellner and Santucci 2010). The nephrostomy can be unilateral, with a tube and drainage bag on one side and the other kidney continuing to drain through the ureter into the bladder. Alternatively, bilateral tubes may be inserted, with a tube and drainage bag on each side and with minimal urine draining through the ureters into the bladder.

Figure 5.15 **Nephrostomy tube.**

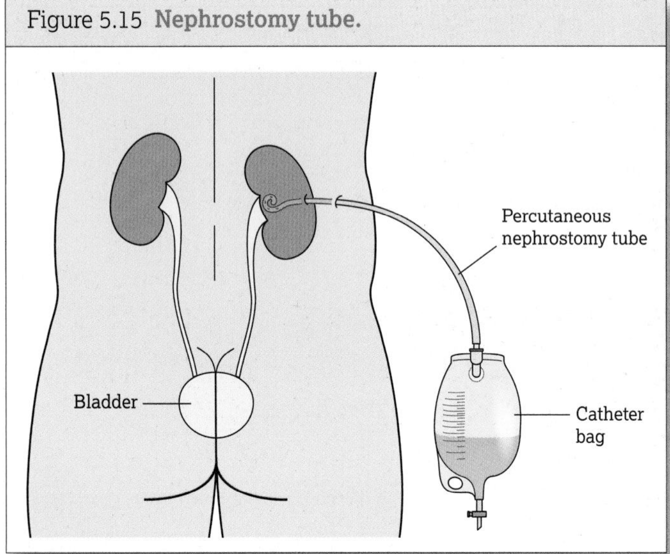

In most cases a nephrostomy is temporary and will be removed when the obstruction has resolved, the obstruction can be bypassed with a stent or the therapeutic intervention has been completed. Rarely, a nephrostomy will be a permanent or semi-permanent solution when bypassing the obstruction is not possible or when it is inadvisable.

EVIDENCE-BASED APPROACHES

Rationale

The decision to perform a percutaneous nephrostomy is taken by the patient's medical/surgical team in discussion with the radiologist. Indications for a nephrostomy include:

- relief of urinary obstruction (the most common reason for insertion, characterized by any of the following: rising creatinine, acute renal failure, loin pain, nausea and vomiting, fever, urosepsis)
- urinary diversion (for example, following a ureteral injury, ureteral fissure/fistula, haemorrhagic cystitis)
- access for therapeutic interventions (for example, stone removal, access for antegrade stent insertion, removal of foreign body such as a broken ureteric stent, delivery of medications, ureteral biopsy)
- diagnostic testing (for example, antegrade pyelography or a ureteral perfusion test) (Dagli and Ramchandani 2011, Ramchandani et al. 2003).

The medical/surgical team will be guided by the urologist when making the decision as a retrograde stent insertion or ureteroscopy may be alternatively indicated for the patient. In general, a retrograde approach is preferred as it has a lower associated morbidity and when a retrograde approach is possible for the patient, a nephrostomy is contraindicated.

Other contraindications include:

- coagulation conditions that increase the tendency to bleed
- anticoagulant use (Patel et al. 2012).

Principles of care

The principles of care for a patient with a nephrostomy tube are similar to those for a patient with an indwelling catheter. Accurate measurement of urine output from each of the indwelling tubes is required and should be recorded separately (usually marked Left/Right/Urethral) and with a total output also recorded.

Good wound site care is essential to avoid exit site infection. Flushing of the nephrostomy should be avoided where possible to avoid introducing infection and potentially causing pyelonephritis. Where flushing of the nephrostomy tube is required, this should be performed by appropriately trained staff with 5 mL of 0.9% sodium chloride using an aseptic technique.

Anticipated patient outcomes

Whether the nephrostomy is short or long term, it is anticipated that the patient will have an uneventful episode of care. The nephrostomy tube will continue to drain urine without occlusion, the patient will remain free from infection and their fluid balance will be maintained.

LEGAL AND PROFESSIONAL ISSUES

The nurse looking after the patient must have an understanding of the principles, anatomy and indications for a nephrostomy tube. All staff managing a patient with a nephrostomy tube should be appropriately trained and working within their scope of practice. If formal competencies are required at the place of employment, these must be met prior to managing the patient's care.

Removal of the nephrostomy tube should be performed by a trained member of staff and under the instruction of the medical/surgical team. If there is a stent *in situ*, the nephrostomy tube should be removed under X-ray or ultrasound guidance to avoid misplacement of the ureteric stent.

PRE-PROCEDURAL CONSIDERATIONS

If this is a long-term nephrostomy, the patient and/or carer should be taught to change both the drain site dressing and the drainage bag on a regular basis. If self-care and independence are not possible, the patient should be referred to the community nursing team.

The recommended dressing is one that supports the nephrostomy tube to prevent accidental tugging and also secures the tube to the patient's skin. There are several drain-specific types available including Drain-Guard, Drain-Fix and OPSITE Post-Op Visible drain dressing. When selecting the dressing, it is important to consider the comfort factor for the patient as the dressing is directly on the patient's back when lying down and sitting against a chair.

To perform the dressing change and drainage bag change, the patient will need to be sitting upright on a stool, couch or a bed with their back facing towards you. The dressing change and drain removal are best performed from behind, so preparing the patient well and good communication are essential. If the patient is unable to sit upright, then positioning the patient on their side in the bed is an alternative with the patient's back facing towards you. Again the procedure is performed from behind the patient.

POST-PROCEDURAL CONSIDERATIONS AND COMPLICATIONS

In between bag changes, the nephrostomy bag should be emptied when it becomes three-quarters full (see Procedure guideline 5.9: Urinary catheter bag: emptying). Where appropriate, the patient or carer should be taught how to do this.

If the kidney has been obstructed the patient may enter a phase of diuresis. This is characterized by high-volume outputs from the nephrostomy tube (polyuria). Close monitoring of the patient's fluid balance and vital signs is required. The patient's intake (intravenous or oral) should closely match the output. A closely monitored and adjusted fluid balance will prevent deterioration in the patient's condition associated with rapid fluid loss.

The patient is at risk of pyelonephritis from the foreign body puncturing the kidney. The patient should be monitored for signs of infection/sepsis, for example loin pain, elevated temperature, fever/chills, purulent urine output or deterioration in their vital signs. A urine specimen should be taken when infection is suspected. In such cases, medical advice should be sought and the patient treated accordingly. Ensuring the drain site remains clean and dry is essential to prevent infection and flushing of the nephrostomy tube should be avoided. Drainage bags should be changed every 5–7 days. Ensure good hand hygiene when handling the drain and exit site and when emptying the drainage bag. Nephrostomy tubes should be changed every 3 months.

Procedure guideline 5.13 Nephrostomy tube: weekly dressing and bag change

Essential equipment

- 0.9% sodium chloride
- Drainage bag and leg straps (with appropriate connector if needed)
- Non-sterile gloves
- Dressing pack with gauze
- Disposable plastic apron
- Drain fixation dressing (e.g. Drain Fix, Drain-Guard or OPSITE Post-Op Visible drain dressing)
- Bactericidal alcohol handrub
- Blunt disposable clamps
- Alcohol (chlorhexidine) wipe
- Adhesive remover
- Micropore tape

Pre-procedure

Action	Rationale
1 Explain and discuss the procedure with the patient.	To ensure that the patient understands the procedure and gives his/her valid consent (NMC 2013, **C**).
2 Screen the bed.	To ensure patient privacy. To allow dust and airborne organisms to settle before the field is exposed (NMC 2015, **E**).
3 Wash hands using bactericidal soap and water or bactericidal alcohol handrub.	To reduce risk of infection (Fraise and Bradley 2009, **E**).
4 Put on a disposable plastic apron.	To reduce risk of cross-infection from micro-organisms on uniform/clothing (Fraise and Bradley 2009, **E**).
5 Prepare the trolley, placing all equipment required on the bottom shelf.	The top shelf acts as a clean working surface.
6 Take the trolley to the patient's bedside, disturbing screens as little as possible.	To minimize airborne contamination (Fraise and Bradley 2009, **E**).
7 Assist the patient onto the edge of the bed/trolley sitting in an upright position with their back exposed.	To enable access to the nephrostomy site. **E**

(continued)

Procedure guideline 5.13 Nephrostomy tube: weekly dressing and bag change *(continued)*

Procedure

Action	Rationale
8 Keeping the drain secure with one hand, carefully remove existing drain fixation dressing and inspect incision site. Check suture remains intact.	To assess skin for signs of infection, inflammation and overgranulation. The suture should remain intact to ensure the drain remains secure. **E**
9 Pour a small amount of adhesive remover onto a gauze square. Keeping the drain secure with one hand, use the adhesive remover to remove any dressing residue from the drain tubing (check manufacturer's guidance to ensure this is safe for use on a drain).	Removing the sticky residue from the tubing minimizes the risk of infection. **E**
10 Clean hands with soap and water and a bactericidal alcohol handrub.	Hands may have become contaminated by handling the outer packs and the old dressing (Fraise and Bradley 2009, **E**).
11 Put on non-sterile gloves.	To reduce risk of cross-infection (Fraise and Bradley 2009, **E**).
12 Clean the drain site with 0.9% sodium chloride, working from the drain outwards. Gently remove any encrustation. Allow the site to dry.	This is performed at least weekly to reduce micro-organisms present and to remove exudate, blood and wound debris from around the site and the device, which may be a medium for bacterial growth, and also to prevent overgranulation (NICE 2012; RCN 2011, **C**).
13 When the site is dry, apply a sterile drain fixation dressing according the manufacturer's guidelines (e.g. Drain Fix or OPSITE Post-Op Visible drain dressing). 'Window frame' the edges of the dressing to prevent it rucking up by using surgical tape around each edge of the dressing.	To improve security of the nephrostomy drain and enable patient mobility. **E**
14 Clean hands with soap and water and a bactericidal alcohol handrub.	Hands may have become contaminated by handling the outer packs and the old dressing (Fraise and Bradley 2009, **E**).
15 Gently clamp nephrostomy tube using blunt disposable clamps.	To prevent leakage of urine. **E**
16 Disconnect the drainage bag, and connector if attached, from the nephrostomy tube.	This is performed every 5–7 days or according to manufacturer's guidelines. **E**
17 Clean connector hub with alcohol-impregnated chlorhexidine wipe.	To minimize risk of infection. **E**
18 Apply new sterile drainage bag, and connector if required, to the nephrostomy tube, being careful not to touch the hubs and unclamp the drain. Urine should begin to flow.	To enable clean passage of urine and to minimize contamination from bacteria within the drainage bag (Pellowe and Pratt 2004; Pomfret 2006). **E**
19 Apply leg strap or waist strap according to patient preference to secure the bag to the patient. Be careful to ensure that the tube is not taut nor pulling at the exit site.	To enable independent mobility and maintain patient dignity. To maintain tube security. **E**

Post-procedure

Action	Rationale
20 Dispose of waste in an orange plastic clinical waste bag and seal the bag before moving the trolley.	To prevent environmental contamination. Orange is the recognized colour for clinical waste (DEFRA 2005, **C**).
21 Draw back the curtains once the patient has been covered.	To maintain the patient's dignity (NMC 2015, **C**).
22 Record information in relevant documents; this should include: • date and time of procedure • procedure/s performed • dressing and bag type used • condition of skin • any problems/concerns during procedure • any swabs/samples taken during the procedure (e.g. exit site swab or urine sample) • any referrals made following the procedure • a review date for next dressing/bag change.	To provide a point of reference or comparison in the event of later queries (NMC 2010, **C**).

Problem-solving table 5.4 **Prevention and resolution (Procedure guideline 5.13)**

Problem	Cause	Action	Prevention
Wound site infection.	Foreign body puncturing the skin.	Monitor patient for signs of infection, e.g. purulent discharge, exit site erythema, pain/itching, elevated temperature. Send swab for MC&S when indicated. Seek medical advice. Treat patient according to medical advice.	Maintain good exit site care. Change dressing and check site at least every 7 days. Ensure good hand hygiene.
Nephrostomy tube falls out.	Locking mechanism on drain has failed. Retaining suture has become loose. Drain fixation dressing has fallen off.	Seek urgent medical assistance. Nephrostomy tube will need to be replaced by physician.	Ensure that all the elements securing the nephrostomy are well situated. Check the locking mechanism on the drain is in the 'lock' or 'drain' position. Check the retaining suture is intact during weekly dressing changes. Be careful to correctly apply and secure the drain fixation dressing.
Nephrostomy tube stops draining.	No urine output. Blocked tube. Kinked tube.	Check patient's vital signs and seek urgent medical assistance if patient is unwell. Ensure there are no kinks in the tube that have occluded flow of urine and straighten tube. If the tube may be blocked with debris, flush tube with 5 mL NaCl using aseptic technique to unblock.	Monitor urine output and vital signs. Escalate concerns to the medical team. Carefully secure the drain and tubing to prevent kinking.

Altered faecal elimination

This section focuses on altered faecal elimination, including diarrhoea and constipation, and considers a range of pharmacological and non-pharmacological strategies to manage these conditions. Also reviewed in this section is the care required to support a patient with a bowel stoma.

Diarrhoea

DEFINITION

The term diarrhoea originates from the Greek for 'to flow through' (Bell 2004) and can be characterized according to its onset and duration (acute or chronic) or by type (e.g. secretory, osmotic or malabsorptive). Diarrhoea can also be defined in terms of stool frequency, consistency, volume or weight (Metcalf 2007). The World Health Organization (2014) defines diarrhoea as the passage of three or more loose stools per day, or more frequent than is normal for the individual.

RELATED THEORY

Diarrhoea is a serious global public health problem, in particularly in low-income and middle-income countries due to poor sanitation. There are almost 1.7 billion cases of diarrhoeal disease each year, with many people dying (WHO 2014). The disease pathogens are most commonly transmitted via the faecal–oral route (Ejemot-Nwadiaro et al. 2008). Diarrhoea should be classified according to time (acute or chronic) and the characteristics of the stools (see Bristol Stool Chart, Figure 5.4) (Baldi et al. 2009).

Acute diarrhoea

Acute diarrhoea is very common, usually self-limiting, generally lasting less than 2 weeks and often requires no investigation or treatment (Hall 2010, Shepherd 2000). Causes of acute diarrhoea include:

- dietary indiscretion (eating too much fruit, alcohol misuse)
- allergy to food constituents
- infective:
  - travel associated
  - viral
  - bacterial (usually associated with food)
  - antibiotic related.

One of the most common causes of acute diarrhoea in the adult population worldwide is viral gastroenteritis resulting from norovirus. Its low infectious dose, resistance to extreme temperatures as well as many household cleaning products, along with viral shedding, before and after symptoms are apparent, have resulted in this virus being prolific during colder months and becoming widely known as the winter vomiting bug (Krenzer 2012).

Chronic diarrhoea

Chronic diarrhoea generally lasts longer than 2–4 weeks (Metcalf 2007) and may have more complex origins. Chronic causes can be divided as follows (Thomas et al. 2003).

- *Colonic*: colonic neoplasia, ulcerative colitis and Crohn's disease, microscopic colitis.
- *Small bowel*: small bowel bacterial overgrowth, coeliac disease, Crohn's disease, Whipple's disease, bile acid malabsorption,

disaccharidase deficiency, mesenteric ischaemia, radiation enteritis, lymphoma, giardiasis.
- *Pancreatic*: chronic pancreatitis, pancreatic carcinoma, cystic fibrosis.
- *Endocrine*: hyperthyroidism, diabetes, hypoparathyroidism, Addison's disease, hormone-secreting tumours.
- *Other causes*: laxative misuse, drugs, alcohol, autonomic neuropathy, small bowel resection or intestinal fistulas, radiation enteritis.

PRE-PROCEDURAL CONSIDERATIONS

Assessment

The cause of diarrhoea needs to be identified before effective treatment can be instigated. This may include clinical investigations such as stool cultures for bacterial, fungal and viral pathogens or a more formal medical evaluation of the gastrointestinal tract (Kornblau et al. 2000).

Ongoing nursing assessment is essential for ensuring individualized management and care. The lack of a systematic approach to assessment and poor documentation cause problems in effective management of diarrhoea (Cadd et al. 2000, Smith 2001). Nurses need to be aware of contributing factors and be sensitive to patients' beliefs and values in order to provide holistic care. A comprehensive assessment is therefore essential and should include the following.

- History of onset, frequency and duration of diarrhoea: patient's perception of diarrhoea is often related to stool consistency (Metcalf 2007).
- Consistency, colour and form of stool, including the presence of blood, fat and mucus. Stools can be graded using a scale such as the Bristol Stool Chart (see Figure 5.4), where diarrhoea would be classified as types 6 or 7 (Longstreth et al. 2006).
- Associated symptoms: pain, nausea, vomiting, fatigue, weight loss or fever.
- Physical examination: check for gaping anus, rectal prolapse and prolapsed haemorrhoids (Nazarko 2007).
- Recent lifestyle changes, emotional disturbances or travel abroad.
- Fluid intake and dietary history, including any cause-and-effect relationships between food consumption and bowel action.
- Regular medication, including antibiotics, laxatives, oral hypoglycaemics, appetite suppressants, antidepressants, statins, digoxin or chemotherapy (Nazarko 2007).
- Effectiveness of antidiarrhoeal medication (dose and frequency).
- Significant past medical history: bowel resection, pancreatitis, pelvic radiotherapy.
- Hydration status: evaluation of mucous membranes and skin turgor.
- Perianal or peristomal skin integrity: enzymes present in faecal fluid can cause rapid breakdown of the skin (Nazarko 2007).
- Stool cultures for bacterial, fungal and viral pathogens: to check for infective diarrhoea (Pellatt 2007). Treatment may not be commenced until results are available except if the patient has been infected by *Clostridium difficile* in the past.
- Blood tests: full blood count, urea and electrolytes, liver function tests, vitamin B_{12}, folate, calcium, ferritin, erythrocyte sedimentation rate (ESR) and C-reactive protein.
- Patient's preferences and own coping strategies including non-pharmacological interventions and their effectiveness (Cadd et al. 2000, Chelvanayagam and Norton 2004, King 2002, Kornblau et al. 2000).

All episodes of acute diarrhoea must be considered potentially infectious until proven otherwise. The risk of spreading the infection to others can be reduced by adopting universal precautions such as wearing of gloves, aprons and gowns, disposing of all excreta immediately and, ideally, nursing the patient in a side room with access to their own toilet (King 2002). Advice should always be sought from the infection control team. At this stage nursing care should also include educating patients about careful hand washing.

Diarrhoea can have profound physiological and psychosocial consequences for a patient. Severe or extended episodes of diarrhoea may result in dehydration, electrolyte imbalance and malnutrition. Patients not only have to cope with increased frequency of bowel movement but may have abdominal pain, cramping, proctitis and anal or perianal skin breakdown. Food aversions may develop or patients may stop eating altogether as they anticipate subsequent diarrhoea following intake. Consequently, this may lead to weight loss and malnutrition. Fatigue, sleep disturbances, feelings of isolation and depression are all common consequences for those experiencing diarrhoea. The impact of severe diarrhoea should not be underestimated; it is highly debilitating and may cause patients on long-term therapy to be non-compliant, resulting in a potentially life-threatening problem (Kornblau et al. 2000).

Once the cause of diarrhoea has been established, management should be focused on resolving the cause and providing physical and psychological support for the patient. Most cases of chronic diarrhoea will resolve once the underlying condition is treated, for example drug therapy for Crohn's disease or dietary management for coeliac disease. Episodes of acute diarrhoea, usually caused by bacteria or viruses, generally resolve spontaneously and are managed by symptom control and the prevention of complications (Shepherd 2000).

> Learning Activity 5.3
>
> **Learning in practice: Diarrhoea**
>
> In your clinical area, find out what the local procedures are for caring for a patient with suspected infective diarrhoea.
>
> - Where is the procedure located?
> - Who should be informed?
> - What are the guidelines for how and where the patient should be cared for?

Pharmacological support

The treatment for diarrhoea depends on the cause.

Antimotility drugs

Antimotility drugs such as loperamide or codeine phosphate may be useful in some cases, for example in blind loop syndrome and radiation enteritis. These drugs reduce gastrointestinal motility to relieve the symptoms of abdominal cramps and reduce the frequency of diarrhoea (Shepherd 2000). It is important to rule out any infective agent as the cause of diarrhoea before using any of these drugs, as they may make the situation worse by slowing the clearance of the infective agent.

Antibiotics

In the case of bacterial diarrhoea, treatment with antibiotics is recommended only in patients who are very symptomatic and show signs of systemic involvement (Metcalf 2007). Not uncommonly, *Salmonella* can become resistant to commonly used antimicrobial agents such as amoxicillin (Metcalf 2007). When dealing with antibiotic-associated diarrhoea, most patients will notice a cessation of their symptoms with discontinuation of the antibiotic therapy. If diarrhoea persists, it is important to exclude pseudomembranous colitis by performing a sigmoidoscopy and sending a stool for cytotoxin analysis. However, over recent years there has been increasing evidence supporting the use of probiotics in cases of diarrhoea associated with antibiotics (McFarland 2007). Researchers believe that probiotics restore the microbial balance in the intestinal tract previously destroyed by inciting antibiotics (Hickson et al. 2007). There are a variety of probiotic products available and their effectiveness appears to be related to the strain of bacteria causing the diarrhoea (Avadhani and Miley 2011, Hickson et al. 2007, McFarland 2007).

Fluid replacement

The prevention and/or correction of dehydration is the first step in managing an episode of diarrhoea. Adults normally require 1.5–2 L of fluid in 24 hours. The person who has diarrhoea will require an additional 200 mL for each loose stool. Dehydration can be corrected by using intravenous fluids and electrolytes or by oral rehydration solutions. The extent of dehydration dictates whether a patient can be managed at home or will need to be admitted to hospital (Nazarko 2007). Nursing care should also include monitoring signs or symptoms of electrolyte imbalance, such as muscle weakness and cramps, hypokalaemia, tachycardia and hypernatraemia (Metcalf 2007).

Non-pharmacological support

Maintaining dignity

Preserving the patient's privacy and dignity is essential during episodes of diarrhoea. The nurse has an important role in minimizing the patient's distress by adjusting language and using terms that are appropriate to the individual to reduce embarrassment (Smith 2001) and by listening to the patient's preferences for care (Cadd et al. 2000). Additionally, the use of deodorizers and air fresheners to remove the smell caused by offensive diarrhoea contributes to the person's dignity. Stoma deodorants are thought to be more effective and samples can be obtained from company representatives (Nazarko 2007).

Skin care

It is important that the patient has easy access to clean toilet and washing facilities and that requests for assistance are answered promptly. Skin care is also essential to prevent bacteria present in faecal matter from destroying the skin's cellular defences and causing skin damage. This is particularly important with diarrhoea since it has high levels of faecal enzymes that come into contact with the perianal skin (Gray et al. 2012, Le Lievre 2002, Ripley 2007). The anal area should be gently cleaned with warm water immediately after every episode of diarrhoea. Frequent washing of the skin can alter the pH and remove protective oils from the skin. Products aimed at maintaining healthy peristomal skin should be used to protect perianal skin in patients with diarrhoea (Nazarko 2007). Soap should be avoided, unless it is an emollient, to avoid excessive drying of the skin and gentle patting of the skin is preferred for drying to avoid friction damage. Talcum powder should not be used and barrier creams should be applied sparingly, gently layered on in the direction of the hair growth rather than rubbed into the skin (Le Lievre 2002). The use of incontinence pads should be carefuly considered in a person with severe episodes of diarrhoea. This particular material does not absorb fluid stools, protect the skin from damage or contain smells.

Faecal collection devices may leak, so are most useful for patients cared for in bed (Nazarko 2007, Wilson 2008). This type of device is fitted over the anus and fluid stools drain into a drainage bag similar to a drainable stoma bag. It is imperative that such devices are fitted by appropriately trained, competent healthcare professionals and that both local policies and manufacturer's instructions are followed to ensure this equipment is used in an appropriate and safe manner (Rees and Sharpe 2009) (Figure 5.16).

Diet

A diet rich in fibre, or 'roughage', can cause diarrhoea. In such cases individuals should be advised to reduce their intake of foods including cereals, fruit and vegetables and space it out over the day (Nazarko 2007). Chilli and other spices can irritate the bowel and should be avoided. Sorbitol (artificial sweetener), beer, stout and high doses of vitamins and minerals should also be avoided.

Figure 5.16 **Faecal management system.**
***Source:* Reproduced with permission from ConvaTec Ltd.**

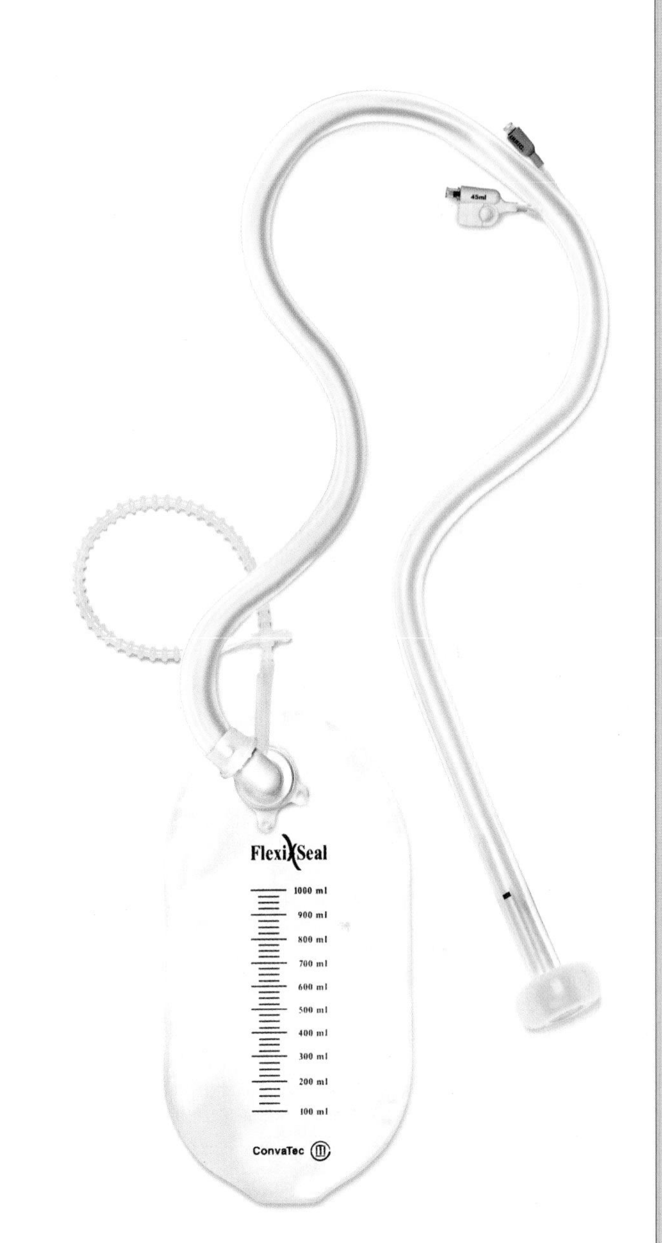

Learning Activity 5.4 Case study: Diarrhoea

Mrs Stone is a 44-year-old woman with Crohn's disease who has been suffering from severe diarrhoea for the last 10 days and has been admitted to your ward with dehydration. She reports having at least 12 episodes of diarrhoea a day (type 7 using the Bristol Stool Chart).

1 What precautions should be taken?
2 What information would you want to include in your assessment of her diarrhoea?

See the end of the chapter for the answers.

Faecal incontinence

Faecal incontinence is a clinical symptom associated with diarrhoea (Nazarko 2007) which has been defined as the uncontrolled passage of solid or liquid faeces at socially inappropriate times and places (Kenefick 2004). When it is not possible to treat the cause of the diarrhoea, a care plan should be created to manage incontinence and prevent complications (NICE 2007).

Factors that can contribute to the development of faecal incontinence include (Nazarko 2007):

- damage or weakness of the anal sphincter: obstetric damage, haemorrhoidectomy, sphincterotomy or degeneration of the internal anal sphincter muscle
- severe diarrhoea
- faecal loading (impaction): immobility, lack of fluids
- neurological conditions: spinal cord injury, Parkinson's disease
- cognitive deficits.

Diarrhoea can potentially disrupt a person's well-being. Community nurses and hospital-based specialist nurses have an essential role in supporting those affected by this condition. Diagnosis, treatment and management of diarrhoea and potential faecal incontinence can take place at home where individuals are more familiar with the environment.

Constipation

DEFINITION

Constipation results when there is a delayed movement of intestinal content through the bowel. It has been described as persistently difficult, infrequent or incomplete defaecation, which may or may not be accompanied by hard, dry stools (Norton 2006). Constipation is a subjective disorder, being perceived differently by different people owing to the wide variety of bowel habits among healthy people (Woodward 2012). Consequently, there is a lack of consensus amongst both healthcare professionals and the general public as to what actually constitutes constipation (Kyle 2011b, Norton 2006, Perdue 2005).

ANATOMY AND PHYSIOLOGY

The rectum is very sensitive to rises in pressure, even of 2–3 mmHg, and distension will cause a perineal sensation with a subsequent desire to defaecate. A co-ordinated reflex empties the bowel from mid-transverse colon to the anus. During this phase the diaphragm, abdominal and levator ani muscles contract and the glottis closes. Waves of peristalsis occur in the distal colon and the anal sphincter relaxes, allowing the evacuation of faeces (Tortora and Derrickson 2011). The stimulus to defaecate varies in individuals according to habit, and if a decision is made to delay defaecation, the stimulus disappears and a process of retroperistalsis occurs whereby the faeces move back into the sigmoid colon (Perdue 2005). If these natural reflexes are inhibited on a regular basis, they are eventually suppressed and reflex defaecation is inhibited, resulting in such individuals becoming severely constipated.

RELATED THEORY

It has been estimated that up to 27% of a given population experience constipation (Longstreth et al. 2006) with an average prevalence across Europe of 17.1% (Peppas et al. 2008).

Constipation occurs when there is either a failure of colonic propulsion (slow colonic transit) or a failure to evacuate the rectum (rectal outlet delay) or a combination of these problems (Norton 2006, Woodward 2012).

The management of constipation depends on the cause and there are numerous possible causes, with many patients being affected by more than one causative factor (Figure 5.17). While constipation is not life-threatening, it does cause a great deal of distress and discomfort. Particularly, constipation can be associated with abdominal pain or cramps, feelings of general malaise or fatigue and feelings of bloatedness. Nausea, anorexia, headaches, confusion, restlessness, retention of urine, faecal incontinence and halitosis may also be present in some cases (Fritz and Pitlick 2012, Kyle 2011b).

The effective treatment of constipation relies on the cause being identified by thorough assessment. Constipation can be categorized as primary or secondary (Perdue 2005). Primary constipation has no pathological cause (RCN 2012b). Factors that lead to the development of primary, or idiopathic, constipation are extrinsic or lifestyle related and include:

- an inadequate diet (low fibre)
- poor fluid intake
- a lifestyle change
- ignoring the urge to defaecate.

Secondary constipation is attributed to another disorder, whether this be metabolic, neurological or psychological; there is an identifiable cause for the constipation (RCN 2012b). Examples of disease processes that may result in secondary constipation include anal fissures, colonic tumours, irritable bowel syndrome or conditions such as Parkinson's disease. Constipation may also result as a side-effect of certain medications, such as opioid analgesics (RCN 2012b, Woodward 2012).

Bowel obstruction and ileus

Bowel obstruction occurs when the passage of contents through the bowel lumen is inhibited, either by mechanical (anatomical) or non-mechanical causes. The alternative term 'ileus' is sometimes used to describe the failure of passage of intestinal contents in the absence of any mechanical obstruction (Morton and Fontaine 2013).

Intestinal obstructions are caused by a physical narrowing or internal blockage of the gut lumen, extrinsic compression of the bowel, or a disruption or failure in motility. In cancer patients, malignant bowel obstruction can be either partial or complete, with acute or gradual onset of symptoms (Letizia and Norton 2003).

Obstruction can occur at a single site or, in the case of disseminated intra-abdominal disease, such as intra-abdominal carcinomatosis, in multiple sites (Lynch and Sarazine 2006).

Intestinal obstruction is a potentially devastating complication for the patient, with a vast number of possible clinical causes, and is a condition which can rapidly progress to cause life-threatening problems (Shih et al. 2003). Intestinal obstruction precipitates a cascade of pathophysiological events which lead to complex and unpleasant symptoms. Thoughtful nursing assessment and evaluation, and meticulous symptom control, can make an important contribution to improving the experience of the patient in bowel obstruction.

EVIDENCE-BASED APPROACHES

Assessment

Taking a detailed history from the patient is pivotal in establishing the appropriate treatment plan. It is therefore of vital importance that nurses adopt a proactive preventive approach to the assessment and management of constipation. Kyle et al. (2005a, Kyle 2011b) have developed, refined and tested a constipation risk assessment tool, now known as the Norgine Risk Assessment Tool (NRAT). This assesses a range of risk factors that appear consistently within relevant literature on the development of constipation, including:

- nutritional intake/recent changes in diet
- fluid intake
- immobility and lack of exercise
- medication, for example analgesics, antacids, iron supplements, tricyclic antidepressants

Figure 5.17 **Classification of constipation.**

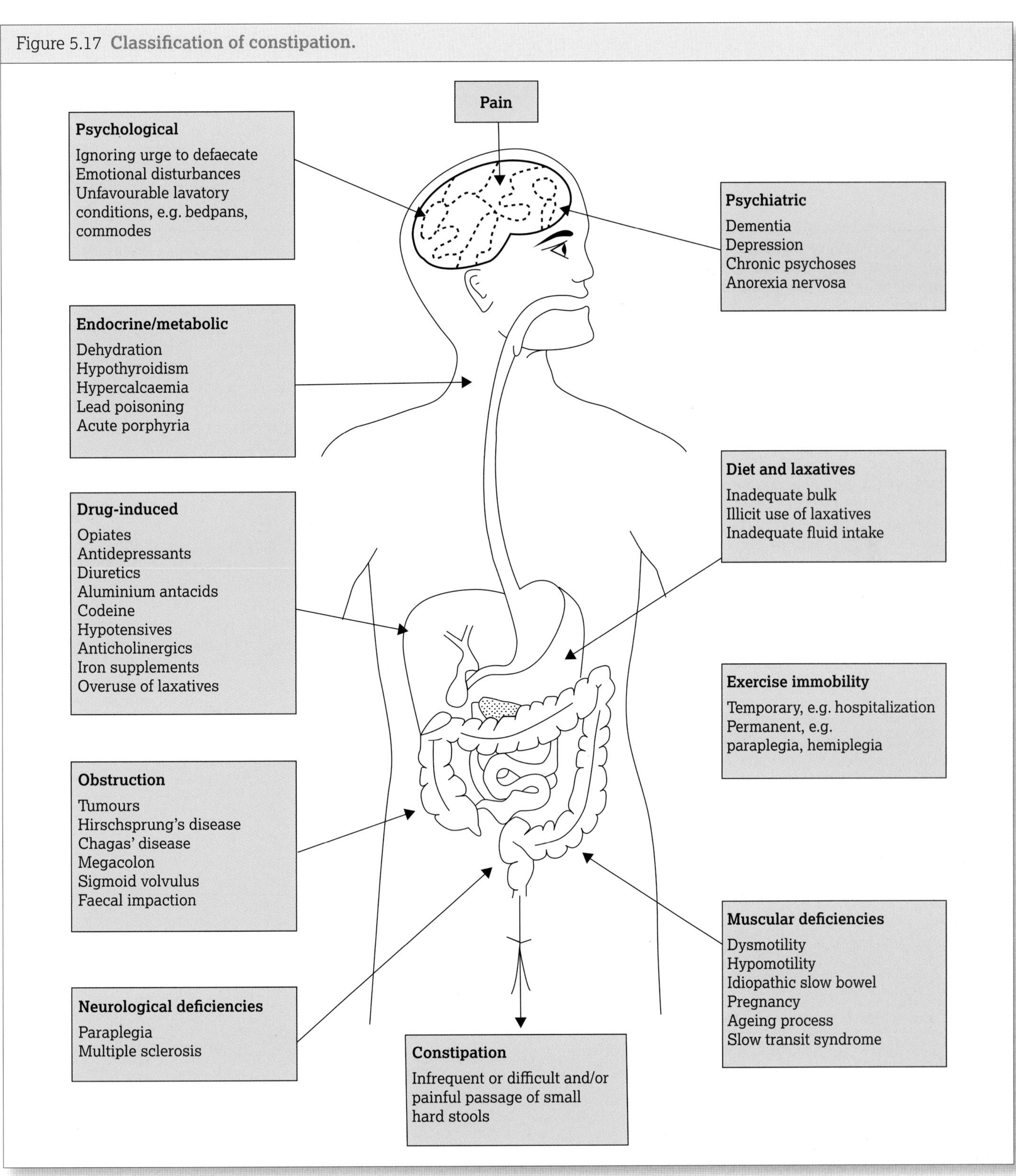

- toileting facilities, for example having to use shared toilet facilities, commodes or bedpans
- medical conditions, for example inflammatory bowel disease, irritable bowel syndrome, colorectal cancer, diabetes and neurological conditions such as multiple sclerosis or muscular dystrophy.

In addition to the identification of these risks/contributing factors, it is important to take a careful history of a patient's bowel habits, taking particular note of the following.

- Any changes in the patient's usual bowel activity. How long have these changes been present and have they occurred before?

- Frequency of bowel action.
- Volume, consistency and colour of the stool. Stools can be graded using a scale such as the Bristol Stool Chart (see Figure 5.4) where constipation would be classified as types 1 or 2 (Longstreth et al. 2006).
- Presence of mucus, blood, undigested food or offensive odour.
- Presence of pain or discomfort on defaecation.
- Use of oral or rectal medication to stimulate defaecation and its effectiveness.

A digital rectal examination (DRE) can also be performed, providing the nurse has received suitable training or instruction to perform it competently. This procedure can be used to assess the contents of the rectum and anal sphincter tone and to identify conditions which may cause discomfort such as haemorrhoids, anal fissures or rectal prolapse (Hinrichs et al. 2001, Kyle 2011c, Peate 2003, RCN 2012b). See 'Digital rectal examination' below for further information.

Additional investigations such as an abdominal X-ray may be necessary to exclude bowel obstruction (Christer et al. 2003, Kyle et al. 2005a, Thompson et al. 2003).

Over recent years, international criteria (the Rome Criteria) have been developed and revised (Longstreth et al. 2006) which can help to more accurately and consistently define constipation. According to the Rome III Criteria, an individual who is diagnosed with constipation should report having at least two of the following symptoms within the last 3 months where those symptoms began at least 6 months prior to diagnosis (Longstreth et al. 2006, Norton 2006).

- Straining for at least 25% of the time.
- Lumpy or hard stool for at least 25% of the time.
- A sensation of incomplete evacuation for at least 25% of the time.
- A sensation of anorectal obstruction or blockage for at least 25% of the time.
- Manual manoeuvres used to facilitate defaecation at least 25% of the time (e.g. manual evacuation).
- Less than three bowel movements a week.
- Loosestools are rarely present without the use of laxatives.

The myth that daily bowel evacuation is essential to health has persisted through the centuries. It is thought that less than 10% of the population have a bowel evacuation daily (Getliffe and Dolman 2007). This myth has resulted in laxative abuse becoming one of the most common types of drug misuse in the Western world. The annual cost to the NHS of prescribing medications to treat constipation is in the region of £45 million (DH 2005).

Given that there is such a wide normal range, it is important to establish the patient's usual bowel habit and the changes that may have occurred. Many patients are too embarrassed to discuss bowel function and will often delay reporting problems, despite the sometimes severe impact these symptoms have on their quality of life (Cadd et al. 2000). Generally complaints will be either that the patient has diarrhoea or is constipated. These should be seen as symptoms of some underlying disease or malfunction and managed accordingly. The nurse's priority is to effectively assess the nature and cause of the problem, to help find appropriate solutions and to inform and support the patient. This requires sensitive communication skills to dispel embarrassment and ensure a shared understanding of the meanings of the terms used by the patient (Smith 2001).

Pharmacological support

Laxatives

Laxatives can be defined simply as substances that cause evacuation of the bowel by a mild action (Mosby 2006). A laxative with a mild or gentle effect is also known as an aperient and one with a strong effect is referred to as a cathartic or purgative. Purgatives should be used only in exceptional circumstances, that is, where all other interventions have failed, or when they are prescribed for a specific purpose. The aim of laxative treatment is to achieve comfortable rather than frequent defaecation and, wherever possible, the most natural means of bowel evacuation should be employed, with preference given to use of oral laxatives where appropriate (Perdue 2005). The many different laxatives available may be grouped into types according to the action they have (Table 5.4, Table 5.5).

Table 5.4 **Types of laxative**

Type of laxative	Example	Brand names and sources
Bulk producers	Dietary fibre Mucilaginous polysaccharides Methylcellulose	Bran, wholemeal bread, Fybogel (ispaghula), Normacol (sterculia)
Stool softeners	Synthetic surface active agents, liquid paraffin	Agarol, Dioctyl, Petrolager, Milpar
Osmotic agents	Sodium, potassium and magnesium salts	Magnesium sulphate, milk of magnesia, lactulose
Stimulant laxatives	Sodium picosulphate, glycerine	Senna, Senokot, bisacodyl, Dulcolax, co-danthrusate, Picolax, glycerol

Table 5.5 **Classification of laxatives**

Type of laxative	How it works	Name of drug	Special notes for patients
Bulk forming	These drugs act by holding onto water so the stool remains large and soft and encourages the gut to move	Fybogel	This is to be avoided if patient's bowel activity is not normal or their fluid intake is limited
Stimulant	Will cause water and electrolytes to accumulate in the bowel and will stimulate the bowel to move	Senna tablet/liquid Bisacodyl tablet/ suppositories	This group of drugs is to be avoided if the bowel is not moving very well as they can cause abdominal cramps

Type of laxative	How it works	Name of drug	Special notes for patients
Mixed stimulant and softener	2-in-1 preparations	Co-danthramer liquid and capsules available Docusate tablets	This drug may cause the urine to change colour Mild stimulant
Softeners	Attract and retain water in the bowel	Milpar (liquid paraffin and magnesium hydroxide) Docusate Arachis oil enema	If the patient is allergic to nuts, tell the nurse or doctor as an arachis oil enema should be avoided
Osmotic	Act in the bowel by increasing stimulation of fluid secretion and movement in the bowel	Lactulose Movicol Phosphate enema Microlax enema	Can cause bloating, excess wind and abdominal discomfort
5-HT4 receptor agonists (prokinetic agents)	Enhance gut motility by mimicking the effects of serotonin on the gut wall	Prucalopride	This is not a laxative. It causes an increase in gut motility resulting in an increase in bowel movement
Peripheral opioid receptor antagonists	Bind to peripheral opioid receptors and so reverse opioid-induced constipation	Methylnaltrexone bromide	This is a subcutaneous injection that is only given in advanced stages of illness, in consultation with a specialist palliative care team, where oral laxatives can no longer be taken by mouth

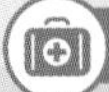 Learning Activity 5.5

Learning in practice: Constipation

Within your clinical area, take a look at how many patients are prescribed laxatives.

- What are the most common types of laxatives used?
- Why do you think this is?
- From your observations of practice, what non-pharmacological approaches are used to manage constipation?
- How effective are these?

BULK-FORMING LAXATIVES

Bulk-forming agents work by increasing the amount of fibre and therefore water retained in the colon, increasing faecal mass and stimulating peristalsis (Peate 2003, Woodward 2012). Ispaghula husk (Isogel, Regulan) and sterculia (Normacol) both trap water in the intestine by the formation of a highly viscous gel which softens faeces, increases weight and reduces transit time. These agents need plenty of fluid in order to work (2–3 litres per day), so their appropriateness for older patients should be questioned (Hinrichs et al. 2001, Perdue 2005). They also take a few days to exert their effect (Woodward 2012) so are not suitable to relieve acute constipation. Furthermore, bulk-forming laxatives are contraindicated in some patients, including those who have bowel obstruction, faecal impaction, acute abdominal pain and reduced muscle tone, or those who have had recent bowel surgery.

Increasing the bulk may produce side-effects including flatulence and bloating (Woodward 2012), worsen impaction, lead to increased colonic faecal loading or even intestinal obstruction and in some cases may increase the risk of faecal incontinence. Other potentially harmful effects include malabsorption of minerals, calcium, iron and fat-soluble vitamins, and reduced bioavailability of some drugs.

STOOL SOFTENERS

Stool-softening preparations, such as docusate sodium and glycerol (glycerine) suppositories, act by lowering the surface tension of faeces which allows water to penetrate and soften the stool (Hinrichs et al. 2001, Peate 2003).

Liquid paraffin acts as a lubricant as well as a stool softener by coating the faeces and allowing easier passage. However, its use should be avoided as there are a number of problems associated with this preparation. It interferes with the absorption of fat-soluble vitamins and can also cause skin irritation and changes to the bowel mucosa, while accidental inhalation of droplets of liquid paraffin may result in lipoid pneumonia (BNF 2014).

Overall, there is little evidence to support the use of stool softeners and so this group of laxatives are no longer recommended in the treatment of constipation (Woodward 2012).

OSMOTIC LAXATIVES

Osmotic laxatives, such as lactulose or macrogols (polyethylene glycol), increase the amount of water within the large bowel either through osmosis or by retaining the water they were administered with (BNF 2014). Lactulose is a semi-synthetic disaccharide which draws water into the bowel through osmosis, resulting in a looser stool. However, it can be metabolized by colonic bacteria which not only reduces the osmotic effect but also produces gas which can result in abdominal cramps and flatulence, thereby causing discomfort as well as delaying the osmotic effect by as much as 3 days (BNF 2014, Woodward 2012). By contrast, polyethylene glycol is an inert polymer that is iso-osmotic and binds to water molecules, so acts by retaining the water it is diluted with when administered (BNF 2014, Woodward 2012). Both lactulose and polyethylene glycol are commonly used in the treatment of constipation. In a recent Cochrane review, it was recommended that polyethylene glycol is used in preference to lactulose (Lee-Robichaud et al. 2010) as it resulted in more frequent bowel motions, softer stools and a reduced need for additional laxative product.

Magnesium and phosphate preparations also exert an osmotic effect on the gut. They have a rapid effect, so fluid intake is important as patients may experience diarrhoea and dehydration.

These preparations should be avoided in elderly patients and those with renal or hepatic impairment (BNF 2014).

STIMULANT LAXATIVES

Laxatives including bisacodyl, dantron and senna stimulate the nerve plexi in the gut wall, increasing peristalsis and promoting the secretion of water and electrolytes in the small and large bowel to improve stool consistency (Peate 2003, Rogers 2012, Woodward 2012). Stimulant laxatives can cause abdominal cramping, particularly if the stool is hard, and so a stool softener may be recommended for use in combination with this group of drugs (BNF 2014, Connolly and Larkin 2012). Other adverse effects with high doses of stimulant laxatives include electrolyte disturbances in frail older people and loose stools (Rogers 2012, Woodward 2012).

Preparations containing dantron are restricted to certain groups of patients, such as the terminally ill, as some studies on rodents have indicated a potential carcinogenic risk (BNF 2014). Dantron preparations should be avoided in incontinent patients, especially those with limited mobility, as prolonged skin contact may cause irritation and excoriation (BNF 2014).

5-HT4 RECEPTOR AGONISTS (PROKINETIC AGENTS)

5-HT4 receptor agonists are not laxatives but enhance gut motility by mimicking the effects of serotonin on the gut wall. Serotonin is usually released when the gut mucosa is stimulated following a meal and its attachment to 5-HT4 receptors triggers a co-ordinated contraction and relaxation of the gut smooth muscle known as the peristaltic wave. Prokinetic agents, such as prucalopride, mimic this action, thereby increasing peristalsis and increasing stool frequency (Rogers 2012, Woodward 2012).

PERIPHERAL OPIOID RECEPTOR ANTAGONISTS

Methylnaltrexone bromide is a parenteral preparation which is administered by subcutaneous injection. It is a peripherally acting selective antagonist of opioid binding to the mu-receptor, thus reversing peripherally mediated opioid-induced constipation. As this preparation does not cross the blood–brain barrier, it does not interfere with the centrally mediated analgesic effects of opioids (Connolly and Larkin 2012, Rogers 2012, Thomas et al. 2008, Toner and Claros 2012). The indications for use are opioid-induced constipation in patients with advanced illness receiving palliative care and who are unable to take oral laxatives. It is necessary to exclude bowel obstruction prior to their use and they should be used under the advice of a palliative care team (Connolly and Larkin 2012).

Non-pharmacological support

Diet

Dietary manipulation may help to resolve mild constipation, although it is much more likely to help prevent constipation from recurring. Increasing dietary fibre increases stool bulk, which in turn improves peristalsis and stool transit time (Rogers 2012). The current recommended daily intake of dietary fibre for an adult is 18 g (British Nutrition Foundation 2012).

There are two types of fibre: insoluble fibre is contained in foods such as wholegrain bread, brown rice, fruit and vegetables and soluble fibre is contained in foods such as oats, pulses, beans and lentils. It is recommended that fibre should be taken from a variety of both soluble and insoluble foods and eaten at times spread throughout the day (Denby 2006, Food Standards Agency 2006). Care should be taken to increase dietary fibre intake gradually as bloating and abdominal discomfort can result from a sudden increase, particularly in the older person and those with slow-transit constipation (Getliffe and Dolman 2007, Rogers 2012).

Dietary changes need to be made in combination with other lifestyle changes. There is little evidence to support the benefit of increasing fluid intake for constipation, but there is arguably a benefit in encouraging people to drink the recommended daily fluid intake of at least 2.0 litres (Fritz and Pitlick 2012, Rogers 2012). There is a need for further studies to examine the role of dietary manipulation in the management of constipation, particularly the function of dietary fibre and fluid intake.

Positioning

Patients should be advised not to ignore the urge to defaecate and to allow sufficient time for defaecation. It is important that the correct posture for defaecation is adopted; crouching or a 'crouch-like' posture is considered anatomically correct (Denby 2006, Woodward 2012) and the use of a footstool by the toilet may enable patients to adopt a better defaecation posture (Getliffe and Dolman 2007, NICE 2007, RCN 2012b, Woodward 2012) (Figure 5.18). The use of the bedpan should always be avoided if possible as the poor posture adopted while using one can cause extreme straining during defaecation.

Exercise

Where possible, patients should be encouraged to increase their level of exercise; physical activity has been found to have a positive effect on peristalsis, particularly after eating (Thompson et al. 2003). Therapies such as homoeopathy and reflexology can also be utilized (Getliffe and Dolman 2007).

Other treatments

Biofeedback is a behaviour modification technique that encourages bracing of the abdominal wall and relaxation of the pelvic floor muscles to achieve effective defaecation. It is reported to be effective in 70% of patients (Koch et al. 2008), but more so in people who have a problem with evacuation rather than slow transit constipation (Rao et al. 2010, Rogers 2012, Woodward 2012).

Rectal irrigation is being increasingly offered as a treatment for chronic constipation, particularly where biofeedback has not worked, as well as faecal incontinence. It involves instilling lukewarm water into the rectum using a rectal catheter with the aim of ensuring the rectum, sigmoid and descending colon are emptied of faeces (Rogers 2012, Woodward 2012).

Overall, lifestyle changes and laxatives (see Table 5.4) are the most commonly used treatments for constipation. In general, laxatives should be used as a short-term measure to help relieve an episode of constipation as long-term use can perpetuate constipation and create dependence, and Emmanuel (2004) suggests that they lose their effect over time. The development of newer aperients broadens the treatment options, particularly for those patients with chronic constipation that has not responded to lifestyle modification or traditional laxatives.

Learning Activity 5.6 **Case study: Constipation**

Mr Jones, aged 32 years, is recovering from orthopaedic surgery for which he has been on bed rest. While on the ward he has suffered from constipation. He would like to know what he should do to avoid getting constipated when he goes home.

What advice would you give to Mr Jones?

See the end of the chapter for the answers.

Enemas

DEFINITION

An enema is the administration of a substance in liquid form into the rectum, either to aid bowel evacuation or to administer medication (Higgins 2006) (Figure 5.19).

Figure 5.18 **Correct positioning for opening your bowel.** *Source:* **Reproduced by kind permission of Ray Addison, Nurse Consultant in Bladder and Bowel dysfunction, and Wendy Ness, Colorectal Nurse Specialist. Produced as a service to the medical profession by Norgine Pharmaceuticals Ltd.**

Correct position for opening your bowels

Step one

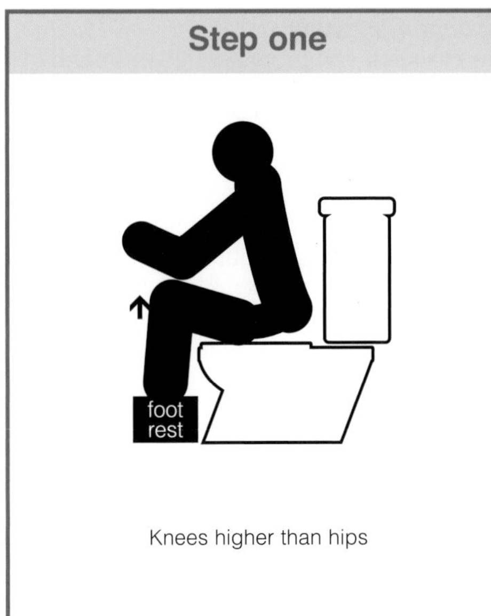

Knees higher than hips

Step two

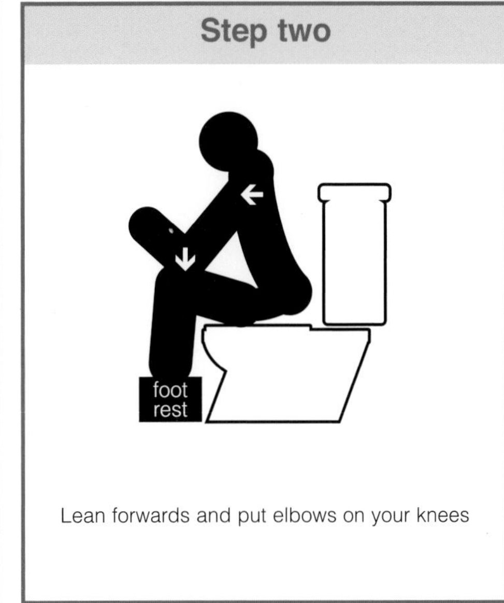

Lean forwards and put elbows on your knees

Step three

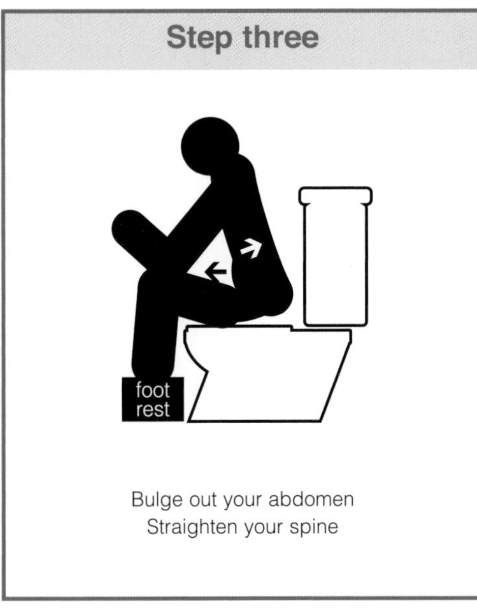

Bulge out your abdomen
Straighten your spine

Correct position

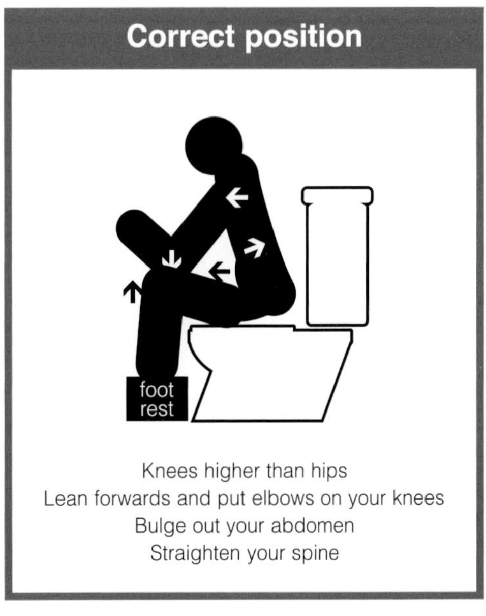

Knees higher than hips
Lean forwards and put elbows on your knees
Bulge out your abdomen
Straighten your spine

EVIDENCE-BASED APPROACHES

Rationale

Indications

Enemas may be prescribed for the following reasons.

- To clean the lower bowel before surgery, X-ray examination of the bowel using contrast medium or endoscopy examination.
- To treat severe constipation when other methods have failed.
- To introduce medication into the system.
- To soothe and treat irritated bowel mucosa.
- To decrease body temperature (due to contact with the proximal vascular system).
- To stop local haemorrhage.
- To reduce hyperkalaemia (calcium resonium).
- To reduce portal systemic encephalopathy (phosphate enema).

Figure 5.19 **Enema.**

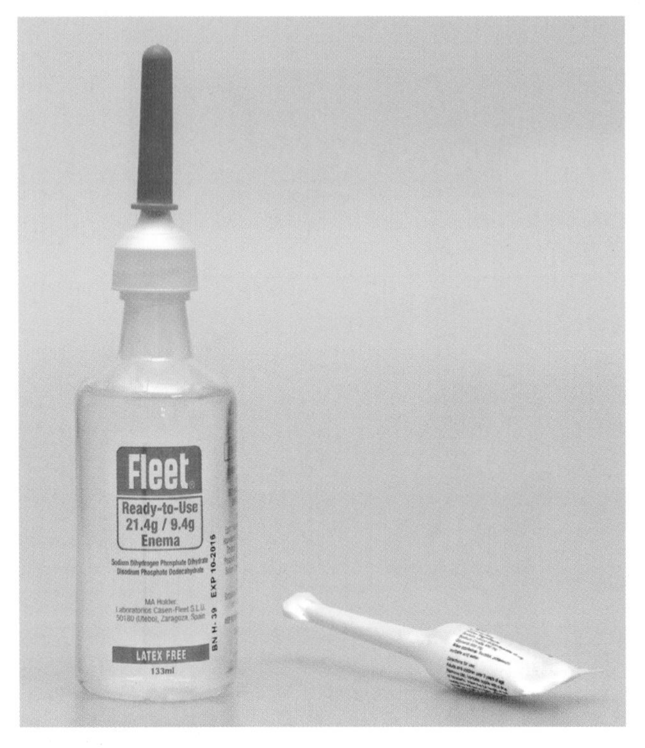

Contraindications

Enemas are contraindicated under the following circumstances.

- In paralytic ileus.
- In colonic obstruction.
- Where the administration of tap water or soap and water enemas may cause circulatory overload, water intoxication, mucosal damage and necrosis, hyperkalaemia and cardiac arrhythmias.
- Where the administration of large amounts of fluid high into the colon may cause perforation and haemorrhage.
- Following gastrointestinal or gynaecological surgery, where suture lines may be ruptured (unless medical consent has been given).
- Frailty.
- Proctitis.
- The use of microenemas and hypertonic saline enemas in patients with inflammatory or ulcerative conditions of the large colon.
- Recent radiotherapy to the lower pelvis unless medical consent has been given (Davies 2004).

LEGAL AND PROFESSIONAL ISSUES

Enema administration must be performed by a practitioner with the appropriate knowledge and skills and where it is within their scope of professional practice to carry out this procedure.

PRE-PROCEDURAL CONSIDERATIONS

Evacuant enemas

An evacuant enema is a solution introduced into the rectum or lower colon with the intention of it being expelled, along with faecal matter and flatus, within a few minutes. The osmotic activity increases the water content of the stool so that rectal distension follows and induces defaecation by stimulating rectal motility.

The following solutions are often used.

- Phosphate enemas with standard or long rectal tubes in single-dose disposable packs. Although these are often used for bowel clearance before X-ray examination and surgery, there is little evidence to support their use due to the associated risks and contraindications. Davies (2004) and Bowers (2006) highlight the risk of phosphate absorption resulting from pooling of the enema due to lack of evacuation and also the risk of rectal injury caused by the enema tip. Studies have found that if evacuation does not occur, patients may suffer from hypovolaemic shock, renal failure and oliguria. When using this type of enema, it is vital that good fluid intake is encouraged and maintained.
- Dioctyl sodium sulphosuccinate 0.1% and sorbitol 25% in single-dose disposable packs are used to soften impacted faeces.
- Sodium citrate 450 mg, sodium alkylsulphoacetate 45 mg and ascorbic acid 5 mg in single-dose disposable packs.

Retention enemas

A retention enema is a solution introduced into the rectum or lower colon with the intention of being retained for a specified period of time. Two types of retention enema have been most commonly used: arachis oil enemas (which are contraindicated in patients with nut allergies) and prednisolone enemas. These work by penetrating faeces, increasing the bulk and softness of stools. Classified as stool softeners, there is little evidence to support the use of this group of laxatives in the treatment of constipation (Woodward 2012).

All types of enemas need to be prescribed and checked against the prescription before administration. It is essential that the implications and procedure are fully explained to the patient, so as to relieve anxiety and embarrassment.

Procedure guideline 5.14 **Enema administration**

Essential equipment

- Disposable incontinence pad
- Disposable apron and gloves
- Rectal tube and funnel (if not using a commercially prepared pack)
- Solution required or commercially prepared enema
- Gauze squares
- Commode or bedpan if required
- Lubricating gel

Pre-procedure

Action	Rationale
1 Explain and discuss the procedure with the patient.	To ensure that the patient understands the procedure and gives their valid consent (NMC 2013, **C**).
2 Wash hands.	For infection prevention and control (Fraise and Bradley 2009, **E**).

Action	Rationale
3 Draw curtains around the patient or close the door to ensure privacy.	To avoid unnecessary embarrassment and to promote dignified care (NMC 2015, **C**).
4 Allow patient to empty bladder first if necessary.	A full bladder may cause discomfort during the procedure (Higgins 2006, **E**).
5 Ensure that a bedpan, commode or toilet is readily available.	In case the patient feels the need to expel the enema before the procedure is completed. **P**
Procedure	
6 Warm the enema to room temperature by immersing in a jug of hot water.	Heat is an effective stimulant of the nerve plexi in the intestinal mucosa. An enema at room temperature or just above will not damage the intestinal mucosa. The temperature of the environment, the rate of fluid administration and the length of the tubing will all have an effect on the temperature of the fluid in the rectum (Higgins 2006, **E**).
7 Assist the patient to lie on the left side, with knees well flexed, the upper knee higher than the lower one, and with the buttocks near the edge of the bed.	This allows ease of passage into the rectum by following the natural anatomy of the colon. In this position, gravity will aid the flow of the solution into the colon. Flexing the knees ensures a more comfortable passage of the enema nozzle or rectal tube (Higgins 2006, **E**).
8 Place a disposable incontinence pad beneath the patient's hips and buttocks.	To reduce potential infection caused by soiled linen. To avoid embarrassing the patient if the fluid is ejected prematurely following administration. **P**
9 Wash hands and put on disposable gloves.	For infection prevention and control (Fraise and Bradley 2009, **E**).
10 Place some lubricating gel on a gauze square and lubricate the nozzle of the enema or the rectal tube.	This prevents trauma to the anal and rectal mucosa which reduces surface friction (Higgins 2006, **E**).
11 Expel excessive air from tge enema and introduce the nozzle or tube slowly into the anal canal while separating the buttocks. (A small amount of air may be introduced if bowel evacuation is desired.)	The introduction of air into the colon causes distension of its walls, resulting in unnecessary discomfort for the patient. The slow introduction of the lubricated tube will minimize spasm of the intestinal wall (evacuation will be more effectively induced due to the increased peristalsis). **C**
12 Slowly introduce the tube or nozzle to a depth of 10.0–12.5 cm.	This will bypass the anal canal (2.5–4.0 cm in length) and ensure that the tube or nozzle is in the rectum. **C**
13 If a retention enema is used, introduce the fluid slowly and leave the patient in bed with the foot of the bed elevated by 45° for as long as prescribed.	To avoid increasing peristalsis. The slower the rate at which the fluid is introduced, the less pressure is exerted on the intestinal wall. Elevating the foot of the bed aids retention of the enema by the force of gravity. **C**
14 If an evacuant enema is used, introduce the fluid slowly by rolling the pack from the bottom to the top to prevent backflow, until the pack is empty or the solution is completely finished.	The faster the rate of flow of the fluid, the greater the pressure on the rectal walls. Distension and irritation of the bowel wall will produce strong peristalsis which is sufficient to empty the lower bowel (Higgins 2006, **E**).
15 If using a funnel and rectal tube, adjust the height of the funnel according to the rate of flow desired.	The forces of gravity will cause the solution to flow from the funnel into the rectum. The greater the elevation of the funnel, the faster the flow of fluid. **E**
16 Clamp the tubing before all the fluid has run in.	To avoid air entering the rectum and causing further discomfort. **E**
17 Slowly withdraw the tube or nozzle.	To avoid reflex emptying of the rectum. **E**
18 Dry the patient's perineal area using gauze squares.	To promote patient comfort and avoid excoriation. **P**
19 Ask the patient to retain the enema for 10–15 minutes before evacuating the bowel.	To enhance the evacuant effect. **C**
20 Ensure that the patient has access to the nurse call system, is near to the bedpan, commode or toilet, and has adequate toilet paper.	To enhance patient comfort and safety. To minimize the patient's embarrassment. **P**
Postprocedure	
21 Remove and dispose of equipment, gloves and apron.	

(continued)

Procedure guideline 5.14 Enema administration *(continued)*

Action	Rationale
22 Wash hands.	For infection prevention and control (Fraise and Bradley 2009, **E**).
23 Record in the appropriate documents that the enema has been given, its effects on the patient and its results (colour, consistency, content and amount of faeces produced), using the Bristol Stool Chart (see Figure 5.4).	To monitor the patient's bowel function (Gill 1999, **C**).
24 Observe patient for any adverse reactions.	To monitor the patient for complications (Peate 2003, **C**).

Problem-solving table 5.5 Prevention and resolution (Procedure guideline 5.14)

Problem	Cause	Prevention	Action
Unable to insert the nozzle of the enema pack or rectal tube into the anal canal.	Tube not adequately lubricated. Patient in an incorrect position. Patient unable to relax anal sphincter. Patient apprehensive and embarrassed about the situation.	Ensure patient is relaxed and in the correct position.	Apply more lubricating jelly. Ask the patient to draw knees up further towards the chest. To ensure the patient is relaxed before inserting the nozzle or rectal tube. Ask the patient to take deep breaths and 'bear down' as if defaecating.
Unable to advance the tube or nozzle into the anal canal.	Spasm of the canal walls.	Ask the patient to take slow deep breaths to help them relax.	Wait until spasm has passed before inserting the tube or nozzle more slowly, thus minimizing spasm.Ensure adequate privacy and give frequent explanations to the patient about the procedure.
Unable to advance the tube or nozzle into the rectum.	Blockage by faeces. Blockage by tumour.		Withdraw tubing slightly and allow a little solution to flow and then insert the tube further. If resistance is still met, stop the procedure and inform a doctor.
Patient complains of cramping or the desire to evacuate the enema before the end of the procedure.	Distension and irritation of the intestinal wall produces strong peristalsis sufficient to empty the lower bowel.	Encourage the patient to retain the enema.	Stop instilling the enema fluid and wait with the patient until the discomfort has subsided.
Patient unable to open bowels after an evacuant enema.	Reduced neuromuscular response in the bowel wall.		Inform the doctor that the enema was unsuccessful and reassure the patient.

Suppositories

DEFINITION

A suppository is a solid or semi-solid, bullet-shaped pellet that is prepared by mixing a medication with a wax-like substance that melts once inserted into the rectum (Galbraith et al. 2007).

EVIDENCE-BASED APPROACHES

Rationale

Indications

The use of suppositories is indicated under the following circumstances.

- To empty the bowel prior to certain types of surgery and investigations.
- To empty the bowel to relieve acute constipation or when other treatments for constipation have failed.
- To empty the bowel before endoscopic examination.
- To introduce medication into the system.
- To soothe and treat haemorrhoids or anal pruritus.

Contraindications

The use of suppositories is contraindicated when one or more of the following pertain.

- Chronic constipation, which would require repetitive use.
- Paralytic ileus.

- Colonic obstruction.
- Malignancy of the perianal region.
- Low platelet count.
- Following gastrointestinal or gynaecological operations, unless on the specific instructions of the doctor.

Methods of administration of suppositories

The use of suppositories dates back to about 460 BC. Hippocrates recommended the use of cylindrical suppositories of honey smeared with ox gall (Hurst et al. 1969). The torpedo-shaped suppositories commonly used today came into being in 1893, when it was recommended that they were inserted apex (pointed end) first (Moppett 2000).

This practice was questioned by Abd-el-Maeboud et al. (1991) who suggested that suppositories should be inserted blunt end first. The rationale for this is based on anorectal physiology; if a suppository is inserted apex first, the circular base distends the anus and the lower edge of the anal sphincter fails to close tightly. The normal squeezing motion (reverse vermicular contraction) of the anal sphincter therefore fails to drive the suppository into the rectum. These factors can lead to anal irritation and rejection of the suppository (Moppett 2000, Pegram et al. 2008). The research study by Abd-el-Maeboud et al. (1991) was very small but remains the only research evidence supporting this practice and consequently a common-sense approach is suggested (Bradshaw and Price 2006). A distinction can be made between suppositories administered for constipation, requiring a local effect, and those given to achieve a systemic effect.

In the management of constipation, a suppository placed against the bowel wall, rather than within faecal matter, enables body heat to soften the suppository. This requires an accurate insertion technique which may be better achieved by inserting the suppository apex first (Kyle 2009). However, Kyle (2009) goes on to suggest that patients may find it more acceptable to self-administer suppositories blunt end first as the sucking action means there is no need to insert the finger into the anal canal. Suppositories for systemic use are best absorbed by the lower rectum. Here venous drainage avoids the portal circulation moving to the inferior vena cava quickly, resulting in a more rapid therapeutic effect (Kyle 2009). There is a need for further research in this area but until such work is carried out, expert opinion such as Kyle (2009) and common sense should guide practice.

PRE-PROCEDURAL CONSIDERATIONS

Pharmacological

There are several different types of suppository available. Retention suppositories are designed to deliver drug therapy, for example analgesia, antibiotic, non-steroidal anti-inflammatory drug (NSAID). Those designed to stimulate bowel evacuation include glycerine, bisacodyl and sodium bicarbonate. Lubricant suppositories, for example glycerine, should be inserted directly into the faeces and allowed to dissolve. They have a mild irritant action on the rectum and also act as faecal softeners (BNF 2014). However, stimulant types, such as bisacodyl, must come into contact with the mucous membrane of the rectum if they are to be effective as they release carbon dioxide, causing rectal distension and thus evacuation.

Procedure guideline 5.15 **Suppository administration**

Essential equipment

- Disposable incontinence pad
- Disposable apron and gloves
- Gauze squares or tissues
- Lubricating gel
- Suppository(ies) as required (check prescription before administering any suppository)
- Bedpan or commode if required

Pre-procedure

Action	Rationale
1 Explain and discuss the procedure with the patient. If you are administering a medicated suppository, it is best to do so after the patient has emptied their bowels.	To ensure that the patient understands the procedure and gives their valid consent (NMC 2013, **C**). To ensure that the active ingredients are not prevented from being absorbed by the rectal mucosa and that the suppository is not expelled before its active ingredients have been released (Moppett 2000, **E**).
2 Wash hands.	To ensure the procedure is as clean as possible and for infection control reasons (Fraise and Bradley 2009, **E**).
3 Draw curtains around the patient or close the door.	To ensure privacy and dignity for the patient (NMC 2015, **C**).
4 Ensure that a bedpan, commode or toilet is readily available.	In case of premature ejection of the suppositories or rapid bowel evacuation following their administration. **P**

Procedure

Action	Rationale
5 Assist the patient to lie on the left side, with the knees flexed, the upper knee higher than the lower one, with the buttocks near the edge of the bed.	This allows ease of passage of the suppository into the rectum by following the natural anatomy of the colon (Galbraith et al. 2007; Pegram et al. 2008). Flexing the knees will reduce discomfort as the suppository is passed through the anal sphincter (Moppett 2000, **E**).

(continued)

Procedure guideline 5.15 **Suppository administration *(continued)***

Action	Rationale
6 Place a disposable incontinence pad beneath the patient's hips and buttocks.	To avoid unnecessary soiling of linen, leading to potential infection and embarrassment to the patient if the suppositories are ejected prematurely or there is rapid bowel evacuation following their administration. **E**
7 Wash hands and put on apron and gloves.	For infection prevention and control (Fraise and Bradley 2009, **E**).
8 Place some lubricating jelly on a gauze square and lubricate the blunt end of the suppository if it is being used to obtain systemic action. Separate the patient's buttocks and insert the suppository blunt end first, advancing it for about 2–4 cm. Repeat this procedure if a second suppository is to be inserted.	Lubricating reduces surface friction and thus eases insertion of the suppository and avoids anal mucosal trauma. The suppository is more readily retained if inserted blunt end first (Abd-el-Maeboud et al. 1991, **R2b**). The anal canal is approximately 2–4 cm long. Inserting the suppository beyond this ensures that it will be retained (Abd-el-Maeboud et al. 1991, **R2b**; Pegram et al. 2008, **E**).
9 Once the suppository(ies) has been inserted, clean any excess lubricating jelly from the patient's perineal area using gauze squares.	To ensure the patient's comfort and avoid anal excoriation (Moppett 2000, **E**).
10 Ask the patient to retain the suppository(ies) for 20 minutes, or until they are no longer able to do so. If a medicated suppository is given, remind the patient that its aim is not to stimulate evacuation and to retain the suppository for at least 20 minutes or as long as possible.	This will allow the suppository to melt and release the active ingredients. Inform patient that there may be some discharge as the medication melts in the rectum (Henry 1999, **E**).
Post-procedure	
11 Remove and dispose of equipment, gloves and apron. Wash hands.	For infection prevention and control (Fraise and Bradley 2009, **E**).
12 Record that the suppository(ies) have been given, the effect on the patient and the result (amount, colour, consistency and content, using the Bristol Stool Chart, Figure 5.4), if appropriate, in the relevant documents.	To monitor the patient's bowel function (Gill 1999, **C**) and to maintain accurate records (NMC 2009, **C**).
13 Observe patient for any adverse reactions.	To monitor for any complications (Peate 2003, **E**).

Digital rectal examination

DEFINITION

A digital rectal examination (DRE) is an invasive procedure that can be carried out, as part of a nursing assessment, by a Registered Nurse who can demonstrate competence to an appropriate level in accordance with the NMC *Code of Conduct* (NMC 2015, RCN 2012b). The procedure involves the nurse inserting a lubricated gloved finger into the rectum.

EVIDENCE-BASED APPROACHES

Rationale

Indications

This examination can be performed in the following circumstances.

- To establish whether faecal matter is present in the rectum and, if so, to assess the amount and consistency.
- To ascertain anal tone and the ability to initiate a voluntary contraction and to what degree.
- To teach pelvic floor exercises.
- To assess anal pathology for the presence of foreign objects.
- Prior to administering rectal medication to establish the state of the rectum.
- To establish the effects of rectal medication.
- To administer suppositories or enema prior to endoscopy.
- To determine the need for digital removal of faeces (DRF) or digital rectal stimulation and evaluating bowel emptiness.
- To assess the need for rectal medication and to evaluate its efficacy in certain circumstances, for example in patients who have diminished anal/rectal sensation.
- For digital stimulation to trigger defaecation by stimulating the rectoanal reflex (Weisner and Bell 2004).
- To establish anal and rectal sensation (RCN 2012b).

LEGAL AND PROFESSIONAL ISSUES

As DRE is an invasive and intimate procedure, it is important that consent is obtained from the patient prior to it being performed (Kyle 2011c, Steggall 2008). A DRE should form part of the bowel assessment, rather than being a stand-alone procedure (Kyle 2011c), and can be undertaken by Registered Nurses who demonstrate competency in this procedure, possessing the knowledge, skills and abilities required for lawful, safe and effective practice (RCN 2012b).

As nursing roles develop, nurse specialists and nurse practitioners are increasingly involved in areas of care that necessitate undertaking DRE as part of a physical assessment or procedure. Such instances may include:

- the assessment of prostate size, consistency, mobility and anatomical limits

- during procedures such as the placement of a rectal probe/sensor prior to urodynamic studies or the placement of catheters used in the treatment of constipation or anismus
- prior to using transanal irrigation
- the placement of an endoscope prior to colonoscopy or sigmoidoscopy (RCN 2012b).

PRE-PROCEDURAL CONSIDERATIONS

Specific patient preparation

Before carrying out a DRE, the perineal and perianal area should be checked for signs of rectal prolapse, haemorrhoids, anal skin tags, fissures or lesions, foreign bodies, scarring, infestations or a gaping anus. The condition of the skin should be noted, as should the type and amount of any discharge or leakage. If any of these abnormalities are seen, a DRE should not be carried out until advice is taken from a specialist nurse or medical practitioner (RCN 2012b, Steggall 2008).

Precautions

Special care should be taken in performing DRE in patients whose disease processes or treatments in particular affect the anus or bowel mucosa. These conditions include (RCN 2012b):

- active inflammation of the bowel, for example ulcerative colitis
- recent radiotherapy to the pelvic area
- rectal/anal pain
- rectal surgery or trauma to the anal/rectal area in the last 6 weeks
- obvious rectal bleeding – consider possible causes for this
- spinal cord injury patients with an injury at or above the sixth thoracic vertebra, because of the risk of autonomic dysreflexia
- patients with known allergies, for example latex
- patients with a known history of abuse
- tissue fragility related to age, radiation or malnourishment.

Procedure guideline 5.16 **Digital rectal examination**

Essential equipment

- Disposable incontinence pad
- Disposable apron and gloves (check if patient allergic to latex)
- Lubricating gel
- Gauze squares or tissues
- Bedpan or commode if required

Preprocedure

Action	Rationale
1 Explain and discuss procedure with the patient.	To ensure that the patient understands the procedure and gives their valid consent (NMC 2013, **C**).
2 Ensure privacy.	To avoid unnecessary embarrassment to the patient and to promote dignity and privacy (NMC 2015, **C**).
3 Ensure that a bedpan, commode or toilet is readily available.	DRE can stimulate the need for bowel movement (Weisner and Bell 2004, **E**).

Procedure

Action	Rationale
4 Assist the patient to lie in the left lateral position with knees flexed, the upper knee higher than the lower knee, with the buttocks towards the edge of the bed.	This allows ease of digital examination into the rectum by following the natural anatomy of the colon (RCN 2012b, **C**). Flexing the knees reduces discomfort as the examining finger passes the anal sphincter (Kyle et al. 2005b, **C**).
5 Place a disposable incontinence pad beneath the patient's hips and buttocks.	To reduce potential infection caused by soiled linen. To avoid embarrassing the patient if faecal staining occurs during or after the procedure. **E**
6 Wash hands with bactericidal soap and water or bactericidal alcohol handrub and put on disposable gloves.	For infection prevention and control (Fraise and Bradley 2009, **E**).
7 Observe anal area prior to the insertion of the finger into the anus for evidence of skin soreness, excoriation, swelling, haemorrhoids, rectal prolapse and infestation.	May indicate incontinence or pruritus. Swelling may be indicative of possible mass or abscess. Abnormalities such as bleeding, discharge or prolapse should be reported to medical staff before any examination is undertaken (RCN 2012b, **C**).
8 Palpate the perianal area starting at 12 o'clock, clockwise to 6 o'clock and then from 12 anticlockwise to 6 o'clock.	To assess for any irregularities, swelling, indurations, tenderness or abscess in the perianal area (RCN 2012b, **C**).
9 Place some lubricating gel on a gauze square and gloved index finger. Inform the patient you are about to proceed.	To minimize discomfort as lubrication reduces friction and to ease insertion of the finger into the anus/rectum. Lubrication also helps minimize anal mucosal trauma (Kyle et al. 2005b, **C**). Informing the patient assists with co-operation with the procedure (NMC 2015, **C**).

(continued)

Procedure guideline 5.16 Digital rectal examination *(continued)*

Action	Rationale
10 Prior to insertion, encourage the patient to breathe out or talk and/or place gloved index finger on the anus for a few seconds prior to insertion. On insertion of finger, assess anal sphincter control; resistance should be felt.	To prevent spasm of the anal sphincter on insertion (RCN 2012b, **C**). Gently placing a finger on the anus initiates the anal reflex, causing the anus to contract and then relax (RCN 2012b, **C**). Digital insertion with resistance indicates good internal sphincter tone, poor resistance may indicate the opposite (RCN 2012b, **C**).
11 With finger inserted in the anus, sweep clockwise then anticlockwise, noting any irregularities.	Palpating around 360° enables the nurse to establish if there is any swelling or tenderness within the rectum (RCN 2012b, **C**; Steggall 2008, **E**).
12 Digital examination may feel faecal matter within the rectum; note consistency of any faecal matter.	May establish loaded rectum and indicate constipation and the need for rectal medication (RCN 2012b, **C**).
13 Clean anal area after the procedure.	To prevent irritation and soreness occurring. Preserves patient dignity and personal hygiene.
Postprocedure	
14 Remove gloves and apron and dispose of equipment in appropriate clinical waste bin. Wash hands with bactericidal soap and water.	For infection prevention and control (Fraise and Bradley 2009, **E**).
15 Assist patient into a comfortable position and offer bedpan, commode or toilet facilities as appropriate.	To promote comfort. **P**
16 Document findings and report to appropriate members of the multidisciplinary team.	To ensure continuity of care and ensure appropriate corrective action may be initiated (RCN 2012b, **C**).

Digital removal of faeces

DEFINITION

Digital removal of faeces (DRF) is an invasive procedure involving the removal of faeces from the rectum using a gloved finger. This should only be performed when necessary and after individual assessment (RCN 2012b).

RELATED THEORY

Managing bowel problems such as constipation and prolonged bowel evacuation in patients following spinal cord injury requires a multimodality approach. This includes dietary fibre, digital stimulation, enemas, suppositories, stool softeners and abdominal massage (Addison and White 2002). Digital stimulation is a method of initiating the defaecation reflex by dilating the anus, with either a finger or an anal dilator (Weisner and Bell 2004), but is only useful if the rectum is full.

Autonomic dysreflexia (AD) is unique to patients with spinal cord injury at the sixth thoracic vertebrae or above. It is an abnormal response from the autonomic nervous system to a painful (noxious) stimulus perceived below the level of spinal cord injury (Harrison 2000, Powell and Rigby 2000, RCN 2012b). Distended bowel caused by constipation or impaction can lead to autonomic dysreflexia and therefore it is important that an effective programme of bowel management is established and followed (Harrison 2000). Acute AD may occur in response to digital intervention. It is therefore important that all healthcare professionals carrying out digital interventions on individuals with spinal cord injury are aware of the signs and symptoms of headache, flushing, sweating, nasal obstruction, blotchiness above the lesion and hypertension. The most significant symptom is the rapid onset of a severe headache; should this occur, the intervention must be stopped immediately (RCN 2012b).

EVIDENCE-BASED APPROACHES

Rationale

Advances in oral, rectal and surgical treatments have reduced the need for digital removal of faeces to be performed; however, for certain groups of patients, such as those with spinal injuries, spina bifida or multiple sclerosis, this procedure may be the only suitable bowel-emptying technique, forming a long-standing, integral part of their bowel routine (Kyle et al. 2005b, RCN 2012b).

Digital removal of faeces can be distressing, painful and dangerous. In particular, stimulation of the vagus nerve in the rectal wall can slow the patient's heart, in addition to the risk of bowel perforation and bleeding (Kyle et al. 2005b).

Indications

Indications for assisted evacuation of bowels (digital removal of faeces or digital stimulation) include:

- faecal impaction/loading
- incomplete defaecation
- inability to defaecate
- when other bowel-emptying techniques have failed or are unsuitable
- neurogenic bowel dysfunction
- patients with spinal cord injury (RCN 2012b).

Patients are at risk of rectal trauma if these procedures are not performed with care or knowledge. The nurse should be aware of any conditions that may contraindicate performance of these procedures (see 'Digital rectal examination, Precautions').

LEGAL AND PROFESSIONAL ISSUES

Digital removal of faeces should be performed by Registered Nurses who demonstrate competency in this procedure, possessing the knowledge, skills and abilities required for lawful, safe and effective practice (RCN 2012b). In addition, they should ensure that their employer has defined policies and procedures for undertaking this role (RCN 2012b, Withell 2000). If appropriate, the patient and their personal carer may wish for the carer to maintain their established programme of bowel management (Harrison 2000).

PRE-PROCEDURAL CONSIDERATIONS

Specific patient preparations

If this procedure is used as an acute intervention, the patient's pulse rate should be recorded before and during the process. Patients with a spinal cord injury should also have their blood pressure measured before, during and after the procedure. A baseline blood pressure measurement should be available for comparison (RCN 2012b). Every time the procedure is performed, the consistency of the stool should be noted before continuing. If the stool is hard and dry, lubricant suppositories should be inserted and left for 30 minutes before commencing. If the stool is too soft to remove effectively, consider delaying the procedure for 24 hours to allow further water reabsorption to occur.

During the procedure the nurse should observe the patient for signs of:

- distress, pain or discomfort
- bleeding
- autonomic dysreflexia: hypertension, bradycardia, headache, flushing above the level of the spinal injury, sweating, pallor below the level of spinal injury, nasal congestion (Harrison 2000, RCN 2012b)
- collapse (RCN 2012b).

Procedure guideline 5.17 **Digital removal of faeces**

Essential equipment

- Disposable incontinence pad
- Receiver and/or yellow bag
- Specimen pot (if required)
- Bedpan or commode (if appropriate)
- Tissues or topical swabs
- Disposable apron and gloves (check if patient is allergic to latex)
- Lubricating gel

Preprocedure

Action	Rationale
1 Explain and discuss procedure with the patient.	To ensure that the patient understands the procedure and gives their valid consent (NMC 2013, **C**).
2 Draw curtain around the patient or close the door to ensure privacy.	To avoid unnecessary embarrassment to the patient.
3 In spinal cord injury patients who are at risk of AD, a blood pressure reading should be taken prior to the procedure. A baseline blood pressure reading should be available for comparison. For such patients where this procedure is routine and tolerance is well established, this is not required (RCN 2012b, **C**).	In spinal cord injury, stimulus below the level of injury may result in symptoms of AD including headache and hypertension (Kyle et al. 2005b; RCN 2012b, **C**).
Procedure	
4 Assist the patient to lie in the left lateral position with knees flexed, the upper knee higher than the lower knee, with the buttocks towards the edge of the bed.	This allows ease of digital insertion into the rectum, by following the natural anatomy of the colon (RCN 2012b). Flexing the knees reduces discomfort as the finger passes the anal sphincter (Kyle et al. 2005b, **C**).
5 Place a disposable incontinence pad beneath the patient's hips and buttocks.	To reduce potential infection caused by soiled linen. To avoid embarrassing the patient if faecal staining occurs during or after the procedure.
6 Wash hands with bactericidal soap and water or bactericidal alcohol handrub and put on disposable apron and gloves.	For infection prevention and control (Fraise and Bradley 2009, **E**).
7 Place some lubricating gel on a gauze square and gloved index finger.	To minimize discomfort as lubrication reduces friction and to ease insertion of the finger into the anus/rectum. Lubrication also helps minimize anal mucosal trauma (Kyle et al. 2005b, **C**).
8 Inform the patient you are about to proceed.	Assists with patient co-operation with the procedure (NMC 2015, **C**).
9 In spinal cord injury patients, observe for signs of AD throughout the procedure (RCN 2012b, **C**).	In spinal cord injury, stimulus below the level of injury may result in symptoms of AD, including hypertension (Kyle et al. 2005b, **C**).

(continued)

Procedure guideline 5.17 Digital removal of faeces *(continued)*

Action	Rationale
10 Observe anal area prior to the insertion of the finger into the anus for evidence of skin soreness, excoriation, swelling, haemorrhoids or rectal prolapse.	May indicate incontinence or pruritus. Swelling may be indicative of possible mass or abscess. Abnormalities such as bleeding, discharge or prolapse should be reported to medical staff before any examination is undertaken (RCN 2012b, **C**).
11 Proceed to insert finger into the anus/rectum. Proceed with caution in those patients with spinal cord injury.	The majority of spinal cord injury patients will not experience any pain (Kyle et al. 2005b, **C**).
12 If the stool is type 1 (see Figure 5.4), remove one lump at a time until no more faecal matter is felt.	To relieve patient discomfort (Kyle et al. 2005b, **C**).
13 If a solid faecal mass is felt, split it and remove small pieces until no more faecal matter is felt. Avoid using a hooked finger to remove faeces.	To relieve patient discomfort (Kyle et al. 2005b, **C**). Use of a hooked finger may cause damage to the rectal mucosa and anal sphincter (RCN 2012b).
14 If faecal mass is too hard to break up, or more than 4 cm across, stop the procedure and discuss with the multidisciplinary team.	To avoid unnecessary pain and damage to the anal sphincter. The patient may require the procedure to be carried out under anaesthetic (Kyle et al. 2005b, **C**).
15 As faeces is removed, it should be placed in an appropriate receiver.	To assist in appropriate disposal and reduce contamination or cross-infection risk.
16 Encourage patients who receive this procedure on a regular basis to have a period of rest or, if appropriate, to assist using the Valsalva manoeuvre.	Patient and nurse education is required to use this technique safely and so further guidance should be sought before introducing this manoeuvre as it may lead to complications such as haemorrhoids (Kyle et al. 2005b, **C**).
17 Wash and dry the patient's anal area and buttocks.	To ensure patient feels comfortable and clean. **P**
Post-procedure	
18 Remove gloves and apron and dispose of equipment in appropriate clinical waste bin. Wash hands.	For prevention and control of infection (Fraise and Bradley 2009, **E**).
19 Assist patient into a comfortable position.	To promote comfort. **P**
20 In spinal cord injury patients, take a blood pressure reading.	In spinal cord injury, stimulus below the level of injury may result in symptoms of AD, including hypertension (Kyle et al. 2005b, **C**).
21 Document findings and report to appropriate members of the multidisciplinary team.	To ensure continuity of care and enable appropriate actions to be initiated (RCN 2012b, **C**).

Stoma care

DEFINITION

Stoma is a word of Greek origin meaning mouth or opening (Taylor 2005).

RELATED THEORY

Every year approximately 11,000 new colostomies, 9000 new ileostomies and 2000 new urostomies are formed in the UK (Welser et al. 2009). The most common underlying conditions resulting in the need for stoma surgery are colorectal cancer, bladder cancer, ulcerative colitis and Crohn's disease. Other causes of stoma surgery include:

- pelvic cancer, for example gynaecological cancer
- trauma
- neurological damage
- congenital disorders
- diverticular disease
- familial polyposis coli
- intractable incontinence
- fistula
- radiation bowel disease
- bowel perforation (Burch 2011a, Taylor et al. 2012).

TYPES OF STOMA

Colostomy

A colostomy may be formed from any section of the large bowel. Its position along the colon will dictate the output and consistency of faeces. Therefore an understanding of the anatomy and physiology is essential to fully care for stoma patients.

The most common site for a colostomy is on the sigmoid colon. This will produce a semi-solid or formed stool and is generally positioned in the left iliac fossa and is flush to the skin (Burch 2011a). Stomas formed higher up along the colon will produce a slightly more liquid stool. A colostomy tends to act on average 2–3 times per day, but this can vary between individuals.

Colostomies can either be permanent (end) (Figure 5.20, Figure 5.21) or temporary (loop) (Figure 5.22, Figure 5.23). Permanent (end) colostomies are often formed following removal of rectal cancers, as in abdominoperineal resections of the rectum, whereas a temporary (loop) colostomy may be formed to divert the faecal output, to allow healing of a surgical join (anastomosis) or

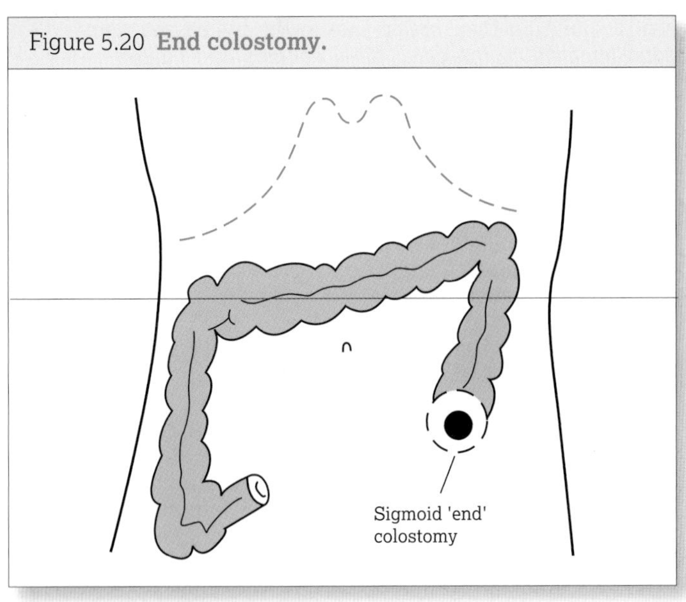

Figure 5.20 **End colostomy.**

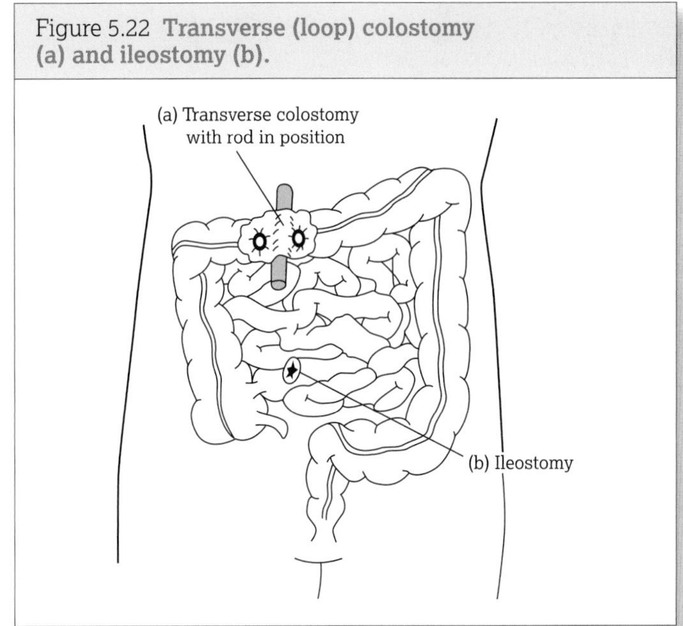

Figure 5.22 **Transverse (loop) colostomy (a) and ileostomy (b).**

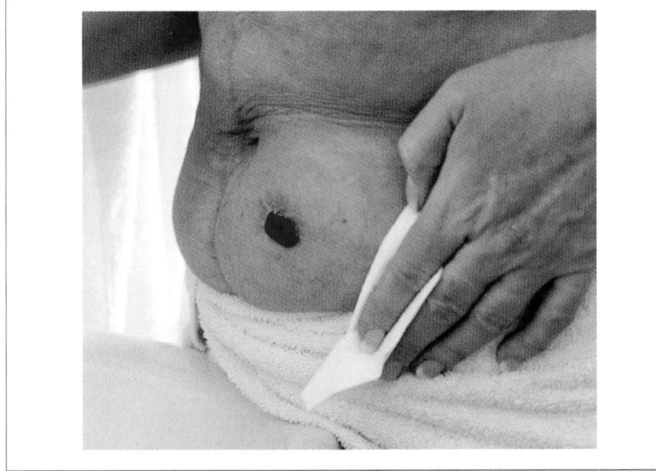
Figure 5.21 **End colostomy.**

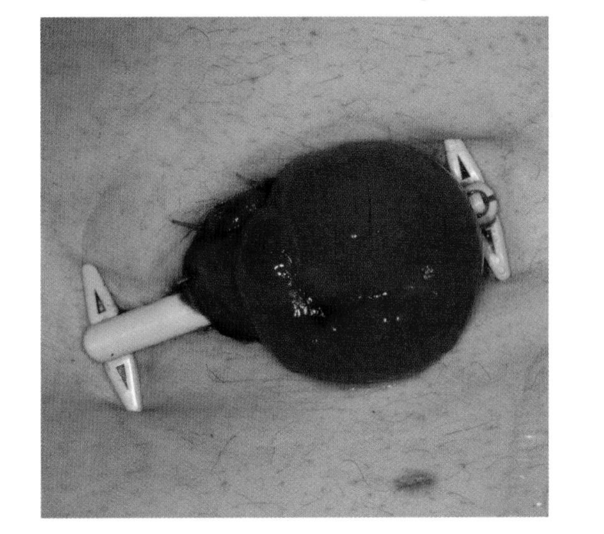
Figure 5.23 **Loop colostomy with bridge *in situ*.**

repair, or to relieve an obstruction or bowel injury (Taylor 2005). Permanent colostomies were the most commonly formed stoma but the number of temporary stomas is increasing, most of which are ileostomies rather than colostomies (IMS 2008).

As is evident from Figures 5.21 and 5.23, end and loop colostomies are very different in appearance. An end colostomy tends to be flush to the skin and sutured to the abdominal wall and consists of an end-section of bowel, whereas a loop colostomy is larger. During the perioperative period, it is supported by a stoma bridge or rod (see Figure 5.23).This is placed under the section of bowel and generally left in place for 3–10 days following surgery and then removed (Wright and Burch 2008).

Ileostomy

Ileostomies are formed when a section of ileum is brought out onto the abdominal wall. This is generally positioned at the end of the ileum on the right iliac fossa, but can be anywhere along the ileum. Consequently, the output tends to be looser, more liquid stool, as waste is being eliminated before the water is absorbed from the large bowel (colon). Due to the more acidic, abrasive nature of the stool at this stage, a spout is formed with this type of stoma. The ileum is everted to form a spout which allows the effluent to drain into an appliance, without coming into contact with the peristomal skin (Burch 2011b) (Figure 5.24). This prevents skin breakdown and allows for better management. The average output from an ileostomy is 200–600 mL per day.

Ileostomies can also be either permanent (end) (see Figure 5.24) or temporary (loop). Permanent ileostomies are often formed following total colectomies (removal of the entire colon). Loop ileostomies are increasingly common and are often formed to allow healing of a surgical join (anastomosis) or an ileoanal pouch (IMS 2008, Taylor 2005). These are sometimes held in place by a stoma bridge or rod. Refer to Procedure guideline 5.19: Stoma bridge or rod removal for more information on bridge/rod care and removal.

Figure 5.24 **End ileostomy.** ***Source:*** **Reproduced with permission from Dansac Ltd.**

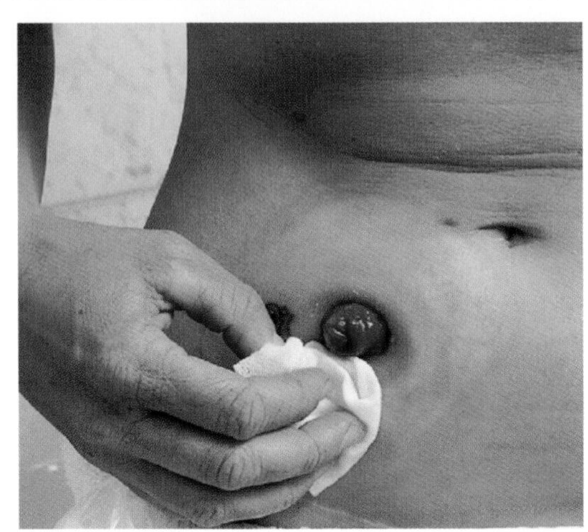

Urostomy/ileal conduit

An ileal conduit is the most common form of urostomy; the colon (colonic conduit) may also be used. Urostomy comes from the Greek words *uros* meaning urine and *stoma* meaning mouth or opening (Nazarko 2008). Approximately 1500 urostomies were formed in the UK in 2006 (Burch 2008).

A section of bowel is isolated, along with its mesentery vessels, and the remaining ends of the bowel are anastomosed to restore continuity. The isolated section is mobilized, the proximal end is closed and the ureters, once resected from the bladder, are implanted at this end. The distal end is brought out onto the surface of the abdominal wall and everted to form a spout (see Figure 5.24), as in an ileostomy (Fillingham and Fell 2004). Urine from a urostomy will contain mucus from the bowel used in its construction (Taylor 2005).

EVIDENCE-BASED APPROACHES

Stoma care has developed greatly over the years. Although an evidence base for this does exist, it mainly centres around clinical practice and experience.

Stoma care is very individual and requires full holistic patient assessment. The primary aim is to promote patient independence by providing care and advice on managing the stoma, therefore allowing the patient to continue with all the necessary activities of daily living.

Rationale

Indications

Stoma care is essential:

- to collect faeces or urine in an appropriate appliance
- to achieve and maintain patient comfort and security
- to support psychological adaptation and independence.

LEGAL AND PROFESSIONAL ISSUES

As already discussed, stoma care is primarily based on experience and therefore the development of skills. It is a fundamental area of nursing practice that all Registered Nurses should have the competency to undertake. It has recently been recognized that many of the core nursing skills in stoma care are being carried out by healthcare assistants and carers. Therefore there is an increasing demand for education in this area. Stoma care often develops due to nurses who have an interest in this area and then further build on their skills. Due to the increasing demand for good effective stoma care, many courses and conferences now exist to improve patient care and enhance professional knowledge and skills.

PRE-PROCEDURAL CONSIDERATIONS

Equipment

Many of the appliances now available are very similar in style, colour and efficiency and often there is very little to choose between them when the time comes for the ostomate to decide what to wear.

The aim of good stoma care is to return patients to their place in society. One of the ways in which this can be facilitated is to provide them with a safe, reliable appliance. This means that there should be no fear of leakage or odour and the appliance should be comfortable, unobtrusive, easy to handle and disposable. The ostomate should be allowed a choice from the management systems available. It is also important to identify and manage problems with the stoma or peristomal skin at an early stage.

When choosing the appropriate management system for the new ostomate, factors which need to be considered include:

- type of stoma
- type of effluent
- patient's cognitive ability
- manual dexterity
- lifestyle
- condition of peristomal skin
- siting of stoma
- patient preference (Kirkwood 2006).

Appliances

Stoma appliances are made from an odour-proof plastic film. They adhere to the peristomal skin using an adhesive hydrocolloid base or flange (Williams 2011). Appliances may be opaque or clear and often have a soft backing to absorb perspiration. They usually have a built-in integral filter containing charcoal to neutralize any odour. The type of appliance used will depend on the type of stoma and effluent expected. Refer to Figure 5.25 to assist with appliance selection.

CHOOSING THE RIGHT SIZE

It is important that the flange of the appliance fits snugly around the stoma within 0.3 cm of the stoma edge (Kirkwood 2006). This narrow edge is left exposed so that the appliance does not rub on the stoma. Stoma appliances usually come with measuring guides to allow for choice of size. During the initial weeks following surgery, the oedematous stoma will gradually reduce in size and the appliance needs to be adapted accordingly.

FEAR OF MALODOUR

Appliances usually have a built-in integral filter containing charcoal to neutralize any odour when flatus is released; therefore, smell is only noticeable when emptying or changing an appliance. There are also various deodorizers that come in the form of drops or powders that may be put into the pouch or sprays, which can be sprayed into the air just before changing or emptying the pouch (Burch and Sica 2005). The individual should be reassured that any problems with odour or leakage will be investigated and that in most circumstances the problem will be solved with alternative appliances or accessories.

Drainable pouches are used when the effluent is fluid or semi-formed, in the case of an ileostomy or transverse colostomy (Figure 5.26a). These pouches have specially designed filters, which are less likely to become blocked or leak faecal fluid. They need to be emptied regularly and the outlet rinsed carefully and then closed with a clip or 'roll-up' method. They may be left on for up to 3 days.

Figure 5.25 **Flow chart for choosing appliances: International Ostomy Forum Group (2006) Observation Index.** *Source:* **Reproduced with permission from Dansac Ltd.**

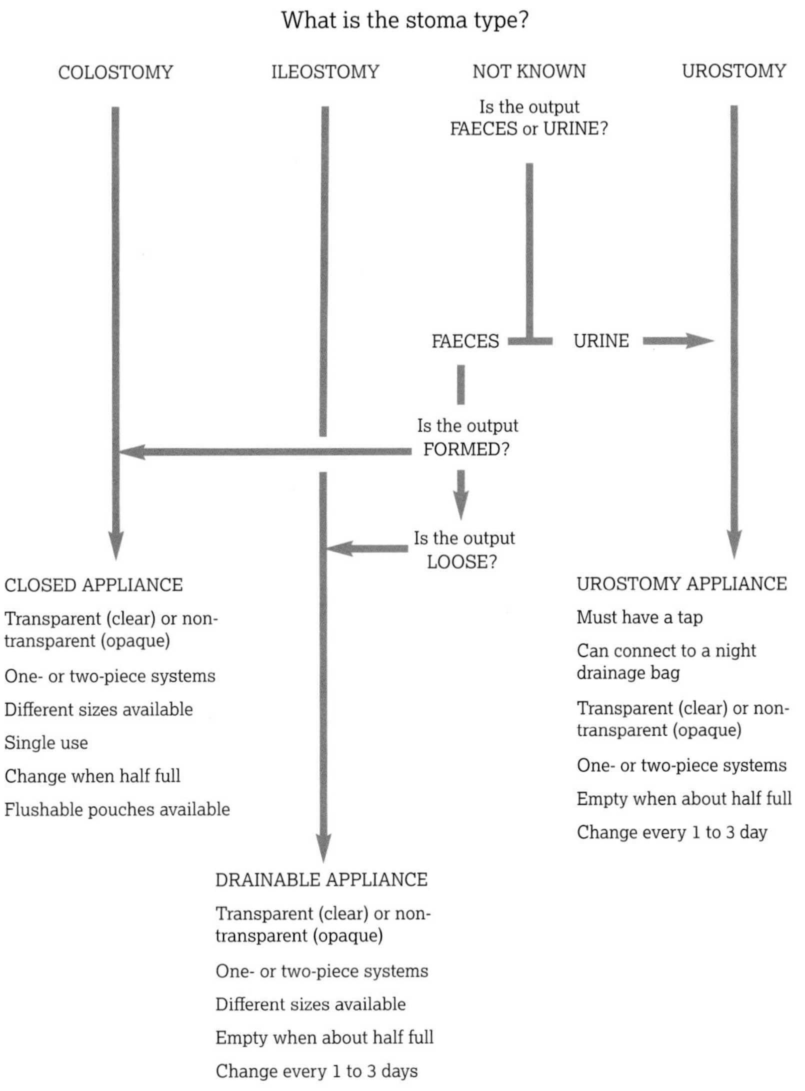

Urostomy pouches have a drainage tap for urine and should be emptied regularly (Figure 5.26b). They can be attached to a large bag and tubing for night drainage. These pouches can remain on for up to 3 days.

Closed pouches are mainly used when formed stool is expected, for example sigmoid colostomy (Figure 5.26c). They have a flatus filter and need to be changed once or twice a day.

ONE- OR TWO-PIECE SYSTEMS

All types of pouch (closed, drainable or with a tap) fall into one of two broad categories: one-piece or two-piece systems (Burch 2011b). Redmond et al. (2009) report that the majority of individuals with a stoma in the UK choose a one-piece system.

- *One-piece*: this comprises a pouch attached to an adhesive wafer that is removed completely when the pouch is changed. This is an easier system for an ostomate with dexterity problems, such as arthritis or peripheral neuropathy, to handle.
- *Two-piece*: this comprises a wafer onto which a pouch is clipped or stuck. It can be used with sore and sensitive skin because when the pouch is removed, the flange is left intact and so the skin is left undisturbed.

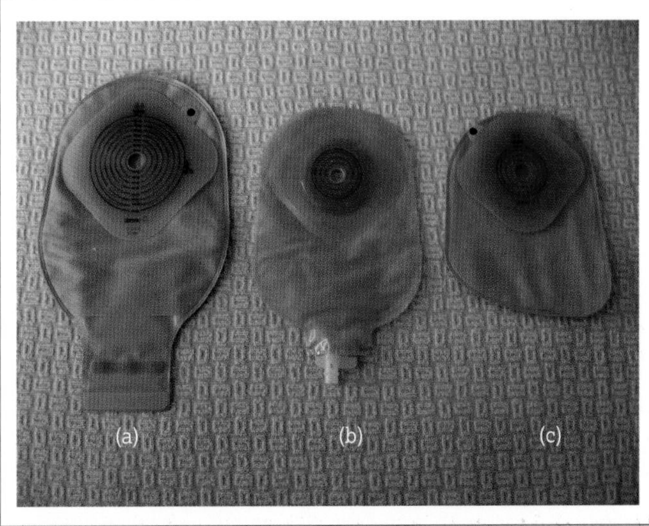

Figure 5.26 **Stoma equipment. (a) Drainable bowel stoma pouch. (b) Urostomy pouch. (c) Closed bag.**

PLUG SYSTEM

Patients with colostomies may be able to stop the effluent by inserting a plug into the stoma lumen. This plug swells in the moist environment and behaves as a seal so that faeces can be passed at a more convenient time (Burch 2011a, Durnal et al. 2011).

Solutions for skin and stoma cleaning

Warm water is sufficient for skin and stoma cleaning. If patients choose to use a mild soap, it is important that all soap residue is removed as this may interfere with pouch adhesion. Detergents, disinfectants and antiseptics cause dryness and irritation and should not be used. The stoma is not a wound or a lesion and should be regarded as a resited urethra or anus.

See Table 5.6 for a summary of products used in managing problems associated with a stoma.

Deodorants

AEROSOLS

Use: To absorb or mask odour. *Method*: One or two puffs into the air before emptying or removing appliance. *Examples*: Limone, Naturcare, FreshAire.

DROPS AND POWDERS

Use: For deodorizing bag contents. *Method*: Before fitting pouch or after emptying and cleaning drainable pouch, squeeze tube two or three times. *Examples*: Ostobon deodorant powder, Nodor S drops, Saltair No-roma.

Pre-operative assessment and care

Pre-operative care can be divided into two sections: physical and psychological.

Physical

Firstly, physical care consists of surgical preparation, which can be in the form of bowel preparation where patients are required to take laxatives to cleanse their bowel prior to surgery. This arguably improves surgical visibility and prevents contamination. This depends on the surgeon's preference and needs to be checked with the patient's surgical team on admission.

Many hospitals now carry out enhanced recovery programmes for colorectal patients. This involves intensive input pre-operatively, where selected patients are required to take nutritional drinks and develop skills in changing a stoma bag. This will improve recovery and management and consequently reduce hospital stay.

Table 5.6 **A summary of products used for problems associated with stoma**

Accessory	Product example	Use	Precautions
Creams	Chiron barrier cream (ABPI 1999)	Sensitive skin as a protective measure	Grease from creams can prevent adherence of the appliance
Protective films	Cavilon no sting barrier film, LBF	To prevent irritation and give protection	If contains alcohol, avoid on broken skin
Protective wafers	Stomahesive	To cover and protect skin	Allergies (rare)
Seals/washers	Cohesive seals Hollister barrier rings	Provide skin protection around the stoma. Useful to fill gaps and dips in skin	Allergies (rare)
Pastes	Stomahesive adapt paste	Useful to fill gaps and dips in skin and provide a smoother surface for applying the pouch	If contains alcohol, avoid on broken skin Should not be used as a solution to an ill-fitting pouch
Protective paste	Orabase paste	Protect raw, sore areas	
Powders	Ostoseal protective powder	Protect sore, wet areas and aid healing	Can sometimes affect adherence
Adhesive preparations	Saltair solution	To improve adherence of product	Should not be used as a solution to an ill-fitting pouch
Adhesive removers	Appeel Adhesive remover aerosols	Aids removal of pouch if patient experiencing pain when pouch removed	Some contain alcohol and should not be used on broken skin
Stoma baseplate securing tape	Hydroframe	To improve patient security. Useful for patients with parastomal hernias	Should not be used as a solution to an ill-fitting pouch
Thickening agents	Gel-X capsules, Ostosorb gel	To help solidify loose stoma output	If output is loose, cause should be investigated
Convex devices	Adapt ring convex inserts, soft seal	Useful for retracted stomas	Bruising and ulceration if used incorrectly
Aerosols	Limone, FreshAire	To mask and absorb odour	Avoid patient associating aerosol spray with stoma
Drops and powders	Nodor S Drops	Deodorizing bag contents	

Finally, stoma siting is one of the most important elements of pre-operative care as the site of the stoma can have a huge impact on post-operative quality of life. Appropriate siting of a stoma minimizes future difficulties such as the stoma interfering with clothes or skin problems caused by leakage of the appliance (Cronin 2012). Stoma siting should be carried out by a nurse who has been deemed competent to do so.

Psychological

Psychological preparation of the individual facing stoma surgery should begin as soon as surgery is considered, preferably by utilizing the skills of a trained stoma care nurse. It is important that the information and discussions are tailored to the individual's needs, taking into account their level of anxiety and distress (Cronin 2012).

It is important that patients meet all members of the multidisciplinary team who are involved in their care and that they fully understand the need for the stoma surgery. This needs to be explained in order to obtain informed consent. It is beneficial if the patient is met in preassessment or at home prior to surgery to discuss the implications of stoma care and the patient's own role in rehabilitation. At this point it is also helpful to provide the patient with written information and access to self-help support groups.

Stoma counselling is ideally carried out by the specialist stoma care nurse involved in the patient's care but all nurses involved in the care of patients undergoing a stoma should be aware of the impact of having a stoma on:

- body image
- family relationships
- sexual relationships
- depression and anger
- fears and concerns.

It is often beneficial to provide patients with some patient information/literature to take home. This gives them an opportunity to digest the information and write down any questions that they have. There are many different aids available, such as information booklets, samples of various products, diagrams, DVDs and websites. These help to reinforce and clarify the verbal information given to the patient.

Specific patient preparation

Patient education

Patients undergoing stoma formation have to make major physical and psychological adjustments following surgery. If surgery is elective, patient education should begin in the pre-operative period (Cronin 2012, O'Connor 2005). Adequate pre- and post-operative support is mandatory to improve quality of life for stoma patients. Individual holistic patient assessment is key as it is important to identify appropriate teaching strategies for each patient. One of the most important ways in which a nurse can support the patient is to teach them stoma care, ensuring independence before discharge (Burch 2011a, Burch and Sica 2005). It is important that the patient is able to independently change their stoma bag, recognize problems and obtain support and supplies once discharged home. Providing patients with adequate information and input helps to promote patient decision making by allowing them control (Henderson 2003).

All healthcare professionals are required to wear disposable gloves and apron when changing an appliance and this practice should be explained to patients so that they do not feel it is just because they have a stoma that these precautions are being taken (Cronin 2012).

Procedure guideline 5.18 **Stoma bag change**

This procedure may also be applied when teaching a patient how to care for their stoma.

Essential equipment

- Clean tray holding:
  - Tissues, wipes
  - New appliance
  - Measuring device/template
  - Scissors
  - Disposal bags for used appliances, tissues and wipes
  - Relevant accessories, for example adhesive remover, protective film, seals/washers
- Bowl of warm water
- Soap (if desired)
- Jug for contents of appliance
- Gloves and apron

Pre-procedure

Action	Rationale
1 Explain and discuss the procedure with the patient.	To ensure that the patient understands the procedure and gives their valid consent (NMC 2013, **C**).
2 Ensure that the patient is in a suitable and comfortable position where they will be able to watch the procedure, if well enough. A mirror may be used to aid visualization.	To allow good access to the stoma for cleaning and for secure application of the stoma bag. The patient will become familiar with the stoma and will also learn about the care of the stoma by observing the nurse. **E**
3 Use a small protective pad to protect the patient's clothing from drips if the effluent is fluid and apply gloves and apron.	Avoids the necessity for renewing clothing or bedclothes and demoralization of the patient as a result of soiling. **E**

(continued)

Procedure guideline 5.18 Stoma bag change *(continued)*

Procedure

Action	Rationale
4 If the bag is of the drainable type, empty the contents into a jug before removing the bag.	For ease of handling the appliance and prevention of spillage. **E**
5 Remove the appliance slowly. Peel the adhesive off the skin with one hand while exerting gentle pressure on the skin with the other.	To reduce trauma to the skin (Burch 2011b, **C**).
6 Fold appliance in two to ensure no spillage and place in disposal bag.	To ensure safe disposal according to environmental policy (DEFRA 2005, **C**).
7 Remove excess faeces or mucus from the stoma with a damp tissue.	So that the stoma and surrounding skin are clearly visible. **E**
8 Examine the skin and stoma for soreness, ulceration or other unusual phenomena. If the skin is unblemished and the stoma is a healthy red colour, proceed.	For the identification of complications or the treatment of existing problems. **E**
9 Wash the skin and stoma gently until they are clean.	To promote cleanliness and prevent skin excoriation. **E**
10 Dry the skin and stoma gently but thoroughly.	The appliance will attach more securely to dry skin. **E, C**
11 Measure the stoma and cut appliance, leaving 3 mm clearance. Apply a clean appliance.	Appliance should provide skin protection. The aperture should be cut just a little larger than the stoma so that effluent cannot cause skin damage (Kirkwood 2006, **C**).

Post-procedure

Action	Rationale
12 Dispose of soiled tissues, used appliance, gloves and apron in a disposal bag and place it in an appropriate plastic bin (in the patient's home, the bag should be placed in a plastic bag, tied and disposed of in a rubbish bag).	To ensure safe disposal. **E**
13 Wash hands thoroughly using bactericidal soap and water or bactericidal alcohol handrub.	To prevent spread of infection by contaminated hands (Fraise and Bradley 2009, **E**).

Procedure guideline 5.19 Stoma bridge or rod removal

Essential equipment

- Clean tray holding:
  - Tissues
  - New appliances
  - Disposal bags for used appliances and tissues
  - Relevant accessories, for example belt
- Bowl of warm water
- Soap if desired
- Jug for contents of appliance
- Gloves and apron

Pre-procedure

Action	Rationale
1 Explain and discuss the procedure with the patient.	To ensure that the patient understands the procedure and gives their valid consent (NMC 2013, **C**).
2 Ensure the patient is in a suitable and comfortable position.	To allow good access to the stoma for cleaning and for secure application of stoma bag. **E**
3 Apply gloves and apron.	To reduce risk of cross-infection (Fraise and Bradley 2009, **E**).
4 If the bag is of the drainable type, empty the contents into a jug before removing the bag.	For ease of handling the appliance and prevention of spillage. **E**

Procedure

5 Remove the appliance. Gently peel the adhesive off the skin with one hand while exerting gentle pressure on the skin with the other.	To reduce trauma to the skin (Burch 2011a, 2011b, **C**).
6 Remove excess faeces or mucus from the stoma with a damp tissue.	So that the stoma and surrounding skin are clearly visible. **E**
7 Slide the bridge gently to one side to ensure the mobile wing of the bridge is away from the stoma. Turn this wing so that it becomes flush with the bridge. Gently slide the bridge through the stoma loop (see **Action figure 7**).	To prepare bridge for removal. **E**
8 Fold the bridge in half so that it appears in a 'C' shape. Gently slide the bridge through the stoma loop (see **Action figure 7**).	
9 Examine the skin and stoma for soreness, ulceration or other unusual phenomena. If the skin is unblemished and the stoma is a healthy red colour, proceed.	For the prevention of complications or the treatment of existing problems. **E**
10 Wash the skin and stoma gently until they are clean.	To promote cleanliness and prevent skin excoriation. **E**
11 Dry the skin and stoma gently but thoroughly.	The appliance will attach more securely to dry skin. **E**
12 If the skin is red and/or broken, apply barrier cream. If the stoma is not a healthy red colour, inform medical and/or stoma care nurse.	To promote skin healing. **E**
13 Apply a clean appliance.	To contain effluent from the stoma. **E**
14 Dispose of soiled tissues, the bridge, the used appliance, gloves and apron.	To prevent environmental contamination. **E**
15 Wash hands with bactericidal soap and water or bactericidal alcohol handrub.	To reduce risk of cross-infection (Fraise and Bradley 2009, **E**).

Action Figure 7 Removal of stoma bridge/rod.

POST-PROCEDURAL CONSIDERATIONS

Initial and ongoing care

Post-operative stoma care

In theatre, an appropriately sized transparent drainable appliance should be applied, which should be left on for approximately 2 days. For the first 48 hours post-operatively, the stoma should be observed for signs of ischaemia or necrosis, and stoma colour (a pink and healthy appearance indicates a good blood supply), size and output should be noted, as should the presence of any devices, such as ureteric stents or bridge with a loop stoma (Kirkwood 2006).

Table 5.7 recommends the most appropriate bag type to use on each type of stoma and the expected output. The drainable appliance should always be emptied frequently, gas should be allowed to escape and the appliance should not be allowed to get more than half full with effluent. If the appliance becomes too full, leaks may occur and the weight from the effluent or the pressure from gas may cause the appliance to fall off. A leak-proof, odour-resistant well-fitted appliance does much to promote patient confidence at this time (Kirkwood 2006). The first time a bowel stoma acts, the type, appearance, quantity and consistency of the matter passed should be recorded; this includes any flatus that may be passed (Kirkwood 2006).

Immediately post-operatively, patients would not be expected to perform their own stoma care but, if appropriate, teaching that would have begun pre-operatively should be recommenced within the first 24–48 hours following surgery. During appliance changes, observations should be made of the following.

- *Stoma:* colour, size and general appearance: oedematous, flush with abdomen, retracted.
- *Peristomal skin:* presence of any erythema, broken areas, rashes.

Table 5.7 **Decision tool to use when selecting appropriate bag/pouch**

Type of stoma	Expected post-operative output	Recommended bag to be used	Expected stoma output on discharge	Recommended bag to be used on discharge
Colostomy	Haemoserous fluid Flatus Liquid/loose stool	Clear drainable bag	Soft formed stool Bowel action 1–3 times a day	Closed opaque bag
Ileostomy	Haemoserous fluid Liquid/loose stool Flatus	Clear drainable bag	Loose stool Approximately >600 mL per day	Opaque drainable bag
Urostomy	Urine Mucus	Clear drainable bag with tap	Urine 0.5 mL/kg/h	Opaque drainable bag with tap

- *Stoma/skin margin (mucocutaneous margin):* sutures intact, tension on sutures, separation of stoma edge from skin (mucocutaneous separation).

Any abnormalities should be reported to the stoma care nurse and medical staff (Burch 2004, Kirkwood 2006). Viewing the stoma may be difficult for the patient, who may be very aware of other people's reaction to it. The patient's reaction to their stoma should be observed and recorded.

Colostomy function

In the first few days, a sigmoid colostomy will produce haemoserous fluid and wind. By day 5 there should be some faecal fluid and then by day 7–14, semi-formed stool. A closed appliance may then be used. Rarely a stoma may be formed in the transverse colon, usually as a result of an emergency procedure (Cronin 2012), and in such cases only a small amount of water will be reabsorbed from the faecal matter, so the stool is less formed. Therefore a drainable pouch will be required.

Patients with a sigmoid colostomy (ostomates) should generally be advised to have a balanced and mixed diet. To avoid constipation, ostomates are advised to take adequate oral fluids and fibre in the form of '5-a-day' fruit and vegetables (Burch 2011c). If either constipation or loose stool is a problem, then dietary intake should be reviewed. Ostomates may find that their colostomy is usually active at particular times of the day, but ultimately the only means of gaining control with a sigmoid colostomy is by using a plug system or by regular irrigation. Stoma care nurses will need to assess patients for their suitability for either using a plug system or irrigation.

Ileostomy function

For the first few days the stoma will produce haemoserous fluid and wind. By days 5–10 there will be brown faecal matter. The fluid output after surgery can be as much as 1500 mL/24 hours but this will gradually reduce to 500–850 mL/24 hours as the bowel settles down (Black 2000). It is important that fluid balance recordings are made and serum electrolytes are measured as patients are at risk of sodium and/or magnesium depletion (Burch 2004). Sometimes the output from a stoma remains high (>1000 mL/24 hours), which may be due to the amount of small bowel removed at surgery or an underlying bowel condition; these patients require careful management. Patients who continue to have a high output from their stoma may need to be managed by specialist teams which include gastroenterologists, dietitians and stoma care nurses in order to provide ongoing support (Slater 2012).

The effluent from an ileostomy takes on a porridge-like consistency when a normal intake of food is established (Burch 2011c). A drainable appliance is therefore used. The effluent contains enzymes, which will excoriate the skin (Burch 2011b), so if the pouch leaks, it must be changed promptly to prevent skin breakdown. The effluent cannot be controlled but may vary throughout the day. Patients with ileostomies often find that the output is thicker first thing in the morning and after meals, or the output is looser with reduced dietary intake (Burch 2011c). Sometimes medication which reduces peristaltic action, for example codeine or loperamide, may be used to control excessive watery output. If using loperamide, this should be taken half an hour to an hour before food in order to achieve an optimal effect.

Urostomy/ileal conduit function

Urine will dribble from the stoma every 20–30 seconds and it starts draining immediately. Normal output is 1500 mL/24 hours, but may be less after periods of reduced fluid intake, for example at night. Urinary stents (fine-bore catheters) may be in place from the ureters past the anastomosis and out of the stoma. They are placed to maintain patency and protect the suturing until primary healing is completed (Black 2000). Stents are left *in situ* for 7–10 days.

Body image

Stoma formation creates many issues for the patient and many struggle with body image. Studies suggest that this is often overlooked (Opus 2010). The circumstances in which the stoma is formed will influence psychological recovery (Black 2000). Communication is key and it is important to allow the patient and family to discuss their concerns and anxieties. Therefore stoma care nurses play a vital role in supporting the patient and family. It is important to promote patient independence and acceptance.

Diet

All patients should be encouraged to eat a wide variety of foods and drink 1.5–2 litres of fluids each day. Our digestive system reacts in an individual way to different foods and so it is important that patients try a wide range of foods on several occasions and that none should be specifically avoided (Burch 2011c). Patients can then make decisions about different foods based on their own experience of their own reaction. Explanations should be given of how the gut functions, how it has been changed since surgery and the effects certain foodstuffs may cause.

Colostomy and ileostomy formation means the loss of the anal sphincter so passage of wind cannot be controlled. High-fibre foods such as beans and pulses produce wind as they are broken down in the gut; hence individuals who eat large quantities of these foodstuffs may be troubled by wind. There are several non-food causes of wind, such as chewing gum, eating irregularly and drinking fizzy drinks, which should be considered before blaming a particular food. Eating yoghurt or drinking buttermilk may help reduce wind for these patients. Green vegetables, pulses and spicy food are examples of foods that may cause colostomy and ileostomy output to increase or become watery. Boiled rice, smooth peanut butter, apple sauce and bananas are some of the foods that may help thicken stoma output (Black 2000, Burch 2011c).

Some foods, for example tomato skin and pips, may be seen unaltered in the output from an ileostomy. Celery, dried fruit, nuts and potato skins are some of the foods which can temporarily block ileostomies (Black 2000, Burch 2011c). The blockage is usually related to the amount eaten and the offending food can be tried at another time in small quantities, ensuring it is chewed well and not eaten in a hurry.

There are no dietary restrictions with a urostomy. It must be stressed, however, that an adequate fluid intake must be maintained to minimize the risk of urinary tract infection due to a shortened urinary tract.. The recommended fluid intake for all individuals is 1.5–2.0 litres per day (Burch 2011c). Fluid intake should be increased in hot weather or at times when there is an increase in sweating, for example with exercise or fever. Patients should be made aware of certain foods that may cause a change to the usual character of the urine. For example, beetroot, radishes, spinach and some food dye may discolour urine; some drugs may also have this effect, for example metronidazole, nitrofurantoin. Similarly, following consumption of asparagus or fish, urine may develop a strong odour.

Fear of malodour

This is a common fear for patients with bowel stomas, often based on hearsay or experience with other ostomates in hospital or the community. Appliances are odour free when fitted correctly. Flatus may be released via charcoal filters and deodorizers are available. The individual must be reassured, however, that any problems that occur post-operatively will be investigated, with a good possibility of their being solved by such means as the use of alternative appliances (Black 2000, Burch 2004).

Sex and the ostomate

The possibility of sexual impairment for both men and women after stoma surgery depends on the nature of the operation and the ensuing damage to the nerves and tissues involved. The psychological impact of the surgery and its effect on the individual's body image must also be taken into consideration. Surgery that results in physical sexual disability will have psychological repercussions, while some sexual difficulties may be of psychological origin (Black 2004). Impairment may be permanent or temporary. In the latter case, resolution of the difficulty may take anything up to 2 years. Pre- and post-operative counselling should be offered for both patient and partner.

All patients may experience loss of libido and sexual desire. Ejaculatory disturbances occur following cystectomy so men facing this surgery should be offered sperm banking prior to surgery. Erectile dysfunction is a common complication of pelvic surgery and there are a number of treatment options available. These include oral medications (sildenafil, tadalafil, vardenafil), sublingual apomorphine, intraurethral and intracavernosal alprostadil, vacuum devices and penile implants (Ashford 1998, Kirby et al. 1999, Newey 1998).

Female patients may experience dyspareunia; this may be due to narrowing or shortening of the vagina, a reduction in the volume of vaginal secretions or changes in genital sensations (Black 2004). The use of a lubricant, adopting different positions during lovemaking or encouraging greater relaxation by extending foreplay may help resolve painful intercourse (Black 2004).

Planning for discharge

Discharge planning for the patient with a stoma should commence once the patient is admitted. It is important to set a provisional discharge date and set realistic goals with the patient. Prior to discharge, ideally the patient should have returned to their prior level of independence, be eating a normal diet and should be competent in stoma care. Family or close friends are likely to require support and information so that they are in a position to help the ostomate and this should be provided as much as possible before discharge. If family or close friends are involved during all stages of stoma surgery, and patients are well informed, they are better able to adapt to life with a stoma (Cronin 2012).

Acceptance of the stoma is a gradual process and, on discharge from hospital, patients may only be beginning to adapt to life with a stoma. Indeed, in a survey of patients following stoma formation (n = 100), 56% felt that support was needed for the first 6 months, indicating the ongoing need for professional advice and support for a substantial amount of time after stoma surgery (Taylor et al. 2012).

Continuity of care for these patients is crucial. Effective communication and collaboration between healthcare professionals are key to psychological adaptation and successful rehabilitation (Borwell 2009).

> **Learning Activity 5.7**
>
> **Scenario: Stoma care**
>
> You have been allocated to care for a patient who has had a sigmoid colostomy formed.
>
> What physical and psychosocial issues should you consider prior to their discharge?
>
> See the end of the chapter for the answers.

Follow-up support

The patient should be discharged home with:

- weeks of stoma supplies
- contact details of community stoma care nurse
- prescription details of products being used
- information on delivery company, if relevant.

The patient should be discharged with an adequate supply of stoma products until a prescription is obtained from the general practitioner. Written reminders should also be provided on how to care for the stoma, how to obtain supplies of appliances, and any other information that may be required. The patient should have details of non-medical stoma clinics, details about the relevant agencies and information about voluntary associations. Arrangements should also be made for a home visit from the stoma care nurse and/or the community nurse (Cronin 2005). Figure 5.27 provides an example of a discharge checklist.

Obtaining supplies

All NHS patients with a permanent stoma are entitled to free prescriptions for their stoma care products, and should complete the relevant forms for exemption from payment. Appliances can then be obtained from the local chemist, free home delivery services or directly from the appropriate manufacturers.

COMPLICATIONS

As a healthcare professional providing support and care to stoma patients, it is important to be able to distinguish normal from abnormal. The observational index (Figure 5.28) provides a reference guide to use when observing, recording and reporting. If any of the complications are noted, it is important to ensure that the medical team and/or stoma care nurse is informed. Advice on how to manage these problems should be obtained from your specialist stoma care nurse. Early recognition of problems and complications can prevent more serious complications later.

Figure 5.27 **An example of a stoma discharge checklist.**

		Tick Box	Date, Signature & Print Name
1.	Planned date of discharge: ___________________________	Yes ☐ No ☐	
2.	Is the patient independent with stoma care	Yes ☐ No ☐	
3.	Community stoma care nurse informed	Yes ☐ No ☐	
4.	Community nurses informed if necessary	Yes ☐ No ☐ N/A ☐	
5.	Date of first home visit by community stoma care nurse	**Date:**	
6.	Patient given contact details of community stoma care nurse Nurse's NAME: ________________________________ Contact telephone number: ___________________________	Yes ☐ No ☐	
7.	If patient has chosen to use a delivery company, company informed and first order placed	Yes ☐ No ☐	
8.	Out-patient appointment made: ___________________________	Yes ☐ No ☐	
9.	Patient given two weeks supply of stoma products	Yes ☐ No ☐	

Figure 5.28 **Ostomy observational index.** ***Source:*** **Reproduced with permission from Dansac Ltd.**

Ostomy Forum Observation index

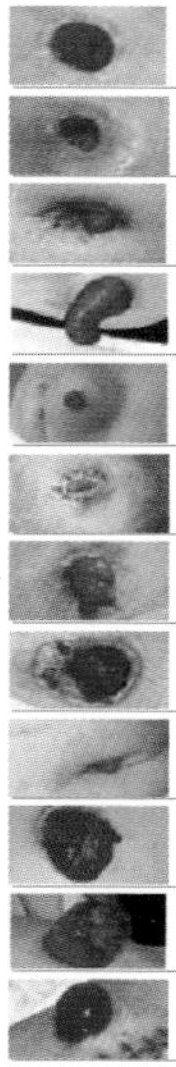

Stoma	Status	
A	Normal	above skin level
B	Flush	mucosa level with the skin
C	Retracted	below skin level
D	Prolapsed	notable increasing length of stoma
E	Hernia	bowel entering parastomal space
F	Stenosis	tightening of stoma orifice
G	Granulomes	nodules/granulation on stoma
H	Separation	mucocutaneous separation
I	Recessed	stoma in a skin fold or a crease
J	Necrosis	lack of blood supply causing partial or complete tissue death
K	Laceration	mucosa that is jagged/torn or ulcerated due to trauma
L	Oedematous	gross swelling of the stoma
Z	Others	

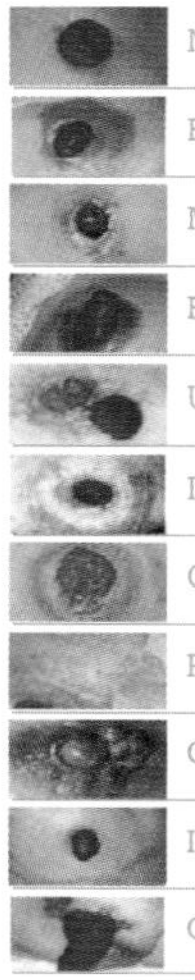

Skin	Condition	
A	Normal	as rest of skin
B	Erythema	red
C	Macerated	excoriated; moist
D	Eroded	excoriated; moist and bleeding
E	Ulcerated	skin defect reaching in to subcutaneous layer
F	Irritated	irritant causing skin to be inflamed, sore, itchy and red
G	Granuloma	nodules/over granulation tissue on skin
H	Predisposing factors	underlying diseases, e.g. eczema and psoriasis
I	CPD*	greyish, nodules on skin, often caused by urine
J	Infected	e.g. fungus, folliculitis
Z	Others	e.g. Pyoderma gangrenosum

* Chronic Papillomatous Dermatitis

Output	Consistency	
A	Normal	For patient and stomatype
B	Fluid	
C	Thick	
D	Solid	
E	Hard	
F	High output	Uro>2500ml/24 hrs Ileo>1500ml/24 hrs
G	Too low output	Uro<1200ml/24 hrs Ileo<500ml/24 hrs
H	Excessive flatus	
I	Excessive odour	
J	Excessive mucus production	
K	Blood	
L	Non functioning stoma	(e.g sub-ileus)
Z	Others	

(continued)

Figure 5.28 **Ostomy observational index.** ***Source:*** **Reproduced with permission from Dansac Ltd.** ***(continued)***

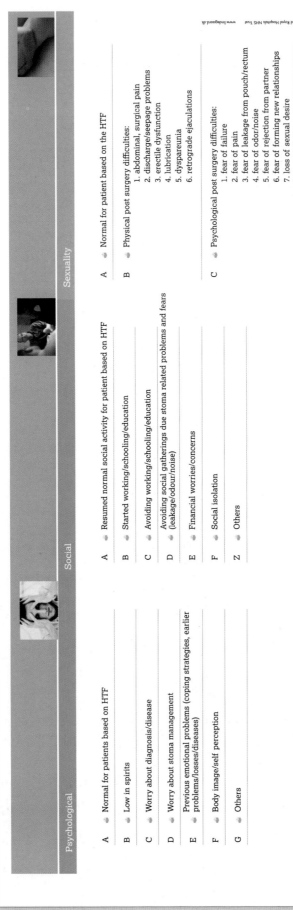

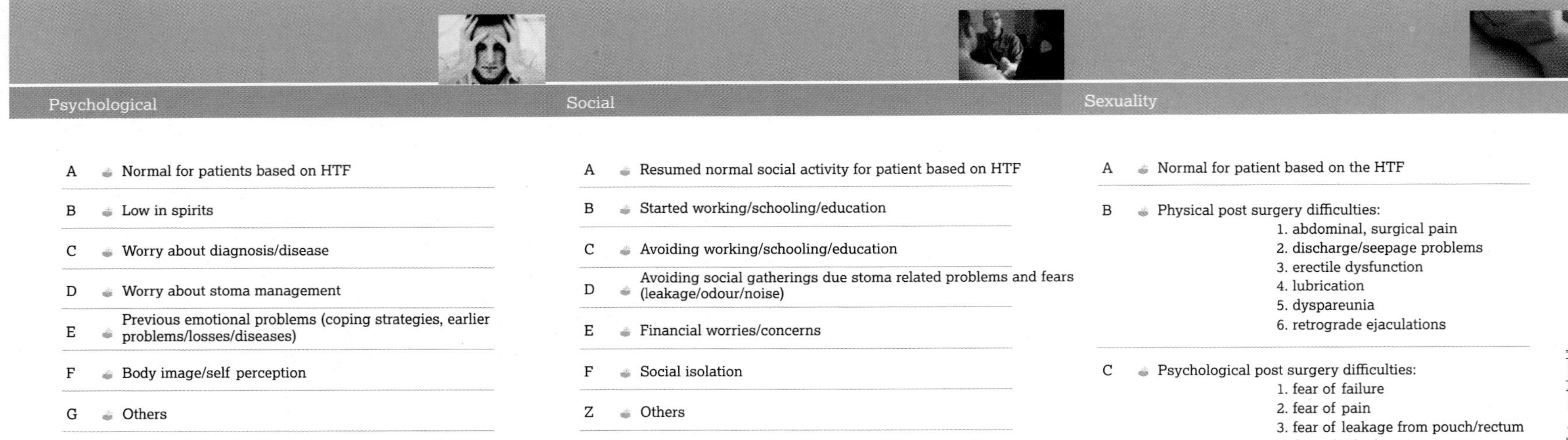

Psychological

- A Normal for patients based on HTF
- B Low in spirits
- C Worry about diagnosis/disease
- D Worry about stoma management
- E Previous emotional problems (coping strategies, earlier problems/losses/diseases)
- F Body image/self perception
- G Others

Social

- A Resumed normal social activity for patient based on HTF
- B Started working/schooling/education
- C Avoiding working/schooling/education
- D Avoiding social gatherings due stoma related problems and fears (leakage/odour/noise)
- E Financial worries/concerns
- F Social isolation
- Z Others

Sexuality

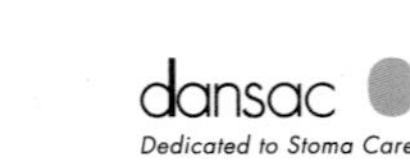

- A Normal for patient based on the HTF
- B Physical post surgery difficulties:
  1. abdominal, surgical pain
  2. discharge/seepage problems
  3. erectile dysfunction
  4. lubrication
  5. dyspareunia
  6. retrograde ejaculations
- C Psychological post surgery difficulties:
  1. fear of failure
  2. fear of pain
  3. fear of leakage from pouch/rectum
  4. fear of odor/noise
  5. fear of rejection from partner
  6. fear of forming new relationships
  7. loss of sexual desire
- Z Other

dansac
Dedicated to Stoma Care

Learning for practice

After studying this chapter, list five key points you have learnt about elimination that you will be able to apply to your clinical practice.

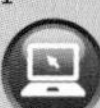

For further learning exercises visit **www.royalmarsdenmanual.com/student**.

Now Test Yourself

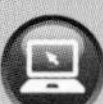

This section provides a range of exercises/activities to further test your learning. For additional exercises visit **www.royalmarsdenmanual.com/student**.

What have you learnt?

1 Thinking about incontinence and skin care.
- **A** What is the name of the skin condition that may occur as a consequence of incontinence?
- **B** What are the most recent recommendations for the prevention and treatment of this condition?

2 What percentage of men between the ages of 65 and 74 are affected by urinary incontinence?
- **A** 10%
- **B** 13%
- **C** 14%
- **D** 15%

3 List five indications for urinary catheterization.

4 Which of the following have been identified as having a direct association with the development of urinary tract infections?
- **A** Maintaining a closed drainage system
- **B** The insertion technique and use of aseptic conditions
- **C** Length of time a catheter remains *in situ*
- **D** Competence of the practitioner performing the procedure
- **E** All of the above

5 What is the usual solution recommended for use as bladder irrigation and why?

6 What are the three main causes of acute diarrhoea?

7 Laxatives are frequently used in the treatment of constipation. Match up the following examples with their appropriate category.

Category	Example by brand name
Bulk producer	Milpar
Stool softener	Senna
Osmotic agent	Fybogel
Stimulant laxative	Lactulose

8 What is the difference between an evacuant enema and a retention enema? Give an example of each.

9 Following stoma formation, what should you observe immediately post-operatively about the following:
- **A** Stoma
- **B** Stoma output
- **C** Peristomal skin
- **D** Stoma/skin margin

10 When selecting a stoma appliance for a patient who has undergone a formation of a loop colostomy, what factors should you consider?
- **A** Dexterity of the patient, consistency of effluent, type of stoma
- **B** Patient preference, type of stoma, consistency of effluent, state of peristomal skin, dexterity of the patient
- **C** Patient preference, lifestyle, position of stoma, consistency of effluent, state of peristomal skin, dexterity of patient, type of stoma
- **D** Cognitive ability, lifestyle, patient dexterity, position of stoma, state of peristomal skin, type of stoma, consistency of effluent, patient preference

See the end of the chapter for the answers.

Key points

- Elimination is a sensitive issue. Nurses must respect the privacy and dignity of the patient when carrying out procedures of an intimate nature, such as assisting with the use of a commode or bedpan.
- The causes of vomiting are often multifactorial. Thorough assessment of the risk factors, precipitating factors and alleviating factors is the key to identifying effective strategies for managing this symptom.
- There are a range of strategies available to manage urinary incontinence. Nurses must be aware of the indications for urinary catheterization and factors to consider prior to the procedure, including informing the patient, selection of device, prevention of infection and other complications, and ongoing care and support.
- Nurses have a key role to play in the management of diarrhoea and constipation in terms of both pharmacological and non-pharmacological support. It is therefore important to understand the possible causes as well as how to accurately assess and manage these conditions.
- With the number of stomas being formed each year, it is important to understand the rationale for different types of stoma (colostomy, ileostomy and ileal conduit/urostomy) and the rationale for each being formed. Nurses have a key role in the pre-operative preparation, post-operative care and effective ongoing support and discharge for this group of patients.

Websites

Colostomy Association:
www.colostomyassociation.org.uk

Ileostomy and internal pouch support group:
www.iasupport.org

Medic-Alert Foundation:
www.medicalert.org.uk

Sexual Dysfunction Association:
www.sexualdysfunctionassociation.com

Urostomy Association:
www.uagbi.org

REFERENCES

Abd-el-Maeboud, K.H., el-Naggar, T., el-Hawi, E.M., et al. (1991) Rectal suppository: commonsense and mode of insertion. *Lancet*, 338(8770), 798–800.

Abraham, J. (2008) Acupressure and acupuncture in preventing and managing postoperative nausea and vomiting in adults. *Journal of Perioperative Practice*, 18(12), 543–551.

Addison, R. (2000) Fluid intake: how coffee and caffeine affect continence. *Nursing Times*, 96(40) (Suppl), 7–8.

Addison, R. & Mould, C. (2000) Risk assessment in suprapubic catheterisation. *Nursing Standard*, 14 (36), 43–46.

Addison, R. & White, M. (2002) Spinal injury and bowel management. *Nursing Times*, 98 (4), 61.

Andreessen, L., Wilde, M.H, Herendeen, P. (2012) Preventing catheter-associated urinary tract infections in acute care: the bundle approach. *Journal of Nursing Care Quality*, 27(3), 209–217.

Ashford, L. (1998) Erectile dysfunction. *Professional Nurse*, 13(9), 603–608.

Association of British Pharmaceutical Industry. (1999) *ABPI Compendium of Data Sheets and Summaries of Product Characteristics 1999–2000.* London: Datapharm Publications.

Avadhani, A. & Miley, H. (2011) Probiotics for prevention of antibiotic-associated diarrhea and Clostridium difficile-associated disease in hospitalized adults – a meta-analysis. *Journal of the American Academy of Nurse Practitioners*, 23(6), 269–274.

Baldi, F., Bianco, M.A., Nardone, G., et al. (2009) Focus on acute diarrhoeal disease. *World Journal of Gastroenterology*, 15(27), 3341–3348.

Bardsley, A. (2005) Use of lubricant gels in urinary catheterisation. *Nursing Standard*, 20(8), 41–46.

Bardsley, A. (2009) Coated catheters – reviewing the literature. *Journal of Community Nursing*, 23(2), 15–17.

Bardsley, A. & Kyle, G. (2008) The use of gloves in uretheral catheterisation. *Continence UK*, 2(1), 65–68.

Beeckman, D., Schoonhoven, L., Verhaeghe, S., et al. (2009) Prevention and treatment of incontinence-associated dermatitis: literature review. *Journal of Advanced Nursing*, 65(6), 1141–1154.

Bell, S. (2004) Investigations and management of chronic diarrhoea in adults. In: Norton, C. & Chelvanayagam, S. (eds) *Bowel Continence Nursing.* Beaconsfield: Beaconsfield Publishers, pp. 92–102.

Bell, M.A. (2010) Severe indwelling urinary catheter-associated urethral erosion in four elderly men. *Ostomy Wound Management* 56(12), 36–39.

Bennett, S. (2009) Antiemetics, uses, mode of action and prescribing rationale. *Nurse Prescribing*, 7(2), 63–70.

Bernard, M.S., Hunter, K.F. & Moore, K.N. (2012) A review of strategies to decrease the duration of indwelling urethral catheters and potentially reduce the incidence of catheter-associated urinary tract infections. *Urologic Nursing*, 32(1), 29–37.

Bierman, S. & Carigan, M. (2003) The prevention of adverse events associated with urinary tract catherterization. *Managing Infection Control*, September, 43–49.

Black, P. (2000) Practical stoma care. *Nursing Standard*, 14(41), 47–53; quiz 54–45.

Black, P.K. (2004) Psychological, sexual and cultural issues for patients with a stoma. *British Journal of Nursing*, 13 (12), 692–697.

BNF (2014) *British National Formulary 67.* London: Pharmaceutical Press.

Booth, F. (2009) Ensuring penile sheaths do their job properly. *Nursing & Residential Care*, 11(11), 550.

Booth, F. & Lee, L. (2005) A guide to selecting and using urinary sheaths. *Nursing Times*, 101(47), 43–44, 46.

Borwell, B. (2009) Continuity of care for the stoma patient: psychological considerations. *British Journal of Community Nursing*, 14(8), 326, 328, 330–321.

Bowers, B. (2006) Evaluating the evidence for administering phosphate enemas. *British Journal of Nursing*, 15(7), 378–381.

Bradshaw, A. & Price, L. (2006) Rectal suppository insertion: the reliability of the evidence as a basis for nursing practice. *Journal of Community Nursing*, 16(1), 98–103.

British Nutrition Foundation (2012) *Dietary Fibre – How Much Fibre Do We Eat?* London: British Nutrition Foundation. Available at: www.nutrition.org.uk/nutritionscience/nutrients/dietary-fibre?start=4

Burch, J. (2004) The management and care of people with stoma complications. *British Journal of Nursing*, 13(6), 307–308, 310, 312, 314–318.

Burch, J. (2008) Nutrition for people with stomas 1: overview of issues. *Nursing Times*, 104(48), 24–25.

Burch, J. (2011a) Resuming a normal life: holistic care of the person with an ostomy. *British Journal of Community Nursing*, 16(8), 366–373.

Burch, J. (2011b) Peristomal skin care and the use of accessories to promote skin health. *British Journal of Nursing*, 20(7), S4, S6, S8–S10.

Burch, J. (2011c) Providing information and advice on diet to stoma patients. *British Journal of Community Nursing*, 16(10), 479–480, 482, 484.

Burch, J. & Sica, J. (2005) Stoma care accessories: an overview of a crowded market. *British Journal of Community Nursing*, 10(1), 24–31.

Cadd, A., Keatinge, D., Henssen, M., et al. (2000) Assessment and documentation of bowel care management in palliative care: incorporating patient preferences into the care regimen. *Journal of Clinical Nursing*, 9(2), 228–235.

Campos de Carvalho, E., Martins, F.T. & dos Santos, C.B. (2007) A pilot study of a relaxation technique for management of nausea and vomiting in patients receiving cancer chemotherapy. *Cancer Nursing*, 30(2), 163–167.

Chelvanayagam, S. & Norton, C. (2004) Nursing assessment of adults with faecal incontinence. In: Norton, C. & Chelvanayagam, S. (eds) *Bowel Continence Nursing.* Beaconsfield: Beaconsfield Publishers, pp.45–62.

Christer, R., Robinson, L. & Bird, C. (2003) Constipation: causes and cures. *Nursing Times*, 99(25), 26–27.

Chung, C., Chu, M., Paoloni, R., O'Brien, M. & Demel, T. (2007) Comparison of lignocaine and water-based lubricating gels for female urethral catheterization: a randomized controlled trial. *Emergency Medicine Australasia*, 19(4), 315–319.

Clifford, E. (2000) Urinary catheters: reducing the incidence of problems. *Community Nurse*, 6(4), 35–36.

Connolly, M. & Larkin, P. (2012) Managing constipation: a focus on care and treatment in the palliative setting. *British Journal of Community Nursing*, 17(2), 60, 62–64, 66–67.

Cronin, E. (2005) Best practice in discharging patients with a stoma. *Nursing Times*, 101(47), 67–68.

Cronin, E. (2012) What the patient needs to know before stoma siting: an overview. *British Journal of Nursing*, 21(22), 1304, 1306–1308.

Cutts, B. (2005) Developing and implementing a new bladder irrigation chart. *Nursing Standard*, 20(8), 48–52.

Dagli, M. & Ramchandani, P. (2011) Percutaneous nephrostomy: technical aspects and indications. *Seminars in Interventional Radiology*, 28(4), 424–437.

Davies, C. (2004) The use of phosphate enemas in the treatment of constipation. *Nursing Times*, 100(18), 32–35.

Davis, M.P. & Walsh, D. (2000) Treatment of nausea and vomiting in advanced cancer. *Supportive Care in Cancer*, 8(6), 444–452.

DEFRA (2005) *Hazardous Waste Regulations: List of Wastes Regulations 2005*. London: Department for Environment, Food and Rural Affairs.

Denby, N. (2006) The role of diet and lifestyle changes in the management of constipation. *British Journal of Community Nursing*, 20(9), 20–24.

Devore, E.E., Townsend, M.K., Resnick, N.M., et al. (2012) The epidemiology of urinary incontinence in women with type 2 diabetes. *Journal of Urology*, 188(5), 1816–1821.

DH (2003) *Winning Ways: Working Together to Reduce Healthcare Associated Infection in England*. London: Department of Health.

DH (2005) *Prescription Cost Analysis: England 2004*. London: HMSO. Available at: www.dh.gov.uk/prod_consum_dh/groups/dh_digitalassets/@dh/@en/documents/digitalasset/dh_4107626.pdf (archived)

Dikken, C. & Wildman, K. (2013) Control of nausea and vomiting caused by chemotherapy. *Cancer Nursing Practice*, 12(8), 24–29.

Doherty, W. (2006) Male urinary catheterisation. *Nursing Standard*, 20(35), 57–63; quiz 64.

Doughty, D., Junkin, J., Kurz, P., et al. (2012) Incontinence-associated dermatitis: consensus statements, evidence-based guidelines for prevention and treatment, and current challenges. *Journal of Wound, Ostomy and Continence Nursing*, 39(3), 303–315; quiz 316–307.

Durnal, A.M., Maxwell, T.R., Kiran, R.P. & Kommala, D. (2011) International study of a continence device with 12 hour wear times. *British Journal of Nursing*, 20(16), S4–S11.

Eastwood, L. (2009) Safe and secure – improving practice in the UK. *Journal of Community Nursing*, 23(5), 30–32.

Ejemot-Nwadiaro, R.I., Ehiri, J.E., Meremikwu, M.M., Critchley, J.A. (2008) Hand washing for preventing diarrhoea. *Cochrane Database of Systematic Reviews*. Available at: http://onlinelibrary.wiley.com/doi/10.1002/14651858.CD004265.pub2/pdf

Emmanuel, A. (2004) *Constipation*. In: Norton, C. & Chelvanayagam, S. (eds) *Bowel Continence Nursing*. Beaconsfield: Beaconsfield Publishers.

Evans, A., Painter, D. & Feneley, R. (2001) Blocked urinary catheters: nurses' preventive role. *Nursing Times*, 97(1), 37–38.

Fader, M., Pettersson, L., Brooks, R., et al. (1997) A multicentre comparative evaluation of catheter valves. *British Journal of Nursing*, 6(7), 359, 362–354, 366–357.

Fillingham, S. & Douglas, J. (2004) *Urological Nursing*, 3rd edn. Edinburgh: Baillière Tindall.

Fillingham, S. & Fell, S. (2004) Urological stomas. In: Fillingham, S. & Douglas, J. (eds) *Urological Nursing*, 3rd edn. Edinburgh: Baillière Tindall, pp.207–225.

Forristal, H. & Maxfield, J. (2004) Prostatic problems. In: Fillingham, S. & Douglas, J. (eds) *Urological Nursing*, 3rd edn. Edinburgh: Baillière Tindall, pp.161–184.

Fraise, A. P. & Bradley, T. (2009) *Aycliffe's Control of Healthcare-associated Infections: A Practical Handbook*, 5th edn. London: Hodder Arnold.

Fritz, D. & Pitlick, M. (2012) Evidence about the prevention and management of constipation: implications for comfort part 1. *Home Healthcare Nurse*, 30(9), 533–540; quiz 540–532.

FSA (2006) *Starchy Foods – Fibre*. Available at: www.eatwell.gov.uk/healthydiet/nutritionessentials/starchfoods/

Galbraith, A., Bullock, S., Manias, E., et al. (2007) *Fundamentals of Pharmacology: An Applied Approach for Nursing and Health*, 2nd edn. Harlow: Prentice Hall.

Geraghty, J. (2011) Introducing a new skin-care regimen for the incontinent patient. *British Journal of Nursing*, 20(7), 409–415.

Getliffe, K. & Dolman, M. (2007) *Promoting Continence: A Clincal and Research Approach*, 3rd edn. Edinburgh: Baillière Tindall.

Gilbert, R. (2006) Taking a midstream specimen of urine. *Nursing Times*, 102(18), 22–23.

Gill, D. (1999) Stool specimen 1. Assessment. *Nursing Times*, 95(25), suppl 1–2.

Godfrey, H. & Evans, A. (2000) Management of long-term urethral catheters: minimizing complications. *British Journal of Nursing*, 9(2), 74–76, 78–81.

Grasso, M.G. & Taylor, F. (1996) Techniques in percutaneous renal access. In: Sosa, R.E. & Albala, D.M. (eds) *Textbook of Endourology*. London: Saunders.

Gray, M., Bliss, D.Z., Doughty, D.B., et al. (2007) Incontinence-associated dermatitis: a consensus. *Journal of Wound, Ostomy and Continence Nursing*, 34(1), 45–54.

Gray, M., Beeckman, D., Bliss, D.Z., et al. (2012) Incontinence-associated dermatitis: a comprehensive review and update. *Journal of Wound, Ostomy and Continence Nursing*, 39(1), 61–74.

Hall, V. (2010) Acute uncomplicated diarrhoea management. *Practice Nursing*, 21(3), 118–122.

Hambridge, K. (2013) Assessing the risk of post-operative nausea and vomiting. *Nursing Standard*, 27(18), 35–43.

Harrison, P. (2000) *Managing Spinal Injury: Critical Care. The Initial Management of People with Actual or Suspected Spinal Cord Injury in High Dependency and Intensive Care*. Milton Keynes: Spinal Injury Association.

Hart, S. (2008) Urinary catheterisation. *Nursing Standard*, 22(27), 44–48.

Head, C. (2006) Insertion of a urinary catheter. *Nursing Older People*, 18(10), 33–36; quiz 37.

Henderson, S. (2003) Power imbalance between nurses and patients: a potential inhibitor of partnership in care. *Journal of Clinical Nursing*, 12(4), 501–508.

Henry, C. (1999) The advantages of using suppositories. *Nursing Times*, 95(17), 50–52.

Hickson, M., D'Souza, A.L., Muthu, N., et al. (2007) Use of probiotic Lactobacillus preparation to prevent diarrhoea associated with antibiotics: randomised double blind placebo controlled trial. *BMJ*, 335(7610), 80.

Higgins, D. (2006) How to administer an enema. *Nursing Times*, 102(20), 24–25.

Hinrichs, M., Huseboe, J., Tang, J.H., et al. (2001) Research-based protocol. Management of constipation. *Journal of Gerontological Nursing*, 27(2), 17–28.

Hohenfellner, M. & Santucci, R.A. (2010) *Emergencies in Urology*. New York: Springer.

Hurst, A.F., Hunt, T. & British Society of Gastroenterology (1969) *Selected Writings of Sir Arthur Hurst (1879–1944)*. London: British Society of Gastroenterology.

IMS (2008) *New Stoma Patients Audit – Great Britain*. Sittingbourne: Institute of Medical Sciences.

Jahn, P., Beutner, K. & Langer, G. (2012) Types of indwelling urinary catheters for long-term bladder drainage in adults, *Cochrane Database of Systematic Reviews*. Available at: http://onlinelibrary.wiley.com/doi/10.1002/14651858.CD004997.pub3/pdf

Jenkins, S.C. (1998) Digital guidance of female urethral catheterization. *British Journal of Urology*, 82(4), 589–590.

Johnson, J.R., Kuskowski, M.A. & Wilt, T.J. (2006) Systematic review: antimicrobial urinary catheters to prevent catheter–associated urinary tract infection in hospitalized patients. *Annals of Internal Medicine*, 144(2), 116–126.

Kelly, B. & Ward, K. (2013) Nausea and vomiting in palliative care. *Nursing Times*, 109(39), 16–19.

Kenefick, N.J. (2004) The epidemiology of faecal incontinence. In: Norton, C. & Chelvanayagam, S. (eds) *Bowel Continence Nursing*. Beaconsfield: Beaconsfield Publishers, pp.14–23.

King, D. (2002) Determining the cause of diarrhoea. *Nursing Times*, 98(23), 47–48.

Kirby, R.S., Carson, C.C. & Goldstein, I. (1999) *Erectile Dysfunction: A Clinical Guide*. Oxford: Isis Medical Media.

Kirkwood, L. (2006) Postoperative stoma care and the selection of appliances. *Journal of Community Nursing*, 20(3), 12–18.

Koch, S.M., Melenhorst, J., van Gemert, W.G. & Baeten, C.G. (2008) Prospective study of colonic irrigation for the treatment of defaecation disorders. *British Journal of Surgery*, 95(10), 1273–1279.

Kornblau, S., Benson, A.B., Catalano, R., et al. (2000) Management of cancer treatment-related diarrhea. Issues and therapeutic strategies. *Journal of Pain and Symptom Management*, 19(2), 118–129.

Krenzer, M.E. (2012) Viral gastroenteritis in the adult population: the GI peril. *Critical Care Nursing Clinics of North America*, 24(4), 541–553.

Kunin, C.M. (1997) *Urinary Tract Infections: Detection, Prevention, and Management*, 5th edn. Baltimore: Williams & Wilkins.

Kyle, G. (2009) Practice questions: solving your clinical dilemmas. *Nursing Times*, 105(2), 16.

Kyle, G. (2011a) The use of urinary sheaths in male incontinence. *British Journal of Nursing*, 20(6), 338.

Kyle, G. (2011b) Risk assessment and management tools for constipation. *British Journal of Community Nursing*, 16(5), 224, 226–230.

Kyle, G. (2011c) Digital rectal examination. *Nursing Times*, 107(12), 18–19.

Kyle, G., Prynn, P., Oliver, H., et al. (2005a) The Eton Scale: a tool for risk assessment for constipation. *Nursing Times*, 101(18), 50–51.

Kyle, G., Oliver, H. & Prynn, P. (2005b) *The Procedure for the Digital Removal of Faeces Guidelines 2005*. Uxbridge: Norgine.

Lay, K. (2012) Continence care. *Nursing Standard*, 27(12), 59–60.

Le Lievre, S. (2002) An overview of skin care and faecal incontinence. *Nursing Times*, 98(4), 58–59.

Leaver, R.B. (2007) The evidence for urethral meatal cleansing. *Nursing Standard*, 21(41), 39–42.

Lee-Robichaud, H., Thomas, K., Morgan, J., et al. (2010) Lactulose versus Polyethylene Glycol for Chronic Constipation. *Cochrane Database of Systematic Reviews*. Available at: http://onlinelibrary.wiley.com/doi/10.1002/14651858.CD007570.pub2/pdf

Letizia, M. & Norton, E. (2003) Successful management of malignant bowel obstruction. *Journal of Hospice and Palliative Nursing*, 5(3), 152–160.

Longstreth, G.F., Thompson, W.G., Chey, W.D., et al. (2006) Functional bowel disorders. *Gastroenterology*, 130(5), 1480–1491.

Lynch, B. & Sarazine, J. (2006) A guide to understanding malignant bowel obstruction. *International Journal of Palliative Nursing*, 12(4), 164–166, 168–171.

Madeo, M. & Roodhouse, A.J. (2009) Reducing the risks associated with urinary catheters. *Nursing Standard*, 23(29), 47–55; quiz 56.

Magnall, J. & Watterson, L. (2006) Principles of aseptic technique in urinary catheterisation. *Nursing Standard*, 21(8), 49–56.

McCarthy, K. & Hunter, I. (2001) Importance of pH monitoring in the care of long-term catheters. *British Journal of Nursing*, 10(19), 1240–1247.

McFarland, L.V. (2007) Diarrhoea associated with antibiotic use. *BMJ*, 335(7610), 54–55.

Metcalf, C. (2007) Chronic diarrhoea: investigation, treatment and nursing care. *Nursing Standard*, 21(21), 48–56; quiz 58.

Metheny, NA., Meert, K.L. (2004) Monitoring feeding tube placement. *Nutrition in Clinical Practice* 19(5) 487–495.

Moharari, R.S., Khajavi, M.R., Khademhosseini, P., et al. (2008) Sterile water as an irrigating fluid for transurethral resection of the prostate: anesthetical view of the records of 1600 cases. *Southern Medical Journal*, 101(4), 373–375.

Moppett, S. (2000) Which way is up for a suppository? *Nursing Times*, 96(19), 12–14.

Morton, P.G. & Fontaine, D.K. (eds) (2013) *Critical Care Nursing: A Holistic Approach*, 10th edn. Philadelphia: Lippincott Williams and Wilkins.

Mosby (2006) *Mosby's Dictionary of Medicine, Nursing & Health Professions*, 7th edn. St. Louis, MO: Mosby Elsevier.

Moslemi, M.K. & Rajaei, M. (2010) An improved delivery system for bladder irrigation. *Therapeutics and Clinical Risk Management*, 6, 459–462.

Mulhall, A.B., King, S.U., Lee, K., et al. (1993) Maintenance of closed urinary drainage systems: are practitioners more aware of the dangers? *Journal of Clinical Nursing*, 2(3), 135–140.

Murphy, C., Fader, M. & Prieto, J. (2014) Interventions to minimise the initial use of indwelling urinary catheters in acute care: a systematic review. *International Journal of Nursing Studies*, 51(1), 4–13.

Nazarko, L. (2007) Managing diarrhoea in the home to prevent admission. *British Journal of Community Nursing*, 12(11), 508–512.

Nazarko, L. (2008) Caring for a patient with a urostomy in a community setting. *British Journal of Community Nursing*, 13(8), 354–361.

Nazarko, L. (2009) Providing effective evidence-based catheter management. *British Journal of Nursing*, 18(7), S4–S12.

Nazarko, L. (2010) Effective evidence-based catheter management: an update. *British Journal of Nursing*, 19(15), 948–953.

Nazarko, L. (2012) Intermittent self-catheterisation: past, present and future. *British Journal of Community Nursing*, 17(9), 408–412.

Nethercliffe, J.M. (2012) Unrinary incontinence. In: Dawson, C. & Nethercliffe, J. (eds) *ABC of Urology*, 3rd edn. Chichester: Wiley, pp.14–18.

Newey, J. (1998) Causes and treatment of erectile dysfunction. *Nursing Standard*, 12(47), 39–40.

Ng, C. (2001) Assessment and intervention knowledge of nurses in managing catheter patency in continuous bladder irrigation following TURP. *Urologic Nursing*, 21(2), 97–108.

NHS Supply Chain (2008). Available at: https://my.supplychain.nhs.uk/catalogue/browse/160/urological-catheters-and-valves

NHSQIS (2004) *Urinary Catheterisation and Catheter Care: Best Practice Statement*. Scotland: NHS Quality Improvement. Available at: www.healthcareimprovementscotland.org/his/idoc.ashx?docid=feaef66c-08e3-4168-ae5c-85eba638ae8b&version=-1

NICE (2007) *Faecal Incontinence: The Management of Faecal Incontinence in Adults, CG49*. London: National Institute for Health and Clinical Excellence. Available at: http://www.nice.org.uk/guidance/cG49

NICE (2012) *Infection: Prevention and Control of Healthcare-Associated Infections in Primary and Community Care, CG139*. London: National Institute for Health and Clinical Excellence. Available at: www.nice.org.uk/nicemedia/live/13684/58656/58656.pdf

Nicol, M. (2008) *Essential Nursing Skills*, 3rd edn. London: Mosby Elsevier.

NMC (2010) *Record Keeping: Guidance for Nurses and Midwives*. London: Nursing and Midwifery Council. Available at: www.nmc-uk.org/Documents/NMC-Publications/NMC-Record-Keeping-Guidance.pdf

NMC (2013) *Consent*. London: Nursing and Midwifery Council. Available at: www.nmc-uk.org/Nurses-and-midwives/Regulation-in-practice/Regulation-in-Practice-Topics/consent/

NMC (2015) *The Code: Standards of Conduct, Performance and Ethics for Nurses and Midwives*. London: Nursing and Midwifery Council. Available at: www.nmc-uk.org/Documents/Standards/The-code-A4-20100406.pdf

Norton, C. (1996) *Nursing for Continence*, 2nd edn. Beaconsfield: Beaconsfield Publishers.

Norton, C. (2006) Constipation in older patients: effects on quality of life. *British Journal of Nursing*, 15(4), 188–192.

NPSA (2009) *Minimising Risks of Suprapublic Catheter Insertion (Adults Only) NPSA/2009/RRR005*. London: National Patient Safety Agency. Available at: www.nrls.npsa.nhs.uk/EasySiteWeb/getresource.axd?AssetID=60311&type=full&servicetype=Attachment

NPSA (2011) *Reducing the Harm Caused by Misplaced Nasogastric Feeding Tubes in Adults, Children and Infants: Patient Safety Alert NPSA/2011/PSA002*. London: National Patient Safety Agency. Available at: www.nrls.npsa.nhs.uk/resources/?entryid45=129640

O'Connor, G. (2005) Teaching stoma-management skills: the importance of self-care. *British Journal of Nursing*, 14(6), 320–324.

Opus (2010) Pre and post op steps to improve body image. *Gastrointestinal Nursing*, 8(2), 34.

Ostaszkiewicz, J. & Paterson, J. (2012) Nurses' advice regarding sterile or clean urinary drainage bags for individuals with a long-term indwelling urinary catheter. *Journal of Wound, Ostomy and Continence Nursing*, 39(1), 77–83.

Patel, I.J., Davidson, J.C., Nikolic, B., et al. (2012) Consensus guidelines for periprocedural management of coagulation status and hemostasis risk in percutaneous image-guided interventions. *Journal of Vascular and Interventional Radiology*, 23(6), 727–736.

Peate, I. (2003) Nursing role in the management of constipation: use of laxatives. *British Journal of Nursing*, 12(19), 1130–1136.

Peate, I., Nair, M. & Wild, K. (2014) *Nursing Practice: Knowledge and Care*. Oxford: John Wiley & Sons.

Pegram, A., Bloomfield, J. & Jones, A. (2008) Safe use of rectal suppositories and enemas with adult patients. *Nursing Standard*, 22(38), 39–41.

Pellatt, G.C. (2007) Clinical skills: bowel elimination and management of complications. *British Journal of Nursing*, 16(6), 351–355.

Pellowe, C. & Pratt, R. (2004) Catheter-associated urinary tract infections: primary care guidelines. *Nursing Times*, 100(2), 53–55.

Peppas, G., Alexiou, V.G., Mourtzoukou, E., et al. (2008) Epidemiology of constipation in Europe and Oceania: a systematic review. *BMC Gastroenterology*, 8, 5.

Perdue, C. (2005) Managing constipation in advanced cancer care. *Nursing Times*, 101(21), 36–40.

Plowman, R., Graves, N., Esquivel, J., et al. (2001) An economic model to assess the cost and benefits of the routine use of silver alloy coated urinary catheters to reduce the risk of urinary tract infections in catheterized patients. *Journal of Hospital Infection*, 48 (1), 33–42.

Pomfret, I.J. (1996) Catheters: design, selection and management. *British Journal of Nursing*, 5(4), 245–251.

Pomfret, I. (2002) Back to basics: an introduction to continence issues. *Journal of Community Nursing*, 16(7), 37–41.

Pomfret, I. (2004) Urinary catheters and associated UTI's. *Journal of Community Nursing*, 18(9), 15–19.

Pomfret, I. (2006) Which Urinary System is Right for You? *Charter Continence Care*. Peterborough: Coloplast.

Pomfret, I. (2007) Urinary catheterisation: selection and clinical management. *British Journal of Community Nursing*, 12(8), 348–354.

Potter, J. (2007) Male urinary incontinence – could penile sheaths be the answer? *Journal of Community Nursing*, 21(5), 40–42.

Powell, M. & Rigby, D. (2000) Management of bowel dysfunction: evacuation difficulties. *Nursing Standard*, 14(47), 47–51.

Pratt, R.J., Pellowe, C.M., Wilson, J.A., et al. (2007) epic2: National evidence-based guidelines for preventing healthcare-associated infections in NHS hospitals in England. *Journal of Hospital Infection*, 65 (Suppl 1), S1–S64.

Ramchandani, P., Cardella, J.F., Grassi, C.J., et al. (2003) Quality improvement guidelines for percutaneous nephrostomy. *Journal of Vascular and Interventional Radiology*, 14(9 Pt 2), S277–S281.

Rao, S.S., Valestin, J. & Schulze, K. (2010) Long term efficacy of biofeedback therapy for dyssynergic defaecation: randomised controlled trial. *American Journal Gastroenterology*, 105(4), 890–896.

RCN (2011) *Guidance on Pin Site Care. Report on Recommendations from the 2010 Consensus Project on Pin Site Care*. London: Royal College of Nursing. Available at: www.rcn.org.uk/__data/assets/pdf_file/0009/413982/004137.pdf

RCN (2012a) *Catheter Care – RCN Guidance for Nurses*. London: Royal College of Nursing. Available at: www.rcn.org.uk/__data/assets/pdf_file/0018/157410/003237.pdf

RCN (2012b) *Management of Lower Bowel Dysfunction, including DRE and DRF: RCN Guidance for Nurses*. London: Royal College of Nursing. Available at: www.rcn.org.uk/__data/assets/pdf_file/0007/157363/003226.pdf

Redmond, C., Cowin, C., Parker, T. (2009) The experience of faecal leakage among ileostomists. *British Journal of Nursing*, 18(17), S14–S17.

Rees, J. & Sharpe, A. (2009) The use of bowel management systems in the high-dependency setting. *British Journal of Nursing*, 18(7), S19–S20, S22, S24.

Rew, M. (2005) Caring for catheterized patients: urinary catheter maintenance. *British Journal of Nursing*, 14 (2), 87–92.

Richardson, J., Smith, J.E., McCall, G., et al. (2007) Hypnosis for nausea and vomiting in cancer chemotherapy: a systematic review of the research evidence. *European Journal of Cancer Care*, 16(5), 402–412.

Rigby, D. (2009) An overview of suprapubic catheter care in community practice. *British Journal of Community Nursing*, 14(7), 278–284.

Ripley, K. (2007) Skin care in patients with urinary of faecal incontinence. *Primary Health Care*, 17(4), 29–34.

Robinson, J. (2001) Urethral catheter selection. *Nursing Standard*, 15 (25), 39–42.

Robinson, J. (2004) A practical approach to catheter-associated problems. *Nursing Standard*, 18(31), 38–42.

Robinson, J. (2006) Continence: sizing and fitting a penile sheath. *British Journal of Community Nursing*, 11(10), 420–427.

Robinson, J. (2008) Insertion, care and management of suprapubic catheters. *Nursing Standard*, 23(8), 49–56.

Rogers, J. (2012) How to manage chronic constipation in adults. *Nursing Times*, 108(41), 12, 14, 16 passim.

Rollins, H (1997) A nose for trouble. *Nursing Times* 93(49): 66–67.

Saint, S. & Lipsky, B.A. (1999) Preventing catheter-related bacteriuria: Should we? Can we? How? *Archives of Internal Medicine*, 159(8), 800–808.

Saint, S., Veenstra, D.L., Sullivan, S.D., et al. (2000) The potential clinical and economic benefits of silver alloy urinary catheters in preventing urinary tract infection. *Archives of Internal Medicine*, 160(17), 2670–2675.

Scholtes, S. (2002) Management of clot retention following urological surgery. *Nursing Times*, 98(28), 48–50.

Schumm, K. & Lam, T.B. (2008) Types of urethral catheters for management of short-term voiding problems in hospitalised adults. *Cochrane Database of Systematic Reviews*. Available at: http://onlinelibrary.wiley.com/doi/10.1002/14651858.CD004013.pub3/pdf

Shepherd, M. (2000) Treating diarrhoea and constipation. *Nursing Times*, 96(6 Suppl), 15–16.

Shih, S.C., Jeng, K.S., Lin, S.C., et al. (2003) Adhesive small bowel obstruction: how long can patients tolerate conservative treatment? *World Journal of Gastroenterology*, 9(3), 603–605.

Simpson, L. (2001) Indwelling urethral catheters. *Nursing Standard*, 15(46), 47–53.

Slater, R. (2012) Managing high-output stomas. *British Journal of Nursing*, 21(22), 1309–1311.

Smith, S. (2001) Evidence-based management of constipation in the oncology patient. *European Journal of Oncology Nursing*, 5(1), 18–25.

Steggall, M. J. (2008) Digital rectal examination. *Nursing Standard*, 22(47), 46–48.

Stensballe, J., Tvede, M., Looms, D., et al. (2007) Infection risk with nitrofurazone-impregnated urinary catheters in trauma patients: a randomized trial. *Annals of Internal Medicine*, 147(5), 285–293.

Stewart, E. (1998) Urinary catheters: selection, maintenance and nursing care. *British Journal of Nursing*, 7(19), 1152–1161.

Stoller, M. (2004) Retrograde instrumentation of the urinary tract. In: Tanagho, E.A., McAninch, J.W. & Smith, D.R. (eds) *Smith's general urology*. 16th edn. New York: Lange Medical Books/McGraw-Hill, pp.163–174.

Stothers, L. & Friedman, B. (2011) Risk factors for the development of stress urinary incontinence in women. *Current Urology Reports*, 12(5), 363–369.

Taylor, C. (1997) Constipation and diarrhoea. In: Bruce, L. & Finlay, T. (eds) *Nursing in Gastroenterology*. Edinburgh: Churchill Livingstone, pp.27–54.

Taylor, C., Lopes de Azevedo-Gilbert, R. & Gabe, S. (2012) Rehabilitation needs following stoma formation: a patient survey. *British Journal of Community Nursing*, 17(3), 102, 104, 106–107.

Taylor, P. (2005) An introduction to stomas: reasons for their formation. *Nursing Times*, 101(29), 63–64.

Thibodeau, G.A. & Patton, K.T. (2010) *Anatomy & Physiology*, 7th edn. St. Louis, MO: Mosby Elsevier.

Thomas, J., Karver, S., Cooney, G.A., et al. (2008) Methylnaltrexone for opioid-induced constipation in advanced illness. *New England Journal of Medicine*, 358(22), 2332–2343.

Thomas, P.D., Forbes, A., Green, J., et al. (2003) Guidelines for the investigation of chronic diarrhoea, 2nd edition. *Gut*, 52(Suppl 5), v1–15.

Thompson, M.J., Boyd-Carson, W., Trainor, B., et al. (2003) Management of constipation. *Nursing Standard*, 18(14–16), 41–42.

Toner, F. & Claros, E. (2012) Preventing, assessing, and managing constipation in older adults. *Nursing*, 42(12), 32–39; quiz 40.

Tortora, G. J. & Derrickson, B.H. (2011) *Principles of Anatomy & Physiology*, 13th edn. Hoboken, NJ: John Wiley & Sons.

Twycross, R. & Back, I. (2004) Nausea and vomiting in advanced cancer. *European Journal of Palliative Care*, 13, 715–721.

Twycross, R.G., Wilcock, A. & Stark Toller, C. (2009) *Symptom Management in Advanced Cancer*, 4th edn. Nottingham: Palliativedrugs.com Ltd.

Warren, A. & King, L. (2008) A review of the efficacy of dexamethasone in the prevention of postoperative nausea and vomiting. *Journal of Clinical Nursing*, 17 (1), 58–68.

Weisner, P. & Bell, S. (2004) Bowel dysfunction: assessment and management in the neurological patient. In: Norton, C. & Chelvanayagam, S. (eds) *Bowel Continence Nursing*. Beaconsfield: Beaconsfield Publishers.

Wells, M. (2008) Managing urinary incontinence with BioDerm external continence device. *British Journal of Nursing*, 17 (9), s24–29.

Welser, M., Riedlinger, I., Prause, U. (2009) A comparative study of two-piece ostomy appliances. *British Journal of Nursing*, 18(9), 530–538.

WHO (2014) *Health Topics: Diarrhoea*. Available at: www.who.int/topics/diarrhoea/en/

Williams, J. (2011) Stoma appliances: it's all about the bag! *British Journal of Nursing*, 20(9), 534.

Wilson, L.A. (2005) Urinalysis. *Nursing Standard*, 19(35), 51–54.

Wilson, M. (2008) Diarrhoea and its possible impact on skin health. *Nursing Times*, 104(18), 49–52.

Winn, C. (1998) Complications with urinary catheters. *Professional Nurse*, 13(5 Suppl), S7–S10.

Withell, B. (2000) A protocol for treating acute constipation in the community setting. *British Journal of Community Nursing*, 5(3), 110–117.

Woodward, S. (1997) Complications of allergies to latex urinary catheters. *British Journal of Nursing*, 6(14), 786–793.

Woodward, S. (2005) Use of lubricant in female urethral catheterization. *British Journal of Nursing*, 14(19), 1022–1023.

Woodward, S. (2007) The BioDerm external continence device: evidence and assessment for use. *British Journal of Neurosceince Nursing*, 3(12), 580–584.

Woodward, S. (2012) Assessment and management of constipation in older people. *Nursing Older People*, 24(5), 21–26.

Woodward, S. (2013) Catheter valves: a welcome alternative to leg bags. *British Journal of Nursing*, 22(11), 650, 652–654.

Woollons, S. (1996) Urinary catheters for long-term use. *Professional Nurse*, 11(12), 825–829, 832.

Wright, S. & Burch, J. (2008) Pre and post operative care. In: Burch, J. (ed) *Stoma Care*. Oxford: John Wiley & Sons, pp.119–141

Yates, A. (2004) Crisis management in catheter care. *Journal of Community Nursing*, 18(5), 28–31.

Young, A.E., Macnaughton, P.D., Gaylard, D.G., et al. (1994) A case of latex anaphylaxis. *British Journal of Hospital Medicine*, 52(11), 599–600.

Answers

Learning Activity 5.2 **Scenario: Urinary catheterization**

You have been asked to catheterize a female patient (under supervision) who has been found to have urinary retention.

1 What factors should you consider prior to the procedure?
- Reason for catheterization.
- Type of catheter, size of catheter.
- Drainage system required (e.g. standard bag, urometer, leg bag).
- Essential equipment required.
- Informing the patient and gaining consent.

2 What steps can you take to minimize the risk of the patient developing a catheter-associated urinary tract infection?
- Ensure the catheter is an appropriate type and size.
- Maintain an aseptic technique.
- Use a lubrication gel with antiseptic properties to reduce the risk of trauma.
- Ensure that you feel confident to undertake the procedure, if not discuss this with your mentor/supervisor.
- Once inserted, maintain a closed drainage system.

3 What should you do after the procedure?
- Measure the volume of urine drained.
- Dispose of all your equipment safely.
- Ensure the patient is comfortable.
- Document the procedure within the patient's notes.

Learning Activity 5.4 **Case study: Diarrhoea**

Mrs Stone is a 44-year-old woman with Crohn's disease who has been suffering from severe diarrhoea for the last 10 days and has been admitted to your ward with dehydration. She reports having at least 12 episodes of diarrhoea a day (type 7 using the Bristol Stool Chart).

1 What precautions should be taken?
- Universal precautions.
- Nurse in a side room (ideally).
- Discuss with infection control team.
- Patient education.

2 What information would you want to include in your assessment of her diarrhoea?
- History of onset, frequency, medical history.
- Colour, consistency, form of stool.
- Stool cultures, blood tests.
- Any associated symptoms. For example, pain, vomiting, fatigue.
- Fluid and food intake.
- Current management strategies (pharmacological, non-pharmacological).
- Coping strategies.

3 What nursing interventions is she likely to require?
- Infection prevention and control.
- Fluid management.
- Dietary management.
- Anti-motility medication once infective causes have been excluded.
- Additional medication to control the inflammation caused by the Crohn's disease.
- Pain management.
- Support and information.

Learning Activity 5.6 **Case study: Constipation**

Mr Jones, aged 32 years, is recovering from orthopaedic surgery for which he has been on bed rest. While on the ward he has suffered from constipation. He would like to know what he should do to avoid getting constipated when he goes home.

What advice would you give to Mr Jones?

- Fluids – drink the recommended daily intake of a minimum of 2 litres.
- Exercise – physical activity, particularly after food, can enhance peristalsis.
- Diet – gradually increasing dietary fibre increases stool bulk, improving peristalsis and transit time.

Learning Activity 5.7 **Scenario: Stoma care**

You have been allocated to care for a patient who has had a sigmoid colostomy formed.

What physical and psychosocial issues should you consider prior to their discharge?

- Stoma supplies and prescription information.
- Level of independence with stoma.
- Stoma care nurse contact details.
- Dietary advice.
- Support at home.
- Lifestyle adaptation.
- Physical and sexual activity.

Now Test Yourself **What have you learnt?**

1 Thinking about incontinence and skin care.
  A What is the name of the skin condition that may occur as a consequence of incontinence?
    - Incontinence-associated dermatitis.

  B What are the most recent recommendations for the prevention and treatment of this condition?
    - Perineal cleansing, moisturization and application of a skin protectant.

2 What percentage of men between the ages of 65 and 74 are affected by urinary incontinence?
  A 10%
  B 13%
  C 14%
  D 15%

3 List five indications for urinary catheterization.
  - See the list of indications within the section 'Urinary catheterization, Rationale' for the answers.

4 Which of the following have been identified as having a direct association with the development of urinary tract infections?
  A Maintaining a closed drainage system
  B The insertion technique and use of aseptic conditions
  C Length of time a catheter remains *in situ*
  D Competence of the practitioner performing the procedure
  E All of the above

5 What is the usual solution recommended for use as bladder irrigation and why?
  - 0.9% sodium chloride. It is isotonic so does not affect the body's fluid and electrolyte balance, which enables large volumes of solution to be used if necessary.

6 What are the three main causes of acute diarrhoea?
  - Diet
  - Allergies
  - Infections

7 Laxatives are frequently used in the treatment of constipation. Match up the following examples with their appropriate category.

Category	Example by brand name
Bulk producer **(Fybogel)**	Milpar
Stool softener **(Milpar)**	Senna
Osmotic agent **(Lactulose)**	Fybogel
Stimulant laxative **(Senna)**	Lactulose

8 What is the difference between an evacuant enema and a retention enema? Give an example of each.
  - An evacuant enema is a solution introduced into the rectum with the intention of it being expelled, along with faecal matter and flatus within a few minutes (phosphate enema).
  - A retention enema is a solution introduced into the rectum with the intention of it being retained for a period of time (arachis oil enema).

  More information on the action of these different enemas is provided in the section on 'Enemas'.

9 Following stoma formation, what should you observe immediately post-operatively about the following?
  A Stoma. Colour, size, appearance, presence of other devices (e.g. bridge)
  B Stoma output. Volume, colour
  C Peristomal skin. Broken areas, rashes, erythema
  D Stoma/skin margin. Sutures intact, evidence of separation of stoma edge from skin

10 When selecting a stoma appliance for a patient who has undergone a formation of a loop colostomy, what factors should you consider?
  A Dexterity of the patient, consistency of effluent, type of stoma
  B Patient preference, type of stoma, consistency of effluent, state of peristomal skin, dexterity of the patient
  C Patient preference, lifestyle, position of stoma, consistency of effluent, state of peristomal skin, dexterity of patient, type of stoma
  D Cognitive ability, lifestyle, patient dexterity, position of stoma, state of peristomal skin, type of stoma, consistency of effluent, patient preference

Moving and positioning

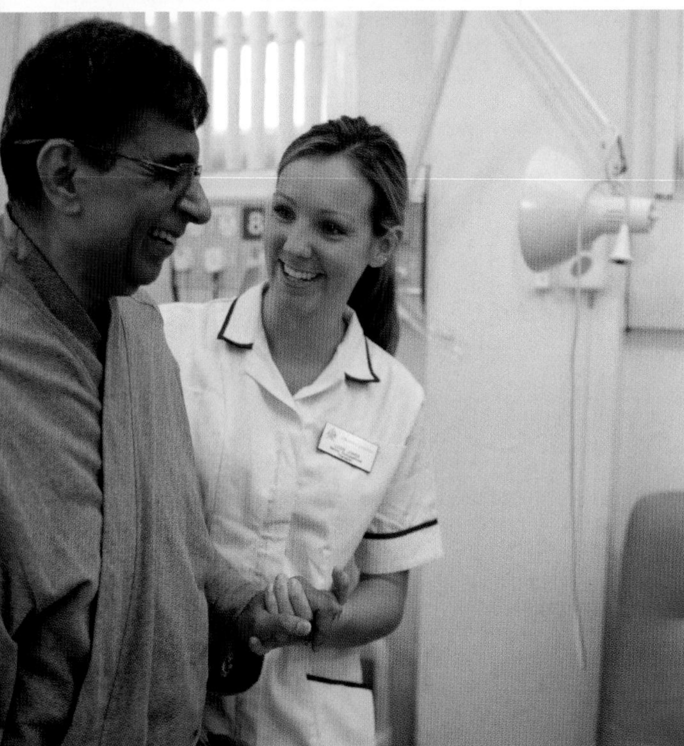

By reading this chapter and undertaking the learning activities within it, you should be able to:

1 Identify the key considerations regarding moving and positioning.

2 Demonstrate an understanding of the principles of moving and positioning, whether the patient is in bed, sitting, or preparing to mobilize.

3 Consider optimal moving and positioning, including modifications for patients with different clinical needs.

Procedure guidelines

The Royal Marsden Manual of Clinical Nursing Procedures: Student Edition, Ninth Edition. Edited by Lisa Dougherty, Sara Lister and Alexandra West-Oram

Overview

The aim of this chapter is to provide guidance on various aspects of moving and positioning patients, acknowledging the need to be clinically effective and, where possible, evidence based. It relates to moving and positioning of adults and does not specifically cover positioning of children or neonates.

The main objectives of the chapter are to:

1 outline the general considerations regarding moving and positioning
2 provide guidance on the principles of moving and positioning whether the patient is in bed, sitting or preparing to mobilize
3 consider optimal moving and positioning including modifications for patients with different clinical needs.

The principles of moving and positioning will relate to the effect on the patient, but the practitioner needs to ensure that they consider their own position regarding the safety aspects of manual handling. For recommendations and further information on safe manual handling, refer to government (HSE 1992, 2012) and local trust policies, the manual handling advisor or the physiotherapist (PT).

In this chapter the general principles of moving and positioning will be discussed first, followed by considerations of positioning for patients with specific clinical needs, which will require modification or additional considerations of the general principles. The first specific clinical area covered will be moving and positioning of unconscious patients and patients with an artificial airway. Following this, there will be a section looking at additional considerations and modifications for patients with different respiratory requirements. The next section of the chapter will relate to the specific moving and positioning needs of patients with a neurological problem, including the management of patients with spinal cord compression. The final clinical area to be considered will relate to moving and positioning considerations and modifications for upper and lower limb amputees.

Moving and positioning: general principles

DEFINITION

The verb 'to position' is defined as 'a way in which someone or something is placed or arranged' (Pearsall 2010). In medical terms, 'position' relates to body position or posture. Moving and positioning lie within the broader context of manual handling, which incorporates 'transporting or supporting a load (including lifting, putting down, pushing, pulling, carrying or moving) by hand or bodily force' (HSE 1992).

ANATOMY AND PHYSIOLOGY

The human body is a complex structure relying on the musculoskeletal system to provide support and also to assist in movement. The musculoskeletal system is an integrated system consisting of bones, muscles and joints.

Whilst bones provide the structural framework for protecting vital organs and providing stability, skeletal muscles maintain body alignment and help movement (Tortora and Derrickson 2011). In order for skeletal muscles to provide these functions, they often cross at least one joint and attach to the articulating bones that help form the joint so that when a muscle contracts, movement of a joint can occur in one direction. Muscles tend to work in synergy with each other (rather than in isolation) not just to create but also to control the movement. The ability of a muscle to either contract or to extend assists their function (Figure 6.1). However, muscles will waste if not used and can also become shortened if not stretched regularly.

Joints are supported not just by the muscles but also by ligaments which are strong connective tissue structures attached either side of the joint, for example the knee joint (Figure 6.2). Ligaments can also become shortened if they are maintained in one position repeatedly or over a long period of time, which can then lead to problems maintaining full joint movement.

EVIDENCE-BASED APPROACHES

Rationale

Moving and positioning are important aspects of patient care because together they can affect the patient physically, physiologically and psychologically. They have a major impact on the patient's recuperation and well-being and can address impairments in order to maximize function.

Optimum positioning is a good starting point to maximize the benefit of other interventions such as bed exercises, breathing exercises, assisting rest and mobility in order to facilitate recovery and enhance function. However, although it is important, it must not be seen in isolation and is just one aspect of patient management within the context of preventative, rehabilitative, supportive and palliative rehabilitation models (Dietz 1981) where the overall goal is to assist independence.

It is important to frequently evaluate the effect that moving and positioning have on the individual with different pathologies to ensure that the intervention is helping to achieve the desired result or goal. This relates to considering whether the moving and positioning procedure is being clinically effective and, where possible, is evidence based.

There are several points to consider with regard to the clinical effectiveness of moving and positioning.

- Is the timing right for moving the patient? For example, is the pain relief adequate?
- Is it being carried out in the correct way? This relates to manual handling with regard to preventing trauma to both the patient and the practitioner. It is well known that nurses have a high incidence of work-related musculoskeletal injuries (Nelson et al. 2008) so that approved patient handling techniques are essential for safe practice.
- Is the required position taking into account all the pertinent needs of the patient? This emphasizes the need to consider the patient in a holistic manner and take into account any co-morbidities as well as the primary focus that is being addressed.
- Is it achieving the desired or preventing a detrimental result?

Indications

Assistance in moving and positioning is indicated for patients who have difficulty moving or require periods of rest when normal function is impaired.

Contraindications

There are no general contraindications for moving and positioning. The severity of an illness may leave no choice except bedrest, but the rest alone is rarely beneficial.

Patients who are clinically unstable may also need medical attention prior to any moving or change in position.

Principles of care

The principles of positioning are based on patterns of posture which maximize function with the minimal amount of effort (Gardiner 1973). The control of body posture includes the alignment of body segments to each other and to the supporting surface (Edwards and Carter 2002). These basic principles of

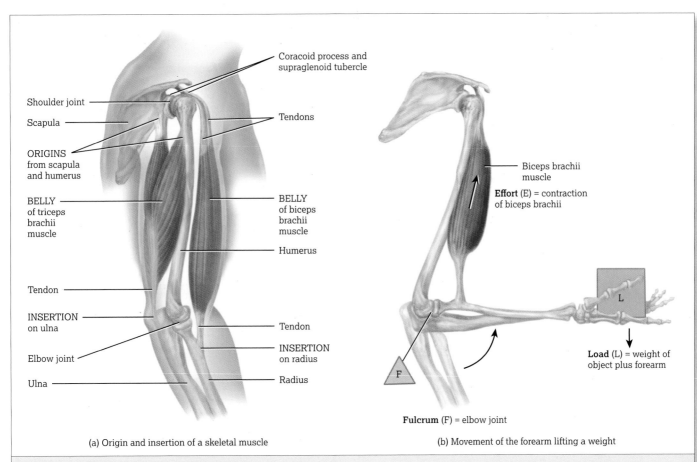

(a) Origin and insertion of a skeletal muscle

(b) Movement of the forearm lifting a weight

Figure 6.1 **Relationship of skeletal muscles to bones: origin and insertion of skeletal muscle.** ***Source:*** **Tortora and Derrickson (2011). Reproduced with permission from John Wiley & Sons.**

Figure 6.2 **Anterior view of the right knee (tibiofemoral) joint.** ***Source:*** **Tortora and Derrickson (2011). Reproduced with permission from John Wiley & Sons.**

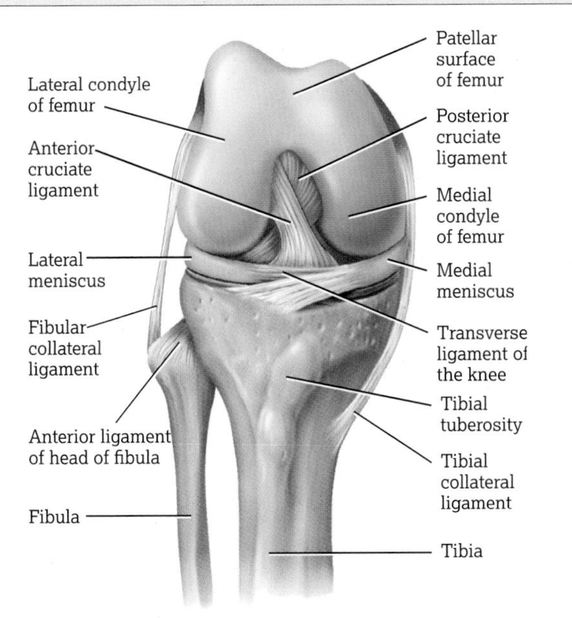

positioning can be applied regardless of a patient's pathology. The aim is to reduce impairment, facilitate function and alleviate symptomatic discomfort and to assist future rehabilitation where appropriate.

The main principles underpinning all interventions regarding patient positioning and mobilization focus on the short- and long-term goals of rehabilitation and management for each specific patient. It is imperative that a thorough assessment is carried out prior to any intervention in order to plan appropriate goals of treatment. It may be necessary to compromise on one principle, depending on the overall goal. For example, for the palliative patient, it may be that the primary aim of any intervention is to facilitate comfort at the cost of reducing function. Regular reassessment is necessary to allow for modification of plans to reflect changes in status.

Effects of bedrest/decreased mobility

Learning Activity 6.1

Check your knowledge: Complications of decreased mobility

- Make a list of the complications of decreased mobility.
- How many did you come up with? Compare this with those listed within this section.
- Think about the different nursing interventions used to minimize the risk of each complication occurring.

Patients with acute medical conditions and decreased mobility are at risk of developing secondary complications of bedrest such as pulmonary embolus (PE) (Riedel 2001), deep vein thrombosis (DVT) or respiratory infection (Convertino et al. 1997). Historically patients complaining of pain, dyspnoea, neurological dysfunction and fatigue were advised to rest. However, inactivity can cause a variety of problems including:

- deconditioning of many of the body's systems (particularly cardiorespiratory and musculoskeletal)
- deterioration of symptoms
- fear of movement
- loss of independence
- social isolation (Creditor 1993, Hanks 2010).

Therefore, patients should be encouraged or assisted to mobilize or change position, at frequent intervals. The use of rehabilitation programmes in the patient with critical illness has the potential to decrease time on the critical care unit, shorten overall hospital stay and prevent readmission (Thomas 2009). Early referral to therapy services is advantageous.

If bedrest is unavoidable then the following factors should be taken into account:

- patient comfort and adequate support
- avoidance of the complications of prolonged bedrest
- the optimum frequency of position change.

Active movements, as advised by the physiotherapist, should be practised where possible in order to:

- maintain full joint range
- maintain full muscle length and extensibility
- assist venous return
- maintain sensation of normal movement (Adam and Forrest 1999).

Active ankle movements (Figure 6.3) are to be encouraged to assist the circulation, as failure to exercise the calf muscle for prolonged periods may result in limited or poor blood circulation in the lower leg and increases the risk of DVT (O'Donovan et al. 2006).

Risk assessment

There is an absolute requirement to assess the risks arising from moving and handling patients that cannot reasonably be avoided (CSP 2014). Once the risk of not moving the patient is deemed to be greater than moving the patient (see previous rationale), consider the following (TILE).

T *Task/operation*: achieving the desired position or movement.

I *Individual*: this refers to the handler/s. In patient handling, this relates to the skills, competencies and physical capabilities of the handlers. It is also important to consider health status, gender, pregnancy, age and disability. It is also important to consider the competency and abilities of all staff involved with the task.

L *Load*: in the case of patient handling, the load is the patient. The aim of rehabilitation is where possible to encourage patients to move for themselves or contribute towards this goal. This may mean that additional equipment is needed. For assistance with regard to this, liaise with the physiotherapist and/or occupational therapist.

E *Environment*: before positioning or moving the patient, think about the space, placement of equipment and removal of any hazards.

Other factors, for example any line attached to the patient, must also be considered when undertaking a risk assessment. The key points to consider are summarized in Box 6.1.

Figure 6.3 **(a) Ankle in dorsiflexion (DF). (b) Ankle in plantarflexion (PF).**

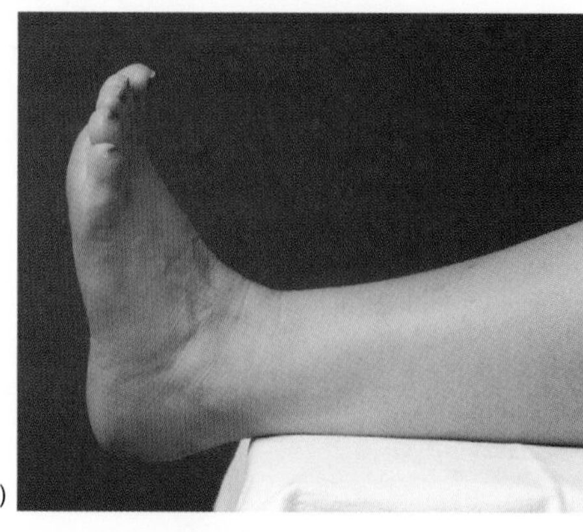

(a)

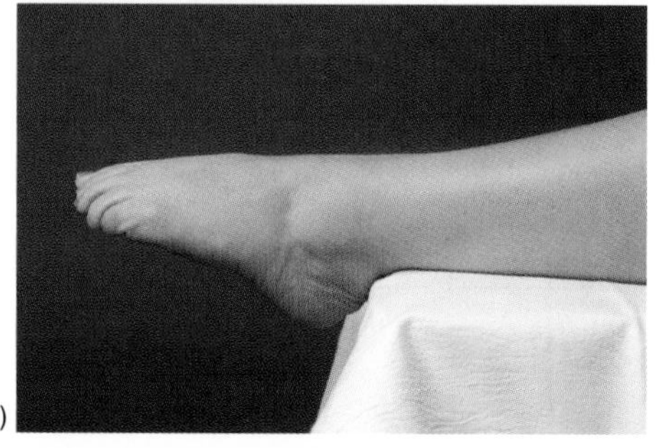

(b)

Box 6.1 **Risk assessment**

1 Assess the patient clinically.
2 Consider realistic clinical goals and functional outcomes in discussion with the patient and ascertain the level at which the patient will be able to participate in the task.
3 Consider whether the proposed intervention involves hazardous manual handling and reduce the hazard by:
   a adapting the technique
   b introducing equipment. Studies advocate the use of assistive devices to promote safer patient handling for patients with complex needs following assessment (Nelson et al. 2006, Rockefeller 2008), with a positive impact on patient outcomes with no detrimental effect on staff handling following assessment (Nelson et al. 2008)
   c seeking advice/assistance from appropriately skilled colleagues.
4 Risk assessment should be an ongoing process and be constantly updated.
5 After the procedure, document the risk assessment in the communication section of the patient's care plan, being sure to include the date, the number of staff involved and the equipment needed to perform the task. Also document any changes in the patient's condition, such as skin redness. It is important to also document the intended duration of time for which the patient should be maintained in this new position.

Source: CSP (2014). Reproduced with permission from The Chartered Society of Physiotherapy (www.csp.org.uk).

Effective use of therapeutic handling in the context of the use of a comprehensive competency-based training tool can benefit patient outcome, enabling balance and motor training in early rehabilitation with minimal risk to staff (Mehan et al. 2008). Where there is any doubt about patients with complex needs, seek advice from the PT or the occupational therapist (OT) for assessment. Once a risk assessment has been carried out, this needs to be recorded prior to proceeding with any manual handling intervention (CSP 2014).

Consent must be obtained before any intervention is started. Consent is the voluntary and continuing permission of the patient to receive a particular treatment based on an adequate knowledge of the purpose, nature and likely risks of the treatment, including the likelihood of its success and any alternatives to it. Permission given under any unfair or undue pressure is not consent (NMC 2013). This principle reflects the right of patients to determine what happens to their own bodies, and is a fundamental part of good practice (DH 2009).

LEGAL AND PROFESSIONAL ISSUES

For recommendations and further information on safe manual handling, refer to professional guidance (CSP 2014), government and local trust policy (HSE 1992) and the manual handling advisor or PT. This is particularly relevant when handling complex, high-risk situations.

PRE-PROCEDURAL CONSIDERATIONS

Before positioning or moving the patient consider the following factors.

Assessment

Learning Activity 6.2 Case study: What are the risk factors for developing pressure sores?

An 86-year-old gentleman has just been admitted onto your ward. He had a fall at home last night resulting in a fractured neck of the femur. You have been asked to assess his risk of developing pressure sores.

1 What are his main risk factors for developing a pressure sore at this time?
2 What tool could you use to assess this risk?
3 What manual handling aids might you require to assist this patient with repositioning?

See the end of the chapter for the answers.

Pressure/skin care

All clinical staff should be aware of the risk factors for developing pressure sores. These include age, malnutrition, immobility, loss of sensation, vascular disease and acute illness. The risk of skin damage when the patient is positioned or moved will be increased by factors including incontinence, profuse perspiration and obesity (Hickey and Powers 2009). Direct pressure to the skin and friction during movement of patients are two of the most common causes of injury to the skin that can lead to pressure ulcers. Sometimes a scoring system such as Norton or Waterlow is used to identify patients at risk. These are helpful but should only be used as an aide mémoire for staff and not replace clinical judgement (RCN 2001). Any patient with a pressure sore or who is thought to be at risk of developing one should be positioned with the use of pressure-relieving equipment such as specialist mattresses and cushions. Additional use of pillows/towels may be required depending on individual assessment.

Wounds

Consider the location of wounds and injuries when selecting a comfortable position. Ideally positions should avoid pressure on or stretching of any wounds and consideration should be given to the timing of dressing changes, which ideally should be done prior to positioning to avoid disturbing the patient twice.

Sensation

Take extra care in positioning patients with decreased sensation as numbness and paraesthesia (abnormal skin sensation) may result in skin damage as the patient is unaware of pressure or chafing. These patients may not be able to adjust their position or alert nursing staff so it is very important to check the patient's skin regularly for areas of redness or breakdown.

Oedema/swelling

Where possible, swollen limbs should not be left dependent but be supported on pillows/footstool as elevation will help to maximize venous return and minimize further swelling. Oedema may result in pain, fragile skin or loss of joint movement.

Pain

Ensure the patient has optimal pain relief before moving. Patients who are pain free at rest may need additional analgesic cover before movement. It is important to allow adequate time for any pain medication to take effect.

Weakness

Consider the patient's ability to maintain the position. Additional support may be required in the form of pillows or towels to maintain the desired posture.

Limitations of joint and soft tissue range (contractures)

Soft tissue changes and contractures occur through disuse in normal muscle (Jones and Moffatt 2002). As a result, restrictions in joint range may mean that positions need to be modified or become inappropriate.

If there is the potential for any joint or soft tissue restrictions then liaise with the PT or OT regarding any specific exercises or positions necessary for the patient to avoid developing contractures. This may affect position choice or may involve incorporating appropriate splinting to maintain muscle length.

Communication and involvement with the multidisciplinary team (MDT) will assist rehabilitation interventions as treatment could be incorporated during positional changes. This potentially allows for more physical assistance in moving the patient without involving other staff, allows collaborative working such as changing sheets, repositioning and assessment of pressure areas, and will minimize unnecessary disturbance of the patient (Hough 2001).

Fracture or suspected fracture

Patients with unstable fractures or suspected fractures should not be moved and the area should be well supported. A change of position could result in pain, fracture displacement and associated complications. Patients with osteoporosis or metastatic bony disease with unexplained bony pain should be treated as having a suspected fracture. Osteoporosis refers to a reduction in the quantity and quality of bone due to loss of both bone mineral and protein content. Risk factors for osteoporosis increase with age and include being female, Caucasian and postmenopausal, having a low body mass index (BMI), a positive family history of osteoporosis, a sedentary lifestyle and smoking. Before an osteoporotic lesion becomes apparent radiologically, at least 50% of bone mass must be lost so that pain may precede radiological changes (McGarvey 1990).

Altered tone

Tone can be altered by positioning with either positive or negative consequences. Further information on moving and handling patients with either neurological impairment or who are unconscious is outlined later in this chapter.

Spinal stability

It is important to establish spinal stability before positioning or moving the patient. The specifics of moving and positioning a patient with spinal cord compression are discussed later in this chapter.

Medical devices associated with treatment

Care should be taken to avoid pulling on lines or causing occlusion if the patient has a catheter, intravenous infusion, venous access device or drain. Pulling on devices may cause pain and/or injury to the patient and be detrimental to care. Prior to any moving or positioning procedure, ensure that any electrical pumps have been disconnected and sets are untangled and flowing freely. Once the moving or positioning procedure has been completed, ensure all devices are reconnected.

Medical status/cardiovascular instability

The defining parameter for mobilization is that the patient's oxygen transport system is capable of increasing the oxygen supply to meet metabolic demand (Pryor and Prasad 2008). Patients who are medically unstable may become more unstable during movement. Therefore, patients who are acutely unwell should be monitored carefully during and after any change of position or when mobilizing.

Fatigue

Fatigue can be a distressing symptom, so advice and help should be given to the patient about how to pace their everyday activities. Barsevick et al. (2002) describe energy conservation as 'the deliberate planned management of one's personal energy resources in order to prevent their depletion'. Therefore, prioritizing activities may help to avoid engaging in tasks that are unnecessary or of little value (Cooper 2006).

Cognitive state

It is important to explain to the patient the reasons for moving and positioning appropriate to their level of understanding. Always explain what will happen step by step and give clear instructions to the patient to enable them to participate in the movement.

It is known that impaired cognition (the mental process involved in gaining knowledge and comprehension) and depression are intrinsic risk factors for falls in older people (DH 2001).

Privacy and dignity

In order to maintain privacy and dignity during positioning, ensure the environment is as private as possible by shutting the door and/or the curtains prior to moving the patient (CSP 2014). It may be appropriate to ask visitors to wait outside. The process of uncovering the patient may make them feel vulnerable and/or distressed, so keep them covered as much as is practically possible during the procedure. Make sure catheter bags and drains are hung as discreetly as possible under the patient's bed/chair.

Patient explanation/instruction

Explain to the patient the reasons for changing their position and where possible gain their verbal consent. If patients are fully informed of the planned change in position they may be able to participate with the manoeuvre and reduce the need for assistance.

Documentation/liaison with MDT

It is important to check to see if there are any instructions or indications regarding positioning or moving the patient in their documentation. If unsure then check with the MDT as this may provide guidance on what positions are more appropriate and any special precautions that need to be considered prior to moving and positioning.

Recent initiatives have looked at specific areas to improve patient care following the publication of *High Impact Actions for Nursing and Midwifery* in 2009 (RCM et al. 2009). One area identified in this report is falls prevention with the aim of demonstrating a reduction in the number of falls in older people within NHS care.

Risk assessment: prevention of falls

The National Patient Safety Agency reported 152,000 falls in England and Wales in acute hospitals in 2009, 26,000 in mental health trusts and 28,000 in community hospitals. The number of falls is set to rise in line with increasing numbers of older and frail people with more complex health needs (RCM et al. 2009).

DEFINITION

A fall is a sudden, unintentional change in position causing an individual to land at a lower level, on an object, the floor or the ground other than as a consequence of sudden onset of paralysis, epileptic seizure or overwhelming external force.

Falls are the most common cause of serious injury in older people, and of hospital attendance and are the most common precipitating event for care home admission (NICE 2013). Falls may result in a loss of confidence or independence which, in turn, may lead to a need for increased or extended support from statutory health and social care agencies (Ward et al. 2010). Preventing falls in the older person has been well described in national guidance and all prevention programmes should include particular reference to the care of the older person (Age UK 2013, Becker et al. 2003, Oliver et al. 2007, Ward et al. 2010).

The causes of falls are complex and elderly hospital patients are particularly likely to be vulnerable to falling due to medical conditions including delirium, cardiac, neurological or musculoskeletal conditions, side-effects from medication or problems with their balance, strength or mobility. Problems such as reduced or poor memory can create a greater risk of falls when someone is out of their normal environment and on a hospital ward, as they are less able to see and avoid any hazards. Continence problems can mean patients are vulnerable to falling whilst making urgent journeys to the toilet. However, patient safety has to be balanced with independence, rehabilitation, privacy, and dignity – a patient who is not allowed to walk alone will very quickly become a patient who is unable to walk alone. Addressing inpatient falls and fall-related injuries is therefore a challenge for all healthcare organizations (NPSA 2010, Patient Safety First 2009).

The prevention of falls is complex and, as with many other types of risk assessment and prevention, a systematic multiprofessional approach is recommended. Individual needs and the different environmental factors associated with different settings – for example, home, care home or hospital – will need to be assessed regularly.

Many interventions have been demonstrated to reduce the incidence of falls, including exercise programmes, identification bracelets, alarm systems and risk assessments (Ward et al. 2010). Part of the Chief Nursing Officer for England's programme of 'High Impact Actions for Care' includes 'Staying Safe – Preventing Falls' (Ward et al. 2010), the aim of which is to demonstrate a year-on-year reduction in the number of falls sustained by older people in NHS-provided care. However, patient safety must always be carefully balanced with patient independence and their right to make informed choices (RCM et al. 2009). The following checklist has been developed for healthcare professionals to use on the wards regularly throughout the day to reduce the risk factors for falling.

- Hydration: making sure patients have something to drink.
- Checking toilet needs.
- Ensuring patients have the right footwear.

- Decluttering the area.
- Making sure patients can reach what they need, such as the call bell.
- Making sure bedrails are correctly fitted.
- Ensuring patients have an appropriate walking aid, if applicable.

It is the responsibility of all staff to undertake regular inspections of their work areas to determine when factors are causing a falls risk and take appropriate action. All staff should be trained in how to reduce/prevent falls within their areas. Every patient should be provided with a clear orientation to the ward and ward layout and their individual needs considered. Clear signage to key areas such as bathrooms and toilets is important, especially to elderly patients who may become easily disorientated outside their familiar environment.

It is the responsibility of all staff to report any environmental hazards within their working areas and to ensure that spillages are removed and appropriate signage is used to warn people of hazards.

 Learning Activity 6.3

Learning in practice: Falls prevention

Take a look at the checklist for falls prevention (above).

- Considering your clinical area, what measures are currently taken to prevent falls occcurring throughout the day and night?
- What can you do, within your own scope of practice, to help reduce the risk of patient falls?

RISK FACTORS

It is important to consider the risk of falls when undertaking a manual handling risk assessment on patient admission. The patient's risk of falls should be reconsidered either at weekly intervals or if the patient experiences a fall.

Falls generally occur due to a complex interaction of diverse risk factors and situations. Over 400 risk factors associated with falling have been reported (NHS Centre for Reviews and Dissemination 1996), but these can be broadly divided into intrinsic (person-related), extrinsic (environment-related) and behavioural (activity-related) risk factors (Connell and Wolf 1997, Stalenhoef et al. 2002).

Intrinsic risk factors

- Previous fall/fracture/stumbles and trips
- Impaired balance and gait/restricted mobility
- Medical history of Parkinson's disease, stroke, arthritis, cardiac abnormalities
- Fear of falling
- Medication including polypharmacy, psychotropic medication
- Dizziness
- Postural hypotension
- Syncope
- Reduced muscle strength
- Foot problems
- Incontinence
- Cognitive impairment
- Impaired vision
- Low mood
- Pain

Extrinsic risk factors

- Stairs and steps
- Clutter and tripping hazards, for example rugs, flexes
- Floor coverings
- Poor lighting, glare, shadows
- Lack of appropriate adaptations such as grab rails, stair rails
- Low furniture
- No access to telephone or alarm call system
- Poor heating
- Thresholds and doors
- Difficult access to property, bins, garden, uneven ground
- Inappropriate walking aids
- Pets

Behavioural risk factors

- Limited physical activity/exercise
- Poor nutrition/fluid intake
- Alcohol intake
- Carrying, reaching, bending, risk-taking behaviour such as climbing on chairs, use of ladders; footwear

In order to reduce the risk, it is important to investigate every fall that does occur and understand the circumstances surrounding it. A useful way of analysing falls is to categorize them and to map areas on the ward or areas in the hospital where more than one patient has fallen. Common themes can then be identified and strategies can be implemented to reduce the risk.

Positioning the patient: in bed

EVIDENCE-BASED APPROACHES

Rationale

Falls from the bed are common and this must be considered when positioning a patient in bed.

Equipment

Sliding sheets are used to assist patients to roll or change position in bed. Due to the slippery surface of the slide sheet fabric, friction is reduced and it is easier to move or relocate the patient with very minimal effort or discomfort.

Procedure guideline 6.1 **Positioning the patient: supine**

Essential equipment

- Pillows/towels
- Sliding sheets/manual handling equipment if indicated following risk assessment in accordance with local manual handling policy
- Bed extension for tall patients

Pre-procedure

Action	Rationale
1 Explain and discuss the procedure with the patient.	To ensure that the patient understands the procedure and gives their valid consent (NMC 2013, **C**).

(continued)

Procedure guideline 6.1 Positioning the patient: supine *(continued)*

Action	Rationale
2 Wash hands thoroughly or use an alcohol-based handrub.	To reduce the risk of contamination and cross-infection (Fraise and Bradley 2009, **E**).
3 Ensure that the bed is at the optimum height for handlers. If two handlers are required try to match handlers' heights as far as possible.	To minimize the risk of injury to the practitioner (Smith 2011, **C**).
Procedure	
4 *Either:*	
Place one pillow squarely under the patient's head. For patients with an airway or who have had recent head and neck surgery, take care not to occlude or displace tubes or increase pressure to vulnerable areas.	To support the head in a neutral position and to compensate for the natural lordosis (anatomical concavity) of the cervical spine. **E** To ensure the airway is patent. **E** To increase patient support and comfort. **E**
Or:	
Use two pillows in a 'butterfly' position so that two layers of pillow support the head with one layer of pillow under each shoulder.	This may be necessary for the patient with pain, breathlessness (see 'Moving and positioning of the patient with respiratory compromise') or an existing kyphosis (anatomical convexity of the spine). **E**
Or:	
Use a folded towel under the patient's head if this provides natural spinal alignment.	To prevent excessive neck flexion. **E**
5 Ensure the patient lies centrally in the bed.	To ensure spinal and limb alignment. **E** To reduce the risk of falls by ensuring the patient is not too close to the edge of the bed. **E**
6 Place pillows and/or towels under individual limbs to provide maximum support for the patient with painful, weak or oedematous limbs.	To ensure patient comfort. **E, P**
7 Ensure the patient's feet are fully supported by the mattress. For taller patients use a bed extension if required.	To ensure patient comfort. **E**
8 Place a pillow at the end of the hospital bed to support the ankles at 90° of flexion if the patient has weakness or is immobile around the ankle.	To ensure patient comfort. **E** To prevent loss of ankle movement. **E**

Positioning the patient: sitting in bed

EVIDENCE-BASED APPROACHES

Rationale

Indications

Patients should be encouraged to sit up in bed periodically if their medical condition prevents them from sitting out in the chair. If the patient is unable to participate fully in the procedure, manual handling equipment should be used to help achieve the desired position. Attention should also be given to sitting posture. Poor posture is one of the most common causes of low back pain which may frequently be brought on by sitting for a long time in a poor position (McKenzie 2006) as it causes increased pressure in the disc (Claus et al. 2008).

Contraindications

Post lumbar puncture, patients should lie flat to prevent dural headache in accordance with local policy.

Spinal instability

Refer to 'Moving and positioning of the patient with actual or suspected spinal cord compression or spinal cord injury' (Procedure 6.14: Log rolling for suspected/confirmed cervical spinal instability).

Procedure guideline 6.2 Positioning the patient: sitting in bed

See Figure 6.4.

Essential equipment

- Pillows
- Manual handling equipment may be required, for example sliding sheets or a hoist, depending on local policy

Pre-procedure

Action	Rationale
1 Explain and discuss the procedure with the patient.	To ensure that the patient understands the procedure and gives their valid consent (NMC 2013, **C**).

Figure 6.4 **Sitting up in bed.**

2 Wash hands thoroughly or use an alcohol-based handrub.	To reduce the risk of contamination and cross-infection (Fraise and Bradley 2009, **E**).
3 Ensure that the bed is at the optimum height for handlers. If two handlers are required try to match handlers' heights as far as possible.	To minimize the risk of injury to the practitioner (Smith 2011, **C**).
Procedure	
4 Ask the patient to sit up in the centre of the bed. The angle at which the patient sits may be influenced by pain, fatigue, abdominal distension or level of confusion/agitation.	To reduce the risk of falls by ensuring the patient is not too close to the edge of the bed. To encourage haemodynamic (physical factors that govern blood flow) stability. **E** To enable effective breathing patterns, maximizing basal expansion (Pryor and Prasad 2008, **R4**). To assist in functional activities such as eating and drinking. **E**
5 Ask the patient to position their hips in line with the hinge of the automatic mattress elevator or backrest of the bed.	To ensure good postural alignment, that is, flexing at the hip when sitting up in bed. **E** To prevent strain on the spine. **E**
6 Place a pillow under the patient's knees or use the electrical control of the bed to slightly bend the patient's knees. Extra care should be taken if the patient has a femoral line or is on haemofiltration (a renal replacement therapy usually used to treat acute renal failure).	To reduce strain on the lumbar spine. **E** To maintain the position. **E**
7 Place a pillow under individual or both upper limbs for patients with a chest drain, upper limb weakness, trunk weakness, surgery involving shoulder/upper limb/breast/thorax, fungating wounds involving axilla, breast and shoulder, upper limb/truncal lymphoedema or fractures involving ribs or upper limbs.	To provide upper limb support. **E** To maintain trunk alignment. **E** To encourage basal expansion (Pryor and Prasad 2008, **E**).

Positioning the patient: side-lying

EVIDENCE-BASED APPROACHES

Rationale

Indications

This can be a useful position for patients with:

- compromised venous return, for example; pelvic/abdominal mass, pregnancy
- global motor weakness
- risk of developing pressure sores
- unilateral pelvic or lower limb pain
- altered tone (see 'Moving and positioning the patient with neurological impairment')
- fatigue
- chest infection, for gravity-assisted drainage of secretions
- lung pathology (see 'Moving and positioning the patient with respiratory compromise')
- abdominal distension, for example ascites (intraperitoneal accumulation of a watery fluid), bulky disease, to optimize lung volume (see 'Moving and positioning the patient with respiratory compromise').

Contraindications

Suspected or actual spinal fracture or instability.

Procedure guideline 6.3 **Positioning the patient: side-lying**

See Figure 6.5.

Essential equipment

- Pillows
- Manual handling equipment may be required following risk assessment, for example sliding sheets or a hoist, depending on local policy

Pre-procedure

Action	Rationale
1 Explain and discuss the procedure with the patient.	To ensure that the patient understands the procedure and gives their valid consent (NMC 2013, **C**).
2 Wash hands thoroughly or use an alcohol-based handrub.	To reduce the risk of contamination and cross-infection (Fraise and Bradley 2009, **E**).
3 Ensure that the bed is at the optimum height for handlers. If two handlers are required try to match handlers' heights as far as possible.	To minimize the risk of injury to the practitioner (Smith 2011, **C**).

Procedure

Action	Rationale
4 Place one or two pillows in a 'butterfly' position under the patient's head, ensuring the airway remains patent. Extra care should be taken for those patients with a tracheostomy, central lines or recent head and neck surgery.	To support the head in mid-position. **E** To support shoulder contours. **E**
5 Ask/assist the patient to semi-flex the lowermost leg at the hip and the knee. Extra care should be taken with the degree of flexion for those patients who have hip or knee pain or loss of movement, fracture involving the femur or pelvis, leg oedema, femoral lines or other venous access devices. Ensure the patient is lying centrally in the bed.	To support the patient in a stable position and prevent rolling. **E** To reduce the risk of falls by ensuring the patient is not too close to the edge of the bed. **E**
6 *Either:* Ask/assist the patient to semi-flex the uppermost leg at the hip and knee. Use a pillow for support under the leg placed on the bed. *Or:* Place a pillow between the patient's knees.	To prevent lumbar spine rotation. **E** To support the pelvic girdle. **E** To aid pressure care. **E**
7 Place the underneath arm in front with scapula protracted, i.e. pushed forward position (this would not be appropriate for patients with shoulder pathology). Extra care should be taken with patients with low tone in the affected arm, swollen arms or who have access lines in that arm.	To promote patient comfort. **E** To promote shoulder alignment. **E** To provide additional support and comfort. **E**

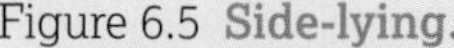

Figure 6.5 **Side-lying.**

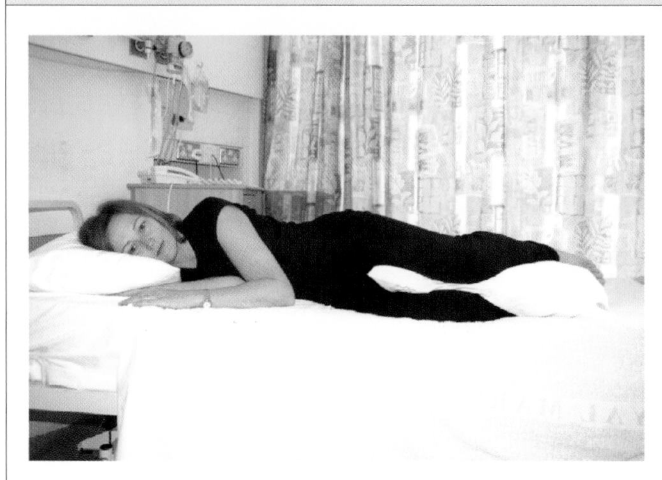

Procedure guideline 6.4 **Positioning the patient: lying down to sitting up**

See Figures 6.6, 6.7 and 6.8.

Essential equipment

- Manual handling equipment may be required dependent on risk assessment, for example sliding sheets or a hoist, depending on local policy

Pre-procedure

Action	Rationale
1 Explain and discuss the procedure with the patient.	To ensure that the patient understands the procedure and gives their valid consent (NMC 2013, **C**).
2 Wash hands thoroughly or use an alcohol-based handrub.	To reduce the risk of contamination and cross-infection (Fraise and Bradley 2009, **E**).
3 Ensure that the bed is at the optimum height for patients or handlers. If two handlers are required try to match handlers' heights as far as possible.	To minimize the risk of injury to the practitioner (Smith 2011, **C**).
Procedure	
4 Ask the patient to bend both knees and turn their head towards the direction they are moving (see Figure 6.6). Abdominal wounds should be supported by the patient's hands. Extra care should be taken with patients who have joint pathology, oedema, ascites or positional vertigo (dizziness or giddiness).	To assist the patient to roll using their bodyweight. **E**
5 Ask patient to reach towards the side of the bed with the uppermost arm and roll on to their side.	
6 Ask the patient to bend their knees and lower their feet over the edge of the bed.	
7 Ask the patient to push through the underneath elbow and the upper arm on the bed to push up into sitting (see Figure 6.7). As the patient sits up, monitor changes in pain or dizziness which could indicate postural hypotension or vertigo. Be aware that the patient with neurological symptoms or weakness may not have safe sitting balance and may be at risk of falling.	To help to lever the patient into a sitting position using the weight of their legs. **E**
8 Achieve upright sitting position with appropriate alignment of body parts (see Figure 6.8).	To ensure safe sitting position achieved. **E**

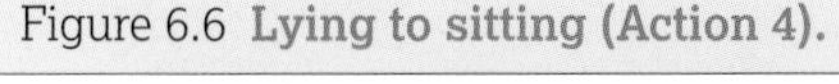

Figure 6.6 **Lying to sitting (Action 4).**

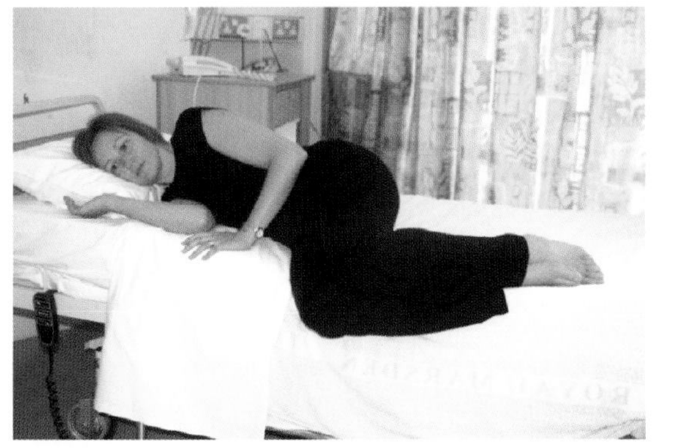

Figure 6.7 **Lying to sitting (Action 7).**

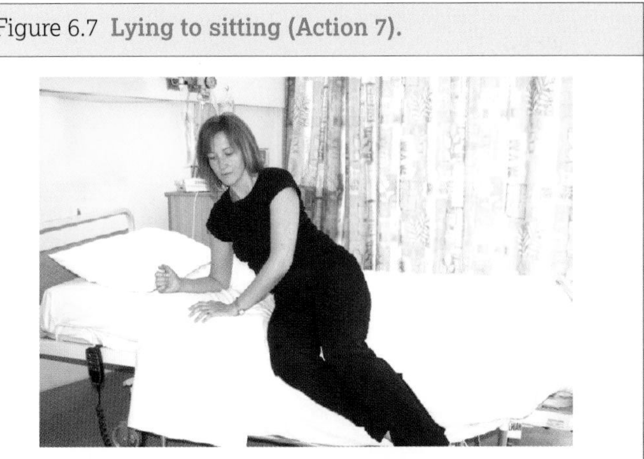

Figure 6.8 **Lying to sitting (Action 8).**

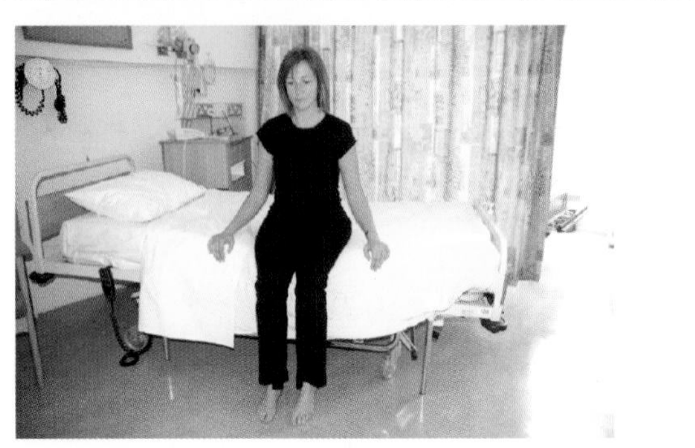

Positioning the patient: in a chair/wheelchair

PRE-PROCEDURAL CONSIDERATIONS

Equipment

Pressure cushion

This is a piece of equipment designed to evenly redistribute the weight of a patient to provide pressure relief for those who are vulnerable to skin breakdown. It is an effective aid to increasing patients' sitting tolerance. There are various types available and they are usually provided by the OT specific to the needs of the patient.

Procedure guideline 6.5 **Positioning the patient: in a chair/wheelchair**

Essential equipment

- Upright chair with arms that provide support from the elbow to wrist – if using a wheelchair, make certain that the chair has been measured where possible by an OT to ensure correct fit and position of the foot rests
- Manual handling equipment may be required following risk assessment, for example a hoist, depending on local policy
- Pillows/rolled-up towel
- Footstool if the patient has lower limb oedema (swelling)
- Pressure cushion

Procedure

Action	Rationale
1 Place a pressure cushion in the chair and ask the patient to sit well back in the chair. They should have a maximum 90° angle at their hips and knee joints. The patient may not be able to achieve this position if they have pain, abdominal distension or hip/back pain. It may be necessary to refer the patient to the OT for chair raises, a specialized cushion or appropriate seating if a comfortable or safe position cannot be achieved.	Patients with reduced mobility are at greater risk of pressure skin damage. To provide a stable base of support for balance and reduce the risk of falls. **E** To ensure good body alignment. **E** To achieve a safe sitting position. **E**
2 Place a pillow or rolled-up towel in the small of the patient's back as is comfortable for the patient.	To allow the patient's back to be supported in a good position. **E**
3 Ensure the patient's feet are resting on the floor or supported surface. Use pillows or a rolled-up towel to provide support under the feet if necessary. Make sure the patient's feet are supported on the foot rests if using a wheelchair.	To provide postural alignment and support the lumbar spine. **E**
4 If the patient has lower leg oedema, use a foot stool, ensuring the whole leg and foot are supported and avoiding hyperextension (defined as an excessive extension of a limb or joint) at the knees.	To improve venous drainage. **E**
5 Discourage the patient from crossing their legs.	To reduce risk of developing a DVT (O'Donovan et al. 2006, **R4**).

Moving the patient from sitting to standing

PRE-PROCEDURAL CONSIDERATIONS

If the patient stands from the side of a hospital bed, it is helpful to raise the bed slightly. This reduces the work of standing for the patient, ensuring that the hips are level or higher than the knees with the feet in contact with the floor.

A physiotherapy referral may be appropriate.

Procedure guideline 6.6 **Moving from sitting to standing: assisting the patient**

See Figures 6.9 and 6.10.

Essential equipment

- Walking aid if required (if previously issued by physiotherapist)
- Suitable non-slip, well-fitting, supportive and flat footwear (if not available then bare feet are preferable to socks or stockings which may slip) (Figure 6.11)

Procedure

Action	Rationale
1 Ask the patient to lean forward and 'shuffle' (by transferring their weight from side to side) and bring their bottom closer to the front of the chair or edge of the bed (see Figure 6.9).	To bring the patient's weight over their feet. **E**
2 Ask the patient to move their feet back so they are slightly tucked under the chair with their feet hip width apart.	To provide a stable base prior to moving. **E**
3 Instruct the patient to lean forward from their trunk.	To help initiate movement. **E** To facilitate a normal pattern of movement. **E**
4 Instruct the patient to push through their hands on the arms of the chair or surface on which they are sitting as they stand (see Figure 6.10). Encourage a forward and upward motion whilst extending their hips and knees.	To minimize energy expenditure. **E**
5 Once standing, ask the patient to stand still for a moment to ensure balance is achieved before attempting to walk.	To ensure safe static standing and reduce the risk of falling **E**

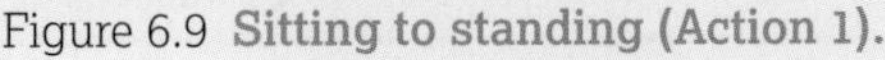

Figure 6.9 **Sitting to standing (Action 1).**

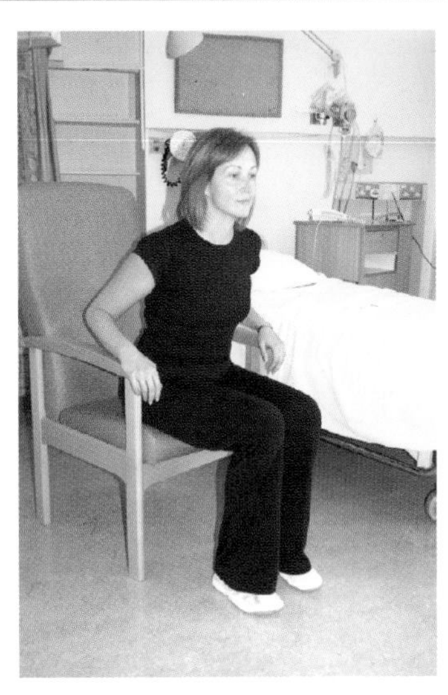

Figure 6.10 **Sitting to standing (Action 4).**

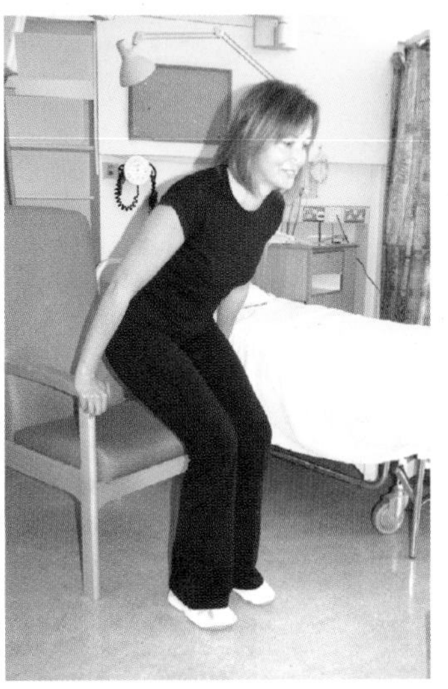

Figure 6.11 **Examples of a supportive shoe.**

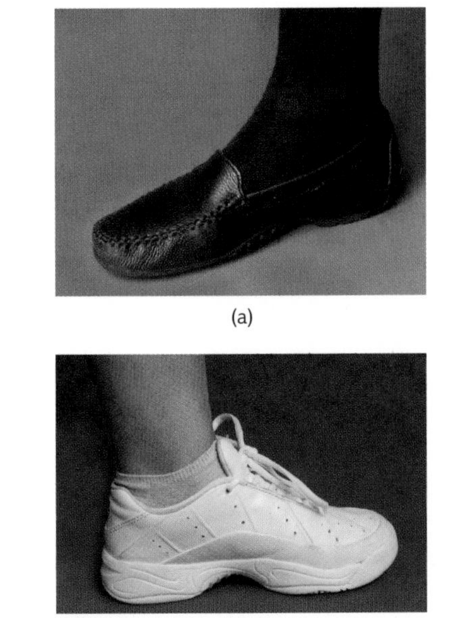

(a)

(b)

Walking

'Walking requires alternating support on one leg and then the other' (Gillis 1989).

Patients may use a variety of different walking aids to help them mobilize. All aids are designed to improve balance and therefore reduce the risk of falls.

It is assumed that patients will take equal amounts of bodyweight through both legs, defined as being fully weight bearing (FWB). If a patient has to be non-weight bearing (NWB) or partially weight bearing (PWB) this will be due to bone or joint pathology, e.g. fracture, joint instability, inflammation or infection. Restrictions in weight bearing should always be clearly documented and communicated by the medical staff. Weight bearing will also be affected by pain, weakness, sensory changes and confidence. If the patient has difficulty mobilizing, appears unsafe or is at risk of falling for any reason, refer for physiotherapy assessment.

Procedure guideline 6.7 **Assisting the patient to walk**

Essential equipment

- Walking aid if required (if previously issued by physiotherapist)
- Suitable non-slip, well-fitting, supportive and flat footwear (if not available then bare feet are preferable to socks or stockings which may slip) (see Figure 6.11)

Procedure

Action	Rationale
1 Stand next to and slightly behind the patient. If patient requires support, place your arm nearest the patient lightly around their pelvis. Your other hand should hold the patient's hand closest to you. Observe changes in pain as the patient walks.	To give appropriate support. **E** To assess patient safety and reduce the risk of falls. **E** To increase patient confidence. **E,P**
2 Give verbal supervision/cueing as required to achieve safe walking.	To provide encouragement. **E** To ensure patient safety. **E**

A physiotherapist will assess and issue the patient with an appropriate walking aid. All patients should be given verbal and written instructions on their use. If they are unsure please refer to the patient information sheets for instructions.

Learning Activity 6.4

Scenario: Assisting the patient to walk

On the ward, you have been asked to assist a female patient, who is currently seated in her chair, to walk to the toilet.

What factors should you consider prior to undertaking this activity?

See the end of the chapter for the answers.

Problem-solving table 6.1 **Prevention and resolution (Procedure guidelines 6.1, 6.2, 6.3, 6.4, 6.5, 6.6 and 6.7)**

Problem	Cause	Prevention	Action
Increase in pain/ nausea.	Change in posture and position of joints and soft tissues. Patients who are symptom-controlled at rest may suffer incidental pain when moving.	Pre-procedural symptom control. Ongoing assessment of symptoms and adjustment of medication.	Assist the patient to move slowly and offer support and reassurance where needed.
Change in medical status.	Change in position may cause a drop in blood pressure or trigger cardiovascular instability.	Monitor carefully.	Always have two people present if the patient is at risk of cardiovascular instability. Be prepared to return to original position.
Bowel/bladder elimination.	Change in position may stimulate bladder and bowels.	Put pads and pants on the patient before moving, where appropriate.	It may be necessary to stop and clean the patient before continuing to move or position.

Problem	Cause	Prevention	Action
Increase in loss of fluid, e.g. wound.	Change in position may cause breakdown of primary healing or increase in muscular activity which may increase fluid loss.	Give support to wounds during movement where possible.	Stop and alert medical team for assessment.
Loss of consciousness, fainting.	Change in position may cause decrease in blood pressure.	Allow adequate time for the patient to adjust to a more upright position. Sit patient up in bed and then sit over the edge of the bed and allow time for positional adjustment in blood pressure before attempting to stand.	Call for help and follow emergency procedure. Refer to local procedure for managing a falling patient.
Fall.	Multifactorial.	Risk assessment and planning.	Call for help and follow emergency procedure. Refer to local procedure for managing a falling patient.
Poor adherence to/toleration of sitting position.	Discomfort, reduced tolerance, cognitive issues.	Use pillows/towels to ensure patient is well supported and comfortable. A timed goal often helps with patient compliance. Start with a short time, for example 30 minutes, and build up the time slowly. Always tell the patient how long they are aiming to sit out for and make sure the call bell is within reach.	Combine sitting out with a meal time as this can help the patient to eat more easily and also help to distract the patient from the length of time they have to sit out.
Inability to maintain the position.	Patients who are weak and/ or fatigued may be at risk of slipping or falling.	Careful positioning of towels and pillows may be needed to maintain a central safe posture in the chair.	Observe the patient regularly.

 Learning Activity 6.5

Learning in practice: Manual handling equipment

Make a list of all the manual handling equipment that is available within your clinical area.

- Are there any other aids that you feel may better help you to assist patients moving and repositioning?
- Who in your clinical area might you discuss this with?

Moving and positioning the unconscious patient

DEFINITION

Consciousness is a state of awareness of self, environment and one's response to that environment. To be fully conscious means that the individual appropriately responds to the external stimuli. An altered level of consciousness represents a decrease in this full state of awareness and response to environmental stimuli (Boss 1998).

ANATOMY AND PHYSIOLOGY

Physiological changes in the unconscious patient

Unconsciousness is a physiological state in which the patient is unresponsive to sensory stimuli and lacks awareness of self and the environment (Hickey 2009). There are many central nervous system conditions that can result in the patient being in an unconscious state. The depth and duration of unconsciousness span a broad spectrum of presentations from fainting, with a momentary loss of consciousness, to prolonged coma lasting several weeks, months or even years. The physiological changes that occur in unconscious patients will depend on the cause of unconsciousness, the length of immobility while unconscious, outcome and quality of care. Also drugs, for example some muscle relaxants such as those used in intensive care, can contribute to muscle weakness, raised intraocular and intracranial pressure, electrolyte imbalances and airway tone (Booij 1996). Unconsciousness can lead to problematic changes for patients which have implications for nursing interventions, including moving and positioning.

EVIDENCE-BASED APPROACHES

Principles of care

The general principles of care already mentioned earlier in the chapter are relevant to this section. However, there are some other general principles that also should be considered for these patients.

Sedation

In the critically ill patient, sedation is an essential part of the management. In addition to managing the primary neurological problem, the nurse must also incorporate a rehabilitation framework to maintain intact function, prevent complications and disabilities, and restore lost function to the maximum possible.

Communication

There is evidence that unconscious patients are aware of what is happening to them and can hear conversations around them (Jacobson and Winslow 2000, Lawrence 1995). It is therefore important to tell them what is going to happen; that they are going to be moved, and explain the procedure just as it would be explained to a conscious patient.

Immobility

The human body is designed for physical activity and movement. Therefore any lack of exercise, regardless of reason, can result in multisystem deconditioning, anatomical and physiological changes. Guidance from a physiotherapist for passive exercises early in the period of unconsciousness may help in the prevention of further complications. There is, however, no evidence to justify the inclusion of regular passive movements within the standard management of a patient's care. Intervention should be specific to the patient's presentation (Harrison 2000, Pryor and Prasad 2008).

The risk of deep vein thrombosis and pulmonary embolism is increased in the unconscious patient. This is due to several factors including blood pooling in the legs, hypercoagulability and prolonged pressure from immobility in bed (Hickey and Powers 2009).

EFFECTS OF IMMOBILITY OF MUSCLE

- *Decreased muscle strength:* the degree of loss varies with the particular muscle groups and the degree of immobility. The antigravitational muscles of the legs lose strength twice as quickly as the arm muscles and recovery takes longer.
- *Muscle atrophy*: this means loss of muscle mass. When the muscle is relaxed, it atrophies about twice as rapidly as in a stretched position. Increased muscle tone prevents complete atrophy so patients with upper motor neurone disease lose less muscle mass than those with lower motor neurone disease (Hickey and Powers 2009). For more information see 'Moving and positioning the neurological patient with tonal problems'.

Respiratory function

Due to the immobility of the unconscious patient, there is an increased threat of developing respiratory complications such as atelectasis, pneumonia, aspiration and airway obstruction. Respiratory assessment should be carried out prior to moving and changing position in order to provide a baseline that can be referred to following the procedure. The assessment should include checking patency of the airway, monitoring the rate, pattern and work of breathing, use of a pulse oximeter (an instrument for measuring the proportion of oxygenated haemoglobin in the blood) and measuring blood gases to assess adequacy of gaseous exchange.

Patients may require mechanical ventilation for the following reasons.

- Inability to ventilate adequately, for example post-anaesthesia or inspiratory muscle fatigue or weakness.
- Inability to protect own airway or presenting with upper airway obstruction.
- Ability to breathe adequately but may be inadvisable depending on diagnosis, for example with an acute head injury.

Mechanical ventilation may be required for days, weeks or even months (MacIntyre and Branson 2009). It is worth remembering that mechanically ventilated patients often cannot express any sort of preference for certain body positions. If the patient is intubated with an endotracheal tube, they are at increased risk of developing nosocomial infections (Hickey and Powers 2009) so it is important that lung volumes and respiratory mechanics should be continuously monitored (Hickey and Powers 2009). For more information see 'Moving and positioning the patient with respiratory compromise'.

Cardiovascular function

Immobility can cause changes in cardiovascular function, for example increased cardiac workload, decreased cardiac output and decreased blood pressure. In addition, the positioning of the unconscious patient will cause central fluid shift, from the legs to the thorax and head, so the head of the unconscious patient with raised intracranial pressure may need to be elevated to at least 30° (Hickey and Powers 2009).

Changes in cardiovascular function may be secondary to neurological changes so the patient's neurological function should be monitored. Hypovolaemia, which is a blood disorder consisting of a decrease in the volume of circulating blood, sepsis or cardiogenic shock, which occurs when there is failure of the pump action of the heart resulting in reduced cardiac output, are other factors that should be considered. This is because they will cause cardiovascular instability and should be treated accordingly (Geraghty 2005).

Moving and positioning the patient with an artificial airway

DEFINITION

Some patients, whether unconscious or not, may not be able to maintain a 'safe' airway and therefore may require an artificial airway to support the respiratory system. Patients may have a particular airway depending upon their individual need and presentation. The different airways include:

- nasal
- endotracheal
- tracheostomy.

For more detailed information regarding these and other specific care issues and including anatomy and physiology, see Chapter 9: Respiratory care.

EVIDENCE-BASED APPROACHES

Principles of care

Maintaining a patent artificial airway

When moving patients with an artificial airway, it is important to maintain neutral head and neck alignment within the movement plane. It is sensible to have one member of staff in sole charge of looking after the patient's artificial airway to avoid risks of trauma, dislodgement and occlusion and, if ventilated, prolonged disconnection from oxygen source. Changing position will also alter the neck musculature so it is important to ensure the tracheostomy tapes are tied securely before and after moving the patient.

With newly formed tracheostomies there is an increased risk of dislodgement 7–10 days following the procedure as the surrounding fascia and muscle need to repair to form the tract (Hough 2001). During this time it is important to have the following equipment by the patient's bedside:

- tracheal dilators
- two spare tracheostomy tubes, one a size smaller
- tracheostomy tapes
- spare inner cannula
- inner tube cleaners, oxygen supply and tracheostomy mask
- humidification
- suction equipment
- Ambu-bag.

These are essential in case the patient's airway is compromised (for guidance on how to use this equipment see Chapter 9: Respiratory care).

Emergency situations

The three most significant life-threatening emergency situations with a tracheostomy tube are blockage, displacement and haemorrhage. These are discussed in more depth in Chapter 9: Respiratory care. If any of these occur whilst moving your patient, stop and call for assistance immediately.

Staff should not be moving a patient with a tracheostomy, particularly a new tracheostomy, unless they are experienced in managing these emergency situations or working alongside someone who is.

LEGAL AND PROFESSIONAL ISSUES

Consent

If an individual is unconscious, an understanding of the Mental Capacity Act 2005 is essential.

PRE-PROCEDURAL CONSIDERATIONS

It is important to ensure regular positional changes, as with any patient unable to move themselves (Harrison 2000), to help maintain pressure areas and reduce complications of prolonged bedrest. Ideally, the patient should be moved 2 hourly and positions alternated between side-lying and supine.

It is important to consider fitting antiembolic stockings on the patient if appropriate and in line with local trust policy. These help reduce the risk of venous thromboembolism (Geraghty 2005). See Chapter 13: Perioperative care.

Equipment

Artificial airway

If the patient has a tracheostomy, ensure the appropriate equipment is at the bedside (see Chapter 9: Respiratory care) and the tracheostomy tapes are tightly secured.

Procedure guideline 6.8 **Positioning the unconscious patient or patient with an airway in supine**

See Figures 6.12, 6.13, 6.14.

Essential equipment

- Manual handling equipment may be required following risk assessment, for example sliding sheets or a hoist, depending on local policy
- Pillows
- Towels
- Splints
- Bed extension for tall patients
- At least three members of staff to move patient; refer to local trust policy
- If patient has artificial airway, one extra staff member to be in charge of airway
- Appropriate emergency airway equipment at bedside in line with local trust policy

Pre-procedure

Action	Rationale
1 Explain the procedure to the patient. If the patient is alert and has an airway, ensure they understand the procedure and give their valid consent.	To inform the patient of the procedure, even if unconscious (NMC 2013, **C**).
2 Wash hands thoroughly or use an alcohol-based handrub.	To reduce the risk of contamination and cross-infection (Fraise and Bradley 2009, **E**).
3 Ensure that the bed is at the optimum height for handlers. If two handlers are required try to match handlers' heights as far as possible.	To minimize the risk of injury to the practitioner (Smith 2011, **C**).
4 It is important to document the patient's vital signs prior to moving.	This will provide a baseline for any changes that may occur during the moving or positioning procedure.
Procedure	
5 Head: maintain proper alignment of head and neck; support with pillow or towel roll.	Helps to maintain a patent airway. **P**
6 Elevate the head of the bed by 30°.	Helps reduce the risk of nosocomial pneumonia (Drakulovic et al. 1999, **R1b**; Methany and Frantz 2013, **E**). This facilitates the drainage of secretions from the oropharynx, minimizes the risk of aspiration, assists the maintenance of adequate cerebral perfusion pressure and promotes an effective breathing pattern (Hickey and Powers 2009, **E**).
7 Body: position in alignment with spine (utilize towels and pillows).	This helps to maintain correct alignment of the body and minimize complications such as contractures. It will also help to maintain musculoskeletal function (Geraghty 2005, **E**).
8 Limbs:	
Upper:	
Support arms and wrists on pillows and towels (see Figure 6.12) or splints (see Figure 6.13); flex the arms at the elbow.	To prevent shoulder drag and wrist drop (Geraghty 2005, **E**).
Lower:	
Place a pillow between the knees, use pillows or splints to flex the ankles parallel to the feet, align the hips with the head (see Figure 6.14).	To prevent skin breakdown and foot drop (Geraghty 2005, **E**). To prevent internal rotation of the upper leg (Hickey and Powers 2009, **E**).

(continued)

Figure 6.12 **Hand resting on towel.**

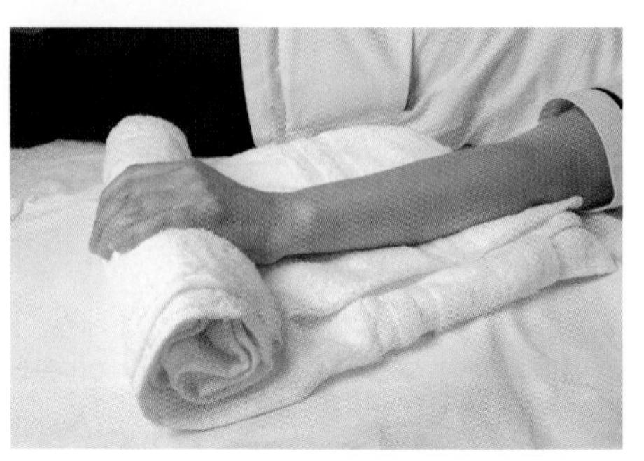

Figure 6.13 **Hand resting in splint.**

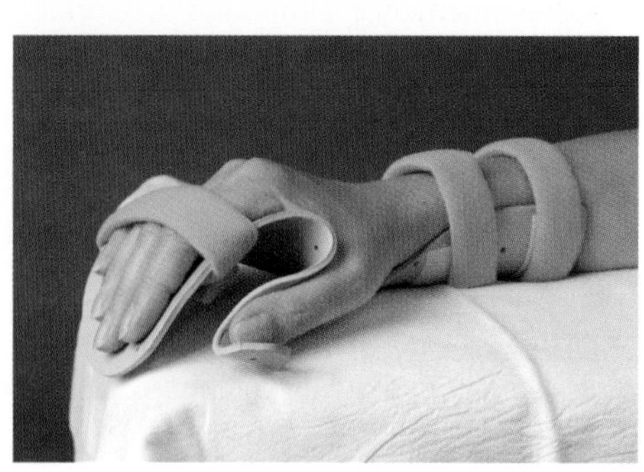

Figure 6.14 **Foot resting in splint.**

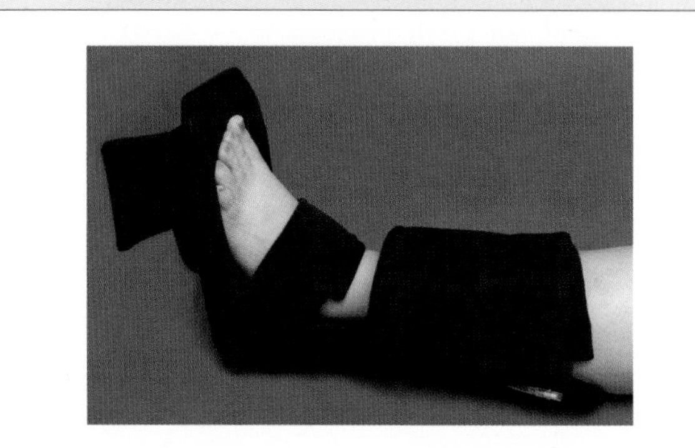

Post-procedure

9 Monitor colour, temperature and pulses of the limbs.	To enhance pulmonary function, prevent atelectasis and hypostatic pneumonia (Geraghty 2005, **E**) and to help preserve musculoskeletal function and prevent deep vein thrombosis (Hickey and Powers 2009, **E**).

Procedure guideline 6.9 **Positioning the unconscious patient or patient with an airway in side-lying**

Essential equipment

- Manual handling equipment may be required following risk assessment, for example sliding sheets or a hoist, depending on local policy
- Pillows
- Towels
- Splints
- Bed extension for tall patients
- Minimum of three members of staff to move patient
- If patient has artificial airway, one extra staff member to be in charge of airway, and appropriate emergency equipment at bedside in line with local trust policy

Pre-procedure

Action	Rationale
1 Explain the procedure to the patient. If the patient is alert and has an airway, ensure they understand the procedure and are aware of what is going on.	To inform the patient of the procedure, even if unconscious (NMC 2013, **C**).
2 Wash hands thoroughly or use an alcohol-based handrub.	To reduce the risk of contamination and cross-infection (Fraise and Bradley 2009, **E**).

Action	Rationale
3 Ensure that the bed is at the optimal height for patients or handlers. If two handlers are required try to match handlers' heights as far as possible.	To minimize the risk of injury to the practitioner (Smith 2011, **C**).
Procedure	
4 Place one or two pillows in 'butterfly' position under the patient's head, ensuring the airway remains patent. Extra care should be taken for those patients with a tracheostomy, central lines or recent head and neck surgery.	To support the head in mid-position. **E** To support shoulder contours. **E**
5 Ask/assist the patient to semi-flex the lowermost leg at the hip and the knee. Extra care should be taken with the degree of flexion for those patients who have hip or knee pain or loss of movement, fracture involving the femur or pelvis, leg oedema, femoral lines or other venous access devices.	To support the patient in a stable position and prevent rolling. **E**
6 *Either:* Ask/assist the patient to semi-flex the uppermost leg at the hip and knee. Use a pillow to support under the leg placed on the bed. *Or:* Place a pillow between the patient's knees.	To prevent lumbar spine rotation. **E** To support the pelvic girdle. **E** To aid pressure care. **E**
7 Place the underneath arm in front with scapula protracted (this may not be appropriate for patients with shoulder pathology). Extra care should be taken with patients with low tone in the affected arm, swollen arms or who have access lines in that arm.	To promote patient comfort. **E** To promote shoulder alignment. **E** To provide additional support and comfort. **E**

Problem-solving table 6.2 **Prevention and resolution (Procedure guidelines 6.8 and 6.9)**

Problem	Cause	Prevention	Action
Change in medical status.	With any change in position, transient changes in vital signs also occur.	It is essential, due to the patient's inability to communicate, that any changes in respiratory and cardiovascular status are closely monitored with any positional change or intervention (Harden 2008, Hough 2001).	If oxygen saturation (SaO_2) drops and does not return to its usual value within 5 minutes, or heart rate (HR) increases or decreases by over 10 bpm and does not settle, the patient should be returned gently to the previous position (Hough 2001).
Joint muscle trauma.	Joints and muscles of the unconscious patient are relatively unprotected and prone to trauma (Pryor and Prasad 2008).	Ensure upon changing position that all limbs are in appropriate positions and not overstretched.	Once repositioned, ensure limbs are well supported.
Risk of excess pressures on body parts.	Body parts, such as ears, positioned without due care and attention.	Also if patient is in side-lying, ensure the ear is not twisted under the head (Hough 2001).	Move patient's head to change position of ear to a more comfortable position.
Artificial airway patency blocked.	Change of position of neck or of airway.	Ensure endotracheal/tracheostomy tube is secure. This may involve checking the cuff pressure and the endotracheal/tracheostomy ties (see Chapter 9: Respiratory care) as movement will alter the soft tissue distribution which will impact on these. Monitor vital signs closely to ensure return to normal values within 5 minutes of position change (Hough 2001).	Call for assistance immediately. Refer to Chapter 9: Respiratory care for more specific guidance on emergency management of the airway.

POST-PROCEDURAL CONSIDERATIONS

The general principles of care mentioned earlier in the chapter are relevant to this section. However, there are also some other general principles that need to be considered for these patients. It is important to ensure regular positional changes as with any patient unable to move themselves (Harrison 2000) to help maintain pressure areas and reduce complications of prolonged bedrest. Ideally, the patient should be moved 2 hourly and positions alternated between side-lying and supine.

Documentation
Alterations in level of consciousness, in cardiovascular and respiratory systems will also need to be recorded.

Learning Activity 6.6 **Case study: Moving the unconscious patient**

Ms Jones is a 56-year-old woman who has been unconscious and intubated in the intensive care unit (ICU) for the last three days following a road traffic collision. You are looking after her today along with one of the members of the ICU nursing team and have been asked to help turn the patient from lying on her right side to a supine position.

1 What are the main considerations prior to repositioning Ms Jones?
2 How many staff are required to move Ms Jones?
3 What equipment is required to assist in moving her safely?
4 What should the team be considering during the procedure?
5 What should be done after Ms Jones is repositioned?

See the end of the chapter for the answers.

Moving and positioning the patient with respiratory compromise

DEFINITION
The causes of respiratory compromise may be multifactorial and should be established before undertaking positioning interventions. Compromise may be due to medical intervention (e.g. side-effects of medication), metabolic, surgical or primary respiratory pathologies. The guidelines regarding principles of moving and positioning are applicable to these patients but particular observation is required regarding their response to the intervention.

ANATOMY AND PHYSIOLOGY
Both skeletal and muscular structures that make up the thoracic cage and surround the lungs play a vital role in respiration (see Chapter 9: Respiratory care). Compromise of one or more of these (e.g. abdominal muscle dysfunction due to abdominal surgery, ascites or deconditioning) may lead to an alteration in normal respiratory function and the ability to generate an effective cough (Hodges and Gandevia 2000).

EVIDENCE-BASED APPROACHES

Principles of care
The main aim of positioning management of the patient with respiratory symptoms is to:

- maximize ventilation/perfusion (V/Q) matching
- minimize the work of breathing (WOB)
- maximize the drainage of secretions.

In many instances, positioning, as outlined above, may enhance medical management by the use of the effects of gravity upon the cardiovascular and respiratory systems. This may reduce the need for more invasive intervention (Jones and Moffatt 2002) such as mechanical ventilation. Therefore, the most advantageous positioning should be integrated into the overall 24-hour plan, and positions that may have an adverse effect should be avoided (Bott et al. 2009).

The general principles of care mentioned earlier in the chapter are all relevant to this aspect of care.

Positioning to maximize ventilation/perfusion matching

DEFINITION
For optimal gaseous exchange to take place, it is necessary that the air and the blood are in the same area of lung at the same time. Matching of these is expressed as a ratio of alveolar ventilation to perfusion (V/Q). A degree of mismatch can occur either due to adequate ventilation to an underperfused area (dead space) or inadequate ventilation to a well-perfused area (shunt) (West 2012).

ANATOMY AND PHYSIOLOGY
The function of the lungs is to exchange oxygen and carbon dioxide between the blood and atmosphere. Oxygen from the atmosphere comes into close contact with blood via the alveolar capillary membrane. Here it diffuses across into the blood and is carried around the body. The amount of oxygen that reaches the blood depends on the rate and depth of the breath, the compliance of the chest and any airway obstruction (Lumb and Nunn 2010).

In a self-ventilating individual in the upright position, ventilation will be preferential in the dependent regions as:

- the apex of the lung is more inflated and therefore has less potential to expand
- the bases of the lung are compressed by the weight of the lungs and the blood vessels and therefore have more potential to inflate.

Perfusion to the alveoli is approximately equal to that of the systemic circulation but as the pressure is far less, the distribution is gravity dependent. The variability in the distribution of perfusion throughout the lung is far greater than that of ventilation (West 2012).

EVIDENCE-BASED APPROACHES

Principles of care
In a self-ventilating upright position, V/Q is not exactly matched even in a healthy lung but is regarded as optimal in the bases (Figure 6.15) as there is the greatest perfusion and ventilation. Similarly in a side-lying position, the effect of gravity alters the distribution of perfusion and ventilation so that the dependent area of lung, that is, the bottom of the lung, has the best V/Q ratio (West 2012).

In a patient receiving mechanical ventilation, especially in a mandatory mode (where the ventilator rather than the patient initiates and terminates the breath), the distribution of ventilation and perfusion will alter (Figure 6.16). As ventilation is driven by a positive pressure, rather than the negative pressure when self-ventilating, air will take the path of least resistance. Ventilation will therefore be optimal in the apex of the lungs in the upright position or the non-dependent/uppermost lung in side-lying. This can, however, be altered further in the presence of lung pathology. Perfusion will remain preferentially delivered to the bases (in the upright position) or the dependent/lowermost lung (in side-lying) and have a higher gradient (variability from apex to bases) than in self-ventilating patients as the positive pressure displaces blood from areas of highest ventilation. These two situations mean that the V/Q ratio of those receiving mechanical ventilation can have a higher degree of mismatch. Strategies such as positive

Figure 6.15 **Effect of gravity on the distribution of ventilation and perfusion in the lung in the upright and lateral positions.** *Source:* **Hough (2001). Reproduced with permission from Oxford University Press.**

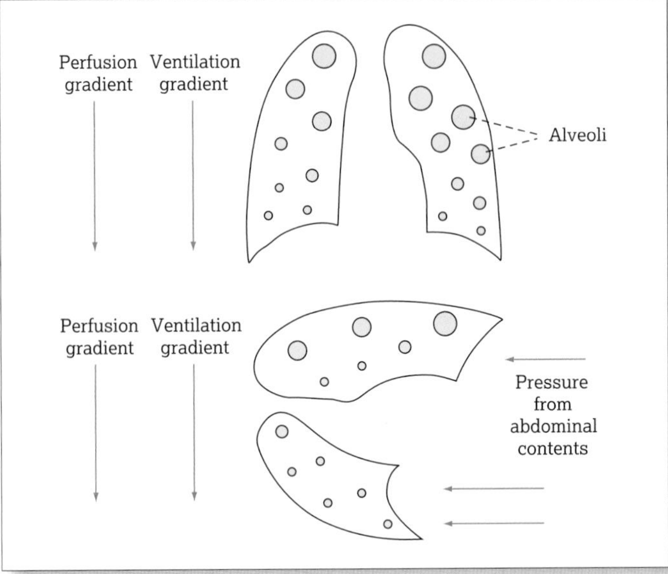

Figure 6.16 **Effect of controlled mandatory ventilation on ventilation and perfusion gradients. In contrast to spontaneous respiration, the perfusion gradient increases downwards and the ventilation gradient is reversed.** *Source:* **Hough (2001). Reproduced with permission from Oxford University Press.**

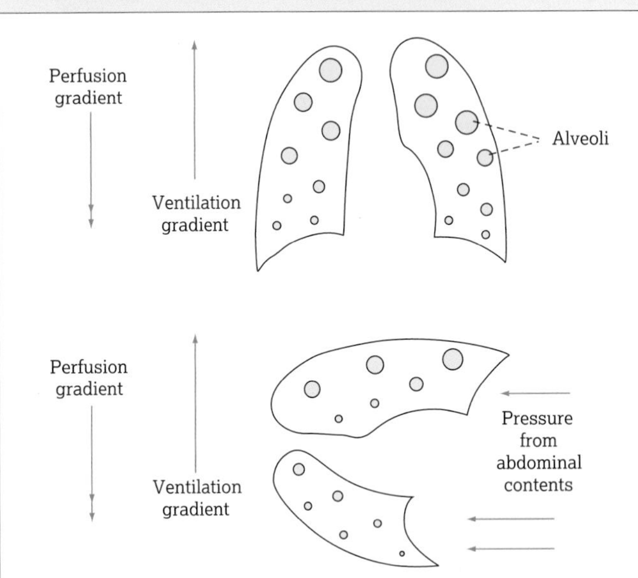

end-expiratory pressure (PEEP) and a higher oxygen delivery will help to overcome this (West 2012).

PRE-PROCEDURAL CONSIDERATIONS

The general principles of care mentioned earlier in the chapter are all relevant to this section. However, there are also some other general principles that need to be considered for these patients.

Pharmacological support

Oxygen requirements

Repositioning can cause a temporary fall in oxygen saturation or a raised respiratory rate. If the fall is greater than 4% or recovery time is protracted, supplemental oxygen delivery may be required for several minutes before, during and after moving.

Procedure guideline 6.10 Positioning the patient to maximize V/Q matching with unilateral lung disease in a self-ventilating patient

Essential equipment

- Pillows/towels
- Sliding sheets/manual handling equipment if indicated following risk assessment in accordance to local manual handling policy
- Bed extension for tall patients

Pre-procedure

Action	Rationale
1 Explain and discuss the procedure with the patient.	To ensure that the patient understands the procedure and gives their valid consent (NMC 2013, **C**).
2 Wash hands thoroughly or use an alcohol-based handrub.	To reduce the risk of contamination and cross-infection (Fraise and Bradley 2009, **E**).
3 Ensure that the bed is at the optimum height for handlers. If two handlers are required try to match handlers' heights as far as possible.	To minimize the risk of injury to the practitioner (Smith 2011, **C**).
Procedure	
4 Position in side-lying on the unaffected side. Refer to the general principles of moving and positioning the patient in side-lying (see Procedure guideline 6.3: Positioning the patient: side-lying).	Ventilation and perfusion are both preferentially distributed to the dependent areas of lung.

Procedure guideline 6.11 Positioning the patient to maximize V/Q matching for widespread pathology in a self-ventilating patient

Essential equipment

- Pillows/towels
- Sliding sheets/manual handling equipment if indicated following risk assessment in accordance with local manual handling policy
- Bed extension for tall patients

Pre-procedure

Action	Rationale
1 Explain and discuss the procedure with the patient.	To ensure that the patient understands the procedure and gives their valid consent (NMC 2013, **C**).
2 Wash hands thoroughly or use an alcohol-based handrub.	To reduce the risk of contamination and cross-infection (Fraise and Bradley 2009, **E**).
3 Ensure that the bed is at the optimum height for handlers. If two handlers are required try to match handlers' heights as far as possible.	To minimize the risk of injury to the practitioner (Smith 2011, **C**).
Procedure	
4 Position the patient in high sitting as discussed in the general principles of moving and positioning of the patient in sitting in bed or chair (see Procedure guideline 6.2: Positioning the patient: sitting in bed and Procedure guideline 6.5: Positioning the patient: in a chair/wheelchair).	The effects of shunting mean perfusion will best match ventilation in high supported sitting (Dean 1985, **R4, E**).

Problem-solving table 6.3 Prevention and resolution (Procedure guidelines 6.10 and 6.11)

Problem	Cause	Prevention	Action
Reduced oxygen saturations. This will be evident by looking at the saturation level on the oximeter (measures the proportion of haemoglobin in the blood), if present, or by observing the patient's colour and work exerted by breathing.	Movement causes an increase in oxygen demand from the tissues. If this is not matched by adequate delivery then saturation levels will be lower.	Preoxygenate prior to movement if patient is requiring high levels of oxygen or is ventilated.	Increase the concentration of oxygen delivered until satisfactory saturations are achieved. Aim to reduce this as much as possible but consider that a higher level of oxygen may be required in the altered position. If this is still not tolerated, return the patient to previous position.
Raised or tense shoulders/ increased effort in breathing.	Use of accessory muscles to assist with respiration.	Use pillows/towels to support upper limbs in positions where they are not able to actively fix and thereby alter their function.	Reassurance to patient. Increase oxygen concentration until respiratory rate returns to normal. If position remains poorly tolerated, return to the previous position.

Positioning to minimize the work of breathing

ANATOMY AND PHYSIOLOGY

At rest, inspiration is an active process whereas expiration is passive. The main muscle involved in inspiration is the diaphragm (Figure 6.17). The diaphragm contracts, thereby increasing the volume of the thoracic cavity. Additionally, the external intercostals work by pulling the sternum and ribcage upwards and outwards, likened to a pump and bucket handle (Figure 6.18). When increased ventilation is required (e.g. with exercise or in disease), the accessory muscles (scalenes and sternocleidomastoid) assist with this process (Lumb and Nunn 2010).

If this situation is prolonged, as in respiratory disease, the diaphragm activity reduces and the accessory muscles have to do a higher proportion of the work. This can be observed in a patient who adopts a posture of raised shoulders.

Although expiration should be passive in normal conditions, the internal intercostals and muscles of the abdominal wall (transversus abdominis, rectus abdominis and the internal and external obliques) are utilized in times of active expiration to push the diaphragm upwards, reducing the volume of the thoracic cavity and forcefully expelling air. This can be observed clinically when the abdominal wall visibly contracts and pulls in the lower part of the ribcage during expiration (Lumb and Nunn 2010).

EVIDENCE-BASED APPROACHES

Principles of care

Many people suffering with long-term breathlessness adopt positions that will best facilitate their inspiratory muscles (Bott et al. 2009). The aim of any position is to restore a normal rate

Figure 6.17 **The diaphragm as seen from the front. Note the openings in the vertebral portion for the inferior vena cava, oesophagus and aorta.**

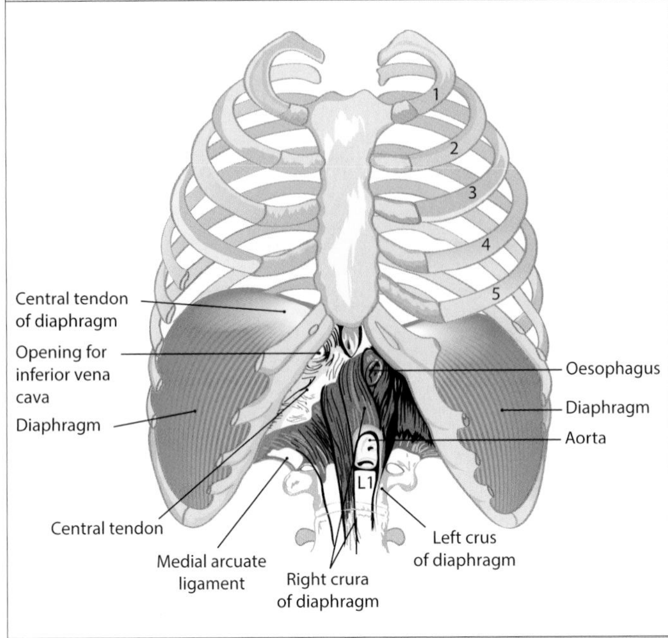

Figure 6.18 **Movement of chest wall on inspiration. (a) The upper ribs move upwards and forwards, increasing the anteroposterior dimension of the thoracic cavity. As a result, the sternum also rises forwards. (b) The lower ribs move like bucket handles, increasing the lateral dimension of the thorax.** ***Source:*** **Aggarwal and Hunter (2007). Reproduced with permission from BMJ Publishing Group Ltd.**

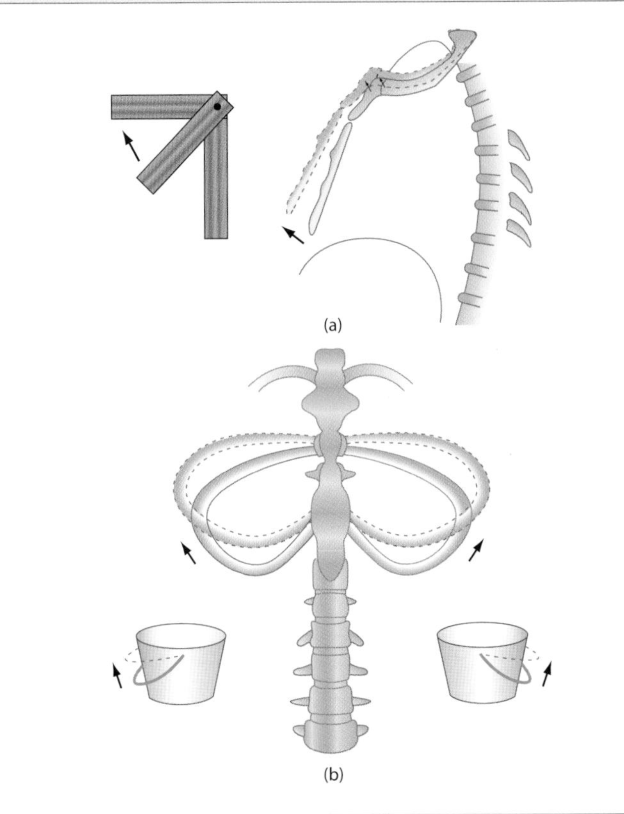

and depth of breathing in order to achieve efficient but adequate ventilation (Box 6.2 [citing Figure 6.19]).

PRE-PROCEDURAL CONSIDERATIONS

The general procedural considerations mentioned earlier in the chapter are all relevant to this section. However, there are also some other general principles that need to be considered for these patients.

Pharmacological support

Administering nebulizers

If prescribed, administering nebulizers approximately 15 minutes prior to moving will help to dilate the airways, making breathing more efficient and ensuring better oxygen delivery to the blood.

Oxygen requirements

Repositioning can cause a temporary fall in oxygen saturation or a raised respiratory rate. If the fall is greater than 4% or recovery time is protracted, supplemental oxygen delivery may be required for several minutes before, during and after moving.

Non-pharmacological support

Pacing

It may be necessary to allow the patient time to rest during the process of getting into a new position to limit the exertion and therefore increased respiratory demand.

Environment

A breathless patient may be anxious about carrying out a task that could exacerbate their breathlessness. By reducing additional stressors such as noise and a cluttered environment, this can be minimized.

Positioning to maximize the drainage of secretions

ANATOMY AND PHYSIOLOGY

The trachea branches into two bronchi, one to each lung (Figure 6.20). Each main bronchus then divides into lobar and then segmental bronchi (upper, middle and lower on the right, upper and lower on the left), each one branching into two or more segmental bronchi with a smaller and smaller diameter, until they reach the bronchioles and finally the alveoli (Tortora and Derrickson 2011).

The walls of the airways are lined with epithelium which contains cilia. The cilia constantly beat in a co-ordinated movement, propelling the mucus layer towards the pharynx.

Box 6.2 **Positioning to minimize the work of breathing**

There are certain resting positions that can help reduce the work of breathing, as shown in Figure 6.19.

1 High side-lying (see Figure 6.19a)
2 Forward lean sitting (see Figure 6.19b)
3 Relaxed sitting (see Figure 6.19c)
4 Forward lean standing (see Figure 6.19d)
5 Relaxed standing (see Figure 6.19e)

These positions serve to:

- support the body, reducing the overall use of postural muscle and oxygen requirements
- improve lung volumes
- optimize the functional positions of the respiratory (thoracic and abdominal) muscles (Dean 1985).

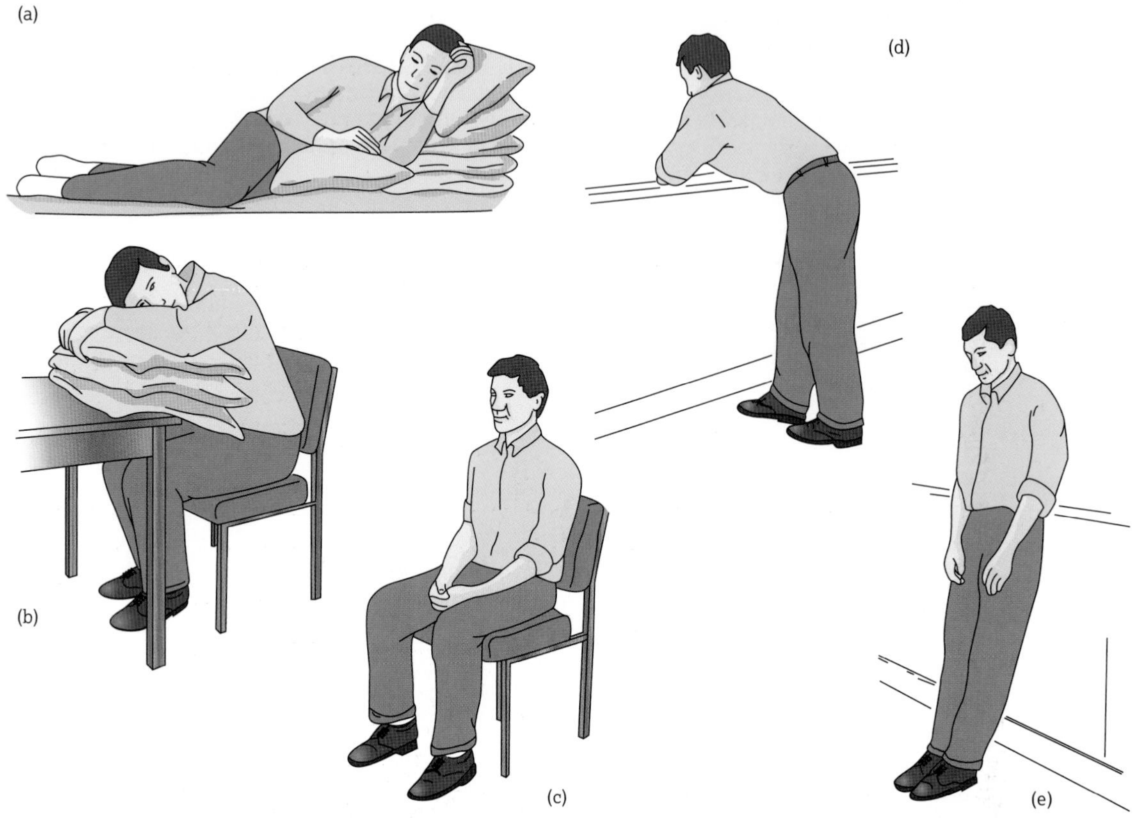

(a) (b) (c) (d) (e)

Figure 6.19 **Positions to support breathing.**

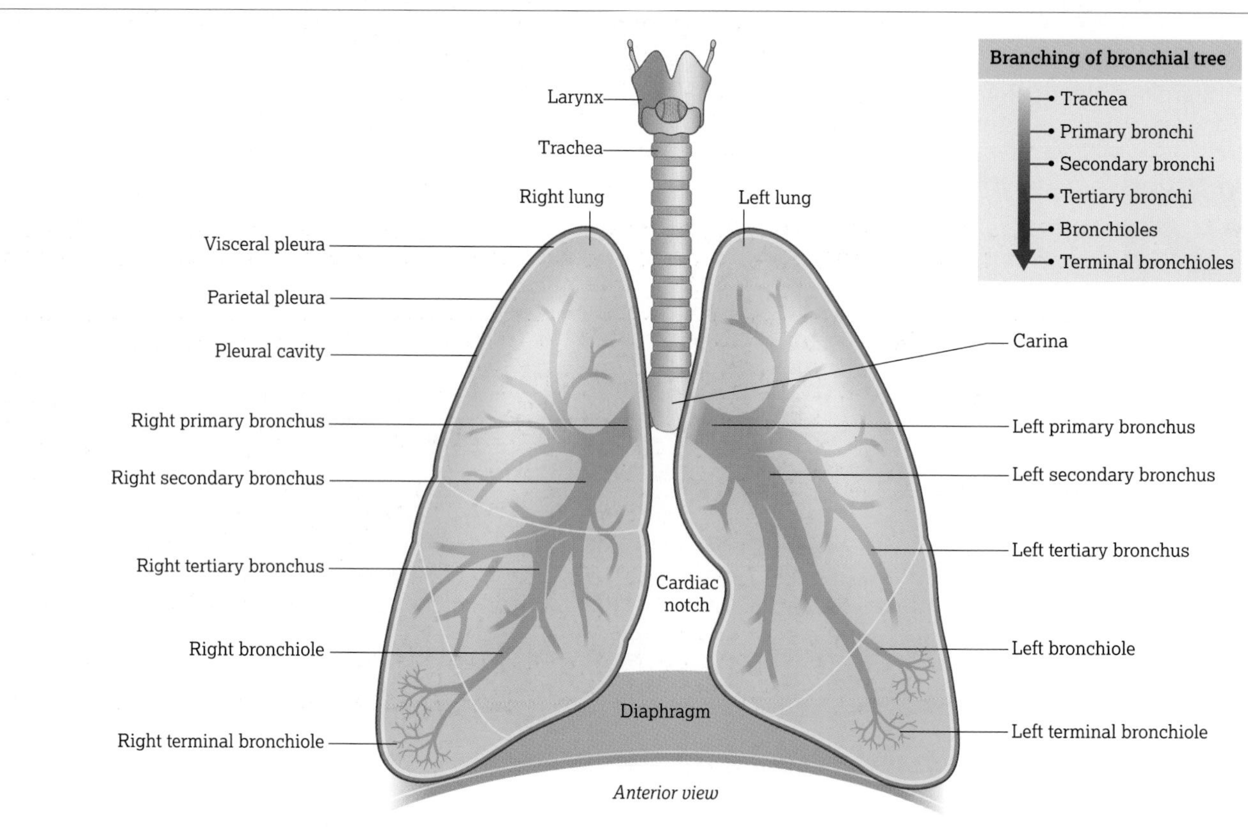

Figure 6.20 **The bronchial tree.** ***Source:*** **Peate et al. (2014). Reproduced with permission from John Wiley & Sons.**

The mucus layer traps any dust particles/foreign objects which can then be transported along the 'mucociliary escalator', an important part of the lungs' defence mechanism. An increased volume of mucus is produced in response to airway irritation and in some disease states (Lumb and Nunn 2010).

A reduced ability to effectively remove this mucus can lead to an increased bacterial load and therefore may compromise respiratory functioning by causing airway obstruction. Consequently leading to segmental atelectasis or lobar collapse, long term this can lead to chronic inflammation and airway destruction (Lumb and Nunn 2010).

PRE-PROCEDURAL CONSIDERATIONS

The general principles of care mentioned earlier in the chapter and the preprocedural considerations to minimize the work of breathing are all relevant to this section. However, there are also some other preprocedural considerations that need to be taken into account for these patients.

Procedure guideline 6.12 Positioning to maximize the drainage of secretions

Essential equipment

- Pillows/towels
- Sliding sheets/manual handling equipment if indicated following risk assessment in accordance with local manual handling policy
- Bed extension for tall patients

Pre-procedure

Action	Rationale
1 Explain and discuss the procedure with the patient.	To ensure that the patient understands the procedure and gives their valid consent (NMC 2013, **C**).
2 Wash hands thoroughly or use an alcohol-based handrub.	To reduce the risk of contamination and cross-infection (Fraise and Bradley 2009, **E**).
3 Ensure that the bed is at the optimum height for handlers. If two handlers are required try to match handlers' heights as far as possible.	To minimize the risk of injury to the practitioner (Smith 2011, **C**).

Procedure

Action	Rationale
4 Auscultate the chest.	To determine most affected area and therefore area to be treated. **E**
5 Position patient with segment to be drained uppermost.	Use gravity to facilitate drainage of secretions. Bronchopulmonary segment needs to be perpendicular to gravity. **E**
6 Leave to drain for 10 minutes if tolerated.	Suggested optimal duration (Fink 2002, **R**).
7 Physiotherapy techniques such as breathing/manual techniques may be carried out whilst in position.	To further assist the removal of secretions. **E**

Problem-solving table 6.4 Prevention and resolution (Procedure guideline 6.12)

Problem	Cause	Prevention	Action
Reduced oxygen saturations. This will be evident by looking at the saturation level on the oximeter, if present, or by observing the patient's colour and work exerted by breathing.	Movement causes an increase in oxygen demand from the tissues. If this is not matched by adequate delivery then saturation levels will be lower. Positions to drain secretions may not comply with positions to match V/Q.	Preoxygenate prior to movement if patient is requiring high levels of oxygen or is ventilated.	Increase the concentration of oxygen delivered until satisfactory saturations are achieved. Aim to reduce this as much as possible but consider that a higher level of oxygen may be required in the altered position. If this is still not tolerated, return the patient to previous position.
Large volume of secretions/increased audible secretions/coughing.	Drainage of distal secretions into more proximal airway.	Clear airway prior to movement. Regular airway clearance following movement.	Clear airway of any secretions either by coughing or suctioning.

Non-pharmacological support

Humidification

Drainage of secretions will be optimized if the patient and therefore the mucus layer and cilia are well hydrated. This can be ensured by adequate humidification (see Chapter 9: Respiratory care).

The problem-solving, post-procedural considerations and complications in general principles of moving and positioning patients and respiratory compromise also apply to these patients. Refer to relevant sections in this chapter.

Moving and positioning the patient with neurological impairment

The general principles of positioning discussed earlier can be applied for this group of patients. However, the complexity of these patients highlights the difficulty of a uniform approach to overall management. Therefore, this section will look at some of the variations in presentation of this patient group and suggest some principles to be considered when positioning these patients.

This will cover recommendations for assisting patients presenting with physical neurological symptoms affecting their central nervous systems (CNS) and peripheral nervous systems (PNS) as a consequence of their disease or treatment itself. These may include:

- hemiparesis (weakness or paralysis affecting one half of the body, also known as hemiplegia) or monoparesis (weakness or paralysis affecting one limb)
- hemi-aesthesia (sensory loss affecting one half of the body, also known as paraesthesia)
- peripheral motor/sensory neuropathies (dysfunction or pathology affecting one or more peripheral nerves resulting in altered movement or sensation)
- spinal cord compression/injury.

DEFINITION

Neurological insult through disease or illness can cause damage to patients' central, peripheral and autonomic nervous systems, affecting the relay of messages along nerve pathways and preventing normal motor and sensory function. Sequelae associated with neurological deficit include altered muscle tone, abnormal movement patterns, sensory, cognitive (the mental processes involved in gaining knowledge and comprehension, including thinking, knowing, remembering, judging, problem solving, imagination, perception and planning), perceptual (interpretation of sensation into meaning) and speech and language problems.

ANATOMY AND PHYSIOLOGY

The nervous system is a complex organ which allows us to automatically and volitionally adjust to internal and external environments. This maintains equilibrium of body systems and enables effective, efficient motor and cognitive function. It can be considered in three main areas: central nervous system, peripheral nervous system and autonomic nervous system (ANS). The CNS consists of two parts: the brain and spinal cord. The brain consists of four lobes (frontal, temporal, parietal and occipital), the midbrain, pons, medulla oblongata and cerebellum. Each has individual and joint roles, and interconnects with the others via a complex system of pathways producing automatic and volitional movement and cognitive function. These connect with every part of the body via the PNS, consisting of cranial and spinal nerves which carry motor (efferent) and sensory (afferent) fibres (see Chapter 11: Observations). The ANS, made up of sympathetic and parasympathetic components, regulates structures not under conscious control, for example arterial blood pressure, gastrointestinal motility and secretion, urinary bladder emptying, sweating, body temperature, and is activated mainly by centres in the brainstem, spinal cord and hypothalamus. Illness, disease and/or side-effects of treatment can affect any or all of these systems which will have implications for clinical practice and patient management.

RELATED THEORY

Disease or damage to the central or peripheral nervous system can lead to temporary or permanent complex physical, cognitive, psychological and psychosocial problems (BNOS/DH 2011, Carr et al. 2008, Formica et al. 2011, Lindsay et al. 2011, NICE 2006). These may include:

- weakness – unilateral, bilateral or global
- altered muscle tone
- sensory changes
- balance problems
- perceptual problems
- visual problems
- cognitive problems
- dysphagia (an impairment of swallowing that may involve any structures from the lips to the gastric cardia)
- dysphasia (an acquired communication disorder that impairs a person's ability to process language in verbal or written forms. It does not affect intelligence but does affect how someone can use language either temporarily or permanently. It does not include speech impairments caused by damage to the muscles involved with speech – that is dysarthria)
- dysarthria (a speech disorder resulting from motor weakness, inco-ordination or stiffness of muscles used for speaking)
- autonomic dysfunction
- behavioural changes.

If a person with a neurological presentation is unable to move, they are deprived of the physical benefits of movement (Box 6.3) and are at risk of developing secondary complications including joint contractures.

Effective management of patients with neurological impairment requires holistic assessment including consideration of altered tone, abnormal patterns of movement, joint protection and prevention of soft tissue changes and contractures.

Altered tone and abnormal patterns of movement

Tone is defined clinically as 'the resistance that is encountered when the joint of a relaxed patient is moved passively' (Britton and Ng 1998). Alterations in tone will affect functional recovery in patients with neurological problems and require careful management. This can be through positioning, splinting if required and oral and focal pharmacological intervention (Barnes 2008).

Increased tone and spasticity are disorders of spinal proprioceptive reflexes. Spasticity is defined as:

> 'a motor disorder characterised by a velocity dependent increase in tonic stretch reflexes (muscle tone) with exaggerated tendon jerks, resulting from hyperexcitability of the stretch reflex, as one component of the upper motor neurone syndrome.' (Barnes 2008, p.1)

Normal movement is dependent on a neuromuscular system that can receive, integrate and respond appropriately to multiple intrinsic and extrinsic stimuli. Key components include:

- normal postural tone
- reciprocal innervation of muscles
- sensory-motor feedback and feedforward mechanism (Duff et al. 2012)
- balance reactions (Edwards 2002b)
- biomechanical properties of muscle (Edwards 1998).

Where any of these components are altered through CNS or PNS disease, abnormal movement patterns will exist which will affect the patient's functional ability. Positioning and active movement

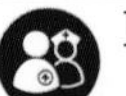
Box 6.3 **The physical benefits of movement**

- Sensorimotor appreciation.
- Posture and balance control.
- Maintenance of joint and soft tissue range of movement.
- Maximization of functional independence.
- Minimization of tonal changes such as spasticity (Hawkins et al. 1999).
- Cardiorespiratory fitness (Convertino et al. 1997).

are key in managing the influence of altered tone and abnormal patterns of movement in the recovery of motor control in patients with neurological problems.

Joint protection

Positioning is suggested as a strategy to prevent pain and to prevent loss of range of movement for patients with low tone (hypotonia), particularly around the shoulder (Ada et al. 2005, Dean et al. 2000, Kaplan 1995). This aims to prevent the patient's functional deterioration (Gloag 1985). Dean et al. (2000) identified that these complications often prevent a patient's full participation in rehabilitation, contributing to poor upper limb functional outcome. Several factors were described for this.

- Glenohumeral subluxation due to lack of muscular activity around the shoulder.
- Trauma to the shoulder complex through unsuitable exercise.
- Trauma through inappropriate handling of the patient by staff during transfers.

Dean et al. (2000) acknowledged that consistency in education is essential to address these common problems. Ada et al. (2005) recommended that patients with little upper limb function in the early stages after a stroke undergo a programme of positioning of the affected shoulder. Their study showed statistical significance in maintaining shoulder range when compared with patients who received standard upper limb care of arm support and exercise only. Such specific joint positioning requires assessment by the physiotherapist for each individual patient.

Soft tissue changes and contractures

Joint range and subsequent function are at risk with increased tone (hypertonia). Restriction in the range of movement is not always simply due to increased tone of the relevant muscles. The surrounding soft tissues, tendons, ligaments and the joints themselves can develop changes leading to an increased likelihood of them being maintained in a shortened position (Barnes 2008). Adaptation of the mechanical properties of muscle also contributes to increased tone in patients with hypertonia (O'Dwyer et al. 1996). It is possible, but not proven, that maintaining a joint through a full range of movement may prevent the longer-term development of soft tissue contractures (Barnes 2008).

Professionals agree that positioning is a key element in the rehabilitation and management of patients with neurological deficit (Davies 2000, Edwards and Carter 2002, Raine et al. 2009, Stokes and Stack 2012). An optimal position is not always possible due to variables such as the patient's medical condition and presence of contractures (Edwards 1998). There appears to be an overall lack of consensus in clinicians' actual practice regarding the key components of the positions necessary to limit the onset of spasticity (Chatterton et al. 2001, Jackson 1998, Mee and Bee 2007). However, prevention of complications is an important aim (Bobath 1990, Davies 2000, Edwards and Carter 2002, Mee and Bee 2007, Raine et al. 2009). Stokes and Stack (2012) describe positioning in bed and Pope (2002) details positioning in sitting with principles of optimum alignment to prevent secondary complications such as pain, and to optimize function such as socialization. Edwards (1998) recommends a variety of postures especially for patients with hypertonia.

EVIDENCE-BASED APPROACHES

Principles of care

The general principles of care mentioned earlier in the chapter are all relevant to this section. However, there are some additional principles that need to be considered for these patients. For those with acute and long-standing neurological issues, principles of moving and positioning can be applied at any time along their treatment trajectory from undertaking rehabilitation, experiencing deteriorating function or those requiring palliative management. Posture and postural control will be affected in these patients. 'Posture' describes the biomechanical alignment and orientation of the body to the environment (Duff et al. 2012), whilst 'postural control' provides orientation and balance (Lundy-Ekman 2007). Positional influences in the patient with neurological impairment may affect spinal, pelvic and shoulder girdle alignment with risk of soft tissue shortening due to the following potential problems.

- Flattened lumbar spine.
- Extended thoracic spine.
- Pelvis tilted backwards.
- Retracted hip.
- Elevated shoulder, retracted scapula.
- Feet tend toward plantarflexion (Duff et al. 2012).

Therefore, additional considerations should be applied for the neurological patient with severe tonal management issues. These should always be discussed with the physiotherapist.

PRE-PROCEDURAL CONSIDERATIONS

The general principles of moving and positioning patients can be applied when assisting those with complex neurological impairment. Patients with neurological impairment may be able to participate in usual transfer techniques but risk assessment will consider several additional factors. This section will identify considerations for staff in their decision making. Where there is any doubt when moving patients with complex needs, guidance should be sought from a physiotherapist/occupational therapist.

Risk management

Patients with neurological deficits may vary in their presentation on a daily basis. The additional considerations for positioning and moving patients with neurological impairment are listed in Box 6.4.

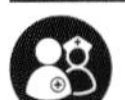

Box 6.4 **Considerations for moving patients with neurological impairment**

- Variations in tone, for example flaccidity or spasm.
- Cognitive problems including attention deficit.
- Behavioural problems.
- Communication problems.
- Variable client ability, for example 'on/off' periods for patients with Parkinson's disease and patients with changing presentations, for example multiple sclerosis, degenerative conditions.
- Sensory and proprioceptive problems, including reduced midline awareness.
- Pain/altered sensitivity.
- Decreased balance and co-ordination.
- Visual disturbance.
- Varying ability over 24 hours, for example, fatigue at the end of the day, at night.
- Effects of medication.
- Varying capability of the patient according to the experience and/or skill mix of handler(s).
- Post-surgery, presence of tracheotomy, chest and other drains.
- Traumatic and non-traumatic spinal injury – risk of spinal instability.
- Importance of maintaining privacy and dignity.

Source: CSP (2014). Reproduced with permission from The Chartered Society of Physiotherapy (www.csp.org.uk).

Equipment

Splints and orthoses

In advanced spasticity, it is often the soft tissue changes that contribute most to subsequent disability, such as limb deformity leading to poor function and problems with regard to hygiene, positioning, transferring and feeding and making the individual prone to pressure sores (O'Dwyer et al. 1996). Therapeutic splinting may maintain and assist function (Edwards 1998, Raine et al. 2009, Shumway-Cook and Woollacott 2012).

An orthosis or splint is an external device designed to apply, distribute or remove forces to or from the body in a controlled manner in order to control body motion and prevent alteration in the shape of body tissues (see Figure 6.13 and Figure 6.14). The aim is to compensate for weak or absent muscle function or to resist unopposed action of spastic muscle (Charlton 2009). They may help gain alignment for proximal and truncal activity (Raine et al. 2009) and enable more balanced and efficient walking (Hesse 2003). As with all therapeutic interventions, they should only be used after detailed assessment and based on sound clinical reasoning.

If a splint or an orthosis is required, then this will normally be provided and fitted by a physiotherapist and/or occupational therapist. They will also give instructions on how to use it.

Seating

Appropriate seating is also advocated as an adjunct to management for effective postural support (Kirkwood and Bardsley 2001, Pope 2002, Raine et al. 2009). Occupational therapists and physiotherapists will consider this for management of patients with complex needs and provide appropriate seating if required.

Environment and positioning

Problems of perception (interpretation of sensation into meaningful forms) are considered to be one of the main factors limiting functional motor recovery following stroke (Verheyden and Ashburn 2012). These can affect patients with disease or illness affecting their CNS. Here, the patient fails to respond appropriately to stimuli presented on their hemiplegic side, the contralateral side to the brain lesion (Verheyden and Ashburn 2012). Environmental factors such as correct positioning are essential for ensuring optimal level of function for each individual (Edwards 2002a, Pope 2002). Clinical management strategies include:

- addressing the patient from the affected side
- deliberate placement of items of interest to the patient on that side (with appropriate assistance to access those items, e.g. drinks)
- advice to carers to position themselves on the patient's affected side whilst talking to them in order to orientate them to their affected side
- positioning the patient on their affected side, enabling function with their sound side.

Limited evidence exists to suggest the benefit of these approaches (Verheyden and Ashburn 2012). However, it is recognized as a useful treatment adjunct for these patients, through promotion of sensory awareness/appreciation, including perception and body image and enabling function (Edwards and Carter 2002, Grieve and Gnanasekaran 2008, Raine et al. 2009, Stokes and Stack 2012).

Rehabilitation opportunity

Patients with neurological illness or disease present with an assortment of clinical symptoms. Positioning can assist in their holistic management and allow future opportunity for rehabilitation where their illness or disease allows. For example,the Department of Health (DH 2013) identifies the importance of early rehabilitation for patients with cancer.

Procedure guideline 6.13 **Positioning the neurological patient with tonal problems**

Essential equipment

- Pillows or towels (as guidance or basic positioning)

Optional equipment

- Hand/foot resting splint if required
- Resting splint if required

Medicinal products

- Analgesia as required
- Antispasmodics as required

Pre-procedure

Action	Rationale
1 Explain the procedure to the patient.	To ensure that the patient understands the procedure and gives their valid consent (NMC 2013, **C**).
2 Wash hands thoroughly or use an alcohol-based handrub.	To reduce the risk of contamination and cross-infection (Fraise and Bradley 2009, **E**).
3 Ensure that the bed is at the optimum height for handlers. If two handlers are required try to match handlers' heights as far as possible.	To minimize the risk of injury to the practitioner (Smith 2011, **C**).

Procedure

Action	Rationale
4 Follow basic advice for positioning the patient in supine, side-lying and sitting in bed as described in the above procedure guidelines for positioning patients.	To promote alignment of body segments and support against gravity for patients with high or low tone resulting in asymmetrical posture (Edwards and Carter 2002, **E**; Stokes and Stack 2012, **R4**). To ensure patient comfort. **E**

Action	Rationale
5 Consider and apply possible modifications as specified below for the supine (**Action figure 5**).	To control pelvic and spinal alignment. **E**
• Place pillow under hemiplegic hip for alignment.	To optimize patient comfort. **E**
• Place additional pillows or wedge under knees and/or head.	To maintain joint and soft tissue range (ACPIN 1998, **C**, **E**; Barnes 2001, **R4**; Edwards 1998, **E**).
6 Place pillow to support feet in neutral/plantargrade position. • Apply foot resting splint, ankle foot orthosis (AFO) (**Action figure 6** and see Figure 6.14) if recommended to weak foot and ankle. NB: Ensure the splint is fitted correctly. • Place pillow under weak arm. • Apply resting splint for hand/forearm if required.	To maintain soft tissue and joint range (Duff et al. 2012, **E**; Edwards 1998, **E**).
7 Consider and apply possible modifications as specified below for side-lying (**Action figure 5b**). • Place pillow under head and in front of trunk. • Place pillow in front of trunk. • Place patient's affected arm on pillow. Apply resting splint for hand/forearm if required.	To support the patient's affected shoulder and upper limb due to a risk of trauma, pain, muscle and soft tissue shortening (Ada et al. 2005, **R2b**; Dean et al. 2000, **R2b**). To reduce the influence of asymmetrical posturing of head and trunk in patients with high or low tone. **E** May be effective in maintaining opposing trunk muscles. **E** To maintain soft tissue and joint range (Barnes 2001, **R4**; Duff et al. 2012, **E**; Edwards 1998, **E**).

Post-procedure

Action	Rationale
8 The general principles of care mentioned earlier in the chapter are all relevant to this section.	
9 For patients requiring use of an external splint to maintain joint position and range, skin condition must be closely monitored.	To monitor skin integrity and pressure care. **E**

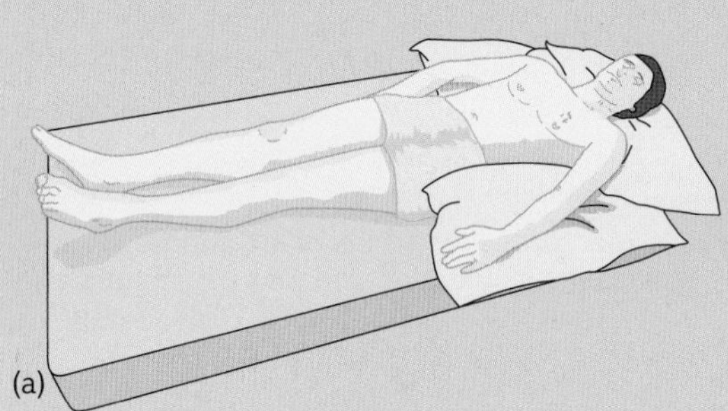
(a)

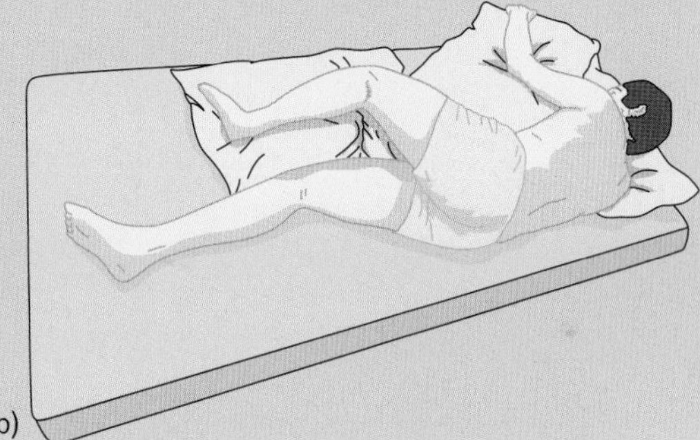
(b)

Action Figure 5 Positioning the patient with neurological weakness. (a) Supine: affected arm supported on pillow. (b) Side-lying: affected arm supported on pillow.

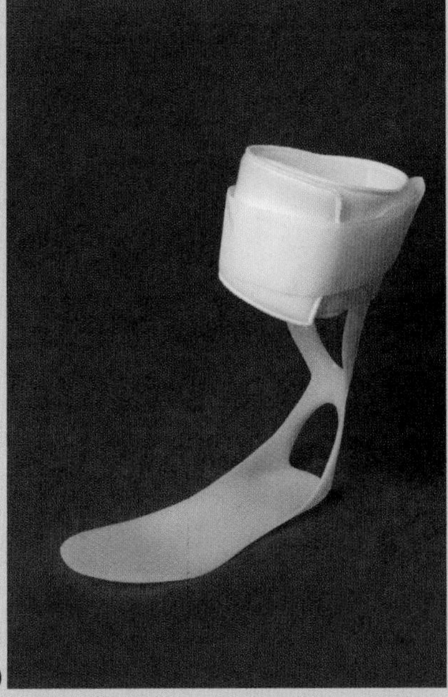
(a)

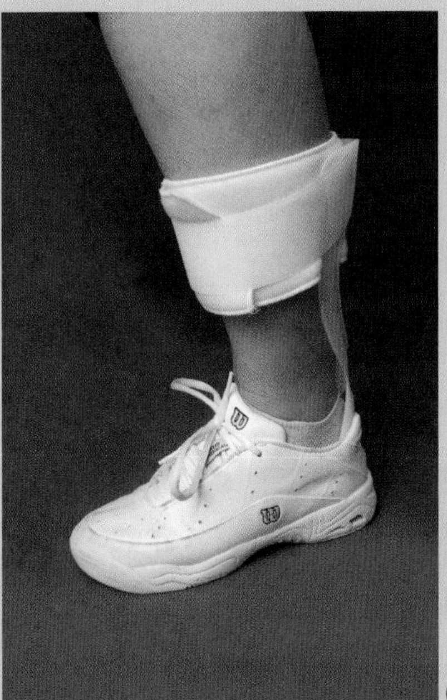
(b)

Action Figure 6 (a) Ankle foot orthosis (AFO). (b) Ankle foot orthosis *in situ*.

Problem-solving table 6.5 Prevention and resolution (Procedure guideline 6.13)

Problem	Cause	Prevention	Action
Unable to position patient's legs in bed due to increased tone – legs remain 'stiff'.	Abnormal tone (high or low) affecting limbs secondary to CNS involvement (cortical/ spinal).	Assess for other noxious stimuli which may increase tone in patients with CNS disease. Ensure pain control. Ensure bowel management. Ensure effective catheter drainage. Assess for infection.	Use leg flexion position in bed control. **And/or:** Position small folded pillow/rolled towel under patient's knees. Avoid contact of patient's feet against end of bed – this can stimulate increased tone in legs. Liaise with physiotherapist.
Unable to achieve comfortable position for patient with CNS involvement. Patient's limbs may demonstrate persistent increased tone despite positioning.	Possible causes: • inadequate pain control • inadequate antiepilepsy medication • other noxious stimuli.	Assess for other noxious stimuli which may increase tone in patients with CNS disease. Ensure pain control. Ensure bowel management. Assess for infection.	Reassess patient. Ensure adequate analgesia. Ensure adequate antiepilepsy medication. Consider a medical review.
Patient's arm remains flexed/unable to position in bed.	Abnormal tone (high or low) affecting limbs due to CNS involvement.		Position small flat pillow under patient's affected arm to provide support **Or:** Position small flat pillow across patient's abdomen to support both upper limbs. Use of resting splint if indicated for patient management – liaise with physiotherapist and/or occupational therapist.
Patent is unaware of affected side.	Sensory/motor inattention.		Ensure patient's environment is made available to them. Ensure affected limbs are supported by pillows/folded/rolled towel as required (refer to positioning for patients with neurological deficits).

POST-PROCEDURAL CONSIDERATIONS

Ongoing care

Where the patient requires use of a splint to maintain joint range and position, skin integrity must be closely monitored (see Chapter 14: Wound management), including skin/pressure care, and any adverse effects treated accordingly following assessment. The instructions for the use of the splint (usually provided by the PT or OT) should specify the recommended length of time that the splint should be applied and the periods of rest from wear. If skin integrity is compromised due to pressure from the splint, it should be reviewed by the dispensing professional before continuing with its use.

Moving and positioning the patient with actual or suspected spinal cord compression or spinal cord injury

DEFINITION

Spinal cord compression or injury is when the function of the spinal cord becomes compromised.

ANATOMY AND PHYSIOLOGY

The spinal cord is about 45 cm in length and extends from the base of the brain, surrounded by the vertebrae, to the pelvis. Nerves situated within the spinal cord, called upper motor neurones (UMNs), carry the messages between the brain and spinal nerves along the spinal tract. Spinal nerves are classified as lower motor neurones (LMNs). Spinal nerves branch out from the spinal cord at each vertebral level to communicate with specific areas of the body.

Following damage to the spinal cord through traumatic vertebral displacement or tumour/oedema growth, 'spinal shock' may occur, which is a temporary suppression of spinal cord activity caused by oedema at and below the level of the lesion in spinal cord injury. Within the confines of the vertebral canal, the oedematous cord is compressed against the surrounding bone. A complex series of physiological and biochemical reactions occur due to resulting oedema and vascular damage. Circulation of blood and oxygen is disrupted; ischaemic tissue necrosis follows with an immediate cessation of conductivity within the spinal cord neurones. This can persist for 2–6 weeks (Harrison 2000).

RELATED THEORY

Spinal cord compression or injury encompasses the following.

- *Traumatic spinal cord injury (SCI).* This is damage or trauma to the spinal cord that results in loss of or impaired function

causing reduced mobility or feeling. The spinal cord does not have to be severed in order for a loss of functioning to occur. Common causes include trauma (for example, car accident, gunshot, falls, sports injuries) or disease (for example, transverse myelitis, polio, spina bifida, Friedreich's ataxia). It is estimated that 500–700 people sustain traumatic SCI in the UK each year (Harrison 2000).
- *Primary/benign spinal cord compression (PSCC).*
- *Degenerative conditions.* These include osteoporosis, which is a reduction in the quantity and quality of bone, and spondylosis, a degenerative osteoarthritis of the joints between the centre of the spinal vertebrae and/or neural foramina (Mann et al. 2000).
- *Haematoma* (Kalina et al. 1995).
- *Primary tumours.* These include intradural extramedullary tumours (neurofibromas, meningiomas: Lohani and Sharma 2004), intramedullary tumours (ependymomas) and low-grade astrocytomas (Britton and Ng 1998).
- *Metastatic spinal cord compression (MSCC).* This is an oncological emergency, defined as compression of the dural sac and its contents (spinal cord and cauda equina) by an extradural mass (Loblaw et al. 2003). Causes include:
  - direct soft tissue extension from vertebral bony metastases
  - tumour growth through intravertebral foramina (e.g. from retroperitoneal tumours or paravertebral lymphadenopathy)
  - compression due to bony collapse
  - intramedullary metastases (rare).

The true incidence of MSCC is unknown due to current restrictions in detection rate and coding systems in the UK (NICE 2008). Postmortem evidence indicates it is present in 5–10% of patients with advanced cancer.

Classification
Spinal cord compression (SCC) is classified as either stable or unstable.

- *Stable:* this is where spinal alignment is intact with no further risk of progression of neurological symptoms as the spine is still able to maintain and distribute weight appropriately.
- *Unstable:* this is where spinal fractures/lesions pose a risk of spinal cord injury and potentially irreversible neurological symptoms due to (potential) abnormal movement at the fracture site. Additionally, it can be further classified as complete or incomplete.
- *Complete spinal cord injury:* when the cord 'loses all descending neuronal control below the level of the lesion' (Lundy-Ekman 2007, p.230).
- *Incomplete spinal cord injury:* when 'the function of some ascending and/or descending fibres is preserved within the spinal cord' (Lundy-Ekman 2007, p.230).

Clinical presentation
Clinical presentation of SCC is dependent on the location of the compression, the duration of its presence and consequently the level of neural function that is spared. The patient presents with loss of all voluntary movement and sensation below the level of the injury/lesion. There is also progressive loss of sympathetic and parasympathetic activity throughout the area (Harrison 2000).

In SCC, early diagnosis is crucial in order to at best prevent and otherwise minimize irreversible neurological damage. Common symptoms include:

- back pain and/or radicular pain – nerve root symptoms resulting in pain or loss of sensation within a dermatome
- limb weakness
- difficulty walking
- sensory loss
- cauda equina signs (saddle anaesthesia, bladder or bowel dysfunction)
- sexual dysfunction (NICE 2008).

Stable spine
The general principles of care mentioned earlier in the chapter are all relevant to this group of patients. However, patients need to be assessed for adequate pain control prior to moving and positioning, and care should be taken to avoid excessive rotation of the spine when turning.

Unstable spine
For patients with an unstable spine or severe mechanical pain suggestive of spinal instability, specific instructions for moving must be followed until bony and neurological stability is radiologically confirmed (Harrison 2000, NICE 2008). This is to ensure spinal alignment and reduce the risk of further spinal damage and potential loss of function (Harrison 2000, NICE 2008).

'Careful handling, positioning and turning can prevent secondary cord damage during transfer and movements for patients with spinal cord injury' (Harrison 2000). Procedure guideline 6.1: Positioning the patient: supine, Procedure guideline 6.3: Positioning the patient: side-lying and Procedure guideline 6.13: Positioning the neurological patient with tonal problems, are relevant to moving patients with metastatic spinal cord compression. However, this patient group will require additional considerations to enable safe practice without compromising their clinical condition. These may include: 231

- lateral surface transfer, for example bed to trolley using a PAT lateral transfer board. Manual support of the patient's head and neck should be given for any flat surface transfer (Harrison 2000). This ensures appropriate spinal alignment and patient comfort
- log rolling for personal/pressure care for patients with unstable SCC.

EVIDENCE-BASED APPROACHES

Rationale
When moving and turning the patient with confirmed/suspected spinal instability who is being nursed flat, log rolling must be used. This is a technique to maintain neutral spinal alignment. It is an essential method to enable the patient to use a slipper pan and also to maintain pressure areas through regular turning every 2–3 hours (NICE 2008). Patients should only be moved with adequate numbers of staff who have been fully trained in moving patients with spinal cord compression/injury. Differing methods are recommended dependent on the level of the lesion/injury (Harrison 2000).

- Cervical and thoracic lesions (T4 and above):
  - pelvic twist for pressure care
  - log roll with five people required.
- Thoracolumbar lesions:
  - log roll with four people required (Harrison 2000).

Contraindications
The pelvic twist is contraindicated in the presence of thoracolumbar or pelvic injury/damage and pre-existing spinal deformity or rigidity, for example ankylosing spondylitis (Harrison 2000).

Principles of care
The general principles of care mentioned earlier in the chapter are all relevant to individuals with SCC. However, there are some other factors that need to be considered for these patients. Early and accurate diagnosis and, if appropriate, treatment are necessary to optimize neurological functioning. Timely referral to rehabilitation services is imperative for assessment, appropriate intervention and thorough discharge planning to enable smooth transition back into the community (NICE 2008). Active rehabilitation may be postponed until the medical team has confirmed that the patient's spine is stable. However, there is a significant role for

members of the rehabilitation team in the management of these patients in terms of:

- assessment of motor recovery
- minimizing further complications such as chest infections which may arise as a result of prolonged bedrest
- effective, co-ordinated discharge planning. The positioning and moving needs of these patients are often complex and so discharge planning may be lengthy and multifaceted, requiring ongoing support and rehabilitation in the community to optimize functional independence (Miller and Cooper 2010).

For patients with complex symptoms, e.g. spinal instability, weakness, sensory impairment, refer to the physiotherapist.

PRE-PROCEDURAL CONSIDERATIONS

Patients may be able to assist with moving, positioning and transfers depending on:

- spinal stability
- pain
- level of lesion
- muscle power
- sensory impairment
- exercise tolerance
- patient confidence.

Pain management: pharmacological and non-pharmacological

As already discussed, spinal and radicular pain can be an indicator of SCC in the first instance but, in relation to moving and handling, it can also be suggestive of changes in neurology once gradual sitting and mobilization commence (NICE 2008). Implementation of a pain assessment chart can enable continuity of care, allowing accurate assessment and evaluation of all pharmacological (i.e. non-steroidal anti-inflammatory drugs, opiates, bisphosphonates and epidural) and non-pharmacological interventions (i.e. relaxation and therapeutic management).

Equipment

Spinal brace/cervical collar

Where there is confirmed or risk of spinal instability due to vertebral injury or collapse, patients will require external spinal support. This may be in the form of a spinal brace or collar. A properly fitted hard collar (Figure 6.21) must be used when there is suspicion of spinal instability (Harrison 2000, NICE 2008). This is available from surgical appliances/orthotics or some physiotherapy departments. Manufacturer's product details and care instructions are provided upon issue. Staff should be guided by medical advice and local policy.

Figure 6.21 **Hard collar *in situ*.**

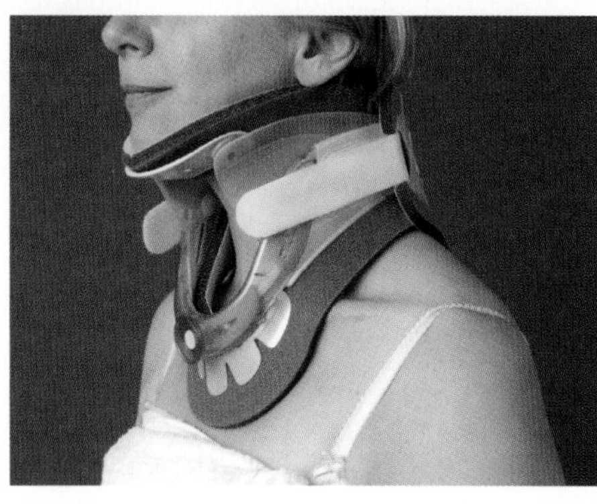

Moving and handling aids

Patients may be able to assist with transfers using transfer boards, standing aids, mobility aids, frames, crutches and sticks. If they are unable to assist, there is a variety of moving and handling aids, for example lateral patient transfer boards, hoists and standing hoists, which maintain the safety of both the patient and the carer (HSE 1992). For lesions affecting the cervical and thoracolumbar spine or where injuries make turning difficult, an electric turning bed can be used (Harrison 2000).

Assessment and recording tools

The focus of an initial neurological assessment is to establish the level of cord injury and act as a baseline against which future improvements or declines may be compared (Harrison 2000). Standard assessments, including pain, motor and sensory charts, should be used as a baseline and updated with any change in a patient's presentation. Assessments will depend on local policy and may include:

- American Spinal Injury Association (ASIA) Spinal Cord Injury Classification (ASIA 2002)
- ASIA Spinal Cord Injury Impairment Scale (ASIA 2002)
- Spinal Cord Independence Measure (SCIM III) (Catz and Itzkovich 2007, Catz et al. 2007, Itzkovich et al. 2007)
- pain assessment chart, for example visual analogue scale (Tiplady et al. 1998)
- manual handling risk assessment
- pressure ulcer assessment, refer to Chapter 14: Wound management.

Procedure guideline 6.14 **Log rolling for suspected/confirmed cervical spinal instability**

See Figure 6.22.

Essential equipment

- Pillows – minimum of four
- Collar or spinal brace
- A minimum of five people is needed to move a person with cervical spinal instability

Optional equipment

- Slipper pan
- Clean sheets
- Hygiene equipment
- Continence pads
- Pressure care

Action	Rationale
Pre-procedure	
1 Explain and discuss the procedure with the patient.	To ensure that the patient understands the procedure and gives their valid consent (NMC 2013, **C**).
2 Wash hands thoroughly or use an alcohol-based handrub.	To reduce the risk of contamination and cross-infection (Fraise and Bradley 2009, **E**).
3 Ensure that the bed is at the optimum height for handlers. If two or more handlers are required try to match handlers' heights as far as possible.	To minimize the risk of injury to the practitioner (Smith 2011, **C**).
4 Ensure there are sufficient personnel available to assist with the procedure (minimum five for patients with cervical spinal instability).	Four staff to maintain spinal alignment and one to perform personal/pressure care check during the procedure (Harrison 2000, **C**).
Procedure	
5 Assess patient's motor and sensory function.	To provide a baseline to compare against after the procedure (Harrison 2000, **C**).
6 Lead practitioner stabilizes the patient's neck, supporting the patient's head.	To co-ordinate and lead log roll. **E** To take responsibility for providing instructions and ensuring all other practitioners are ready before commencing the manoeuvre (Harrison 2000, **C**).
7 Ideally, the lead practitioner's hands should offer support for the entire cervical curve from the base of the skull to C7.	To immobilize patient's head. **E** To ensure spinal alignment is monitored throughout the procedure (Harrison 2000, **C**).
8 The second practitioner stands at the thorax and positions their hands over the patient's lower back and shoulder.	To ensure the lower spine remains aligned (Harrison 2000, **C**).
9 The third practitioner stands at the hip area and places one hand on the patient's lower back and the other under the patient's upper thigh.	To prevent movement at thoracolumbar site (Harrison 2000, **C**).
10 The fourth practitioner stands at the patient's lower leg and places one hand under knee and the other under ankle.	To ensure the lower spine remains aligned (Harrison 2000, **C**).
11 Ensure there is a fifth person standing on the opposite side of bed.	To position the equipment or take care of hygiene needs. **E** To assess upper back and occiput. This needs to be carried out once a day to check pressure areas (Harrison 2000, **C**).
12 The lead practitioner holding the head provides clear instructions to the team; for example, 'We will roll on three: One, two, three'.	To ensure co-ordinated approach to the move. **E**
13 Each practitioner remains in place whilst the necessary action is performed.	
14 The person holding the head then provides clear instructions to return to supine.	To complete the move. **E**
15 In order to leave the patient in a lateral position:	
(a) All practitioners must stay in place until the practitioner holding the patient's head confirms neutral spine alignment.	To ensure the lower spine remains aligned (Harrison 2000, **C**). To ensure patient comfort. **E**
(b Position patient between 30° and 50° lateral tilt.	To ensure pressure care. **E** To prevent excessive pressure being exerted on lower trochanter (Harrison 2000, **C**).
(c) The fifth person places a pillow lengthwise behind the patient from shoulder to hip.	To ensure the lower spine remains aligned (Harrison 2000, **C**). To ensure patient comfort. **E**
(d) The fifth person places a pillow under the patient's upper thigh lengthwise from hip to foot.	To ensure the lower spine remains aligned (Harrison 2000, **C**). To ensure patient comfort. **E**
(e) The fifth person places pillow between foot and end of bed.	To ensure the lower spine remains aligned (Harrison 2000, **C**). To ensure patient comfort. **E**
Post-procedure	
16 Reassess and record neurological symptoms.	To ensure clinical status maintained (Harrison 2000, **C**).

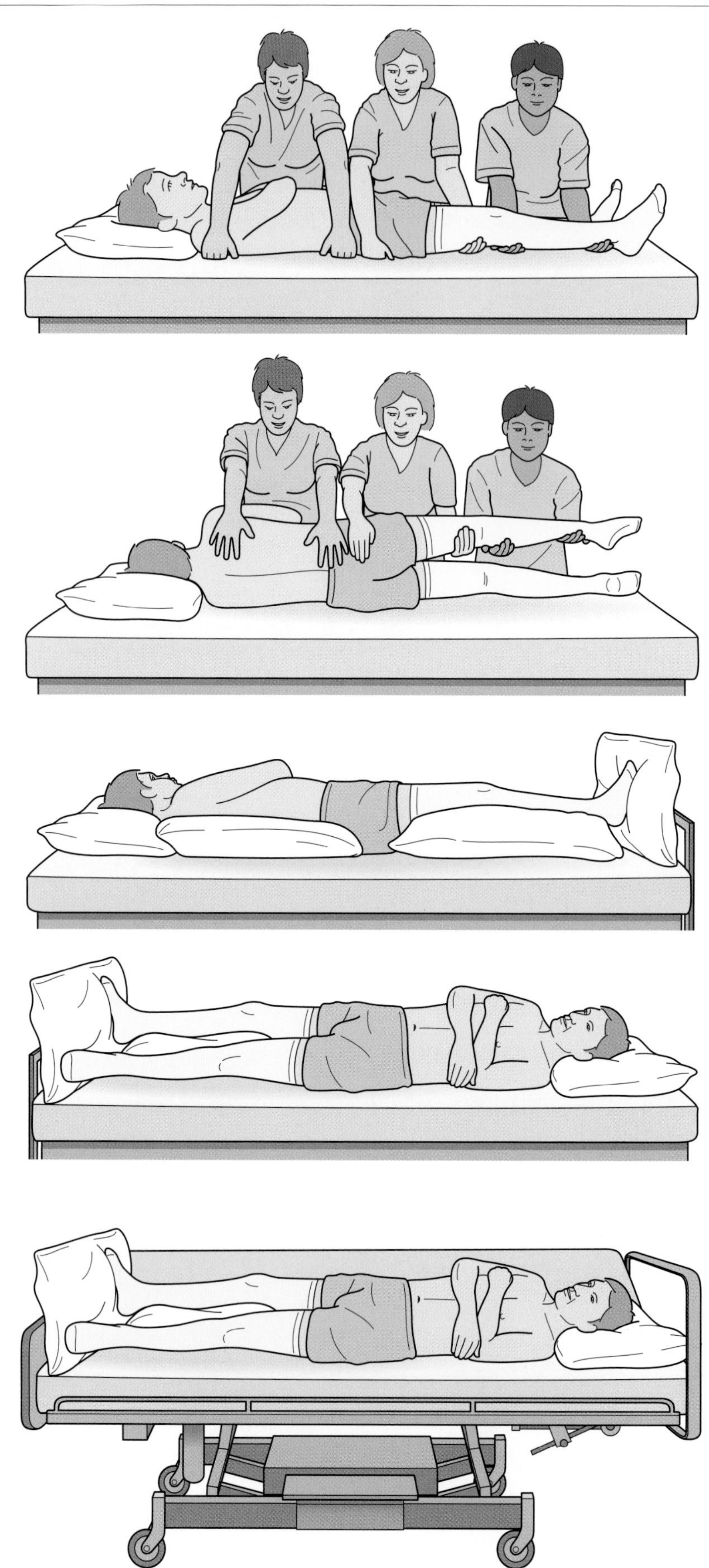

Figure 6.22 Log rolling and positioning of patient with spinal cord compression or injury. *Source:* Adapted from SIA (2000). Reproduced with permission from the Spinal Injuries Association (www.spinal.co.uk/).

Procedure guideline 6.15 Log rolling for suspected/confirmed thoracolumbar spinal instability

Essential equipment

- Pillows
- Collar or spinal brace

Optional equipment

- Slipper pan
- Clean sheets
- Hygiene equipment
- Pads
- Pressure care

Pre-procedure

Action	Rationale
1 Explain and discuss the procedure with the patient.	To ensure that the patient understands the procedure and gives their valid consent (NMC 2013, **C**).
2 Wash hands thoroughly or use an alcohol-based handrub.	To reduce the risk of contamination and cross-infection (Fraise and Bradley 2009, **E**).
3 Ensure that the bed is at the optimum height for patients or handlers. If two handlers are required try to match handlers' heights as far as possible.	To minimize the risk of injury to the practitioner (Smith 2011, **C**).
4 Ensure there are sufficient personnel available to assist with the procedure (minimum four for patients with thoracolumbar spinal instability).	Three staff to maintain spinal alignment and one to perform personal/pressure care check during the procedure (Harrison 2000, **C**).
5 Assess patient's motor power and sensation as per local documentation agreement.	For assessment before and after log roll (Harrison 2000, **C**).

Procedure

Action	Rationale
6 The lead practitioner stands at the patient's thorax and positions hands over the patient's lower back and shoulder.	To co-ordinate and lead log-roll. **E** To take responsibility for providing instructions and ensuring all other practitioners are ready before commencing the manoeuvre (Harrison 2000, **C**). To ensure the lower spine remains aligned (Harrison 2000, **C**).
7 The second practitioner stands at the hip area. Place one hand on the patient's lower back and the other under the patient's upper thigh.	To prevent movement at thoracolumbar site (Harrison 2000, **C**).
8 The third practitioner stands at the patient's lower leg. Place hands under knee and ankle.	To ensure the lower spine remains aligned (Harrison 2000, **C**).
9 Ensure there is a fourth person standing on the opposite side of bed.	To position the equipment or take care of hygiene needs. **E** To assess upper back and occiput. **E** To be carried out once a day to check pressure areas (Harrison, 2000 **C**).
10 The lead practitioner provides clear instructions to the team, for example 'We will roll on three: One, two, three'.	To ensure co-ordinated approach to the move. **E**
11 Each practitioner remains in place whilst the necessary action is performed.	
12 The person holding the head then provides clear instructions to return to supine.	To complete the move. **E**
13 In order to leave the patient in a lateral position:	
(a) All practitioners must stay in place until the practitioner holding the patient's head confirms neutral spine alignment.	To ensure the lower spine remains aligned (Harrison 2000, **C**). To ensure patient comfort. **E**
(b) Position patient between 30° and 50° lateral tilt.	To ensure pressure care. **E** To prevent excessive pressure being exerted on lower trochanter (Harrison 2000 **C**).
(c) The fourth person places pillow lengthwise behind patient from shoulder to hip.	To ensure the lower spine remains aligned (Harrison 2000, **C**). To ensure patient comfort. **E**
(d) The fourth person places pillow under patient's upper thigh lengthwise from hip to foot.	To ensure the lower spine remains aligned (Harrison 2000, **C**). To ensure patient comfort. **E**
(e) The fourth person places pillow between foot and end of bed.	To ensure the lower spine remains aligned (Harrison 2000, **C**). To ensure patient comfort. **E**

(continued)

Procedure guideline 6.15 **Log rolling for suspected/confirmed thoracolumbar spinal instability *(continued)***

Post-procedure

Action	Rationale
14 Reassess and record neurological symptoms. In the event of a worsening of pain or neurological symptoms, reassessment by medical team.	To ensure clinical status maintained (Harrison 2000, **C**).

POST-PROCEDURAL CONSIDERATIONS

Ongoing care

Reassessment by the medical team will be necessary in the event of an increase in pain or neurological symptoms.

Documentation

Any changes in (neurological) presentation and/or function must be documented both prior to and following any procedure.

Problem-solving table 6.6 **Prevention and resolution (Procedure guidelines 6.14 and 6.15)**

Problem	Cause	Prevention	Action
1 **Autonomic dysreflexia (mass reflex):** • Severe hypertension (abrupt rise in blood pressure) – systolic blood pressure can easily exceed 200 mmHg. • Bradycardia. • Pounding headache. • Flushed or blotchy appearance of skin above the level of lesion. • Profuse sweating above the level of lesion. • Pallor below the level of lesion. • Nasal congestion. • Non-drainage of urine.	Overstretching of bladder or rectum (urinary obstruction being the most common cause). Ingrown toenail or other painful stimuli. Fracture (#) below level of lesion. Pressure sore/burn/scald/ sunburn. UTI/bladder spasm. Renal or bladder calculi. Visceral pain or trauma. Pregnancy/delivery. DVT/PE. Severe anxiety/emotional distress (Lundy-Ekman 2007, Harrison 2000).	Closely monitor urinary drainage. Ensure effective bowel management regime.	THIS IS A MEDICAL EMERGENCY: Identify or eliminate the most common (most lethal) cause of autonomic dysreflexia, which is non-drainage of urine. If this is not the cause, then proceed to investigate alternative causes according to the list given. Reassure the patient throughout because anxiety increases the problem. Remove the noxious stimulus, for example recatheterize immediately in the event of a blocked catheter. Do not attempt a bladder washout because there is no guarantee that the fluid will be returned. If possible, sit the patient up, or tilt the bed head up, to induce some element of postural hypotension. If symptoms remain unresolved after removal of noxious stimulus, or if the noxious stimulus cannot be identified, administer a proprietary chemical vasodilator, such as sublingual glyceryl trinitrate (GTN) or captopril 25 mg, sublingually. (*Note*: Nifedipine capsules, which were previously recommended for use in treating or preventing autonomic dysreflexia, are being withdrawn as they have been implicated in episodes of severe hypotension.) Record blood pressure and give further reassurance. Monitor patient's condition. Refer to local spinal injuries unit (SIU) for a specialist opinion/referral (Harrison 2000).
2 **Orthostatic hypotension**	Loss of sympathetic vasoconstriction. Loss of muscle-pumping action for blood return.	Antiembolic stockings. Careful assessment and monitoring during early mobilization/ upright positional changes.	Medical review.

Problem	Cause	Prevention	Action
3 Pain Increased pain on movement to the extent that it is perceived by the patient as severe or does not reverse with rest.	Potential extension of spinal cord compression.	Ensure patients with unstable spine are moved appropriately.	Nurse patient flat. Reassess spinal stability prior to further movement (NICE 2008).
4 Respiratory function Reduced respiratory function in patient with cervical level SCC.	Ineffective use of main respiratory muscles for effective ventilation for tetraplegic patients with lesions at C3 and above. Most patients with tetraplegia (paresis/paralysis of arms, trunk, lower limbs and pelvic organs) at C4 and below are able to make sufficient respiratory effort to avoid the need for mechanical ventilation. They will, however, require oxygen therapy (Harrison 2000).	Ensure effective GI clearance/management – constipation and impaction of the bowel are a common complication of SCI management. This may place undue pressure on the diaphragm and lessen breathing space for effective respiratory function (Harrison 2000). Closely monitor respiratory function during any procedure.	Ensure appropriate head/neck support as required – collar/cervicothoracic brace for unstable cervical spinal involvement – during any moving and positioning, but if patients respiratory function decreases contact medical team urgently.
5 Cardiac syncope, i.e. fainting with unconsciousness of any cardiac cause	A cervical collar applied too tightly may cause cardiac syncope (Harrison 2000).	Ensure appropriate fit of cervical collar.	Check cervical collar is not too tight. Liaise with orthotist/PT.
6 Cardiac syncope: 2° hypoxia following initial injury. 2° turning to left side.	Sustained hypoxia increases vagal activity with a high risk of cardiac syncope (Harrison 2000). Turning the patient on to their left side for prolonged periods can increase vagal stimulation and may induce cardiac syncope. This problem is not usual during routine turning or twisting to the left side for pressure relief.	Avoid turning the patient on to their left side for prolonged periods (e.g. during a back wash or sheet change). Turning the patient onto their right side does not have the same effect.	Administer high concentrations of oxygen and atropine (Harrison 2000). Measure dynamic trend of the patient's observations (Harrison 2000).

Learning Activity 6.7

Check your knowledge:
Moving the patient with actual or suspected spinal cord compression or spinal cord injury

1 List four conditions that may result in spinal cord injury or spinal cord compression.
2 What are three common symptoms of spinal cord compression?
3 What are two techniques that should be used to move and reposition this group of patients?

See the end of the chapter for the answers.

COMPLICATIONS

There are a number of potential long-term complications that may occur during or after moving and positioning SCC/SCI patients. These are due to initial injury, the subsequent effects of changes in bowel and bladder functions and paralysis, that is, complete loss of motor function, associated with their disease or injury through autonomic and peripheral nervous system dysfunction, and those associated with bedrest.

1 *Spinal shock:* following initial injury/lesion development, spinal shock can occur due to the loss of vasomotor tone throughout the paralysed areas of the body.
   This is most pronounced in cases of tetraplegia. Patients present with hypotension, bradycardia and poikilothermia, that is, having a body temperature that varies with the temperature of its surroundings. This is due to a temporary/permanent loss of reflexes and muscle tone/control potentially leading to a compromised cardiac output. The patient must be closely monitored throughout and following any procedure or transfer, as recommended by medical staff.
2 *Autonomic dysfunction:* following injury/lesion development, secondary effects occur due to autonomic dysfunction, a potential complication for all patients with complete spinal cord lesions above the level of T6 (see Problem-solving table 6.6).
   a *Autonomic dysreflexia:* a mass reflex due to excessive activity of the sympathetic nervous system elicited by noxious stimuli below the level of the lesion.

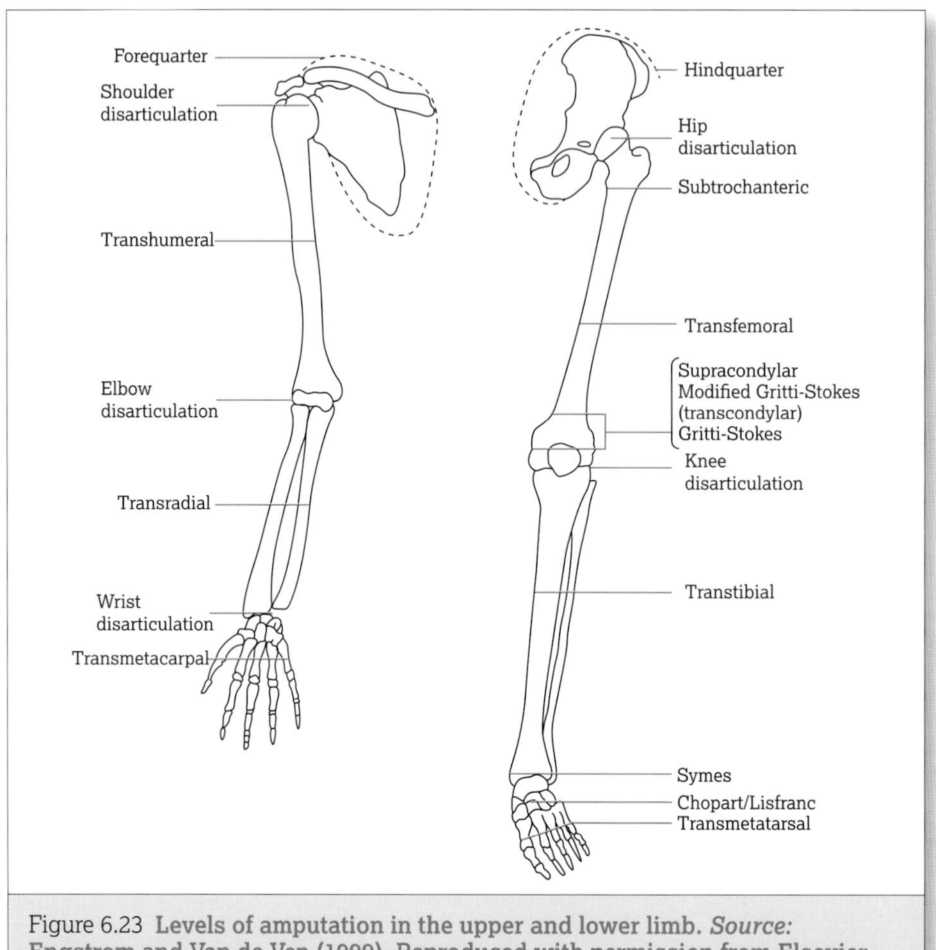

Figure 6.23 **Levels of amputation in the upper and lower limb.** ***Source:*** **Engstrom and Van de Ven (1999). Reproduced with permission from Elsevier.**

This is a medical emergency; unresolved, it can cause fatal cerebral haemorrhage. Patients present with severe hypertension (abrupt rise in blood pressure), systolic blood pressure that can easily exceed 200 mmHg, bradycardia, 'pounding' headache, flushed or blotchy appearance of skin above the level of lesion, profuse sweating above the level of lesion, pallor below the level of lesion, nasal congestion, non-drainage of urine.

b *Orthostatic hypotension:* extreme fall in blood pressure on assuming an upright position (systolic >20 mmHg, diastolic >10 mmHg). More common in tetraplegia than quadriplegia (Krassioukov et al. 2009, Lundy-Ekman 2007).

c *Poor thermoregulation:* compensatory sweating above the level of lesion and loss of ability to shiver below the level of lesion.

Patients should avoid exposure to excessive heat/cold temperatures; peripheral vasodilation means that the patient's core temperature can soon equal the environmental temperature through circulatory conduction – poikilothermia. Ensure that the patient's body temperature is maintained at an appropriate level during all procedures, treatments, investigations and transfers. Active warming should be undertaken cautiously for fear of causing skin damage (Harrison 2000).

3 *Pressure care:* risk to skin integrity and the development of pressure sores due to a lack of movement, poor circulation and altered sensation.

4 *Circulation:* risk of DVT due to the loss of vasomotor tone throughout the paralysed areas of the body. Application of thigh-length thromboembolic deterrent (TED) stockings can replace some of the lost muscle resistance, as well as reducing the risk of DVT (Harrison 2000).

Moving and positioning the patient with an amputation

DEFINITION

Amputation refers to the loss of a part or whole of a limb normally as a result of trauma or vascular disease but can also be a result of malignancy or congenital deficiency (Figure 6.23). The majority of amputations are as a result of vascular disease affecting the older population who are likely to have co-morbidities.

RELATED THEORY

The level of the amputation and the surgical technique can affect both the cosmetic appearance as well as the potential functional ability for the individual.

> 'There are certain levels of amputation that provide a residual limb suitable for a prosthetic fitting, function and cosmesis. Cosmetic appearance will depend to some extent on the level of the amputation and what prosthetic options this leaves. It is essential that one of these levels is selected rather than the boundary of the dead or diseased tissue with the viable tissue.' (Engstrom and van de Ven 1999, p.6)

EVIDENCE-BASED APPROACHES

Rationale

Indications

Any patient who has had an upper or lower limb amputation in order to:

- prevent problems arising as a consequence of reduced mobility
- maintain range of movement and muscle strength in order to rehabilitate the patient early post-operatively and to regain maximum function as soon as possible
- help decrease phantom (sensation in the part of the extremity that has been amputated) and residual limb pain.

Contraindications (with regard to certain positions)

Leaving the limb on the amputated side unsupported as this can:

- exacerbate pain
- hinder wound healing
- increase stump oedema.

Principles of care

The main goals of moving and positioning with regard to amputee management are to:

- maximize function by preventing contractures (particularly if the patient's goal is prosthetic rehabilitation)
- help to control stump oedema in order to assist wound healing
- assist the regaining of functional independence as soon as possible.

There are also two important points to consider when assisting an amputee patient.

- First, any level of amputation, either of an upper or lower limb, will alter the patient's centre of gravity, potentially resulting in decreased balance. This in turn will increase the risk of falls for these patients.
- Second, body symmetry and posture will be altered which can also affect balance and may lead to poor postural habits that will hinder recovery and function.

Where possible, the process of positioning starts at the pre-operative stage for amputation as a result of vascular problems or malignancy. In this situation the affected limb is often painful and the patient is frequently less able to mobilize. As a result, the patient may adopt positions of comfort that can lead to contractures. These positions are often maintained post amputation due to comfort and habit but are also due to changes in muscle balance (Engstrom and van de Ven 1999). For example, above-knee amputees may adopt a flexed and abducted position of their stump due to an alteration in muscle balance and pain but this can lead to contracture over time if not corrected.

Contractures can profoundly affect the potential for prosthetic rehabilitation and overall function so early correct positioning is paramount in this cohort of patients (Munin et al. 2001).

Pre-operatively, patients should also be encouraged to keep as mobile as possible within pain limits to reduce the effects of deconditioning.

Pain, including phantom limb pain, can be a major problem with these patients in the early post-operative stages.

In order to ensure that everyone works together towards a common goal, the British Association of Chartered Physiotherapists in Amputee Rehabilitation (BACPAR 2006) recommends a comprehensive assessment by key professionals to establish rehabilitation goals. This assessment should be carried out as soon as possible following the decision to amputate and will need to undergo regular review. Nurses play a vital role at all stages providing technical and physical care, including wound care and assisting in personal hygiene (Kelly and Dowling 2008) which will all impact on the patient's rehabilitation.

The general principles of care mentioned earlier in the chapter are all relevant to these patients. However, particular attention should be given to any possible balance issues for both upper limb and lower limb amputations as previously mentioned. Following lower limb amputation, patients should be mobilized with caution, particularly if a prosthetic assessment is planned. This is because standing for long periods or hopping can:

- negatively influence stump oedema and wound healing
- overtire a patient, particularly elderly patients or those who are physically deconditioned prior to the amputation
- encourage the patient to adopt poor gait patterns due to excessive weight bearing on the remaining limb, leading to difficulty with prosthetic rehabilitation.

PRE-PROCEDURAL CONSIDERATIONS

Equipment

Stump board

This will be required when sitting out in a wheelchair to ensure that the limb is fully supported and help prevent knee flexion contractures for below-knee (transtibial) amputees (Figure 6.24). 239

Wheelchair and seating cushion

Where possible, occupational therapists will assess and provide a wheelchair and a suitable cushion for lower limb amputees. If a patient has a bilateral lower limb amputation, they will need a specially adapted wheelchair with the wheels set back in order to provide sufficient stability.

Figure 6.24 Two designs of stump board. (a) An adjustable stump board: the angle can be varied for comfort. (b) A fixed stump board: this slides underneath the wheelchair cushion. *Source:* Engstrom and Van de Ven (1999). Reproduced with permission from Elsevier.

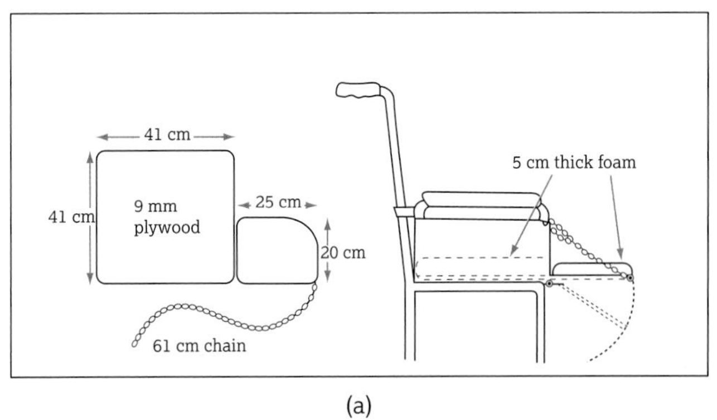

(a)

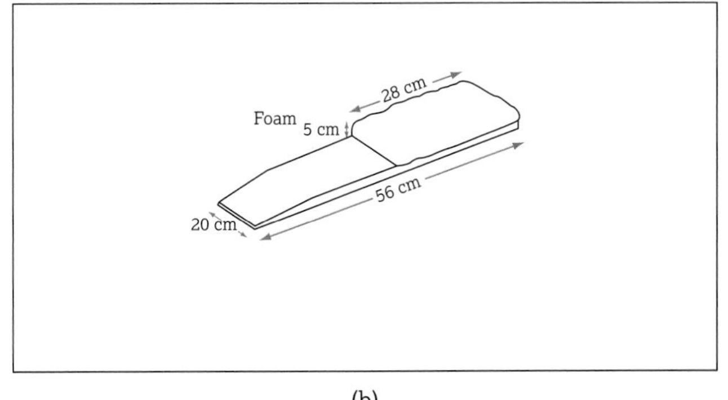

(b)

Procedure guideline 6.16 Positioning the pre-operative and post-operative amputation patient

Essential equipment

- Stump board (for below-knee amputees sitting out in wheelchair)
- Pillows
- Hoists and appropriate amputee and rehabilitation slings or sliding sheets may be required if the patient presents as a manual handling risk

Pre-procedure

Action	Rationale
1 Explain and discuss the procedure with the patient.	To ensure that the patient understands the procedure and gives their valid consent (NMC 2013, **C**).
2 Wash hands thoroughly or use an alcohol-based handrub.	To reduce the risk of contamination and cross-infection (Fraise and Bradley 2009, **E**).
3 Ensure that the bed is at the optimum height for the patient and handlers. If two handlers are required try to match handlers' heights as far as possible.	To minimize the risk of injury to the practitioner and patient (Smith 2011, **C**).
Procedure	
Upper limb amputee	
4 Ensure patient is maintaining full range of motion of all remaining joints of the upper limb by encouraging active movements of the limb.	To prevent contractures in case of possible prosthetic rehabilitation and functional use. **E**
Below-knee amputee	
5 Maintain knee extension.	
• In bed: do not place a towel or pillow under the knee unless it is supporting the whole of the stump; that is, do not encourage the knee to be maintained in a flexed position. • In chair: use a stump board on the wheelchair if one has been issued. If the patient is sitting out in the chair then support the amputation with a footstool and pillows.	To prevent knee flexion contracture. **E** To assist stump oedema management. **E** To promote healing. **E** To support knee joint. **E** To prevent excessive knee flexion. **E** To aid stump oedema management (White 1992, **R4**, **E**). To protect the residual limb. **E**
Above-knee amputee	
6 Maintain hip in a neutral position.	To maintain hip extension. **E**
• In bed: ensure the patient is periodically lying supine. *Or:*	To prevent hip flexion contracture. **E**
• Consider prone-lying or side-lying with the hip in neutral position.	To avoid shortening of hip flexors and abductors. **E**
• In sitting: ensure that the patient does not place a towel or pillow under stump.	To prevent excessive hip flexion. **E**

Problem-solving table 6.7 Prevention and resolution (Procedure guideline 6.16)

Problem	Cause	Prevention	Action
Painful stump following transfer or change of position.	Fear of movement. Pressure on distal end of stump over wound. Stump dependent, leading to increased oedema and reduced blood flow. Unsupported stump.	Reassure patient. Ensure that stump is well supported following change in position. Ensure adequate analgesia prior to movement and support stump wherever possible during the procedure.	Explain procedure to patient prior to moving position. Ensure that there is no pressure over the wound site following the procedure.
Wound breakdown.	Unsupported stump during movement. Infection. Vascular insufficiency.	Ensure that stump is well supported during and following change in position.	Ensure that there is no pressure over the wound site following the procedure. Seek medical review.

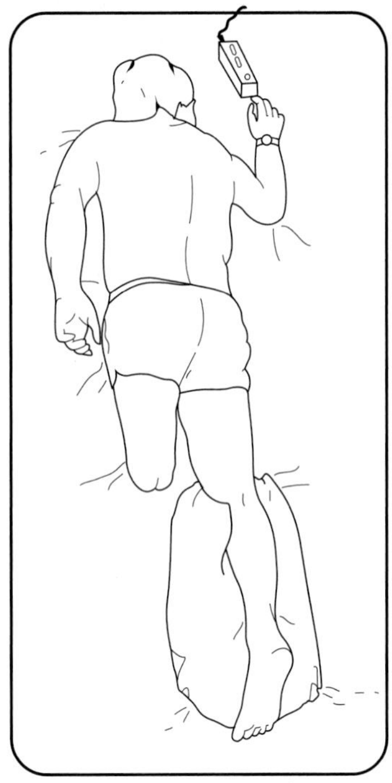
No pillows or one pillow
Arms positioned wherever comfortable for patient
Residual limb lying flat (with knee straight if t/t) No pillow
Nurse call bell placed within patient's reach
Head turned to sound side
Patient wearing a watch to time the period of lying prone
Both hips completely flat on bed
Remaining leg supported on a pillow to prevent toes from digging into bed
Footboard and bedclothes turned right back out of the way
Points to remember
1. To roll prone, the amputee must turn towards the unaffected side, the nurse ensuring that the residual limb is lowered gently.
2. Intially the amputee lies prone for about 10 minutes.
3. The amputee should then build up to lying prone for 30 minutes three times a day.

Figure 6.25 **The correct position for prone lying (t/t denotes transtibial).** ***Source:*** **Engstrom and Van de Ven (1999). Reproduced with permission from Elsevier.**

POST-PROCEDURAL CONSIDERATIONS

Mobilization following amputation

The same principles apply as outlined earlier in the chapter. The main considerations following both upper and lower limb amputation are balance and pain issues. If a lower limb amputee has a prosthesis, ensure that this is correctly applied and fitted prior to standing and mobilizing the patient.

COMPLICATIONS

1 *Limb contracture* can occur due to:
  a immobility
  b alteration in muscle balance around the joints
  c pain
  d habit.

  In order to help prevent limb contracture, the patient will require adequate analgesia to control pain. It is also important to help patients increase awareness of the positions they adopt with their stump, particularly those which may lead to limb contracture. The physiotherapist may recommend that the patient adopts certain positions for periods during the day to help prevent contractures, such as prone-lying for above-knee amputees (Figure 6.25).

2 *Ongoing phantom limb pain.* This can be a persistent problem and will need referral to the pain team for appropriate management.

3 *Wound infection or delayed healing.* Review by medical team for appropriate management.

Learning for practice

After studying this chapter, list five key points you have learnt about moving and positioning that you will be able to apply to your clinical practice.

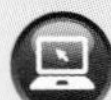 For further learning exercises visit **www.royalmarsdenmanual.com/student**.

Now Test Yourself

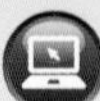

This section provides a range of exercises/activities to further test your learning. For additional exercises visit **www.royalmarsdenmanual.com/student**.

What have you learnt?

1 What is the clinical benefit of active ankle movements?
   A Assist with circulation
   B Maintain joint range
   C Lower the risk of DVT
   D All of the above

2 In the context of assessing risks prior to moving and handling, what does 'T-I-L-E' stand for?
   A Task – individual – lift – environment
   B Task – intervene – load – environment
   C Task – intervene – load – equipment
   D Task – individual – load – environment

3 If your patient is unable to reposition themselves, how often should their position be changed?
   A 1-hourly
   B 2-hourly
   C 3-hourly
   D As often as possible

4 You have been asked to reposition a patient, who already has a pressure sore, on a pressure-relieving mattress. What factors should you consider prior to moving the patient?
   A Which position will cause least pain and disruption to the wound
   B Need for pain relief, location of the pressure sore, overall skin integrity, any swelling, weakness, loss of sensation, gaining verbal consent
   C Whether pain relief is required prior to moving and gaining verbal consent
   D Need for pain relief prior to moving, location of the pressure sore, overall skin integrity

5 You are caring for a patient with dementia who has a recent history of falls. What are three interventions you could use to reduce this risk?

6 In a self-ventilating upright position, gaseous exchange (ventilation/perfusion ratio) is regarded as optimal in which of the following?
   A The apex of each lung
   B The bases of the lungs
   C The left lung
   D The right lung

7 In normal breathing, what is the main muscle(s) involved in inspiration?
   A The lungs
   B The diaphragm
   C The intercostals
   D All of the above

8 If a patient is prescribed nebulizers, how long before moving should these be administered?
   A 1 minute
   B 5 minutes
   C 15 minutes
   D 30 minutes

9 What are three important considerations before moving someone with a neurological impairment?

10 In spinal cord injury patients, what is the most common cause of autonomic dysreflexia (a sudden rise in blood pressure)?
   A Bowel obstruction
   B Urinary obstruction
   C Fracture below the level of the spinal lesion
   D Pressure sore

See the end of the chapter for the answers.

Key points

- The principles of moving and positioning will relate to the effect on the patient, but the practitioner needs to ensure that they consider their own position regarding the safety aspects of manual handling.
- Inactivity can cause a variety of problems; patients should therefore be encouraged, or assisted, to move and change position at frequent intervals.
- There is an absolute requirement to assess the risks that arise from moving and handling patients, which cannot reasonably be avoided.
- It is important to consider the risk of falls when undertaking a manual handling risk assessment. There are many interventions which have been demonstrated to reduce the incidence of falls.
- Patients with different clinical needs (for example, patients who are unconscious or have a spinal cord injury) are likely to require some modifications to the general principles of safe moving and handling.

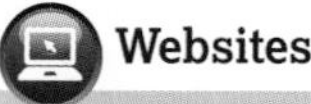

http://spinal.co.uk
www.asia-spinalinjury.org
http://guidance.nice.org.uk/CG75

REFERENCES

ACPIN (1998) *Clinical Practice Guidelines on Splinting Adults with Neurological Dysfunction.* London: Chartered Society of Physiotherapy.

Ada, L., Goddard, E., McCully, J., et al. (2005) Thirty minutes of positioning reduces the development of shoulder external rotation contracture after stroke: a randomized controlled trial. *Archives of Physical Medicine and Rehabilitation*, 86(2), 230–234.

Adam, S. & Forrest, S. (1999) ABC of intensive care: other supportive care. *BMJ*, 319(7203), 175–178.

Age UK (2013) *Staying Steady Guide.* London: Age UK. Available at: www.ageuk.org.uk/Documents/EN-GB/information-guides/AgeUKIG14_staying_steady_inf.pdf?dtrk=true

Aggarwal, R. & Hunter, A. (2007) How exactly does the chest wall work? *Student BMJ*, 15.

ASIA (2002) *Impairment Scale.* Atlanta, GA: American Spinal Injury Association.

BACPAR (2006) *Clinical Guidelines for the Pre and Post Operative Physiotherapy Management of Adults with Lower Limb Amputation.* London: Chartered Society of Physiotherapy.

Barnes, M.P. (2001) Spasticity: a rehabilitation challenge in the elderly. *Gerontology*, 47(6), 295–299.

Barnes, M.P. (2008) An overview of the clinical management of spasticity. In: Barnes, M.P. & Johnson, G.R. (eds) *Upper Motor Neurone Syndrome and Spasticity: Clinical Management and Neurophysiology*, 2nd edn. Cambridge: Cambridge University Press, pp 1–9.

Barsevick, A.M., Whitmer, K., Sweeney, C., et al. (2002) A pilot study examining energy conservation for cancer treatment-related fatigue. *Cancer Nursing*, 25(5), 333–341.

Becker, C., Kron, M., Lindemann, U., et al. (2003) Effectiveness of a multifaceted intervention on falls in nursing home residents. *Journal of the American Geriatrics Society*, 51(3), 306–313.

BNOS/DH (2011) *National Guidelines for the Management of Rare CNS Tumours.* Available at: www.bnos.org.uk/documents/rare_tumours_guidelines/CNS%20Lymphoma%20Guidelines.pdf

Bobath, B. (1990) *Adult Hemiplegia: Evaluation and Treatment*, 3rd edn. Oxford: Heinemann.

Booij, L. (1996) Fundamentals of anaesthesia and acute medicine. In: *Neuromuscular Transmission.* London: BMJ Books, pp.124–159.

Boss, B.J. (1998) Nursing management of adults with common neurologic problems. In: *Adult Health Nursing*, 3rd edn. St Louis, MO: Mosby, pp.904–947.

Bott, J., Blumenthal, S., Buxton, M., et al. (2009) Guidelines for the physiotherapy management of the adult, medical, spontaneously breathing patient. *Thorax*, 64(Suppl 1), i1–i51.

Britton, J. & Ng, V. (1998) Clinical neuro-imaging. In: Guerrero, D. (ed) *Neuro-Oncology for Nurses.* London: Whurr, pp.81–123.

Carr, J., Finlay, P., Pearson, D., et al. (2008) Multi-professional management of patients with neurological and associated conditions. In: Rankin, J., Robb, K., Murtagh, N., Cooper, J. & Lewis, S. (eds) *Rehabilitation in Cancer Care.* Oxford: John Wiley & Sons, pp.88–112.

Catz, A. & Itzkovich, M. (2007) Spinal Cord Independence Measure: comprehensive ability rating scale for the spinal cord lesion patient. *Journal of Rehabilitation and Research Development*, 44(1), 65–68.

Catz, A., Itzkovich, M., Tesio, L., et al. (2007) A multicenter international study on the Spinal Cord Independence Measure, version III: Rasch psychometric validation. *Spinal Cord*, 45(4), 275–291.

Charlton, P.T. (2009) Orthotic management. In: Lennon, S. & Stokes, M. (eds) *Pocketbook of Neurological Physiotherapy.* Edinburgh: Churchill Livingstone, pp.261–272.

Chatterton, H.J., Pomeroy, V.M. & Gratton, J. (2001) Positioning for stroke patients: a survey of physiotherapists' aims and practices. *Disability and Rehabilitation*, 23(10), 413–421.

Claus, A., Hides, J., Moseley, G.L., et al. (2008) Sitting versus standing: does the intradiscal pressure cause disc degeneration or low back pain? *Journal of Electromyography and Kinesiology*, 18(4), 550–558.

Connell, B.R. & Wolf, S.L. (1997) Environmental and behavioral circumstances associated with falls at home among healthy elderly individuals. Atlanta FICSIT Group. *Archives of Physical Medicine and Rehabilitation*, 78(2), 179–186.

Convertino, V.A., Bloomfield, S.A. & Greenleaf, J.E. (1997) An overview of the issues: physiological effects of bed rest and restricted physical activity. *Medicine and Science in Sports and Exercise*, 29(2), 187–190.

Cooper, J. (2006) *Occupational Therapy in Oncology and Palliative Care*, 2nd edn. Chichester: John Wiley & Sons.

Creditor, M.C. (1993) Hazards of hospitalization of the elderly. *Annals of Internal Medicine*, 118(3), 219–223.

CSP (2014) *Guidance in Manual Handling for Chartered Physiotherapists*, 4th edn. London: Chartered Society of Physiotherapy.

Davies, P.M. (2000) *Steps to Follow: The Comprehensive Treatment of Adult Hemiplegia.* Berlin: Springer-Verlag.

Dean, C.M., Mackey, F.H. & Katrak, P. (2000) Examination of shoulder positioning after stroke: a randomised controlled pilot trial. *Australian Journal of Physiotherapy*, 46(1), 35–40.

Dean, E. (1985) Effect of body position on pulmonary function. *Physical Therapy*, 65(5), 613–618.

DH (2001) *National Service Framework for Older People.* London: Department of Health.

DH (2009) *Reference Guide to Consent for Examination or Treatment*, 2nd edn. London: Department of Health.

DH (2013) *Living With and Beyond Cancer: Taking Action to Improve Outcomes.* London: Department of Health. Available at: www.gov.uk/government/uploads/system/uploads/attachment_data/file/181054/9333-TSO-2900664-NCSI_Report_FINAL.pdf

Dietz, J.H. (1981) *Rehabilitation Oncology.* Chichester: John Wiley & Sons.

Drakulovic, M.B., Torres, A., Bauer, T.T., et al. (1999) Supine body position as a risk factor for nosocomial pneumonia in mechanically ventilated patients: a randomised trial. *Lancet*, 354(9193), 1851–1858.

Duff, S.V., Shumway-Cook, A. & Woollacott, M.H. (2012) Clinical management of the patient with reach, grasp and manipulation disorders. In: Shumway-Cook, A. & Woollacott, M.H. (eds) *Motor Control: Translating Research into Clinical Practice*, 4th edn. Philadelphia: Lippincott Williams and Wilkins, pp.552–594.

Edwards, S. (1998) Physiotherapy management of established spasticity in spasticity rehabilitation. In: Shean, G. (ed) *Spasticity Management.* London: Churchill Communications Europe Ltd, pp.71–90.

Edwards, S. (2002a) Abnormal tone and movement as a result of neurological impairment. In: Edwards, S. (ed) *Neurological Physiotherapy: A Problem-Solving Approach*, 2nd edn. Edinburgh: Churchill Livingstone, pp.63–86.

Edwards, S. (2002b) An analysis of normal movement as the basis for the development of treatment techniques. In: Edwards, S. (ed) *Neurological Physiotherapy: A Problem-Solving Approach*, 2nd edn. Edinburgh: Churchill Livingstone, pp.35–68.

Edwards, S. & Carter, P. (2002) General principles of treatment. In: Edwards, S. (ed) *Neurological Physiotherapy: A Problem-Solving Approach*, 2nd edn. Edinburgh: Churchill Livingstone, pp.121–154.

Engstrom, B. & van de Ven, C. (1999) *Therapy for Amputees*, 3rd edn. Edinburgh: Churchill Livingstone.

Fink, J.B. (2002) Positioning versus postural drainage. *Respiratory Care*, 47(7), 769–777.

Formica, V., Del Monte, G., Giacchetti, I., et al. (2011) Rehabilitation in neuro-oncology: a meta-analysis of published data and a mono-institutional experience. *Integrative Cancer Therapies*, 10(2), 119–126.

Fraise, A.P. & Bradley, C. (2009) *Ayliffe's Control of Healthcare-Associated Infection: A Practical Handbook*, 5th edn. London: Hodder Arnold.

Gardiner, M.D. (1973) *The Principles of Exercise Therapy*, 3rd edn. London: Bell.

Geraghty, M. (2005) Nursing the unconscious patient. *Nursing Standard*, 20(1), 54–64.

Gillis, M.K. (1989) Observational gait analysis. In: *Physical Therapy.* Philadelphia: Lippincott, pp.670–695.

Gloag, D. (1985) Rehabilitation after stroke: 1 What is the potential? *BMJ (Clin Res)*, 290(6469), 699–701.

Grieve, J.I. & Gnanasekaran, L. (2008) *Neuropsychology for Occupational Therapists: Cognition in Occupational Performance*, 3rd edn. Oxford: Blackwell Publishing.

Hanks, G.W.C. & Ovid Technologies. (2010) *Oxford Textbook of Palliative Medicine*, 4th edn. Oxford: Oxford University Press.

Harden, B. (2008) *Respiratory Physiotherapy: An On-Call Survival Guide*, 2nd edn. Oxford: Elsevier Health Sciences.

Harrison, P. (2000) *Managing Spinal Injury: Critical Care. The Initial Management of People with Actual or Suspected Spinal Cord Injury in High Dependency and Intensive Care.* Milton Keynes: Spinal Injury Association.

Hawkins, S., Stone, K. & Plummer, L. (1999) An holistic approach to turning patients. *Nursing Standard*, 14(3), 51–56.

Hesse, S. (2003) Rehabilitation after stroke: evaluation, principles of therapy, novel treatment approaches and assistive devices. *Topics in Geriatric Medicine*, 19(2), 109–126.

Hickey, J.V. (2009) Neurological assessment. In: Hickey, J.V. (ed) *The Clinical Practice of Neurological and Neurosurgical Nursing*, 6th edn. Philadelphia: Wolters Kluwer/Lippincott Williams and Wilkins Health, pp.154–180.

Hickey, J.V. & Powers, M.B. (2009) Management of patients with a depressed state of conciousness. In: Hickey, J.V. (ed) *The Clinical Practice of Neurological and Neurosurgical Nursing*, 6th edn. Philadelphia: Wolters Kluwer/Lippincott Williams and Wilkins Health, pp.336–351.

Hodges, P.W. & Gandevia, S.C. (2000) Changes in intra-abdominal pressure during postural and respiratory activation of the human diaphragm. *Journal of Applied Physiology*, 89(3), 967–976.

Hough, A. (2001) *Physiotherapy in Respiratory Care: An Evidence-Based Approach to Respiratory and Cardiac Management*, 3rd edn. Cheltenham: Nelson Thornes.

HSE (1992) *Manual Handling Operations Regulations 1992*. London: HMSO.

HSE (2012) *Manual Handling at Work: A Brief Guide*. Sudbury: Health and Safety Executive. Available at: www.hse.gov.uk/pubns/indg143.pdf

Itzkovich, M., Gelernter, I., Biering-Sorensen, F., et al. (2007) The Spinal Cord Independence Measure (SCIM) version III: reliability and validity in a multi-center international study. *Disability and Rehabilitation*, 29(24), 1926–1933.

Jackson, J. (1998) Specific treatment techniques. In: *Neurological Physiotherapy*. London: Mosby, pp.299–311.

Jacobson, A.F. & Winslow, E.H. (2000) Caring for unconscious patients. *American Journal of Nursing*, 100(1), 69.

Jones, M. & Moffatt, F. (2002) *Cardiopulmonary Physiotherapy*. Oxford: BIOS.

Kalina, P., Drehobl, K.E., Black, K., et al. (1995) Spinal cord compression by spontaneous spinal subdural haematoma in polycythemia vera. *Postgraduate Medical Journal*, 71(836), 378–379.

Kaplan, M.C. (1995) Hemiplegic shoulder pain – early prevention and rehabilitation. *Western Journal of Medicine*, 162(2), 151–152.

Kelly, M. & Dowling, M. (2008) Patient rehabilitation following lower limb amputation. *Nursing Standard*, 22(49), 35–40.

Kirkwood, C.A. & Bardsley, G.I. (2001) Seating and positioning in spasticity. In: *Upper Motor Neurone Syndrome and Spasticity: Clinical Management and Neurophysiology*. Cambridge: Cambridge University Press, pp.122–141.

Krassioukov, A., Eng, J.J., Warburton, D.E., et al. (2009) A systematic review of the management of orthostatic hypotension after spinal cord injury. *Archives of Physical Medicine and Rehabilitation*, 90(5), 876–885.

Lawrence, M. (1995) The unconscious experience. *American Journal of Critical Care*, 4(3), 227–232.

Lindsay, K.W., Bone, I., Fuller, G., et al. (2011) *Neurology and Neurosurgery Illustrated*, 5th edn. Edinburgh: Churchill Livingstone.

Loblaw, D.A., Laperriere, N.J. & Mackillop, W.J. (2003) A population-based study of malignant spinal cord compression in Ontario. *Clinical Oncology*, 15(4), 211–217.

Lohani, B. & Sharma, M.R. (2004) Patterns in spinal tumours in Nepal: a clinico-radiological study. *Nepal Journal of Neuroscience*, 1, 113–119.

Lumb, A.B. & Nunn, J.F. (2010) *Nunn's Applied Respiratory Physiology*, 7th edn. London: Elsevier.

Lundy-Ekman, L. (2007) Motor neurons. In: *Neuroscience: Fundamentals for Rehabilitation*, 3rd edn. St Louis, MO: Saunders Elsevier, pp.188–242.

MacIntyre, N.R. & Branson, R.D. (2009) *Mechanical Ventilation*, 2nd edn. St Louis, MO: Saunders Elsevier.

Mann, F.A., Kubal, W.S. & Blackmore, C.C. (2000) Improving the imaging diagnosis of cervical spine injury in the very elderly: implications of the epidemiology of injury. *Emergency Radiology*, 7(1), 36–41.

McGarvey, C.L. (1990) *Physical Therapy for the Cancer Patient*. New York: Churchill Livingstone.

McKenzie, R. (2006) *Treat Your Own Back*, 6th rev edn. New Zealand: Spinal Publications.

Mee, L.Y. & Bee, W.H. (2007) A comparison study on nurses' and therapists' perception on the positioning of stroke patients in Singapore General Hospital. *International Journal of Nursing Practice*, 13(4), 209–221.

Mehan, R., Mackenzie, M. & Brock, K. (2008) Skilled transfer training in stroke rehabilitation: a review of use and safety.. including commentary by Sparkes V. *International Journal of Therapy and Rehabilitation*, 15(9), 382–389.

Methany, N.A. & Frantz, R.A. (2013) Head-of-bed elevation in critically ill patients: a review. *Critical Care Nurse*, 33(3), 53–67.

Miller, J. & Cooper, J. (2010) The contribution of occupational therapy to palliative medicine. In: Doyle, D., Cherny, N.I., Christakis, N.A., Fallon, M., Kasasa, S. & Portenoy, R.K (eds) *Oxford Textbook of Palliative Medicine*. 4th edn. Oxford: Oxford University Press, pp.206–213.

Munin, M.C., Espejo-De Guzman, M.C., Boninger, M.L., et al. (2001) Predictive factors for successful early prosthetic ambulation among lower-limb amputees. *Journal of Rehabilitation Research and Development*, 38(4), 379–384.

Nelson, A., Matz, M., Chen, F. *et al.* (2006) Development and evaluation of a multifaceted ergonomics program to prevent injuries associated with patient handling tasks. *International Journal of Nursing Studies*, 43(6), 717–733.

Nelson, A., Collins, J., Siddharthan, K., et al. (2008) Link between safe patient handling and patient outcomes in long-term care. *Rehabilitation Nursing*, 33(1), 33–43.

NHS Centre for Reviews and Dissemination (1996) Preventing falls and subsequent injury in older people. *Effective Health Care*, 2(4), 1–16. Available at: www.york.ac.uk/inst/crd/EHC/ehc24.pdf

NICE (2006) *Guidance on Cancer Services: Improving Outcomes for People with Tumours of the Brain and Central Nervous System*. London: National Institute for Health and Clinical Excellence. Available at: www.nice.org.uk/nicemedia/pdf/CSG_brain_needsassessment.pdf

NICE (2008) *CG75 Metastatic Spinal Cord Compression: Full Guideline*. London: National Institute for Health and Clinical Excellence. Available at: www.nice.org.uk/nicemedia/live/12085/42668/42668.pdf

NICE (2013) *Falls: Assessment and Prevention of Falls in Older People, CG161*. London: National Institute for Health and Care Excellence. Available at: www.nice.org.uk/nicemedia/live/14181/64088/64088.pdf

NMC (2013) *Consent*. London: Nursing and Midwifery Council. Available at: www.nmc-uk.org/Documents/Standards/The-code-A4-20100406.pdf

NPSA (2010) *Slips, Trips and Falls in Hospital Update*. London: National Patient Safety Agency. Available at: www.nrls.npsa.nhs.uk/resources/?entryid45=74567

O'Donovan, K.J., Bajd, T., Grace, P.A., et al. (2006) An investigation of recommended lower leg exercises for induced calf muscle activity. Proceedings of the 24th IASTED International Conference on Biomedical Engineering. Innsbruck, Austria, ACTA Press.

O'Dwyer, N.J., Ada, L. & Neilson, P.D. (1996) Spasticity and muscle contracture following stroke. *Brain*, 119(5), 1737–1749.

Oliver, D., Connelly, J.B., Victor, C.R., et al. (2007) Strategies to prevent falls and fractures in hospitals and care homes and effect of cognitive impairment: systematic review and meta-analyses. *BMJ*, 334(7584), 82.

Patient Safety First (2009) *The 'How To' Guide for Reducing Harm from Falls*. London: Patient Safety First. Available at: www.patientsafetyfirst.nhs.uk/ashx/Asset.ashx?path=/Intervention-support/FALLSHow-to%20Guide%20v4.pdf

Pearsall, J. (2010) *The Concise Oxford Dictionary*, 10th edn. Oxford: Oxford University Press.

Peate, I., Nair, M., Wild, K. (2014) *Nursing Practice: Knowledge and Care*. Oxford: John Wiley & Sons.

Pope, P. (2002) Postural management and special seating. In: Edwards, S. (ed) *Neurological Physiotherapy: A Problem Solving Approach*, 2nd edn. Edinburgh: Churchill Livingstone, pp.189–218.

Pryor, J.A. & Prasad, S.A. (2008) *Physiotherapy for Respiratory and Cardiac Problems: Adults and Paediatrics*, 4th edn. Edinburgh: Churchill Livingstone Elsevier.

Raine, S., Meadows, L. & Etherington-Lynch, M. (2009) *Bobath Concept. Theory and Clinical Practice in Neurological Rehabilitation*. Oxford: John Wiley & Sons.

RCM, RCN, DH, et al. (2009) *High Impact Actions for Nursing and Midwifery*. London: NHS Institute for Improvement and Innovation. Available at: www.institute.nhs.uk/images//stories/Building_Capability/HIA/NHSI%20High%20Impact%20Actions.pdf

RCN (2001) *Presure Ulcer Risk Assessment and Prevention*. London: Royal College of Nursing. Available at: www.rcn.org.uk/__data/assets/pdf_file/0003/78501/001252.pdf

Riedel, M. (2001) Acute pulmonary embolism 1: pathophysiology, clinical presentation, and diagnosis. *Heart*, 85(2), 229–240.

Rockefeller, K. (2008) Using technology to promote safe patient handling and rehabilitation. *Rehabilitation Nursing*, 33(1), 3–9.

Shumway-Cook, A. & Woollacott, M.H. (eds) (2012) *Motor Control: Translating Research into Clinical Practice*, 4th edn. Philadelphia: Lippincott Williams and Wilkins.

SIA (2000) *Managing Spinal Injury: Critical Care*. London: Spinal Injuries Association. Available at: www.spinal. co.uk/pdf/SIA%20Critical%20care.pdf

Smith, J., National Back Exchange & BackCare (2011) *The Guide to the Handling of People: A Systems Approach*, 6th edn. Teddington, Middx: BackCare.

Stalenhoef, P.A., Diederiks, J.P., Knottnerus, J.A., et al. (2002) A risk model for the prediction of recurrent falls in community-dwelling elderly: a prospective cohort study. *Journal of Clinical Epidemiology*, 55(11), 1088–1094.

Stokes, M. & Stack, E. (2012) *Physical Management for Neurological Conditions*, 3rd revised edn. Edinburgh: Elsevier.

Thomas, A.J. (2009) Exercise intervention in the critical care unit – what is the evidence? *Physical Therapy Reviews*, 14(1), 50–59.

Tiplady, B., Jackson, S.H., Maskrey, V.M., et al. (1998) Validity and sensitivity of visual analogue scales in young and older healthy subjects. *Age and Ageing*, 27(1), 63–66.

Tortora, G.J. & Derrickson, B.H. (2011) *Principles of Anatomy and Physiology*, 13th edn. Hoboken, NJ: John Wiley & Sons.

Verheyden, G. & Ashburn, A. (2012) *Stroke*. In: Stokes, M. & Stack, E. (eds) *Physical Management for Neurological Conditions*, 3rd revised edn. Edinburgh: Elsevier, pp.2–28.

Ward, J.A., Harden, M., Gibson, R.E., et al. (2010) A cluster randomised controlled trial to prevent injury due to falls in a residential aged care population. *Medical Journal of Australia*, 192(6), 319–322.

West, J.B. (2012) *Respiratory Physiology: The Essentials*, 9th edn. Philadelphia: Lippincott Williams and Wilkins.

White, E.A. (1992) Wheelchair stump boards and their use with lower limb amputees. *British Journal of Occupational Therapy*, 55(5), 174–178.

Answers

Learning Activity 6.2 Case study: What are the risk factors for developing pressure sores?

An 86-year-old gentleman has just been admitted onto your ward. He had a fall at home last night resulting in a fractured neck of the femur. You have been asked to assess his risk of developing pressure sores.

1 What are his main risk factors for developing a pressure sore at this time?
- His age, fractured hip and resulting lack of mobility.

2 What tool could you use to assess this risk?
- Norton or Waterlow.

3 What manual handling aids might you require to assist this patient with repositioning?
- Sliding sheets, hoist, additional pillows (depending on desired position) (see Procedure guidelines 6.1 and 6.2).

Learning Activity 6.4 Scenario: Assisting the patient to walk

On the ward, you have been asked to assist a female patient, who is currently seated in her chair, to walk to the toilet.

What factors should you consider prior to undertaking this activity?
- Any restrictions to her mobility (e.g. recent surgery, IV lines/ pumps/stands)?
- Is she fully weight bearing?
- Is she wearing appropriate footwear?
- Does she have a walking aid that should be used to assist with her mobility?
- Do you need assistance to carry out this activity?

Learning Activity 6.6 Case study: Moving the unconscious patient

Ms Jones is a 56-year-old woman who has been unconscious and intubated in the intensive care unit for the last three days following a road traffic collision. You are looking after her today along with one of the members of the ICU nursing team and have been asked to help turn her from lying on her right side to a supine position.

1 What are the main considerations prior to repositioning Ms Jones?
- Maintaining her airway.
- Ensuring she is repositioned at least 2-hourly.

2 How many staff are required to move Ms Jones?
- At least four members of staff (one to be in charge of airway).

3 What equipment is required to assist in moving her safely?
- Manual handling equipment.
- Pillows and towels to ensure a comfortable position.

4 What should the team be considering during the procedure?
- Communicating with Ms Jones, explaining the procedure.
- Checking and maintaining skin integrity.

5 What should be done after Ms Jones is repositioned?
- Monitor colour, temperature and pulses of the limbs.
- Document that the procedure has been carried out, within the patient's records.

For the full procedure, refer to Procedure guideline 6.8: Positioning the unconscious patient or patient with an airway in supine.

Learning Activity 6.7 Check your knowledge: Moving the patient with actual or suspected spinal cord compression or spinal cord injury

1 List four conditions that may result in spinal cord injury or spinal cord compression.
- For example: degenerative conditions, traumatic spinal cord injury, haematoma, primary tumours.

2 What are three common symptoms of spinal cord compression?
- For example: back pain, limb weakness, bladder dysfunction.

3 What are two techniques that should be used to move and reposition this group of patients?
- Lateral surface transfer, log rolling.

Now Test Yourself What have you learnt?

1 What is the clinical benefit of active ankle movements?
A Assist with circulation
B Maintain joint range
C Lower the risk of DVT
D All of the above

2 In the context of assessing risks prior to moving and handling, what does 'T-I-L-E' stand for?
A Task – individual – lift – environment
B Task – intervene – load – environment
C Task – intervene – load – equipment
D Task – individual – load – environment

3 If your patient is unable to reposition themselves, how often should their position be changed?
A 1-hourly
B 2-hourly
C 3-hourly
D As often as possible

4 You have been asked to reposition a patient, who already has a pressure sore, on a pressure-relieving mattress. What factors should you consider prior to moving the patient?
A Which position will cause least pain and disruption to the wound
B Need for pain relief, location of the pressure sore, overall skin integrity, any swelling, weakness, loss of sensation, gaining verbal consent
C Whether pain relief is required prior to moving and gaining verbal consent
D Need for pain relief prior to moving, location of the pressure sore, overall skin integrity

5 You are caring for a patient with dementia who has a recent history of falls. What are three interventions you could use to reduce this risk?

For example: hydration, declutter, walking aids, exercise programmes, identification bracelets, risk assessments, alarm systems

6 In a self-ventilating upright position, gaseous exchange (ventilation/perfusion ratio) is regarded as optimal in which of the following?
A The apex of each lung
B The bases of the lungs
C The left lung
D The right lung

7 In normal breathing, what is the main muscle(s) involved in inspiration?
A The lungs
B The diaphragm
C The intercostals
D All of the above

8 If a patient is prescribed nebulizers, how long before moving should these be administered?
A 1 minute
B 5 minutes
C 15 minutes
D 30 minutes

9 What are three important considerations before moving someone with a neurological impairment?

For example: variations in tone, communication/behavioural/sensory problems, variable ability (such as on/off periods for patients with Parkinson's disease)

10 In spinal cord injury patients, what is the most common cause of autonomic dysreflexia (a sudden rise in blood pressure)?
A Bowel obstruction
B Urinary obstruction
C Fracture below the level of the spinal lesion
D Pressure sore

Nutrition, fluid balance and blood transfusion

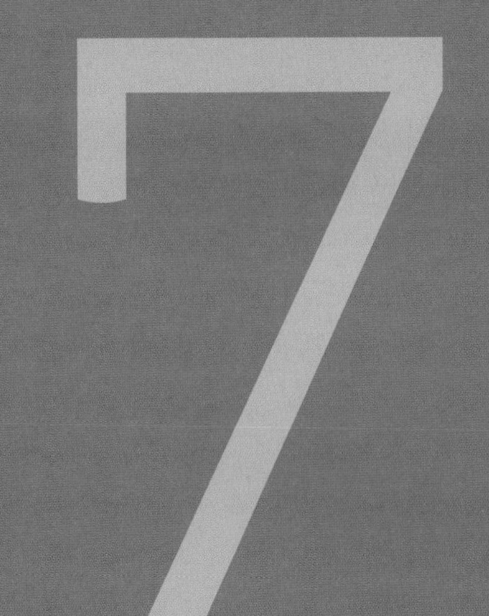

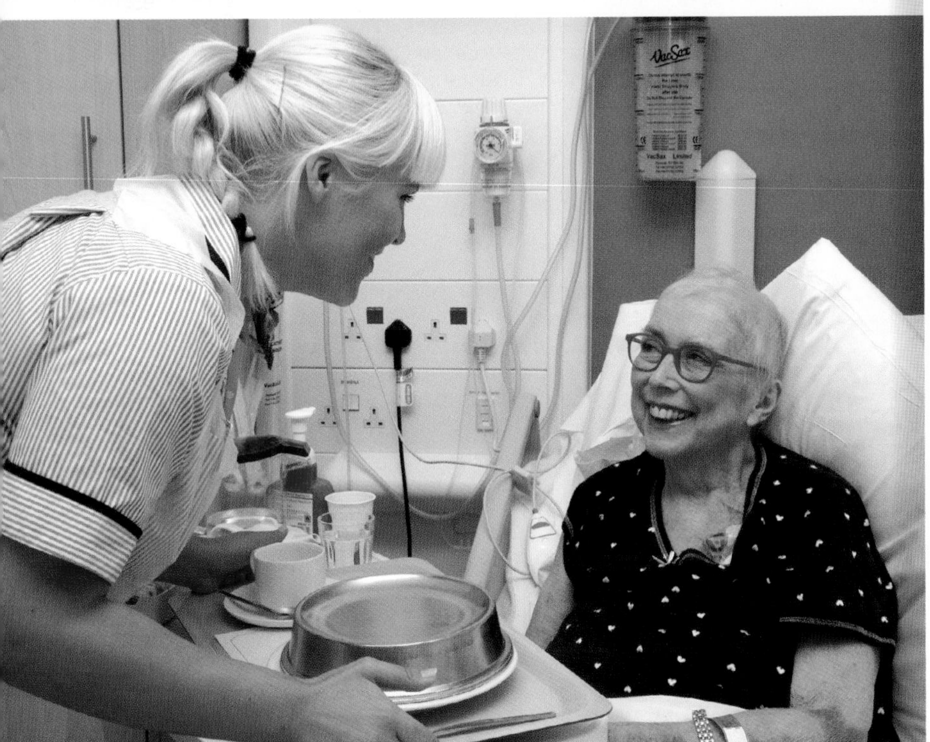

By reading this chapter and undertaking the learning activities within it, you should be able to:

1 Gain insight and understanding about the significant role that fluid and nutrition play in body composition.

2 Identify the critical importance of maintaining an accurate record of fluid balance.

3 Review different methods of nutritional assessment in order to identify patients who are malnourished or at risk of malnutrition.

4 Identify various strategies to ensure that patients' fluid and nutritional needs can be met, through oral, enteral and parenteral routes of nutrition, fluid or blood products.

Procedure guidelines

The Royal Marsden Manual of Clinical Nursing Procedures: Student Edition, Ninth Edition. Edited by Lisa Dougherty, Sara Lister and Alexandra West-Oram

Overview

Good nutrition, the supply of optimal nutrients and fluid to meet requirements, is an essential component of health, with poor nutrition contributing to ill health and prolonged recovery from illness or disease. It is therefore crucial that the nutritional status of all patients is assessed and considered during the whole of the patient's care. This chapter addresses how fluid and nutrition can influence body composition, how to identify patients who are malnourished or at risk of malnutrition and, most importantly, how the patient's nutritional needs can be met.

The provision of food and fluids to patients is an integral part of basic care. In normal circumstances, adequate nutritional intake enables the body to maintain homeostasis of body composition and function but in disease states this balance can be altered. The majority of patients will achieve adequate nutrition through the oral route of diet and fluids but, for some, additional artificial nutritional support or products such as blood will be required to maintain optimal body composition and function. This chapter describes how the patient's needs can be assessed and met through oral, enteral and parenteral routes of nutrition, fluid or blood products.

Fluid balance

DEFINITION

In the human homeostatic state, the intake of fluids equals fluid excreted from the body, thereby maintaining optimal hydration. In nursing practice, this term refers to the procedure of measuring fluid input and output to determine fluid balance (Marieb and Hoehn 2010, Scales and Pilsworth 2008).

ANATOMY AND PHYSIOLOGY

Body composition

The human body is made up of approximately 60% water (this varies with age, gender and percentage of fatty tissue) (Rhoda and Porter 2011, Scales and Pilsworth 2008, Tortora and Derrickson 2011). Bodily water/fluid is essential to life and vital for:

- controlling body temperature
- the delivery of nutrients and gases to cells
- the removal of waste
- acid/base balance
- the maintenance of cellular shape (Baumberger-Henry 2008).

Total body water is distributed between two main compartments: intracellular fluid (ICF, within the cell) and extracellular fluid (ECF, outside the cell). ECF is further divided into the intravascular space, within the blood vessels (known as plasma), the interstitial space which surrounds the cells and the transcellular space. The transcellular space contains specialized fluids such as cerebrospinal fluid; these do not readily exchange fluid with other compartments so are rarely considered in fluid management (Bishop 2008, Rhoda and Porter 2011).

Bodily fluid is a composition of water and a variety of dissolved solutes which Marieb and Hoehn (2010) classify as electrolytes and non-electrolytes. Non-electrolytes include glucose, lipids, creatine and urea and are molecules that do not dissociate in solution and have no electrical charge. Electrolytes such as potassium, sodium, chloride, magnesium and bicarbonate all dissociate in solution into charged ions that conduct electricity. Concentration of these solutes varies depending on the compartment in which they are contained; for example, ECF has a high sodium content (135–145 mmol/L) and is relatively low in potassium (3.5–4.5 mmol/L) and ICF is the reverse – high in potassium but lower in sodium (Tortora and Derrickson 2011). The movement and distribution of fluid and solutes between compartments are controlled by the semi-permeable phospholipid cellular membranes that separate them (Baumberger-Henry 2008).

Transport and movement of water and solutes

Water can readily and passively pass across the membrane and does so by osmosis (Table 7.1) in response to changing solute concentrations (Tortora and Derrickson 2011). The amount of solute in solution determines the osmolarity – the higher the solute concentration, the higher the osmolarity; this is also referred to as the osmotic pressure (or pull). Electrolytes move across the membrane via the protein channels, some by diffusion (see Table 7.1) and also via a passive mode of transport where solutes move towards an area of low solute concentration. Sodium and potassium are an exception to this rule, as they are required to move against the concentration gradient in order to preserve higher intravascular sodium concentrations. Energy is utilized to pump sodium out of the cell via the protein channels and pump potassium back into the cell, known as the sodium/potassium pump (see Table 7.1).

The movement of water and solutes out of the intravascular space and into the interstitial space is dependent on opposing osmotic and hydrostatic pressures (Scales and Pilsworth 2008). Hydrostatic pressure is caused by the pumping action of the heart and the diameter (resistance) of the vessels/capillaries forcing water and molecules that are small enough to pass through the membrane out of the vessel and into the interstitial fluid. Within the vascular system, only the capillaries have semi-permeable membranes and this is where 'filtration' occurs. At the arteriole end of the capillary, the hydrostatic pressure exceeds the osmotic pressure, moving solutes out of the plasma and into the interstitial space. At the venous end, hydrostatic pressure is reduced and the osmotic pressure within the vessel (plasma) is higher so water is pulled back into the vessel and circulating volume (Tortora and Derrickson 2011). The osmotic pressure is provided by plasma proteins that are too large to pass through the membrane even under pressure. Oedema can result if the membranes become permeable to protein; osmotic pressure is then reduced, resulting in excess of water moving into the interstitial space. Pulmonary oedema is caused by this mechanism at the site of the lungs. Sepsis or a systemic inflammatory response is an example of a condition where the capillary membranes become more permeable to protein.

Osmolarity and fluid balance

Sodium is the most influential electrolyte in fluid balance and is the primary cation (positively charged ion) of the ECF. The concentration of sodium in the ECF has the most profound effect on its osmolarity and therefore water balance (Rhoda 2011). If ECF osmolarity increases (for example, with increased intake of sodium, reduced fluid intake, increased loss of fluid), osmoreceptors of the hypothalamus detect very slight changes (1–2% increase) in plasma osmolarity (Marieb and Hoehn 2010) and trigger the thirst response which in turn encourages oral fluid intake in an attempt to restore the balance (Figure 7.1).

Hormonal mechanisms and the kidneys are highly influential in fluid and electrolyte balance and again are also triggered in response to changing osmolarity and/or plasma volumes. Antidiuretic hormone (ADH) is released from the posterior pituitary gland (in response to stimulus of the osmoreceptors in the hypothalamus) (Tortora and Derrickson 2011) and acts on the tubules and collecting ducts of the kidneys, inhibiting water excretion and encouraging water reabsorption. If plasma osmolarity falls (indicating water excess), these mechanisms are suppressed by a negative feedback loop; the osmoreceptors are no longer stimulated. This in turn inhibits ADH release; renal tubules no longer conserve water and thirst is reduced, leading to a reduction of oral intake and restoration of balance. ADH is also released in the renin-angiotensin response to a reduction in blood pressure (detected by baroreceptors in blood vessels); more detailed information on this mechanism can be found in Chapter 11: Observations.

Table 7.1 **Molecule transport modes**

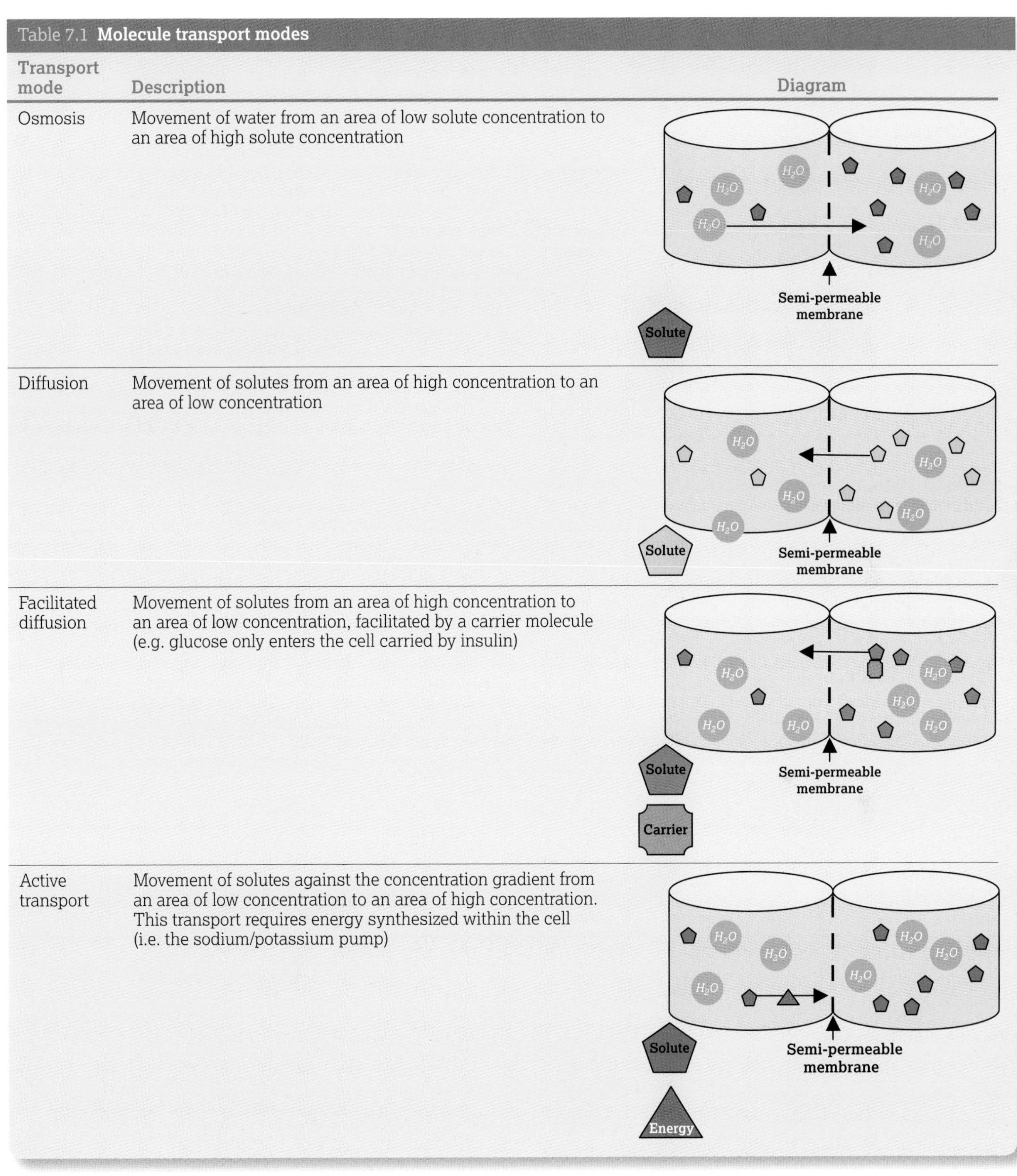

Transport mode	Description	Diagram
Osmosis	Movement of water from an area of low solute concentration to an area of high solute concentration	
Diffusion	Movement of solutes from an area of high concentration to an area of low concentration	
Facilitated diffusion	Movement of solutes from an area of high concentration to an area of low concentration, facilitated by a carrier molecule (e.g. glucose only enters the cell carried by insulin)	
Active transport	Movement of solutes against the concentration gradient from an area of low concentration to an area of high concentration. This transport requires energy synthesized within the cell (i.e. the sodium/potassium pump)	

Aldosterone is a mineralocorticoid secreted by the adrenal cortex in response to increased osmolarity and/or decreased blood pressure (part of the renin-angiotensin system). It acts on the renal tubules, initiating the active transport of sodium (and hence water) from the tubules and collecting ducts back into the plasma and circulating volume (Baumberger-Henry 2008).

These homeostatic mechanisms are very effective in maintaining fluid and electrolyte balance in health and act to compensate for fluid imbalances to ensure effective cellular function. However, these compensatory mechanisms are not sustainable and will eventually fail if ill health or imbalance persists. For example, in continued haemorrhage, the body will compensate by conserving water and vasoconstricting vessels in an attempt to increase blood pressure and volume. Failure to replace lost fluids, improve volume and therefore perfusion will eventually lead to cellular and organ dysfunction which in turn lead to organ failure and possible death (Goldstein 2012).

Dehydration is a particular concern in ill health as often fluid intake is reduced (poor appetite, nil by mouth, nausea) and often coincides with an increased output (vomiting, diarrhoea, haemorrhage,

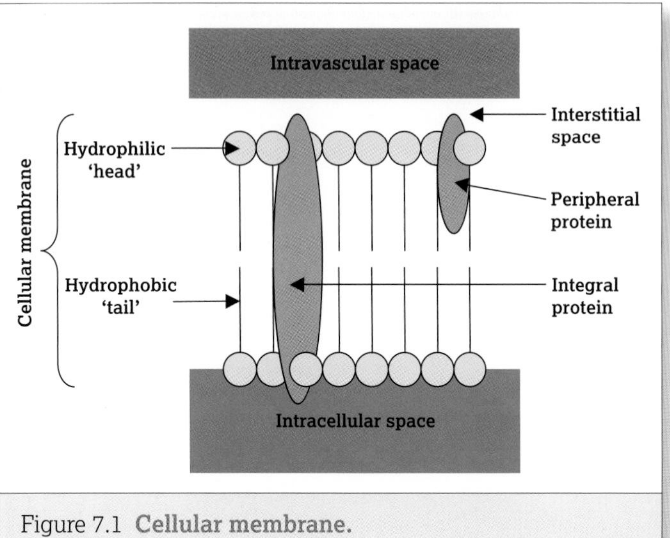

Figure 7.1 **Cellular membrane.**

drains, fever). The elderly are at particular risk of dehydration as the effectiveness of the thirst response diminishes with age (Mentes 2006, Welch 2010). When the osmolarity of the ECF increases, it encourages water out of the cell into the ECF, which eventually leads to cellular dehydration, impaired metabolism, disturbed cellular shape and impaired cellular function (Tortora and Derrickson 2011).

If the osmolarity of the ECF falls, water moves into the cell. If this continues, it will lead to water toxicity, causing cells to expand and eventually burst. Care should therefore be taken when administering intravenous fluids (Powell-Tuck et al. 2011), as fluids that are of lower osmolarity than ECF (hypotonic) will cause a shift of water into the cells. Conversely, hypertonic solutions will cause a shift of fluid from the cells, causing dehydration. Maintenance fluids should usually be isotonic (have the same osmolarity as ECF) (Sheppard and Wright 2006).

EVIDENCE-BASED APPROACHES

Fluid and electrolyte balance monitoring and management are integral and vital to nursing care (Jevon and Ewens 2007). The fluid balance chart serves as a non-invasive tool to monitor fluid status and guides the prescription and administration of intravenous fluids (Tang and Lee 2010).

Fluid balance charting allows healthcare professionals to carefully monitor the fluid input and output and calculate the fluid balance. This is usually measured over a 24-hour period (Jevon and Ewens 2007). A positive fluid balance indicates that the input has exceeded the output, and a negative fluid balance indicates the reverse, that is, the output has exceeded the input. Although a fluid balance chart is a good indication of fluid balance, it is not an exact measurement, for several reasons. Some losses are insensible such as those from perspiration, respiratory secretions and immeasurable bowel losses. The calculation of fluid balance also relies heavily on the accurate measuring, charting and calculating of input, output and overall balance. For such measurements to be taken accurately, additional interventions such as catheterization may be required. The benefit of accurate fluid balance measurement in the critically or acutely unwell patient must be considered to outweigh the risks associated with such interventions (Callum et al. 1999, NICE 2007, 2013a). Table 7.2 identifies routes and sources of fluid intake and output.

Although a very useful tool, fluid balance charting should not be used in isolation. When considering fluid and electrolyte balance, additional triggers such as physical assessment and monitoring plasma levels of electrolytes should be integral to the observation and care of a patient with actual or potential fluid and electrolyte imbalances (NICE 2007, 2013a, Shepherd 2011).

Nursing assessment is discussed in detail in Chapter 2: Assessment and discharge and the assessment of a patient's fluid status should be an integral part of any admission and subsequent daily assessments, particularly if the patient is critically ill and/or a fluid deficit has been identified. See Table 7.3 for details of what should be included in a fluid status assessment.

Table 7.2 **Fluid intake and output**

Intake	Output
Oral	**Urine**
Food and drinks *Normally 2000 mL/per day*	*Normally approx 1500 mL/per day*
Parenteral/intravenous	**Faeces**
Maintenance fluids, intravenous infusion, intermittent drugs, flushes *Additional to or replaces oral intake*	*Normally approx 100 mL/per day*
Enteral	**Perspiration**
Nasal gastric/nasal jejunostomy, percutaneous gastric jejunostomy feed, flushes *Additional to or replaces oral intake*	*Normally approx 200 mL/day* **Gastric secretions** Vomit, nasal gastric/gastrostomy drainage *Additional to normal output* **Wounds and drains** *Additional to normal output* **Insensible losses** Perspiration, respiratory secretions *Additional to normal output*

Source: Sheppard and Wright (2006). Reproduced with permission from Elsevier.

Table 7.3 **Assessment of fluid status**

Assessment		Indications	
Symptoms	**Usual findings**	**Fluid deficit**	**Fluid overload**
History			
To establish any condition, medication or lifestyle that may contribute to or predispose the patient to a fluid imbalance	Differs for each patient	For example, chronic or acute diarrhoea, medication such as diuretics, poor oral fluid intake	Ingestion of too much water/fluid, renal failure/dysfunction
Thirst *Ask the patient*	Occasional; resolved by taking an oral drink	Unusually thirsty	No thirst, normal
Mucosa and conjunctiva *Inspect*	Usually moist and pink	Dry and whitened mucosa, dry conjunctiva and 'sunken' eyeballs	Moist, pink and glistening
Clinical signs			
Heart rate	Usual resting 60–100 bpm	Raised	Normal or raised
Peripheral pulse character	Radial pulse is felt just under the skin at the wrist, light palpation with two or three fingers	Thready, difficult to palpate	Bounding, easy to palpate
Blood pressure	Patient's own normal should be used as a guide	Blood pressure will fall if blood volume falls beyond compensatory mechanisms. Patient may experience postural hypotension	Rise in blood pressure, or may remain normal
Central venous pressure	3–10 mmHg	Low	Raised
Respiratory rate	12–20 breaths/min	High, to meet increased oxygen demands of compensatory mechanisms	High, if overload present
Capillary refill	Usually 2–3 seconds	Slower	Faster
Urine output	0.5–1 mL/kg	Low	Increase, if good renal function
Lung sounds, auscultation	Vesicular breath sounds, 'rustling' heard mainly on inspiration	Normal	Additional sounds (crackles) may indicate fluid overload
Skin turgor	Following a gentle pinch, the fold of skin should return to normal	Skin will take much longer to 'bounce' back to normal. Unreliable in elderly who may have lost some elasticity of their skin	May be normal; however, may be oedematous therefore skin remains dented/pinched
Serum electrolyte levels			
Sodium	135–145 mmol/L	Raised	Lowered
Potassium	3.5–5 mmol/L	May be lowered if cause of fluid deficit is gastrointestinal losses	Normal
Urea	2.5–6.4 mmol/L	Decreased	Normal
Creatinine	Male: 63–116 μmol/L		
	Female: 54–98 μmol/L	Normal, but eventually rises with prolonged poor renal perfusion	Normal
	This is a basic examination of serum electrolytes in fluid balance. There are several conditions and treatments that may affect these so they should not be used in isolation to assess or treat fluid imbalance.		
Serum osmolarity	275–295 mosmol/kg	Increased	Decreased
Urine osmolarity	50–1400 mosmol/kg	Increased	Decreased
Daily weight	A person's daily weight should be fairly stable; large losses or gains in weight may indicate fluid imbalance	Reduced each day	Increased each day
Temperature	36.5–37.5°C	May be elevated and this may also contribute to the fluid deficit (increased insensible losses)	Normal

Source: Adapted from Adam and Osbourne (2006), Epstein et al. (2003), Flanagan et al. (2007), Levi (2005).

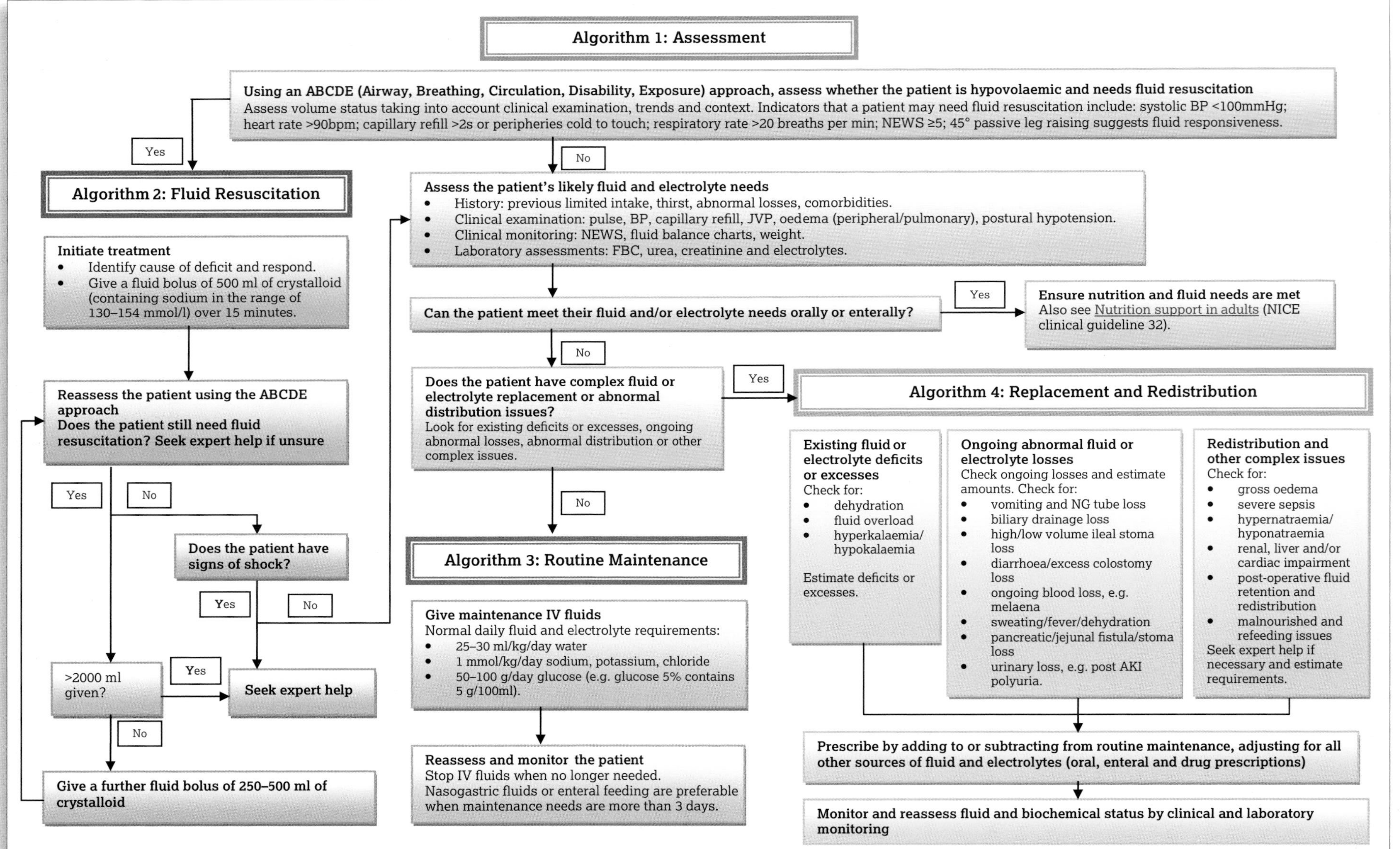

Algorithm 1: Assessment
Using an ABCDE (Airway, Breathing, Circulation, Disability, Exposure) approach, assess whether the patient is hypovolaemic and needs fluid resuscitation
Assess volume status taking into account clinical examination, trends and context. Indicators that a patient may need fluid resuscitation include: systolic BP <100mmHg; heart rate >90bpm; capillary refill >2s or peripheries cold to touch; respiratory rate >20 breaths per min; NEWS ≥5; 45° passive leg raising suggests fluid responsiveness.
Yes
No
Algorithm 2: Fluid Resuscitation
Initiate treatment
• Identify cause of deficit and respond.
• Give a fluid bolus of 500 ml of crystalloid (containing sodium in the range of 130–154 mmol/l) over 15 minutes.
Reassess the patient using the ABCDE approach
Does the patient still need fluid resuscitation? Seek expert help if unsure
Yes
No
Does the patient have signs of shock?
Yes
No
>2000 ml given?
Yes
No
Seek expert help
Give a further fluid bolus of 250–500 ml of crystalloid
Assess the patient's likely fluid and electrolyte needs
• History: previous limited intake, thirst, abnormal losses, comorbidities.
• Clinical examination: pulse, BP, capillary refill, JVP, oedema (peripheral/pulmonary), postural hypotension.
• Clinical monitoring: NEWS, fluid balance charts, weight.
• Laboratory assessments: FBC, urea, creatinine and electrolytes.
Can the patient meet their fluid and/or electrolyte needs orally or enterally?
Yes
Ensure nutrition and fluid needs are met
Also see Nutrition support in adults (NICE clinical guideline 32).
No
Does the patient have complex fluid or electrolyte replacement or abnormal distribution issues?
Look for existing deficits or excesses, ongoing abnormal losses, abnormal distribution or other complex issues.
Yes
No
Algorithm 3: Routine Maintenance
Give maintenance IV fluids
Normal daily fluid and electrolyte requirements:
• 25–30 ml/kg/day water
• 1 mmol/kg/day sodium, potassium, chloride
• 50–100 g/day glucose (e.g. glucose 5% contains 5 g/100ml).
Reassess and monitor the patient
Stop IV fluids when no longer needed.
Nasogastric fluids or enteral feeding are preferable when maintenance needs are more than 3 days.
Algorithm 4: Replacement and Redistribution
Existing fluid or electrolyte deficits or excesses
Check for:
• dehydration
• fluid overload
• hyperkalaemia/hypokalaemia
Estimate deficits or excesses.
Ongoing abnormal fluid or electrolyte losses
Check ongoing losses and estimate amounts. Check for:
• vomiting and NG tube loss
• biliary drainage loss
• high/low volume ileal stoma loss
• diarrhoea/excess colostomy loss
• ongoing blood loss, e.g. melaena
• sweating/fever/dehydration
• pancreatic/jejunal fistula/stoma loss
• urinary loss, e.g. post AKI polyuria.
Redistribution and other complex issues
Check for:
• gross oedema
• severe sepsis
• hypernatraemia/hyponatraemia
• renal, liver and/or cardiac impairment
• post-operative fluid retention and redistribution
• malnourished and refeeding issues
Seek expert help if necessary and estimate requirements.
Prescribe by adding to or subtracting from routine maintenance, adjusting for all other sources of fluid and electrolytes (oral, enteral and drug prescriptions)
Monitor and reassess fluid and biochemical status by clinical and laboratory monitoring

Figure 7.2 **Algorithm for IV fluid therapy in adults.** *Source:* **NICE (2013a). Reproduced with permission from NICE (www.nice.org.uk/cg174).**

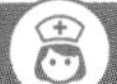 Learning Activity 7.1

Scenario: Assessing fluid status

You have been asked to assess a 79-year-old woman who has just been admitted to the ward following a fall at home. You, and other members of the team, are concerned that she may be dehydrated.

1 What particular questions can you ask to help determine her fluid status?
2 When carrying out her vital signs, what may indicate dehydration and why?
3 Which blood results may be abnormal, indicating dehydration?
4 Are there any other clinical indications of dehydration that you can think of?

See the end of the chapter for the answers.

Throughout the literature, it is recognized that fluid balance monitoring is often poorly performed by nurses (Bennett 2010, Mooney 2007, Shepherd 2011, NICE 2013a). Alexander and Allen (2011) identify barriers to accurate monitoring of fluid status and suggest that nurses must have a good understanding of the concepts involved in fluid balance in order to recognize or anticipate imbalances. They suggest the use of a fluid management policy to guide both nursing and medical staff and to standardize practice. NICE (2013a) offer guidance on the management of the adult patient in hospital receiving IV fluids; suggesting history taking, full clinical assessment, review of current medications, fluid balance charts and laboratory investigations are all required in order to fully assess the need for IV fluid and/or electrolyte administration.

Understanding of the physiological mechanisms and potential implications will ensure fluid balance charting is carried out with knowledge and thought. Stewart et al. (2009) suggest that these assessment skills should be 'core' for any healthcare professional caring for inpatients. More recently, the British Consensus Guidelines on Intravenous Fluid Therapy for Adult Surgical Patients (Powell-Tuck et al. 2011) and NICE guidance on intravenous fluid therapy in adults (NICE 2013a) has highlighted detrimental effects of fluid overload and therefore the importance of accurate fluid balance monitoring. Recommendations included the need for improved accuracy and for medical staff to review these charts regularly and prior to prescribing any intravenous fluids. Tang and Lee (2010) highlight the implications of incorrect fluid balance calculations (by nurses and doctors), which may lead to under- or overprescribing of fluid administration and therefore affect patient outcome. They suggested that these charts are counterproductive and dangerous unless completed correctly.

NICE (2013a) recommend all patients receiving IV fluids require at least daily assessment of their fluid status and that clinicians are mindful of the electrolyte content of the IV fluids they prescribe.

Within fluid management, and particularly fluid resuscitation, there is an ongoing debate surrounding the benefits of the use of colloids over crystalloid for fluid replacement. Perel and Roberts (2007) conducted a systematic review of the evidence and concluded that there is no apparent benefit to the patient when using colloid rather than crystalloid. Bayer et al. (2012) performed a prospective sequential analysis on the use of both colloid and crystalloid in fluid resuscitation in the septic patient; they found that shock reversal was achieved equally fast with both types of fluid replacement and there was only a marginal reduction in the volume required when using colloid. The UK Adult Resuscitation Guidelines (Resuscitation Council 2005) agree that there is no benefit in choosing colloid over crystalloid but they do recommend that dextrose is avoided due to the redistribution of fluid from the intravascular space and because it may cause hyperglycaemia. Dellinger et al. (2012) provide detailed guidelines on the management of sepsis and recommend crystalloid as the first choice in fluid resuscitation (Dellinger et al. 2012).

This ongoing debate has led to a wide variation in practice across trusts and even departments. NICE (2013a) have offered clear, standardized guidance with regard to IV fluid administration for the adult patient in hospital (excluding patients with diabetes, severe liver or renal disease, pregnant women and patients under the age of 16 years). A summary and useful form of this guidance can be found in the 'Algorithms for IV fluid therapy in adults' produced by NICE (2013a). See Figure 7.2.

Synthetic colloid fluids containing hydroxyethyl starch have previously been utilized in fluid replacement. However, the benefits of these over the risks have come under scrutiny (Antonelli and Sandroni 2013) and it was decided by the European Medicines Agency (2013) that production and use of these be suspended.

Rationale

Indications

Any patient who has shown signs or symptoms of a fluid imbalance or who has undergone surgery or acute illness that has led to critical care admission should have their fluid intake and output monitored and fluid balance calculated on an hourly basis (Mooney 2007, Tang and Lee 2010). The decision to monitor fluid balance should be a multidisciplinary one; however, it is the responsibility of the bedside nurse to ensure this is done accurately.

LEGAL AND PROFESSIONAL ISSUES

The Code (NMC 2015) clearly states that clear and accurate records must be kept; this includes fluid balance charts (Figure 7.3). Nurses should have an understanding of the mechanisms of fluid balance and identify potential imbalances and the problems associated with them.

PRE-PROCEDURAL CONSIDERATIONS

In order to monitor fluid balance, both input and output must be accurately measured. Below are procedural guidelines for measuring input and output. If the patient is awake, able to take oral fluids and is mobile, they must be educated about the fact that their fluid balance is being monitored and each drink must be recorded, as should each episode of passing urine, bowel motion or vomiting and so on. It is helpful to provide a cup with markings showing volume.

It is important to note that patients may have other means of urine output, for example an ileal conduit, ureteric stents, suprapubic catheterization, neobladder. The same concepts can be utilized to measure the output, by attaching a urometer to the catheter or urostomy bag.

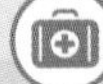 Learning Activity 7.2

Learning in practice: Fluid balance charts

Take a look at the fluid balance charts in use within your clinical area.

- How accurately are the charts completed?
- Can you think of any strategies to improve their accuracy?

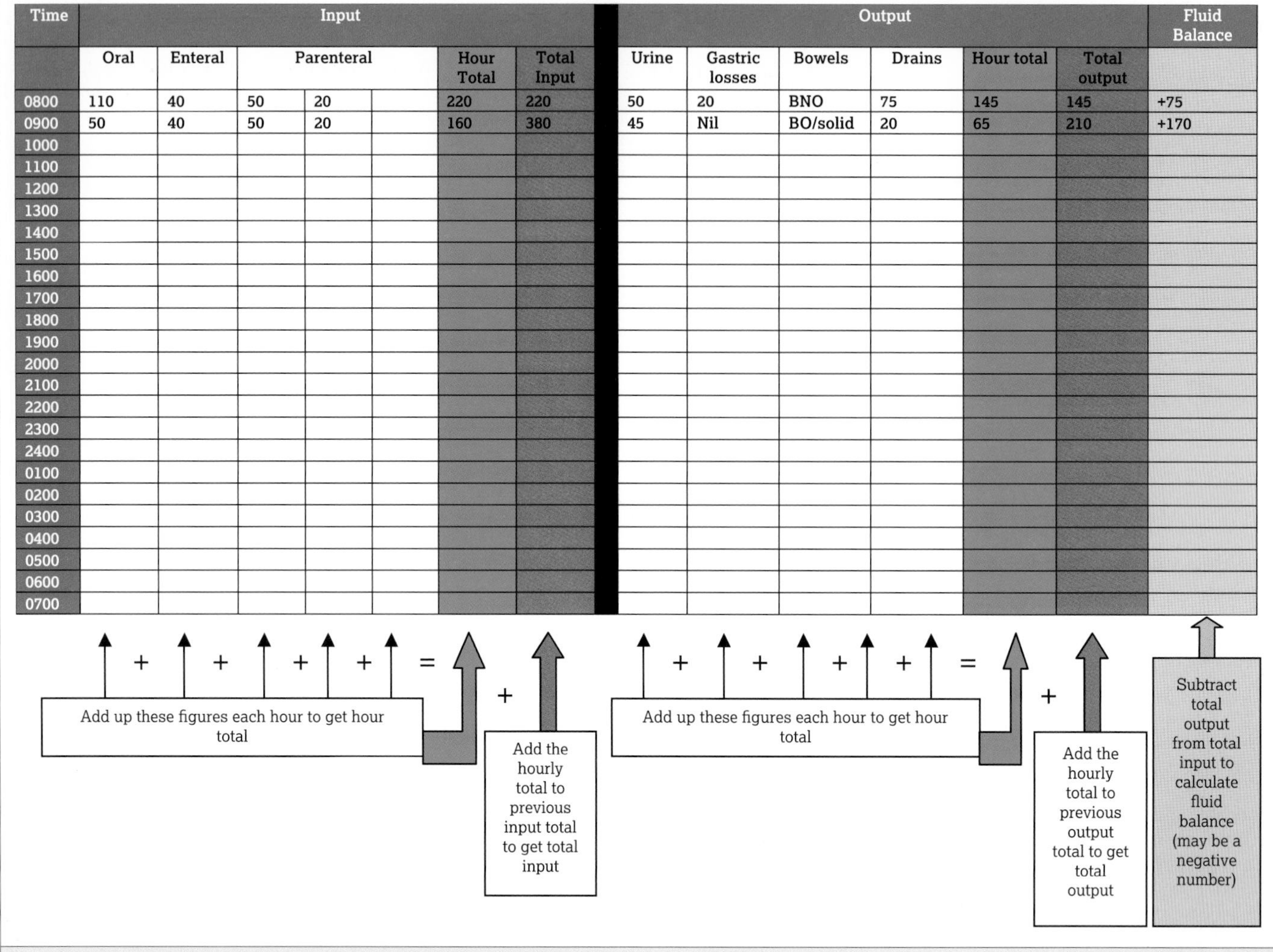

Time	Input							Output						Fluid Balance
	Oral	Enteral	Parenteral			Hour Total	Total Input	Urine	Gastric losses	Bowels	Drains	Hour total	Total output	
0800	110	40	50	20		220	220	50	20	BNO	75	145	145	+75
0900	50	40	50	20		160	380	45	Nil	BO/solid	20	65	210	+170
1000														
1100														
1200														
1300														
1400														
1500														
1600														
1700														
1800														
1900														
2000														
2100														
2200														
2300														
2400														
0100														
0200														
0300														
0400														
0500														
0600														
0700														

+ + + + =
+
Add up these figures each hour to get hour total
Add the hourly total to previous input total to get total input
+ + + + =
+
Add up these figures each hour to get hour total
Add the hourly total to previous output total to get total output
Subtract total output from total input to calculate fluid balance (may be a negative number)

Figure 7.3 **Example of a fluid balance chart.**

Procedure guideline 7.1 **Fluid input: measurement**

Essential equipment

- Fluid balance chart
- Appropriate pumps for fluid or feeding

Pre-procedure

Action	Rationale
1 Educate the patient about the fact that their fluid input is being monitored and ask them to alert you to any oral intake.	To ensure the patient is aware of the need to record any oral intake so this can be noted accurately (Baraz et al. 2009, **R4**).
2 Obtain fluid balance chart and document patient's name and the date commenced.	To ensure chart is correctly labelled for the correct patient, allowing accurate documentation (Powell-Tuck et al. 2011, **C**).
3 Ensure pumps available for intravenous fluids, nasogastric/jejunostomy feeds.	To enable accurate hourly record of intake (Reid et al. 2004, **E**).

Procedure

Action	Rationale
4 Measure oral fluid intake hourly, noting it on the fluid balance chart (see Figure 7.3).	To obtain accurate real-time fluid balance status (Sumnall 2007, **E**).
5 Note any enteral or parenteral intake.	To obtain accurate real-time fluid balance status and ensure all possible input considered (Smith and Roberts 2011, **E**).

Action	Rationale
6 Add together the values for oral, enteral and parenteral intake for the hour.	To assess hourly fluid intake (Scales and Pilsworth 2008, **E**).
7 Add this value to the cumulative total for intake (see Figure 7.3).	To assess total intake and enable calculation of the fluid balance (Scales and Pilsworth 2008).
Post-procedure	
8 Once output totals are calculated (see Procedure guideline 7.6: Fluid output: monitoring output from bowels), subtract output from input.	To calculate fluid balance (Powell-Tuck et al. 2011, **C**).
9 Document on chart and in patient's notes.	To ensure accurate documentation (NMC 2010, **C**).

Procedure guideline 7.2 **Fluid output: monitoring/measuring output if the patient is catheterized**

Essential equipment

- Urometer
- Measuring jugs (with volume indicators)
- Non-sterile gloves, apron, goggles
- Bedpan/urinary bottles/commode
- Bile drainage bag/gastrostomy drainage bag
- Scales

Pre-procedure

Action	Rationale
1 Determine sources of fluid output (see Table 7.2) and note them on the fluid balance chart.	To ensure all possibilities have been considered and to ensure accurate (as possible) output determination (Scales and Pilsworth 2008, **E**).
Procedure	
2 Explain to the patient that it is necessary to monitor their urine output and that you will be doing so every hour.	To ensure the patient is not alarmed by frequent observation and that they are kept informed about current care (Bryant 2007, **E**).
3 Attach a urometer to the catheter, using an aseptic technique (see Chapter 3, Procedure guideline 3.10: Aseptic technique example: changing a wound dressing).	To allow accurate assessment of hourly urine output, to prevent cross-infection (Fraise and Bradley 2009, **E**).
4 Each hour, on the hour, note the volume of urine in the urometer, recording this on the fluid balance chart.	To determine urine output and to keep accurate records of this, thus enabling assessment of fluid balance (Scales and Pilsworth 2008, **E**).
5 Empty the urometer into the collection bag (until the bag is full; this will then need emptying).	To ensure urometer is empty for the next hour's determination. **E**
6 Add recorded urine output to the other values for output, giving an hourly total.	To allow for fluid balance determination (see Table 7.2). **E**
Post-procedure	
7 Once all output has been determined, noted on chart and total hourly output calculated, subtract total output from total input.	To calculate hourly fluid balance (Levi 2005, **E**).
8 Document all values on the chart and any other actions relating to your findings in the patient's notes.	To ensure accurate documentation (NMC 2010, **C**).

Procedure guideline 7.3 **Fluid output: monitoring/measuring output if the patient is not catheterized**

Essential equipment

- Measuring jugs (with volume indicators)
- Non-sterile gloves, apron, goggles
- Bedpan/urinary bottles/commode
- Scales

Pre-procedure

Action	Rationale
1 Determine sources of fluid output (see Table 7.2) and note on the fluid balance chart.	To ensure all possibilities have been considered to ensure accurate (as possible) output determination (Scales and Pilsworth 2008, **E**).

(continued)

Procedure guideline 7.3 Fluid output: monitoring/measuring output if the patient is not catheterized *(continued)*

Procedure

Action	Rationale
2 Explain to the patient that it is necessary to measure their urine output.	To ensure that the patient knows that any urine they pass needs to be measured in order to record output and to obtain their co-operation in ensuring accuracy of measurement (Chung et al. 2002, **R4**).
3 Supply the patient with urine bottles and/or bedpans and ask them to use these even if they are able to mobilize to the toilet; ask them to inform you of each episode.	To ensure the urine is kept for measuring and not disposed of (Chung et al. 2002, **R4**).
4 Use protective equipment for bodily fluids when handling used bottle or bedpan.	To prevent cross-infection (Fraise and Bradley 2009, **E**).
5 Place bedpan/bottle on to scales, subtracting appropriate value to compensate for weight of item.	To obtain value of urine in millilitres. **E**
6 If no scales available, use a jug with volume markings; pour urine into jug (using universal precautions), noting level of urine.	To measure urine volume. **E**
7 Once noted, dispose of urine appropriately.	To prevent contamination and/or cross-infection (Fraise and Bradley 2009, **E**).
8 Record value on fluid balance chart, adding this to the rest of the output values for the hour.	To determine fluid output for the hour (Sumnall 2007, **E**).
Post-procedure	
9 Once all output has been determined, noted on chart and total hourly output calculated, subtract total output from total input.	To calculate hourly fluid balance (Levi 2005, **E**).
10 Document all values on the chart and any other actions relating to your findings in the patient's notes.	To ensure accurate documentation (NMC 2010, **C**).

Procedure guideline 7.4 Fluid output: measuring output from drains

Essential equipment

- Measuring jugs (with volume indicators)
- Non-sterile gloves, apron, goggles
- Tape and pen

Pre-procedure

Action	Rationale
1 Determine sources of fluid output (see Table 7.2) and note them on the fluid balance chart.	To ensure all possibilities have been considered to ensure accurate (as possible) output determination (Scales and Pilsworth 2008, **E**).
Procedure	
2 Explain to the patient that the output from the drains will be monitored hourly.	To inform the patient about current care and to ensure they are not alarmed by the frequent observations (Bryant 2007, **E**).
3 If the drain is drainable, empty contents into jug, noting volume; use universal precautions.	To determine volume of fluid drained and prevent cross-infection (Fraise and Bradley 2009, **E**).
4 If it is not possible to drain the fluid out of the bag, use a suitable pen and mark the level the fluid reaches each hour. Date and time each marking.	To determine drainage each hour. To ensure consistency in reading and to communicate to other members of the multidisciplinary team regarding drainage (Sumnall 2007, **E**).
5 Note volume/drainage on fluid balance chart.	To determine drainage each hour (Sumnall 2007, **E**).
6 Add this figure to the rest of the output values for the hour.	To determine accurate total fluid lost each hour (Sumnall 2007, **E**).

Post-procedure

Action	Rationale
7 Once all output has been determined, noted on chart and total hourly output calculated, subtract total output from total input.	To calculate hourly fluid balance (Levi 2005, **E**).
8 Document all values on the chart and any other actions relating to your findings in the patient's notes.	To ensure accurate documentation (NMC 2010, **C**).

Procedure guideline 7.5 Fluid output: monitoring output from gastric outlets, nasogastric tubes, gastrostomy

Essential equipment

- Urometer
- Measuring jugs (with volume indicators)
- Non-sterile gloves, apron, goggles
- Bile drainage bag/gastrostomy drainage bag

Action	Rationale
Pre-procedure	
1 Determine sources of fluid output (see Table 7.2) and note them on the fluid balance chart.	To ensure all possibilities have been considered to ensure accurate (as possible) output determination (Scales and Pilsworth 2008, **E**).
Procedure	
2 Explain to the patient that it is necessary to monitor drainage every hour.	To inform the patient of current care and interventions (Bryant 2007, **E**).
3 Ensure gastric outlet device has a drainage bag attached.	To collect any output for measurement. **E**
4 If instructed, leave the bag open to drain (this may differ depending on condition).	To enable drainage. **E**
5 Drain contents into marked jug every hour (if quantity allows), using universal precautions.	To determine volume and prevent cross-infection (Fraise and Bradley 2009, **E**).
6 Attach a urometer if output is high.	To ensure accurate reading and for ease of measuring. **E**
7 Note volume on fluid balance chart, adding this value to the rest of the output values for that 1 hour.	To enable determination of fluid balance (Sumnall 2007, **E**).
Post-procedure	
8 Once all output has been determined, noted on chart and total hourly output calculated, subtract total output from total input.	To calculate hourly fluid balance (Levi 2005, **E**).
9 Document all values on the chart and any other actions relating to your findings in the patient's notes.	To ensure accurate documentation (NMC 2010, **C**).

Procedure guideline 7.6 Fluid output: monitoring output from bowels

Essential equipment

- Measuring jugs (with volume indicators)
- Scales
- Non-sterile gloves, apron, goggles
- Bedpan/commode
- Rectal tube 'Flexiseal' (if required)

Action	Rationale
Pre-procedure	
1 Determine sources of fluid output (see Table 7.2) and note them on the fluid balance chart.	To ensure all possibilities have been considered to ensure accurate (as possible) output determination (Scales and Pilsworth 2008, **E**).

(continued)

Procedure guideline 7.6 Fluid output: monitoring output from bowels *(continued)*

Procedure

Action	Rationale
2 Explain to the patient that it is necessary to monitor volume of fluid excreted, including that from the bowel, particularly if the stool is loose/watery.	To keep the patient informed about current care and observations, to ensure co-operation in monitoring fluid output (Bryant 2007, **E**).
3 Provide the patient with bedpans, even if able to mobilize to the bathroom; ask them to place the bedpan over the toilet bowl.	To enable inspection and measurement of fluid lost via the bowel. **E**
4 If stool is loose enough, this can be transferred into a jug and the volume measured, or use scales.	To quantify fluid output from stool (Scales and Pilsworth 2008, **E**).
5 If the stool is formed and it is not possible to accurately quantify, still note on fluid balance chart that bowels were opened.	To take into account any insensible losses (Mooney 2007, **E**).
6 A rectal tube may be suitable in some patients; please refer to local policy regarding use of rectal tube. Note any output on the fluid balance chart.	To ensure correct use of tube and to quantify any fluid losses from the bowel. **E**
7 Add losses to the previous losses for the hour.	To calculate hourly fluid output (Sumnall 2007, **E**).
Post-procedure	
8 Once all output has been determined, noted on chart and total hourly output calculated, subtract total output from total input.	To calculate hourly fluid balance (Levi 2005, **E**).
9 Document all values on the chart and any other actions relating to your findings in the patient's notes.	To ensure accurate documentation (NMC 2010, **C**).

Procedure guideline 7.7 Fluid output: monitoring output from stoma sites

Essential equipment

- Measuring jugs (with volume indicators)
- Non-sterile gloves, apron, goggles

Pre-procedure

Action	Rationale
1 Determine sources of fluid output (see Table 7.2) and note them on the fluid balance chart.	To ensure all possibilities have been considered to ensure accurate (as possible) output determination (Alexander et al. 2006, **E**).
Procedure	
2 Explain to the patient that you are monitoring hourly output.	To ensure the patient understands why their stoma is being checked hourly. To ensure they are up to date with current care (Bryant 2007, **E**).
3 Check that the stoma bag is drainable; if not, change (see Chapter 5: Elimination).	To ensure ease of draining bag contents and to reduce the number of times the adhesive flange is removed, in order to protect the skin. **E**
4 Using protective equipment, empty the contents of the stoma bag into the measuring jug, noting volume.	To determine output from stoma for 1 hour and prevent cross-infection (Fraise and Bradley 2009, **E**).
5 Dispose of contents using protective equipment, adhering to local policy.	To ensure correct disposal of contents and prevent cross-infection (Fraise and Bradley 2009, **E**).
6 Note volume of stool on chart; add to other losses for the hour.	To ensure correct documentation of output and allow calculation of fluid balance (NICE 2013a, **C**).
7 Add hourly total (all outputs) to cumulative output (see Figure 7.3).	To enable fluid balance determination (Sumnall 2007, **E**).
Post-procedure	
8 Once all output has been determined, noted on chart and total hourly output calculated, subtract total output from total input.	To calculate hourly fluid balance. **E**
9 Document all values on the chart and any other actions relating to your findings in the patient's notes.	To ensure accurate documentation (NMC 2010, **C**).

Problem-solving table 7.1 **Prevention and resolution (Procedure guidelines 7.1, 7.2, 7.3, 7.4, 7.5, 7.6 and 7.7)**

Problem	Cause	Prevention	Action
Non-compliance/co-operation from patients.	Usually misunderstanding or lack of education regarding importance of monitoring fluid balance.	Effective patient education and teaching.	Determine effective teaching methods, considering individual needs, for example poor hearing, illiteracy. Re-educate the patient, using appropriate means.
Inability to record input due to lack of pumps to regulate intravenous fluids or enteral feeds.	Not available, unable to use, inappropriate.	Request more equipment from appropriate sources, request training.	Calculate drip rates on free-flowing fluids to ensure correct hourly input calculated.
Insensible losses.	Inability to measure some losses.	N/A	Note on chart if perspiration is excessive or if bowels opened and immeasurable, to highlight possible inaccuracy in fluid balance.
Leaking drains.	Inevitable with some drains.	Inevitable with some drains; however, surrounding opening may require further suturing; request surgical review if necessary.	Utilize stoma bag/wound drainage bag to collect drainage, to enable measurement.
Incorrect fluid balance calculation.	Incorrect fluid input determination. Incorrect fluid output determination. Incorrect calculation.	Appropriate teaching and education for nurses performing these procedures, competency checking.	Ensure nurses are educated appropriately, access information and education if unsure of procedure or technique.

POST-PROCEDURAL CONSIDERATIONS

Every hour, the findings of fluid input/output monitoring should be recorded; any deficit or change in fluid balance should be reported. Any imbalance noted will require action and a management plan. The nurse recording the fluid balance should have an appreciation of the importance of fluid imbalance management and should notify the appropriate person.

COMPLICATIONS

Correct fluid balance monitoring is essential in the successful management of actual or potential fluid balance disturbances (Jevon and Ewens 2007). Over- or underestimation of the fluid status could lead to incorrect management, resulting in fluid overload (hypervolaemia), dehydration (hypovolaemia) (Bryant 2007, Tang and Lee 2010) and/or electrolyte disturbances, all of which will ultimately lead to organ dysfunction.

Fluid overload/hypervolaemia

Underestimating the fluid balance may lead to continued or increased administration of IV fluids, which if monitored incorrectly could result in circulatory overload. Excess IV fluid administration is not the only cause of circulatory overload, which can also result from acute renal failure, heart failure and intake of excessive sodium (Welch 2010).

In health, homeostatic mechanisms exist to compensate and redistribute excess fluids but, in ill health, these mechanisms are often inadequate, leading to increasing circulatory volumes. As the volume within the circulatory system rises, so does the hydrostatic pressure which, when excessive, results in leaking of fluid from the vessels into the surrounding tissues. This is evident as oedema, initially apparent in the ankles and legs or buttocks and sacrum if the patient is in bed. This can progress to generalized oedema, where even the tissues surrounding the eyes become puffy and swollen.

A bounding pulse and an increased blood pressure are also signs of fluid overload, as is an increased cardiac output and raised central venous pressure.

One of the most dangerous symptoms of fluid overload is pulmonary oedema, which occurs when the hydrostatic pressure within the vessels causes congestion within the pulmonary circulation, increasing the hydrostatic pressure there and causing fluid to leak into the lungs and pulmonary tissues (Casey 2004). This presents with respiratory symptoms, including shortness of breath, increased respiratory rate, a cough (Welch 2010), often associated with pink frothy sputum, and finally reduced oxygen saturations due to inadequate gaseous exchange at the alveolar level (Casey 2004). Left untreated, this can be fatal as the lungs are failing to provide essential cells and organs with oxygen; this would eventually lead to organ dysfunction and then failure.

Cardiac dysfunction can result from fluid overload, not only from the reduced availability of oxygen to the cardiac cells due to the pulmonary oedema, but also from the increase in volume causing the cardiac muscle to stretch, leading to cell damage and possible inability to contract effectively (Treacher 2009).

Treatment of hypervolaemia would involve restricting fluid intake, monitoring electrolytes and using diuretics in an attempt to offload some of the excess fluid (Thomsen et al. 2012). Vasodilators may also be considered to reduce the pressure in the vessels. If these mechanisms fail, it may be necessary to use renal replacement therapy to drive the fluid out of the circulation.

In some cases fluid overload is part of the disease process. However, with effective monitoring and fluid balance recording and assessment, it may be possible to avoid the devastating complications.

Hypovolaemia/dehydration

Dehydration refers to a negative fluid balance, when the fluid output exceeds the fluid intake (Jevon 2010). Overestimation of the fluid balance may lead to inadequate replacement of lost fluids. Dehydration can, however, be caused by a loss of fluids to 'third spaces' such as ascites or lost due to a reduction in colloid osmotic pressure (hypoalbuminaemia) (Casey 2004), losses which are not easy to account for. Fluid balance charts should therefore always be used in association with physical assessment of the patient, weight measurement and laboratory results.

There are three categories of dehydration (Mentes 2006) – isotonic, hypertonic and hypotonic – each related to the type of fluid and solutes lost. Isotonic describes the loss of both water and sodium from the ECF; hypertonic is excessive loss of water only, which leads to a rise in ECF sodium, causing a shift in fluid from the intracellular space to the extracellular. Hypotonic dehydration results from excessive sodium loss, particularly with the overuse of diuretics (Welch 2010).

Dehydration can ultimately cause a reduction in circulating volume (Tortora and Derrickson 2011). As with any change in a homeostatic state, the body in health has the ability to compensate but in ill health these mechanisms are often inadequate. Untreated dehydration will quickly lead to a drop in blood pressure and a rise in heart rate (to compensate for the fall in blood pressure). A fall in blood pressure will firstly lead to inadequate renal perfusion, causing a rise in metabolites, acidosis, acute renal failure and eventual toxaemia. Untreated, other organs will suffer from underperfusion, possibly resulting in ischaemia, organ dysfunction and eventual organ failure (Sumnall 2007).

Additional signs and symptoms of dehydration are thirst, weight loss, decreased urine output, dry skin and mucous membranes, fatigue and increased body temperature (Goertz 2006).

Treatment of dehydration includes the replacement of lost fluid and electrolytes but caution must be exercised. If the dehydration is mild, slower fluid replacement is advised, in order to prevent further complications in shifts in electrolytes. However, if hypovolaemia exists with the signs and symptoms of circulatory shock, low blood pressure and organ dysfunction, aggressive fluid replacement is advised (Jevon 2010, NICE 2013a).

Acute kidney injury

Acute kidney injury (which can be due to a multitude of causes) is a common feature in the acutely or critically unwell patient and will require even more careful approaches to monitoring and maintenance of fluid balance (Goldstein 2012). The National Confidential Enquiry into Patient Outcome and Death (NCEPOD 2009) reviewed the care delivered to patients with acute kidney injury and found that 50% received suboptimal care. NICE responded to these findings by producing guidance for the prevention, detection and management of acute kidney injury (NICE 2013b). The relevant recommendations from this guidance include the need for reliable monitoring of urine output and early recognition of oliguria. These guidelines reinforce the need for accurate and reliable fluid balance monitoring along with healthcare professionals understanding the implications of the findings.

Nutritional status

DEFINITION

Nutritional status refers to the state of a person's health as determined by their dietary intake and body composition. Nutritional support refers to any method of giving nutrients which encourages an optimal nutritional status. It includes modifying the types of foods eaten, dietary supplementation, enteral tube feeding and parenteral nutrition (NCCAC 2006).

ANATOMY AND PHYSIOLOGY

The normal process of ingestion of food or fluids is via the oral cavity to the gastrointestinal tract.

Swallowing is a complex activity with voluntary and reflexive components. It is usually described as having four stages and requires intact anatomy and sensorimotor functioning of the cranial nerves (Bass 1997, Butler and Leslie 2012, Logemann 1998). The stages start with the oral preparatory stage which is influenced by the sight and smell of food. Food or liquid is placed in the mouth and the lips are closed. After chewing and mixing with saliva, it forms a cohesive mass (bolus) that is held on the centre of the tongue. The oral stage of the swallow is initiated as food is moved through the oral cavity towards the pharynx. These swallowing stages are voluntary.

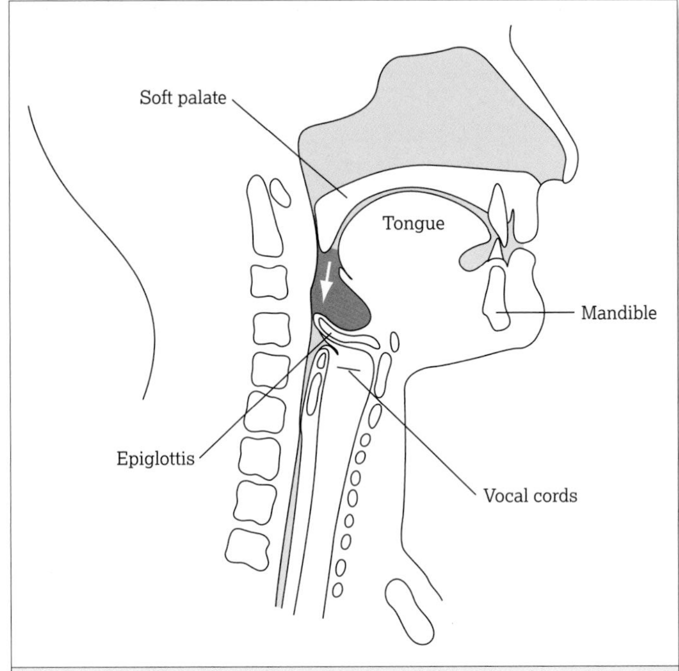

Figure 7.4 **Pharyngeal stage of swallowing.**

The pharyngeal stage of swallowing, which is involuntary (Figure 7.4), occurs as the food bolus crosses the mandible/tongue base as the palate closes, sealing entry to the nasal cavity and reducing risk of nasal regurgitation. Movement of the tongue base and posterior pharyngeal wall squeezes the bolus down the pharynx. Involuntary movements of the larynx (voice box), vocal cords and epiglottis protect the airway and open the cricopharyngeus. The bolus travels from the cricopharyngeus to the gastro-oesophageal junction and peristaltic action then transfers the bolus down the oesophagus (Atkinson and McHanwell 2002, Butler and Leslie 2012).

The gastrointestinal tract is the site where food is ingested, digested and absorbed, thus enabling nutrients to be used by the body for growth and maintenance of body functions. Food ingested is moved along the gastrointestinal tract by peristaltic waves through the oesophagus, stomach, small intestine and large intestine. The passage of food and fluid through the gastrointestinal tract is dependent on the autonomic nervous system, gut hormones such as gastrin and cholecystokinin, the function of exocrine glands such as the parotid, pancreas and liver and psychological aspects such as anxiety. Sphincters situated between the stomach and duodenum, the ileocaecal valves and the anal sphincter also regulate the rate of passage of food and fluids through the tract (Barrett 2014).

Before food can be absorbed, it must be digested and broken down into molecules that can be transported across the intestinal epithelium which line the gastrointestinal tract. This process is dependent on digestive enzymes secreted by the pancreas and lining of the intestinal tract which act on specific nutrients. Bile, from the liver, is required to emulsify fat, thus enabling it to be broken down by digestive enzymes. The absorption of nutrients is dependent on an active, or energy-dependent, transport across the intestinal epithelium lining the digestive tract. Villi, finger-like projections, increase the surface area of the small intestine to aid absorption.

Most nutrients are absorbed from the small intestine although some require specific sites within the gastrointestinal tract; for example, vitamin B_{12} is absorbed in the terminal ileum. Mucosa shed into the lumen of the intestine is broken down and absorbed along with fluid and electrolytes secreted into the lumen during the process of digestion. The volumes of fluid secreted into the gut are large and may amount to 8–9 litres a day when combined with an oral intake of 1.5–2 litres daily. The majority of fluid is reabsorbed in the small intestine with the remainder being absorbed in the large intestine. Bacteria in the large intestine metabolize non-starch polysaccharides (dietary fibre), increasing faecal bulk and producing short chain fatty acids which are absorbed and metabolized for energy (Brownlee 2011).

RELATED THEORY

Bodyweight is the most widely used measure of nutritional status in clinical practice. However, whilst weight provides a simple, readily obtainable and usually fairly precise measure, it remains a one-dimensional metric and as such has limitations. In contrast, an understanding of anatomy and physiology and in particular the changes that can occur in body composition, in addition to frank weight gain or loss, provides valuable clinical insight (Thibault et al. 2012). In the so-called 'two-compartment' model of body composition, bodyweight is described in terms of, firstly, fat-free mass, that is bones, muscles and organs, which includes the hepatic carbohydrate energy store glycogen, and secondly, fat mass or adipose tissue (Thibault et al. 2012). In health, water constitutes up to 60% of total bodyweight. It is distributed throughout the fat-free and fat compartments with approximately two-thirds present as intracellular and one-third as extracellular fluid. Thus, a healthy 70 kg male comprises 42 kg of water which amounts to 60% of total bodyweight. This is made up of 28 litres of intracellular fluid and 14 litres of extracellular fluid. The same 'typical' male contains approximately 12 kg of muscle, also referred to as lean body mass, and 12 kg of fat (Geissler and Powers 2005).

Body composition and nutritional status are closely linked and are dependent upon a number of factors, including age, sex, metabolic requirements, dietary intake and the presence of disease. Depletion of lean body mass occurs in both critical illness and injury and negatively affects functional and immune function and can be associated with increased mortality and length of hospital stay (Carlsson et al. 2013, Jensen et al. 2012, Pichard et al. 2004). Lean body mass tends to decrease with age (Hickson 2006). Shifts in body water compartments are readily observed in conditions such as ascites and oedema (Bedogni et al. 2003). Both of these conditions result from an abnormally increased extracellular water compartment and, despite a gain in total bodyweight, are indicative of worsening outcome.

The physiological characteristics of the different body compartments can be exploited by various assessment tools and techniques to determine changes indicative of nutritional risk (Bedogni et al. 2006). Such changes are masked if weight alone is used as the sole measurement.

EVIDENCE-BASED APPROACHES

Rationale

Nutritional support, to maintain or replete body composition, should be considered for anybody unable to maintain their nutritional status by taking their usual diet (NCCAC 2006). These include the following.

- Patients unable to eat their usual diet (e.g. because of anorexia, mucositis, taste changes or dysphagia) should be given advice on modifying their diet.
- Patients unable to meet their nutritional requirements, despite dietary modifications, should be offered oral nutritional supplements.
- Patients unable to take sufficient food and dietary supplements to meet their nutritional requirements should be considered for an enteral tube feed.
- Patients unable to eat at all should have an enteral tube feed. Reasons for complete inability to eat include carcinoma of the head and neck area or oesophagus, surgery to the head or oesophagus, radiotherapy treatment to the head or neck, fistulae of the oral cavity or oesophagus or dysphagia due to cerebrovascular accident (CVA).
- Parenteral nutrition (PN) may be indicated in patients with a non-functioning or inaccessible gastrointestinal (GI) tract who are likely to be 'nil by mouth' for 5 days or longer. Reasons for a non-functioning or inaccessible GI tract include bowel obstruction, short bowel syndrome, gut toxicity following bone marrow transplantation or chemotherapy, major abdominal surgery, uncontrolled vomiting and enterocutaneous fistulae. Enteral nutrition should always be the first option when considering nutritional support.

Patients in any group may have an increased requirement for nutrients due to an increased metabolic rate, as found in those with burns, major sepsis, trauma or cancer cachexia (Bozzetti 2001, Thomas and Bishop 2007, Todorovic and Micklewright 2011). Patients should have nutritional requirements estimated prior to the start of nutritional support and should be monitored regularly.

Methods of assessing of nutritional status

Before the initiation of nutritional support, the patient must be assessed. The purpose of assessment is to identify whether a patient is undernourished, the reasons why this may have occurred and to provide baseline data for planning and evaluating nutritional support (NCCAC 2006). It is helpful to use more than one method of assessing nutritional status. For example, a dietary history may be used to assess the adequacy of a person's diet but does not reflect actual nutritional status, whereas percentage weight loss does give an indication of nutritional status. However, percentage weight loss taken in isolation gives no idea of dietary intake and likelihood of improvement or deterioration in nutritional status (NCCAC 2006).

Bodyweight and weight loss

Body Mass Index (BMI) or comparison of a patient's weight with a chart of ideal bodyweight gives a measure of whether the patient has a normal weight, is overweight or underweight, and may be calculated from weight and height using the following equation.

$$\text{BMI} = \frac{\text{Weight (kg)}}{\text{Height (m)}^2}$$

Tables are available to allow the rapid and easy calculation of BMI (BAPEN 2003a). These comparisons, however, are not a good indicator of whether the patient is at risk nutritionally, as an apparently normal weight can mask severe muscle wasting.

Of greater use is the comparison of current weight with the patient's usual weight. Percentage weight loss is a useful measure of the risk of malnutrition.

$$\%\text{Weight loss} = \frac{\text{Usual weight} - \text{Actual weight}}{\text{Usual weight}} \times 100$$

A patient would be identified as malnourished if they had any of the following:

- BMI less than 18.5 kg/m^2
- unintentional weight loss greater than 10% within the last 3–6 months

- BMI less than 20 kg/m^2 and unintentional weight loss greater than 5% within the last 3–6 months (NCCAC, 2006).

Sick children should have their weight and height measured frequently. It may be useful to measure on a daily basis (Shaw and Lawson 2007). These measurements must be plotted onto centile charts. A single weight or height cannot be interpreted as there is much variation of growth within each age group. It is a matter of concern if a child's weight begins to fall across the centiles or if the weight plateaus.

Obesity and oedema may make interpretation of bodyweight difficult; both may mask loss of lean body mass and potential malnutrition (Pennington 1997).

Accurate weighing scales are necessary for measurement of bodyweight. Patients who are unable to stand may require sitting scales or hoist scales.

It is often not appropriate to weigh palliative care patients who may experience inevitable weight loss as disease progresses. Psychologically, it may be difficult for patients to see that they are continuing to lose weight (Shaw 2011). Measures of nutritional status such as clinical examination and current food intake may still be used in addition to measures of bodyweight.

Learning Activity 7.3 **Case study: Assessing nutritional status**

John Goody is a 44-year-old man with a history of Crohn's disease. He has just been admitted for bowel surgery following worsening of his GI symptoms and significant weight loss over the last 4–5 months. John reports that 6 months ago he weighed 12st 7lb (79.4 kg). He has just been weighed on admission today and he now weighs 68 kg (10st 10lb). His height is 1.88 m (6ft 2in). On examination his clothing appears to be very loose fitting. He tells you that he has lost so much weight that his wedding ring falls off his finger now and he notices some of his bones are sticking out more than they used to. His face appears drawn and he seems to be a little slow in responding to questions.

1. Using the formula provided within this section, calculate John's current body mass index (BMI).
2. Now calculate his percentage weight loss.
3. Based on your calculations, is John malnourished?
4. What other signs/symptoms of malnourishment does John have?

See the end of the chapter for the answers.

Skinfold thickness and bio-electrical impedance

Skinfold thickness measurements can be used to assess stores of body fat. They are rarely used in routine nutritional assessment due to the insensitivity of the technique and the variation between measurements made by different observers. They are more appropriate for long-term assessments or research purposes and the technique should only be used by practitioners who are practised in using skinfold thickness calipers because of the potential for intra-investigator variation in results (Durnin and Womersley 1974).

Bio-electrical impedance analysis (BIA) is a simple, non-invasive and relatively inexpensive technique for measuring body composition (Janssen et al. 2000). This technique works well in healthy individuals but may be of limited use in some hospital patients with abnormal hydration status (for example, severe dehydration or ascites) and is also less reliable at the extremes of BMI ranges (Kyle et al. 2004, Leahy et al. 2012).

Clinical examination

Observation of the patient may reveal signs and symptoms indicative of nutritional depletion.

- *Physical appearance*: emaciated, wasted appearance, loose dentures, teeth or clothing/jewellery .
- *Oedema*: will affect weight and may mask the appearance of muscle wastage. May indicate plasma protein deficiency and is often a reflection of the patient's overall condition rather than a measure of nutritional status.
- *Mobility*: weakness and impaired movement may result from loss of muscle mass.
- *Mood*: apathy, lethargy and poor concentration can be features of undernutrition.
- *Pressure sores and poor wound healing*: may reflect impaired immune function as a consequence of undernutrition and vitamin deficiencies (Thomas and Bishop, 2007).

Specific nutritional deficiencies may be identifiable in some patients. For example, thiamine deficiency characterized by dementia is associated with high alcohol consumption. Rickets is seen in children with vitamin D deficiency.

A more structured approach can be taken by using an assessment tool such as Subjective Global Assessment (SGA) or patient-generated SGA (PG-SGA) (Bauer et al. 2002). This involves a systematic evaluation of muscle and fat sites around the body and assessment for oedema in the ankles or sacral area in immobile patients. Such an assessment can be used to determine whether the patient is malnourished and can be repeated to assess changes in nutritional status.

Dietary intake

Nutrient intake can be assessed by a diet history (Thomas and Bishop 2007). A 24-hour recall may be used to assess recent nutrient intake and a food chart may be used to monitor current dietary intake. A diet history may also be used to provide information on food frequency, food habits, preferences, meal pattern, portion sizes, the presence of any eating difficulty and changes in food intake (Omran and Morley 2000, Reilly 1996). A food chart on which all food and fluid taken is recorded is a useful method for monitoring nutritional intake, especially in the hospital setting or when dietary recall is not reliable (Thomas and Bishop 2007).

Biochemical investigations

Biochemical tests carried out on blood may give information on the patient's nutritional status. The most commonly used are as follows.

- *Plasma proteins*: changes in plasma albumin may arise due to physical stress, changes in circulating volume, hepatic and renal function, shock conditions and septicaemia. Plasma albumin and changes in plasma albumin are not a direct reflection of nutritional intake and nutritional status as it has been shown that they may remain unchanged despite changes in body composition (NCCAC 2006). In addition, albumin has a long half-life of 21 days, so it cannot reflect recent changes in nutritional intake. It may be useful to review serum albumin concentrations in conjunction with C-reactive protein (CRP), which is an acute-phase protein produced by the body in response to injury or trauma. CRP greater than 10 mg/L and serum albumin less than 30 g/L suggest 'illness' (Elia 2001). Prealbumin and retinol binding protein levels are more sensitive measures of nutrition support, reflecting recent changes in dietary intake rather than nutritional status. However, they may be expensive to measure and are not measured routinely in hospital.
- *Haemoglobin*: this is often below haematological reference values in malnourished patients (men 13.5–17.5 g/dL, women 11.5–15.5 g/dL). This can be due to a number of reasons, such as loss of blood from circulation, increased destruction of red blood cells or reduced production of erythrocytes and haemoglobin, for example due to dietary deficiency of iron or folate.

- *Serum vitamin and mineral levels:* clinical examination of the patient may suggest a vitamin or mineral deficiency. For example, gingivitis may be due to a deficiency of vitamin C. Goitre is associated with iodine deficiency, and muscle weakness and cramps may be caused by magnesium deficiency (Thomas and Bishop 2007). Serum vitamin and mineral levels are rarely measured routinely, as they are expensive and often cannot be performed by hospital laboratories.
- *Immunological competence*: total lymphocyte count may reflect nutritional status (Gibson 2005) although levels may also be depleted with malignancy, chemotherapy, zinc deficiency, age and non-specific stress (Thomas and Bishop 2007).

If a patient is considered to be malnourished by one or more of the above methods of assessment then referral to a dietician should be made immediately (NCCAC 2006).

Methods for calculation of nutritional requirements

The body requires protein, energy, fluid and micronutrients such as vitamins, minerals and trace elements to function optimally. Nutritional requirements should be estimated for patients requiring any form of nutritional support to ensure that these needs are met.

Energy requirements may be calculated using equations such as those derived by Henry (2005), which take into account weight, age, sex, activity level and clinical injury, for example post surgery, sepsis or ventilator dependency. An easier and more appropriate method is to use bodyweight and allowances based on the patient's clinical condition (Table 7.4). Careful adjustments may be necessary in cases of oedema or obesity, in order to avoid overfeeding (Horgan and Stubbs 2003).

Fluid and nitrogen (or protein) requirements can be calculated in a similar way. If additional nitrogen is being given in situations where losses are increased, for example due to trauma, GI losses or major sepsis, then additional energy intake is required to assist in promoting a nitrogen balance. Improvement in nitrogen balance is the single nutritional parameter most consistently associated with improved outcome, and the primary goal of nutrition support should be the attainment of nitrogen balance (Gidden and Shenkin 2000). Additional fluid of 500–750 mL is necessary for every 1°C rise in temperature in pyrexial patients (Thomas and Bishop 2007).

Vitamin and mineral requirements calculated as detailed in the Committee on Medical Aspects of Food Policy (COMA) Report 41 on dietary reference values (COMA and DH 1991) apply to groups of healthy people and are not necessarily appropriate for those who are ill. A patient deficient in a vitamin or mineral may benefit from additional supplements to improve a condition. Macronutrient and micronutrient requirements for children are also listed in the COMA Report. Calculations are usually done with the reference nutrient intake (RNI). The child's actual bodyweight, not the expected bodyweight, is used when calculating requirements. This is to avoid excessive feeding.

Table 7.4 **Guidelines for estimation of patient's daily energy and protein requirements (per kilogram bodyweight) (guidelines not always appropriate for patients who are severely ill)**

Factor	Measurement
Energy (kcal)	25–35
Energy (kJ)	105–146
Protein (g)	0.8–1.5
Fluid (mL)	35 (18–60 years) 30 (>60 years) (plus 2–2.5 mL per °C in temperature above 37°C)

Source: Todorovic and Micklewright (2011). Reproduced with permission from PENG – Parenteral and Enteral Nutrition Group (www.peng.uk.com) of the British Dietetic Association (www.bda.uk.com).

Methods for measuring height and weight of an adult patient

Taking an accurate height and weight of a patient is an essential part of nutrition screening. Accurate measurements of bodyweight may also be required for estimating body surface area and calculating drug dosages, such as for anaesthesia and chemotherapy. All patients should have height and weight measured on admission to hospital and weight should be measured at regular intervals during their hospital stay according to local policy and individual clinical need.

PRE-PROCEDURAL CONSIDERATIONS

Check that the patient is able to stand or sit on the appropriate scales. The patient should remove outdoor clothing and shoes before being weighed and having height measured.

When obtaining a height measurement, check that the patient is able to stand upright whilst the measurement is taken. For patients who are unable to stand then height may be determined by measuring ulna length and using conversion tables. If neither height nor weight can be measured or obtained, BMI can be estimated using the mid upper arm circumference (MUAC) (BAPEN 2003a). It may not be possible to weigh patients who cannot be moved or are unable to sit or stand. Alternative methods to obtain weight should be explored, for example bed scales which can be placed under the wheels of the bed, scales as an integral part of a bed or a patient hoist with weighing facility.

Equipment

Scales

Scales (either sitting or standing) must be calibrated and positioned on a level surface. If electronic or battery scales are used then they must be connected to the mains or have appropriate working batteries prior to the patient getting on the scales.

Stadiometer

These are devices for measuring height and may be mounted on weighing scales or wall mounted.

Tape measure

Required if estimating height from ulna length or MUAC. The tape measure should use centimetres, be disposable or made of plastic that can be cleaned with a detergent wipe between patient uses.

Assessment tools

Identification of patients who are malnourished or at risk of malnutrition is an important first step in nutritional care. There are a number of screening tools available which consider different aspects of nutritional status. National screening initiatives have demonstrated that 28% of patients admitted to hospital were found to be at risk of malnutrition – high risk (22%) and medium risk (6%) (BAPEN 2009). Particular diagnoses, such as cancer, increase the risk of malnutrition.

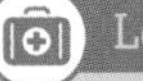 Learning Activity 7.4

Learning in practice: Nutritional assessment

Is a nutritional screening tool used within your clinical area? Have a look at the tool.

- What aspects of nutritional status does the tool assess?
- What do the results/score indicate?
- How easy is the tool to use?
- Is there guidance provided to indicate what interventions should be taken depending on the patient's result/score?

Procedure guideline 7.8 Measuring the weight and height of the patient

Essential equipment

- Scales
- Stadiometer (preferably fixed to the wall)

Optional equipment

- Tape measure

Pre-procedure

Action	Rationale
1 Position the scales for easy access and apply the brakes (if appropriate).	To ensure that the patient can get on and off the scales easily and to avoid accidents should the scales move. **E**
2 Ask the patient to remove shoes and outdoor garments. The patient should be wearing light indoor clothes only (see **Action figure 2**).	Outdoor clothes and shoes will add additional weight and make it difficult to obtain an accurate bodyweight. **E**
Procedure	
3 Ensure that the scales record zero, then ask the patient to stand on scales (or sit if using sitting scales). Ask the patient to remain still and check that the patient is not supporting any weight on any object, for example wall, stick or feet on the floor.	To record an accurate weight (NMC 2010, **C**).
4 Note the reading on the scale and record immediately, taking care that it is legible. Check with the patient that the weight reflects their expected weight and that the weight is similar to previous weights recorded. This may require conversion of weight from kg to stones and pounds or vice versa.	To check that the weight is correct. If the weight is not as expected then the patient should be reweighed. **E**
5 Ensure that the patient has removed their shoes and then ask them to stand straight with heels together. If the stadiometer is wall mounted, the heels should touch the heel plate or the wall. With a freestanding device the person's back should be toward the measuring rod.	Shoes will provide additional height and make the measurement inaccurate. **E** To ensure that the patient is standing upright. If the person does not have their back against the measuring rod then the measuring arm may not reach the head. **E**
6 The patient should look straight ahead and with the bottom of the nose and the bottom of the ear in a parallel plane. The patient should be asked to stretch to reach maximal height.	To ensure an accurate height is measured. **E**
7 Record height to the nearest millimetre.	To record an accurate measurement of the patient's height (NMC 2010, **C**).
8 To estimate the height of a patient from ulna length, ask the patient to remove long-sleeved jacket, shirt or top.	To be able to access their left arm for measurement purposes. **E**
9 Measure between the point of the elbow (olecranon process) and the midpoint of the prominent bone of the wrist (styloid process) on the left side if possible (**Action figure 9**).	To obtain measurement of the length of the ulna. **E**
10 Estimate the patient's height to the nearest centimetre, using a conversion table.	To estimate the patient's height (BAPEN 2003a, **C**).
11 Estimate BMI from MUAC, ask the patient to remove long-sleeved jacket, shirt or top.	To be able to access their left arm for measurement purposes (BAPEN 2003a, **C**).
12 Measure the distance between the top of the shoulder (acromion) and the point of the elbow (olecranon process) – identify the midpoint between the two points and mark the arm (**Action figure 12a, 12b**).	To obtain measurement of the mid upper arm circumference. **E**
13 As the patient to let the arm hang loosely by their side and with a tape measure, measure the circumference of the arm at the midpoint (**Action figure 13**).	To obtain accurate measurement of the mid upper arm circumference. **E**
14 Document the measurement.	To record an accurate measurement of MUAC (BAPEN 2003a, **C**).
15 Estimate the patient's BMI using a conversion table.	To estimate the patient's BMI (BAPEN 2003a, **C**).
Post-procedure	
16 Document height and weight, or estimated BMI, in patient's notes.	To record the accurate measurement of patient's height and weight (NMC 2010, **C**).

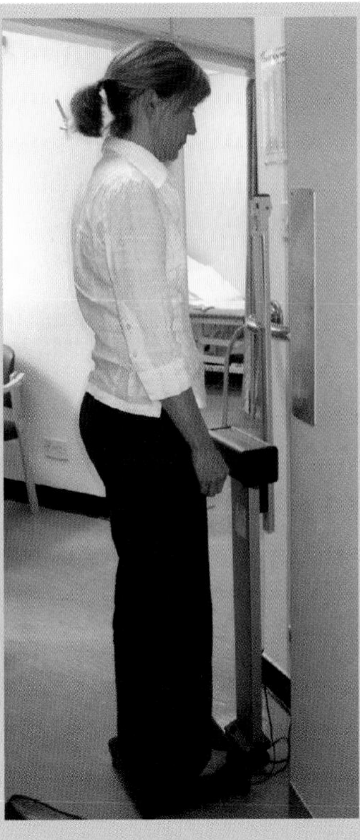

Action Figure 2 Weighing a patient.

Action Figure 9 Measure between the point of the elbow (olecranon process) and the midpoint of the prominent bone of the wrist (styloid process).

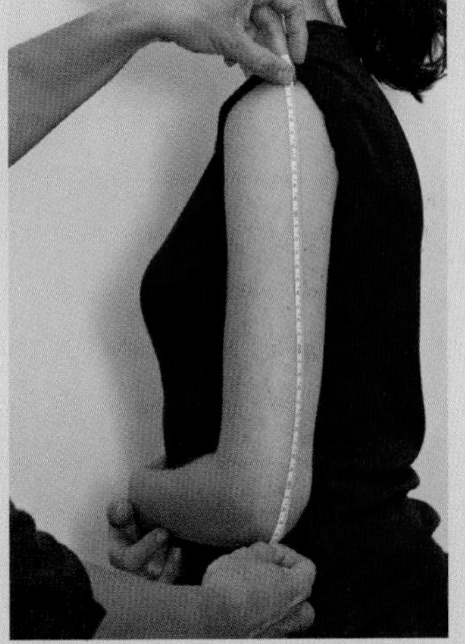

Action Figure 12a Identify the midpoint between the two points.

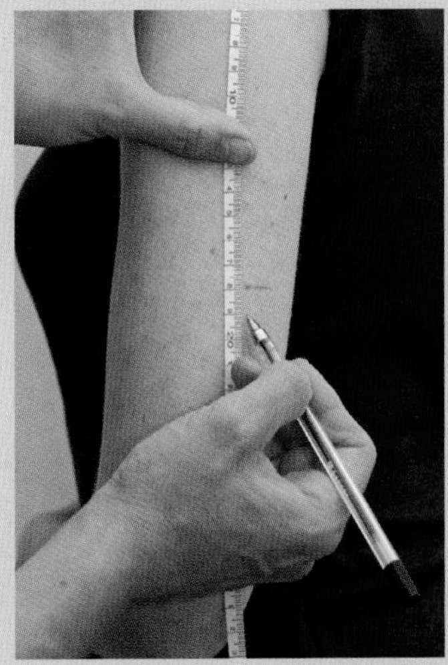

Action Figure 12b Mark the arm.

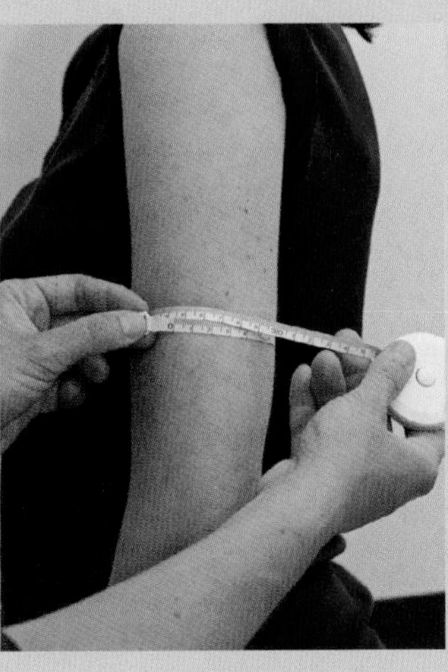

Action Figure 13 Measure the circumference of the arm at the midpoint using a tape measure.

Problem-solving table 7.2 **Prevention and resolution (Procedure guideline 7.8)**

Problem	Cause	Prevention	Action
Patient unable to stand on scale.	Poorly positioned scales. Patient balance not sufficient.	Check with patient prior to asking them to stand on scales if they are able to do so. Offer sitting scales if necessary.	Ensure both sitting and standing scales are available in the hospital.
Weight obtained appears too low.	Patient may have put pressure on scales prior to them reaching zero.	Ensure zero is visible before patient touches scales.	Check weight with patient once obtained. Reweigh patient to check correct weight.
Weight obtained appears too high.	Patient may be wearing outdoor clothes or shoes or be carrying a bag, drainage bag and so on. Patient may have fluid retention, for example oedema or ascites.	Ensure that the patient is wearing light indoor clothes before standing on the scales. Check whether patient has fluid retention. Ask patient to empty any drainage bags.	Check weight with patient once obtained. Reweigh patient to check correct weight.
Patient is unable to stand.	Patient is unwell or has physical disability.	Discuss the procedure with patient before undertaking height measurement.	Consider estimating height from ulna measurement.

All patients who are identified as at risk of malnutrition should undergo a nutritional assessment. Subjective global assessment (SGA) and patient-generated SGA (PG-SGA) are comprehensive assessment tools that necessitate more time and expertise to carry out than most screening tests. Some more simple screening tools, including the Malnutrition Universal Screening Tool (MUST) (BAPEN 2003a), based on the patient's BMI, weight loss and illness score, are less time consuming. Other tools may be specific to the patient's age or diagnosis (Kondrup et al. 2003). The most important feature of using any screening tool is that patients identified as requiring nutritional assessment or intervention have a nutritional care plan initiated and are referred to the dietician for further advice if appropriate.

POST-PROCEDURAL CONSIDERATIONS

Consideration must be given to the patient's weight and whether this reflects a change in their clinical condition. The weight may be being used as part of a nutritional screening or assessment or for planning of treatment, for example medication. Any significant changes should be interpreted in the light of potential changes in body composition and incorporated into the patient's care plan. For example, a loss of weight may require further questioning about dietary intake and the commencement of a nutritional care plan.

After taking a measurement of height, it is useful to check with the patient that the figure obtained is approximately the height expected. However, it is important to consider that patients may report a loss in height with increasing years. A cumulative height loss from age 30 to 70 years may be about 3 cm for men and 5 cm for women and by age 80 years it increases to 5 cm for men and 8 cm for women (Sorkin et al. 1999).

Provision of nutritional support: oral

EVIDENCE-BASED APPROACHES

Rationale

An essential part of providing diet for a patient is to ensure that the patient is able to consume the food and fluid in a safe and pleasant environment. Some patients may require assistance with feeding or drinking and a system should be in place to ensure that these patients receive the required attention at each mealtime and beverage service, as well as adaptive cutlery or crockery if appropriate. Choice should be encouraged, preferably from a menu. Ideally the menu should be coded to assist patients to select suitable options such as high energy, soft, vegetarian, etc. Meals should be available for patients requiring gluten-free, halal, kosher or texture-modified choices.

It is essential that meals are appetising and strictly comply with any dietary restriction relevant to the patient. For example, those with food allergies, texture modifications, religious or cultural dietary requirements need to be clearly identified with the senior ward nurse, before assistance with feeding commences. Eating and drinking are pleasurable experiences and the psychosocial aspect of this cannot be overestimated. The inability to participate in mealtimes can be socially isolating (Ekberg et al. 2002). Research has highlighted that dysphagia also affects carers due to the impact on social activity and can lead to permanent changes in lifestyle. (Patterson et al. 2012).

Patient-centred care requires respect and involvement of the patient in the process of feeding (Care Quality Commission 2010). Supporting the dignity of the patient throughout the process is also imperative to its success and acceptance.

Provision of food and nutrition in a hospital setting

Good nutritional care, adequate hydration and enjoyable mealtimes can dramatically improve the general health and well-being of patients who are unable to feed themselves, and can be particularly relevant to older people (Nutrition Summit Stakeholder Group and DH 2007). Unfortunately, it is evident that assistance with meals for those that require it does not always occur. In the summary of the results for the 2011 national inpatients survey, 15% described the hospital food as 'poor', an increase over 13% in 2010. Of those needing help to eat their meals, 19% did not receive this (Care Quality Commission 2010).

Many factors, including being in hospital, need to be taken into consideration when planning nutritional support. Clinical benchmarking (DH 2010) and clinical initiatives such as protected mealtimes aim to address common problems that patients experience whilst in hospital that impact on food intake.

The *Essence of Care Benchmark for Food and Drink* (DH 2010) sets the standard for best practice with regard to the provision of food and drink in hospital. The document states that people must be enabled to consume food and drink (orally) which meets their needs and preferences. Ten factors affecting intake and benchmarks of best practice are identified to support optimal provision and monitoring of food and drink. These are shown in Box 7.1. The Department of Health and the Nutrition Summit Stakeholder Group have worked together to produce an action plan based on the 10 key characteristics of good nutritional care in hospitals. These are outlined in Box 7.2.

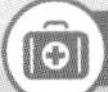 Learning Activity 7.5

Learning in practice: Providing food in hospital

Visit the following website which provides an overview of the latest hospital inpatient survey results for food (p. 6). http://www.cqc.org.uk/sites/default/files/inpatient_survey_national_summary.pdf

- What can you learn from this report about hospital food?
- How can you help patients to have a better choice of food?
- How can you help to ensure that patients get the assistance they need to eat their food?

The hospital inpatient survey is undertaken annually. Visit http://www.cqc.org.uk/content/surveys to find the most up-to-date survey results.

Modification of diet

There are various publications providing initial advice for people requiring modification of diet, such as *Have You Got a Small Appetite?* (National Advisory Group for Elderly People/British Dietetic Association n.d.). See also Table 7.5.

Dietary supplements

If patients are unable to meet their nutritional requirements with food alone then they may require dietary supplements. These may be used to improve an inadequate diet or as a sole source of nutrition if taken in sufficient quantity.

Sip feeds

These come in a range of flavours, both sweet and savoury, and are presented as a powder in a packet or ready prepared in a can, bottle or carton. Sip feeds contain whole protein, hydrolysed fat and carbohydrates. Most are called 'complete feeds' since they provide all protein, vitamins, minerals and trace elements to meet requirements if a prescribed volume is taken (Thomas and Bishop 2007). Others may be aimed at specific needs, for example high protein.

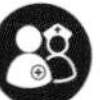 Box 7.1 **Food and nutrition benchmark ('*food*' includes drinks)**

Agreed patient/client-focused outcome: patients/clients are enabled to consume food (orally) which meets their individual needs.

Indicators/information that highlight concerns which may trigger the need for benchmarking activity:

- Patient satisfaction surveys
- Complaints figures and analysis
- Audit results: including catering audit, nutritional risk assessments, documentation audit, environmental audit (including dining facilities)
- Contract monitoring, for example wastage of food, food handling and/or food hygiene training records
- Ordering of dietary supplements/special diets
- Audit of available equipment and utensils
- Educational audits/student placement feedback
- Litigation/Clinical Negligence Scheme for Trusts
- Professional concern
- Media reports
- *Sustainable Food and the NHS* (King's Fund 2005), *Food and Nutritional Care in Hospitals* (Council of Europe 2003)

Factor	Benchmark of best practice
1 Promoting health	*People* are encouraged to eat and drink in a way that promotes health
2 Information	*People* and carers have sufficient information to enable them to obtain their food and drink
3 Availability	*People* can access food and drink at any time according to their needs and preferences
4 Provision	*People* are provided with food and drink that meets their individual needs and preferences
5 Presentation	*People*'s food and drink are presented in a way that is appealing to them
6 Environment	*People* feel the environment is conducive to eating and drinking
7 Screening and assessment	*People* who are screened on initial contact and identified as at risk receive a full nutritional assessment
8 Planning, implementation, evaluation and revision of care	*People*'s care is planned, implemented, continuously evaluated and revised to meet individual needs and preferences for food and drink
9 Assistance	*People* receive the care and assistance they require with eating and drinking
10 Monitoring	*People*'s food and drink intake is monitored and recorded

Other factors which may influence food intake, such as treatments, surgery and medications, also need to be taken into account when planning nutritional support, as clinical experience shows that these may have a deleterious effect on appetite and the ability to maintain an adequate nutritional intake, although rehabilitation therapy can be helpful in increasing intake.

Source: DH (2010).

Box 7.2 **Ten key characteristics of good nutritional care in hospitals**

- All patients are screened on admission to identify those who are malnourished or at risk of becoming malnourished. All patients are rescreened weekly.
- All patients have a care plan which identifies their nutritional care needs and how they are to be met.
- The hospital includes specific guidance on food services and nutritional care in its clinical governance arrangements.
- Patients are involved in the planning and monitoring arrangements for food service provision.
- The ward implements protected mealtimes to provide an environment conducive to patients enjoying and being able to eat their food.
- All staff have the appropriate skills and competencies needed to ensure that patients' nutritional needs are met. All staff receive regular training on nutritional care and management.
- Hospital facilities are designed to be flexible and patient centred with the aim of providing and delivering an excellent experience of food service and nutritional care 24 hours a day, every day.
- The hospital has a policy for food service and nutritional care which is patient centred and performance managed in line with home country governance frameworks.
- Food service and nutritional care are delivered to the patient safely.
- The hospital supports a multidisciplinary approach to nutritional care and values the contribution of all staff groups working in partnership with patients and users.

Energy supplements

CARBOHYDRATES

Glucose polymers in powder or liquid form contain approximately 350 kcal (1442 kJ) per 100 g and 187–299 kcal (770–1232 kJ) per 100 mL respectively. Powdered glucose polymer is virtually tasteless and may be added to anything in which it will dissolve, for example milk and other drinks, soup, cereals and milk pudding; liquid glucose polymers may be fruit flavoured or neutral (Thomas and Bishop 2007). Such supplements would be used to increase the energy content of the diet.

FAT

Fat may be in the form of long-chain triglycerides (LCT) or medium-chain triglycerides (MCT) and comes as a liquid which can be added to food and drinks. These oils provide 416–772 kcal (1714–3181 kJ) per 100 mL; the oils with a lower energy value are presented in the form of an emulsion and those with a higher energy value are presented as pure oil (Thomas and Bishop 2007).

Mixed fat and glucose polymer solutions and powders are available and provide 150 kcal per 100 mL or 486 kcal per 100 g, depending on the relative proportion of fat and carbohydrates in the product.

Products containing MCT are used in preference to those containing LCT where a patient suffers from GI impairment causing malabsorption. Patients require specific advice about their use to ensure that they are introduced into the diet slowly and GI tolerance is assessed (Thomas and Bishop 2007).

Always check with the manufacturer for the exact energy content of products.

Note: products containing a glucose polymer are unsuitable for patients with diabetes mellitus.

Table 7.5 **Suggestions for modification of diet**

Eating difficulty	Dietary modification
Anorexia	Serve small meals and snacks, for example twice-daily snack options
	Make food look attractive with garnish
	Fortify foods with butter, cream or cheese to increase energy content of meals
	Use alcohol, steroids, megestrol acetate or medroxyprogesterone as an appetite stimulant
	Encourage food that patient prefers
	Offer nourishing drinks between meals. In hospital consider a 'cocktail' drinks round
Sore mouth	Offer foods that are soft and easy to eat
	Avoid dry foods that require chewing
	Avoid citrus fruits and drinks
	Avoid salt and spicy foods
	Allow hot food to cool before eating
Dysphagia	Offer foods that are soft and serve with additional sauce or gravy
	Some foods may need to be blended: make sure food is served attractively
	Supplement the diet with nourishing drinks between meals
Nausea and vomiting	Have cold foods in preference to hot as these emit less odour
	Keep away from cooking smells
	Sip fizzy, glucose-containing drinks
	Eat small frequent meals and snacks that are high in carbohydrate (e.g. biscuits and toast)
	Try ginger drinks and ginger biscuits
Early satiety	Eat small, frequent meals. In hospital, access an 'out-of-hours' meal service
	Avoid high-fat foods which delay gastric emptying
	Avoid drinking large quantities when eating
	Use prokinetics, for example metoclopramide, to encourage gastric emptying

Protein supplements

These come in the form of a powder and provide 55–90 g protein per 100 g. Protein supplement powders may be added to any food or drink in which they will dissolve, for example milk, fruit juice, soup, milk pudding.

Energy and protein supplements are not used in isolation as these would not provide an adequate nutritional intake. They are used in conjunction with sip feeds and a modified diet. The detailed nutritional compositions of dietary supplements are available from the manufacturers.

Specialist supplements

Supplements designed for specific patient groups are also available, for example, aimed at dementia, chronic obstructive pulmonary disease, renal or dysphagia patients.

Vitamin and mineral supplements

When dietary intake is poor, a vitamin and mineral supplement may be required. This can often be given as a one-a-day tablet supplement that provides 100% of the dietary reference values. Care should be taken to avoid unbalanced supplements or those containing amounts larger than the dietary reference value (FSA and Expert Group on Vitamins and Minerals 2003). Excessive doses of vitamins and minerals may be harmful, particularly as some vitamins and minerals are not excreted by the body when taken in amounts exceeding requirements. Additionally, vitamins and minerals may interact with medication to influence its efficacy; for example, vitamin K may influence anticoagulants such as warfarin.

Patients being discharged from hospital on nutritional supplements

It is important to ensure that patients who require continued oral nutritional supplements in the community are discharged with a suitable supply. The decision on choice of supplement will usually be with the prescriber and should be based on clinical need and patient acceptability. Where more than one suitable option is available, the ease of use in a community setting, likely compliance and the impact on primary care budgets may be factors to be weighed up in the choice of supplement.

Anticipated patient outcomes

It is anticipated that feeding an adult will ensure safe delivery of the meal, in a comfortable environment which the patient feels is a pleasurable and positive experience, promoting adequate nutritional care.

LEGAL AND PROFESSIONAL ISSUES

Protected mealtimes should be in place on the wards, whereby all non-essential clinical activities have been discontinued and a calm environment exists (Age Concern 2006). The use of protected mealtimes within hospitals is strongly encouraged by the National Patient Safety Agency which encourages trusts to have an appropriate policy in place to monitor its implementation on the wards and to have a structure in place to report patients missing meals via the local risk management system (NPSA 2007). The Care Quality Commission carried out a dignity and nutrition inspection programme in 2012, and found that protected mealtimes was one of the contributing factors in encouraging support for patients to eat and drink sufficient amounts in hospitals, achieving the standard of 'meeting people's nutritional needs' (Care Quality Commission 2013).

PRE-PROCEDURAL CONSIDERATIONS

Sufficient staff need to be available to support those who need help. Patients who require assistance should be identified through screening and a discreet signal should be evident to identify that further assistance is required, for example a red tray, a coloured serviette or a red sticker (Bradley and Rees 2003).

Assessment and recording tools

Food record charts can provide the essential information that forms the basis of a nutritional assessment and help to determine subsequent nutritional care. They are therefore a valuable resource for dieticians, nurses and ultimately the patient (Freeman 2002). They can be used to assess whether the patient is eating and drinking enough, thereby enabling action to be taken to encourage intake in those who have a reduced dietary intake.

The objective is to quantify the amount of food and drink (including oral nutritional supplements) consumed by a patient over an agreed time period and, although open to error, it has been demonstrated that this type of record keeping provides more accurate information than methods involving recall (Kroke et al. 1999). In hospital, a patient's intake frequently changes as a result of disease, symptoms, medication, unfamiliar surroundings and food availability. It is frequently not evident how much a patient is eating, particularly on busy wards with regular staff changes.

All screening, including food charts, should be linked to a care plan and documented in the patient's notes (DH 2010, Freeman, 2002, NPSA 2009a). If there is noted weight loss, concerns expressed by staff or from relatives regarding the patient's nutritional intake, particularly where there are difficulties observed with eating and drinking, close monitoring of oral intake is essential. The only exception to this is when a patient is receiving end-of-life care and it has been clarified with the clinical team that active nutritional support is not appropriate.

Food charts should be available on all wards and should be simple to complete. It is often preferable to include on the chart household measures such as tablespoons, slice of bread or hospital portions, to assist with the speed of completion.

Training should be given on how the chart should be completed and preferably should be undertaken by the dietician or the specialist nutrition nurse, as this will facilitate understanding of the rationale and continuity of recording and improve accuracy. Charts need to be carefully completed over a minimum and consecutive 2- or 3-day period or longer if requested by the dietician. Some research suggests that information should be collected over at least 7 days in order to estimate protein and energy intake to within ±10% (Bingham 1987).

Specific patient preparations

Before commencing assistance, please discuss this with the patient in order that they understand and consent to assistance being provided. When verbal communication is not possible, non-verbal agreement needs to be obtained wherever possible. Try to engage the patient in the feeding process and interpret and record any preferences or dislikes they may express regarding the meal process.

Make sure the patient has the opportunity to visit the bathroom and wash or clean their hands with an antiseptic wipe and to undertake any appropriate mouthcare prior to eating. Establish whether any medication is to be administered prior to or after feeding which will facilitate the feeding and digestive process. Individual symptoms should be assessed; for example, if patients are nauseous they may benefit from the prescribing of antiemetics or prokinetic agents. Patients who have pancreatic insufficiency may require pancreatic enzyme replacements. All drugs should be correctly prescribed on the drug chart. The timing in relation to feeding is important and antiemetics should be given approximately 30 minutes prior to meal service. Any special equipment, such as cutlery or non-slip mats, that is required for assisting the patient with the meal should be provided. This may require referral to an occupational therapist for an assessment.

Procedure guideline 7.9 Feeding an adult patient

Essential equipment

- A clean table or tray
- Equipment required to assist the patient such as adequate drinking water, adapted cups, cutlery and napkin
- A chair for the nurse or carer to sit with the patient

Pre-procedure

Action	Rationale
1 Explain and discuss feeding with the patient.	To ensure that the patient understands the procedure and gives their valid consent (NMC 2013).
2 Wash hands, put on apron.	To ensure that the procedure is as clean as possible (Fraise and Bradley 2009, **E**).
3 Ensure that the patient is comfortable, that is, they have an empty bladder, clean hands, clean mouth and, if applicable, clean dentures. Ensure there are no unpleasant sights or smells that would put the patient off eating.	To make the mealtime a pleasant experience (Age Concern 2006, **E**).
4 Ensure the nurse or carer is positioned in front or to the side of the patient and sat at the patient's level to assist with feeding.	To enable the patient and helper to see each other and to assist communication. **E**
5 Ensure that the patient is sitting upright in a supported midline position, preferably in a chair, if it is safe and appropriate, and at a table.	To facilitate swallowing and protect the airway. **E**
6 Protect the patient's clothing with a napkin.	To maintain dignity and cleanliness. **E**

Procedure

Action	Rationale
7 Assist the patient to take appropriate portions of food at the correct temperature but encourage self-feeding. Tailor the size of each mouthful to the individual patient. If possible, each hot course of a meal should be served individually and items which may change in consistency, such as ice cream, served separately.	To make the mealtime a pleasant experience. To maintain textures of foods. To ensure that swallowing is not compromised if the patient feels that they must hurry with the meal (Samuels and Chadwick 2006, **E**).
8 Allow the patient to chew and swallow foods before the next mouthful. Avoid hovering with the next spoonful.	To maintain the dignity of the patient. **E**
9 Avoid asking questions when the patient is eating, but check between mouthfuls that the food is suitable and that the patient is able to continue with the meal.	To reduce the risk of aspirating, which may be increased if speaking whilst eating. **E**
10 Use the napkin to remove particles of food or drink from the patient's face.	To maintain dignity and cleanliness. **E**
11 Ask the patient when they wish to have a drink. Assist the patient to take a sip. Support the glass or cup gently so that the flow of liquid is controlled or use a straw if this is helpful. Take care with hot drinks to avoid offering these when too hot to drink.	To give the opportunity for the patient to swallow. Hot liquids may scald the patient. **E**
12 If the food appears too dry, ask the patient if they would like some additional gravy or sauce added to the dish.	To facilitate chewing and swallowing (Wright et al. 2008, **E**).
13 Observe patient for coughing, choking, wet or gurgly voice, nasal regurgitation or effortful swallow. See Table 7.6 for details of problems that may be experienced by patients.	May indicate aspiration, laryngeal penetration or weakness in muscles required for swallowing (Leslie et al. 2003, **E**).
14 Encourage the patient to take as much food as they feel able to eat, but do not press if they indicate that they have eaten enough.	To improve nutritional intake but also maintain patient dignity and choice (Wright et al. 2008, **E**).

Post-procedure

Action	Rationale
15 After the meal assist the patient to meet hygiene needs, for example, wash hands and face and clean teeth.	To maintain cleanliness and dignity. **E**

Table 7.6 **Difficulties that may be experienced by patients during eating and drinking and their potential implications**

Difficulty experienced	Implications
Coughing and choking during and after eating and/or drinking	Indicates laryngeal penetration or aspiration (Smith Hammond 2008)
Wet or gurgly voice quality	Indicates laryngeal penetration or aspiration (Leslie et al. 2003)
Drooling/excess oral secretions	Indicates less frequent swallowing and is associated with dysphagia (Langmore et al. 1998). May result from poor lip seal
Nasal regurgitation	Indicates impaired velopalatal seal (Leslie et al. 2003)
Food/drink pooling in mouth	Indicates lack of oral sensation from intraoral flaps or may be a sign of cognitive impairment (Logemann 1998)
Swallow is effortful	May indicate weakness in muscles required for swallowing (Logemann et al. 2008)
Respiration rate on eating/drinking is increased	Increased respiration rate may be associated with risk of aspiration (Leslie et al. 2003)
Signs of recurrent chest infections and pyrexia	This may indicate aspiration pneumonia as a consequence of dysphagia (Leslie et al. 2003b)
Patient report of swallowing problems	Patients can be very accurate in self-diagnosis of dysphagia (Pauloski et al. 2002)
Patient reports food sticking	Patients can be very accurate in self-diagnosis of dysphagia (Pauloski et al. 2002)
Additional time required to eat a meal	Taking a long time to eat may indicate dysphagia (Leslie et al. 2003)
Avoidance of certain foods	Patients will avoid food items that they find difficult to swallow (Leslie et al. 2003)
Weight loss	Patients may eat less due to difficulty swallowing (Leslie et al. 2003)
Poor oral hygiene	Aspiration of secretions in those with poor oral hygiene may result in aspiration pneumonia (Langmore 2001)

POST-PROCEDURAL CONSIDERATIONS

Education of patient and relevant others

It is important that volunteers, family members or visitors who wish to assist the patient with feeding are familiar with and trained in the processes listed in Procedure guideline 7.9: Feeding an adult patient (NPSA 2009b). This is to ensure that the family is confident and can safely and effectively assist the patient.

Documentation

It is essential that the plate is not removed before wastage has been recorded and this is relayed to the ward catering staff prior to meal service commencement. If the patient has not managed a reasonable amount of their meal, this needs to be addressed later in the afternoon or evening. It is also important to ascertain whose responsibility it is for completion of the charts to avoid confusion, that is, nurse, healthcare assistant, ward catering staff or patient, as this will vary across institutions. These charts can be used by the dietician or healthcare professional to effectively assess the patient's meal pattern and nutrition intake. Some patients may be able to complete the record themselves if given guidance on what is required. All food record charts that have been reviewed by a healthcare professional should be signed and dated on completion of review.

Difficulties arise when the food chart data are not accurately completed or reviewed, during which time malnutrition and its consequences continue, rather than being quickly identified and addressed.

If there is strong concern about the quantity of food that has been consumed by the patient, this must also be verbally relayed to the nurse in charge, ward dietician and possibly the clinician.

Nutritional management of patients with dysphagia

DEFINITION

Dysphagia is an impairment of swallowing that may involve any structure from the lips to the gastric cardia (Leslie et al. 2003).

EVIDENCE-BASED APPROACHES

Rationale

Indications

Patients who are at high risk of dysphagia are summarized in Box 7.3.

Goals of clinical assessment

Some patients who are eating and drinking may experience dysphagia. It is important to correctly ascertain the presence of dysphagia and the factors contributing to its possible aetiology. Such patients may be at risk of aspiration and subsequent chest infections and therefore require a referral to a speech and language therapist for a full assessment (Roe 2012). Patients require a nutritional assessment from a dietician with consideration of possible enteral tube feeding if the patient is unable to maintain an adequate nutritional intake or is at risk of aspiration. A suitable swallowing rehabilitation programme should be developed. Patients undergoing surgery or radiotherapy for head and neck cancer should have a baseline clinical swallowing evaluation before treatment (Lazarus 2000, NICE 2004, Patterson and Wilson 2011).

Box 7.3 **Patient groups at high risk of dysphagia**

- Head and neck cancer patients undergoing surgery and/or radiotherapy/chemoradiotherapy. The risk of dysphagia is increased with multimodal therapy. Side-effects from treatment may affect swallow function, such as xerostomia (dry mouth), odynophagia (pain on swallowing), thick oral secretions, nausea, candidiasis, taste changes, mucositis, fatigue, fibrosis and trismus (reduced mouth opening). Nutritional support with enteral tube feeding may be required.
- Patients with neurological involvement including brain tumours or metastases, other co-morbid neurological disorders, for example cerebrovascular accident, multiple sclerosis, motor neurone disease, Parkinson's disease, myasthenia gravis. Such patients may also have cognitive or behavioural issues which can affect their mood, motivation, feeding and appetite.
- Patients with lung cancer and vocal cord paralysis and respiratory disorders such as chronic obstructive pulmonary disease, including mechanically ventilated patients.
- Tracheostomy patients may present with swallowing problems although frequently their medical diagnosis is the primary cause of dysphagia.
- Gastrointestinal patients may present with oropharyngeal or oesophageal dysphagia.
- Any other patient with significant generalized weakness or other co-morbidities, including palliative care patients.
- Patients with psychogenic dysphagia.
- Laryngectomy patients and particularly pharyngolaryngectomy and pharyngolaryngo-oesophageal patients. Some patients may experience dysphagia due to altered anatomy after surgery.

Source: Adapted from Donzelli et al. (2005), Leder and Ross (2000), Lewin et al. (2001), Roe (2005), Roe et al. (2007), Royal College of Speech and Language Therapists (2006).

Principles of care

Care will be influenced by the timing of patient referral dependent on their disease and treatment status. Management of the dysphagic patient will be tailored to individual needs and they will require regular reviews to ensure that intervention and management decisions remain appropriate. The nature of the dysphagia may persist, recur or worsen depending on the patient's treatment or disease.

Treatment options may include normal diet with specifically targeted therapy techniques, modified diet, combination of alternative feeding and limited oral intake or nil by mouth. For patients with oropharyngeal dysphagia, dysphagia food texture descriptors have been developed and updated to provide industry and in-house caterers with detailed guidance on categories of food texture, thereby enhancing patient safety (NPSA 2012). For patients undergoing radiotherapy for head and neck cancer, it may be appropriate to implement a programme of prophylactic swallowing exercises (Cappell et al. 2009, Paleri et al. 2014).

Close liaison between the nursing staff, dieticians and members of the MDT is essential. The speech and language therapist (SLT) may recommend that the patient adopts certain compensatory swallow techniques to reduce the risk of aspiration or eliminate discomfort. Exercises or swallow techniques may be given to the patient to rehabilitate their swallow (Lazarus et al. 2002, Lewin et al. 2001, Logemann et al. 1997). It is important for nurses to participate in educational programmes for patients and carers in order to improve awareness of the implications of dysphagia. Nurses may be required to supervise patients with oral intake and encourage their participation with regard to therapy exercises, and reduce other risk factors by encouraging good mouthcare and independent feeding.

Methods of assessment

Clinical swallow assessment

In any patient presenting with a new onset of dysphagia, a medical review is necessary as this may be the first indicator of a change in disease or condition. A subsequent specialist SLT referral is then necessary. The SLT will take a full comprehensive case history including subjective reports, medical, physical and mental status. Surgical and/or disease details will be determined, including where the patient is on the care pathway, for example pre-operative, post-operative, receiving treatment, medication or palliative care. An examination of the oral cavity and cranial nerve assessment will be carried out to evaluate motor and sensory function associated with swallowing (Figure 7.5). Food and drink trials may be carried out by the SLT. The clinical swallowing evaluation may include tests such as the 100 mL Water Swallow Test (Patterson and Wilson 2011).

Instrumental swallowing evaluation

Following an initial assessment, the SLT may recommend instrumental assessments to evaluate in detail the nature and extent of any swallowing disorder. Silent aspiration is a particular issue and in the absence of any overt clinical signs of aspiration or relevant medical history (such as frequent chest infections), instrumental evaluation will be the most appropriate way to identify the problem and its cause. The SLT can implement a range of compensatory strategies during these assessments to optimize swallowing function and minimize the risk of aspiration where possible, By observing swallowing biomechanics, SLTs will be able to define rehabilitation targets. A number of instrumental assessments of swallowing are available but videofluoroscopy (modified barium swallow) and fibreoptic endoscopic evaluation of swallowing (FEES) are the most commonly utilized (Roe 2012). Videofluoroscopy takes place in the X-ray department and involves use of radio-opaque contrast mixed with food (Logemann 1998). FEES involves use of an endoscope passed transnasally, allowing a view of the swallow process while a patient eats and drinks (Langmore 2001). These assessments should be selected on a

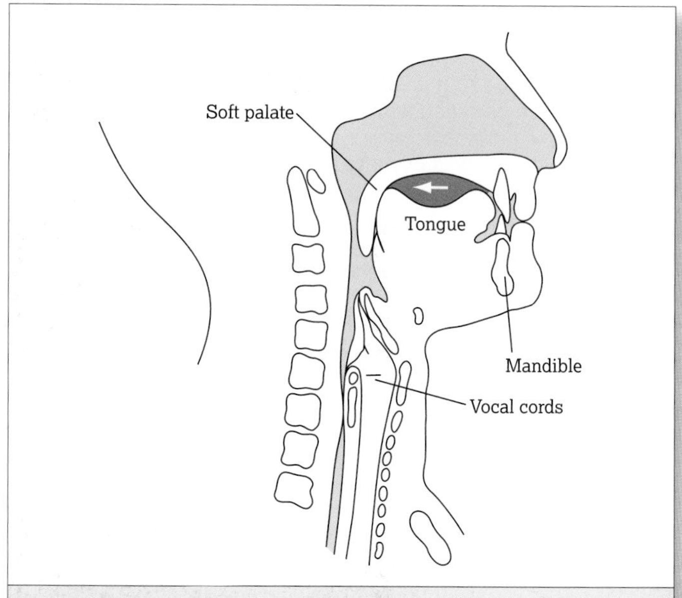

Figure 7.5 **Oral stage of swallowing.**

patient-by-patient basis and in the knowledge that each method has its own particular advantages and limitations (Roe 2012).

Anticipated patient outcomes

Early identification of dysphagia and appropriate management is an essential part of patient care. Appropriate management aims to reduce the incidence of aspiration and the risk of aspiration pneumonia and to help maintain adequate nutrition. If it is not addressed appropriately, it can lead to malnutrition, weight loss and dehydration, aspiration and aspiration pneumonia, low mood and reduced quality of life (Gaziano 2002). Ultimately it may result in increased length of hospital stay (Low et al. 2001). Ensuring the patient has a clear understanding of their swallowing difficulty is essential and may help them to become motivated rehabilitation partners (Roe and Ashforth 2011).

Enteral tube feeding

DEFINITION

Enteral tube feeding refers to the delivery of a nutritionally complete feed (containing protein, fat, carbohydrate, vitamins, minerals, fluid and possibly dietary fibre) directly into the gastrointestinal tract via a tube. The tube is usually placed into the stomach, duodenum or jejunum via either the nose or direct percutaneous route (NCCAC 2006).

RELATED THEORY

Enteral feeding tubes allow direct access to the gastrointestinal tract for the purposes of feeding. A nasogastric or nasojejunal tube is placed via the nose and passed down the oesophagus with the feeding tip ending in the stomach (gastric) or small intestine (jejunum) respectively. A gastrostomy tube is placed directly into the stomach allowing infusion of nutrients into the stomach or, alternatively, such tubes may have a jejunal extension passing through the pylorus, allowing feeding into the jejunum (small intestine). A jejunostomy tube allows direct access to the jejunum for feeding. The choice of appropriate tube should be based on the method of insertion and the associated risks, length of time feeding is required, function of the gastrointestinal tract, the physical condition of the patient and body image issues relating to the visibility of the feeding tube, after discussion with the patient. The feeding regimen, care of the tube and stoma will depend on the enteral feeding tube inserted and should be undertaken within the care of a multiprofessional team (Majka et al. 2013, NCCAC 2006).

EVIDENCE-BASED APPROACHES

Rationale

While the majority of patients will be able to meet their nutritional requirements orally, there is a group of individuals who will require enteral tube feeding either in the short term or on a more permanent basis.

The primary aim of enteral tube feeding is to:

- avoid further loss of bodyweight
- correct significant nutritional deficiencies
- rehydrate the patient
- stop the related deterioration of quality of life of the patient due to inadequate oral nutritional intake (Loser et al. 2005).

Indications

Indications for enteral tube feeding are as follows:

- patient is unable to meet nutritional needs through oral intake alone
- the gastrointestinal tract is accessible and functioning
- it is anticipated that intestinal absorptive function will meet all nutritional needs (NCCAC, 2006).

PRE-PROCEDURAL CONSIDERATIONS

Equipment: types of enteral feed tubes

Nasogastric/nasoduodenal/nasojejunal

Nasogastric feeding is the most commonly used enteral tube feed and is suitable for short-term feeding, that is, 2–4 weeks (NCCAC 2006). Nasogastric tubes must be radio-opaque throughout their length and have externally visible length markings (NPSA 2011). Fine-bore feeding tubes should be used whenever possible as these are more comfortable for the patient than wide-bore tubes. They are less likely to cause complications such as rhinitis, oesophageal irritation and gastritis (Payne-James et al. 2001). Polyurethane or silicone tubes are preferable to polyvinylchloride (PVC) as they withstand gastric acid and can stay in position longer than the 10–14-day lifespan of the PVC tube (Payne-James et al. 2001). The initial placement of a nasogastric tube should be confirmed with an abdominal X-ray (unless placed under radiological guidance) (NCCAC 2006).

Gastrostomy

A gastrostomy may be more appropriate than a nasogastric tube when enteral tube feeding is anticipated to be greater than 4 weeks. It avoids delays in feeding and discomfort associated with tube displacement (NCCAC 2006).

A gastrostomy tube may be placed endoscopically (percutaneous endoscopically placed gastrostomy; PEG) or radiologically (radiologically inserted gastrostomy; RIG). They are made from polyurethane or silicone and are therefore suitable for short- or long-term feeding. A flange, flexible dome, inflated balloon or pigtail sits within the stomach and holds the tube in position.

For long-term feeding (i.e. longer than 1 month), a gastrostomy tube may be replaced with a button which is made from silicone. The entry site for feeding is flush with the skin, making it neat and less obvious than a gastrostomy tube. This is more cosmetically acceptable, especially for teenagers or patients who are physically active, but does require a certain amount of manual dexterity from the patient (Thomas and Bishop 2007). The button is held in place by a balloon or dome inside the stomach (Griffiths 1996). Percutaneous endoscopically placed gastrostomy tubes may be placed while the patient is sedated, thereby avoiding the risks associated with general anaesthesia. However, patients who have compromised airways may require general anaesthesia and appropriate consideration for maintenance of the airway (see Chapter 9: Respiratory care).

Certain groups of patients are not suitable for endoscopy; in these cases a RIG can be used. They are indicated for oesophageal patients with bulky tumours where it would be difficult to pass an endoscope and also for head and neck patients whose airway would be obstructed by an endoscope. There is also documented risk of the endoscope seeding the tumour to the gastrostomy site when it pulls the tube past a bulky tumour, although this is a rare complication (Pickhardt et al. 2002).

Jejunostomy

A jejunostomy is preferable to a gastrostomy if a patient has undergone upper GI surgery or has severe delayed gastric emptying; in some cases it can be used to feed a patient with pyloric obstruction (Thomas and Bishop 2007). Fine-bore feeding jejunostomy tubes may be inserted surgically or laparoscopically with the use of a jejunostomy kit, which consists of a needle-fine catheter. The use of needles and an introducer wire allows a fine-bore polyurethane catheter to be inserted into a loop of jejunum. Alternatively, some gastrostomy tubes allow the passage of a fine-bore tube through the pylorus and into the jejunum. A double-lumen tube allows aspiration of stomach contents whilst feed is administered into the small intestine.

Table 7.7 **Methods of administering enteral feeds**

Feeding regimen	Advantages	Disadvantages
Continuous feeding via a pump	Easily controlled rate	Patient connected to the feed for majority of the day
	Reduction of gastrointestinal (GI) complications	May limit patient's mobility
Intermittent feeding via gravity or a pump	Periods of time free of feeding Flexible feeding routine May be easier than managing a pump for some patients	May have an increased risk of GI symptoms, for example early satiety Difficult if outside carers are involved with the feed
Bolus feeding	May reduce time connected to feed Very easy Minimum equipment required	May have an increased risk of GI symptoms May be time consuming

Enteral feeding equipment

The administration of enteral feeds may be as a bolus, intermittent or continuous infusion, via gravity drip or pump assisted (Table 7.7). There are many enteral feeding pumps available which vary in their flow rates from 1 to 300 mL per hour. The following systems may be used for feeding via a pump or gravity drip.

- Feed is decanted into plastic bottles or PVC bags. The administration set may be an integral part of the bag or may be supplied separately. The feed is sterile until opened and decanting feed into reservoirs will increase the risk of contamination from handling (Payne-James et al. 2001). Generally this method is only used for feeds that require reconstitution with water. Malnourished and immunocompromised patients are particularly at risk from contamination and infection so this method of administration should be avoided where possible.
- The 'ready-to-hang' system has a plastic bottle or pack attached directly to the administration set. The bottles and packs are available in different types of feeds and sizes for flexibility. This is a closed sterile system which has been shown to be successful in preventing exogenous bacterial contamination (Payne-James et al. 2001).
- For powdered feeds that require reconstitution with water, the feed is decanted into plastic bottles or PVC bags. The administration set may be an integral part of the bag or may be supplied separately. The feed is sterile until opened and decanting feed into reservoirs will increase the risk of contamination of the feed from handling (Payne-James et al. 2001). Malnourished and immunocompromised patients are particularly at risk from contamination and infection so this method of administration should be avoided where possible.

Enteral feeds

Commercially prepared feeds should be used for nasogastric, gastrostomy or jejunostomy feeding. Available in liquid or powder form, they have the advantage of being of known composition and are sterile when packaged. Enteral feeds can be nutritionally complete when given in the advised quantity and can be used as a sole source of nutrition or to supplement the patient's oral intake (Lochs et al. 2006).

Whole protein/polymeric feeds

These contain protein, lipid in the form of LCTs and carbohydrate and so require digestion (Lochs et al. 2006). They may provide 1.0–1.5 kcal/mL (see manufacturer's specifications). As the energy density of the feed increases, so does the osmolarity. Hyperosmolar feeds tend to draw water into the lumen of the gut from the bloodstream and can contribute to diarrhoea if given too rapidly. Fibre may be beneficial for maintaining gut ecology and function, rather than promoting bowel transit time (Thomas and Bishop 2007).

Feeds containing medium-chain triglycerides

In some whole-protein feeds, a proportion of the fat or LCTs may be replaced with MCTs. The feed often has a lower osmolarity and is therefore less likely to draw fluid from the plasma into the gut lumen. MCTs are transported via the portal vein rather than the lymphatic system. These feeds are suitable for patients with fat malabsorption and maybe steatorrhoea (Cummings 2000).

Elemental/peptide feeds

These contain free amino acids, short-chain peptides or a combination of both as the nitrogen source. They are often low in fat or may contain some fat as MCTs. Glucose polymers provide the main energy source. These feeds require little or no digestion and are suitable for patients with impaired GI function, maldigestion or malabsorption (Thomas and Bishop 2007). They are hyperosmolar and low in residue.

Special application feeds

These feeds have altered nutrients for particular clinical conditions. Low-protein and low-mineral feeds may be used for patients with liver or renal failure. High-fat, low-carbohydrate feeds may be used for ventilated patients because less carbon dioxide is produced per calorie intake compared with a low-fat, high-carbohydrate feed. Very high-energy and high-protein feeds may be used where nutritional requirements are exceptionally high, for example burns, severe sepsis. These feeds contain approximately double the amount of energy and protein compared to standard whole-protein feeds (Thomas and Bishop 2007).

Paediatric feeds

These are designed for children 1–12 years old and/or 8–45 kg in weight. The protein, vitamin and mineral profile is suitable for children. Generally they are lower in osmolarity than adult feeds. The whole-protein/polymeric feeds are based on cow's milk but are lactose free. Some of these feeds may contain dietary fibre. These feeds provide 1.0–1.5 kcal/mL for children who require additional energy and protein in a smaller volume. Protein hydrolysed feeds and elemental feeds are used in conditions such as food allergies or malabsorption. The osmolarity of these feeds is higher than whole-protein feeds. They need to be introduced carefully (Thomas and Bishop 2007).

Immune-modulating feeds

There is evidence to show that the addition of glutamine, arginine or omega-3 fatty acids, if given pre-operatively, may benefit post-surgical GI patients by reducing the risk of post-operative infections. These specialized liquids may be given pre- or post-operatively (Braga et al. 2002, Weimann et al. 2006).

Up-to-date information on the exact composition of dietary supplements and enteral feeds can be obtained from the manufacturers.

Administration of enteral tube feed

PRE-PROCEDURAL CONSIDERATIONS

Prior to using enteral feeding tubes for medication or feed administration, it is vital to know where in the gastrointestinal tract the tube tip lies. This may be difficult in patients who have tubes placed in other organs or where there is little visible difference externally between gastrostomy, gastrojejunostomy or jejunostomy tubes. Where available, the tube size, type, insertion date and method should be clearly documented. If this information is unavailable, the tube should be aspirated and the pH used to differentiate between gastric or small bowel placement. If there are sutures securing the external fixator to the patient's abdomen, these should not be removed until it has been confirmed that they are not required to keep the tube in position.

Procedure guideline 7.10 Enteral feeding tubes: administration of feed

Essential equipment

- 50 mL enteral or catheter-tipped syringe
- Commercial ready-to-hang feed

Optional equipment

- Tap water or sterile water (for jejunostomy tubes or for patients who are immunosuppressed) (NICE 2003). Water should be fresh and kept covered

Pre-procedure

Action	Rationale
1 Explain and discuss the procedure with the patient.	To ensure that the patient understands the procedure and gives their valid consent (NMC 2013, **C**).

Procedure

Action	Rationale
2 Check the date on the feed container.	To ensure that the feed has not passed its expiry date. **E**
3 Shake the feed container gently.	To ensure the feed is evenly dispersed, therefore reducing the risk of blocking the giving set. **E**
4 Take a new giving set from a sealed package and ensure that the roller clamp/tap is closed.	To avoid accidental spillage of feed from end of administration set. **E**
5 Screw the giving set tightly onto the feed container.	In order to pierce the seal on the container and maintain a sealed system (Matlow et al. 2006, **C**).
6 Hang the container upside down from the hook on a drip stand.	To avoid backflow of intestinal contents into the feed container (Matlow et al. 2006, **E**).
7 Open the roller clamp/tap and prime the feed to the end of the giving set. (Follow instructions for individual pump.)	This ensures that air is not fed into the stomach when feeding commences. **E**
8 Feed the giving set into the pump as directed by the manufacturer's instructions.	To connect the giving set to the pump device. **E**
9 Set the rate of the feed as directed by the manufacturer's instructions and according to the patient's feeding regimen.	To ensure the correct rate of feed is administered. **E**
10 Set the dose of the feed as directed by the manufacturer's instructions and according to the patient's feeding regimen.	To ensure that the correct dose of feed is administered. **E**
11 Flush the feeding tube with a minimum of 30 mL of water or sterile water in an enteral syringe by attaching to the end of the feeding tube. Depress the plunger on the syringe slowly.	To ensure the patency of the feeding tube (BAPEN 2003b, **C**).
12 Remove the end cover from the giving set and connect to the feeding tube.	To ensure that the feed is delivered via the enteral feeding tube. **E**
13 Commence administration of feed.	To ensure that the feed is delivered via the enteral feeding tube. **E**

Post-procedure

Action	Rationale
15 Dispose of any equipment that is no longer required.	To reduce the chance of equipment being reused and to reduce cross-contamination with new equipment. **E**
14 Document the time that the feed commenced and the rate of administration.	To ensure accurate documentation of nutritional and fluid intake (NMC 2010, **C**).

Problem-solving table 7.3 **Prevention and resolution (Procedure guideline 7.10)**

Problem	Cause	Prevention	Action
Pump alarms with 'occlusion' or 'empty'.	The feed may have finished. There may be a blockage in the giving set or feeding tube.	Ensure the feed container was shaken well before feeding. Ensure the giving set was not bent when feeding was commenced. Ensure that the roller clamp/tap is fully open. Flush the feeding tube as directed before commencing.	Straighten any kinks in the giving set. Ensure that the giving set is fixed correctly around the rotor. Open the roller clamp/tap fully. Check that the feeding tube is not blocked. Disconnect from the feeding tube and run the feed into a container; if feed runs and there is no alarm, this indicates that the pump is working properly and the feeding tube is probably blocked.
Pump alarms with 'low battery'.	This indicates that the pump battery needs to be recharged and that there is approximately 30 minutes of power remaining.	Keep pump plugged in and charged.	Connect to the mains power and continue to feed.
Unable to prime giving set.	The roller clamp/tap may not be fully open. There may be a fault with the giving set. If a drip chamber is present then feed may not have run into this.	Ensure that the roller clamp/tap is fully open when beginning to prime the giving set.	Open the roller clamp/tap fully. Squeeze some feed into the drip chamber if applicable. Try with a new giving set.
Continuous audio alarm and all visual displays go blank.	The pump may require servicing.	Ensure it is serviced regularly.	Send to equipment library or manufacturers for servicing.

POST-PROCEDURAL CONSIDERATIONS

Immediate care

As soon as the feed commences, check that it appears to be running without problems and is at the correct rate. Monitor this regularly throughout the feed administration.

Monitor the patient for signs of nausea/abdominal discomfort within the first hour and every 2–4 hours during feed administration. This may not be possible if the feed is given overnight and the patient is asleep.

Ongoing care

If appropriate, the patient should be taught how to follow the procedure of setting up the enteral feeding equipment. They should be confident with the maintenance of the equipment and be aware of how to troubleshoot.

COMPLICATIONS

Aspiration

This may occur due to regurgitation of feed, poor gastric emptying or incorrect placement of a nasogastric tube. The risk of this can be reduced by:

- the use of prokinetics which encourage gastric emptying, for example metoclopramide
- checking the position of the tube before feeding
- ensuring the patient has their head at a 45° angle during feeding. If the patient is in bed then this can be achieved through raising the head of the bed and ensuring the patient has sufficient pillows for support (Thomas and Bishop 2007).

Nausea and vomiting

This could be caused by a number of factors. It could be related to disease or a side-effect of treatment or a medication such as antibiotics or analgesia. A combination of poor gastric emptying and rapid infusion rates could also stimulate nausea and vomiting. Nausea and vomiting can be better controlled through the use of antiemetics, a reduction in the infusion rate or a change from bolus to intermittent feeding.

Diarrhoea

This could be a result of:

- medications such as antibiotics, chemotherapy or laxatives
- disease or treatment, for example pancreatic insufficiency, bile acid malabsorption
- gut infection, for example *Clostridium difficile*
- poor tolerance to the feed.

Antidiarrhoeal agents could be used if a person is experiencing diarrhoea as a side-effect of medication. If possible, an alternative medication should be found that does not cause diarrhoea. In the case of antibiotics, these should be stopped as soon as possible (Thorson et al. 2008). When the diarrhoea is disease related, the underlying problem should be treated; that is, if a person has pancreatic insufficiency they should be provided with a pancreatic enzyme supplement and/or peptide-based feed.

Avoiding microbiological contamination of the feed or equipment will help to reduce the risk of diarrhoea. This will involve keeping the equipment clean and, when feeding, maintaining a sealed system.

A stool sample should be sent to check for any gut infection. If the sample is found to be positive then the infection should be treated appropriately.

If all the above have been ruled out, the dietician can review the osmolarity, fibre content and infusion rate (Todorovic and Micklewright 2011).

Constipation

Constipation could be caused by inadequate fluid intake, immobility, bowel obstruction or the use of opiates or other medications causing gut stasis.

Methods to improve symptoms of constipation include:

- checking fluid balance and increasing fluid intake if necessary
- providing laxatives/bulking agents
- if possible, encouraging mobility
- if in bowel obstruction, discontinuing enteral feeding (Todorovic and Micklewright 2011).

Abdominal distension

This could be caused by poor gastric emptying, rapid infusion of feed, constipation or diarrhoea. Possible ways to improve distension include:

- gastric motility agents
- reducing the rate of infusion
- encouraging mobility if possible
- treating constipation or diarrhoea.

Blocked tube

Blockage can be a result of inadequate flushing or failure to flush the feeding tube or administration of inappropriate medications via the tube.

Enteral feeding tubes: administration of medication

EVIDENCE-BASED APPROACHES

Rationale

Indications

- Patients requiring medications who are not able to take oral preparations due to dysphagia.
- Where possible, medications should be administered in liquid or soluble form. Alternatively, some preparations can be given in sublingual form.

Contraindications

- Not all medications can be administered through an enteral tube due to risk of blockage.
- If the medication has an enteric coating or is a slow-release preparation, it should not be crushed.
- Some medications may be harmful to the administrator and advice from a pharmacist is required.
- If a number of different medications are required, always administer separately. Do not mix medications unless advised to do so by a pharmacist.

Procedure guideline 7.11 **Enteral feeding tubes: administration of medication**

Essential equipment

- 50 mL enteral syringe
- Mortar and pestle or tablet crusher if tablets are being administered (BAPEN 2003b)

Optional equipment

- Tap water or sterile water (for jejunostomy tubes or for patients who are immunosuppressed) (NICE 2003). Water should be fresh and kept covered

Action	Rationale
Pre-procedure	
1 Check whether patient can take medication orally, whether medication is necessary or if it can be temporarily suspended.	If patient can take medication orally this reduces the risk of tube blockage (BAPEN 2003b, **C**).
2 Consider whether an alternative route can be used, for example buccal, transdermal, topical, rectal or subcutaneous.	If patient can take medication via an alternative route this reduces the risk of tube blockage (BAPEN 2003b, **C**).
3 Check drug is absorbed from the site of delivery.	Some drugs may not be absorbed directly from the jejunum (BAPEN 2003b, **C**).
4 Clean hands with bactericidal soap and water or alcohol-based handgel. Put on non-sterile gloves.	To minimize cross-infection and protect the practitioner from gastric/intestinal contents (Fraise and Bradley 2009, **E**).
Procedure	
5 Stop the enteral feed and flush the tube with at least 30 mL of water (sterile water for jejunostomy administration), using an enteral syringe.	To clear the tube of enteral feed as this may cause a blockage or interact with medications. Sterile water should be used for jejunostomy tubes as the water is bypassing the protective acidic environment of the stomach. **E**
Where there is an absolute contraindication for medicine to be taken with feed:	
6 Stop the feed 1–2 hours before and 2 hours after administration (this will depend on the drug); for example, for phenytoin administration, stop feed 2 hours before and for 2 hours after.	To avoid interaction with enteral feed. **E**
7 Consult with the dietician to prescribe a suitable feeding regimen.	To ensure that the patient's nutritional requirements are met in the time available around medicine administration (BAPEN 2003b, **C**).

(continued)

Procedure guideline 7.11 Enteral feeding tubes: administration of medication *(continued)*

Action	Rationale
8 Prior to preparation, check with the pharmacist which medicines should never be crushed.	Some medications are not designed to be crushed. These include: *modified-release tablets*: absorption will be altered by crushing, possibly causing toxic side-effects *enteric-coated tablets*: the coating is designed to protect the drug against gastric acid *cytotoxic medicines*: this will risk exposing the practitioner to the drug (BNF 2014, **C**).
9 Prepare each medication to be given separately. Volumes greater than 10 mL may be drawn up in a 50 mL syringe and administered via the tube. For small volumes (less than 10 mL) follow step 12. *Either:* *Soluble tablets:* dissolve in 10–15 mL water. *Or:* *Liquids:* shake well. For thick liquids mix with an equal volume of water. *Or:* *Tablets:* crush using a mortar and pestle or tablet crusher and mix with 10–15 mL water.	To avoid interaction between different medications and to ensure solubility (BAPEN 2003b, **C**).
10 Never add medication directly to the enteral feed.	To avoid interaction between medicines and feed (BAPEN 2003b, **C**).
11 Administer the medication through the tube via a 50 mL syringe. Do not use a three-way tap or syringe tip adaptor. Rinse the tablet crusher or mortar with 10 mL water, draw up in a 50 mL syringe, and flush this through the tube.	To ensure the whole dose is administered (BAPEN 2003b, **C**). To ensure that intravenous syringes are not connected to an enteral feeding system (NPSA 2011, **C**).
12 If volumes of less than 10 mL are required, the dose should be measured in a 10 mL oral syringe. The plunger of a 50 mL syringe should be removed and the 50 mL syringe connected with the enteral tube. The dose should then be administered into the barrel of the 50 mL syringe and the 10 mL syringe rinsed with water, which should also be administered via the barrel of the 50 mL syringe.	To ensure the whole dose is administered (BAPEN 2003b, **C**).
13 If more than one medicine is to be administered, flush between drugs with at least 10 mL of water to ensure that the drug is cleared from the tube.	To avoid interactions between medicines (BAPEN 2003b, **C**).
14 Flush the tube with at least 30 mL of water following the administration of the last drug.	To avoid medicines blocking the enteral tube (BAPEN 2003b, **C**).
15 If the patient is on fluid restriction or for a paediatric patient, consult the dietician and pharmacist about the quantity of water to be given before and after medication.	To ensure that the patient does not exceed their fluid restriction or requirements (BAPEN 2003b, **C**).
Post-procedure	
16 Remove and dispose of any equipment.	To reduce the risk of cross-infection. **E**
17 Record the administration on the prescription chart.	To maintain accurate records (NMC 2010, **C**).

Problem-solving table 7.4 Prevention and resolution (Procedure guideline 7.11)

Problem	Cause	Prevention	Action
Tube became blocked with medication.	Medication had not been administered in the correct composition and/or the tube was not flushed adequately.	Ensure that the guidance from the pharmacist is followed correctly. Ensure that the tube is flushed before and after administration.	See local guidance and the Professional edition of *The Royal Marsden Manual of Clinical Nursing Procedures*
Unable to administer required medication.	It is in a form that cannot be crushed or dissolved.	Ensure that the pharmacist and medical team are aware that all medications need to be administered via an enteral tube.	Contact the medical team or pharmacist to seek advice on an alternative medication.

POST-PROCEDURAL CONSIDERATIONS

Immediate care

The tube patency should be checked to ensure that the medication has not caused a blockage. This could be done by flushing the tube.

The patient should be monitored to ensure that there are no side-effects of the medication administered.

Ongoing care

In order to avoid complications and ensure optimal nutritional status, it is important to monitor the following in patients on enteral tube feeds:

- oral intake
- bodyweight
- urea and electrolytes
- blood glucose
- full blood count
- fluid balance
- tolerance to feed, for example nausea, fullness and bowel activity
- quantity of feed taken
- care of tube
- care of stoma site (where appropriate).

Education of the patient and relevant others

If the patient is going home with the enteral tube in place, it should be ensured that the patient is educated and confident with administering their medication. If this is not possible then the patient should be referred to a healthcare professional, such as a community nurse, who can undertake this aspect of care.

Home enteral feeding

Some patients who are established on tube feeding in hospital also require enteral tube feeding at home. A multidisciplinary approach is needed for a successful discharge, usually involving a dietician, doctor, ward nurse, community nurse and general practitioner. The patient's circumstances and the ability of the patient or carers to manage the feed must be considered when discharge is being planned. Adequate time should be allowed in the hospital setting for patients to become fully accustomed to the techniques of feed administration and care of the feeding tube, prior to discharge home. Patients should also be given written information to reinforce the education they receive prior to discharge (BAPEN 2003a).

Support in the form of the general practitioner, community nurse and community dietetic services should be established before discharge. A multidisciplinary discharge meeting may be of benefit to both the patient and the professionals involved. Many of the commercial feed companies organize for the patient's feed and equipment to be delivered to their home, after consultation with the local community services (BAPEN 2003b). The hospital or community dietician can arrange this. Early notification of discharge is essential as it usually takes a minimum of 7 days to set this up.

Termination of enteral tube feeding

It is important to ensure that an individual is able to meet their nutritional requirements orally prior to termination of the feed. Enteral tube feeding may be discontinued when oral intake is established (NCCAC 2006). It may be useful to maintain an overnight feed while the patient is establishing oral intake.

Transfusion of blood and blood components

DEFINITION

Blood transfusion is the administration of a blood component- or plasma-derived product to the patient (Gray et al. 2007). Blood is a raw material from which different therapeutic products are made (McClelland 2007).

ANATOMY AND PHYSIOLOGY

ABO and Rh blood groups

In 1901, Landsteiner discovered that human blood groups existed and developed the ABO system which marked the start of safe blood transfusion (Bishop 2008). There are four principal blood groups: A, B, AB and O. Each group relates to the presence or absence of surface antigens on the red blood cells and antibodies in the serum which dictate blood compatibility (Table 7.8).

People with the blood group **AB** have red cells with A and B surface antigens, but they do not have any anti-A or anti-B immunoglobulin M (IgM) antibodies in their serum. Therefore, they are able to receive blood from any group, but can only donate to other people from group AB.

People with group **O** red cells do not have either A or B surface antigens but they do have anti-A and anti-B IgM antibodies in their serum. They are only able to receive blood from group **O**, but can donate to A, B, O and AB groups.

People with group **A** red cells have type A surface antigens, and they have anti-B IgM antibodies in their serum. They are only able to receive blood from groups **A** or **O** and can only donate blood to people from A and AB groups.

People with group **B** red cells have type B surface antigens and they have anti-A IgM antibodies in their serum. They are therefore only able to receive blood from groups **B** or **O** and can only donate blood to people from B and AB groups.

In addition to the ABO system, the Rh blood group was discovered in 1940; again, these are surface antigens and they are another essential system used in transfusion therapy (Mollison et al. 1997). The Rh D antigen is the most immunogenic of the Rh antigens (Porth 2005). Approximately 85% of Caucasians have the D antigen and are therefore Rh positive and 15% lack the D antigen and are Rh negative (Daniels 2013). There has now been identification of several hundreds of red cell transfusion-related antigens, and antibody production can happen after contact with non-self blood antigens, usually due to transfusion or pregnancy (Zwaginga and van Ham 2013).

RELATED THEORY

Blood group incompatibility

The transfusion of ABO incompatible red cells can lead to intravascular haemolysis where the recipient's IgM antibodies

Table 7.8 **Red cell compatibility**

Group	Antigens	IgM antibodies	Compatible donor for	Compatible recipient of
A	A	Anti-B	A	A
			AB	O
B	B	Anti-A	B	B
			AB	O
AB	A and B	None	AB	A
				B
				AB
				O
O	None	Anti-A	A	O
		Anti-B	B	
			AB	
			O	

bind to the corresponding surface antigens of the transfused cells (McClelland 2007). Complement activation results in lysis of the transfused cells and the haemoglobin that is released precipitates renal failure, with the fragments of the lysed cells activating the clotting pathways, which in turn leads to the development of disseminated intravascular coagulation (DIC) (Mollison et al. 1997). Transfusion of Rh D-positive cells to a Rh D-negative individual will result in immunization and the appearance of anti-D antibodies in at least 30% of recipients (Daniels 2013). If the person is immunized then on any subsequent exposure to D antigen-positive red cells, extravascular haemolysis occurs when rhesus antibody-coated red cells are destroyed by macrophages in the liver and spleen (McClelland 2007). This can present as a severe immediate or delayed haemolytic transfusion reaction (Daniels 2013).

A patient's Rh status is of particular importance if they are female and of child-bearing potential requiring a transfusion and during pregnancy. Immunization can happen by two processes: transfusion of D-positive cells into someone who is D negative or in pregnancy when transplacental passage of fetal red cells exposes the mother to D-positive cells. When the mother is Rh D negative and the developing fetus is Rh D positive, the exposure to fetal blood can stimulate anti-D activation in the mother. Anti-D is one of the red cell antibodies which can cross the placenta and cause haemolysis of the fetal blood which results in haemolytic disease of the fetus and newborn (HDFN) (McClelland 2007, Norfolk 2013).

Blood groups in haemopoietic stem cell transplantation

The human leucocyte antigen (HLA) is used to determine compatibility for organ transplantation, including bone marrow and peripheral blood stem cells. However, because ABO blood groups and HLA tissue types are determined genetically, it is not uncommon to find a suitable HLA donor who is ABO and/or Rh incompatible with the recipient. In such circumstances, major transfusion reactions can be avoided by red cell and/or plasma depletion of the donor cells in the laboratory before reinfusion (Mollison et al. 1997). However, collection of peripheral stem cells by apheresis usually results in a product that is already significantly red cell depleted and so further red cell depletion in the laboratory is not necessary (McKenna and Clay 2005).

EVIDENCE-BASED APPROACHES

The transfusion of blood components is a complex multistep process involving personnel from diverse backgrounds with differing levels of knowledge and understanding. Errors made in the process of transfusion present a significant risk to patients.

Although there is little evidence to support the efficacy of set procedures to manage this risk, current professional opinion has been provided by the British Committee for Standards in Haematology (BCSH) in collaboration with the Royal College of Nursing (RCN) and the Royal College of Surgeons of England (RCS) (BCSH 2009, Gray and Illingworth 2005). As a result of this guidance, every hospital should have a policy for the administration of blood and blood components, including identification of the patient, blood sampling, special blood requirement requests, processing of blood samples, the storage, collection and transportation of blood components, administration of blood components and the care and monitoring of the transfused patient. Furthermore, hospitals are also required to manage and report any adverse events or near misses, with a statutory requirement to hold a record of every step of the transfusion process, including the final fate of each blood product, for 30 years (James 2005). Only staff authorized to do so should be involved at any stage in the transfusion process.

Nurses in the UK are normally the healthcare professionals ultimately responsible for the bedside check and arguably have the final opportunity to prevent errors occurring when patients receive blood transfusions (Wilkinson and Wilkinson 2001). Errors in the requesting, collection and administration of blood components (red cells, platelets and plasma concentrates) lead to significant risks for patients. Since its launch in 1996, the Serious Hazards of Transfusion (SHOT) scheme has continually shown that 'wrong blood into patient' episodes are a frequently reported transfusion hazard. These wrong blood incidents are mainly due to human error arising from misidentification of the patient during blood sampling, blood component collection and delivery or administration which can lead to life-threatening haemolytic transfusion reactions and other significant morbidity (BCSH 2009). In the 2013 SHOT report (Bolton-Maggs et al. 2014) the cumulative data submitted since 1996 were analysed to assess likelihood of preventability. It was found that half of all reports are adverse events caused by human error, such as assuming patient identity and not following the correct checking processes. See Figure 7.6.

The National Comparative Audits (NCA) of bedside transfusion practice (2003, 2005, 2009 and 2011) show that patients continue to be placed at risk of avoidable complications of transfusion through misidentification and inadequate monitoring.

Rationale

Blood transfusion is an essential part of modern medicine and potentially a life-saving intervention. However, its use should be appropriate and limited when possible through the following strategies: early diagnosis and treatment of conditions that may eventually require a transfusion, optimal patient management using evidence- based approaches to transfusion and assessing the possibility of alternative treatments such as pharmacological interventions, good surgical and anaesthetic techniques (WHO 2011).

Recent publications and legislation have created greater awareness of the need to continue to improve transfusion practice in many ways. Blood and blood components are no longer regarded as safe unlimited resources. There are risks inherent in transfusion practice and therefore unnecessary exposure to blood components should be avoided. This is of particular importance for patients who may only have one transfusion in their lifetime, such as surgical patients. However, all patients should only receive a transfusion when it is absolutely necessary. Furthermore, the appropriate use of components is essential for the conservation of blood supplies. Regularly updated guidance on the safe appropriate use of blood and blood components is available online at www.transfusionguidelines.org.uk and these should be consulted in collaboration with local hospital and blood transfusion service guidelines.

Indications for red cells

Anaemia is defined as a haemoglobin concentration in blood that is below the expected value, when age, gender, pregnancy and certain environmental factors, such as altitude, are taken into consideration. In general, anaemia is a consequence of one or more of the following generic causes:

- increased loss of red blood cells
- decreased production of red blood cells
- increased destruction of red blood cells
- increased demand for red blood cells
- increased production of abnormal red blood cells

which may be due to nutritional deficits, blood loss, kidney disease, medication or chronic diseases (Fields and Meyers 2006, Moftah 2005). The cause of anaemia should be ascertained and possible effective treatment options explored, such as treatment of iron deficiency before the patient is transfused with red cells (BCSH 2001).

A minimum transfusion trigger has not been well established because of the variability of patient co-morbidities and anaemia tolerance. Evidence suggests that most patients can safely tolerate anaemia of 70 g/L of Hb in the absence of active bleeding (Tolich 2008). A systematic review of the evidence for restrictive

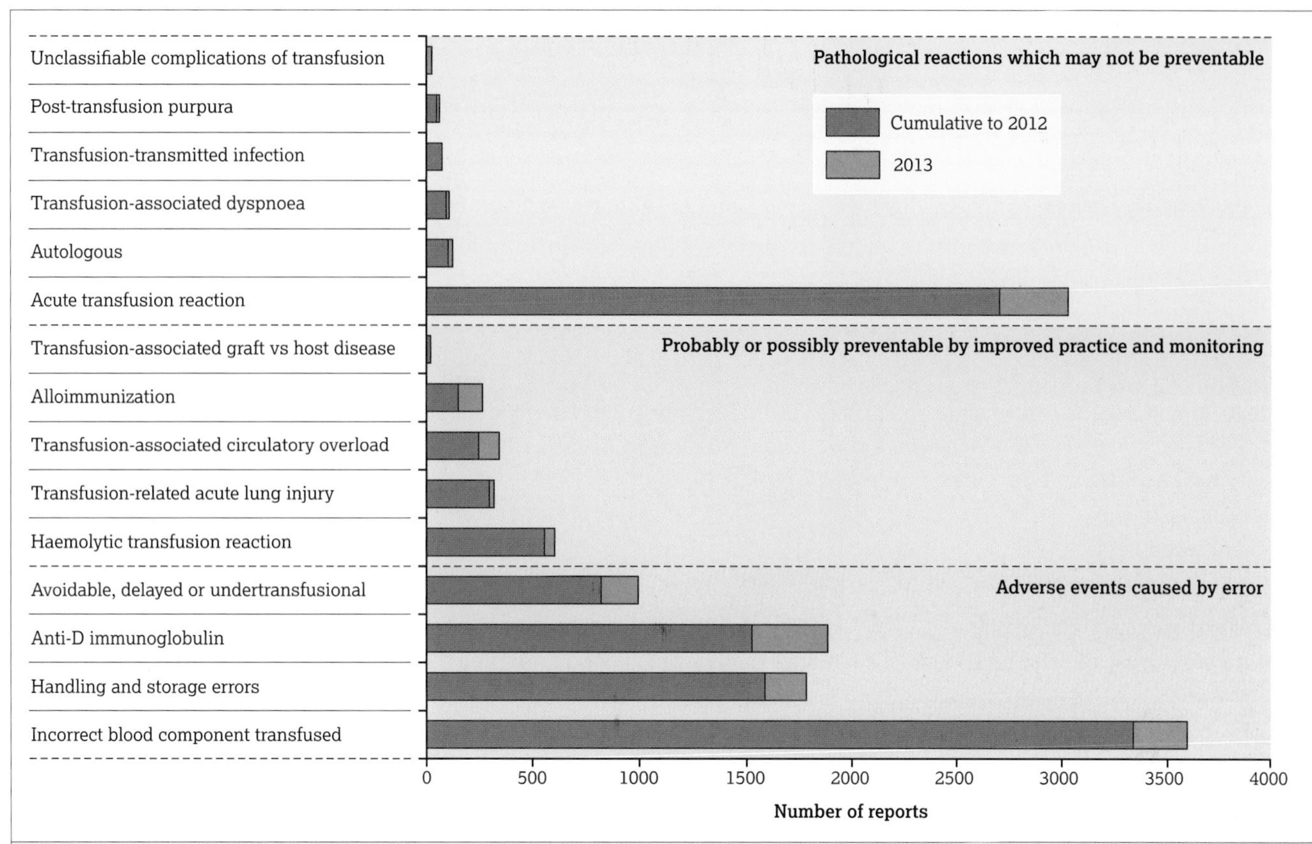

Figure 7.6 **Cumulative data for SHOT categories 1996/7–2013, n=13,141.** ***Source:*** **Adapted from Bolton-Maggs et al. (2014). Reproduced with permission from SHOT (www.shotuk.org).**

red cell transfusions practice concluded that the evidence was in favour of restrictive transfusion triggers in the majority of patients and that a haemoglobin threshold of 70 or 80 g/L lowers the number of red cells units transfused. The review also concluded that restrictive transfusion thresholds had no adverse associations with mortality, cardiac morbidity and length of hospital stay (Carson et al. 2012). However, surveys of the UK population show that most blood recipients are relatively elderly; many will have cardiovascular disease and may be less tolerant of low haemoglobin levels than younger, fitter patients. In this group of patients, consider adopting a higher transfusion trigger of 80 g/L (BCSH 2001). Patients who have cardiovascular disease, renal disease, low albumin concentration or are of low weight (in particular, the elderly and children) may also be more susceptible to congestive cardiac failure due to volume overload when blood and other fluids are infused (McClelland 2007, Norfolk 2013). There were six patient deaths reported to SHOT in 2010 which were attributed to overtransfusion and transfusion-associated cardiac overload (TACO). One of the recommendations from the SHOT report 2010 was that the existing BCSH guidelines for the administration of blood components should be supplemented with advice on how to prevent TACO. This addendum to the guidelines was published in August 2012 and makes several recommendations such as only transfusing single units of red cells when possible, assessment of fluid balance and reducing the amount of blood transfused in low bodyweight patients (BCSH 2012a).

Indications for platelets

Platelet transfusions are indicated in the prevention and treatment of haemorrhage in patients with thrombocytopenia or platelet function defects (BCSH 2003). Thrombocytopenia can be defined as a platelet count below the normal range for the population and this is usually considered to be between 150 and 450 × 10^9/L (Sekhon and Roy 2006). Thrombocytopenia is usually due to either decreased platelet production or increased destruction. Not all thrombocytopenic patients require a platelet transfusion and in some cases it may be contraindicated. Patients who have chronic stable thrombocytopenia due to such conditions as myelodysplasia and aplastic anaemia often do not require a transfusion and do not experience haemorrhage even with platelet counts below 10 × 10^9/L (BCSH 2003). In prophylactic situations there are various thresholds, depending on the reason for the transfusion and presence of risk factors for bleeding; see Table 7.9 for adult thresholds for transfusion and Table 7.10 for paediatric thresholds.

In all cases of prophylactic platelet transfusions, the patient should receive one adult therapeutic dose (one pool or pack) and then be reassessed. Giving double dose platelet transfusions does not decrease the risk of the patient bleeding (Slichter et al. 2010). There should be careful assessment of the need for a platelet transfusion as the effectiveness and the platelet rise following the transfusion will start to reduce as the number of platelet transfusions increases (Slichter et al. 2010), and following the transfusion, the platelet effectiveness should be evaluated by checking the increment. One adult dose of platelets in a 70-kg adult typically gives a rise of 20–40 × 10 ^{9}/L and the sample to check the count can be taken 10 minutes after completion of the transfusion (O'Connell et al. 1988).

Blood donation and testing

All blood donated in the UK is given voluntarily and without remuneration. The successful selection of a donor must protect them from any harm that may be caused by the donation

Table 7.9 Indications for use of platelet transfusions in adults

Indication	Transfusion indicated (threshold provided)/not indicated
Routine prophylactic use	
Reversible bone marrow failure	10×10^9/L
Chronic bone marrow failure, peripheral destruction/consumption, abnormal platelet function	Not indicated
Prophylactic use in the presence of risk factors for bleeding (e.g. sepsis, antibiotic treatment, abnormalities of haemostasis)*	
Reversible/chronic bone marrow failure	20×10^9/L
Peripheral destruction/consumption, abnormal platelet function	Not indicated
Prophylactic use pre-procedure except eyes or brain	
Reversible/chronic bone marrow failure and platelet destruction/consumption if urgent/other therapy failed	
Bone marrow aspirate and trephine	Not indicated
Epidural anaesthesia	80×10^9/L
All other procedures†	50×10^9/L
Abnormal platelet function	
Bone marrow aspirate and trephine	Not indicated
All other procedures in selected patients if alternative therapy failed/contraindicated	Not possible to state threshold
Prophylactic use pre-procedure involving eyes or brain	
Reversible/chronic bone marrow failure and platelet destruction/consumption if urgent/other therapy failed	100×10^9/L
Abnormal platelet function in selected patients if alternative therapy failed/contraindicated	Not possible to state threshold
Therapeutic use	
Massive transfusion, all patient indication categories except platelet function defects where not possible to state threshold‡	75×10^9/L
For patients with multiple trauma or central nervous system injury	100×10^9/L

Source: NCA Platelet Working Group (2012). Reproduced with permission from National Comparative Audit Platelet Working Group at NHS Blood and Transplant (http://hospital.blood.co.uk/safe_use/platelet_education_resources).
*BCSH guidelines for multiple myeloma recommend a threshold count of 30 with bortezomib treatment.
BCSH guidelines for aplastic anaemia recommend a threshold count of 30 during treatment with anti-thymocyte globulinand a threshold count of 20 if pregnant or fever.
†American Society for Hematology immune throbocytopeniaguidelines recommend a threshold count of 80 for major surgery.
‡Thrombotic thrombocytopenic purpura and heparin-induced throbocytopenia platelet transfusion contraindicated unless life-threatening haemorrhage.

Table 7.10 Differences/additions to indications in Table 7.9 for neonates and older children

Indication	Transfusion indicated (threshold provided)/not indicated
Routine prophylaxis in neonates	
Stable preterm or term infant	20×10^9/L
Sick preterm or term infant	30×10^9/L
Small preterm infant	Higher threshold, not specified
Neonatal alloimmune thrombocytopenia	30×10^9/L
Prophylactic use for children in the presence of risk factors	
Additional risk factors include severe mucositis, local tumour infiltration, platelet count likely to fall to $<10 \times 10^9$/L before next evaluation, anticoagulation therapy	20×10^9/L
Severe hyperleucocytosis or DIC with induction therapy for leukaemia	40×10^9/L
DIC	20×10^9/L
Prophylactic pre-procedure	
ECMO	100×10^9/L
Lumbar puncture or indwelling line insertion in children	40×10^9/L

Source: NCA Platelet Working Group (2012). Reproduced with permission from National Comparative Audit Platelet Working Group at NHS Blood and Transplant (http://hospital.blood.co.uk/safe_use/platelet_education_resources).
DIC, disseminated intravascular coagulation; ECMO, extracorporeal membrane oxygenation.

process and also protect the possible recipient of components derived from the donor's blood. Donors of blood for therapeutic use should be in good health; if there is any doubt about their suitability, the donation should be deferred and they should be fully assessed by a designated medical officer. All donors of blood or its components (via apheresis) should be assessed in accordance with the Joint UKBTS/NIBSC Professional Advisory Committee (JPAC) donor selection guidelines (JPAC 2013). The assessment of fitness to donate includes a questionnaire relating to general health, lifestyle, past medical history and medication. Donation may be temporarily or permanently deferred for a variety of reasons including cardiovascular disease, central nervous system diseases, malignancy and some infectious diseases, all of which are detailed in the JPAC (2013) guidelines. Donors are also screened for risk of exposure to transmissible infectious diseases, and specific guidance is provided for donors receiving therapeutic drugs.

Prevention of transmission of infection is determined by donor selection criteria and laboratory testing. In the UK, all blood donations are tested for infections which could be passed on to the recipient. However, concern about transfusion-related variant Creutzfeldt–Jakob disease (vCJD) transmission is now supported by clinical evidence (Ludlam and Turner 2006) and in 2011 a prototype blood test for diagnosis of vCJD in symptomatic individuals was developed by the Medical Research Council (MRC) Prion Unit. It is hoped that this will lead to the development of a screening test for asymptomatic vCJD prion infection (Edgeworth et al. 2011). At present, donor exclusion criteria remain an important precautionary measure for all infection including vCJD (Cervenakova and Brown 2004). Since April 2004 all individuals who have received a blood component since January 1980 are excluded from donating blood due to the risk of transmitting vCJD (DH 2013). When a donor has been successfully screened, they must validate the information they have provided and record that they have given consent to proceed.

Cell salvage and autologous transfusion

Since the 1980s there has been interest in autologous transfusion (blood and blood components collected from an individual and intended solely for subsequent autologous transfusion to that same individual) (Blood Safety and Quality Regulations 2005). This has largely been attributed to high-profile infection risks: human immunodeficiency virus (HIV), hepatitis C and more recently vCJD (James and Harrison 2002). However, autologous transfusion is not risk free, with 42 cases of adverse events being reported to SHOT in 2011, all related to intraoperative and post-operative cell salvage (SHOT 2011a). Autologous transfusion is contraindicated in certain circumstances. Furthermore, there has been significant concern about the efficacy of some methods (Carless et al. 2004, Henry et al. 2002). Three principal methods of autologous transfusion exist.

PRE-OPERATIVE AUTOLOGOUS DONATION (PAD)

This technique is rarely undertaken and not currently recommended unless the clinical circumstances are exceptional, such as the patient has a rare blood group and allogeneic blood would be difficult to obtain (BCSH 2007). This requires the patients to donate up to four units of blood whilst simultaneously taking iron supplements in the month preceding surgery. However, the efficacy of this method has been questioned by systematic review (Henry et al. 2002) and it is only indicated in very specific circumstances such as patients with very rare blood types, patients donating bone marrow and fit patients who have a significant fear of receiving allogeneic blood products such that it is preventing them from seeking necessary surgery (James 2004). This technique can only be carried out in organizations licensed as blood establishments by the Medicines and Healthcare Products Regulatory Agency (MHRA).

ACUTE NORMOVOLAEMIC HAEMODILUTION (ANH)

This technique is not currently encouraged and the effectiveness of the procedure is unproven (McClelland 2007). It involves the donation of up to three units of blood immediately prior to surgery. The patient is then given crystalloids to dilute the circulating volume. This method is only indicated for surgery where considerable blood loss is expected on the principle that the number of red cells lost will be reduced and the patient's autologous whole blood can be returned after surgery.

INTRAOPERATIVE CELL SALVAGE (ICS)

Blood loss during surgery is collected, anticoagulated, filtered and held in a sterile reservoir. The collected blood is then processed, washed and suspended in 0.9% sodium chloride for return. Although ICS is not without risks, such as embolism, bacterial contamination and enhanced inflammatory responses through reinfusion of inflammatory mediators (Harrison 2004), it has been recommended as the most effective form of autologous transfusion to assist in the conservation of blood supplies (James 2004). Cell salvage has been shown to be effective in reducing the requirement for perioperative allogeneic blood transfusion in orthopaedic, cardiac and vascular surgery (Carless et al. 2010). The effectiveness of intraoperative cell salvage to minimize a patient's exposure to allogeneic blood is dependent on the amount of blood lost during surgery. However, if this blood can be retrieved and reinfused, thus preventing a transfusion, then it has been shown to be an effective strategy which should be widely available (Thompson 2005).

POST-OPERATIVE CELL SALVAGE

Where there is a predictable blood loss following elective surgery, the blood is collected in the wound drain and then reinfused to the patient through special equipment. The blood can be passed through a filter incorporated into the cell salvage post-operative equipment or washed before returning to the patient and this has become almost routine for some surgical practice (Hamer 2005a, McClelland 2007). The main surgical area of use is orthopaedic surgery, in particular replacement knee surgery, and is safe and clinically beneficial (Hamer, 2005b).

Several cases have been reported to SHOT (2011a) where the autologous blood had not been labelled with the correct patient identification and in some cases this had not been noted by staff in the clinical area prior to reinfusion (SHOT 2011a). SHOT highlighted that it is still critical to maintain correct patient identification in autologous transfusion. In 2006 a UK cell salvage group was founded to support the implementation of cell salvage; more information and advice can be found on the Better Blood Transfusion Appropriate Use of Blood Toolkit at www.transfusionguidelines.org.uk.

Blood component donation

Donors of blood components by automated apheresis are subject to the same selection criteria used for donating whole blood and any exception to this must be decided by a designated medical officer. Apheresis can be used to collect plasma, red cells and platelets. Leucopheresis procedures are used for the collection of granulocytes, lymphocytes and peripheral blood progenitor cells (James 2005). Over 80% of the platelets issued in the UK are now from single donor, apheresis collection as part of a Department of Health requirement to reduce the risk of vCJD transmission (NHSBT 2011, SaBTO 2009).

Appropriate use of donated blood components

Donated blood components are a precious gift; they are not a limitless resource and must be used appropriately. The BCSH has guidelines in place for the use of red cell, platelet, fresh frozen plasma (FFP), cryoprecipitate and cryosupernatant transfusions, available on the BCSH website: www.bcshguidelines.com.

The decision to transfuse must be based on a thorough clinical assessment of the patient and their individual needs. Each blood component should only be given after careful consideration, when there is valid clinical indication or when there are no alternative treatment options available (Oldham et al. 2009).

Blood and blood components have varying shelf-lives and storage requirements. The range of components currently available, indications for use and recommendations for administration are listed in Table 7.11. Clinical indications for use are also provided by the BCSH (BCSH 2012b, Murphy et al. 2001, O'Shaughnessy et al. 2004).

Anticipated patient outcomes

Blood component transfusion can be a life-saving and life-enhancing treatment when used appropriately and when patients are cared for safely and by knowledgeable, skilled practitioners (Oldham et al. 2009).

LEGAL AND PROFESSIONAL ISSUES

Blood safety and quality in the UK

Approximately 3.4 million blood products are administered in the UK every year (SHOT 2011a). The transfusion of blood and its components is usually safe and uneventful; however, there are associated risks and there have been significant developments over recent years to improve the quality and safety of transfusion practice in the UK. The Blood Safety and Quality Regulations came into effect in February 2005 and were fully implemented on 8 November 2005. These Regulations cover the collecting, testing, processing, storing and distributing of blood and blood components (Blood Safety and Quality Regulations 2005). The official government agency with jurisdiction for these regulations is the MHRA.

The principal requirements of these Regulations in relation to transfusion practice are as follows.

- *Traceability*: there must be a full audit trail from the donor to the recipient so hospitals must have a system to record and retain information on the fate of each unit of blood/blood component for a period of 30 years.
- *Haemovigilance*: an organized surveillance procedure relating to serious adverse or unexpected events or reactions. The reporting of such events can be done via the online Serious Adverse Blood Reactions and Events (SABRE) system which is maintained by the MHRA. This will usually be done by a designated member of laboratory staff or transfusion practitioner and therefore clinical staff must ensure that all incident reporting is conducted in line with hospital policy.

The Blood Safety and Quality Regulations (2005) defines such events as follows.

- A **serious adverse event** is defined as an unintended occurrence associated with the collection, testing, processing, storage and distribution of blood or blood components that might lead to death or life-threatening, disabling or incapacitating conditions for patients or which results in, or prolongs, hospitalization or morbidity.
- A **serious adverse reaction** is defined as an unintended response in a donor or in a patient associated with the collection or transfusion of blood components that is fatal, life-threatening, disabling or incapacitating, or which results in or prolongs hospitalization or morbidity (Blood Safety and Quality Regulations 2005).

Prior to these regulations, Better Blood Transfusion initiatives aimed to ensure that such guidance became an integral part of NHS care, making blood transfusion safer, ensuring that all blood used in clinical practice is necessary and improving the information both patients and the public receive about blood transfusion (DH 2007). Therefore it is a key requirement that all staff involved in the process of transfusion maintain their awareness of all appropriate guidance.

Competencies

The transfusion of any blood component carries with it the potential for reaction and risk (SHOT 2005). All staff involved in the transfusion of blood and/or blood components must have the knowledge and skills to ensure the process is completed safely. Therefore, the nurse caring for those receiving transfusion therapy must do so within his or her sphere of competence, always acting to minimize risk to the patient (NMC 2015).

Practitioners must understand the theory and reasoning behind the necessity to follow the correct transfusion procedures and practices (Pirie and Gray 2007). In November 2006, the NPSA, the Chief Medical Officer's National Blood Transfusion Committee (NBTC) and SHOT, working in collaboration, developed strategies aimed at ensuring that blood transfusions are carried out safely, and issued the Safer Practice Notice (SPN) No. 14, *Right Patient, Right Blood*. One of the key action points in this Notice was for all NHS and independent sector organizations involved in administering blood transfusions to develop and implement an action plan for competency-based training and assessments for all staff involved in blood transfusions. In 2009, BCSH recommended that blood components must only be administered by a registered healthcare professional who has been trained and competency assessed to NPSA SPN 14 standard and that all staff involved in transfusion in the clinical area must have a minimum of a 2 yearly training (BCSH 2009).

There are three key principles which underpin every stage of the blood component transfusion process:

- patient identification
- documentation
- communication (BCSH 2009).

Consent

In 2010 the Advisory Committee on the Safety of Blood, Tissues and Organs (SaBTO) undertook a public consultation on consent for blood transfusion. A total of 14 recommendations were published following the consultation (SaBTO 2011). They recommended that a valid consent for transfusion should be obtained and documented in the patient's record by the healthcare professional. SaBTO has also recommended that those patients who could not be consented before the transfusion should receive information retrospectively. The Good Practice Guidance (SaBTO 2011) outlines that retrospective information can be given at any point during the hospital stay but recommends that it is incorporated in the discharge procedure. The retrospective information should include the risk of a transfusion-transmitted infection and inform the patient that, as they have received a blood component, they can no longer donate blood (SaBTO 2011).

Providing the patient with information before a procedure and ascertaining that the patient understands the procedure and has consented to it is the responsibility of the healthcare professional carrying out the procedure as well as those prescribing it (NMC 2013). A blood component transfusion must be treated as any prescribed medicine; that is, patients (or guardian) must be informed of the indication for the transfusion, advised of the risks and benefits, of alternatives to blood transfusion including autologous transfusion (BCSH 2009), be given the opportunity to ask questions and have the right to refuse to receive it in accordance with local and national guidance (NMC 2013). One of the key objectives of the HSC 2007/001 Better Blood Transfusion was to improve information provided to patients and to ensure that those who are likely to receive a blood transfusion will be well informed of their choices. There are a number of information leaflets issued by the NHS Blood and Transplant Service for both patients and healthcare professionals. Guidance is also available from SaBTO (2011) to ensure that patients have standardized information prior to a transfusion and outlines all the key information that should be provided.

Patients have the right to refuse transfusion and to be treated with respect. Staff must be sensitive to individual patient needs,

Table 7.11 **Blood, blood components and blood products used for transfusion**

Type	Description	Indications	Cross-matching	Shelf-life	Average infusion time	Technique	Special considerations
Red cells in optimal additive solutions (SAGM)*	Red cells with plasma removed: 100 mL additive fluid used as replacement to give optimal red cell preservation; haematocrit 60–65% leuco-depleted	Correction of anaemia	ABO and Rh compatible (not necessarily identical)	35 days at 2–6°C	1–2 hours/unit Transfusion to be completed within 4 hours of component's removal from storage	Give via a blood administration set	If more than half blood volume is replaced with red cells in SAGM, use of FFP should be considered to replace clotting factors
Washed red blood cells	Red cells centrifuged and resuspended twice in 0.9% sodium chloride Leuco-depleted	Correction of anaemia where patient may react to plasma components, for example in IgA deficiency	As above	Prepared by non-sterile process, used within 24 hours Closed system preparation, used within 72 hours	1–2 hours/unit	As above	–
Frozen red blood cells	Red cells of very rare phenotype Leuco-depleted	To treat patients with very rare antibody	As above	Stored frozen cells: up to 10 years Use within 12 hours of thawing	2–3 hours/unit	As above	–
White blood cells (buffy coat or apheresed granulocytes)†	Mainly granulocytes obtained by leucophoresis or by 'creaming off' the white blood cell layer from fresh blood	To treat patients with life-threatening granulocytopenia	As above	24 hours after preparation Stored at room temperature	60–90 minutes/unit	Administer via a blood administration set	White blood cell infusion induces fever, may cause hypotension, rigors and confusion Treat symptoms and reassure patient
							White cell component is always irradiated to prevent initiation of transfusion-associated graft-versus-host disease (TA-GVHD)
							Do not give to patients receiving amphotericin B. Indications for granulocyte transfusions should be when possible benefits are thought to outweigh considerable hazards of the treatment option

(continued)

Table 7.11 **Blood, blood components and blood products used for transfusion** ***(continued)***

Type	Description	Indications	Cross-matching	Shelf-life	Average infusion time	Technique	Special considerations
Platelets*	Platelets in 200–300 mL plasma May be pooled from 5 donors or apheresed from a single donor Leuco-depleted	To treat thrombocytopenia either for prophylaxis to prevent bleeding or therapeutically to treat bleeding	No cross-matching necessary	Up to 7 days after collection Storage is at 22°C, with continuous gentle agitation	20–30 minutes/unit	Administration using a platelet or blood component administration set Use a new set for each transfusion Do not use micro-aggregate filters	General guide to use: use in chronic bone marrow failure for routine prophylaxis is not indicated Platelets are not clinically indicated for a bone marrow aspirate and trephine regardless of the cause of thrombocytopenia. See Tables 7.9 and 7.10
Fresh frozen plasma	Citrated plasma separated from whole blood	To treat multi-factor deficiencies associated with severe bleeding and/or DIC FFP is not indicated in DIC without bleeding or for the immediate reversal of warfarin	No cross-matching necessary	3 years at <–25°C Once thawed, kept at 4°C, to be used as soon as possible but within 24 hours	15–45 minutes/unit (approx. 250 mL), more rapid infusion may be indicated in major haemorrhage	Administer rapidly via a blood administration set	FFP should be considered if patient has received more than half their blood volume in red cells, to prevent dilutional hypocoagulability The dose given is based on the patient's weight
Albumin 4.5% (HAS)	Solution of albumin from pooled plasma in a buffered, stabilized 0.9% sodium chloride diluent Supplied in 250 mL or 500 mL bottle	To treat hypovolaemic shock or hypoproteinaemia due to burns, trauma, surgery or infection Sourced outside UK to reduce risk of transmission of vCJD	Unnecessary Not blood group specific	5 years at room temperature Kept in dark	30–60 minutes/unit	Administer via a standard solution administration set	The solution should be crystal clear with no deposits
Albumin 20% (HAS)	Heat-treated, aqueous, chemically processed fraction of pooled plasma	To treat hypovolaemic shock or hypoproteinaemia due to burns, trauma, surgery or infection To maintain appropriate electrolyte balance	Unnecessary	5 years at room temperature Kept in dark	30–60 minutes/unit	Administer via a blood administration set undiluted or diluted with 0.9% sodium chloride or 5% glucose solution Slower administration is advised if a cardiac disorder is present to avoid gross fluid shift	The solution should be crystal clear with no deposits

Type	Description	Indications	Cross-matching	Shelf-life	Average infusion time	Technique	Special considerations
Cryoprecipitate	Cold-insoluble portion of plasma recovered from FFP: rich in factor VIII, von Willebrand's factor and fibrinogen	Hypofibrinogenaemia, in acute DIC with bleeding and surgery prophylaxis with fibrinogen <1.5 g/L Sever liver disease with bleeding and in cases of massive transfusion.	No cross-matching necessary	3 years at <–25°C Use immediately after thawing	Available as single donor units or as pooled units (5 single donor units), typical adult dose is two pooled packs, administered at 10–20 ml/kg/hr, 30–60 minutes as a pooled unit	Administer via blood administration set	
Solvent detergent treated FFP (SD-FFP) Licensed medicinal product Octaplas®	FFP prepared from pools of donations and the solvent detergent process inactivates bacteria and most encapsulated viruses.	Guidelines recommend use in treating thrombotic thrombocytopenic purpura: patients are plasma-exchanged daily to reduce circulating von Willebrand's factor	No cross-matching necessary	4 years at <–18°C Once thawed transfuse	Time depends on machine; average ±2.5 hours	Via apheresis machine	

DIC, disseminated intravascular coagulation; FFP, fresh frozen plasma; HAS, human albumin solution; INR, international normalized ratio; SAGM, saline, adenine, glucose and mannitol; vCJD, variant Creutzfeldt–Jakob disease.

*Most commonly used blood components.

†See leucocyte depletion.

acknowledging their values, beliefs and cultural background and exploring alternative treatments if appropriate and available (Oldham et al. 2009). There is increasing public concern about blood transfusion safety and the need to accommodate some patients' religious beliefs (John et al. 2008).

Jehovah's Witnesses and other patients who may refuse a blood transfusion

The principles in caring for the patient remain the same regardless of the reason for refusal and there should be a local policy in place to expedite non-blood management for these patients.

The role of blood in Jehovah's Witnesses' spiritual belief is based on scripture and followers are usually well informed on both their beliefs and their rights. Many Jehovah's Witnesses carry information with them regarding any objection and therefore the need to ensure informed consent is very important. Their religious position leads them to refuse red cells, white cells, plasma and platelets. Derivatives of these are seen as a matter of individual patient choice. Staff caring for patients must ensure that they have clearly documented what the patient will accept or refuse and that decisions to consent to or refuse treatment are respected and recorded appropriately (McClelland 2007). Furthermore, in individual circumstances, practitioners should endeavour to consider non-blood or autologous methods as described previously, where appropriate (McClelland 2007). Jehovah's Witness patients usually carry an Advance Directive listing which blood products and autologous procedures are acceptable or not acceptable to them (McClelland 2007, Norfolk 2013). The Jehovah's Witness community has a network of support called the Hospital Liaison Committees (HLCs) and they are available at any time, night and day, to assist with communication between hospital teams and the patient.

Management of massive blood loss

Massive blood loss is defined as a 50% blood volume loss within 3 hours or a rate loss of 150 mL/min (Frakry and Sheldon 1994). Good patient outcomes are dependent on clinical staff recognizing the blood loss early, taking effective action and ensuring efficient communication between the clinical area and the transfusion laboratory (NPSA 2010). To aid the provision of blood in an emergency situation, the majority of hospitals will have an agreed major haemorrhage protocol where all processes required in the provision of emergency blood are clearly stated. This includes how to activate the protocol, what blood component availability will be and how the blood components will be transferred from the laboratory to the clinical area.

In emergency situations, where the need for blood is immediate and the patient's blood group is unknown, it may be necessary to transfuse group O uncross-matched red cells (BCSH 2006). In major haemorrhage situations there is still a need to use group O Rh D-negative blood judiciously as it is a scarce resource. At the earliest opportunity, a sample should be taken from the patient so that blood group determination can take place. Once the laboratory receives the sample, it usually takes no longer than 10 minutes to determine the blood group and then issue group-specific blood (BCSH 2006).

PRE-PROCEDURAL CONSIDERATIONS

Equipment

Intravenous access

Blood components may be administered through a peripheral cannula or via a central venous access device. Where possible, one lumen should be reserved for the taking of blood specimens and blood component administration for the duration of therapy.

Administration sets

All blood components must be transfused through a sterile blood component administration set with an integral mesh filter (170–200 micron). Blood administration sets should be changed at least every 12 hours or after every second unit for a continuing transfusion (Loveday et al. 2014); see local guidance. Administration sets used for blood components must be changed immediately upon suspected contamination or when the integrity of the product or system has been compromised. Platelets and plasma components may be administered through a normal blood administration set or through a platelet set. Platelets should never be administered through an administration set that has previously been used for red cell transfusion or other blood component as this may cause aggregation of platelets in the administration set (McClelland 2007). Administration sets used for blood components must be changed using aseptic technique and observing universal precautions, in line with manufacturer's instructions (RCN 2010).

Infusion devices

Either gravity or electronic infusion devices may be used for the administration of blood components. There are a variety of electronic infusion devices available and it is therefore essential that individuals using any type of infusion device are competent in their use. Only blood component administration sets compatible with the infusion device should be used. Rapid infusion devices that are CE marked may be used when large volumes have to be infused rapidly. Typically, devices can infuse from 6 to 30 L an hour and usually incorporate a blood-warming device (BCSH 2009, McClelland 2007).

Blood-warming devices

The warming of blood and blood components is generally not recommended as it is of limited benefit and can be dangerous. Blood warmers are only indicated when:

- massive, rapid transfusion could result in cooling of cardiac tissue, causing potentially fatal dysrhythmia (McClelland 2007). If the rate of transfusion is greater than 100 mL per minute, blood-warming devices should be used (McClelland 2007)
- transfusion is required by patients with cold agglutination disease (Gray and Illingworth 2005)
- exchange transfusion is indicated in the newborn (Weinstein and Plumer 2007)
- thawing of cryopreserved stem cells prior to transfusion (blood or marrow).

Both water baths and dry heat blood warmers are available. However, whichever device is chosen, the temperature should be maintained below 38°C. Warming in excess of this can cause haemolysis of red cells and can denature proteins and increase the risk of bacterial infection. Blood warmers must always be used and maintained according to the manufacturer's guidelines. Blood components must *never* be warmed by improvisation, such as putting the pack into hot water, in a microwave or on a radiator, as uncontrolled heating can damage the contents of the pack (Gray and Illingworth 2005, McClelland 2007, Norfolk 2013). The use of water baths also increases the risk of bacterial contamination. Therefore certain safety measures must be adhered to.

- Water baths must be drained after each use and must be stored dry and empty.
- The blood warmer should be drained after each use and must be stored dry and empty.
- When needed, they should be refilled with sterile water.
- A protective sterile over-bag to thaw blood and blood products reduces the entry of contaminants through microscopic punctures or breaks in the seal.
- The product should be used immediately after it has been thawed.

All devices should be serviced as per hospital health and safety policies, MHRA and manufacturers' guidelines.

Specific patient preparations

In 2007 the NPSA issued a Safer Practice Notice No. 24, *Standardising Wristbands Improves Patient Safety*, stating that only the following core identifiers should be used on patients' identification bands:

- last name
- first name
- date of birth
- NHS number.

Patients should have their identification confirmed on admission to the unit and one wristband attached to their wrist. If a wristband is removed for any reason, for example to gain intravenous access via a cannula, it is the responsibility of the person removing it to ensure that a correctly completed wristband is then reapplied.

ELECTRONIC SYSTEMS FOR PATIENT IDENTIFICATION AND TRANSFUSION

Wristbands can now hold patient information in an electronic format such as in a bar code or a radiofrequency identification tag (RFID). Electronic systems offer improved security and patient safety (BCSH 2009, Murphy et al. 2009) by removing the elements of human error from the process. At the point of taking a sample for pre-transfusion testing, the patient is identified through the usual process of stating name and date of birth but there is the added safety of scanning the bar code or RFID tag on the wristband.

The electronic systems can be used during collection and administration. During administration, the blood component and the wristband are scanned to confirm that it is the right component for the right patient. The Safer Practice Notice No. 14, *Right Patient, Right Blood*, recommended that all NHS trusts and independent sector organizations responsible for administering blood should risk assess their transfusion procedures and look at the feasibility of using bar codes and other electronic identification and tracking systems for patients, samples and blood components.

The nurse must ensure that the patient has been informed of the proposed transfusion and has had an opportunity to raise any concerns, understands the risks and benefits of the transfusion and has agreed to and is available for the transfusion. Pre-transfusion/baseline observations including blood pressure, temperature, pulse and respiratory rate must be undertaken and documented; also ensure that there is patent venous access prior to administering the transfusion (BCSH 2009).

Pre-transfusion/bedside check

While professional accountability must be taken at every stage by the personnel involved, the final barrier to wrong blood administration is at the bedside. The final link is ensuring the right patient receives the right blood and it is therefore essential that the check is performed thoroughly prior to the transfusion of each component (Oldham et al. 2009).

To ensure that each blood component is used to its full advantage, local hospital policy should be followed with regard to correct handling and storage, transportation and administration of blood components. If unused, the component should be returned to the transfusion laboratory as quickly as possible to maximize the opportunity for it to be used for another patient.

The written order for the blood component must be checked to ensure that it is correctly completed and to ensure that it contains the following information.

- Patient core identifiers.
- Date (and time if appropriate) the blood component is required.
- Type of blood component to be administered.
- Any clinical special transfusion requirements, for example irradiated or administration via a blood warmer.
- Volume or number of units to be transfused (exact number in mL for paediatric transfusions).
- Time over which each unit is to be transfused (exact rate or length of time over which the specified volume is to be transfused for paediatric transfusions).
- Any special instructions, for example concomitant drugs required, such as diuretics.
- Signature of the 'prescriber' (BCSH 2009).

Procedure guideline 7.12 **Blood components: collection and delivery to the clinical area**

Removal of blood components from their storage location continues to be identified as a major source of error in the transfusion process (BCSH 2009). Only those staff who are authorized, trained and competent may remove blood components from storage. A guide to the necessary elements of blood pack labelling is shown in Figure 7.7.

Essential equipment

- Documentation containing the patient's three core identifiers – full name, date of birth and hospital number/unique identifying number – must be held by the person removing the component from storage

Pre-procedure

Action	Rationale
1 Check that the reason for the transfusion has been documented in the patient's notes.	To ensure the transfusion is appropriate and necessary (BCSH 2009, **C**).
2 Check that there is a valid written order for the administration of the component including special requirements – CMV negative or irradiated components.	To ensure the selected component meets the patient's individual requirements (BCSH 2009, **C**).
3 Check the patient is aware of and has 'consented' to the procedure.	To ensure the patient is fully informed (BCSH 2009, **C**).
4 Check the patient is available.	To avoid delays once the component has been removed from storage. **E**
5 Take baseline observations to include blood pressure, temperature, pulse and respiratory rate.	To ensure that any transfusion reaction can be immediately identified, due to changes in baseline (BCSH 2009, **C**), and managed appropriately (SNBTS 2004, **C**).

(continued)

Procedure guideline 7.12 Blood components: collection and delivery to the clinical area *(continued)*

Action	Rationale
6 Check the patient has patent venous access. If not then ensure appropriate device is inserted.	To avoid any delay in commencement of the transfusion and adhere to 'cold chain' requirements (BCSH 2009, **C**).
7 Check the patient is wearing an identification wristband.	To avoid delays in confirming patient identity (BCSH 2009, **C**).
Procedure	
8 Where possible, the same person who will administer the component should collect it from storage.	To minimize the number of people involved in the process (BCSH 2009, **C**).
9 Remove the component (using electronic or manual method) from storage in accordance with trust policy.	To ensure that only authorized, trained and competent staff may collect blood components (BCSH 2009, **C**).
10 Remove one component at a time, unless rapid transportation of large quantities is needed or if blood is being transported to remote areas in specifically designed validated blood transport containers. If large quantities are required this must be discussed with the transfusion laboratory and local procedures followed.	To ensure components are stored in the appropriate conditions. **E**
11 Check the component at the point of removal for correct patient-identifying details. A visual inspection of the component should also be performed to check the expiry date and any signs of leakage, clumping or discoloration.	In order to minimize the risk of incorrectly administering the component to the wrong patient (BCSH 2009, **C**). Expired or damaged products must not be used (McClelland 2007, **E**).
12 Deliver the component to the clinical area where an appropriately trained and competent member of staff should check that the correct blood has been delivered.	To ensure the correct component has been received for the patient, to comply with traceability and cold chain requirements (BCSH 2009, **C**).

Procedure guideline 7.13 Blood component administration

Essential equipment

- Written order for blood component transfusion
- Blood administration set with 170–200 μm macroaggregate filter

Pre-procedure

Action	Rationale
1 Check that the component has been correctly 'prescribed', including any special requirements such as irradiated or CMV-negative blood, and if the patient requires any other medications, for example diuretic, premedication.	To prevent incorrect blood component transfused (IBCT) error: ABO incompatibility or non-irradiated CMV-positive products may cause a fatal reaction if transfused (McClelland 2007, **E**). Negative and positive status should always be written in full and not as + or – as they may get defaced and be incorrectly processed. **E**
2 Check that the patient's baseline vital signs, temperature, pulse, blood pressure and respirations have been recorded.	To ensure that any transfusion reaction can be immediately identified, due to changes in baseline (**E**), and managed appropriately (SNBTS 2004, **C**).
3 Conduct a visual inspection of the component to be used for signs of clumping, discoloration, damage or leaks.	Expired or damaged products must not be used (McClelland 2007, **E**).
4 If there are any discrepancies at this point do not proceed until they have been resolved.	To ensure an IBCT event does not occur. **E**
5 Positively identify the patient by asking them to state the following information. a First name b Surname c Date of birth If the patient is unable to positively identify themselves then verification can be given by a carer or relative. This information must match the wristband exactly.	This is the final check of identity which must be performed next to the patient prior to transfusion and is absolutely vital in minimizing the risk of IBCT errors (BCSH 2009, **C**; SNBTS 2004, **C**).
6 Check the details given against the patient's nameband and the patient details on the blood component.	To minimize the risk of error (SNBTS 2004, **C**).

7 Check that the information on the compatibility label matches the details on the blood component, checking expiry date, unique component donation number, blood group on the component label against the laboratory-produced label. Check special requirements have been met. If there are any interruptions during this checking procedure, the entire process should be restarted from the beginning.	To minimize the risk of error (BCSH 2009, **C**; SNBTS 2004, **C**).
8 If there are any discrepancies at this point do not proceed until they have been resolved.	To ensure an IBCT event does not occur (SHOT 2008, **C**).
Procedure	
9 Prime the set with blood/blood components unless there are concerns about patency of the device, then prime with 0.9% sodium chloride.	Other agents may damage the product components and precipitate transfusion complications (SNBTS 2004, **C**); for example, dextrose should never be used to prime a set or flush the blood administration set following a transfusion as this can cause haemolysis (SNBTS 2004, **C**).
10 Set up infusion via a volumetric infusion pump if appropriate. Check the infusion pump and settings prior to use.	To ensure the pump is in working order (BCSH 2009, **C**). Some older infusion pumps can damage the red cells. Blood administration sets for specific infusion pumps must always be used. If none are available, the standard blood administration set should be used via gravity and the rate monitored as necessary. **E**
11 Set the desired infusion rate as indicated by the blood component being used and the patient's condition. *Either:* *Red cell administration* can range from 5–10 minutes in acute blood loss to the maximum time of 4 hours (from the time the component is removed from storage) in elderly patients (SNBTS 2004). *Or:* *Platelets, fresh frozen plasma and cryoprecipitate* should be transfused over 30–60 minutes and must be completed within 4 hours of puncturing the blood component.	The rate of administration is indicated by the patient's clinical condition (SNBTS 2004, **C**; Weinstein and Plumer 2007, **E**) and/or dictated by current guidelines (SNBTS 2004, **C**).
12 Sign the written order 'prescription' as the person administering the component. The unique component donation number, the date and start time should be recorded in the patient's clinical notes.	To ensure that documentation and traceability requirements are met (BCSH 2009, **C**).
13 Fifteen minutes after the commencement of each component, take and record patient observations – blood pressure, temperature, pulse and respiratory rate. Follow local hospital policy regarding how observations are documented but they should be easily identifiable as being related to the transfusion.	Adverse reactions will often occur during the first 15 minutes of transfusion (Gray and Illingworth 2005, **C**). Complaints of serious anxiety, transfusion site pain, loin pain, backache, fever, skin flushing or urticaria could be indicative of a serious transfusion reaction (McClelland 2007, **E**). In such cases the transfusion should be stopped immediately and urgent medical advice sought (SNBTS 2004, **C**).
14 Observe and monitor the patient throughout the transfusion episode. If there are any concerns, undertake additional observations as appropriate.	To monitor for any adverse reactions (McClelland 2007, **E**).
15 Record the finish time of each unit. All units must be completed within 4 hours of removal from storage.	Continuation of a transfusion beyond 4 hours increases the risk of transfusion reaction and complications (BCSH 2009, **C**).
16 Take and record the patient's observations on completion of each unit, ensuring that post-transfusion observations are performed within 60 minutes of completion of the unit.	To ensure the patient's progress is recorded and acts as a baseline for subsequent units (BCSH 2009, **C**).
Post-procedure	
17 Record the time the transfusion finished and the volume of the component transfused on the patient's fluid balance chart.	To ensure an accurate record of fluid is maintained as fluid balance monitoring can identify fluid overload in at-risk patients (Weinstein and Plumer 2007, **E**).

(continued)

Procedure guideline 7.13 Blood component administration *(continued)*

Action	Rationale
18 Carefully file all transfusion documentation in the patient's clinical record. In line with local policy, return information on the final fate of each blood component to the hospital transfusion laboratory.	To ensure the transfusion episode has been recorded, maintaining the clinical record for patient safety. To comply with Statutory Instrument No. 50 (Blood Safety and Quality Regulations 2005, **C**), where the final fate of all blood components must be held for a duration of 30 years.
19 Return any unused blood components to the laboratory promptly.	To allow unused components to be reallocated if returned in time. Refer to local guidelines. **E**
20 If there is any suspicion of a transfusion reaction then the pack should be returned to the transfusion laboratory with full clinical details. If the transfusion is completed uneventfully then the empty pack and administration set should be disposed of according to local policy.	To ensure transfused bags are available in the event of incident investigation (SNBTS 2004, **C**). Previously it was advocated that empty packs be kept for a period of 48 hours to aid the investigation of severe post-transfusion reactions. The benefits of this are unproven and it is associated with both practical and health and safety concerns (BCSH 2009).
21 For patients receiving ongoing transfusion support, the blood administration set should be changed at least every 12 hours, or after every second unit transfused. Dispose of used set in clinical waste: refer to local guidelines/protocols.	To minimize risk from bacterial contamination (BCSH 2009, **C**; McClelland 2007, **E**; SNBTS 2004, **E**).

Problem-solving table 7.5 Prevention and resolution (Procedure guidelines 7.12 and 7.13)

Problem	Cause	Prevention	Resolution
Patient does not have a nameband.	Nameband has been removed or is no longer legible.	**Always** follow local policy and **never** use secondary identifiers such as bed numbers, notes or request forms that the patient may be carrying (Murphy 2009). If a member of staff removes a patient's identification band, they are then responsible for ensuring that it is replaced.	All inpatients are required to wear a nameband; therefore, replace nameband and reconfirm identity (NPSA 2005).
	Patient is in an outpatient setting.	Follow hospital policy for the identification of patients.	Ensure patient has a correctly completed identification wristband prior to commencing a transfusion.
Unable to obtain verbal confirmation.	Patient unconscious.	Ensure hospital policy for the identification of unconscious patients is followed.	Confirm identity with a relative or second member of staff or use unique patient identifier.
Patient unable to communicate verbally.	Due to disease or language barrier.	Follow hospital policy for the identification of patients unable to confirm their identity verbally. Consider the introduction of photo identification cards. Ensure interpreting services are available if appropriate.	Confirm identity with a relative or second member of staff (SNBTS 2004). Always follow local policy and never use secondary identifiers such as bed numbers, notes or request forms that the patient may be carrying (Murphy 2009).
Infusion slows or stops.	Venous spasm due to cold infusion.	Apply a heat pad prior to the transfusion to reduce venous spasm.	Apply warm compress to dilate the vein and increase the blood flow.
	Occlusion.	Check patency prior to administration. Always use a pulsatile flush ending with a positive pressure flush.	Flush gently with 0.9% sodium chloride and resume infusion. If occlusion persists, consider resiting cannula.
Elevation in temperature of less than 2.0°C after commencing a unit of blood with no other symptoms. Temperature falls if the blood is slowed/stopped.	Febrile non-haemolytic transfusion reaction.	Take history to identify whether patient has had a reaction previously.	Observe the patient's temperature, pulse and blood pressure during the transfusion as indicated. If patient has no other signs and symptoms, give paracetamol and continue the transfusion at a slower rate and observe more frequently (Norfolk 2013).

Compatibility label or tie-on tag

The compatibility label is generated in the hospital transfusion laboratory. It is attached to the blood bag and contains the following patient information: *Surname, First Name(s), Date of Birth, Gender, Hospital Number/Patient Identification Number, Hospital* and *Ward*.
The *blood group, component type* and *date requested* are also included on the label. The *unique donation number* is printed on the compatibility label; this number must match exactly with the number on the blood bag label.

STOP, SEE BACK OF THIS TAG BEFORE TRANSFUSION
NHS
SCOTLAND ©Scottish National Blood Transfusion Service 2005 V9

Donation No: G101 606 597 229 N
Component: Red Cells
Signature 1: Date Given:
Signature 2: Time Given:

Peel off label above and place in patient's Medical Records

Surname: MACDONALD	Forename: MORAG
DOB: 11/07/1956	Gender: FEMALE
25 HILL STREET TOWN CENTRE	
Patient Identity No: 100198E	Date/Time Required: 20/12/2006
Patient Blood Group: O Rh POS	Component: Red Cells
Donation Number: G101 606 597 229 N	
Special Requirements:	

Once transfusion has been started, you must send the completed section below to the Hospital Transfusion Laboratory.
This is a legal requirement

Surname: MACDONALD	Forename: MORAG
Patient Identity No: 100198E	Lab Sample No: 1803905
Donation Number: G101 606 597 229 N	
Component: Red Cells	
Date Given:	Time Given:

I confirm that the above patient received this blood component
Sign and Print Name

Unique donation number

This is the unique number assigned to each blood donation by the transfusion service and allows follow-up from donor to patient. From April 2001 all donations bear the new 14 digit (ISBT 128) donation number
The unique donation number on the blood bag must match exactly the number on the compatibility label

Blood group

Shows the blood group of the component

This does not have to be identical with the patient's blood group but must be compatible

Group O patients must receive group O red cells

Expiry date

The expiry date must be checked – do not use any component that is beyond the expiry date

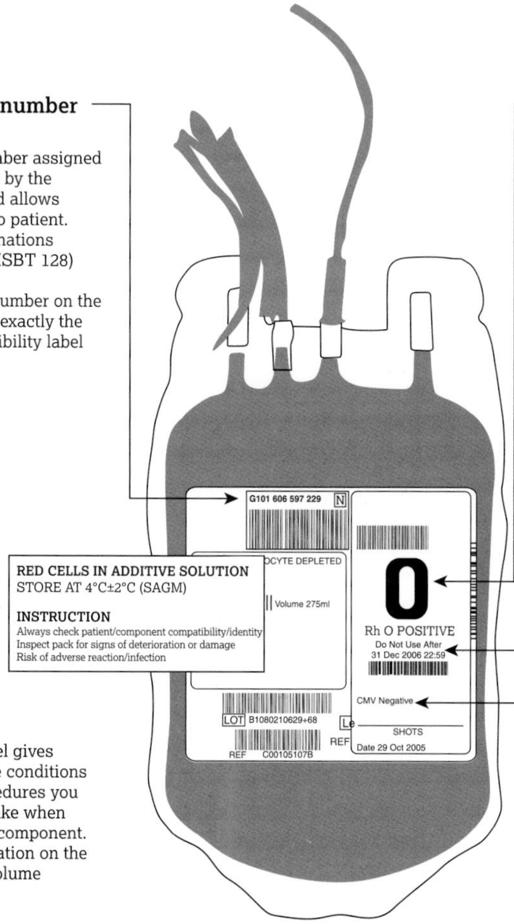

RED CELLS IN ADDITIVE SOLUTION
STORE AT 4°C±2°C (SAGM)

INSTRUCTION
Always check patient/component compatibility/identity
Inspect pack for signs of deterioration or damage
Risk of adverse reaction/infection

Cautionary notes

This section of the label gives instructions on storage conditions and the checking procedures you are required to undertake when administering a blood component. It also includes information on the component type and volume

Special requirements

This shows the special features of the donation, e.g. CMV negative

Figure 7.7 **Blood pack labelling.**

POST-PROCEDURAL CONSIDERATIONS

Immediate care

The patient should be asked to inform a member of staff of any symptoms which may indicate a transfusion-related adverse event, such as feeling anxious, rigors (shivering), flushing, pain or shortness of breath. The patient should be cared for where they can be visually observed and should be shown how to use the nurse call system. The patient should have vital signs monitored as indicated in the Procedure guidelines: however, it may be necessary to take additional observations if clinically indicated, such as if the patient complains of feeling unwell or they develop signs of a transfusion reaction (Gray and Illingworth 2005). Guidance for the initial recognition of transfusion reactions is provided in Table 7.12.

Many drugs may cause a pyretic hypersensitivity reaction (BNF 2014). There is at present insufficient evidence to allow guidance on the co-administration of drugs with red blood cell transfusion. A lack of clinical reporting of reactions in patients cannot be taken to indicate safe practice: adverse reactions may be attributed to other causes, subclinical haemolysis or agglutination may occur undetected and serious adverse effects may be masked by pre-existing illness in the patient (Murdock et al. 2009).

Ongoing care

On completion of a blood transfusion episode, observations to include blood pressure, temperature, pulse and respiratory rate should be taken and recorded. The patient's records should be updated to confirm that the transfusion has taken place, including the volume transfused, whether the transfusion achieved the desired effect (either post-transfusion increment rates or an improvement in the patient's symptoms) and the details of any reactions to the transfusion. If intravenous fluids are prescribed to follow the transfusion, these should be administered through a new administration set appropriate for that infusion. The traceability documentation confirming the fate of the component should be returned to the laboratory (Blood Safety and Quality Regulations 2005).

The SHOT report (2008) emphasizes that, on occasion, transfusion reactions can occur many hours and sometimes days

Table 7.12 **Recognition of transfusion reactions**

Symptoms/signs	Mild	Moderate	Severe
Temperature	Temperature of ≥38°C **AND** rise of 1–2°C from baseline temperature	Temperature of ≥39°C **OR** a rise of ≥2°C from baseline temperature	Sustained febrile symptoms or any new, unexplained pyrexia *in addition* to clinical signs
Rigors/shaking	None	Mild chills	Obvious shaking/rigors
Pulse	Minimal or no change from baseline	Rise in heart rate from baseline of 10 bpm or more NOT associated with bleeding	Rise in heart rate from baseline of 20 bpm or more NOT associated with bleeding
Respirations	Minimal or no change from baseline	Rise in respiratory rate from baseline of 10 or more	Rise in respiratory rate from baseline of 10 or more accompanied by dyspnoea/ wheeze
Blood pressure (hypo/hypertension)	Minor or no change to systolic or diastolic pressure	Change in systolic or diastolic pressure of ≥30 mm/Hg NOT associated with bleeding	Change in systolic or diastolic pressure of ≥30 mm/Hg NOT associated with bleeding
Skin	No change	Facial flushing, rash Urticaria, pruritus	Rash, urticaria *and* periorbital oedema Conjunctivitis
Pain	None	General discomfort or myalgia Pain at drip site	Acute pain in chest, abdomen, back
Urine	Clear Normal output		Haematuria/haemoglobinuria Oliguria, anuria
Bleeding	No new bleeding		Uncontrolled oozing
Nausea	None		Nausea or vomiting
All Green	**STOP the transfusion but leave connected.** Recheck identity of the unit with the patient, inform doctor. If all well, continue at reduced rate **for the next 30 minutes and then** resume at prescribed rate. Continue to monitor the patient carefully and be alert for other symptoms or signs of a transfusion reaction. Antipyretics may be required.		
1 or more Amber	**STOP the transfusion but leave connected**, request urgent clinical review, recheck identity of the unit with the patient, give IV fluids. If symptoms stable or improving over next 15 minutes, consider restarting the unit. Antihistamines and/or antipyretics may be required.		
1 or more Red	**STOP the transfusion and disconnect,** request immediate clinical review, recheck identity of the unit with the patient, give IV fluids, inform the transfusion laboratory, contact the consultant haematologist.		

Note: in all cases where a transfusion reaction is suspected and the transfusion is stopped and disconnected, the implicated unit, complete with giving set, must be returned to the laboratory for further investigation.
Follow your local transfusion policy and contact the transfusion laboratory for further instructions.
Source: Produced by Wales Transfusion Practitioner Group, V2: WBS BBT Team Oct 2012. Based on SHOT (2011b), UK Blood Services (2007) and BCSH Blood Transfusion Task Force (2012).

after the transfusion is completed. Therefore, for patients receiving a transfusion as a day case, it is important to ensure that they are counselled on the possibility of later adverse reactions and that they have access to clinical advice at all times. The BCSH recommends that day-case and short-stay patients are issued with a contact card facilitating 24-hour access to appropriate clinical advice, similar to the scheme used for patients receiving chemotherapy treatments on an outpatient basis (BCSH 2009).

COMPLICATIONS

Bacterial infections

Contamination of blood and blood components can occur during donation, collection, processing, storage and administration. Despite strict guidelines and procedures, the risk of contamination remains. Most common contaminating organisms are skin contaminants such as staphylococci, diphtheroids and micrococci, which enter the blood at the time of venesection (Barbara and Contreras 2009, Provan et al. 2009). Bacterial contamination can lead to severe septic reaction. Two strategies have been implemented by NHSBT to reduce bacterial infections. First, donor arm disinfection and the diversion of the first 30 mL of each donation to reduce contamination of the blood component by the skin plug from venepuncture. Since 1996, 40 bacterial infections have been reported to SHOT, 33 of these related to platelet transfusions (SHOT 2011a). NHSBT implemented bacterial screening in January 2011, and aerobic and anaerobic cultures are performed on each platelet collection (NHSBT 2011).

Viral infections

Viruses transmissible via blood transfusions can be either plasma borne or cell associated (Barbara and Contreras 2009, Williamson et al. 1999). Plasma-borne viruses include hepatitis B, hepatitis C, hepatitis A (rarely), serum parvovirus B19, and human immunodeficiency viruses (HIV-1 and HIV-2). Cell-associated viruses include CMV, Epstein–Barr virus, human T cell leukaemia/lymphoma viruses (HTLV-1/HTLV-2) and HIV-1/HIV-2.

Sepsis

Sepsis occurs when bacteria enter the blood or blood component that is to be infused. Bacteria can enter at any point from the time of collection, during storage through to administration to the patient. Organisms implicated in transfusion-related sepsis include Gram-negative *Pseudomonas*, *Yersinia* and *Flavobacterium* (Provan et al. 2009). Septic reactions usually present with a fever, tachycardia and/or hypotension, and can lead rapidly to systemic inflammatory response syndrome (SIRS) (Porth 2005). This is a serious life-threatening condition, sometimes referred to as septic shock, and requires urgent medical attention.

Transfusion-related acute lung injury (TRALI)

Transfusion-related acute lung injury is most frequently associated with plasma-rich products such as platelets and FFP (Federico 2009). TRALI is usually caused by antileucocyte antibodies reacting against donor leucocytes. In nearly 90% of cases, either HLA or neutrophil-specific antibodies were detected in the donors and most of the donors were multiparous women. The corresponding antigen in the recipient was also found to be important (Chapman et al. 2009). The antigen/antibody reaction can result in 'leucoagglutination'. Leucoagglutinins can in turn become trapped in the pulmonary microvasculature, causing severe respiratory distress without evidence of circulatory overload or cardiac failure (Contreras and Navarrete 2009).

Transfusion-related acute lung injury is defined as dyspnoea with hypoxia and bilateral pulmonary infiltrates during or within 6 hours of transfusion, not due to circulatory overload or other likely causes (Chapman 2009). As the antibodies were mostly found in multiparous women and, as a result of SHOT reports demonstrating that in the majority of cases the donor was female, the National Blood Service developed a strategy to use only the plasma from male donors for FFP and male plasma in pooled platelets (Chapman et al. 2009).

Transfusion-related acute lung injury is usually treated the same as any adult respiratory distress syndrome (ARDS) and therefore patients who develop TRALI may require ventilatory support (SNBTS 2004) and should be treated as an emergency. Diuretics should not be administered as patients are generally hypotensive and hypovolaemic. Although the symptoms resemble ARDS, TRALI is self-limiting and with most patients improving over a 4-day period, without long-term consequences (Federico 2009). As TRALI is donor related, it is essential that cases are reported to the blood transfusion services so that donors can be contacted, investigated for antibodies to HLA and if necessary removed from the donor panel (McClelland, 2007, Norfolk 2013).

Transfusion-related immunomodulation

The infusion of foreign antigen during a packed red blood cell (PRBC) transfusion induces a non-specific immunosuppression, which is known as transfusion-associated immunomodulation. Allogeneic plasma components, white blood cells, fibrin and accumulants from the storage process have all been implicated (Englesbe et al. 2005).

Urticaria

This uncommon reaction is caused by the recipient reacting to protein in the donor plasma (Davies and Williamson 1998). Urticaria is characterized by localized oedematous plaques, hives and itching and is usually mediated by histamines (Porth 2005). Therefore urticarial reactions usually respond well to antihistamines which should be administered once the patient has been assessed and antihistamine therapy has been prescribed (SNBTS 2004). The infusion can then be recommenced; however, if symptoms return, the infusion should be discontinued.

Transfusion reactions

In November 1996 the Serious Hazards of Transfusion (SHOT) scheme was launched. This voluntary and anonymized reporting scheme collects data from participating hospitals across the UK and Ireland. The purpose of SHOT is to collect data on the serious morbidity related to the transfusion of blood and blood products. These data have since been utilized to inform education programmes, policy development and guideline development, ultimately improving hospital transfusion practice (SNBTS 2004).

Although the Blood Safety and Quality Regulations 2005 have now made the reporting of such events via SABRE mandatory, the SHOT scheme remains active and important and has presented yearly retrospective reports of data collected since its inception. These data demonstrate improved performance in recognizing reporting of transfusion-related incidents and continue to generate key recommendations to improve all transfusion practice (SNBTS 2004). Despite significant improvement in the reduction of risk from transfusion-transmitted infection, human error which results in an IBCT – the transfusion of a blood product that is not suitable for or not intended for the recipient – remains the greatest risk to patients (SNBTS 2004). Figures from the 2013 SHOT report confirm 247 cases in this category (Bolton-Maggs et al. 2014).

The prompt management of any adverse transfusion reaction can reduce associated morbidity and can be life saving. Therefore staff caring for patients receiving transfused products must be fully familiar with the immediate management of any suspected reaction. However, specialist advice should always be sought for the diagnosis and ongoing management of transfusion reactions, such as haemolytic, anaphylactic and septic reactions (McClelland 2007, SNBTS 2004).

Minor transfusion reactions

It should always be remembered that the symptoms of a 'minor' transfusion reaction may be the prelude to a major, life-threatening reaction. It is essential that staff take any transfusion reaction seriously. Symptomatic patients should have their vital signs monitored closely and they should be clearly observable. Patients with persistent or deteriorating symptoms should always be managed as a major reaction and urgent medical and specialist support should be sought (McClelland 2007, SNBTS 2004).

Allergic and anaphylactic reactions are more common and more severe with transfusion of FFP and platelets than with red blood cells (Domen and Hoeltge 2003).

Symptoms of minor reactions include a temperature rise of up to 1.5°C, rash without systemic disturbance and moderate tachycardia without hypotension (SNBTS 2004). Such symptoms may be caused by an immunological reaction to components of the blood product. Whilst it may be possible to manage such symptoms and continue with the transfusion, the following action should always be taken (Contreras and Navarrete 2009).

- Stop the transfusion and inform the responsible medical team.
- Confirm the patient's identity and recheck their details against the product compatibility label.
- Antihistamines should be considered for skin rashes or urticarial itch.
- Antipyretic agents can be considered for mild fever.

It may be possible to continue with the transfusion at a reduced rate once the patient's symptoms are controlled; however, it may be necessary to increase the frequency of observations until the transfusion is completed. Some patients who have regular transfusions may experience recurrent febrile reactions and may benefit from an antipyretic premedication. *Note*: aspirin and other non-steroidal anti-inflammatory drugs (NSAIDs) are contraindicated in patients with a thrombocytopenia or coagulopathy (BNF 2014).

Major transfusion reactions

Major transfusion reactions include anaphylaxis, haemolysis and sepsis and may present as a fever of >38.5°C, tachycardia ± hypotension. In such circumstances a severe reaction should always be considered and the transfusion should be stopped until a specialist assessment has been conducted (Box 7.4).

Care should be taken when returning the blood product to the laboratory, to ensure that the product does not leak and that no needles remain attached.

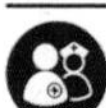

Box 7.4 **Initial management of a suspected transfusion reaction**

- Stop the transfusion and seek urgent medical help.
- Initiate appropriate emergency procedures, for example call resuscitation team.
- Depending on venous access, withdraw the contents of the lumen being used and disconnect the blood product.
- Keep venous access patent.
- Confirm the patient's identity and recheck their details against the product compatibility label.
- Keep the patient and relative informed of all progress and reassure as indicated.
- Initiate close and frequent observations of temperature, pulse, blood pressure, fluid balance.
- Inform the transfusion laboratory and seek the urgent advice of the haematologist for further management.
- Return the transfused product to the laboratory with new blood samples (10 mL clotted and 5 mL ethylenediamine tetra-acetic acid (EDTA)) from the patient's opposite arm (SNBTS 2004) with a completed transfusion reaction notification form (if available) or note the patient's details, the nature and timing of the reaction and details of the component transfused.

Any further products being held locally for the patient should also be returned to the hospital transfusion laboratory for assessment. The events surrounding the reaction should be clearly documented and reported in the following ways.

- Record the adverse event in the patient's clinical record.
- Complete a detailed incident form as per local policy.
- Follow local, regional and national criteria for reporting via SABRE and SHOT.

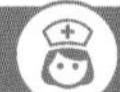

Learning Activity 7.6

Scenario: Minor transfusion reaction

You have been asked to perform a set of observations on a patient who is receiving a blood transfusion (red blood cells). You discover that his temperature has risen from 36.2°C to 37.3°C and his pulse has risen from 84 to 98 bpm.

What would you do next?

See the end of the chapter for the answers.

Acute haemolytic reactions

These are usually directly related to ABO incompatibilities due to an IBCT where antigen/antibody reactions occur when the recipient's antibodies react with surface antigens on the donor red cells. This reaction causes a cascade of events within the recipient which can present with chills/rigors, facial flushing, pain/oozing at the cannula site, burning along the vein, chest pain, lumbar or flank pain, or shock (Gillespie and Hillyer 2001, McClelland 2007). Patients may express a feeling of anxiety or doom, which may be associated with cytokine activity. Haemolytic shock can occur after only a few millilitres of blood have been infused. Treatment is often vigorous to reverse hypotension, aid adequate renal perfusion and renal flow to reduce potential damage to renal tubules, and appropriate therapy for DIC reactions (Provan et al. 2009). It is important to remember that most acute haemolytic reactions are preventable as they are usually caused by human error when taking or labelling pre-transfusion samples, collecting blood components and/or failing to perform a correct identity check of blood pack and patient at the bedside (McClelland 2007, Norfolk 2013) (Figure 7.8).

Acute anaphylactic reactions

These are rare and usually occur after only a few millilitres of blood or plasma have been infused (Weinstein and Plumer 2007) and present with bronchial spasm, respiratory distress, abdominal cramps, shock and potential loss of consciousness.

Circulatory overload (transfusion-associated circulatory overload)

Circulatory overload can occur when blood or any of its components are infused rapidly or administered to a patient with an increased plasma volume, causing hypervolaemia. Patients at risk are those with renal or cardiac deficiencies, the young and elderly (Weinstein and Plumer 2007). Patients with signs of cardiac failure should receive their transfusion slowly with diuretic support (McClelland 2007). The need for concomitant drugs such as diuretics should always be assessed before commencing treatment (SNBTS 2004).

Febrile non-haemolytic reactions

These reactions are due to an immunological response to the transfusion of cellular components such as donor leucocytes. Specific patient groups are at risk of greater sensitization to leucocytes, for example, critically ill patients, those receiving anticancer therapies or patients requiring multiple transfusion therapy (Williamson et al. 1999). Such reactions present with a mild fever (up to 2°C from the baseline), rash without systemic

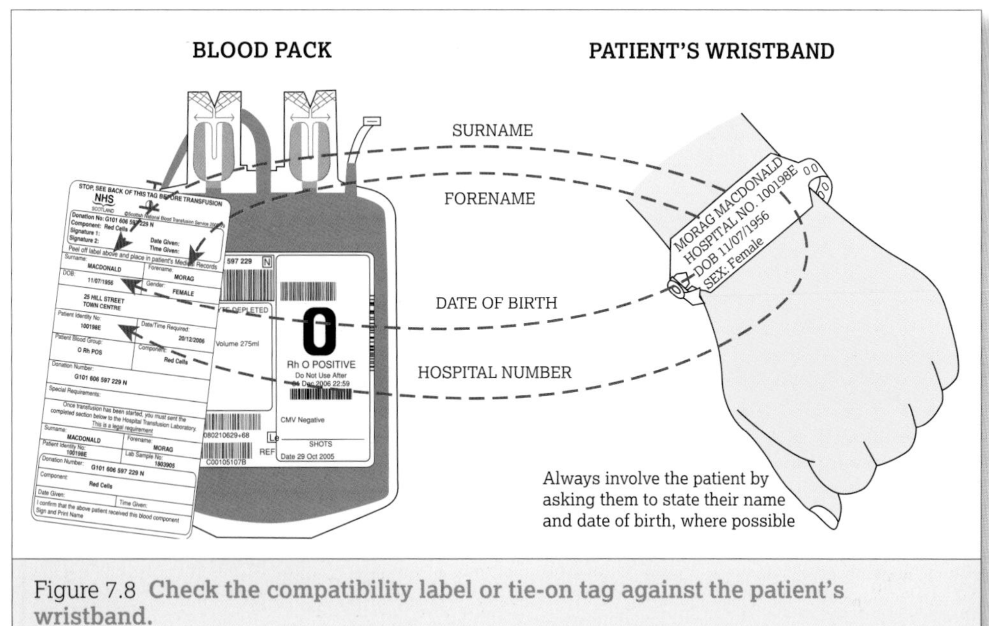

Figure 7.8 **Check the compatibility label or tie-on tag against the patient's wristband.**

disturbance and moderate tachycardia without hypotension (Norfolk 2013, SNBTS 2004).

Hypothermia

Infusing large quantities of cold blood rapidly can cause hypothermia. Patients likely to experience this reaction are those who have suffered massive blood loss due to trauma, haemorrhage, clotting disorders or thrombocytopenia (McClelland 2007). Such reactions present with alteration in vital signs and development of pallor and chills.

Delayed effects

These reactions may occur days, months or even years after transfusion.

Delayed haemolytic reactions

These reactions are caused when immune antibodies react to a foreign antigen. Reactions are classified as primary or secondary. A *primary* reaction is often mild, occurring days or weeks after initial transfusion, and may be indicated by no clinical alteration in haemoglobin following transfusion therapy (Cook 1997a). *Secondary* reactions occur with re-exposure to the same antigen, and on rare occasions may be associated with ABO incompatibilities (Cook 1997a). The patient may present with a fever, mild jaundice and unexplained decrease in haemoglobin value and may require antiglobulin testing (Norfolk 2013).

Hyperkalaemia

Hyperkalaemia is a rare complication associated with trauma and the subsequent infusion of large quantities of blood. Potassium is known to leak out of red cells during storage, thereby increasing circulatory levels in recipients receiving blood products (Cook 1997b). The process is exacerbated if products are kept too long at room temperature or gamma irradiated (Davies and Williamson 1998). From starting the infusion to completion, the infusion should take a maximum of 4 hours (McClelland 2007). The patient may present with irritability, anxiety, abdominal cramps, diarrhoea and weakness in the extremities (Cook 1997b). The patient's medical team should be contacted to assess the patient.

Iron overload

Patients who are dependent on frequent transfusion, such as those with thalassaemic, sickle cell and other transfusion-dependent disorders, can become overloaded with iron (McClelland 2007). A unit of red blood cells contains 250 mg iron, which the body is unable to excrete, and as a result patients receiving large volumes of blood are at risk of iron overload (Davies and Williamson 1998). This can result in poor growth, pigment changes, hepatic cirrhosis, hypoparathyroidism, diabetes, arrhythmia, cardiac failure and death. Chelation therapy through the use of desferrioxamine, which induces iron excretion, minimizes the accumulation of iron (BNF 2014).

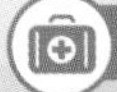 Learning Activity 7.7

Learning in practice: Administration of blood and blood products

In your clinical area, find the local policy for the administration of blood and blood products.

- Review and familiarize yourself with the guidance for monitoring patients who are receiving a blood transfusion.
- How does this compare with what you have learnt/read/been advised?
- Talk through your responsibilities as a student nurse caring for a patient receiving a transfusion with a qualified nursing colleague.

Learning for practice

After studying this chapter, list five key points you have learnt about nutrition that you will be able to apply to your clinical practice.

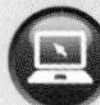 For further learning exercises visit **www.royalmarsdenmanual.com/student**.

Now Test Yourself

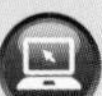

This section provides a range of exercises/activities to further test your learning. For additional exercises visit **www.royalmarsdenmanual.com/student**.

What have your learnt?

1 The human body is made up of approximately what proportion of water?
A 50%
B 60%
C 70%
D 80%

2 Concentration of electrolytes within the body vary depending on the compartment within which they are contained. Extracellular fluid has a high concentration of which of the following?
A Sodium
B Potassium
C Chloride
D Magnesium

3 In order to avoid dehydration or fluid overload when administering maintenance intravenous fluids they should be:
A Hypertonic
B Hypotonic
C Isotonic
D All of the above may be used

4 Which of the following is NOT a clinical sign of fluid overload?
A Bounding pulse
B Decreased blood pressure
C Increased respiratory rate
D Decreased oxygen saturations

5 Nationally, what percentage of patients admitted to hospital are at risk of malnutrition?
A 8%
B 18%
C 28%
D 38%

6 How can patients who need assistance at mealtimes be identified?
A A red sticker
B A colour serviette
C A red tray
D Any of the above

7 What can happen if dysphagia is not managed appropriately? List four possible consequences.

8 People with blood group A are able to receive blood from the following:
A Group A only
B Groups AB or B
C Groups A or O
D Groups A, B or O

9 Errors in the requesting, collection and administration of blood components lead to significant risks for patients. In the SHOT report (2011) what proportion of adverse events were reportedly caused by human error?
A One-quarter
B One-third
C Half
D Two-thirds

10 The three key principles that underpin each stage of the blood component transfusion process are:
A Patient identification, documentation, education
B Patient consent, patient identification, documentation
C Patient identification, documentation, communication
D Documentation, communication, patient consent

See the end of the chapter for the answers.

Key points

- The provision of food and fluids to patients is an integral part of their care. In normal circumstances adequate nutritional intake enables the body to maintain homoeostasis of body composition and function, but in disease states this balance can be altered with negative consequences for the patient.
- Monitoring and reporting a patient's fluid and electrolyte balance is a critical element of nursing care. The calculation of fluid balance relies heavily on the accurate measuring, charting and calculating of input, output and overall balance.
- The body requires protein, energy, fluid and micronutrients such as vitamins, minerals and trace elements to function optimally. Nutritional requirements should be estimated for patients requiring any form of nutritional support to ensure that these needs are met.
- Patients who require assistance to meet their nutritional needs should be identified through screening, and a discreet sign used to identify that further assistance is required, for example a red tray or a red sticker.
- All staff involved in the transfusion of blood and/or blood components must have the knowledge and skills to ensure the process is completed safely. The three key principles which must underpin every stage of the blood component transfusion process are patient identification, documentation and communication (BCSH 2009).

Websites and useful addresses

www.bda.uk.com/resources/Delivering_Nutritional_Care_through_Food_Beverage_Services.pdf

www.bapen.org.uk/ofnsh/OrganizationOfNutritionalSupportWithinHospitals.pdf

www.npsa.nhs.uk/nrls/improvingpatientsafety/cleaning-and-nutrition/nutrition/good-nutritional-care-in-hospitals/nutrition-fact-sheets

www.dh.gov.uk/en/Publicationsandstatistics/Publications/PublicationsPolicyAndGuidance/DH_079931

www.scie.org.uk/publications/guides/guide15/mealtimes

www.bapen.org.uk/pdfs/nsw/nsw07_report.pdf

www.ageuk.org.uk/documents/en-gb/hungry_to_be_heard_inf.pdf?dtrk=true

www.dh.gov.uk/en/Publicationsandstatistics/Publications/PublicationsPolicyAndGuidance/DH_079931

www.dh.gov.uk/en/SocialCare/Socialcarereform/Dignityincare/

www.dh.gov.uk/PolicyandGuidance/HealthandSocialCareTopics/SpecialisedServices

www.espen.org/espenguidelines.html

www.nice.org.uk/nicemedia/pdf/cg032fullguideline.pdf

www.bcshguidelines.com

www.hospital.blood.co.uk

www.mhra.gov.uk

www.shotuk.org

www.transfusionguidelines.org.uk

Age Concern

Telephone: 0800 00 99 66

Website: www.ageuk.org.uk

Patients on Intravenous and Nasogastric Nutrition Therapy (PINNT)

Telephone: 01202 481 625

Website: www.pinnt.com

PINNT is a support group for patients receiving parenteral or enteral nutrition therapy.

REFERENCES

Adam, S.K. & Osborne, S. (2005) *Critical Care Nursing: Science and Practice*, 2nd edn. Oxford University Press, Oxford.

Age Concern (2006) *Hungry To Be Heard*. London: Age Concern. Available at: www.ageuk.org.uk/documents/en-gb/hungry_to_be_heard_inf.pdf?dtrk=true

Alexander, L. & Allen, D. (2011) Establishing an evidence-based inpatient medical oncology fluid balance measurement policy. *Clinical Journal of Oncology Nursing*, 15(1), 23–25.

Alexander, M.F., Fawcett, J.N. & Runciman, P.J. (2006) *Nursing Practice: Hospital and Home: The Adult*, 3rd edn. Edinburgh: Elsevier Churchill Livingstone.

Antonelli, M. & Sandroni, C. (2013) Hydroxyethyl starch for intravenous volume replacement: more harm than benefit. *JAMA*, 309(7), 723–724.

Atkinson, M. & McHanwell, S. (2002) *Basic Medical Science for Speech and Language Therapy Students*. London: Whurr.

BAPEN (2003a) *Malnutrition Universal Screening Tool 'MUST' Report*. Maidenhead: British Association for Parenteral and Enteral Nutrition.

BAPEN (2003b) *Tube Feeding and Your Medicines: A Guide for Patients and Carers*. Maidenhead: British Association for Parenteral and Enteral Nutrition.

BAPEN (2009) *Nutrition Screening Survey in the UK in 2008. Hospitals, Care Homes and Mental Health Units. A report by the BAPEN*. Maidenhead: British Association for Parenteral and Enteral Nutrition. Available at: www.bapen.org.uk/pdfs/nsw/nsw_report2008-09.pdf

Baraz, S., Parvardeh, S., Mohammadi, E. & Broumand, B. (2009) Dietary and fluid compliance: an educational intervention for patients having haemodialysis. *Journal of Advanced Nursing*, 66(1), 60–68.

Barrett, K.E. (2014) *Gastrointestinal Physiology*, 2nd edn. New York: Lange Medical Books/McGraw-Hill.

Bass, N.H. (1997) *The Neurology of Swallowing*, 3rd edn. Boston, MA: Butterworth-Heinemann.

Bauer, J., Capra, S. & Ferguson, M. (2002) Use of scored patient-generated subjective global assessment (PG-SGA) as a nutritional assessment tool in patients with cancer. *European Journal of Clinical Nutrition*, 56(8), 779–785.

Baumberger-Henry, M. (2008) *Quick Look Nursing: Fluids and Electrolytes*, 2nd edn. Sudbury, MA: Jones and Barlett.

BCSH (2001) Guidelines for the clinical use of red cell transfusions. *British Journal of Haematlogy*, 113(1), 24–31.

BCSH (2003) Guidelines for the use of platelet transfusion. *British Journal of Haematology*, 122(1), 10–23.

BCSH (2006) *Guidelines on the Management of Massive Blood Loss*. Available at: www.bcshguidelines.com/documents/massive_bloodloss_bjh_2006.pdf

BCSH (2009) *Guideline on the Administration of Blood Components*, London: British Society of Haematology. Available at: www.bcshguidelines.com/documents/Admin_blood_components_bcsh_05012010.pdf

BCSH (2012a) *Avoidance of Transfusion Associated Circulatory Overload (TACO) and Problems Associated with Over-transfusion: Addendum August 2012*. Available at: www.bcshguidelines.com/documents/BCSH_Blood_Admin_-_addendum_August_2012.pdf

BCSH (2012b) Red cells in critical care. *British Journal of Haematology*, 160(4), 445–464.

BCSH Blood Transfusion Task Force (2012) Guideline on the investigation and management of acute transfusion reactions. Available at: www.bcshguidelines.com

BCSH Blood Transfusion Task Force, Boulton, F.E. & James, V. (2007) Guidelines for policies on alternatives to allogeneic blood transfusion. 1. Predeposit autologous blood donation and transfusion. *Transfusion Medicine*, 17(5), 354–365.

Bedogni, G., Borghi, A. & Battistini, N. (2003) Body water distribution and disease. *Acta Diabetologica*, 40(Suppl 1), S200–S202.

Bedogni, G., Brambilla, A., Bellentani, S. & Tiribelli, C. (2006) The assessment of body composition in health and disease. *Human Ecology*, 14, 21–25.

Bennett, C. (2010) *'At a glance' Fluid Balance Bar Chart*. Available at: www.institute.nhs.uk/resources/nhslive/3155/FBC%20details%20and%20implementation%20notes%20%2015-07-10.doc

Bingham, S.A. (1987) The dietary assessment of individuals: methods, accuracy, new techniques and recommendations. *Nutrition Abstracts and Reviews*, 57, 705–742.

Bishop, E. (2008) Blood transfusion therapy. In: Dougherty, L. & Lamb, J. (eds) *Intravenous Therapy in Nursing Practice*, 2nd edn. Oxford: Blackwell Publishing, pp.377–394.

Blood Safety and Quality Regulations (2005) SI 2005/50. London: Stationery Office. Available at: www.opsi.gov.uk/si/si2005/20050050.htm

BNF (2014) *British National Formulary 67*. London: Pharmaceutical Press.

Bolton-Maggs, P.H.B. (ed), Poles, D., Watt, A. & Thomas, D. on behalf of the Serious Hazards of Transfusion (SHOT) Steering Group. (2014) *The 2013 Annual SHOT Report*. Manchester: SHOT. Available at: www.shotuk.org/wp-content/uploads/74280-SHOT-2014-Annual-Report-V12-WEB.pdf

Bozzetti, F. (2001) Nutrition support in patients with cancer. In: Payne-James, J., Grimble, G. & Silk, D.B. (eds) *Artificial Nutrition Support in Clinical Practice*. 2nd edn. London: Greenwich Medical Media, pp.639–680.

Bradley, L. & Rees, C. (2003) Reducing nutritional risk in hospital: the red tray. *Nursing Standard*, 17(26), 33–37.

Braga, M., Gianotti, L., Vignali, A. & Carlo, V.D. (2002) Preoperative oral arginine and n-3 fatty acid supplementation improves the immunometabolic host response and outcome after colorectal resection for cancer. *Surgery*, 132(5), 805–814.

Brownlee, I.A. (2011) The physiological roles of dietary fibre. *Food Hydrocolloids*, 25, 238–250.

Bryant, H. (2007) Dehydration in older people: assessment and management. *Emergency Nurse*, 15(4), 22–26.

Butler, C. & Leslie, P. (2012) *Anatomy and Physiology of Swallowing*. San Diego, CA: Plural.

Callum, K.G., Gray, A.J., Hoile, R.W., et al. (1999) *Extremes of Age: The 1999 Report of the National Confidential Enquiry into Perioperative Deaths*. London: National Confidential Enquiry into Perioperative Deaths. Available at: www.ncepod.org.uk/pdf/1999/99full.pdf

Cappell, M.S., Inglis, B. & Levy, A. (2009) Two case reports of gastric ulcer from pressure necrosis related to a rigid and taut percutaneous endoscopic gastrostomy bumper. *Gastroenterology Nursing*, 32(4), 259–263.

Care Quality Commission (2010) *Provider Compliance Assessment, Outcome 5 Regulation 14 (Meeting Nutritional Needs)*. London: CQC. Available at: www.cqc.org.uk

Care Quality Commission (2013) *Time to Listen In NHS Hospitals: Dignity and Nutrition Inspection Programme 2012 - National Overview*, Newcastle upon Tyne. Available at: www.cqc.org.uk

Carless, P.A., Moxey, A.J., O'Connell, D. & Henry, D.A. (2004) Autologous transfusion techniques: a systematic review of their efficacy. *Transfusion Medicine*, 14(2), 123–144.

Carless, P.A., Henry, D.A., Moxey, A.J., O'Connell, D., Brown, T. & Fergusson, D.A. (2010) Cell salvage for minimising perioperative allogeneic blood transfusion. *Cochrane Database of Systematic Reviews*, (4), CD001888.

Carlsson, M., Haglin, L., Rosendahl, E. & Gustafson, Y. (2013) Poor nutritional status is associated with urinary tract infection among older people living in residential care facilities. *Journal of Nutrition, Health & Aging*, 17(2), 186–191.

Carson, J.L., Carless, P.A. & Hebert, P.C. (2012) Transfusion thresholds and other strategies for guiding allogeneic red blood cell transfusion. *Cochrane Database of Systematic Reviews*, (4), CD002042.

Casey, G. (2004) Oedema: causes, physiology and nursing management. *Nursing Standard*, 18(51), 45–51.

Cervenakova, L. & Brown, P. (2004) Advances in screening test development for transmissible spongiform encephalopathies. *Expert Review of Anti-Infective Therapy*, 2(6), 873–880.

Chapman, C., Stainsby, D., Jones, H., et al. (2009) Ten years of hemovilgilance reports of transfusion-related acute lung injury in the United Kingdom and the impact of preferential use of male donor plasma. *Transfusion*, 49, 440–452.

Chung, L.H., Chong, S. & French, P. (2002) The efficiency of fluid balance charting: an evidence-based management project. *Journal of Nursing Management*, 10(2), 103–113.

Committee on Medical Aspects of Food Policy & DH (1991) *Dietary Reference Values for Food Energy and Nutrients for the United Kingdom: Report of the Panel on Dietary Reference Values of the Committee on Medical Aspects of Food Policy*, London: HMSO.

Contreras, M. & Navarrete, C. (2009) Immunological complications of blood transfusion. In: Contreras, M. (ed) *ABC of Transfusion*, 4th edn. Oxford: Blackwell Publishing, pp.61–68.

Cook, L.S. (1997a) Blood transfusion reactions involving an immune response. *Journal of Intravenous Nursing*, 20(1), 5–14.

Cook, L.S. (1997b) Nonimmune transfusion reactions: when type-and-cross match aren't enough. *Journal of Intravenous Nursing*, 20(1), 15–22.

Council of Europe (2003) *Food and Nutritional Care in Hospitals: How to Prevent Undernutrition*. Council of Europe, Paris.

Cummings, J.H. (2000) Nutritional management of diseases of the gut. In: Garrow, J.S., James, W.P. & Ralph, A. (eds) *Human Nutrition and Dietetics*, 10th edn. Edinburgh: Churchill Livingstone, pp.547–573.

Daniels, G. (2013) Human blood group systems. In: Murphy, M., Pamphilon, D. & Heddle, N. (eds) *Practical Transfusion Medicine*, 4th edn. Chichester: John Wiley & Sons, pp.21–30.

Davies, S.C. & Williamson, L.M. (1998) Transfusion of red cells. In: Contreras, M. (ed) *ABC of Transfusion*, 3rd edn. London: BMJ Books, pp.10–17.

Dellinger, R.P., Levy, M.M. & Rhodes, A. (2012) Surviving sepsis campaign: international guidelines for management of severe sepsis and septic shock. *Critical Care Medicine*, 41(2), 580–637.

DH (2007) *Better blood tranfusion: safe and appropriate use of blood: HSC 2007/001*. London: Department of Health. Available at: www.dh.gov.uk/prod_consum_dh/groups/dh_digitalassets/documents/digitalasset/dh_080803.pdf

DH (2010) *Essence of Care 2010 Benchmark for Food and Drink*. London: Department of Health. Available at: www.gov.uk/government/uploads/system/uploads/attachment_data/file/216696/dh_125313.pdf

DH (2013) *Measures Currently in Place in the UK to Reduce the Potential Risk of vCJD Transmission via Blood*. London: Department of Health. Available at: www.gov.uk/government/news/measures-currently-in-place-in-the-uk-to-reduce-the-potential-risk-of-vcjd-transmission-via-blood

Domen, R.E. & Hoeltge, G.A. (2003) Allergic transfusion reactions: an evaluation of 273 consecutive reactions. *Archives of Pathology & Laboratory Medicine*, 127(3), 316–320.

Donzelli, J., Brady, S., Wesling, M. & Theisen, M. (2005) Effects of the removal of the tracheotomy tube on swallowing during the fiberoptic endoscopic exam of the swallow (FEES). *Dysphagia*, 20(4), 283–289.

Durnin, J.V. & Womersley, J. (1974) Body fat assessed from total body density and its estimation from skinfold thickness: measurements on 481 men and women aged from 16 to 72 years. *British Journal of Nutrition*, 32(1), 77–97.

Edgeworth, J.A., Farmer, M., Sicilia, A., et al. (2011) Detection of prion infection in variant Creutzfeldt-Jakob disease: a blood-based assay. *Lancet*, 377(9764), 487–493.

Ekberg, O., Hamdy, S., Woisard, V., Wuttge-Hannig, A. & Ortega, P. (2002) Social and psychological burden of dysphagia: its impact on diagnosis and treatment. *Dysphagia*, 17(2), 139–146.

Elia, M. (2001) Metabolic response to starvation, injury and sepsis. In: Payne-James, J., Grimble, G. & Silk, D.B. (eds) *Artificial Nutrition Support in Clinical Practice*, 2nd edn. London: Greenwich Medical Media, pp.1–24.

Englesbe, M.J., Pelletier, S.J., Diehl, K.M., et al. (2005) Transfusions in surgical patients. *Journal of the American College of Surgeons*, 200(2), 249–254.

Epstein, O., Solomons, N.B. & Robins, A. (2003) *Clinical Examination*, 3rd edn. Mosby, Edinburgh.

European Medicines Agency (2013) *Assessment Report for Solutions for Infusion Containing Hydroxyethyl Starch*. Available at: www.ema.europa.eu/docs/en_GB/document_library/Referrals_document/Hydroxyethyl_starch-containing_medicines_107/Recommendation_provided_by_Pharmacovigilance_Risk_Assessment_Committee/WC500154254.pdf

Federico, A. (2009) Transfusion-related acute lung injury. *Journal of Perianesthesia Nursing*, 24(1), 35–37.

Fields, R.C. & Meyers, B.F. (2006) The effects of perioperative blood transfusion on morbidity and mortality after esophagectomy. *Thoracic Surgery Clinics*, 16(1), 75–86.

Flanagan, J., Melillo, K.D., Abdallah, L. & Remington, R. (2007) Interpreting laboratory values in the rehabilitation setting. *Rehabilitation Nursing*, 32 (2), 77–84.

Fraise, A.P. & Bradley, T. (2009) *Ayclliffe's Control of Healthcare – Associated Infections: A Practical Handbook*, 5th edn. London: Hodder Arnold.

Freeman, L. (2002) Food record charts. *Nursing Times*, 98(34), 53–54.

FSA & Expert Group on Vitamins and Minerals (2003) *Safe Upper Levels for Vitamins and Minerals*. Available at: www.food.gov.uk/multimedia/pdfs/vitmin2003.pdf

Gaziano, J.E. (2002) Evaluation and management of oropharyngeal Dysphagia in head and neck cancer. *Cancer Control*, 9(5), 400–409.

Geissler, C. & Powers, H. (2005) *Human Nutrition*, 11th edn. Edinburgh: Elsevier Churchill Livingstone.

Gibson, R. (2005) *Principles of Nutrition Assessment*, 2nd edn. Oxford: Oxford University Press.

Gidden, F. & Shenkin, A. (2000) Laboratory support of the clinical nutrition service. *Clinical Chemistry and Laboratory Medicine*, 38(8), 693–714.

Gillespie, T.W. & Hillyer, D. (2001) Granulocytes. In: Hillyer, C.D. (ed) *Handbook of Transfusion Medicine*. San Diego, CA: Academic, pp.63–68.

Goertz, S. (2006) Gauging fluid balance with osmolality. *Nursing*, 36(10), 70–71.

Goldstein, S.L. (2012) Fluid management in acute kidney injury. *Journal of Intensive Care Medicine*, Nov 14, [Epub ahead of print]

Gray, A., Hearnshaw, K., Izatt, C., Kirwan, M., Murray, S. & Shreeve, K. (2007) Safe transfusion of blood and blood components. *Nursing Standard*, 21(51), 40–47.

Gray, A. & Illingworth, J. (2005) *Right Blood, Right Patient, Right Time: RCN Guidance for Improving Transfusion Practice*. London: Royal College of Nursing. Available at: www.rcn.org.uk/__data/assets/pdf_file/0009/78615/002306.pdf

Griffiths, M. (1996) Single-stage percutaneous gastrostomy button insertion: a leap forward. *Journal of Parenteral and Enteral Nutrition*, 20(3), 237–239.

Hamer, A. (2005a) Intra-operative cell salvage. In: Thomas, D., Thompson, J. & Ridler, B. (eds) *A Manual for Blood Conservation*. Harley, UK: Tfm Publishing Ltd.

Hamer, A. (2005b) Postoperative cell salvage. In: Thomas, D., Thompson, J. & Ridler, B. (eds) *A Manual for Blood Conservation*. Harley, UK: Tfm Publishing Ltd.

Harrison, J. (2004) Getting your back – an update on autologous transfusion. *Blood Matters*, 16, 7–9. Available at: www.blood.co.uk/pdf/publications/blood_matters_16.pdf

Henry, C.J. (2005) Basal metabolic rate studies in humans: measurement and development of new equations. *Public Health Nutrition*, 8(7A), 1133–1152.

Henry, D.A., Carless, P.A., Moxey, A.J., et al. (2002) Pre-operative autologous donation for minimising perioperative allogeneic blood transfusion. *Cochrane Database System Review*, (2), CD003602.

Hickson, M. (2006) Malnutrition and ageing. *Postgraduate Medical Journal*, 82(963), 2–8.

Horgan, G.W. & Stubbs, J. (2003) Predicting basal metabolic rate in the obese is difficult. *European Journal of Clinical Nutrition*, 57(2), 335–340.

James, V. (2004) *A National Blood Conservation Strategy for NBTC and NBS: Report from the Working Party Autologous Transfuion and the Working Party on Alternatives to Transfusion of the NBS Sub-Group on Appropriate Use of Blood.* Available at: www.dh.gov.uk/prod_consum_dh/groups/dh_digitalassets/@dh/@en/documents/digitalasset/dh_4089513.pdf (archived)

James, V. (2005) *Guidelines for the Blood Transfusion Services in the United Kingdom*, 7th edn. London: The Stationery Office.

James, V. & Harrison, J. (2002) The pros and cons of predeposit autologous donation and transfusion. *Blood Matters*, (11), 4–5. Available at: www.blood.co.uk/pdf/publications/blood_matters_11.pdf

Janssen, I., Heymsfield, S.B., Baumgartner, R.N. & Ross, R. (2000) Estimation of skeletal muscle mass by bioelectrical impedance analysis. *Journal of Applied Physiology*, 89(2), 465–471.

Jensen, G.L., Hsiao, P.Y. & Wheeler, D. (2012) Adult nutrition assessment tutorial. *Journal of Parenteral and Enteral Nutrition*, 36(3), 267–274.

Jevon, P. (2010) How to ensure patient observations lead to effective management of oliguria. *Nursing Times*, 106(7), 18–19.

Jevon, P. & Ewens, B. (2007) *Monitoring the Critically Ill Patient*, 2nd edn. Oxford: Blackwell Publishing.

John, T., Rodeman, R. & Colvin, R. (2008) Blood conservation in a congenital cardiac surgery program. *AORN Journal*, 87(6), 1180–1186.

Joint UKBTS/NIBSC Professional Advisory Committee (JPAC) (2013) Care and selection of whole blood and component donors (including donors of pre-deposit autogous blood. In: *Guidelines for the Blood Transfusion Services in the United Kingdom.* London: The Stationery Office.

King's Fund Research Summary (2005) *Sustainable Food and the NHS.* www.kingsfund.org.uk/publications/kings_fund_publications/sustainable_food.html.

Kondrup, J., Allison, S.P., Elia, M., Vellas, B. & Plauth, M. (2003) ESPEN guidelines for nutrition screening 2002. *Clinical Nutrition*, 22(4), 415–421.

Kroke, A., Klipstein-Grobusch, K., Voss, S., et al. (1999) Validation of a self-administered food-frequency questionnaire administered in the European Prospective Investigation into Cancer and Nutrition (EPIC) Study: comparison of energy, protein, and macronutrient intakes estimated with the doubly labeled water, urinary nitrogen, and repeated 24-h dietary recall methods. *American Journal of Clinical Nutrition*, 70(4), 439–447.

Kyle, U.G., Bosaeus, I., De Lorenzo, A.D., et al. (2004) Bioelectrical impedance analysis – part I: review of principles and methods. *Clinical Nutrition*, 23(5), 1226–1243.

Langmore, S.E. (2001) *Endoscopic Evaluation and Treatment of Swallowing Disorders.* New York: Thieme.

Langmore, S.E., Terpenning, M.S., Schork, A. et al. (1998) Predictors of aspiration pneumonia: how important is dysphagia? *Dysphagia*, 13 (2), 69–81.

Lazarus, C.L. (2000) Management of swallowing disorders in head and neck cancer patients: optimal patterns of care. *Seminars in Speech and Language*, 21(4), 293–309.

Lazarus, C., Logemann, J.A., Song, C.W., Rademaker, A.W. & Kahrilas, P.J. (2002) Effects of voluntary maneuvers on tongue base function for swallowing. *Folia Phoniatrica et Logopaedica*, 54(4), 171–176.

Leahy, S., O'Neill, C., Sohun, R. & Jakeman, P. (2012) A comparison of dual energy X-ray absorptiometry and bioelectrical impedance analysis to measure total and segmental body composition in healthy young adults. *European Journal of Applied Physiology*, 112(2), 589–595.

Leder, S.B. & Ross, D.A. (2000) Investigation of the causal relationship between tracheotomy and aspiration in the acute care setting. *The Laryngoscope*, 110(4), 641–644.

Leslie, P., Carding, P.N. & Wilson, J.A. (2003) Investigation and management of chronic dysphagia. *BMJ (Clinical Research Edition)*, 326(7386), 433–436.

Levi, R. (2005) Nursing care to prevent dehydration in older adults. *Australian Nursing Journal*, 13(3), 21–23.

Lewin, J.S., Hebert, T.M., Putnam, J.B. Jr. & DuBrow, R.A. (2001) Experience with the chin tuck maneuver in postesophagectomy aspirators. *Dysphagia*, 16(3), 216–219.

Lochs, H., Allison, S.P., Meier, R., et al. (2006) Introductory to the ESPEN guidelines on enteral nutrition: terminology, definitions and general topics. *Clinical Nutrition*, 25(2), 180–186.

Logemann, J.A. (1998) *Evaluation and Treatment of Swallowing Disorders*, 2nd edn. Austin, TX: PRO-ED.

Logemann, J.A., Pauloski, B.R., Rademaker, A.W. & Colangelo, L.A. (1997) Super-supraglottic swallow in irradiated head and neck cancer patients. *Head & Neck*, 19(6), 535–540.

Logemann , J.A., Pauloski, B.R., Rademaker, A.W. et al. (2008) Swallowing disorders in the first year after radiation and chemoradiation. *Head Neck*, 30 (2), 148–158.

Loser, C., Aschl, G., Hebuterne, X., et al. (2005) ESPEN guidelines on artificial enteral nutrition – percutaneous endoscopic gastrostomy (PEG). *Clinical Nutrition*, 24(5), 848–861.

Loveday, H.P., Wilson, J.A., Pratt, R.J., et al. (2014) epic3: national evidence-based guidelines for preventing healthcare-associated infections in NHS hospitals in England. *Journal of Hospital Infection*, 86(Suppl 1), S1–70.

Low, J., Wyles, C., Wilkinson, T. & Sainsbury, R. (2001) The effect of compliance on clinical outcomes for patients with dysphagia on videofluoroscopy. *Dysphagia*, 16(2), 123–127.

Ludlam, C.A. & Turner, M.L. (2006) Managing the risk of transmission of variant Creutzfeldt Jakob disease by blood products. *British Journal of Haematology*, 132(1), 13–24.

Majka, A.J., Wang, Z., Schmitz, K.R., et al. (2013) Care co-ordination to enhance management of long-term enteral tube feeding: a systematic review and meta-analysis. *Journal of Parenteral and Enteral Nutrition*, 38(1), 40–52.

Marieb, E.N. & Hoehn, K. (2010) *Human Anatomy and Physiology*, 8th edn. San Francisco, CA: Pearson.

Matlow, A., Jacobson, M., Wray, R., et al. (2006) Enteral tube hub as a reservoir for transmissible enteric bacteria. *American Journal of Infection Control*, 34(3), 131–133.

McClelland, D.B. (2007) *Handbook of Transfusion Medicine.* London: The Stationery Office.

McKenna, H. & Clay, M.E. (2005) Haemopoietic stem cell processing and storage. In: Murphy, M.F. & Pamphilon, D.H. (eds) *Practical Transfusion Medicine*, 2nd edn. Oxford: Blackwell Publishing.

Mentes, J. (2006) Oral hydration in older adults: greater awareness is needed in preventing, recognizing, and treating dehydration. *American Journal of Nursing*, 106(6), 40–49.

Moftah, F. (2005) Blood transfusion and alternatives in elderly, malignancy and chronic disease. *Hematology*, 10(Suppl 1), 82–85.

Mollison, P.L., Engelfriet, C.P. & Contreras, M. (1997) *Blood Transfusion in Clinical Medicine*, 10th edn. Oxford: Blackwell Science.

Mooney, G.P. (2007) Fluid balance. *Nursing Times.* Available at: www.nursingtimes.net/nursing-practice/clinical-zones/cardiology/fluid-balance/199391.article#

Murphy, M.F., Staves, J., Davies, A., et al. (2009) How do we approach a major change program using the example of the development, evaluation, and implementation of an electronic transfusion management system. *Transfusion*, 49(5), 829–837.

Murphy, M.F., Wallington, T.B., Kelsey, P., et al. (2001) Guidelines for the clinical use of red cell transfusions. *British Journal of Haematology*, 113(1), 24–31.

NAGE (n.d.) *Have You Got a Small Appetite?* Nutrition Advisory Group for Elderly People of the British Dietetic Association, Rotherham.

National CJD Surveillance Unit (2008) *Creutzfeldt–Jakob Disease Surveillance in the UK.*

NCCAC (2006) *Nutrition Support in Adults: Oral Nutrition Support, Enteral Tube Feeding and Parenteral Nutrition: Clinical Guidance 32.* London: National Collaborating Centre for Acute Care. Available at: www.nice.org.uk/guidance/cg032

NCEPOD (2009) *Adding Insult to Injury.* London: National Confidential Enquiry into Patient Outcome and Death. Available at: www.ncepod.org.uk/2009report1/Downloads/AKI_report.pdf

NHSBT (2011) *Platelet Strategy 2011-2014: 'Delivering for Patients and Donors'.* Available at: www.nhsbt.nhs.uk/download/board_papers/july11/platelet_strategy_board_2011.pdf

NICE (2003) *Infection Control: Prevention and Control of Healthcare-Associated Infections in Primary and Community Care, CG139.* London: National Institute for Health and Clinical Excellence. Available at: www.nice.org.uk/guidance/cg139

NICE (2004) *Improving Outcomes in Head and Neck Cancer.* London: National Institute for Health and Clinical Excellence.

NICE (2007) *Acutely Ill Patients in Hospital: Recognition of and Response to Acute Illness in Adults in Hospital, CG50.* London: National Institute for Health and Clinical Excellence. Available at: www.nice.org.uk/guidance/cg50

NICE (2013a) *Intravenous Fluid Therapy in Adults in Hospital: CG174.* Manchester: National Institute for Health and Care Excellence. Available at: www.nice.org.uk/cg174

NICE (2013b) *Acute Kidney Injury: Prevention, Detection and Management of Acute Kidney Injury up to the Point of Renal Replacement Therapy:*

CG169. Manchester: National Institute for Health and Care Excellence. Available at: www.nice.org.uk/ cg169

NMC (2010) *Record Keeping: Guidance for Nurses and Midwives*. London: Nursing and Midwifery Council. Available at: www.nmc-uk.org/Documents/NMC-Publications/NMC-Record-Keeping-Guidance.pdf

NMC (2013) *Consent*. London: Nursing and Midwifery Council. Available at: www.nmc-uk.org/Nurses-and-midwives/Regulation-in-practice/Regulation-in-Practice-Topics/consent/

NMC (2015) *The Code: Standards of Conduct, Performance and Ethics for Nurses and Midwives*. London: Nursing and Midwifery Council. Available at: www.nmc-uk.org/Documents/Standards/The-code-A4-20100406.pdf

Norfolk, D. (2013) *Handbook of Transfusion Medicine*, 5th edn. London: The Stationery Office.

NPSA (2005) *Reducing the Harm Caused by Misplaced Nasogastric Feeding Tubes: Patient Safety Alert 5*. National Patient Safety Agency, London. Available at: www.nrls.npsa.nhs.uk/resources/ ?entryid45=59794.

NPSA (2007) *Protected Mealtimes Review: Findings and Recommendations Report*. London: National Patient Safety Agency. Available at: www.nrls.npsa.nhs.uk/resources/?entryid45=59806

NPSA (2009a) *10 Key Charateristics of Good Nutritional Care in Hospitals: All Staff Volunteers Have the Appropriate Skills and Competencies and Receive Regular Training: Nutrition Fact Sheet 8*. London: National Patient Safety Agency. Available at: www.nrls.npsa.nhs.uk/resources/?EntryId45=59865

NPSA (2009b) *10 Key Charateristics of Good Nutritional Care in Hospitals: Everyone Using Care Services Has a Personal Care/Support Plan and, Where Possible, Personal Input to Identify Their Nutritional Care and Fluid Needs: Nutrition Fact Sheet 7*. London: National Patient Safety Agency. Available at: www.nrls.npsa.nhs.uk/resources/?EntryId45=59865

NPSA (2010) *Early Detection of Complications after Gastrostomy: Rapid Response Report: NPSA/2010/RRR01*. London: National Patient Safety Agency. Available at: www.nrls.npsa.nhs.uk/resources/?EntryId45=73457

NPSA (2011) *Reducing the Harm Caused by Misplaced Nasogastric Feeding Tubes in Adults, Children and Infants*. London, National Patient Safety Agency. Available from: www.nrls.npsa.nhs.uk/resources/?EntryId45=129640

NPSA (2012) *Dysphagia Diet Food Texture Descriptors*. London: National Patient Safety Agency.

Nutrition Summit Stakeholder Group & DH (2007) *Improving Nutritional Care: A Joint Action Plan from the Department of Health and Nutrition Summit Stakeholders*. London: Department of Health. Available at: www.dh.gov.uk/prod_consum_dh/groups/dh_digitalassets/@dh/@en/documents/digitalasset/dh_079932.pdf (archived)

O'Connell, B., Lee, E.J. & Schiffer, C.A. (1988) The value of 10-minute posttransfusion platelet counts. *Transfusion*, 28(1), 66–67.

O'Shaughnessy, D.F., Atterbury, C., Bolton Maggs, P., et al. (2004) Guidelines for the use of fresh-frozen plasma, cryoprecipitate and cryosupernatant. *British Journal of Haematology*, 126(1), 11–28.

Oldham, J., Sinclair, L. & Hendry, C. (2009) Right patient, right blood, right care: safe transfusion practice. *British Journal of Nursing*, 18(5), 312, 314, 316–320.

Omran, M.L. & Morley, J.E. (2000) Assessment of protein energy malnutrition in older persons, part I: History, examination, body composition, and screening tools. *Nutrition*, 16(1), 50–63.

Paleri, V., Roe, J.W., Strojan, P., et al. (2014) Strategies to reduce long term post chemoradiation dysphagia in patients with head and neck cancer: an evidence based review. *Head & Neck*, I36(3), 431–443.

Pauloski, B.R., Rademaker, A.W., Logemann, J.A. et al. (2002) Swallow function and perception of dysphagia in patients with head and neck cancer. *Head Neck*, 24 (6), 555–565.

Patterson, J. & Wilson, J.A. (2011) The clinical value of dysphagia preassessment in the management of head and neck cancer patients. *Current Opinion in Otolaryngology & Head and Neck Surgery*, 19, 177–181.

Patterson, J.M., Rapley, T. & Carding, P.N. (2012) Head and neck cancer and dysphagia; caring for carers. *Psycho-Oncology*, 22(8), 1815–1820.

Payne-James, J., Grimble, G. & Silk, D. (2001) Enteral nutrition: tubes and techniques of delivery. In: Payne-James, J., Grimble, G. & Silk, D. (eds) *Artificial Nutrition Support in Clinical Practice*, 2nd edn. London: Greenwich Medical Media, pp.281–302.

Pennington, C.R. (1997) Disease and malnutrition in British hospitals. *The Proceedings of the Nutrition Society*, 56(1B), 393–407.

Pichard, C., Kyle, U.G., Morabia, A., Perrier, A., Vermeulen, B. & Unger, P. (2004) Nutritional assessment: lean body mass depletion at hospital admission is associated with an increased length of stay. *American Journal of Clinical Nutrition*, 79(4), 613–618.

Pickhardt, P.J., Rohrmann, C.A. Jr. & Cossentino, M.J. (2002) Stomal metastases complicating percutaneous endoscopic gastrostomy: CT findings and the argument for radiologic tube placement. *American Journal of Roentgenology*, 179(3), 735–739.

Pirie, E.S. & Gray, M.A. (2007) Exploring the assessors' and nurses' experience of formal assessment of clinical competency in the administration of blood components. *Nurse Education in Practice*, 7(4), 215–227.

Porth, C. (2005) *Pathophysiology: Concepts of Altered Health States*, 7th edn. Philadelphia: Lippincott Williams & Wilkins.

Powell-Tuck, J., Gosling, P., Lobo, D.N., et al. (2011) *British Consensus Guidelines on Intravenous Fluid Therapy for Adult Surgical Patients*. Available at: www.bapen.org.uk/pdfs/bapen_pubs/giftasup.pdf

PPSA (2006) *Confirming Feeding Tube Placement: Old Habits Die Hard*. Harrisburg, PA: Pennsylvania Patient Safety Authority.

Provan, D., Singer, C.R., Baglin, T. & Dokal, I. (2009) *Oxford Handbook of Clinical Haematology*, 3rd edn. Oxford: Oxford University Press.

RCN (2010) *Standards for Infusion Therapy*, 3rd edn. London: Royal College of Nursing.

Reid, J., Robb, E., Stone, D., et al. (2004) Improving the monitoring and assessment of fluid balance. *Nursing Times*, 100(20), 36–39.

Reilly, H.M. (1996) Screening for nutritional risk. *Proceedings of the Nutrition Society*, 55(3), 841–853.

Rhoda, K.M. (2011) Developing a plan of care for fluid and electrolyte management. *Support Line*, 33(3), 7–12.

Rhoda, K.M,. & Porter, M.J. (2011) Fluid and electrolyte management: putting a plan in motion. *Journal of Parenteral and Enteral Nutrition*, 35(6), 676–685.

Roe, J.W. (2005) Oropharyngeal dysphagia in advanced non-head and neck malignancy. *European Journal of Palliative Care*, 12(6), 229–233.

Roe, J.W. (2012) *Alternative Investigations*. San Diego, CA: Plural.

Roe, J.W. & Ashforth, K.M. (2011) Prophylactic swallowing exercises for patients receiving radiotherapy for head and neck cancer. *Current Opinion in Otolaryngology & Head and Neck Surgery*, 19(3), 144–149.

Roe, J.W., Leslie, P. & Drinnan, M.J. (2007) Oropharyngeal dysphagia: the experience of patients with non-head and neck cancers receiving specialist palliative care. *Palliative Medicine*, 21(7), 567–574.

Royal College of Speech and Language Therapists (2006) *Communicating Quality 3*. London: Royal College of Speech and Language Therapists.

SaBTO (2009) *Summary of the Seventh Meeting*. Available at: http://webarchive.nationalarchives.gov.uk/+/www.dh.gov.uk/ab/SaBTO/DH_089412?PageOperation=email

SaBTO (2011) *Guidance for Clinical Staff to Support Patient Consent for Blood Transfusion, Advisory Committee on the Safety of Blood, Tissues and Organs*. Available at: http://www.transfusionguidelines.org.uk/transfusion-practice/consent-for-blood-transfusion-1

Samuels, R. & Chadwick, D.D. (2006) Predictors of asphyxiation risk in adults with intellectual disabilities and dysphagia. *Journal of Intellectual Disability Research*, 50(Pt 5), 362–370.

Scales, K. & Pilsworth, J. (2008) The importance of fluid balance in clinical practice. *Nursing Standard*, 22(47), 50–57; quiz 58, 60.

Sekhon, S.S. & Roy, V. (2006) Thrombocytopenia in adults: a practical approach to evaluation and management. *Southern Medical Journal*, 99(5), 491–498; quiz 499–500, 533.

Shaw, C. (2011) *Nutrition and Palliative Care*. Oxford: John Wiley & Sons.

Shaw, V. & Lawson, M. (2007) Nutritional assessment, dietary requirements and feed supplementation. In: Shaw, V. & Lawson, M. (eds) *Clinical Paediatric Dietetics*, 3rd edn. Oxford: Blackwell Publishing, pp.3–20.

Shepherd, A. (2011) Measuring and managing fluid balance. *Nursing Times*, 107(28), 12–16.

Sheppard, M. & Wright, M.M. (2006) *Principles and Practice of High Dependency Nursing*, 2nd edn. Edinburgh: Bailliere Tindall.

SHOT (2005) *Annual Report 2005*. London: Serious Hazards of Transfusion. Available at: www.shotuk.org/wp-content/uploads/2010/03/SHOT-report-2005.pdf

SHOT (2008) *Annual report 2008*. London: Serious Hazards of Transfusion. Available at: http://www.shotuk.org/wp-content/uploads/2010/03/SHOT-Report-2008.pdf

SHOT (2010) *Annual SHOT report 2010*. London: Serious Hazards of Transfusion. Available at: http://www.shotuk.org/wp-content/uploads/2012/07/SHOT-ANNUAL-REPORT_FinalWebVersionBookmarked_2012_06_22.pdf

SHOT (2011a) *Annual SHOT Report 2011*. London: Serious Hazards of Transfusion. Available at: www.shotuk.org/wp-content/uploads/2012/07/SHOT-ANNUAL-REPORT_FinalWebVersionBookmarked_2012_06_22.pdf

SHOT (2011b) Definitions of current categories and what to report. London: Serious Hazards of transfusion. Available at: www.shotuk.org

Slichter, S.J., Kaufman, R.M., Assmann, S.F., et al. (2010) Dose of prophylactic platelet transfusions and prevention of hemorrhage. *New England Journal of Medicine*, 362(7), 600–613.

Smith Hammond, C. (2008) Cough and aspiration of food and liquids due to oral pharyngeal dysphagia. *Lung*, 186 (Suppl 1), S35–S40.

SNBTS (2004) *Better Blood Transfusion Level 1: Safe Transfusion Practice : Self-Directed Learning Pack*. Edinburgh: Effective Use of Blood Group, Scottish National Blood Transfusion Service. Available at: http://www.learnbloodtransfusion.org.uk/

Sorkin, J.D., Muller, D.C. & Andres, R. (1999) Longitudinal change in height of men and women: implications for interpretation of the body mass index: the Baltimore longitudinal study of aging. *American Journal of Epidemiology*, 150(9), 969–977.

Sumnall, R. (2007) Fluid management and diuretic therapy in acute renal failure. *Nursing in Critical Care*, 12(1), 27–33.

Tang, V.C. & Lee, E.W. (2010) Fluid balance chart: do we understand it. *Clinical Risk*, 16, 10–13.

Thibault, R., Genton, L. & Pichard, C. (2012) Body composition: why, when and for who? *Clinical Nutrition*, 31(4), 435–447.

Thomas, B. & Bishop, J. (2007) *Manual of Dietetic Practice*, 4th edn. Oxford: Blackwell Publishing.

Thompson, J. (2005) Intra-operative cell salvage. In: Thomas, D., Thompson, J. & Ridler, B. (eds) *A Manual for Blood Conservation*. Harley, Shropshire: Tfm Publishing Ltd, pp.75.

Thomsen, G., Bezdjian, L., Rodriguez, L. & Hopkins, R.O. (2012) Clinical outcomes of a furosemide infusion protocol in edematous patients in the intensive care unit. *Critical Care Nurse*, 32(6), 25–34.

Thorson, M.A., Bliss, D.Z. & Savik, K. (2008) Re-examination of risk factors for non-*Clostridium difficile*-associated diarrhoea in hospitalized patients. *Journal of Advanced Nursing*, 62(3), 354–364.

Todorovic, V.E. & Micklewright, A. (2011) *A Pocket Guide to Clinical Nutrition*, 4th edn. London: Parenteral and Enteral Nutrition Group (PENG) of the British Dietetic Association.

Tolich, D.J. (2008) Alternatives to blood transfusion. *Journal of Infusion Nursing*, 31(1), 46–51.

Tortora, G.J. & Derrickson, B.H (2011) *Principles of Anatomy and Physiology*, 13th edn. Hoboken, NJ: John Wiley & Sons.

Treacher, D. (2009) Acute heart failure. In: Bersten, A.D. & Soni, N. (eds) *Oh's Intensive Care Manual*, 6th edn. Maryland Heights, MO: Elsevier, pp.259–274.

UK Blood Services (2007) *Handbook of Transfusion Medicine*, 4th edn. Available at: www.transfusionguidelines.org.uk

Vamvakas, E.C. (1999) Risk of transmission of Creutzfeldt-Jakob disease by transfusion of blood, plasma, and plasma derivatives. *Journal of Clinical Apheresis*, 14(3), 135–143.

Weimann, A., Braga, M., Harsanyi, L., et al. (2006) ESPEN guidelines on enteral nutrition: surgery including organ transplantation. *Clinical Nutrition*, 25(2), 224–244.

Weinstein, S.M. & Plumer, A.L. (2007) *Plumer's Principles & Practice of Intravenous Therapy*, 8th edn. Philadelphia: Lippincott Williams & Wilkins.

Welch, K. (2010) Fluid balance. *Learning Disability Practice*, 13(6), 33–38.

WHO (2011) *Global Forum for Blood Safety: Patient Blood Management*. 14–15 March 2011, Dubai, UAE: World Health Organization. Available at: www.who.int/bloodsafety/events/gfbs_01_pbm_concept_paper.pdf

Wilkinson, J. & Wilkinson, C. (2001) Administration of blood transfusions to adults in general hospital settings: a review of the literature. *Journal of Clinical Nursing*, 10(2), 161–170.

Williamson, L.M., Lowe, S., Love, E., et al. (1999) *Serious hazards of transfusion*, SHOT, Manchester. Available at: www.shotuk.org/wp-content/uploads/2010/04/SHOT-Report-1997-98.pdf

Wright, L., Cotter, D. & Hickson, M. (2008) The effectiveness of targeted feeding assistance to improve the nutritional intake of elderly dysphagic patients in hospital. *Journal of Human Nutrition and Dietetics*, 21(6), 555–562.

Zwaginga, J.J. & van Ham, M. (2013) Essential immunology for transfusion medicine. In: Murphy, M., Pamphilon, D. & Heddle, N. (eds) *Practical Transfusion Medicine*, 4th edn. Oxford: John Wiley & Sons.

Answers

Learning Activity 7.1 Scenario: Assessing fluid status

You have been asked to assess a 79-year-old woman who has just been admitted to the ward following a fall at home. You, and other members of the team, are concerned that she may be dehydrated.

- What particular questions can you ask to help determine her fluid status? Consider fluid intake, thirst, unintentional weight loss, urine output, bowels.
- When carrying out her vital signs, what may indicate dehydration and why? Low blood pressure, raised heart rate with peripheral pulse sometimes difficult to palpate, raised respiratory rate (Table 7.3 provides rationale for these changes).
- Which blood results may be abnormal, indicating dehydration? Serum electrolytes: sodium raised, potassium may be lower if the patient has diarrhoea or vomiting, decreased urea, creatinine initially normal but may rise over time.
- Are there any other clinical indications of dehydration that you can think of? Reduced skin turgor, dry conjunctiva, sunken eyeballs, mucous membranes pale.

Learning Activity 7.2 Learning in practice: Fluid balance charts

Take a look at the fluid balance charts in use within your clinical area.

- How accurately are the charts completed?
- Can you think of any strategies to improve their accuracy? Measure the volumes of cups/glasses used on the ward. Ensure a measuring container is always available to avoid statements such as 'out to toilet'.

Learning Activity 7.3 Case study: Assessing nutritional status

John Goody is a 44-year-old man with a history of Crohn's disease. He has just been admitted for bowel surgery following worsening of his GI symptoms and significant weight loss over the last 4–5 months. John reports that 6 months ago he weighed 12st 7lb (79.4 kg). He has just been weighed on admission today and he now weighs 68 kg (10st 10lb). His height is 1.88 m (6ft 2in). On examination his clothing appears to be very loose fitting. He tells you that he has lost so much weight that his wedding ring falls off his finger now and he notices some of his bones are sticking out more than they used to. His face appears drawn and he seems to be a little slow in responding to questions.

1. Using the formula provided within this section, calculate John's current body mass index (BMI).
   - $68 / (1.88)^2 = 19.2$
2. Now calculate his percentage weight loss.
   - $79.4 - 68 / 79.4 = 14.4\%$
3. Based on your calculations, is John malnourished?
   - Yes.
4. What other signs/symptoms of malnourishment does John have?
   - Loose fitting clothes, jewellery, wasted appearance, lethargy.

Learning Activity 7.6 Scenario: Minor transfusion reaction

You have been asked to perform a set of observations on a patient who is receiving a blood transfusion (red blood cells). You discover that his temperature has risen from 36.2°C to 37.3°C and his pulse has risen from 84 to 98 bpm.

What would you do next?

- Stop the transfusion and inform the nurse in charge and the responsible medical team.
- Confirm the patient's identity and re-check their details against the product compatibility label.
- Consider antipyretic agents for mild fever.
- In consultation with the nursing and medical teams, it may be possible to continue with the transfusion at a reduced rate once the patient's symptoms are controlled; however, it may be necessary to increase the frequency of observations.

Now Test Yourself What have you learnt?

1 The human body is made up of approximately what proportion of water?
A 50%
B 60%
C 70%
D 80%

2 Concentration of electrolytes within the body vary depending on the compartment within which they are contained. Extracellular fluid has a high concentration of which of the following?
A Sodium
B Potassium
C Chloride
D Magnesium

3 In order to avoid dehydration or fluid overload when administering maintenance intravenous fluids they should be:
A Hypertonic
B Hypotonic
C Isotonic
D All of the above may be used

4 Which of the following is NOT a clinical sign of fluid overload?
A Bounding pulse
B Decreased blood pressure
C Increased respiratory rate
D Decreased oxygen saturations

5 Nationally, what percentage of patients admitted to hospital are at risk of malnutrition?
A 8%
B 18%
C 28%
D 38%

6 How can patients who need assistance at mealtimes be identified?
A A red sticker
B A colour serviette
C A red tray
D Any of the above

7 What can happen if dysphagia is not managed appropriately? List four possible consequences.
For example: malnutrition, weight loss, dehydration, aspiration, aspiration pneumonia, low mood.

8 People with blood group A are able to receive blood from the following:
A Group A only
B Groups AB or B
C Groups A or O
D Groups A, B or O

9 Errors in the requesting, collection and administration of blood components lead to significant risks for patients. In the SHOT report (2011) what proportion of adverse events were reportedly caused by human error?
A One-quarter
B One-third
C Half
D Two-thirds

10 The three key principles that underpin each stage of the blood component transfusion process are:
A Patient identification, documentation, education
B Patient consent, patient identification, documentation
C Patient identification, documentation, communication
D Documentation, communication, patient consent

Patient comfort and end-of-life care

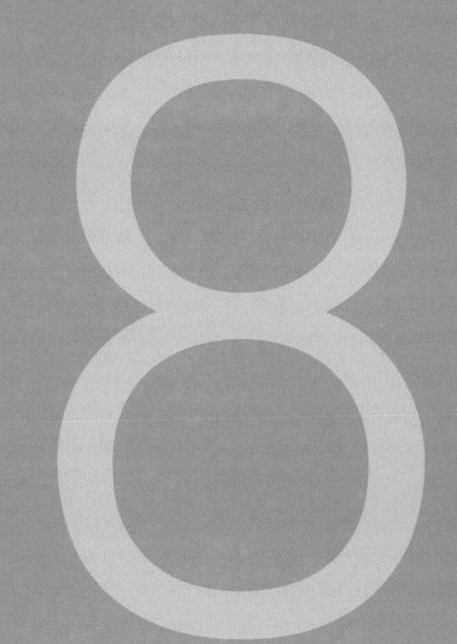

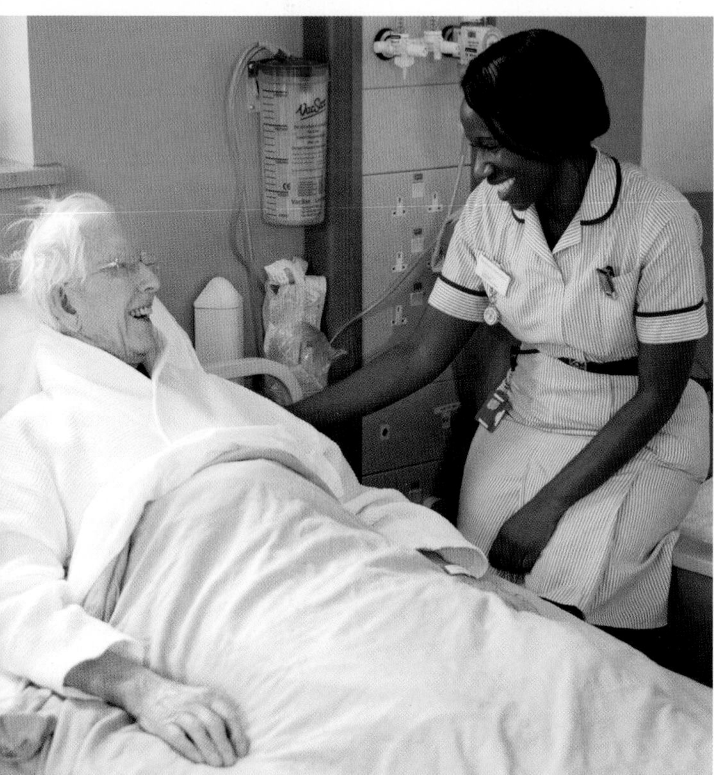

By reading this chapter and undertaking the learning activities within it, you should be able to:

1 Gain insight and understanding about the range of procedures involved in achieving patient comfort.

2 Demonstrate an appreciation of comfort meaning different things to different patients.

3 Identify the different aspects of any procedure that should be considered in order to ensure patient comfort.

4 Identify specific skills, such as observation and non-verbal communication, that are required to address the issue of comfort in vulnerable patients, such as those with dementia or learning difficulties.

Procedure guidelines

The Royal Marsden Manual of Clinical Nursing Procedures: Student Edition, Ninth Edition. Edited by Lisa Dougherty, Sara Lister and Alexandra West-Oram

Overview

The aim of this chapter is to present the many varied procedures that contribute towards the comfort of patients at all times. This ranges from the very specific procedures involved in pain management to those that promote comfort from a wider perspective, such as personal hygiene and end-of-life care.

In ensuring patient comfort, it is necessary to consider aspects of any procedure from the pre-planning stage to the return of the patient to their pre-procedure position.

Comfort will mean different things to different patients. It may involve being in a relaxed state of tolerable pain, disappointment or perhaps satisfaction or physical well-being provided by another person. For the nurse, aspects of care to be considered include discussions prior to undertaking the procedure, gaining consent, ensuring pain control and maintaining privacy and dignity, offering mouthcare as well as paying attention to the patient's immediate environment.

For some patients, for instance those with dementia or learning disabilities, addressing the issue of patient comfort may rely on other skills such as observation, non-verbal communication or working closely with family and carers to help identify and meet the patient's needs.

Personal hygiene

DEFINITION

Maintaining levels of good personal hygiene is essential for all patients during their stay in hospital (Massa 2010). Hygiene is the science of health and its maintenance. Personal hygiene is the self-care by which people attend to such functions as bathing, toileting, general body hygiene and grooming. Hygiene is a highly personal matter determined by individual values and practices. It involves care of the skin, hair, nails, teeth, oral and nasal cavities, eyes, ears, and perianal- and perineal-genital areas (Berman et al. 2010).

ANATOMY AND PHYSIOLOGY

Skin

Being the largest organ of the body, maintaining the skin's integrity is essential to the prevention of infection and the promotion of both physical and psychological health. The skin has several functions.

- Regulation of temperature.
- Physical and immunological protection.
- Excretion and preservation of water balance.
- Sensory perception.
- Communication of feelings.
- Identity, self-perception and body image (Burr and Penzer 2005).

The skin is made up of three layers: epidermis, dermis and deep subcutaneous layer (Figure 8.1).

Epidermis

The epidermis is the outer coating of the skin and contains no blood vessels or nerve endings. The cells on the surface are gradually shed and replaced by new cells which have developed from the deeper layers; this process takes approximately 28 days. The epidermis has hairs, sweat glands and the ducts of sebaceous glands passing through it. It provides an efficient natural barrier (Burr and Penzer 2005).

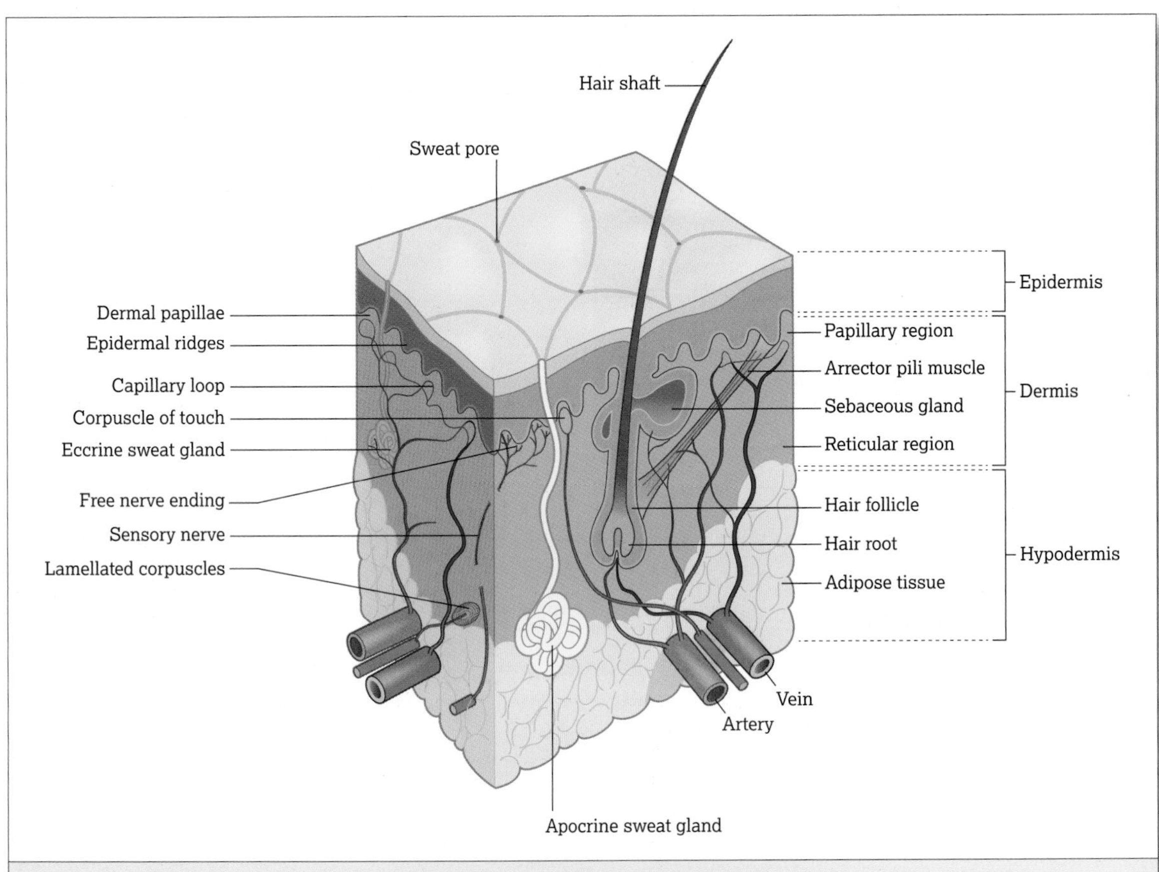

Figure 8.1 **Skin and subcutaneous layer.** ***Source:*** Peate et al. (2014). **Reproduced with permission from John Wiley & Sons.**

Dermis

The dermis is the thicker layer which contains blood and lymph vessels, nerve fibres, sweat and sebaceous glands. It is made up of white fibrous tissue and yellow elastic fibres which give the skin its toughness and elasticity. It provides the epidermis with structural and nutritional support (Holloway and Jones 2005).

Subcutaneous layer

The subcutaneous layer contains the deep fat cells (areolar and adipose tissue) and provides heat regulation for the body. It is also the support structure for the outer layers of the skin (Tortora and Derrickson 2011). Maintaining skin integrity, through good personal hygiene, will allow this complex system to provide an efficient natural barrier to the external environment.

It is important to remember that the skin is a changing organ, affected by internal and external factors, temperature, air humidity and age (Burr and Penzer 2005). It has great ability to adapt to changes in the environment and stimuli but will be affected by ill health and immobility (McLoughlin 2005). Its integrity, continuity and cleanliness are essential to maintaining its physiological functions.

The ageing process can adversely affect the skin structure. Skin tissue becomes thin and less elastic and resistant to trauma and shearing forces. The blood supply is reduced as cells are replaced more slowly, which adversely affects healing. Transmission of stimuli from sensory receptors slows and can lead to damage. The production of natural oils declines and can lead to dry skin which increases the risk of infection and tissue breakdown (Penzer and Finch 2001). Hence extra care should be taken when washing and drying elderly patients; nursing interventions can protect and restore the skin's natural barrier (Bryant and Rolstad 2001).

EVIDENCE-BASED APPROACHES

Personal cleanliness is a fundamental value in society. Often, when patients become unwell they depend on nurses to assist them with meeting their personal hygiene needs. When this occurs, it is important that the nurse observes and assesses the patient's needs on an individual basis.

Some patients may have a long-term need for personal care support, such as those with dementia or a severe learning disability; their family and carers will know them best and are best placed to advise you on how best to provide such personal care.

Hygiene is a personal issue and everyone will have their own individual requirements and standards of cleanliness.The nurse should not impose his or her own standards of cleanliness on the patient or even assume that theirs will match those of the patient. Within the assessment, the patient's religious and cultural beliefs should be taken into account and incorporated into care. When the patient has any degree of cognitive impairment, the approach taken to providing any personal care must consider how the patient is likely to experience that care. For example, a patient who has dementia may not know who you are or what you are doing and so may need to be orientated and talked through the process to prevent them from becoming distressed. Personal hygiene is individual to that person and is also based on family influences, peer groups, economic and social factors (Berman et al. 2010).

In Western culture, privacy is of the utmost importance and considered to be a basic human right. In addition, in some religions like Islam, modesty is crucial and can be challenging to manage in the hospital setting (Hollins 2009). Patients may feel a great deal of embarrassment having to depend on another person to help them with an extremely private act. It is therefore surprising that so little reference is made to this in the literature. However, in the clinical situation the best person to discuss this with is the patient, exploring with them how they want their hygiene needs met and identifying any specific requests they may have related to their culture or religion (Pegram et al. 2007).

Florence Nightingale (1859) first noted the importance of good personal hygiene and the essential role nurses have in maintaining this, to prevent infection and increase well-being. During the delivery of personal hygiene care, the nurse is able to demonstrate a wide range of skills such as assessment, communication, observation and caring for the patient. Within the activity, opportunities may arise for the patient to discuss issues, concerns or fears that they may have regarding admission, treatment, discharge planning or prognosis (Burns and Day 2012). This can be the most significant social interaction of the day for the patient, as the nurse develops a deeper understanding of the patient's personality and needs, providing a personal bond between the nurse and patient (Massa 2010). This relationship offers the nurse an opportunity to encourage the patient to reclaim autonomy and independence within this care need through participation, which can increase patients' feelings of self-worth and dignity.

Delegating personal hygiene to a junior member of the team or a healthcare assistant may mean that vital information about the patients may be missed. It is important that nurses recognize their personal accountability for the care that is provided, but also for delegating care to an appropriate person (RCN 2010). It is crucial that health professionals share their knowledge and any changes identified during procedures; verbal handover and documentation are good tools for this. The world of nursing is ever changing, and there is a risk that activities such as attending to the personal hygiene of patients may become devalued or just another routine (Castledine 2005, Voegeli 2008). The literature supports the enhanced quality of care for patients, when hygiene needs are attended to by qualified/experienced practitioners. Personal hygiene is considered part of the essence of care that nurses should never treat as ritualistic.

Principles of care

Skin care is particularly important to prevent the colonization of Gram-positive and -negative micro-organisms on the skin, which lead to healthcare-associated infection (Parker 2004). By implementing simple personal hygiene measures, the risk of infection can be reduced.

An initial assessment of the skin using observational skills is essential to ascertain the skin's general condition, colour, texture, smell and temperature (Penzer and Finch 2001). Factors that may influence the appearance of the skin are as follows.

- *Nutritional and hydration state*: imbalances will cause loss of elasticity and drying of the skin. Oedema will cause stretching and thinning of the skin (Potter and Perry 2003).
- *Incontinence*: the presence of urine and/or faeces on the skin increases the normal pH of 4.0–5.5 and makes the skin wet, which increases the risk of tissue breakdown and infection (Ersser et al. 2005).
- *Age, health and mobility status*: for example, the presence of pressure ulcers (Smoker 1999, Stockton and Flynn 2009).
- *Treatment therapies*: for example, radiotherapy (skin may become moist and cracked), chemotherapy (some cytotoxic agents such as methotrexate can cause erythematous rashes), and continuous infusions of 5-fluorouracil (5-FU) can cause a condition called palmar-plantar erythrodysaesthesia syndrome, which presents with cracking and epidermal sloughing of the palms and soles (Lokich and Moore 1984). A low platelet count can lead to an increased risk of bruising and a decrease in the white blood cells can influence the rate of healing. Steroids may cause the skin to become papery and fragile.
- *Any concurrent conditions*: for example, eczema, psoriasis, diabetes or stress, can affect the ability of skin to maintain its integrity (Holloway and Jones 2005).

Box 8.1 lists the specific considerations for skin care.

Methods of perineal/perianal care

Meticulous care with the perineal/perianal areas areas is vital, especially for those people who may be prone to infection. Problems can arise from treatment modalities; radiotherapy, for example, can cause fistulas, diarrhoea, constipation and urinary

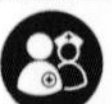

Box 8.1 **Specific considerations for skin care**

- Frail and papery skin should prompt the nurse to take extra care in the bathing process. Patients need to be involved in writing their care plans, ensuring that correct and/or preferred lotions are used; this will maintain the integrity of the skin and prevent the skin from being compromised.
- Areas of red skin. If redness is noted, wound prevention measures need to be implemented to prevent sores and ulcers from developing. These include good pressure-relieving positioning and repositioning and the use of barrier products in the form of creams, ointments and films (Joseph and Clifton 2013).
- Open wounds. When open wounds are present, such as pressure ulcers, abrasions or cuts, preventive measures such as pressure-relieving mattresses should be used to prevent further breakdown (Philips and Buttery 2009) and dressings such as hydrocolloids used where appropriate to promote wound healing (Bouza et al. 2005).
- Intravenous devices and drains. Frequently, patients have intravenous devices and wound drains inserted as part of their therapy and these should be handled with care to prevent the introduction of infection or the 'pulling' of the tubes.

tract infections. Vigilance with cleanliness can prevent some of these problems or reduce their severity. Whenever possible, patients should be encouraged and assisted to perform this care themselves (Downey and Lloyd 2008). If a nurse is performing the care of this area, it is important that informed consent is sought, where possible, and privacy maintained as the patient may be embarrassed or humiliated. Nurse and patient should discuss this procedure together, ensuring that the patient gives agreement to care (NMC 2013).

Ideally, perineal hygiene should be attended to after the general bath or, at the very least, the water and wipes should be changed and cleaned once utilized due to the large colonies of bacteria that tend to live in or around this area (Gooch 1989, Gould 1994). It is generally acknowledged that soap and lotions administered incorrectly to the perineum/perianal area can cause irritation and infection (Ersser et al. 2005, Holloway and Jones 2005).

Methods of hair care

The way a person feels is often related to their appearance, and hair condition and style are usually pertinent to this. Hair care can be complex and so it should be planned and carried out according to the patient's personal preferences.

Washing the hair of a bed-bound patient can be challenging, but there are several ways to manage this as follows.

- Using a special bed tray water aid.
- Using an inflatable shampoo basin.
- Using a dry or no rinse shampoo.
- Using a no rinse shampoo cap (Schiff 2001).

The patient's condition must always be assessed before performing this task as it would not be appropriate for patients with head and neck or spinal injuries. Shampooing frequency depends on the patient's well-being and their hair condition. Referral to a hairdresser may be appropriate.

Grooming the hair provides an ideal opportunity to observe for dandruff, psoriasis, flaky skin and head lice. Head lice are extremely infectious so it is imperative to treat the hair with a medicated shampoo as soon as possible. Hospital policy/protocol should be followed regarding the disposal of infected linen. Towel drying of hair should occur and hairdryers can be used with the consent of the patient (NMC 2013). However, use of a hairdryer may not be appropriate if the patient has had recent alopecia (loss of hair). Hairdryers should be checked for safety in accordance with local policy. Care of the beard and moustache is also important. Excess food can often become lodged here so regular grooming is essential for hygiene and comfort purposes. Beard trimmers can be used as appropriate.

Methods for care of the nails and feet

The feet and nails require special care in order to avoid pain and infection. Poor toe nail condition can affect mobility and compromise independence which can increase length of hospital stay (Dingwall 2010). Finger and toe nails should be kept short and neat; nail clippers are recommended for the trimming of nails and emery boards for filing to prevent jagged edges (Malkin and Berridge 2009). Patients with visual impairment or dexterity problems and those with learning disabilities may require assistance with the trimming and filing of nails. Note that in many healthcare settings, toe nail trimming requires a chiropodist or is contraindicated for patients with diabetes, toe infections or peripheral vascular disease, unless performed by a podiatrist (Malkin and Berridge 2009).

Special attention should be paid to cleaning the feet and in between the toes to avoid any fungal infection (Geraghty 2005). Fungal infections of the skin can be subdivided into two distinct categories: dermatophytes (moulds) and *Candida* (yeasts). A fungal infection occurs where moulds or yeasts begin to live on the keratin of the host individual. This can include the keratin of the nail plate, leading to onycomycosis (fungal nail infection). The term 'athlete's foot', caused by poor foot hygiene associated with excess sweating, infrequent changes of shoes and ineffective washing, is a common misnomer for a fungal foot infection. However, it is a precursor to infection as it provides the ideal environment for dermatophytes and yeasts. In general, fungal infections present as red, itchy, dry and flaky areas of skin and, depending on location, there may also be associated maceration and fissuring. Onycomycosis presents as thickened, discoloured nails which are also crumbly, elevated from the nail bed and malodorous (Roberts and Holdich 2012). Powders and creams are available that help with the treatment of infections and odour management, for example miconazole nitrate 2% for fungal infections (BNF 2014).

Diabetic footcare

Chronic diseases such as diabetes and the long-term use of steroids can result in problems such as pressure ulcers, breakdown of skin integrity and delays in healing.

A patient's whole body is affected by diabetes but in particular, this chronic disease can cause foot complications. Damage to the nerves and blood supply to the feet causes lack of sensation and ischaemia. These problems can lead to diabetic foot ulceration which, if left untreated, can result in amputation or even death (Holt 2013).

The Diabetes UK (2012) campaign 'Putting Feet First' highlights the increasing number of amputations caused by diabetes and calls for better awareness and improved standards of care for people with the disease. The importance of recognizing and acting on a diabetic foot ulcer cannot be overestimated. For nurses, it is not a case of having to know everything, but rather knowing who to call and when that can make the difference (Moakes 2012).

Guidelines published by the National Institute for Health and Clinical Excellence (NICE 2004a) require that all people with diabetes should have an annual foot examination. As a minimum, this should include:

- testing of foot sensation using a 10 g monofilament or vibration test. Without the patient looking, pressure from a monofilament or vibration fork is applied to at least five different areas on the sole of the foot. Decreased sensation at any of the sites tested could be an indication of neuropathy
- palpation of foot pulses
- inspection of any foot deformity and footwear.

Based on the findings of the foot examination, the person would then be classified as low risk, increased risk, high risk or ulcerated foot (Table 8.1). By having this information, patients can be given the appropriate care and screening to avoid any acute diabetic foot episodes (Holt 2013).

When a patient with diabetes has a foot with complications such as sensory neuropathy and poorblood supply, it can be easily damaged. Even a small graze or bruise can cause a foot ulcer to develop. Some causes of foot ulceration are:

- animal scratches
- corn/verruca treatment containing salicylic acid
- footwear
- foreign body in shoe
- hot water bottle used in bed
- ill-fitting hosiery, for example, sock seams
- elastic on stockings
- resting feet on or near a heater or radiator
- scald from bath water (Moakes 2012).

The formation of a foot ulcer is multifactorial.The underlying features of diabetes predispose the person to ulceration. Any altered sensation in the foot may impair recognition of injury to the skin, particularly in individuals who are unable to cut their toe nails adequately, and a mycotic nail may damage the skin of an adjacent toe or the nail bed of the affected toe leading to subungual ulceration. Older people with diabetes may suffer from age-related changes to vision which makes nail care more difficult; bending down to carry out self-checks of the foot may be hampered by reduced mobility, being overweight and loss of dexterity (Roberts and Holdich 2012). Some risk factors for diabetic foot ulcers are as follows.

- Build-up of callus.
- Foot deformity.
- Peripheral arterial disease.
- Peripheral neuropathy.
- Previous amputation.
- Previous ulceration.
- Problems with vision and/or mobility (Drury and Gatling 2005).

Daily foot care checks should be undertaken either by the person with diabetes or a relative/carer and are as follows.

- Check top of foot, bottom of foot, tips of toes, between toes and back of heels.
- Be aware of fragile skin, especially in those who are very old, and of pressure areas if the person is spending a lot of time in one position, for example, in bed or seated.
- Check for pain, but remember absence of pain in those with neuropathy does not mean that all is well.
- Check for foreign bodies in shoes, slippers or sandals.
- Apply emollient all over feet but not in between toes because this may predispose to fungal infection as this is already a moist and warm area.
- Refer for specialist help if needed (Moakes 2012).

When the patient is in a healthcare setting, these checks can be undertaken by a competent healthcare professional. By performing these checks and by touching the feet when applying emollient, problems are much more likely to be detected and treated promptly.

Table 8.1 **Level of risk for developing foot ulcers**

Risk level	Nursing action
Low risk Normal circulation, pulses palpable, normal sensation (feeling in the feet)	Plan care with patient Education and advice on maintaining foot health Assess foot health as part of daily care
Increased risk Evidence of neuropathy, poor or absent pulses	Refer to footcare team or podiatrist Evaluate footwear Offer advice on footcare Assess foot health as part of daily care
High risk Evidence of neuropathy, absent pulses, skin changes, history of previous ulcers	Refer to footcare team or podiatrist Evaluate footwear Assess foot health as part of daily care Perform footcare as part of daily care
Foot ulcerated	Refer to specialist as an emergency and follow planned care accordingly Evaluate and reassess the ulcer on a daily basis

Source: Adapted from NICE (2008).

Methods for care of the ears and nose

Lack of attention to cleaning the ears and nose can lead to impairment of the senses. Usually these small organs require minimal care but observation for a build-up of wax in the ears and deposits in the nose is essential to maintain patency. The outer ear can be cleaned with cotton wool or gauze and warm water (Alexander et al. 2007).

Patients undergoing enteral feeding and/or oxygen therapy should have regular nasal care to avoid excessive drying, excoriation of the delicate air passages and skin breakdown. Gentle cleaning of the nasal mucosa with cotton wool/gauze and water is recommended. Coating the area with a thin water-based lubricant to prevent discomfort can be beneficial, but petroleum jelly is not recommended as a nasal skin barrier when oxygen therapy is in progress as it is highly flammable. These interventions will remove debris and maintain a moist environment (Geraghty 2005).

Patients who have piercing to the ears or nose will require cleaning of the holes to avoid the risk of infection. Gently cleaning around the pierced area with cotton wool/gauze and warm water and then towel drying is recommended. Observe for inflammation or oozing; if this occurs, inform the patient and doctor and seek permission from the patient to remove the device.

PRE-PROCEDURAL CONSIDERATIONS

Non-pharmacological support

Soap

Persistent use of some soaps can alter the pH of the skin and remove the natural oils, leading to drying and cracking (Bryant and Rolstad 2001, Smoker 1999), creating an ideal environment for bacteria to multiply (Holloway and Jones 2005). According to Ersser et al. (2005), patients with dry skin have a 2.5-fold greater likelihood of skin breakdown. Care should be taken with skinfolds and crevices, paying particular attention to thorough drying of the areas and observing for any breaks in the skin. It is recommended that the skin is patted and not rubbed, to reduce damage caused by friction (Ersser et al. 2005).

Emollient therapy

Current evidence recommends a move away from traditional washing using soap and water, and recent research demonstrates that surfactants found in soap are irritant to the skin (Voegeli 2008). Penzer and Finch (2001) and Burr and Penzer (2005) recommend the use of emollient therapy for washing and moisturizing to seal the skin. In a literature review of hygiene practices, the use of soap and water remained common practice but several studies suggest that skin cleansers, for example emollient creams, followed by moisturizing may be less likely to disrupt the skin barrier and have a therapeutic benefit (Ersser et al. 2005). These products allow the patient to have a more active role in their own care, as the products can be left within reach and the patient can initiate the activity without the need to access running water (Collins and Hampton 2003).

Washbowls

Conventional plastic washbowls can harbour bacteria and fungi if they are not cleaned and dried effectively. Research indicates that reusable washbowls, washcloths and water can all pose a serious risk of cross-infection (Johnson et al. 2009, Marchaim et al. 2011). Johnson et al. (2009) also highlight that inadequate storage of reusable washbowls can contribute to the presence of microbial biofilms and place patients at risk of cross-infection. A 2007 study at Salford Royal Hospital showed that when a disposable washbowl was introduced alongside other measures, it helped to reduce the number of cases of *C. difficile* infection by 56% over a 5-month period (Power et al. 2010). Many organizations now utilize single-use maceratable pulp washbowls.

Prepackaged cloths

Bacteria exist in hospital water supplies and hospital staff can transmit bacteria both into and via water. In addition, reusable washcloths can spread harmful bacteria when they are transferred to the basin and returned to the patient. Due to the risk of transmission of Pseudomonas aeruginosa, the DH (2013b) suggests that organizations should consider utilizing single-use wipes when patients are being cared for in augmented specialized care areas, such as:

- those who are severely immunosuppressed because of disease or treatment
- those cared for in units where organ support is necessary, e.g. critical care
- those who have extensive breaches in their dermal integrity and require contact with water as part of their continuing care, e.g. burns units.

Prepackaged cloths impregnated with cleanser and moisturizers are a cost-effective and evidence-based alternative to soap and water (Larson et al. 2004, Sheppard and Brenner 2000). These wipes are designed for single use straight from the packet and the cleansers and emollients delivered via the wipe are formulated to nourish and hydrate the skin without the need for rinsing and drying after use. To enhance patient comfort, the wipes can be warmed before use. Warming must take place in a dedicated heating unit. A specially designed warming cabinet is available which stores multiple packets at the correct temperature to ensure they are ready for use straight from the warmer (Massa 2010).

Cultural and religious factors

The nurse must respect and consider the patient's cultural and religious factors, while maintaining privacy and dignity at all times; for example, some people prefer to sit under running water rather than sitting in a bath (Hollins 2009). Some religions do not allow hair washing or brushing, while others may require the hair to be covered by a turban. Similarly, in some countries facial hair is significant and should never be removed without the patient's/relatives' consent. Always establish any preferences before beginning care (Hollins 2009) (Box 8.2).

Clothing

Effort should be made to encourage and empower patients to dress in their own clothing during the day, where possible, and in their own nightwear to sleep. This increases independence and well-being, encourages normality and promotes dignity. If the patient is too unwell or does not have their own clothing, hospital provision should be made available to protect their modesty (Wilson 2006).

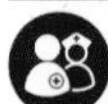

Box 8.2 **Religion-specific considerations related to personal hygiene**

- Those following *Islam* must perform ablution (*wudhu*, to use the Islamic term) before the daily prayer, which is the formal washing of the face, hands and forearms, and so on. One of the criteria for cleanliness is washing after the use of the lavatory. Any traces of urine or faeces must be eliminated by washing with running water, at least. If a bedpan or commode is used, fresh water must be provided for cleansing. The use of toilet tissues for cleaning is not sufficient. With such emphasis on washing and personal hygiene, adhering to the practical teaching of Islam on washing would enhance personal hygiene for the individual and therefore reduce the chance of disease and sickness individually and subsequently for the whole society.
- *Hindus* also place importance on washing before prayer; they believe the left hand should dominate in this process and therefore do not eat with the left hand as it is deemed unclean.
- *Sikhs* place great importance on not shaving or cutting hair, choosing to comb their hair twice a day and washing it regularly. Male Sikhs wear their hair underneath a turban as a sign of respect for God.

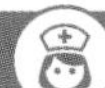

Learning Activity 8.1

Scenario: Bathing a patient

You have been asked to wash a 78-year-old male patient with limited mobility.

What factors should you take into account when considering how to meet his hygiene needs?

See the end of the chapter for the answers.

Bedbathing

A bedbath is not the most effective way of washing patients, and wherever possible they should be encouraged and supported to shower or bathe. However, a bedbath can be performed if it is the only way to meet the patient's hygiene needs (Dingwall 2010).

Before commencing this procedure, read the patient's care plan, manual handling documentation and risk assessment to gain knowledge of safe practice. Prior to each part of the procedure, explain and obtain verbal agreement from the patient (NMC 2013). It is important that the nurse engages in appropriate conversation with the patient. If two nurses are present during bedbathing, the patient should not be excluded. Complex language and terminology should be adapted to meet the needs of the patient and ensure that he or she understands the procedure (Downey and Lloyd 2008). Planned care is negotiated with the patient and is based on assessment of their individual needs. Planned care should be documented and changed according to the patient's needs on a daily basis. Prior to commencing each step, the patient should be offered the opportunity to participate if able to, to encourage dignity, independence and autonomy.

Privacy and dignity must be maintained throughout, doors and curtains kept closed and only opened when absolutely necessary, with the patient's permission.

Procedure guideline 8.1 Bedbathing a patient

Essential equipment

- Disposable apron
- Non-sterile gloves
- Clean bedlinen
- Bath towels
- Laundry skip, applying local guidelines for soiled and/or infected linen
- Flannels, preferably disposable wipes
- Toiletries, as preferred by patient
- Comb/brush
- Equipment for oral hygiene
- Clean clothes
- Disposable or non-disposable washbowl

Optional equipment

- Antiembolic stockings
- Razor
- Scissors/nail clippers
- Emery boards
- Manual handling equipment
- Urinal, bedpan or commode

Pre-procedure

Action	Rationale
1 Assess and plan care with the patient. Note personal preferences, addressing religious and cultural beliefs. Explain each step of the procedure and gain consent.	To plan care and encourage participation and independence (Hollins 2009, **C**; NMC 2013, **E**,**C**; Pegram et al. 2007, **E**).
2 Offer the patient analgesia as appropriate. During the procedure observe for any non-verbal cues such as grimacing or frowning which may suggest that the patient is experiencing pain or discomfort.	To maintain patient comfort throughout the procedure (Downey and Lloyd 2008, **E**).
3 Clear the area of any obstacles, ensuring that the environment is warm. Draw the curtains around the bed or close doors to ensure privacy and dignity. Use available signage as appropriate.	To maintain comfort and a safe environment and promote privacy and dignity (NMC 2015, **C**).
4 Offer the patient the opportunity to use a urinal, bedpan or commode.	To reduce any disruption to procedure and prevent any discomfort (NMC 2015, **C**).
5 Collect all the equipment listed at the beginning of the procedure by the bedside.	To minimize time away from patient during procedure. **E**
6 Clean the washbowl with hot soapy water before use if a non-disposable bowl is being used. Fill the bowl with warm water as close to the patient's bedside as possible. Check the temperature of the water with the patient and adjust it as necessary.	To minimize cross-infection (Fraise and Bradley 2009, **E**; Parker 2004, **C**). To promote patient comfort. **E**
7 Check that the bed brakes are on and adjust the bed to an appropriate height for you to carry out care comfortably.	To prevent the bed moving unexpectedly and to avoid injuring your back (Pegram et al. 2007, **E**).
8 Wash your hands and put on disposable gloves and apron in accordance with local guidelines.	To minimize risk of cross-infection (Fraise and Bradley 2009, **E**; Parker 2004, **C**).

Throughout the procedure

Action	Rationale
9 The linen skip should be positioned and kept near to the bed throughout the procedure.	To reduce the potential dispersal of micro-organisms, dust and skin cells from the linen into the environment (Pegram et al. 2007, **C**).
10 The water used to wash the patient may be changed at any stage during the procedure. For example, if the patient feels the temperature is too hot or cold. Very soapy or dirty water must be changed before proceeding with the wash and water should be changed after washing the genitalia and surrounding area.	To promote patient comfort. **E** To minimize risk of cross-infection (Downey and Lloyd 2008, **E**).
11 Care needs to be taken not to wet drains/dressings and IV devices.	To reduce the risk of infection and prevent any drains or IV catheters from becoming dislodged (Downey and Lloyd 2008, **E**).

Procedure

Action	Rationale
12 Check for hearing aids, spectacles and wrist watches and with permission remove these from the patient, putting them in a safe place.	To ensure that the patient's face is washed thoroughly. **E**
13 Place a towel across the patient's chest.	To protect from splashes and to prepare for drying. **E**

(continued)

Procedure guideline 8.1 Bedbathing a patient *(continued)*

Action	Rationale
14 Ask the patient whether they use soap on their face. The face, neck and ears should be washed, rinsed and dried.	To promote cleanliness and to ensure that the patient's preferences are acknowledged. **E**
15 Hearing aids and spectacles should be cleaned and returned to the patient.	To ensure that the prosthesis is in good working order and free from debris and contaminants (Downey and Lloyd 2008, **E**).
16 Assist the patient with the removal of their upper clothing. The patient should be covered with a bath towel or sheet before folding back the bedclothes. Areas of the body that are not being washed should remain covered.	To maintain the patient's modesty and sustain body temperature (Downey and Lloyd 2015, **E**).
17 Wash, rinse and pat dry the top half of the patient's body, starting with the side furthest away from you.	The rationale for washing the side furthest away first is that any spills will not dampen parts of the body that would have already been washed and dried if carried out the other way round (Pegram et al. 2007, **E**).
During washing, pressure points such as elbows can be checked for redness or skin changes.	To prevent and treat pressure ulcers, ensuring appropriate referrals are made (NMC 2015, **C**).
18 If pyjama trousers are worn, these should be removed, while keeping the patient covered. If worn, antiembolic stockings should also be carefully removed.	To prevent venous emboli and to prevent and treat pressure ulcers, ensuring appropriate referrals are made (NMC 2015, **C**).
19 Wash the patient's legs, rinse and pat them dry, starting with the leg furthest away from you. Check pressure points on the heels for any change to skin integrity.	To prevent and treat pressure ulcers, ensuring appropriate referrals are made (NMC 2015, **C**).
20 Change the water in the bowl and your disposable gloves. Tell the patient that the next step is to wash around the genitalia; ask the patient if they wish to wash this area themselves or gain verbal consent from the patient to do it for them. Using a separate flannel or wipe, wash around the area and then dry it. Remove your gloves, dispose as per hospital policy. When washing this area, remember that female patients are washed from the front to back. The foreskin needs to be drawn back gently when washing the penis of uncircumcised male patients.	To reduce risk of infection and to maintain a safe environment (NMC 2015, **C**; Pegram et al. 2007, **C**).
If the patient has an indwelling catheter, put on clean gloves and wash the tubing, moving the disposable cloth down the tube away from the genitalia area, then dry the tubing. Remove your gloves and dispose of them as per hospital policy.	Disposable flannels/wipes are preferable as this reduces the risk of infection (DH 2013b, **C**).
21 Ensure the patient is covered and has a call bell within easy reach. Change the water and put on clean gloves.	To maintain cleanliness, preserving dignity and privacy (NMC 2015, **C**).
22 Request assistance as necessary to roll the patient on to their side. Cover the areas of the patient that are not being washed. Wash their back. Pressure points of the sacrum, shoulder blades and spine can be assessed at this time. Using disposable flannel or wipe, wash sacral area, then rinse and dry the area. Gloves should be removed and hands decontaminated. Keep the patient on their side while changing the lower bed sheet. Return patient onto their back, ensuring that they remain covered. Apply toiletries as required. Assist the patient to don appropriate clothing.	To prevent and treat pressure ulcers, ensuring appropriate referrals are made (NMC 2015, **C**). Disposable flannels/wipes are preferable as this reduces the risk of infection (DH 2013b,**C**). To minimize risk of cross-infection (Fraise and Bradley 2009, **E**; Parker 2004, **C**).
23 Inspect the patient's finger and toe nails; if necessary clean under the nails using a nail file. Cut or clip finger nails to the top level of the finger, shaping edges with an emery board if necessary. Check feet for any areas of skin dryness, inflammation or calluses. The need for possible podiatry referral should be assessed. Refit antiembolic stocking as necessary, measuring according to local policy. See Chapter 13: Perioperative care, Procedure guideline 13.1: Step-by-step guide to measuring and applying antiembolic stockings.	To enhance positive body image and patient comfort and reduce risk of infection (NMC 2015, **C**)

Action	Rationale
24 Provide appropriate equipment, and assist patient to brush their teeth and/or rinse their mouth.	To maintain good oral hygiene and prevent infection (Fraise and Bradley 2009, **E**; Parker 2004, **C**).
25 Style patient's hair as desired.	To enhance patient comfort, and to promote positive body image (NMC 2015, **C**).
26 Assist male patients with facial shaving, apply chosen shaving foam/soap. Ensure skin is taut; begin shaving from cheeks down to neck in short strokes. Rinse razor as required. Change water and rinse face with clean water (or use electric shaver).	To enhance patient comfort, and to promote positive body image (NMC 2015, **C**).
27 Remake top bedclothes.	
28 Help patient to sit or lie in desired position.	To enhance patient comfort and reduce risk of pressure area breakdown (NMC 2015, **C**).
29 Remove equipment from the patient's bedside; replace the patient's possessions in their appropriate place. Place the locker, bedside table and call bell within the reach of the patient.	To maintain a safe environment and promote patient independence (NMC 2015, **C**).
30 Remove your apron and gloves, disposing of them according to local regulations.	To prevent cross-infection (Loveday et al. 2014, **C**).

Post-procedure

31 Document any changes in planned care.	To provide recorded documentation of care and aid communication to the multiprofessional team (NMC 2010, **C**).

Procedure guideline 8.2 **Washing a patient's hair in bed**

Essential equipment

- Disposable apron
- Non-sterile gloves
- Comb and brush
- Plastic sheet or pad
- Two large towels
- Shampoo tray
- Receptacle for the shampoo water, e.g. bucket
- Basin and jug
- Shampoo and conditioner
- Hair dryer if required
- Washcloth or pad

Pre-procedure

Action	Rationale
1 Assess and plan care with the patient. Note personal preferences, Explain each step of the procedure and gain their consent.	To plan care and encourage participation and independence (Hollins 2009, **C**; NMC 2013, **E**).
2 Determine the type of shampoo to be used.	Arrange for any prescribed care, e.g. medicated shampoo, to be administered (Berman et al. 2010, **E**).
3 Assess the patient's ability to lie flat throughout the procedure.	To ensure patient stability, comfort and safety. **E**
4 Collect all the equipment listed at the beginning of the procedure by the bedside.	To minimize time away from patient during procedure. **E**
5 Clear the area of any obstacles, ensuring that the environment is warm. Draw the curtains around the bed or close doors to ensure privacy and dignity. Use available signage as appropriate.	To maintain comfort and a safe environment and promote privacy and dignity (NMC 2015, **C**).
6 Wash your hands and put on disposable gloves and apron in accordance with local guidelines.	To minimize risk of cross-infection (Fraise and Bradley 2009, **E**; Parker 2004, **C**).

Procedure

7 Remove the pillows from under the patient's head, lower or remove the bed head.	Allows access to the patient and gives the nurse more control during the procedure, thus reducing the risk of water entering the patient's eyes/ears (Dingwall 2010, **E**).

(continued)

Procedure guideline 8.2 Washing a patient's hair in bed *(continued)*

Action	Rationale
8 Place the plastic sheet under the patient's head and tuck a bath towel around their shoulders, bringing it towards their chest.	This will keep the bed and patient dry. This may prevent unnecessary disruption to the patient by having to change bedlinen and clothes. **E**
9 Gently lift the patient's head and slide in the shampoo tray with the U opening under the neck. Place a towel underneath the patient's neck for support.	The shampoo tray allows water drainage into a receptacle and prevents spills onto the floor. Padding supports the muscles of the neck and prevents undue strain and discomfort (Berman et al. 2010; Dingwall 2010, **E**).
10 Fold the top bedding down to the waist and cover the upper part of the patient with a towel.	To maintain patient dignity and prevent them from becoming cold (Berman et al. 2010; Dingwall 2010, **E**).
11 Place the receptacle for the shampoo water on the floor with an absorbent sheet underneath. Put the spout of the shampoo basin over the receptacle.	The receptacle must be lower than the bed to collect used water. Not using an absorbent sheet increases the risk of spills and slips (Dingwall 2010, **E**).
12 Protect the patient's eyes and ears. Place a washcloth over the patient's eyes. Place cotton balls in the patient's ears if indicated.	The washcloth protects the eyes from soapy water. These keep water from collecting in the ear canals (Berman et al. 2010; Dingwall 2010, **E**).
13 Ensure the patient is covered and has a call bell within easy reach. Fill the basin with warm water. Check the temperature of the water with the patient and adjust it as necessary.	To preserve dignity and privacy (NMC 2015, **C**) and patient safety. To promote patient comfort. **E**
14 Fill a jug with water from the basin, carefully wet the patient's hair and make sure the water drains into the receptacle.	To ensure there is minimal spillage of water. **E**
15 Apply a small amount of shampoo to the hair and scalp and gently massage with your fingertips.	Massaging stimulates the blood circulation in the scalp. The pads of the fingers are used so that finger nails will not scratch the scalp (Berman et al. 2010, **E**).
16 Using fresh water from the basin, rinse the hair thoroughly. Start at the top of the head and let the water work its way down to the bottom of the head.	To ensure all the shampoo is removed (Berman et al. 2010, **E**).
17 Apply conditioner if desired and rinse using warm water until the water runs clear.	Soapy residue causes the appearance of soap scum in the hair and the scalp will become irritated and dry (Dingwall 2010, **E**).
18 Squeeze excess water from the hair into the shampoo tray before removal. Gently rub hair dry with a towel. Dry the patient's face.	To facilitate optimal drying of the hair. **E** To ensure patient comfort. **E**
19 Remove any equipment and return the patient back to a comfortable position.	To ensure patient comfort (Berman et al. 2010; Dingwall 2010, **E**).
20 Replace any wet linen and ensure that the patient is appropriately clothed.	To ensure patient comfort and warmth. **E**
21 Style the patient's hair. Use a hair dryer on a cool/warm setting if the patient wishes and if it has had all its safety checks.	To prevent drying of the scalp. Prevents the discomfort of prolonged heat on the scalp (Berman et al. 2010; Dingwall 2010, **E**).
22 Clear away equipment from the patient's bedside. Place the call bell within the reach of the patient.	To maintain a safe environment and promote patient independence (NMC 2015, **C**).
23 Remove your apron and gloves, disposing of them according to local regulations.	To prevent cross-infection (Loveday et al. 2014, **C**).
Post-procedure	
24 Document any changes in planned care.	To provide recorded documentation of care and aid communication to the multiprofessional team (NMC 2010, **C**).

Eye care

DEFINITION

Eye care is the process of assessing, cleaning and/or irrigating the eye, including the instillation of prescribed ocular preparations where applicable; patient education is also included (Stollery et al. 2005, Watkinson and Seewoodhary 2007).

ANATOMY AND PHYSIOLOGY

The eye consists of three main parts: the orbit, the globe (eyeball) and the extrinsic structures.

The orbit

The orbit or socket is formed by seven bones of the skull and is lined with fat; it supports and protects the globe and its accessory structures (blood vessels and nerves) and provides attachments for the ocular muscles (Stollery et al. 2005).

The globe

The globe is approximately 2.5 cm in diameter and can be divided into three layers (Figure 8.2).

- The *outer layer or fibrous tunic* is composed of the transparent cornea and the white sclera. The primary function of the outer layer, in particular the sclera, is protective and it gives shape to the eyeball. The cornea functions as a refracting and protective membrane through which light rays pass on their route to the retina (Watkinson and Seewoodhary 2007).
- The *middle layer or vascular tunic* is composed of the choroid, ciliary body and iris; the globe's vascular supply is provided by the choroid.
- The *inner layer or nervous tunic* is composed of the retina, which contains the light-sensitive cells called the rods and cones. It is responsible for converting light rays into electrical signals that are transmitted to the brain via the optic nerve. This area contains the macula lutea, also known as the yellow spot. The central fovea, the area of highest visual acuity, is also located here, as is the blind spot, the area of no visual field (Watkinson and Seewoodhary 2007).

Figure 8.2 **Horizontal section through the eyeball at the level of the optic nerve. Optic axis and axis of eyeball are included.**

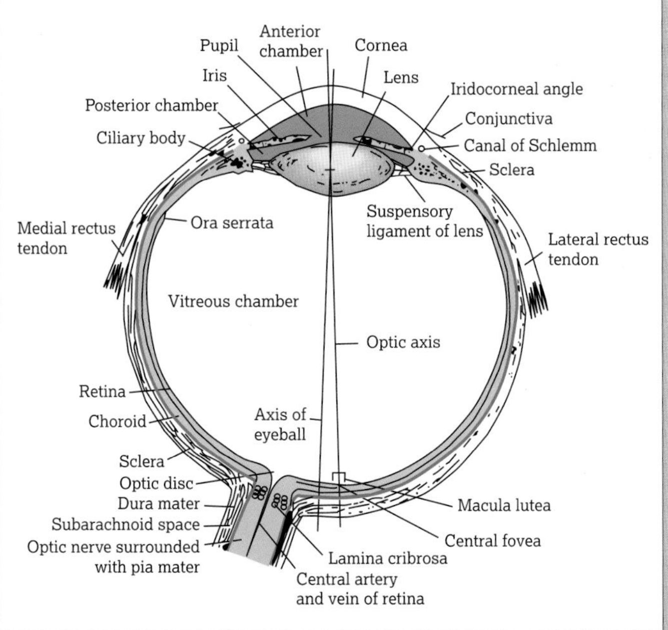

The globe – internally

The globe is divided into two chambers by the lens (Figure 8.3): the anterior cavity, in front of the lens, and the vitreous chamber, behind the lens. The anterior cavity is divided into the anterior chamber and the posterior chamber by the iris. It contains a clear, watery fluid called the aqueous humour. The vitreous chamber is filled with a jelly-like substance called the vitreous body or vitreous humour. The vitreous humour is a clear gelatinous substance which fills the vitreous chamber, which, unlike the aqueous humour, is produced during fetal development and is never replaced (Tortora and Derrickson 2011). Together, these two fluid-filled cavities help maintain the shape of the eyeball and the intraocular pressure (Tortora and Derrickson 2011).

The aqueous humour is continuously secreted by the ciliary process (a part of the ciliary body) located behind the iris. This fluid then permeates the posterior chamber, passing between the lens and the iris, and flows through the pupil into the anterior chamber. From the anterior chamber, the aqueous humour drains into the scleral venous sinus (canal of Schlemm) and is absorbed back into the bloodstream (see Figure 8.3).

The aqueous humour is the principal source of nutrients and waste removal for the lens and cornea, as these structures have no direct blood supply. If the outflow of aqueous humour is blocked, excessive intraocular pressure may develop, leading to the disease process known as glaucoma. This excessive pressure can cause degeneration of the retina, which may result in blindness (Lee 2006).

Extrinsic structures

Extrinsic structures of the eye protect the globe from external injury (Stollery et al. 2005).

- *Eyelashes*: protect the eye from debris.
- *Eyebrows*: prevent moisture, in particular sweat, from flowing into the eye.
- *Eyelids*: the eyelid is made up of complex muscles for eye movement, glands for tear and oil production that serve as a cleansing mechanism against dirt and foreign objects, and sensitive nerves for defence (Watkinson and Seewoodhary 2007).
- *Lacrimal (tear) apparatus*: tears are produced in the lacrimal glands located at the upper, outer edge of the eye. They are excreted onto the upper surface of the globe and wash over the

Figure 8.3 **The anterior cavity in front of the lens is incompletely divided into anterior chamber (anterior to iris) and posterior chamber (behind iris), which are continuous through the pupil. Aqueous humour, which fills the cavity, is formed by ciliary processes and reabsorbed into the venous blood by the canal of Schlemm.**

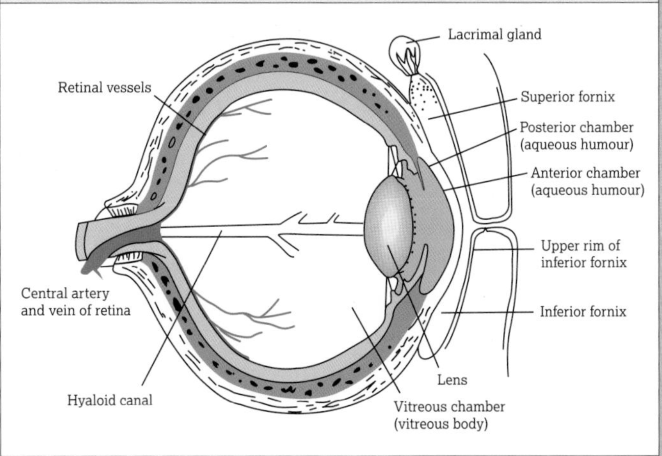

Figure 8.4 **Lacrimal apparatus.**

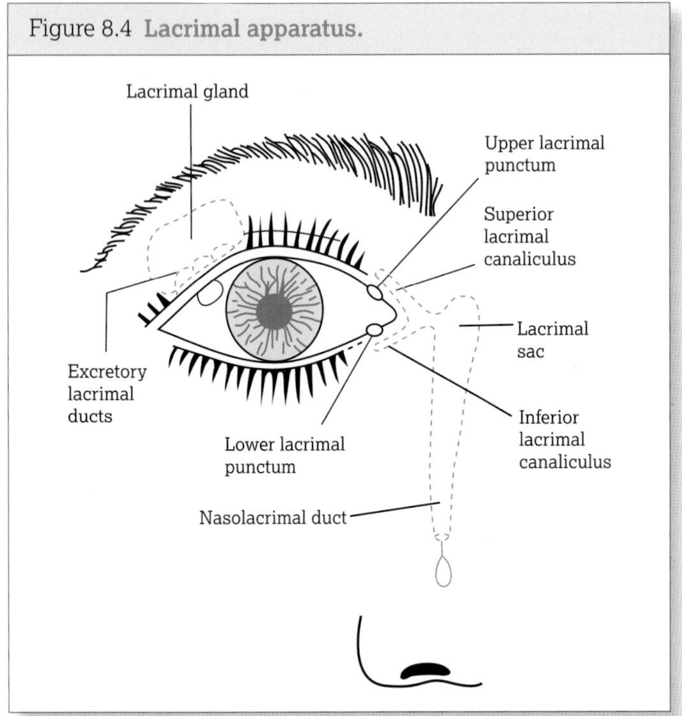

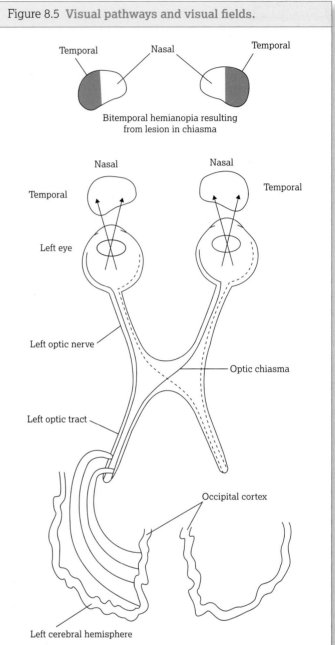

ocular surface by the action of blinking. The function of tears is to clean, moisten and lubricate the ocular surface and eyelids. Tears also provide antisepsis as they contain an enzyme called lysozyme that is able to rupture the cell membranes of some bacteria, leading to their lysis and death (Forrester 2002). The tears collect in the nasal canthus (inner, medial aspect of the eye) from where they drain into the upper and lower lacrimal puncti which drain into the lacrimal sac. From here, the tears pass into the nasolacrimal duct and empty into the nasal cavity (Figure 8.4) (Tortora and Derrickson 2011).

Optic nerve

The optic nerve, which is responsible for vision (cranial nerve II), exits the eye to the side of the macula lutea at an area called the optic disc (see Figure 8.2). This area is sometimes referred to as the anatomical blind spot. The optic nerve passes from the orbit through the optic foramen and into the brain. The two separate optic nerves meet at the optic chiasma and some optic nerve fibres cross over here to the opposite side of the brain. The nerves then continue along the optic tracts and terminate in the thalamus. From there, projections extend to the visual areas in the occipital lobe of the cerebral cortex (Tortora and Derrickson 2011) (Figure 8.5).

An additional blind spot or area of depressed vision, called a scotoma, may be indicative of a brain tumour. In pituitary gland tumours, for example, it is common to develop bilateral defects in the field of vision due to invasion of the optic chiasm (Goodman and Wickham 2005).

The ageing process

The eye changes with age. This process can start in the third decade of life, with most anatomical and physiological changes becoming more prevalent the older a person becomes (Nigam and Knight 2008) (Box 8.3, Box 8.4).

RELATED THEORY

Sight provides us with important sensory input to enable self-care and pleasurable activities such as reading. 'Early detection of changes in the eye is important to enable effective treatment and prevent long-term problems and even blindness' (Holman et al. 2005, p.37).

Figure 8.5 **Visual pathways and visual fields.**

Temporal
Nasal
Temporal
Bitemporal hemianopia resulting from lesion in chiasma
Nasal
Nasal
Temporal
Temporal
Left eye
Left optic nerve
Optic chiasma
Left optic tract
Occipital cortex
Left cerebral hemisphere

Reduced vision or blindness can make the hospital environment very unwelcoming. When caring for patients with eye problems, it is essential to promote a safe, secure environment, where the person is supported and encouraged to communicate their needs effectively.

EVIDENCE-BASED APPROACHES

Rationale

Indications

Eye care may be necessary under the following circumstances.

- After eye surgery to prevent post-operative complications.
- In the care of the unconscious patient to maintain eye integrity.
- To relieve pain and discomfort.
- To prevent or treat infection.
- To prevent or treat injury to the eye, for example to remove sharp objects.

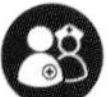 Box 8.3 **Effects of ageing on the eye**

Anatomical changes

- The retro-orbital fat atrophies.
- Eyelid tissues become weak.
- The levator muscle weakens, causing the eyelid to droop which can occlude the upper visual field.

Physiological changes

- *Presbyopia*: the distance from which print can be read increases.
- Reduced flexibility of the lens means it can no longer change shape to focus on close objects quickly.
- *Cataracts*: the lens becomes dense and yellow, affecting colour perceptions; it can become so dense that the lens proteins precipitate, creating a halo effect around bright lights.
- Night vision reduces.
- Diminished central vision caused by cells within the retina dying.
- Dry eyes from reduced tear production.

Source: Adapted from Holman et al. (2005), Nigam and Knight (2008).

- For eye tests such as refraction.
- For screening to detect disease such as glaucoma.
- To treat existing problems such as conjunctivitis.
- To detect drug-induced toxicity at an early stage.
- To maintain contact lenses and care for false eye prostheses.
- To optimize the eye's visual function, especially with age-related degeneration (Boyd-Monk 2005, Cunningham and Gould 1998, Stollery et al. 2005, Watkinson and Seewoodhary 2007).

These indications may present singularly or in combination.

Eye care includes patient education about the eye and surrounding structures as well as health promotion and safety advice to promote quality of life (Watkinson and Seewoodhary 2007).

Principles of care

Eye care is performed to maintain healthy eyes that are moist and infection free. The eye is an important organ and inadequate techniques may lead to the transmission of infection from one eye to the other or the development of irreversible damage to the eye which could lead to loss of sight (Cunningham and Gould 1998). If an infection is present in one eye, this should be cleaned and/or treated last to prevent transmission of infection to the uninfected eye (Holman et al. 2005).

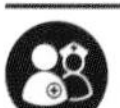 Box 8.4 **Eye conditions common in the older population**

- *Glaucoma*: the optic nerve is damaged by increased pressure in the eye, resulting in reduced visual field and pain.
- *Cataract*: see Box 8.3.
- *Diabetic retinopathy*: blood vessels connected to the retina are damaged by the disease and sight becomes blurred and patchy, and can be totally lost.
- *Age-related macular degeneration*: a chronic disorder of the macula cells in the centre of the retina, a highly sensitive area responsible for detailed central vision. As this degenerates, central vision declines which can lead to blindness.

Source: Adapted from Holman et al. (2005), Watkinson and Seewoodhary (2007).

A clean technique should be used for eye care procedures and an aseptic technique, if deemed necessary, for vulnerable exposed eyes or to reduce the risk of infection (Alexander et al. 2007).

The eye area must be treated gently and unnecessary pressure must be avoided, especially to the globe (Alexander et al. 2007). Low-linting swabs are generally used as lint from other types of swab can become detached and scratch the cornea (Woodrow 2006). The fluids most commonly used for eye care procedures are sterile 0.9% sodium chloride or sterile water for irrigation; however, sterile 0.9% sodium chloride can irritate and sting the sensitive eye area so where possible it is recommended that sterile water is used (Woodrow 2006).

If able, and after appropriate instruction, patients should be encouraged to carry out eye care procedures themselves. However, in the case of post-operative, physically limited or unconscious patients, it is often the nurse who is responsible for eye care.

Consideration should always be given to patients' sight aids, such as glasses and contact lenses (Holman et al. 2005). Assistance may be required to clean these aids and advice regarding the most appropriate method should be sought, preferably from the patient.

For all procedures which involve removal or insertion of contact lenses or prosthetic eyes, the patient should be encouraged to do this themselves as they will have developed their own particular methods. However, the nurse must observe as the patient may still need education to improve their technique. Advice regarding the ideal method of removal and insertion should be sought from the local ophthalmology service or the nursing team in the ophthalmology unit.

Methods of eye assessment

Before beginning any eye care procedure, the eye and surrounding structures should be examined and assessed and then re-examined and reassessed after the intervention. Begin by examining the eye closed, looking carefully at the eyelids, noting any bruising, spasms, inflammation, discharge or crusting (Holman et al. 2005). Look for signs that the eyelids are closed properly, as an inability to close completely could indicate the presence of a cyst or lump that would require further investigation and reporting to the patient's doctor.

Ask the patient to open their eyes and, using a pen torch, look for abnormalities in the conjunctiva such as inflammation, redness or the presence of a discharge; the eye should be clear of clouding and redness (Alexander et al. 2007). Ask the patient whether they are experiencing any pain or photophobia. Any abnormalities need to be reported to the patient's doctor immediately, as eye complications can develop quickly. Any changes should also be documented (Alexander et al. 2007, Holman et al. 2005, NMC 2010).

Methods of eye swabbing

Eye swabbing is performed to clear the outer eye structures of foreign bodies, including discharges, which could be infected matter. The swab should be moistened with sterile water for irrigation and lightly wiped over the eyelid from the nose outward. This process should be repeated with clean gauze until the area is clean of discharge or encrustation.

Methods of eye irrigation

Eye irrigation is usually performed to remove foreign bodies or caustic substances from the eye, for example domestic cleaning agents or medications, particularly cytotoxic material; it should be performed as soon as possible to minimize damage (Stollery et al. 2005). The procedure is also used for pre-operative preparation or to remove infected material.

Using the least volume of sterile water for irrigation necessary will reduce the likelihood of deeper corneal damage which can be a side-effect of the corrosive chemicals due to water's hypotonic nature (Kuckelkorn et al. 2002). The volume required will vary depending on the degree of contamination; copious amounts are needed for corrosive chemicals and smaller volumes for removal of eye secretions. The solution may be directed to the area affected by using a intravenous fluid giving set to ensure a controllable, directable flow of fluid (Marsden 2007, Rodrigues 2009). To avoid physical damage, the tubing should be held approximately 2.5 cm from the eye (Stollery et al. 2005) and directed to the inner canthus. Other irrigation devices include the Morgan lens, an irrigating contact lens that is attached to a giving set to enable hands-free irrigation. Eye wash and eye irrigation stations are commercially available and mix tap water with air for a very soft spray of water (Marsden 2007).

Care of contact lenses

Contact lenses are thin, curved discs made of hard or soft plastic or a combination of both. Hard contact lenses are made of a rigid plastic that does not absorb water or saline solutions and can be worn for a maximum of 12–14 hours continuously. Soft contact lenses are more pliable, retain more water and so can be worn for up to 30 days and cleaned once weekly. Ill-fitting lenses may reduce the tear film between lens and cornea, which may result in oxygen deprivation of the cornea, leading to corneal oedema and blurred vision. Further damage to the corneal epithelial cells may lead to corneal abrasion and pain. Gas-permeable lenses are a combination of both hard and soft plastic; these permit oxygen to reach the cornea, providing greater comfort, and can be left in for several days (Olver and Cassidy 2005).

Most people look after their own contact lenses. Cleaning and storage solutions depend on the type of lenses used; manufacturers provide specific instructions for the care of their products. They should be stored in a container with slots for right (R) and left (L) eye, so they can be worn in the correct eye. Seriously ill patients should have their lenses removed and stored correctly until they can reinsert them. Contact lenses are stored in a sterile solution when they are not in the eye; this helps to lubricate the lens and enable it to glide over the cornea, reducing the risk of injury.

Artificial eyes

These are made of glass or plastic; some are permanently implanted. Most people who have artificial eyes care for them themselves. If the patient is unable to do this, it is recommended that the eye is removed once daily for cleaning; the patient will be able to advise how they would like this done (Alexander et al. 2007). However, if they are unable to do so, advice should be sought from the local ophthalmology service or the nursing team in the ophthalmology unit.

PRE-PROCEDURAL CONSIDERATIONS

Light source

A good light source such as a minor procedure light or bright lamp is necessary to enable careful assessment of the eyes and to avoid damage to the delicate structures.

Position of light source

The light source should be positioned above and behind the nurse. It should never be allowed to shine directly into the patient's eyes, as this will be extremely uncomfortable for the patient (Shaw 2006).

Position of patient

The patient should be sitting or lying with their head tilted backwards and chin pointing upwards. This allows for easy access to the eyes and is usually a good position for patient comfort and compliance (Stollery et al. 2005).

Procedure guideline 8.3 **Eye swabbing**

Essential equipment

- Sterile dressing pack
- Sterile low-linting or lint-free swabs
- Sterile water for irrigation
- Light source

Optional equipment

- Sterile/non-sterile powder-free gloves

Pre-procedure

Action	Rationale
1 Explain and discuss the procedure with the patient. Ask the patient to explain how their eyes feel, if they are able to.	To ensure that the patient understands the procedure and gives their valid consent (NMC 2013). To have a baseline understanding of current problems or changes the patient is experiencing (NMC 2015, **C**).
2 Assist the patient into the correct position:	The patient needs to be discouraged from flinching or making unexpected movements and so should be in the most comfortable, pain-free position possible at the start of the procedure (Shaw 2006, **R5**).
Head well supported and tilted back	To enable access to and assessment of the eyes. **E**
Preferably the patient should be in bed or lying on a couch.	To enable patient comfort. **E**
3 Ensure an adequate light source, taking care not to dazzle the patient.	To enable maximum observation of the eyes without causing the patient harm or discomfort (Shaw 2006, **R5**).
4 Wash hands and put on personal protective equipment.	To reduce the risk of cross-infection (Fraise and Bradley 2009, **E**).

Procedure

Action	Rationale
5 Always treat the uninfected or uninflamed eye first.	To reduce the risk of cross-infection (Fraise and Bradley 2009, **E**).
6 Always bathe lids with the eyes closed first.	To reduce the risk of damaging the cornea and to remove any crusted discharge. **E**
7 Ask the patient to look up and, using a slightly moistened swab, gently swab the lower lid from the inner canthus outwards. Use an aseptic technique for the damaged or postoperative eye.	If the swab is too wet, the solution will run down the patient's cheek. This increases the risk of cross-infection and causes the patient discomfort. Swabbing from the nasal corner outwards avoids the risk of swabbing discharge into the lacrimal punctum or even across the bridge of the nose into the other eye. Aseptic technique reduces the risk of cross-infection (Fraise and Bradley 2009, **E**).

Action	Rationale
8 Ensure that the edge of the swab is not above the lid margin.	To avoid touching the sensitive cornea. **E**
9 Using a new swab each time, repeat the procedure until all the discharge has been removed.	To reduce risk of cross-infection (Fraise and Bradley 2009, **E**).
10 Gently swab the upper lid by slightly everting the lid margin and asking the patient to look down. Swab from the nasal corner outwards and use a new swab each time until all discharge has been removed.	To effectively remove any foreign material from the eye. **E** To reduce the risk of cross-infection (Fraise and Bradley 2009, **E**).
11 Once both eyelids have been cleaned and dried, make the patient comfortable.	To ensure patient comfort. **E**
12 Remove and dispose of equipment.	To keep area clean and reduce risk of cross-infection (Fraise and Bradley 2009, **E**).
13 Wash hands.	To reduce the risk of cross-infection (Fraise and Bradley 2009, **E**).
Post-procedure	
14 Discuss with the patient any changes post procedure; report any adverse effects to the patient's doctor. Record the procedure in the appropriate documents.	To monitor effectiveness of procedure, trends and fluctuations (NMC 2010, **C**).

Procedure guideline 8.4 **Eye irrigation**

Essential equipment

- Sterile dressing pack
- Sterile water for irrigation (in an emergency, tap water may be used)
- Receiver (kidney dish or plastic receptacle)
- Towel
- Plastic cape
- Intravenous fluid giving set and drip stand
- Warm water in a bowl to warm irrigating fluid to tepid temperature
- Low-linting or lint-free swabs
- Light source

Optional equipment

- Anaesthetic drops
- Sterile/non-sterile powder-free gloves

Pre-procedure

Action	Rationale
1 Explain and discuss the procedure with the patient. Ask the patient to explain how their eyes feel, if they are able to.	To ensure that the patient understands the procedure and gives their valid consent (NMC 2013). To have a baseline understanding of current problems or changes the patient is experiencing (Rodrigues 2009, **E**).
2 Wash hands and put on personal protective equipment.	To reduce risk of cross-infection (Fraise and Bradley 2009, **E**).
3 If possible, remove any contact lens (see Procedure guideline 8.7: Contact lens removal: hard lenses and Procedure guideline 8.8: Contact lens removal: soft lenses).	To ensure no reservoir of chemical remains in the eye (Marsden 2006, **E**).
4 Instil anaesthetic drops if required.	To relieve pain and aid irrigation (Duffy 2008, **E**).
5 The patient should sit upright with head supported and tilted to the affected side.	To avoid the solution running either over the nose into the other eye, to avoid cross-infection, or out of the affected eye and down the side of the cheek (Fraise and Bradley 2009, **E**). To reduce risk of cross-infection (Fraise and Bradley 2009, **E**). To prevent washing the discharge down the lacrimal duct or across the cheek (Marsden 2007, **E**).
6 Drape the patient's shoulders with a towel or if available a waterproof cape. Ask the patient to hold the receiver (kidney dish or plastic receptacle) against the cheek below the eye being irrigated.	To protect the patient from getting wet and to collect irrigation fluid as it runs away from the eye (Rodrigues 2009, **E**).

(continued)

Procedure guideline 8.4 Eye irrigation *(continued)*

Action	Rationale
7 Prepare the irrigation fluid to the appropriate temperature by placing in bowl of water until warmed.	Tepid fluid will be more comfortable for the patient. The solution should be poured across the inner aspect of the nurse's wrist to test the temperature (Duffy 2008, **E**).
Hang the irrigation fluid on the drip stand, connect the fluid to the intravenous giving set and prime the line.	To ensure that the irrigation fluid is ready for the procedure (Marsden 2007, **E**).
Procedure	
8 If there is any discharge, proceed as for eye swabbing (see Procedure guideline 8.3: Eye swabbing).	To remove any infected material. **E**
9 Hold the patient's eyelids apart, using your first and second fingers, against the orbital ridge. Do not press on the eyeball.	The patient will be unable to hold the eye open once irrigation commences (Marsden 2007, **E**). To avoid causing the patient discomfort or pain (Alexander et al. 2007, **C**).
10 Warn the patient that the flow of solution is going to start and pour a little onto the cheek first.	To allow time to adjust to the feeling of water flow (Duffy 2008, **E**).
11 Direct the flow of the fluid from the nasal corner outwards (**Action figure 11**). Keep the fluid flow constant by adjusting the giving set roller clamp.	To wash away from the lacrimal punctum and prevent contaminating other eye. **E** To ensure constant flow (Rodrigues 2009, **E**).
12 Ask the patient to look up, down and to either side while irrigating.	To ensure that the whole area, including fornices, is irrigated (Stollery et al. 2005, **E**).
13 Evert upper and lower lids whilst irrigating.	To ensure complete removal of any foreign body. **E**
14 Keep the flow of irrigation fluid constant.	To ensure swift removal of any foreign body (Marsden 2006, **R5**).
15 When the eye has been thoroughly irrigated, ask the patient to close the eyes and use a new swab to dry the lids.	For patient comfort (Rodrigues 2009, **E**).
16 Take the receiver from the patient and dry the cheek.	To prevent spillage of receiver contents and promote patient comfort (Duffy 2008, **E**).
17 Make the patient comfortable.	
Post-procedure	
18 Remove and dispose of equipment.	To keep area clean and reduce risk of cross-infection (Fraise and Bradley 2009, **E**).
19 Wash hands with bactericidal soap and water.	To reduce the risk of cross-infection (Fraise and Bradley 2009, **E**).
20 Document the intervention in the patient's notes.	To maintain accurate records. To provide a point of reference in the event of any queries. To prevent any duplication of treatment (NMC 2010, **C**).
21 Discuss with the patient any changes post procedure; report any adverse effects to the patient's doctor.	To monitor effectiveness of procedure, trends and fluctuations (NMC 2010, **C**).

Action Figure 11 Irrigation of the eye from inner to outer canthus.

Procedure guideline 8.5 **Artificial eye care: insertion**

Essential equipment
- Sterile dressing pack
- Sterile water for irrigation
- Low-linting or lint-free swabs

Optional equipment
- Sterile/non-sterile powder-free gloves
- Extractor

Pre-procedure

Action	Rationale
1 Explain and discuss the procedure with the patient.	To ensure that the patient understands the procedure and gives their consent (NMC 2013, **C**).
2 Wash hands and put on personal protective equipment.	To reduce the risk of cross-infection (Fraise and Bradley 2009, **E**).
Procedure	
3 Wearing non-sterile gloves and with the dominant hand, gently lift up the upper eyelid and pull down the lower eyelid. With the other hand, hold the prosthesis between the thumb and index finger and gently insert it.	To minimize patient discomfort and ensure correct insertion. **E**
Post-procedure	
4 Remove gloves and dispose of equipment.	To keep area clean and reduce risk of cross-infection (Fraise and Bradley 2009, **E**).
5 Wash hands with bactericidal soap and water.	To reduce the risk of cross-infection (Fraise and Bradley 2009, **E**).
6 Document the intervention in the patient's notes.	To maintain accurate records. To provide a point of reference in the event of any queries. To prevent any duplication of treatment (NMC 2010, **C**).

Procedure guideline 8.6 **Artificial eye care: removal**

Essential equipment
- Sterile dressing pack
- Sterile water for irrigation
- Low-linting or lint-free swabs

Optional equipment
- Sterile/non-sterile powder-free gloves
- Extractor

Pre-procedure

Action	Rationale
1 Explain and discuss the procedure with the patient.	To ensure that the patient understands the procedure and gives their consent (NMC 2013, **C**).
2 Wash hands and put on personal protective equipment.	To reduce the risk of cross-infection (Fraise and Bradley 2009, **E**).
Procedure	
3 Wearing non-sterile gloves and with the dominant hand, gently pull the eyelid downwards and exert slight pressure below the eyelid to overcome the suction, enabling the prosthesis to be removed. An extractor may be necessary to gently lever the eye out.	To minimize patient discomfort and trauma to the area (Alexander et al. 2007, **C**, **E**).
4 Rinse and drain the eye socket with sterile water for irrigation.	To remove any loose debris and to minimize damage caused by touch. **E**
5 Clean the eye with sterile water for irrigation.	To prevent the build-up of debris and to reduce the risk of infection (Fraise and Bradley 2009, **E**).
Post-procedure	
6 Remove gloves and dispose of equipment.	To keep area clean and reduce risk of cross-infection (Fraise and Bradley 2009, **E**).
7 Wash hands with bactericidal soap and water.	To reduce the risk of cross-infection (Fraise and Bradley 2009, **E**).
8 Document the intervention in the patient's notes.	To maintain accurate records. To provide a point of reference in the event of any queries. To prevent any duplication of treatment (NMC 2010, **C**).

Procedure guideline 8.7 Contact lens removal: hard lenses

Essential equipment
- Sterile dressing pack
- Contact lens solution
- Low-linting or lint-free swabs
- Apron

Optional equipment
- Sterile/non-sterile powder-free gloves

Action	Rationale
Pre-procedure	
1 Explain and discuss the procedure with the patient.	To ensure that the patient understands the procedure and gives their consent (NMC 2013, **C**).
2 Wash hands and put on apron.	To reduce the risk of cross-infection (Fraise and Bradley 2009, **E**).
Procedure	
3 Wearing non-sterile gloves and using thumb and forefinger, separate the eyelids. Keeping the eyelid stationary, place the index finger on the lens. Gently move the lens to one side of the cornea and pull away (**Action figure 3**).	To minimize corneal trauma (Stollery et al. 2005, **R5**).
4 Store lenses in the appropriate solution as recommended by the manufacturer and ensure lenses are placed in the correct left and right storage pots.	To prevent deterioration and contamination (Stollery et al. 2005, **R5**).
5 Refer to manufacturer's instructions for further storage information, particularly if patient will not be using the lenses for a lengthy period of time.	To prevent deterioration of lens and growth of organisms. **E**
Post-procedure	
6 Remove and dispose of equipment.	To keep area clean and reduce risk of cross-infection (Fraise and Bradley 2009, **E**).
7 Wash hands with bactericidal soap and water.	To reduce the risk of cross-infection (Fraise and Bradley 2009, **E**).
8 Document the intervention in the patient's notes.	To maintain accurate records. To provide a point of reference in the event of any queries. To prevent any duplication of treatment (NMC 2010, **C**).

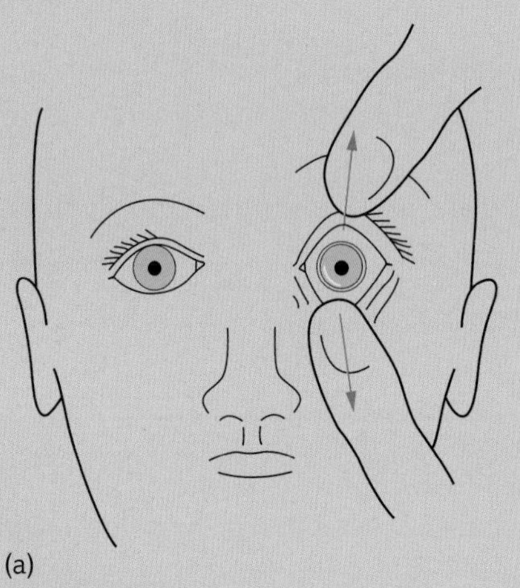

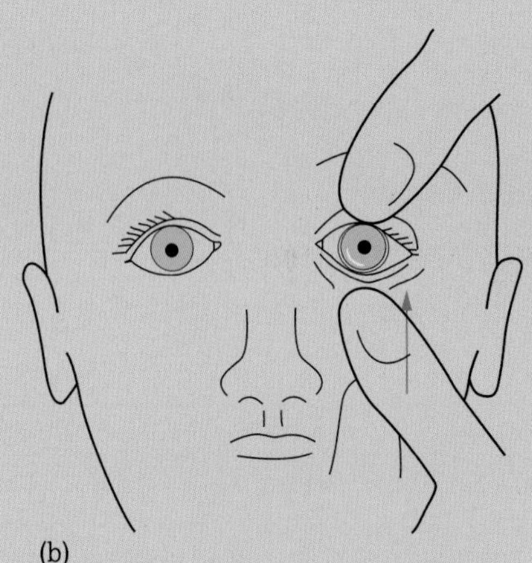

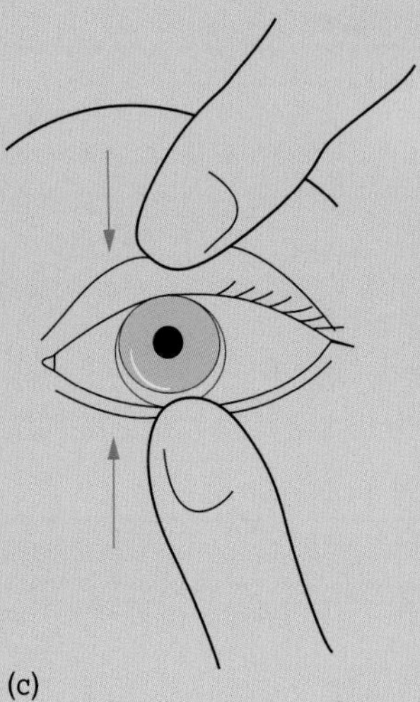

Action Figure 3 Removing hard contact lenses.

Procedure guideline 8.8 Contact lens removal: soft lenses

Essential equipment
- Sterile dressing pack
- Contact lens solution
- Low-linting or lint-free swabs

Optional equipment
- Sterile/non-sterile powder-free gloves

Action	Rationale
Pre-procedure	
1 Explain and discuss the procedure with the patient.	To ensure that the patient understands the procedure and gives their consent (NMC 2013, **C**).
2 Wash hands and put on personal protective equipment.	To reduce the risk of cross-infection (Fraise and Bradley 2009, **E**).
Procedure	
3 Wearing non-sterile gloves, gently pinch the lens between the thumb and index finger (**Action figure 3**).	To encourage the lens to fold together, allowing air to enter underneath the lens for easy removal. **E**
4 Store lenses in the appropriate solution as recommended by the manufacturer and ensure lenses are placed in the correct left and right storage pots.	To prevent deterioration and contamination (Stollery et al. 2005, **E**).
5 Refer to manufacturer's instructions for further storage information, particularly if patient will not be using the lenses for a lengthy period of time.	To prevent deterioration and growth of organisms. **E**
6 Make the patient comfortable.	
Post-procedure	
7 Remove and dispose of equipment.	To keep area clean and reduce risk of cross-infection (Fraise and Bradley 2009, **E**).
8 Wash hands with bactericidal soap and water.	To reduce the risk of cross-infection (Fraise and Bradley 2009, **E**).
9 Document the intervention in the patient's notes.	To maintain accurate records. To provide a point of reference in the event of any queries. To prevent any duplication of treatment (NMC 2010, **C**).

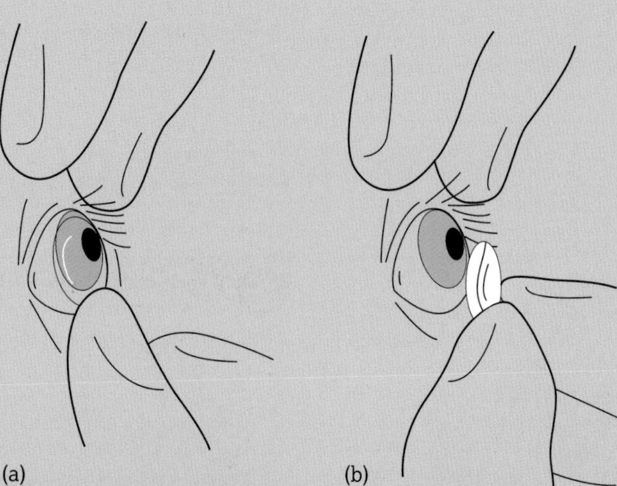

Action Figure 3 (a) Moving a soft lens down the interior part of the sclera. (b) Removing a soft lens by pinching it between the pads of the thumb and index finger.

Ear care

DEFINITION

Ear care encompasses the assessment and cleaning of the ears, including the instillation of prescribed ear drops. The monitoring and maintenance of hearing are also included.

ANATOMY AND PHYSIOLOGY

The ears capture sounds for hearing and maintain balance for equilibrium (Nigam and Knight 2008). The ear has three parts: external, middle and inner (Figure 8.6).

External ear

The external ear is a protective funnel made up of the cartilaginous pinna and external acoustic canal and the eardrum (see Figure 8.6). The external acoustic canal is lined with small hairs and next to it lie the ceruminous glands which produce cerumen or ear wax. The amalgamation of cerumen and hairs prevents foreign objects from entering the ear.

The pinna collects sound waves and delivers them via the external acoustic canal to the tympanic membrane or eardrum which vibrates in harmony (Nigam and Knight 2008, Richardson 2007). The eardrum separates the external and middle ear; it has a slight cone shape and the pointed end sits within the inner ear to assist the funnelling of sounds.

Middle ear

The middle ear is an air-filled chamber. It contains the three smallest bones in the body, the malleus, incus and stapes, collectively known as the auditory ossicles. To one side, it has a thin bony partition that holds two small membrane-covered apertures which are the oval and round windows (Tortora and Derrickson 2011). The auditory ossicles receive vibrations from the tympanic membrane. Vibrations are passed on to the oval window and through to the cochlea in the inner ear; within this process the sound waves are magnified (Alexander et al. 2007, Richardson 2007).

At the bottom of the chamber lies the eustachian tube which connects to the nasopharynx and regulates the pressure in the ear. It is usually closed but yawning or swallowing briefly opens it, allowing air to enter or leave until the pressure in the middle ear equalizes to that of external air pressure (Richardson 2007). When the pressures are equalized, the tympanic membrane vibrates freely as the sound waves hit it. However, if the pressures are not balanced, the individual may experience pain, hearing impairment, tinnitus and vertigo (Tortora and Derrickson 2011).

Figure 8.6 **Internal structure of the ear. *Source:* Tortora and Derrickson (2011). Reproduced with permission from John Wiley & Sons.**

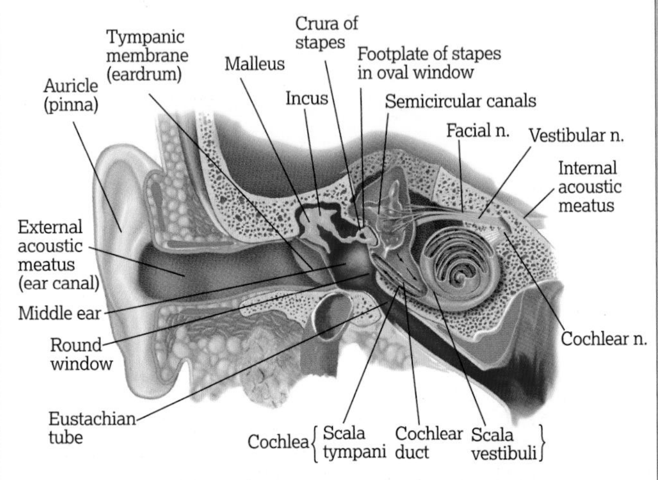

Inner ear

The inner ear is very small and includes the organ of Corti, which is situated inside the snail-shaped cochlea, the three semi-circular canals and vestibular apparatus (see Figure 8.6).

The organ of Corti is the organ for hearing. It is fluid-filled and has a membranous layer that connects to the end of the auditory nerve; the membrane is covered in tiny cells with hair-like projections (Alexander et al. 2007). Sound waves travel through the fluid and are distributed to the hair cells. At this point the sound waves change to impulses which pass along the auditory nerve to the brainstem and cortex, where they are interpreted as sound.

The semi-circular canals and vestibular apparatus maintain balance. These canals are highly sensitive; they contain fluid and hair cells that recognize when the head moves and send signals to the brain to maintain equilibrium. The brain interprets these messages along with visual input from the eyes (Nigam and Knight 2008). Adjustments to the muscles and joints are made in response to the information received (Tortora and Derrickson 2011).

If the inner ear structures are damaged, the patient may develop permanent vertigo or hearing loss (Pullen 2006).

Ear wax impaction

Ear wax (cerumen) is a waxy secretion of glands within the auditory canal, combined with skin scales and hair. As the cerumen dries, it usually falls out of the ear canal but in some circumstances the wax can become impacted (Harkin and Kelleher 2011).

Ear wax impaction is the biggest cause of ear problems; thousands of people in the UK have ear wax removed every week (Harkin and Kelleher 2011) (Box 8.5).

The symptoms of ear wax impaction are:

- dull hearing
- tinnitus
- disturbed balance
- earache
- itchiness in the ear
- reflex cough
- dizziness
- vertigo (Alexander et al. 2007).

RELATED THEORY

Communication and balance can be affected by poor ear hygiene; for example, using cotton buds to clean the ears can result in ear wax impaction which can dull hearing. Hearing loss can develop over time and become less noticeable to the individual and those close to them, as they find alternative ways to cope. Hearing impairment can cause frustration, stress, social isolation, paranoia and depression (Harkin and Kelleher 2011).

It is imperative that nurses notice and investigate when patients don't respond when spoken to or report feeling frustrated when communicating with others (Harkin 2005).There is a high overall incidence of hearing difficulties in people with learning disabilities. These are due to a variety of factors including genetic tendencies to deafness, fragile X syndrome, structural abnormalities within

Box 8.5 **Individuals prone to ear wax impaction**

- Older people.
- Those with learning disabilities – the reason for this is not known.
- Narrow ear canals.
- Hearing aid users.
- Those who use cotton buds to clean the ear as this causes the wax to be pushed further down the canal and can cause injury to the surface of the canal.

Source: Adapted from Aung and Mulley (2002), Harkin (2008), Kraszewski (2008).

the organ and neural complications which can further complicate communication difficulties for this population (Dingwall 2010).

Nurses need to be aware of how ear problems occur so they are able to explore these with patients and identify problems early and provide appropriate patient education. All findings should be documented and handed over to the patient's doctor for further investigation (Box 8.6) such as hearing assessment.

EVIDENCE-BASED APPROACHES

After bathing or showering, the outer ear should be dried with tissue or alcohol-free wipes; nothing should be put into the ear to dry it (Harkin 2008). The ear canal is self-cleaning through jaw movement and epithelial migration action which moves wax and debris up to the outer ear skin (Harkin 2008).

Principles of care

Ear hygiene needs to be carried out carefully to avoid causing damage to the ear. Public awareness of this is low and leads to attempts to remove wax with instruments such as cotton swabs and hairpins (Dingwall 2010). As well as traumatizing the skin, these actions often contribute to increased wax production and impaction (see Box 8.5) and can also impair the self-cleansing mechanism of the organ. Fundamentals of ear hygiene include the following.

- Never insert any implements such as cotton buds into the ear.
- To dry/clean the outside of the ear, use a dry tissue or alcohol-free baby wipe around and behind the ear after the patient has showered/bathed.
- Use a soft disposable damp cloth to gently wipe around the cartilaginous area of the ear.

If there are any signs of inflammation or the patient is complaining of any discomfort:

- keep the ears dry, avoiding any entry of water: shampoo and soaps may be irritating to the skin
- when washing hair, use cotton wool coated in petroleum jelly or ear plugs placed at the entrance to both ear canals.

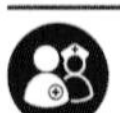

Box 8.6 **Hearing tests for adults**

Pure tone audiometry

Pure tone audiometry (PTA) tests the hearing of both ears. During PTA, a machine called an audiometer is used to produce sounds at various volumes and frequencies (pitches).

Speech perception

The speech perception test, also sometimes known as a speech discrimination test or speech audiometry, involves testing ability to hear words without using any visual information. The words may be played through headphones or a speaker, or spoken by the tester.

Tympanometry

The eardrum should allow as much sound as possible to pass into the middle ear. If sound is reflected back from the eardrum, hearing will be impaired.

During tympanometry, a small tube is placed at the entrance of the ear and air gently blown down it into the ear. The test can be used to confirm whether the ear is blocked, most commonly by fluid.

Whispered voice test

The whispered voice test is a very simple hearing test. It involves the tester blocking one of the participant's ears and testing their hearing by whispering words at varying volumes.

Tuning fork test

A tuning fork produces sound waves at a fixed pitch when it is gently tapped and can be used to test different aspects of hearing.

The tester will tap the tuning fork on their elbow or knee to make it vibrate, before holding it at different places around the participant's head.

Bone conduction test

A bone conduction test is often carried out as part of a routine pure tone audiometry (PTA) test in adults.

Bone conduction involves placing a vibrating probe against the mastoid bone behind the ear. It tests how well sounds transmitted through the bone are heard.

Bone conduction is a more sophisticated version of the tuning fork test, and when used together with PTA, it can help determine whether hearing loss comes from the outer and middle ear, the inner ear, or both (NHS Choices 2013).

Assessment

A good light source such as a bull's eye lamp and head mirror or an operating lamp positioned above and behind the nurse is necessary prior to commencing ear care procedures to enable careful assessment of the ears and to avoid damage to the delicate structures (Alexander et al. 2007). The patient and nurse should be sitting at the same height to examine the outer ear and pinna (Harkin 2008). Any alteration to the appearance of the ear must be reported to the doctor.

Before proceeding with any form of invasive ear care, it is important to undertake careful examination of the ear, taking note of any discharge, redness or swelling, and the amount and texture of any ear wax present, as this will give an indication of the general health of the ear. A small amount of wax should be expected in the ear canal. Its absence may be a sign of a dry skin condition, infection or excessive cleaning that has interfered with the normal wax production (Harkin 2008).

The nurse should discuss with the patient their current level of hearing and after the procedure they should ask the patient if there are any changes so as to monitor the effectiveness of the intervention. Consideration should always be given to a patient's hearing aids and assistance given to clean these. Advice regarding the most appropriate method should be sought, preferably from the patient. Irrigation of the inner ear is sometimes necessary to remove foreign bodies or to clear excessive build-up of ear wax (cerumen) (Harkin 2008).

Poor ear care can cause:

- otitis media
- trauma to the external meatus
- tinnitus
- deafness
- perforation of the tympanic membrane.

Special care should be taken to avoid damage to the aural cavity and eardrum.

Methods of ear wax softener use

Due to the invasive nature of ear irrigation, it is advised that the patient first tries using wax softeners such as olive oil, which may avoid the need for irrigation (Jacobs 2008, Kraszewski 2008). A typical treatment regime for ear wax softening is the instillation of 2–3 drops of olive oil into the ear daily for a 5-day period (Aung and Mulley 2002).

Methods of ear irrigation

Ear irrigation is an invasive procedure that requires good understanding of the anatomy and physiology of the ear and competence with the procedure (Kraszewski 2008).

Box 8.7 **Contraindications to ear irrigation**

- Perforated eardrums.
- Middle ear infection in the previous 6 weeks.
- Mucus discharge.
- *In situ* grommet.
- Cleft palate.
- Acute otitis externa with pain and tenderness to the pinna.
- History of ear surgery (Jacobs 2008).

An electric oral jet irrigator fitted with a special ear irrigator tip is recommended for ear irrigation as the water pressure can be controlled more precisely, along with the direction of the water (Aung and Mulley 2002). The water temperature should be 37°; if too hot or cold, it can cause dizziness or vertigo (Aung and Mulley 2002). The traditional method of irrigation uses a metal water-filled, hand-held syringe but due to the high risk of infection and trauma to the ear, this is no longer recommended practice (Harkin 2008).

Following irrigation, the patient's symptoms should resolve. If the symptoms continue, further treatment may be required and in some cases referral to Ear Nose and Throat (ENT) may be appropriate. Irrigation is not the only method of removing excess earwax. Those patients who have contraindications to ear irrigation (Box 8.7) still require wax removal, and this can be by instrumentation or microsuction. This must only be carried out by a nurse trained to carry out this procedure. This procedure is not readily accessible in primary care so patients are usually referred to local ENT clinics.

Mouth care

DEFINITION

Mouth care is the care given to the oral mucosa, lips, teeth and gums in order to promote health and prevent or treat disease. It involves assessment, correct care and patient education to promote independence (Hahn and Jones 2000).

ANATOMY AND PHYSIOLOGY

Structure of the oral cavity

The mouth consists of the vestibule and the oral cavity (Figure 8.7). The vestibule is the space between the lips and cheeks on the outside and the teeth and gingivae (gums) on the inside. The palate forms the roof of the oral cavity with the base of the tongue forming the floor of the mouth. It is bordered by the alveolar arches, teeth and gums at either side (Cooley 2002). The lips and cheeks are formed of skeletal muscle; the inner part of the cheeks is known as the buccal mucosa and consists of columnar epithelium. The lips are involved in speech and facial expression and keep food within the oral cavity. The cheeks control the location of food as the teeth break it down.

Teeth

Teeth are formed of the crown (the visible part) and the root. The crown is covered in enamel, a hard, dense material which cannot repair itself once damaged. Below the enamel cap, the tooth is formed of a bone-like material called dentine. This extends into the root and surrounds the pulp cavity, which contains nerve fibres, blood vessels and connective tissue. When the pulp cavity extends into the root, it is known as the root canal. Teeth are embedded in alveoli (sockets) in the maxilla and mandible and are held in place by periodontal ligaments and a substance known as cementum. Teeth are important in breaking down and grinding food and are also involved in producing sounds in speech (Marieb 2001).

Tongue

The tongue is a muscular structure extending from its tip (apex) to the posterior attachment in the oropharynx. It houses taste buds and is involved in taste, forming food into a bolus and pushing it to the back of the mouth for swallowing. It is also involved in the articulation of sounds in speech.

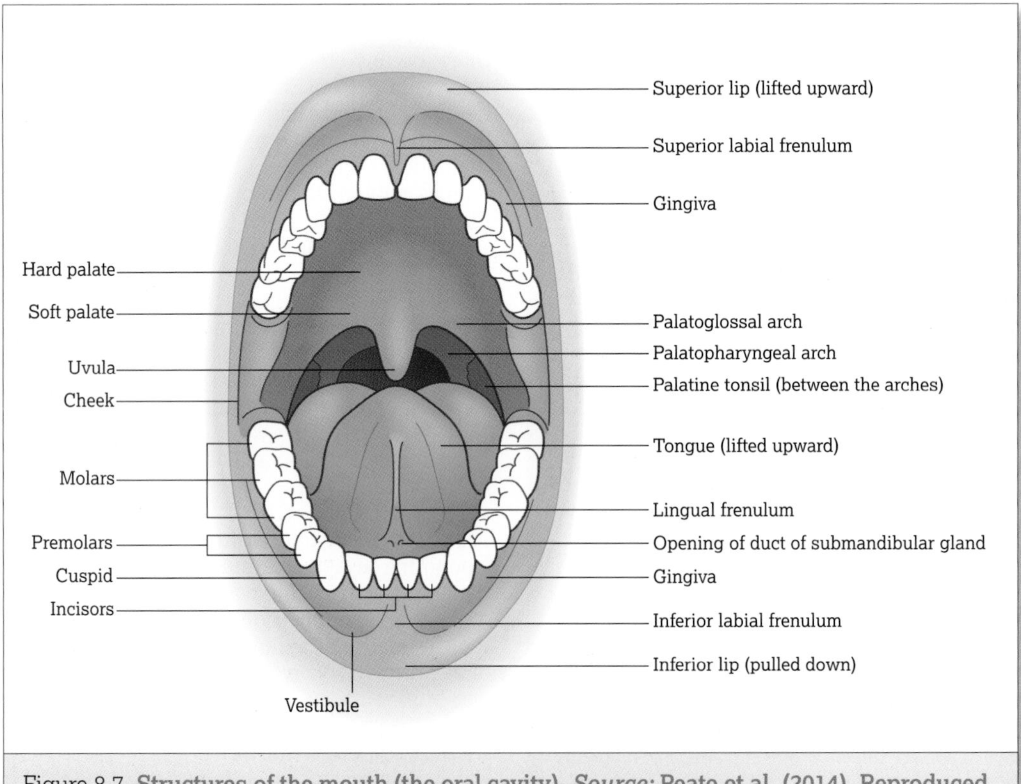

Figure 8.7 **Structures of the mouth (the oral cavity).** ***Source:*** **Peate et al. (2014). Reproduced with permission from John Wiley & Sons.**

Palate

The palate consists of the hard palate anteriorly and the soft palate which is a muscular structure leading to the palatoglossal arches and the uvula. The hard and soft palates are involved in mastication, swallowing and production of speech (Lockhart and Resick 2006).

Saliva

Saliva is produced by the parotid glands (in front of the ears), which produce saliva rich in amylase, the submandibular glands (in the lower part of the floor of the mouth), which produce mucinous saliva, the sublingual glands (in the floor of the mouth between the side of the tongue and the teeth), producing viscous saliva, and many minor salivary glands throughout the oral cavity (Hahn and Jones 2000). One litre of saliva can be produced daily, consisting of mainly water with electrolytes, amylase, proteins such as mucin, lysozyme and IgA and metabolic wastes (Lockhart and Resick 2006). Saliva is slightly acidic and can act as a buffer. It is also important in mastication, taste and speech. It acts as a defence against infection by physically washing debris off teeth and saliva proteins also have an antibacterial action (Hahn and Jones 2000).

RELATED THEORY

Oral health can be defined as 'a state of being free from chronic mouth and facial pain, oral and throat cancer, oral sores, birth defects such as a cleft lip and palate, periodontal (gum) disease, tooth decay and tooth loss and other diseases and disorders that affect the oral cavity' (WHO 2012). Good oral hygiene is essential as poor oral health can affect a patient's ability to eat or taste food, affect verbal and non-verbal communication, limit self-confidence and desire to interact with others and cause pain and infection, in some cases leading to life-threatening illness (Malkin 2009). Evidence has shown that the knowledge and attitudes of caregivers are integral to the delivery of effective oral care. The barriers to providing effective oral care include the view of oral health as a low priority, psychological distress about working inside another person's mouth and the lack of time (Bissett and Preshaw 2011).

Dental decay

Dental decay begins with the formation of a biofilm known as plaque which is made up of sugar, bacteria and other debris on the teeth. Tooth enamel can be damaged due to bacterial action, resulting in a drop in pH around the tooth. Once there is damage to the enamel then the inner dentine can also decay (Cooley 2002). Areas of decay in teeth are known as caries. Plaque can be physically removed by brushing and flossing teeth. If it is not regularly removed, it can harden to form calculus (tartar) which requires dental treatment for removal. Calculus can also disrupt the seal between the gingiva and the tooth, resulting in red, swollen and bleeding gums (gingivitis). This inflammation can progress to the formation of deep pockets of infection, damaging the teeth and underlying bone (periodontitis) (Marieb 2001). Smoking is known to be a risk factor for periodontitis and other factors such as xerostomia can also increase the risk of such problems.

Xerostomia

Xerostomia is the subjective sensation of a dry mouth, which does not always correlate to a reduction in saliva production (Maher 2004). It can be associated with thickened saliva or discomfort which may be burning in nature, leading to difficulty eating or speaking (Davies 2005b). Thirty percent of 65-year-olds have xerostomia and salivary gland hypofunction (Bissett and Preshaw 2011).

Where possible, the cause should be treated; sips of water normally only relieve the problem briefly. Artificial saliva may be helpful and mucin-based salivary substitutes are the most effective, available in gel and spray forms. Production of saliva may be stimulated by use of sugar-free chewing gum but acidic sweets should be avoided as they may cause discomfort and increase the risk of dental caries (Davies 2000). Salivary stimulants such as pilocarpine can also be useful. Studies have also demonstrated that acupuncture can be helpful (Davies 2005b).

Patients with xerostomia must pay careful attention to oral hygiene as they are at increased risk of oral complications such as caries and periodontitis due to loss of the protective effect of saliva (Maher 2004).

EVIDENCE-BASED APPROACHES

Principles of care

The aims of oral care are to:

- keep the oral mucosa and lips clean, soft, moist and intact
- keep natural teeth free from plaque and debris
- maintain denture hygiene and prevent disease related to dentures
- prevent oral infection
- prevent oral discomfort
- maintain the mouth in a state of normal function (Jones 1998).

Box 8.8 lists the recommendations for maintaining oral health.

Within a variety of care settings, patients can find themselves at risk of poor oral health. Patients in particular need of assistance or extra care include those with the following problems.

- Patients who are nil by mouth (including unconscious or ventilated patients).
- Patients who mouth breathe (including those on oxygen therapy or with a nasogastric tube).
- Cancer patients receiving radiotherapy to the head and neck or chemotherapy which can directly affect the oral cavity or result in reduced immunity to infection.
- Patients having oral surgery or who have traumatic injury to the head and neck.
- Older patients.
- Patients with diabetes.
- Patients unable to maintain their own oral hygiene due to physical disability or psychological disorders which could affect motivation.
- Patients with clotting disorders.
- Patients who have dry mouth or gum overgrowth as side-effects of medication (Carpenito-Moyet 2012).

Every patient should have a thorough assessment of the oral cavity. This should begin with a detailed nursing history of the

Box 8.8 **Factors that maintain good oral health**

- Eating a healthy diet, particularly limiting sugary foods and drinks to reduce the build-up of plaque (this includes sugar-containing medicines).
- Stop smoking; it is known to increase the risk of gum disease and oral cancers.
- Limit alcohol consumption: high intake is a known risk factor for oral cancers.
- Have regular dental check-ups.
- Brush teeth for 2 minutes at least twice daily with a fluoride toothpaste and use floss or an interdental brush to clean areas that are hard to reach.
- Look for signs of oral disease; consult a dentist if anything unusual is seen.
- Take care in activities such as contact sports where facial injuries can occur.

Source: DH (2005a).

patient's usual oral hygiene practices. This will help the nurse determine the patient's needs and preferences when planning oral care, and will also establish the level of nursing care required. Examples of those who may need assistance include those with dexterity problems where hand co-ordination may be impaired, those with cognitive impairment, those whose illness may cause them to feel fatigued and those whose illness imposes restrictions on activities (Kozier et al. 2008).

Good assessment is vital before a care plan can be formulated. Assessment should include visual inspection and obtaining a history from the patient. Many factors should be considered when carrying out a full oral assessment (Box 8.9).

Assessment of the oral cavity should include assessment of the lips, tongue, gums and tissues, saliva, natural teeth or dentures, oral cleanliness, and the presence of any dental pain (Chalmers et al. 2005). This is especially important if the patient has cognitive impairment or a learning disability that may prevent them from self-reporting any oral or dental symptoms.

Inspection should be undertaken in good light, gloves should be worn, a pen torch should be available, and any dentures or plates should be removed. It is helpful to have a set order in which areas are examined so nothing is missed. The following areas should be inspected.

- *The lips*: are they dry, cracked or bleeding?
- *The upper and lower labial sulci (inner part of the lip towards the vestibule)*: the lip should be retracted with a gloved finger or tongue depressor.
- *The buccal mucosa on the right and left sides*: is it intact, soft, moist, coated, ulcerated or inflamed?
- *The dorsal surface of the tongue (ask the patient to stick out the tongue)*: is it dry, coated or ulcerated?
- *The ventral surface of the tongue (ask the patient to lift the tongue up and move it from side to side)*: can the patient move it normally?
- *The floor of the mouth should also be inspected*: is the normal saliva pool present, is the saliva watery?
- *The hard and soft palate*: are they intact, ulcerated or red?
- *The gums*: are they inflamed or bleeding?
- *The teeth*: are they present, cared for, loose or stained, is debris present? (Davies 2005a, Hahn and Jones 2000)

Patients with dentures

Patients with dentures should be encouraged or assisted to remove and clean the denture at least daily. The denture should be cleaned over a towel or a water-filled sink to reduce the risk of damage if it is dropped. It should be brushed with a large toothbrush, denture brush or personal nailbrush and a specialized denture paste or cleaner. Toothpaste should never be used as it is too abrasive for dentures. The dentures should be rinsed with water before being replaced in the mouth. Denture wearers are at risk of fungal infections developing under the denture and spreading to the hard palate and should be advised to remove and soak the denture ideally overnight or at least for 1 hour. The denture should be soaked in water or a disinfectant commercial denture soak preparation if you suspect the patient has an oral infection (Frazer et al. 2009). If the denture has metal parts or if infection is present, chlorhexidine 0.2% can be used to disinfect the denture (Sweeney 2005). The denture should be rinsed well before reinsertion. It should be marked with the wearer's name and the storage container should also be marked and should be either disposable or able to be sterilized (Chalmers and Pearson 2005). Denture wearers should also clean any remaining teeth, gums and tongue with a soft toothbrush and fluoride toothpaste. They should also have regular dental check-ups as ill-fitting dentures can cause ulcers or irritation (Clay 2000, Duffin 2008).

Box 8.9 Factors to consider when carrying out an oral assessment

- Usual oral hygiene practice and frequency.
- Regularity of dental visits.
- Oral discomfort or pain.
- Dry mouth.
- Difficulty chewing.
- Difficulty swallowing.
- Difficulty speaking.
- Halitosis (malodorous breath).
- Drooling.
- Presence of dentures and normal care routine.
- Current or past dental problems.
- Other risk factors, for example diabetes, steroid treatment, smoking, alcohol intake, altered nutritional status.

Source: Adapted from Davies (2005a), Malkin (2009).

Patients needing assistance

A variety of patient groups may need assistance. Patients with mental illness or learning disabilities may need encouragement or assistance to maintain their oral hygiene (Doyle and Dalton 2008, Griffiths et al. 2000). Patients with conditions affecting mobility, sight or dexterity may find it difficult to carry out oral hygiene without assistance. Practical aids such as using a mirror and sitting down rather than standing can aid independence. Use of a foam handle aid to make the toothbrush easier to hold (Figure 8.8) or a pump action toothpaste can also help (Holman et al. 2005).

Older patients may be at risk of oral problems due to a natural decline in salivary gland function, wear and tear of teeth, and taking medication with side-effects which can cause oral problems such as dry mouth, taste changes or increased risk

Figure 8.8 **Foam handle to assist with holding a toothbrush.**

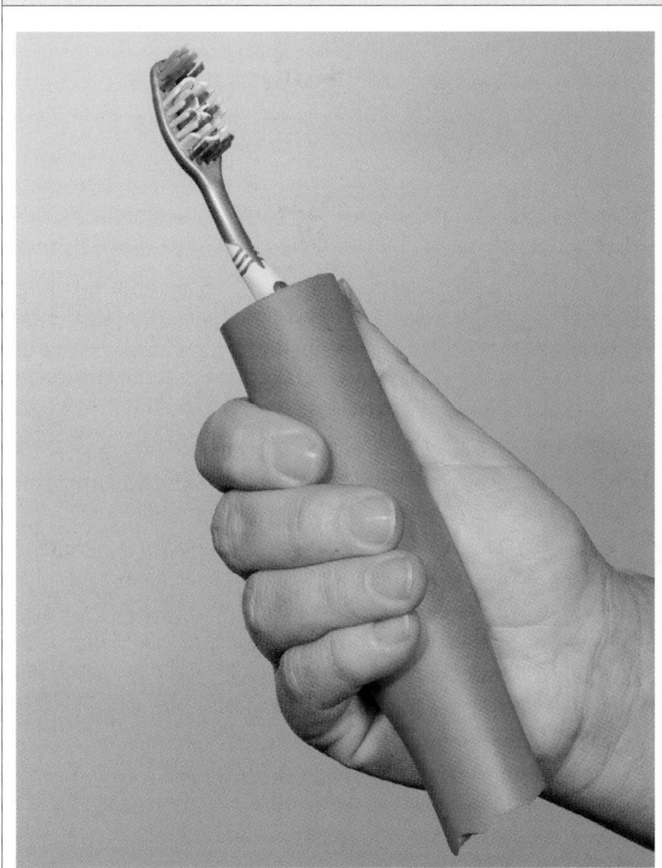

of infection (Chalmers and Pearson 2005, Clay 2000, Fitzpatrick 2000). Regular assessment and assistance with maintaining oral hygiene are recommended (NHSQIS 2004). For the patient who needs assistance, it is recommended that the carer stands behind or to the side of the patient and supports the lower jaw (Sweeney 2005).

Unconscious patients

Unconscious patients require particular interventions to maintain oral hygiene and comfort. For patients who are close to death, there is a lack of evidence relating to oral care and the focus should be on patient comfort. Any interventions causing distress should be stopped; mouthcare can be offered 1–2 hourly but in practice it should be dependent on the need of the individual (Sweeney 2005). Gentle cleaning with a soft toothbrush or foam stick is recommended and a lubricant should be applied to the lips (Dahlin 2004).

In critically ill patients who are unconscious and requiring mechanical ventilation, management is different (Box 8.10). It is well known that aspiration of oropharyngeal flora can cause bacterial pneumonia (Li et al. 2000). Ventilator-associated pneumonia (VAP) is a serious complication which can occur in up to a quarter of ventilated patients and has a mortality of up to 50% (Berry et al. 2007). In critically ill patients the mouth can become colonized within 48 hours of admission to hospital with bacteria that tend to be more virulent than those normally found in the mouth (Grap et al. 2003). The oropharynx can become colonized, as can an artificial airway. This can allow pathogens to travel to the respiratory tract, resulting in pneumonia (Cutler and Davis 2005). It is well recognized that good oral care is essential in critically ill patients to reduce the incidence of VAP.

Other contributing factors to poor oral health in this group of patients include dry mouth related to use of oxygen, mouth breathing and the patient being nil by mouth. The presence of tubes or securing tapes can make it difficult to view and clean the oral cavity. Further research is needed in this area as there is a lack of trial-based evidence to support practice (Munro and Grap 2004).

LEGAL AND PROFESSIONAL ISSUES

Nurses should provide a high standard of care to patients, based on the best evidence available, ensuring they have the necessary skills (NMC 2015). Numerous studies have found that nurses feel they lack knowledge and training about providing oral care (Southern 2007). Although a number of training tools are available, the provision of adequate training before and after registration requires further attention (Doyle and Dalton 2008, NHSQIS 2004). As is the case for all procedures, a full explanation must be given to the patient and verbal consent obtained (NMC 2013). If patients refuse oral care, nurses should try and explore their reasons for refusal. If you suspect a patient lacks capacity to understand the outcome of refusing oral care then you should follow the guidance in the most current version of the Mental Capacity Act.

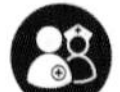

Box 8.10 **Recommendations for oral care in critically ill patients**

- Daily assessment.
- Oral care 2–4 hourly.
- Brushing with a small-headed soft toothbrush and fluoride toothpaste.
- Cleaning the mouth with foam sticks and chlorhexidine mouthwash or gel for patients for whom a toothbrush would be unsuitable, for example bleeding, severe ulcers.
- Use of suction to prevent aspiration.

Source: Adapted from Abidia (2007), Stiefel et al. (2000).

PRE-PROCEDURAL CONSIDERATIONS

Equipment

Toothbrush

The toothbrush is recognized as being the most effective means of removing plaque and debris from the teeth and gums. A small-headed, medium-textured brush is most effective at reaching all areas of the mouth. Powered toothbrushes have been shown to be as effective as manual toothbrushes and may be easier for patients with limited dexterity to use (Robinson et al. 2005). Aids such as foam handles can also be obtained from the occupational therapist to make a manual toothbrush easier to hold (see Figure 8.8). The toothbrush should be allowed to air dry to reduce bacterial contamination and changed every 3 months or sooner if worn (Hahn and Jones 2000). For patients with a sore mouth, a soft or baby toothbrush can be used.

Foam sticks

The foam stick is one of the most common pieces of equipment used in hospital to provide oral care although it is well known that less plaque is removed than with a toothbrush, particularly from less obvious areas of the teeth (Pearson and Hutton 2002). The foam stick should only be used on patients who cannot tolerate use of a toothbrush, such as those with painful or bleeding mouths. Care should be taken that the foam head is securely attached to avoid risk of accidental aspiration (Malkin 2009).

Interdental cleaning

The use of dental floss or other equipment is recommended to clean areas between the teeth which may be difficult to reach with a toothbrush (Huskinson and Lloyd 2009). There is currently limited evidence of the efficacy of flossing although it is generally believed to be beneficial (Berchier et al. 2008). A variety of equipment is available such as dental floss, dental tape, wood sticks or interdental brushes (Figure 8.9). For patients who have limited dexterity, this may be difficult or impossible to carry out. Similarly, in patients with painful mouths or bleeding gums, this type of equipment could cause further discomfort or bleeding and should be avoided.

Oral irrigation devices such as the WaterPik® can also be used for interdental cleaning. Oral irrigation involves a jet of water being used to remove debris and plaque and can be useful for people who find it difficult to use dental floss or tape such as those with

Figure 8.9 **Examples of interdental cleaning products. (a) Disposable flosser. (b) Interdental brush. (c) Dental floss.**

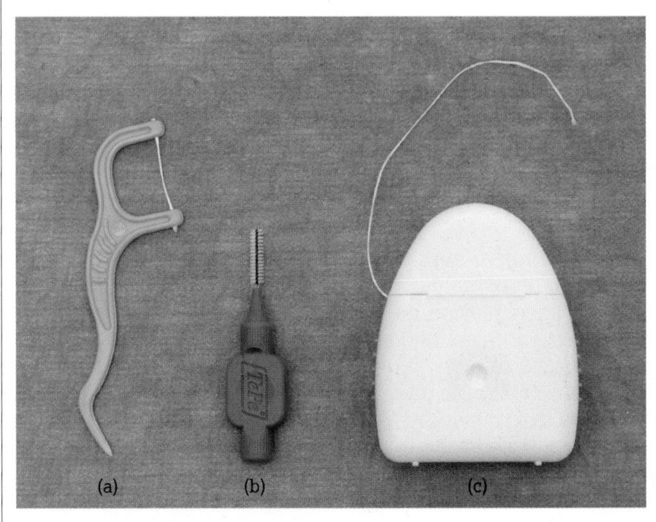

braces. A systematic review of oral irrigation has shown a positive tendency but no overall benefit in reducing plaque over use of a toothbrush alone (Husseini et al. 2008).

Assessment and recording tools

The mouth should be assessed as part of the initial nursing assessment and should be reassessed regularly thereafter (DH 2001, NHSQIS 2004). Frequency of assessment is often based on clinical judgement rather than evidence. For patients at high risk of changes to the condition of the mouth, such as those receiving high-dose chemotherapy, assessment should be carried out daily (Quinn et al. 2008). For elderly patients receiving long-term care, it has been recommended that reassessment takes place on a regular basis. Recommendations for the frequency of assessment vary – monthly (NHSQIS 2004) or quarterly (Sarin et al. 2008) – but all recommend assessment on admission to the care facility and then at regular intervals throughout the year.

The use of an oral assessment tool is recommended to ensure consistency between assessors and to monitor changes. A number of tools have been devised for different patient groups. Tools such as the WHO scale (WHO 1979) or the Oral Assessment Guide (OAG) (Eilers et al. 1988) are commonly used in assessing patients receiving anticancer treatments. Numerous other tools exist to assess oral mucositis, although some lack evidence of validity and reliability. Use of a validated tool is recommended (Huskinson and Lloyd 2009). Several tools have also been designed to meet the needs of elderly patients and those with dementia (Kayser-Jones et al. 1995, Roberts 2001). An example of a tool that can be used with patients in residential care is the Oral Health Assessment Tool (OHAT; Chalmers et al. 2005).

The ideal assessment tool should measure:

- functional changes, for example ability to talk or eat
- physical changes, for example presence of ulcerated areas
- subjective changes, for example pain or dryness.

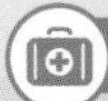

The ideal tool has not yet been developed and it may be necessary to use a combination of tools to make a thorough assessment. Patient education to encourage self-assessment is also recommended (Quinn et al. 2008).

Learning Activity 8.2

Learning in practice: Oral assessment

Thinking about oral assessment in your clinical practice:

- Do you routinely assess a patient's mouth as part of their initial assessment?
- Find a copy of the assessment tool that is routinely used by your Trust. Discuss the use of this tool in your practice area with your mentor/supervising nurse.
- With consent, and referring to Procedure Guideline 8.9: Mouth care, carry out an oral assessment on one of your patients and document your findings. (You will require a tongue depressor, gauze and a pen torch to effectively inspect the oral cavity.)

Pharmacological support

The choice of an oral care agent will be dependent on the aim of care. The agent may be used to remove debris and plaque, prevent superimposed infection, alleviate pain, provide comfort, stop bleeding, provide lubrication or treat specific problems (Dickinson and Porter 2006). A wide variety of agents is available and choice should be determined by the individual needs of the patient and the particular clinical situation together with a detailed nursing assessment. There is ongoing debate on the efficacy of agents presently available and there is insufficient evidence to clearly state the best agents to use in the clinical setting.

Toothpaste

Toothpaste is a paste or gel used with a toothbrush (mechanical or powered) to clean and maintain the health of teeth and gums. It is an abrasive substance that aids in the removal of food from the teeth and dental plaque. Most of the cleaning is achieved from the mechanical action of the toothbrush and not by the toothpaste. Most toothpastes have active ingredients to help prevent tooth and gum disease. Toothpastes are composed of 20–42% water with a variety of other components such as abrasives (remove plaque and stains from the tooth surface), fluoride (prevents cavities) and detergents (surfactants used mainly as a foaming agent). Different types are listed in the Dental Prescribing Formulary.

A pea-sized amount of fluoride toothpaste should be used; fluoride is known to have anticaries activity and can reduce dentine sensitivity. If toothpaste is too abrasive for a patient whose mouth is painful, water alone can be used (Sweeney 2005).

Commercial mouthwash

Over-the-counter mouthwashes are not generally recommended. Many have a high alcohol content which can cause stinging, particularly for patients with sensitive mouths (Milligan et al. 2001).

Bland rinses

Several agents have been used to rinse the mouth, moisten the mucosa and loosen and remove debris. Normal saline has been recommended by a number of authors as part of a patient's oral care. This relatively cheap and generally well-tolerated solution can alleviate discomfort although it is not effective at removing heavy amounts of debris (Milligan et al. 2001). Patients with mucositis can benefit from frequent rinsing of the mouth with warm normal saline to remove debris without causing irritation (Meechan 2005). The use of water has also been suggested to rinse the mouth after meals to remove debris (Sweeney 2005). Its use in critical care has been discouraged due to risk of infection in vulnerable patients, but sterile water may be an alternative (Berry et al. 2007). Sodium bicarbonate has been used in some centres although there is some evidence that patients find it unpleasant to taste and that it can alter pH in the mouth, predisposing to bacterial growth (Wood 2004).

Chlorhexidine gluconate

Chlorhexidine gluconate is an effective antibacterial and antiplaque agent. For the patient who is unable to use a toothbrush, it can provide a chemical method of stopping plaque build-up. As chlorhexidine is released from tissues for up to 12 hours, it only needs to be used twice daily. Chlorhexidine does not remove plaque which is already present so brushing of teeth should continue as far as possible (Sweeney 2005). Foam sticks can be used with chlorhexidine rather than plain water for an antibacterial effect (Huskinson and Lloyd 2009). It is also available as a gel formulation which may be useful for those requiring a non-foaming alternative to toothpaste (patients at risk of aspiration or with swallowing difficulties).

Contraindicated agents

A number of agents widely used in the past for mouth care have been found to have detrimental effects and are no longer recommended. Glycerine and lemon swabs have been used for dry mouth but the acid content can damage tooth enamel and the overall effect is to increase oral dryness (Hahn and Jones 2000). Hydrogen peroxide is also not recommended as it can cause mucosal abnormalities (Berry et al. 2007).

Specific patient pharmacological preparations

Fluoride

Fluoride helps to prevent and arrest tooth decay, especially radiation caries, demineralization and decalcification. High-dose fluoride toothpaste may be recommended for patients with xerostomia (NHSQIS 2004).

Artificial saliva

Saliva substitutes which are mucin based are more effective than those which are carboxymethylcellulose based for relieving dry mouth (xerostomia) (Davies 2005b). Recommendations are to spray several times around the mouth and then to use the tongue to spread the artificial saliva around. It should be used prior to meals and at any other time when the mouth feels dry (Davies 2000).

Coating agents

A coating agent can be used to coat the surface of the mouth, forming a thin protective film over painful oral lesions or mucositis. Oral lesions or mucositis can be caused by medication, disease, oral surgery, stress, traumatic ulcers caused by dental braces and dentures, radiotherapy and chemotherapy. Examples include GelClair, Mugard and Episil. These products should be rinsed around the mouth to form a protective layer over the sore areas, and generally applied 1 hour before eating. Several agents have been used to coat the oral mucosa and they are thought to have a protective effect although there is limited evidence to support their use. Sucralfate has not been shown to be effective in preventing or treating chemotherapy- or radiotherapy-associated oral mucositis (Clarkson et al. 2007, Worthington et al. 2007).

Antifungal agents

Colonization of the mouth with yeast occurs in one-third of the population. In patients receiving steroids or antibiotics, the balance of oral flora can be altered and oral candidiasis (oral thrush) can occur. Predisposing factors also include xerostomia and the presence of dentures. These infections can be treated with either topical or systemic antifungal medications. In debilitated or immunocompromised patients, candidiasis can become a systemic disease.

Antifungal agents are a group of drugs specifically used for the treatment of fungal infections. Oropharyngeal candidiasis can be treated with either topical antifungal agents (e.g. nystatin, clotrimazole, amphotericin B oral suspension) or systemic oral azoles (fluconazole, itraconazole or posaconazole). Length of treatment will depend on the pharmacological agent chosen and should follow recommendations in the *British National Formulary* (most current publication) and local prescribing guidelines.

Topical treatment is normally effective using an antifungal oral suspension or lozenges (Finlay and Davies 2005).

Procedure guideline 8.9 **Mouth care**

Essential equipment

- Small torch
- Plastic cups
- Mouthwash or cleaning solutions
- Appropriate equipment for cleaning
- Clean receiver or bowl
- Paper tissues/gauze
- Wooden spatula
- Small-headed, soft toothbrush
- Toothpaste
- Non-sterile disposable gloves
- Dental floss

Pre-procedure

Action	Rationale
1 Explain and discuss the procedure with the patient. When possible, encourage patients to carry out their own oral care.	To ensure that the patient understands the procedure and gives their valid consent (NMC 2013, **C**). To enable patients to gain confidence in managing their own symptoms (DH 2005a, **C**).
2 Wash hands with soap and water and dry with paper towel or use alcohol handrub. Put on disposable gloves.	To reduce the risk of cross-infection (Fraise and Bradley 2009, **E**).

Procedure

Action	Rationale
3 Prepare solutions required.	Solutions must always be prepared immediately before use to maximize their efficacy and minimize the risk of microbial contamination (Fraise and Bradley 2009, **E**).
4 Carry out oral assessment using an oral assessment tool.	Provides baseline to enable monitoring of mucosal changes and evaluate response to treatment and care (Eilers et al. 1988, **R5**; Sonis et al. 2004, **R5**).
5 (a) Inspect the patient's mouth, including teeth, with the aid of a torch, spatula and gauze, paying special attention to the lips, buccal mucosa, lateral and ventral surfaces of the tongue, floor of the mouth and the soft palate (**Action figure 5**).	The mouth is examined for changes in condition with respect to moisture, cleanliness, infected or bleeding areas, ulcers, and so on. These areas are known to be more susceptible to cytotoxic damage (Sonis et al. 2004, **R5**).
(b) Ask the patient if they have any of the following: taste changes, change in saliva production and composition, oral discomfort or difficulty swallowing.	To assess nutritional deficits, salivary changes and pain secondary to oral changes (Sonis et al. 2004, **R5**).
6 Using a soft, small toothbrush and toothpaste (or foam stick if the gingiva is damaged or susceptible to bleeding), brush the patient's natural teeth, gums and tongue.	To remove adherent materials from the teeth, tongue and gum surfaces (Hitz Lindenmüller and Lambrecht 2011,**E**). Brushing stimulates gingival tissues to maintain tone and prevent circulatory stasis (Clay 2000, **E**; Pearson and Hutton 2002, **R1b**). Foam stick reduces possibility of trauma (Cooley 2002, **E**).

(continued)

Procedure guideline 8.9 Mouth care *(continued)*

Action	Rationale
7 Hold the brush against the teeth with the bristles at a 45° angle. The tips of the outer bristles should rest against and penetrate under the gingival sulcus. Then move the bristles back and forth using horizontal or circular strokes and a vibrating motion (bass sulcular technique), from the sulcus to the crowns of the teeth. A gentle scrubbing action is recommended, using small movements with gentle pressure for 2 minutes (Sweeney 2005). The brush should be placed at a 45° angle against the teeth and overlaying the gum edge to allow cleaning of the gingival margin (Jones 1998). Repeat until all teeth surfaces have been cleaned. Clean the biting surfaces of the teeth by moving the toothbrush back and forth over them in short strokes and brush tongue to remove any debris.	Brushing loosens and removes debris trapped on and between the teeth and gums (DH 2005a, **C**). This reduces the growth medium for pathogenic organisms and minimizes the risk of plaque formation and dental caries (Clay 2000, **E**; Pearson and Hutton 2002, **R1b**).
8 Give a beaker of water to the patient. Encourage patient to rinse the mouth vigorously then spit the contents into a receiver. Paper tissues should be to hand to dry any spillage of water or dribbling.	Rinsing removes loosened debris and toothpaste and makes the mouth taste fresher (Sonis et al. 2004, **R5**).
9 If the patient is unable to rinse and spit, use a rinsed toothbrush to clean the teeth and moistened foam sticks to wipe the gums and oral mucosa. Foam sticks should be used with a rotating action so that most of the surface is used.	To remove debris as effectively as possible (Sonis et al. 2004, **R5**).
10 Floss teeth (unless contraindicated, such as clotting abnormality, thrombocytopenia) once in 24 hours using lightly waxed floss. (a) To floss the upper teeth, use your thumb and index finger to stretch the floss and wrap one end of floss around the third finger of each hand. Move the floss up and down between the teeth from the tops of the crowns to the gum and along the gum lines wherever possible (**Action figure 10**). (b) To floss the lower teeth, use the index fingers to stretch the floss.	Flossing helps to remove debris between teeth. Flossing when patient has abnormal clotting or low platelets may lead to bleeding and predispose the oral mucosa to infection (Clay 2000, **E**; Beck 2004, **E**).
Post-procedure	
11 Discard remaining mouthwash solutions.	To prevent infection (Fraise and Bradley 2009, **E**).
12 Clean the toothbrush and allow it to air dry.	To prevent the risk of contamination (Jones 1998, **E**).
13 Remove gloves. Wash hands with soap and water and dry with paper towel or use alcohol handrub.	To reduce the risk of cross-infection (Fraise and Bradley 2009, **E**).
14 Ensure the patient is comfortable.	

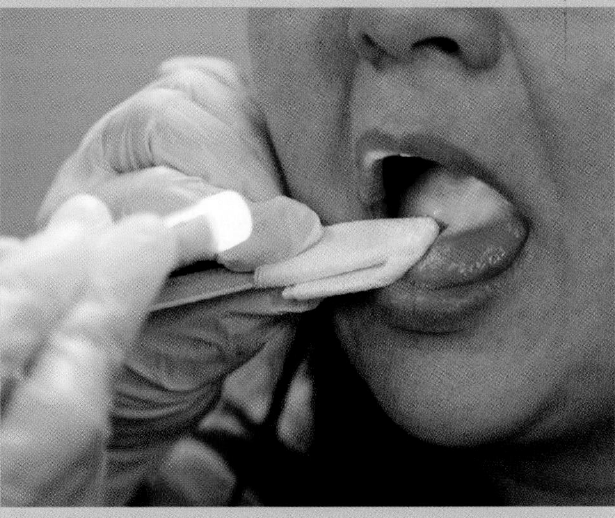

Action Figure 5 Oral assessment using a torch, spatula and gauze.

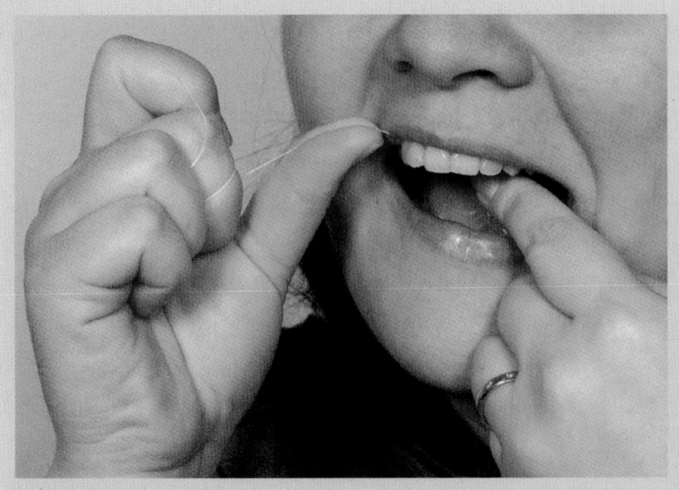
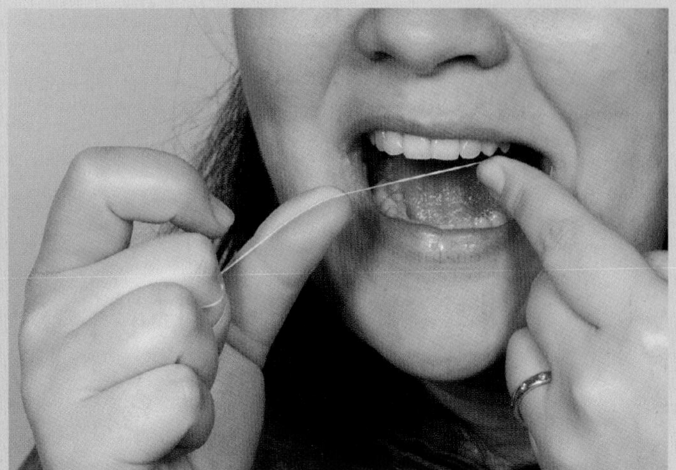

Action Figure 10 Interdental cleaning using dental floss.

Procedure guideline 8.10 **Mouth care for the patient with dentures**

Essential equipment

- Small torch
- Plastic cups
- Mouthwash or cleaning solutions
- Appropriate equipment for cleaning dentures
- Clean receiver or bowl
- Small-headed, soft toothbrush or denture brush
- Denture paste
- Non-sterile disposable gloves
- Denture pot

Pre-procedure

Action	Rationale
1 Explain and discuss the procedure with the patient. When possible, encourage patients to carry out their own oral care.	To ensure that the patient understands the procedure and gives their valid consent (NMC 2013, **C**). To enable patients to gain confidence in managing their own symptoms (DH 2005a, **C**).
2 Wash hands with soap and water and dry with paper towel or use alcohol handrub. Put on disposable gloves.	To reduce the risk of cross-infection (Fraise and Bradley 2009, **E**).
Procedure	
3 Prepare solutions required.	Solutions must always be prepared immediately before use to maximize their efficacy and minimize the risk of microbial contamination (Fraise and Bradley 2009, **E**).
4 If the patient cannot remove their own dentures, remove the lower denture first.	
(a) *Lower denture*: grasp it in the middle and lift it, rotating it gently to remove from the mouth, and place in denture pot.	The lower denture should be removed first to avoid the risk of aspiration (Sweeney 2005, **R5**).
(b) *Upper denture*: remove the upper denture by grasping firmly in the middle and tilting the denture forward while putting pressure on the front teeth to break the seal with the palate. Rotate the denture from side to side to remove it from the mouth and place it in the denture pot.	Removal of dentures is necessary for cleaning of underlying tissues (Sweeney 2005, **R5**).
5 Carry out oral assessment using an oral assessment tool.	Provides baseline to enable monitoring of mucosal changes and evaluate response to treatment and care (Eilers et al. 1988, **R5**; Sonis et al. 2004, **R5**).
6 (a) Inspect the patient's mouth with the aid of a torch, spatula and gauze, paying special attention to the lips, buccal mucosa, lateral and ventral surfaces of the tongue, floor of the mouth and the soft palate (see Procedure guideline 8.9: Mouth care, **Action figure 5**).	The mouth is examined for changes in condition with respect to moisture, cleanliness, infected or bleeding areas, ulcers, and so on. These areas are known to be more susceptible to cytotoxic damage (Sonis et al. 2004, **R5**).
(b) Ask the patient if they have any of the following: taste changes, change in saliva production and composition, oral discomfort or difficulty swallowing.	To assess nutritional deficits, salivary changes and pain secondary to oral changes (Sonis et al. 2004, **R5**).

(continued)

Procedure guideline 8.10 Mouth care for the patient with dentures *(continued)*

Action	Rationale
7 Give a beaker of water to the patient. Encourage patient to rinse the mouth vigorously then spit the contents into a receiver. Paper tissues should be to hand to dry any spillage of water or dribbling.	Rinsing removes loosened debris and makes the mouth taste fresher (Sonis et al. 2004, **R5**).
8 Clean the patient's dentures on all surfaces with a denture brush or toothbrush and soap and water or denture cleaner. Check the dentures for cracks, sharp edges and missing teeth. Rinse them well and return them to the patient.	Cleaning dentures removes accumulated food debris which could be broken down by salivary enzymes to products which irritate and cause inflammation of the adjacent mucosal tissue (Sweeney 2005, **R5**).
9 Dentures should be removed for at least 1 hour but ideally overnight and placed in a suitable cleaning solution.	Dentures can easily become colonized by bacteria. Soaking can disinfect the denture, discouraging bacterial growth (Clay 2000, **E**; Sweeney 2005, **R2b**).
Post-procedure	
10 Discard remaining mouthwash solutions.	To prevent infection (Fraise and Bradley 2009, **E**).
11 Clean the toothbrush or denture brush and allow it to air dry.	To prevent the risk of contamination (Jones 1998, **E**).
12 Remove gloves. Wash hands with soap and water and dry with paper towel or use alcohol handrub.	To reduce the risk of cross-infection (Fraise and Bradley 2009, **E**).
13 Ensure the patient is comfortable.	

Problem-solving table 8.1 Prevention and resolution (Procedure guidelines 8.9 and 8.10)

Problem	Cause	Prevention	Action
Dry mouth (xerostomia).	Oxygen therapy, mouth breathing, nil by mouth.	Humidified oxygen.	Swabbing the mouth with moistened foam stick or encouraging the patient to rinse the mouth with water and spit it out.
Dry mouth (xerostomia).	Salivary gland hypofunction due to disease, drugs or side-effects of radiotherapy or chemotherapy.	Not always possible to prevent.	Good oral hygiene to prevent complications, use of salivary stimulants, for example chewing gum, pilocarpine or saliva substitutes.
Patient unable to tolerate toothbrush.	Pain, for example post surgery. Mucositis.	Consider anaesthetic mouth spray or mouthwash before mouth care. Give regular and/or prn analgesia.	Use foam sticks and chlorhexidine 0.2% to clean the patient's teeth, gums and mucosa; 0.9% sodium chloride rinse can be used if the patient cannot tolerate any form of oral care.
Toothbrush inappropriate or ineffective.	Infected stomatis. Accumulation of dried mucus, new lesions, blood or debris.	As above.	As above and take a swab of any infected areas for culture before giving mouth care.

Pain

DEFINITION

Pain is a complex phenomenon, that has physiological, psychological and social factors that influence the individual patient experience. It is subjective so the patient's perspective is important to understand. It has both a physical and an affective (emotional) component. To reflect this, the International Association for the Study of Pain (IASP 1994) published the following definition of pain: 'An unpleasant sensory and emotional experience associated with actual or potential tissue damage, or described in terms of such damage'. As pain is subjective, another favoured definition for use in clinical practice, proposed originally by McCaffrey (1968) and cited in McCaffrey (2000, p.2), is: 'Pain is whatever the experiencing person says it is, existing whenever the experiencing person says it does'.

ANATOMY AND PHYSIOLOGY

Pain mechanisms (anatomy and physiology) are usually described in terms of nociceptive pain or neuropathic pain. As with acute and chronic pain, it may be common for pain to be both nociceptive and neuropathic in origin rather than purely one or the other.

Figure 8.10 **Processing of sensory input and motor output by the spinal cord. *Source:* Tortora and Derrickson (2011). Reproduced with permission from John Wiley & Sons.**

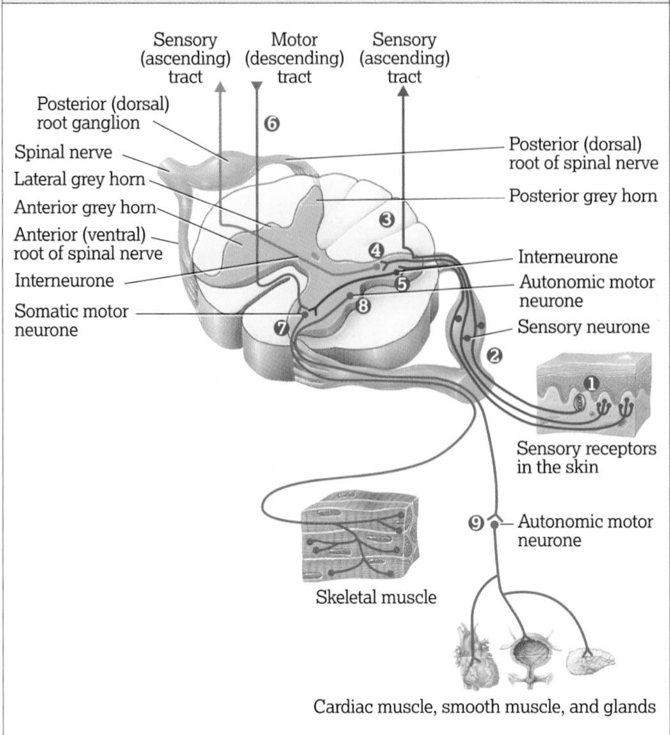

Figure 8.11 **The pain pathway showing key sites for particular analgesic interventions.**

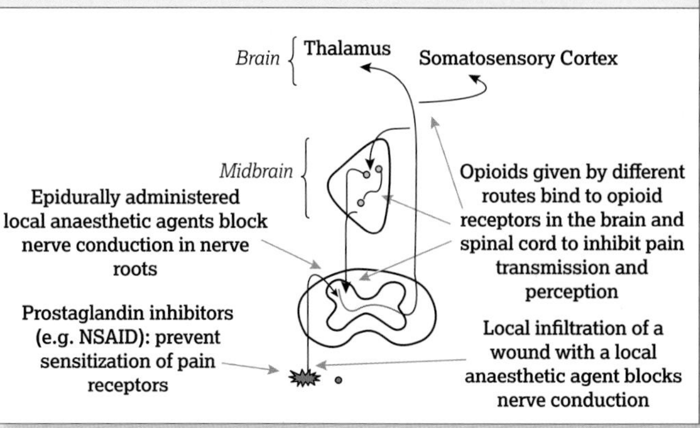

Nociceptive pain

Nociceptive pain is the 'normal' pain pathway that occurs in response to tissue injury or damage (Figure 8.10). It consists of four components: transduction, transmission, perception and modulation. Nociceptors are free nerve endings found at the end of pain neurones. They occur in skin and subcutaneous tissue, muscle, visceral organs, tendons, fascia, joint capsules and arterial walls (Godfrey 2005). Nociceptors respond to noxious thermal stimuli (heat and cold) and mechanical stimuli (stretching, compression, infiltration) and to the chemical mediators released as part of the inflammatory response to tissue injury. These chemical mediators include prostaglandins, bradykinin, substance P, serotonin and adenosine. As a result of this stimulation process, an action potential is generated in the nerve (*transduction*).

The pain signal is then transmitted along the peripheral nervous system (A delta and C fibres) to the central nervous system, arriving at the dorsal horn of the spinal cord. Neurotransmitters are released to allow the pain signal to be transmitted from the endings of the peripheral nerves to the nociceptors in the dorsal horn. The message is then transmitted to the brain where perception of the pain occurs (*transmission*). *Perception* is the end-result of the neuronal activity of pain transmission. The perception of pain includes behavioural, psychological and emotional components as well as physiological processes.

Modulation occurs when the transmission of pain impulses in the spinal cord is changed or inhibited. Modulatory influences on pain perception are complex, involving a gating system which is linked to a descending modulatory pathway. Modulation can occur as a result of a natural release of inhibitory neurotransmitter chemicals that inhibit transmission of pain impulses and therefore produce analgesia. Other interventions, including distraction, relaxation, sense of well-being, heat/cold therapy, massage and TENS, can also help to modulate pain perception. Analgesic medications work by inhibiting some of the chemicals involved in pain transduction and transmission and thus modulating pain perception (Figure 8.11). Pain signals can also be increased by certain factors such as anxiety, fear and low mood/depression.

Neuropathic pain

Neuropathic pain is not pain that originates as part of 'normal' pain pathways. It has been described as pain related to abnormal processing within the nervous system (Mann 2008). Nerve injury or dysfunction can be caused by a range of conditions such as infection, trauma, metabolic disorder, chemotherapy, surgery, radiation, neurotoxins, nerve compression, joint degeneration, tumour infiltration and malnutrition (Mann 2008).

The mechanisms by which neuropathic pain is generated and maintained are not fully understood but the following theories are currently thought to contribute.

- Damage or abnormalities in the nerves change the way that nerves communicate with each other.
- Pain receptors require less stimulation to initiate pain signals both in peripheral nerves and the central nervous system, where it is often referred to as central sensitization.
- Pain transmission is altered from its normal sequence.
- There may be an increase in the release of chemical neurotransmitters.
- There can be increased and chaotic firing of nerves.
- Damaged nerves spontaneously generate impulses in the absence of any stimulation.
- The descending inhibitory systems may also be reduced or lost.

The nervous system changes its structure and function in response to the input it receives, i.e. it is plastic. Plasticity is evident at all levels from the nociceptor to the brain (cortex). These mechanisms result in increased activity or transmission of pain signals despite less input from the peripheral nervous system. Pain can be spontaneous, may be triggered by non-painful stimuli such as touch (allodynia), may be an exaggerated pain response (hyperalgesia) and patients may also experience non-painful sensations such as pins and needles and tingling (paraesthesias).

RELATED THEORY

Many factors influence the expression of pain and may be associated with the patient, the nurse or the clinical environment (organizational aspects) (Carr and Mann 2000). Pain can have many dimensions including physical, psychological, spiritual and sociocultural.

Pain can be categorized into three main types.

- Acute pain – less than 3 months' (12 weeks) duration.
- Persistent or chronic pain – more than 3 months' (12 weeks) duration.
- Cancer pain associated with a malignancy.

There are several ways to categorize the types of pain that occur, for example nociceptive (somatic or visceral) or neuropathic. It is increasingly recognized that acute and chronic pain may represent a continuum rather than being distinct separate entities (Macintyre et al. 2010) and may combine different pain mechanisms and vary in duration.

Acute pain

The IASP has defined acute pain as: 'Pain of recent onset and probable limited duration. It usually has an identifiable temporal and causal relationship to injury or disease' (Ready and Edwards 1992, p.1). Acute pain is produced by a wide range of physiological processes, and includes inflammatory, neuropathic, sympathetically maintained, visceral and cancer pain (Walker et al. 2006). Acute pain serves a purpose by alerting the individual to a problem and acting as a warning of tissue damage or potential tissue damage. If left untreated, it may result in severe consequences; for example, not seeking help for acute abdominal pain may result in an emergency such as appendicitis progressing to peritonitis. Acute pain is short-term pain of less than 12 weeks' duration (British Pain Society 2008). It occurs in response to any type of injury to the body and resolves when the injury heals.

Common causes of acute pain include:

- surgery (e.g. upper or lower abdominal surgery, colorectal surgery, gynaecological surgery, appendicectomy, orthopaedic surgery)
- acute trauma (e.g. work-related injuries, road traffic accidents, sports injuries, head injury, spinal and neck injuries, burns/scalds)
- acute musculoskeletal pain (e.g. acute low back pain, acute joint pain)
- procedural pain or incident pain (e.g. related to a painful procedure such as venepuncture, insertion of catheter or drain or pain as a consequence of a movement or an event, e.g. defecation after anal surgery, ischaemic leg pain associated with intermittent claudication on walking)
- acute visceral pain (e.g. ischaemic heart disease, pancreatitis, cholecystitis, ulcerative colitis, Crohn's disease, cystitis) (Mann and Carr 2006).

Chronic pain

Chronic pain is usually prolonged and defined as pain that exists for more than 3 months, lasting beyond the usual course of the acute disease or expected time of healing (IASP 1996). It is often associated with major changes in personality, lifestyle and functional ability (Orenius et al. 2013). Chronic pain occurs as a result of non-malignant chronic conditions such as neuropathic, musculoskeletal and chronic post-operative pain syndromes or as a result of cancer. Types of chronic pain include the following.

- *Chronic benign pain*: pain that persists for more than 6 months but does not necessarily change over time, for example low back pain.
- *Recurrent acute pain*: acute pain that is associated with chronic conditions, episodes which occur regularly over a period longer than 6 months and potentially over a lifetime, for example migraine and trigeminal neuralgia.
- *Chronic progressive pain*: pain that persists for more than 6 months, originates from a constant cause and is likely to increase in severity, for example degenerative disorders such as osteoporosis (Mackintosh and Elson 2008).

Common causes of chronic pain can be:

- musculoskeletal pain, e.g. degenerative low back pain, osteoarthritis, polymyalgia
- post-traumatic pain, e.g. nerve plexus injury, vertebral crush fractures
- post-surgical pain, e.g. after breast surgery, thoracotomy, vasectomy, hernia repair, amputation
- central pain, e.g. spinal cord damage, central post-stroke pain, multiple sclerosis
- peripheral nerve pain, e.g. peripheral neuropathy, complex regional pain syndrome
- facial pain, e.g. trigeminal neuralgia, temporomandibular joint pain, atypical facial pain
- headaches, e.g. tension headache, migraine, cluster headaches, medication overuse headache
- infection, e.g. post-herpetic neuralgia (PHN), HIV-related pains
- vascular pain, e.g. peripheral vascular disease, Raynaud's, refractory angina
- visceral pain, e.g. pancreatitis, sickle cell pain, interstitial cystitis, endometriosis
- life-limiting conditions, e.g. cancer, end-stage heart failure (Simpson 2008).

Patients with chronic pain often describe variations in the intensity of the pain, either throughout the day or day by day depending on their activities (Nicholas et al. 2003). Within the medical literature, several terms are used to describe the variations in pain including pain flare, episodic pain, exacerbation of pain, transient/transitory pain and breakthrough pain.

Cancer pain management

Pain is a common symptom in patients with cancer (Chapman 2012). Causes of cancer pain can be multifactorial and often are related to the effects of cancer treatment such as surgery, radiotherapy or chemotherapy. In some instances, pain can be caused by the cancer itself such as patients with bone metastases or where the cancer has caused injury to nerves. Cancer pain has been reported as being present in a third of patients undergoing active anticancer treatment with a curative intent. It has also been suggested that patients who have treatment to both cure and for palliation experience pain in 59% of cases, with 64% of patients experiencing pain in advanced disease (van den Beuken-van-Everdingen et al. 2007). Cancer can be both acute and chronic and requires careful assessment and attention to detail, including a detailed history of previously tried medications and responses to these pharmacological interventions. Assessment, treatment plan and review are key in the management of cancer pain.

EVIDENCE-BASED APPROACHES

The ethos of this section will be based on acute and chronic pain management.

Rationale for effective acute pain control

There are several reasons why acute pain needs to be well controlled, not least that patients have a right to expect adequate treatment of pain and that all members of the healthcare team have an ethical obligation to provide it (Audit Commission 1997). It is now known that undertreatment of acute pain coupled with the physiological response to surgery or injury, known as the stress response, can have a number of adverse consequences (Macintyre and Schug 2007).

Pain can have long-lasting effects on the central nervous system, leaving an 'imprint' if pain is poorly controlled, which may mean that future episodes of pain are difficult to control (Carr 2007). Uncontrolled pain can lead to increased anxiety, fear, sleeplessness and muscle tension which further exacerbate pain. It can delay the recovery process by hindering mobilization and deep breathing, which increases the risk of a patient developing a deep vein thrombosis, chest infection or pressure ulcer. Pain can also lead to significant delays in gastric emptying and a reduction in intestinal motility (Macintyre and Schug 2007). With severe pain, activity of the sympathetic nervous system and the neuroendocrine 'stress response' causes platelet activation, changes in regional blood flow and stress on the heart. These can lead to impaired wound healing and myocardial ischaemia (Macintyre and Schug 2007). There is evidence to suggest that in the long term, poorly controlled acute pain may lead to the development of chronic pain. Perkins and Kehlet (2000) established that moderate-to-severe acute post-operative pain was a predictor for developing chronic pain after breast surgery, thoracic surgery and hernia repair.

Methods of pain assessment

Pain assessment is a key step in the process of managing pain and pain should be assessed before any intervention takes place. The aim of assessment is to identify all the factors, physical and non-physical, that affect the patient's perception of pain. A comprehensive clinical assessment is essential to gain a thorough understanding of the patient's pain, select an appropriate analgesic therapy, evaluate the effectiveness of interventions and modify therapy according to the patient's response.

Acute pain assessment

The key components of acute pain assessment are the pain history, measurement of the pain and the response to any intervention (Macintyre and Schug 2007). A pain history in addition to a physical examination can provide important information that will help in understanding the cause of the pain. A pain history should be repeated when there is any sign of an alteration in the nature and intensity of the pain.

Assessment of pre-existing pain

Patients who have been taking regular opioid analgesics for a pre-existing chronic pain problem may require higher doses of analgesia to manage an acute pain episode (Lewis and Williams 2005, Macintyre 2001, Mehta and Langford 2006). It is therefore important to take a history of pre-existing pain and analgesic use so that appropriate analgesic measures can be planned in advance of surgery. This is particularly important for opioid-tolerant patients irrespective of whether opioid tolerance is due to analgesic therapy or recreational opioid drug use (Box 8.11).

Assessment of location and intensity of pain

LOCATION

Many complex surgical procedures involve more than one incision site and the nature and extent of pain at each site may vary. A careful assessment of the location and type of pain is required, because each pain problem may respond to different pain management techniques. Pain location may also help to determine why pain is exacerbated by certain movements or positions (Anderson and Cleeland 2003).

INTENSITY

As part of the assessment process, it is important to assess the intensity of pain. Only then can the effects of any intervention be evaluated and care modified as appropriate. The simplest techniques for pain measurement involve the use of a verbal rating scale, numerical rating scale or visual analogue scale. Patients are asked to match pain intensity to the scale. Three principles apply to the use of these scales.

- The patient must be involved in scoring their own pain intensity. It provides the patient with an opportunity to express their pain intensity and also what it means to them and the effect it has on their lives. This is important because healthcare professionals frequently underestimate the intensity of a patient's pain and effectiveness of pain relief (Drayer et al. 1999, Idvall et al. 2002, Loveman and Gale 2000).
- Pain intensity assessment should incorporate different components of pain. This should include assessment of static (rest) pain and dynamic pain (on sitting, coughing or moving the affected part). For example, in a post-operative patient this is important to prevent complications of delayed recovery such as chest infections and emboli (deep vein thrombosis, pulmonary embolism) and to determine if analgesia is adequate for return of normal function (Hobbs and Hodgkinson 2003, Macintyre and Schug 2007).
- It is important to remember that a complete picture of a patient's pain cannot be derived solely from the use of a pain scale (Lawler 1997). Ongoing communication with the patient is required to uncover and manage any psychosocial factors that may be affecting the patient's pain experience.

Chronic pain assessment

There are many pain assessment tools that have been developed specifically for patients with chronic pain (Mann and Carr 2006). Pain assessment tools should be used to support the diagnosis and to determine the effectiveness of any treatment for the pain. The assessment tool should be easy to use and understand by patients and healthcare professionals (Cox 2010). Assessment tools for chronic pain need to be able to define the pain as well as assess the impact the pain is having on the patient's mood and lifestyle. Unidimensional tools can be suitable for the assessment of acute pain but, in chronic pain, more holistic tools are required to facilitate a better understanding of the nature of the pain. The concept of total pain reminds practitioners that pain is a deeply personal experience and that one of the greatest challenges is for nurses to be able to facilitate the expression for each individual of that particular pain (Krishnasamy 2008). Pain assessment needs to acknowledge these facts and particular attention must be paid to factors that will modulate pain sensitivity (Table 8.2).

Assessment in vulnerable and older adults

Pain assessment in vulnerable adults, for example those with cognitive impairment or dementia, and older adults may require

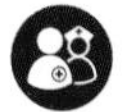

Box 8.11 **Key points for managing acute pain in opioid-dependent patients**

- Good communication: patients at risk should be identified at preassessment and effective communication maintained between preassessment staff, recovery staff and anaesthetist/pain service.
- Formalization of peri- and post-operative pain management plan.
- Use of adjuvant drugs and regional analgesia peri- and post-operatively to spare opioid use.
- Physical dependence requires baseline pre-operative opioids to be maintained to prevent acute withdrawal symptoms.
- Post-operative opioid requirements may vary depending on the effects of surgery.

Source: Bourne (2008). Reproduced with permission from The Association for Perioperative Practice (www.afpp.org.uk).

Table 8.2 **Factors affecting pain sensitivity**

Sensitivity increased	Sensitivity lowered
Discomfort	Relief of symptoms
Insomnia	Sleep
Fatigue	Rest
Anxiety	Sympathy
Fear	Understanding
Anger	Companionship
Sadness	Diversional activity
Depression	Reduction in anxiety
Boredom	Elevation of mood

careful consideration. Older people form the population most likely to have their pain inadequately assessed and especially so for those patients who are elderly and have dementia (Ni Thuathail and Welford 2011). Barriers to effective pain relief for this group of patients include issues such as lack of recognition by the staff that the patient is in pain, insufficient education about pain in this group, misdiagnosis of pain and the lack of use of appropriate assessment tools (McAuliffe et al. 2008). The same can be said for people with learning disabilties. It is not uncommon for assumptions to be made that people with learning disabilities do not experience pain and for their pain to go unassessed (Beacroft and Dodd 2010). Assessing pain in people with learning disabilities may require the use of non-verbal pain assessment tools and working closely with family and carers who may recognize indicators that the person with a learning disability is in pain.

Culture and effects on pain assessment

Individuals are greatly influenced by each other and by the cultural groups they belong to. Ethnic, religious and socio-economic factors all affect the way we live in society. Pain is greatly influenced by cultural factors (Fink and Gates 2006). Some groups are stoical regarding expressions of pain whilst others are more expressive, behaviours that may have been learned in childhood. They key in nursing is to ensure patients are cared for in a culturally comfortable way. The principles that can be applied in this situation include the following.

- Understand the patient as a unique person.
- Explore that patient's experience of illness and pain.
- Perceive pain management from the patient's perspective.
- Promote shared decision making and adapt care where possible to meet the patient's expectations (Narayan 2010).

Learning Activity 8.3 Case study: Pain

James is a 37-year-old man who was admitted to your ward having had knee surgery this morning following an injury he sustained playing football a couple of months ago. It is now early evening; he is using patient-controlled analgesia (PCA), containing morphine, in order to control his pain, and is also receiving regular doses of oral paracetamol and diclofenac (a non-steroidal anti-inflammatory).

James has said he has some pain. The nurse you are working with has asked you to assess James' pain.

1 What tool would you use to do this?
2 What else would you want to find out about his pain?
3 What pharmacological interventions may be appropriate?
4 What non-pharmacological interventions may be appropriate?

See the end of the chapter for the answers.

PRE-PROCEDURAL CONSIDERATIONS

Assessment and recording tools

Accurate pain assessment is a prerequisite of effective control and is an essential component of nursing care. In the assessment process, the nurse gathers information from the patient that allows an understanding of the patient's experience and its effect on their life. The information obtained guides the nurse in planning and evaluating strategies for care. Pain is rarely static; therefore, its assessment is not a one-time process but is ongoing.

Pain assessment can be difficult to achieve. For example, the tendency suggested by both research and clinical practice is for the patient not to report any pain or to do so inadequately or inaccurately, minimizing the pain experience (McCaffery and Beebe 1989). Nurses are influenced by a number of variables when assessing the amount of pain a patient is suffering (Kitson 1994). Pargeon and Hailey (1999) demonstrated that healthcare providers usually over- or underestimate a patient's pain. It has also been suggested that nurses do not possess sufficient knowledge to care for patients in pain (Drayer et al. 1999, McCaffery and Ferrell 1997). A survey of over 3000 nurses (McCaffery and Robinson 2002) demonstrated that nurse education has improved confidence in the pain assessment process but that further education continues to be required in the pharmacology of pain medications and addressing nurses' fears of opioid addiction and respiratory depression, which continue to contribute to the undertreatment of pain.

A variety of pain assessment tools exist to assist nurses to assess pain and plan nursing care. They enable pain to be successfully assessed and monitored (McCaffery and Beebe 1989, Twycross et al. 1996, Walker et al. 1987) and improve communication between staff and patients (Raiman 1986). Higginson (1998, p.150) notes that: 'Taking assessments directly from the patient is the most valid way of collecting information on their quality of life'. Encouraging patients to take an active role in their pain assessment by using pain tools helps to increase their confidence and makes them feel part of the pain management process.

Some degree of caution, however, must be exercised with the use of pain assessment tools. The nurse must be careful to select the tool that is most appropriate for a particular type of pain experience (Box 8.12). For example, it would not be appropriate to use a pain assessment tool designed for use with patients with chronic pain to assess post-operative pain. Furthermore, pain tools should not be used totally indiscriminately. Walker et al. (1987) found that pain tools appeared to have little value in cases of unresolved or intractable pain.

The use of pain assessment tools for acute pain has been shown both to increase the effectiveness of nursing interventions and to improve the management of pain (Harmer and Davies 1998, Scott 1994). Several pain assessment tools are available. Verbal descriptor scales (VDS) are based on numerically ranked words such as 'none', 'mild', 'moderate', 'severe' and 'very severe' for assessing both pain intensity and response to analgesia. Numerical rating scales (NRS) have both written and verbal forms. The written forms are either a vertical or a horizontal line with '0', indicating no pain, located at one end of the line and '10', indicating severe pain, at the other. This type of scale is easily used as a verbal scale of 0–10 if patients are unable to see or focus on a written scale. Although originally published as a line with a scale of 0–10, there are many versions of it (Williamson and Hoggart 2005). Since many of these scales focus on assessing the intensity of pain, it is important that nurses remember to combine their use of these tools with an assessment of the patient's psychosocial needs.

Other pain assessment tools have been developed to capture the multidimensional nature of pain. These specifically measure

Box 8.12 Most commonly used pain assessment tools

The most commonly used pain assessment tools meet the following criteria.

- *Simplicity*: ease of understanding for all patient groups.
- *Reliability*: reliability of the tool when used in similar patient groups; results are reproducible and consistent.
- *Valid*: the tool measures the patient's perception of pain.
- *Sensitivity*: sensitivity of the tool to the patient's pain.
- *Accuracy*: accurate and precise recording of data.
- *Interpretable*: meaningful pain scores or data are produced.
- *Feasibility/practicality*: the degree of effort involved in using the tool is acceptable; a practical tool is more likely to be used by patients.

several features of the pain experience, including the location and intensity of pain, pattern of pain over time, the effect of pain on the patient's daily function and activities, the effect on the patient's mood and the ability to interact and socialize with others. Examples of these include the McGill Pain Questionnaire (MPQ) (Melzack 1975) and the Brief Pain Inventory which has been validated for use in chronic non-cancer pain (Tan et al. 2004). These are more commonly used in chronic pain assessment. Accurate pain assessment and reassessment are crucial to develop an understanding and baseline measure of the pain. The key is to ask appropriate questions which should seek to cover the following areas. The SOCRATES pain assessment framework is a mnemonic commonly used by healthcare professionals.

S – *severity*: none, mild, moderate, severe
O – *onset*: when and how did it start?
C – *characteristic*: is it shooting, burning, aching – ask the patient to describe it
R – *radiation*: does it radiate anywhere else?
A – *additional factors*: what makes it better?
T – *time*: is it there all the time, is there a time of day when it is worse?
E – *exacerbating factors*: what makes it worse?
S – *site*: where is the pain?

In addition to this, questions relating to the following psychosocial elements should also be addressed.

- The effect of pain on mood.
- Are relationships affected by the pain?
- Physical limitations caused by the pain.
- Social effects: has the pain resulted in a loss of work or loss of role?
- Other types of pain affecting the patient.
- Previous treatments for pain and their effects.
- Other co-morbidities.
- Allergies (Mackintosh and Elson 2008).

Neuropathic pain may require a specific assessment tool. Patients may describe spontaneous pain (arising without detectable stimulation) and evoked pain (abnormal responses to stimuli) (Bennett 2001). The Leeds Assessment of Neuropathic Symptoms and Signs (LANSS) pain scale (Bennett 2001) was developed to more accurately assess this type of pain.

In adults with no or mild cognitive impairment, both numerical rating scales (0–10) and verbal descriptor rating scales (no pain, mild, moderate or severe pain) are reliable and valid for patients' self-report of pain intensity. The Mini Mental State Examination is the tool most commonly used to assess mental health status and is frequently used as a precursor to pain assessment (Ni Thuathail and Welford 2011). Older or vulnerable adults with moderate-to-severe cognitive/communication impairment may be able to use pictorial rating scales such as the Pain Thermometer or the Faces Pain Scale (Royal College of Physicians, British Geriatric Society and British Pain Society 2007). For patients with dementia or who may be unable to vocalize, an observational tool that assesses pain behaviours may need to be considered, such as the Abbey Scale (Abbey et al. 2004, Royal College of Physicians, British Geriatric Society and British Pain Society 2007). Similarly for patients who have a learning disability, who cannot communicate their pain verbally, the use of pictorial or non-verbal assessment tools may be appropriate and questioning those around the patient who know them well can be a great asset in assessing the pain needs of the person with a learning disability.

Fixed times for reviewing the pain have been omitted intentionally to allow for flexibility. It is suggested that, initially, the patient's pain is reviewed by the patient and nurse every 4 hours. When a patient's level of pain has stabilized, recordings may be made less frequently, for example 12-hourly or daily. The chart should be discontinued if a patient's pain becomes totally controlled.

Procedure guideline 8.11 **Pain assessment**

Essential equipment

- Select an appropriate assessment tool. For example:
  - in acute pain, consider the use of a verbal or numerical rating scale
  - in chronic pain, consider the use of the British Pain Inventory (BPI)
  - in adults with severe cognitive impairment, consider the use of the Abbey Scale

Pre-procedure

Action	Rationale
1 Explain to the patient the purpose of using the chart.	To ensure that the patient understands the procedure and gives their valid consent and co-operation (NMC 2013, **C**; Sherman et al. 2004, **R4**).
Procedure	
2 Encourage the patient, where appropriate, to identify pain themselves and to describe the character of the pain, if possible.	The body outline (see Figure 8.12) is a tool for the patient to describe their own pain experience (Sherman et al. 2004, **R4**).
3 When it is necessary for the nurse to complete the chart, ensure that the patient's own description of their pain is recorded.	To reduce the risk of misinterpretation. **E**
4 (a) Record any factors that influence the intensity of the pain, for example activities or interventions that reduce or increase the pain such as distractions or a heat pad. (b) Record whether or not the patient is pain free at night, at rest or on movement.	Ascertaining how and when the patient experiences pain enables the nurse to plan realistic goals. For example, relieving the patient's pain during the night and while they are at rest is usually easier to achieve than relief from pain on movement (Davis and McVicker 2000, **E**).
(c) Record frequency of pain, what helps to relieve the pain, what makes the pain worse and how the patient feels when they are in pain.	To gain an understanding of the experience of pain for the patient (Twycross and Wilcock 2001, **R5**).
(d) Determine if there are any associated symptoms when the pain is present, i.e. nausea and vomiting.	To ensure all elements of a pain assessment are explored (Macintyre and Schug 2007, **E**).

(continued)

Procedure guideline 8.11 Pain assessment *(continued)*

Action	Rationale
5 Index each site (Figure 8.12) in whatever way seems most appropriate, for example shading or colouring of areas or arrows to indicate shooting pains.	This enables individual pain sites to be located (Sherman et al. 2004, **R4**).
6 Give each pain site a numerical value according to the pain intensity or the pain scale and note time recorded where possible.	To indicate the intensity of the pain at each site (Turk and Okifuji 1999, **E**).
If cognitive impairment is present then complete an appropriate tool so that the patient does not need to verbalize a pain score.	To ensure that the patient's pain is assessed as well as possible (Abbey et al. 2004, **E**).
7 Record any analgesia given and note route, dose and response.	To monitor efficacy of prescribed analgesia (Twycross and Wilcock 2001, **R5**).
Post-procedure	
8 Record any significant activities that are likely to influence the patient's pain.	Extra pharmacological or non-pharmacological interventions might be indicated (Disorbio et al. 2006, **E**; Turk and Okifuji 1999, **E**).
9 Discuss with the patient an ongoing reassessment plan for pain.	To ensure that the patient is informed regarding ongoing pain assessment and understands when to alert the nurse if needing additional help, for example when there is a change in nature of the pain or when the pain is not responding to the planned treatment or activities of daily living are being inhibited which previously could be maintained (Macintyre and Schug 2007, **E**).

Figure 8.12 **Body diagram used for pain assessment.**

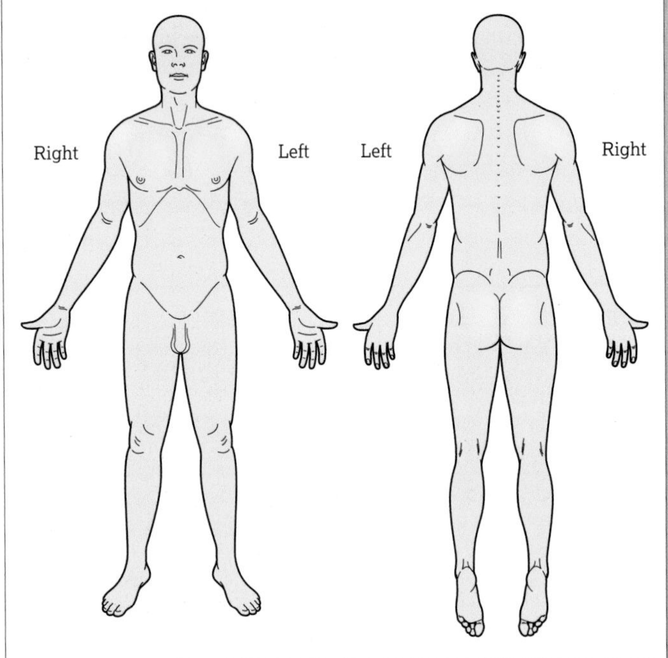

Pain management

EVIDENCE-BASED APPROACHES

Pain management uses a multidisciplinary team approach that matches therapy to the individual patient. In some instances simple analgesia can be sufficient to control pain. Simple or non-opioid analgesics include paracetamol and non-steroidal anti-inflammatory drugs (NSAIDs) used either individually or in combination.

Multimodal analgesia

Multimodal or balanced analgesia involves the use of more than one analgesic compound or method of pain control to achieve additive (or synergistic) pain relief while minimizing adverse effects (Schug and Chong 2009). This allows for lower doses of individual drugs. It combines different analgesics that act by different mechanisms and at different sites in the nervous system. The aim is to achieve greater analgesia than each of the individual drugs could provide alone.

Opioids, non-opioids (such as paracetamol, NSAIDs, cyclo-oxygenase-2-selective inhibitors [COX-2]), local anaesthetics and anticonvulsants are all examples of drugs that may be used as part of a multimodal analgesic approach. An example of multimodal analgesia to manage acute post-operative pain would be a continuous epidural infusion of a combined opioid and local anaesthetic solution in combination with paracetamol and an NSAID (if not contraindicated). Another example would be a continuous peripheral nerve block with paracetamol and an NSAID. Both of these approaches combine different analgesic compounds and analgesic approaches (oral route, epidural route and peripheral nerve block).

A multimodal approach may also include non-pharmacological approaches such as relaxation therapy, imagery, transcutaneous electrical nerve stimulation (TENS) and heat therapy.

Management of persistent chronic and cancer pain

The control of pain is directed by the 'analgesic ladder', which was presented by the World Health Organization (WHO) in 1996 as a guide to the management of persistent cancer pain (Figure 8.13). It is also often used to guide the management of chronic persistent pain. It involves a stepwise approach to the use of analgesics, including non-opioids (step 1), opioids for mild-to-moderate pain (step 2) and opioids for moderate-to-severe pain (step 3). Adjuvant drugs are those that contribute to pain relief but are not primarily indicated for pain management. They can be used at all steps of the ladder. Examples include antidepressant and anticonvulsant drugs, corticosteroids,

Figure 8.13 **The WHO analgesic ladder.**

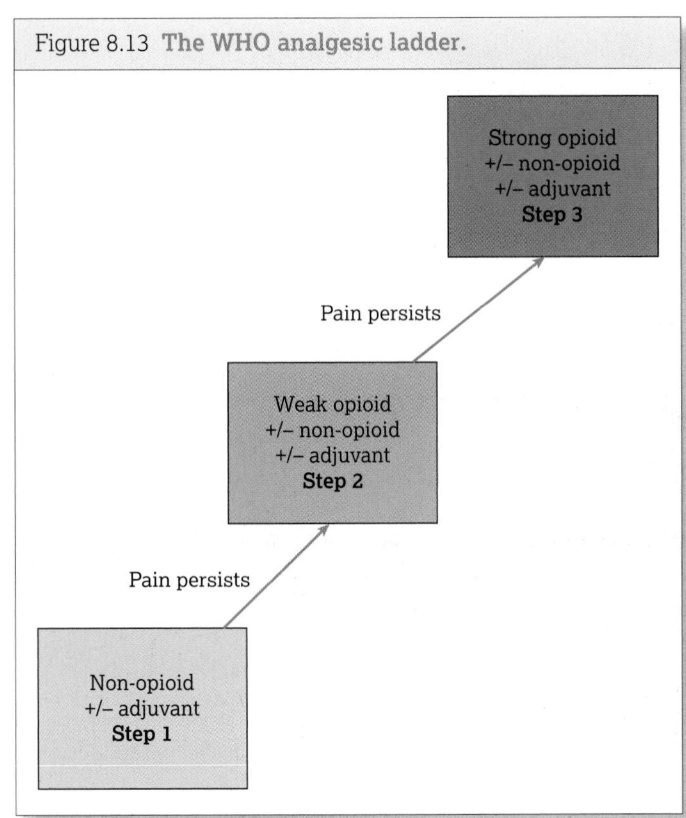

Table 8.3 **The use of adjuvant drugs (co-analgesics)**

Type	Use	Examples
Non-steroidal anti-inflammatory drugs	Bone pain	Diclofenac
	Muscular pain	Naproxen
	Inflammation	Ibuprofen
	Visceral pain	
Steroids	Pressure	Dexamethasone
	Bone pain	Prednisolone
	Inflammation	
	Raised intracranial pressure	
Tricyclic antidepressants	Neuropathic pain	Amitriptyline
Anticonvulsants		Sodium valproate
		Carbamazepine
		Gabapentin
		Pregabalin
Antibiotics	Infection	Flucloxacillin
		Trimethoprim
Benzodiazepines	Anxiety	Diazepam
		Clonazepam
Antispasmodics	Spasms	Baclofen
Bisphosphonates	Bone pain	Sodium clodronate
		Disodium pamidronate
		Zoledronic acid

benzodiazepines, antispasmodics and bisphosphonates. The WHO treatment guide recommends the following five points for the correct use of analgesics.

- Administered orally if appropriate.
- Given at regular intervals.
- Prescribed according to assessment of pain intensity evaluated using a pain intensity scale.
- The dose of the analgesic should be adapted to the individual. There is no standard dose to treat certain types of pain.
- Analgesia should be prescribed with ongoing review, monitoring for effectiveness and side-effects (WHO 1996).

Therefore, some patients who present with severe pain will need to start on step 3 of the ladder; it would not be appropriate to progress through each step in this circumstance. Treatment of chronic/cancer pain does not necessarily begin with step 1, progress to step 2 and follow with step 3 (Eisenberg et al. 2005).

It is important to remember that the patient will experience different types of pain due to different aetiological and physiological changes. Each pain needs to be assessed separately, since the pain may need to be managed in a different manner and one analgesic intervention or route will rarely be sufficient. Often the best practice is to combine different types of analgesia in order to achieve maximum pain control (Table 8.3). It is also important to utilize non-pharmacological interventions at all stages of the treatment plan.

Accurate ongoing assessment is imperative for efficient and effective pain control.

Methods of pain management

Using the WHO analgesic ladder

The analgesic ladder was designed as a framework for the management of chronic pain (see Figure 8.13). There are several drugs available to manage chronic pain and the analgesic ladder allows the flexibility to choose from the range according to the patient's requirements and tolerance (Hanks et al. 2004). For acute pain management, the WHO ladder can be used as a guide in reverse, starting at step 3 for immediate post-operative pain and moving down through step 2 and then step 1 as post-operative pain improves.

STEP 1: NON-OPIOID DRUGS

Examples of non-opioid drugs include paracetamol, aspirin and NSAIDs that are effective for mild-to-moderate pain. These drugs are especially effective for musculoskeletal and visceral pain (Twycross and Wilcock 2001).

STEP 2: OPIOIDS FOR MILD-TO-MODERATE PAIN

Examples of opioids for mild-to-moderate pain include codeine, dihydrocodeine, tramadol and low-dose oxycodone (steps 2 and 3). These drugs are used when adequate pain management is not achieved with non-opioids and are usually used in combination formulations. It is not recommended to administer another analgesic from the same group if the drug being used is not controlling the pain. Uncontrolled pain needs to be assessed and managed with the titration of an opioid by moving up the ladder. The exception to this would be if the patient was experiencing intolerable side-effects on the weak opioid and an alternative drug might be beneficial.

STEP 3: OPIOIDS FOR MODERATE-TO-SEVERE PAIN

Examples of opioids for moderate-to-severe pain include morphine, oxycodone, fentanyl, diamorphine, methadone, buprenorphine, hydromorphone and alfentanil.

Methods of drug delivery

ORAL ANALGESIA

Oral opioids are used less frequently in the immediate post-operative period because many patients are nil by mouth or on restricted oral intake for a period of time. Often this route is used if patients require strong analgesics following discontinuation of epidural or intravenous analgesia. Morphine is an ideal oral preparation because it is available as a tablet (Sevredol) or an elixir (Oramorph). Oxycodone can be given as second-line opioid treatment if patients are allergic/sensitive to or fail to respond to morphine.

INTRAVENOUS ANALGESIA

Continuous intravenous infusions of opioids such as morphine, diamorphine and fentanyl are effective for controlling pain in the immediate post-operative period. Their use is often restricted to critical care units where patients can be closely monitored because of the potential risk of respiratory depression (Macintyre and Schug 2007). Compared with patient-controlled analgesia (PCA), continuous infusions of opioids for acute pain management in a general ward setting resulted in a fivefold increase in the incidence of respiratory depression (Schug and Torrie 1993).

Patient-controlled analgesia is an alternative and safer technique for giving intravenous opioids (usually morphine, diamorphine, fentanyl or oxycodone) in the ward environment (Sidebotham et al. 1997). With PCA, patients self-administer intermittent doses of opioids, by using an infusion pump and timing device. When in pain, the patient presses a button connected to the pump and a set dose of opioid is delivered (usually intravenously but it may also be given subcutaneously) to the patient (Macintyre and Schug 2007).

There are a number of advantages to using PCA.

- PCA is more likely to maintain reasonably constant blood concentrations of the opioid within the analgesic corridor. This is the blood level where analgesia is achieved without significant side-effects. The flexibility of PCA helps to overcome the wide interpatient variation in opioid requirements (Macintyre and Schug 2007).
- PCA allows patients to titrate analgesia against daily variations in the pain stimulus (Tye and Gell-Walker 2000). By using a PCA pump, patients can administer analgesia as soon as pain occurs and titrate the dose according to increases and decreases in the pain stimulus. This is particularly helpful for controlling more intense pain during movement.
- PCA prevents delays in patients receiving analgesics (Chumbley et al. 2002).

Whilst PCA may be very effective for controlling pain for a number of patients undergoing surgery (Macintyre and Schug 2007), it is not suitable for the groups listed in Box 8.13.

EPIDURAL ANALGESIA

Epidural analgesia refers to the provision of pain relief by continuous administration of analgesic pharmacological agents (usually low concentrations of local anaesthetics and opioids) into the epidural space via an indwelling catheter (Macintyre et al. 2010). Giving analgesia epidurally is a particularly valuable technique for the prevention of post-operative pain in patients undergoing major thoracic, abdominal and lower limb surgery, and can sometimes be used to manage the pain associated with trauma. Commonly used opioids for epidural analgesia include fentanyl and diamorphine (Wheatley et al. 2001). Combinations of low concentrations of local anaesthetic agents and opioids have been shown to provide consistently superior pain relief compared with either drug alone (Macintyre and Schug 2007).

Box 8.13 Patients for whom patient-controlled analgesia (PCA) is inappropriate

- Those who are unable to activate the PCA device due to problems with dexterity or visual impairment.
- Those who are unable to understand the concept of PCA, particularly the very young or patients who are confused.
- Those who do not wish to take responsibility for their pain control.

Source: Tye and Gel-Walker (2000). Reproduced with permission from EMAP Publishing Ltd.

SUBCUTANEOUS ANALGESIA

Opioids are often given subcutaneously to manage chronic cancer pain. More recently, there has been an increase in the use of subcutaneous opioids for post-operative pain control. Both PCA and nurse-administered opioid injections of morphine, diamorphine or oxycodone via an indwelling subcutaneous cannula have been used successfully to manage postoperative pain (Macintyre and Schug 2007). An advantage of giving analgesia subcutaneously is that it avoids the problems associated with maintaining intravenous access.

INTRAMUSCULAR ANALGESIA

Until the early 1990s, regular 3–4-hourly intramuscular injections of opioids such as pethidine and morphine were routinely used for the management of post-operative pain. Because alternative techniques such as PCA and epidural analgesia are now available, intramuscular analgesia is used less frequently. Some useful algorithms have been developed to give guidance on titrating intramuscular analgesia (Harmer and Davies 1998, Macintyre and Schug 2007). Absorption via this route may be impaired in conditions of poor perfusion (e.g. in hypovolaemia, shock, hypothermia or immobility). This may lead to inadequate early analgesia (the drug cannot be absorbed properly and reach the systemic circulation and so forms a drug depot) and late absorption of the drug depot (where the drug has remained in the muscular tissue and is absorbed only once perfusion is restored) (Macintyre et al. 2010).

TRANSDERMAL ANALGESIA

Transdermal analgesia is a simple method of giving analgesia. It is convenient, and often very acceptable to patients, particularly those who dislike tablets or have many to take. A number of patch formulations have been developed to allow the delivery of drugs across the skin (such as fentanyl, buprenorphine or local anaesthetics). Disadvantages of giving strong opioids such as fentanyl by this route include inflexibility (the patient usually has to be on a stable dose of an opioid and it takes a long time for a dose increase to take effect) and breakthrough doses must be given by another route (oral, buccal or sublingual).

BUCCAL OR SUBLINGUAL ANALGESIA

Buccal means the analgesia is placed between the upper lip and the lining of the upper gum. A sublingual drug is placed under the tongue. Drugs given by this route pass directly into the systemic circulation and bypass first-pass metabolism. Their speed of onset is often rapid (Stannard and Booth 2004).

PRE-PROCEDURAL CONSIDERATIONS

Pharmacological support

Non-opioid analgesics

PARACETAMOL AND PARACETAMOL COMBINATIONS

The use of non-opioid analgesics such as paracetamol or paracetamol combined with a weak opioid such as codeine is recommended for managing pain following minor surgical procedures or when the pain following major surgery begins to subside (McQuay et al. 1997). Paracetamol can also be given rectally if the oral route is contraindicated. An intravenous preparation of paracetamol is now available and can provide effective analgesia after surgical procedures (Romsing et al. 2002). It is more effective and of faster onset than the same dose given enterally. The use of the intravenous form should be limited to patients in whom the enteral route cannot be used. With regard to dosing schedules for parenteral administration of paracetamol, the dose should be reduced for those who weigh 50 kg or under. For example, patients who weigh 33–50 kg should not exceed a maximum daily dose of 60 mg/kg, not exceeding 3 g. For patients over 50 kg with an additional risk factor for hepatotoxicity, the maximum daily dose should be 3 g in 24 hours and for those patients over 50 kg with no risk factor then the maximum daily dose can be up to 4 g (Bristol-Myers Squibb 2012).

Paracetamol taken in the correct dose of not more than 4 g per day is relatively free of side-effects. When used in combination with codeine preparations, the most frequent side-effect is constipation.

NON-STEROIDAL ANTI-INFLAMMATORY DRUGS

Non-steroidal anti-inflammatory drugs (NSAIDs) have been shown to provide better pain relief than paracetamol combinations for acute pain (McQuay et al. 1997). These drugs can be used alone or in combination with both opioid and non-opioid analgesics. Two commonly used NSAIDs are diclofenac, which can be administered by the oral, parenteral, enteral or rectal route, and ibuprofen, which is available only as an oral or enteral preparation. The disadvantage of both of these is that often side-effects such as coagulation problems, renal impairment and gastrointestinal disturbances limit their use. Newer COX-2-specific NSAIDs have the advantage that they have similar analgesic and anti-inflammatory effects (Reicin et al. 2001) but have no effect on platelets or the gastric mucosa (Rowbotham 2000). As a result, coagulation problems and gastrointestinal irritation are likely to be significantly reduced. However, recently, several of these drugs have been withdrawn from the market due to long-term cardiovascular side-effects and it will take time for newer products with an improved safety profile to re-establish themselves in practice (Macintyre et al. 2010).

A recent meta-analysis has suggested that there is little evidence to suggest that any of these drugs are safe in cardiovascular terms. Compared with placebo, rofecoxib was associated with the highest risk of myocardial infarction and ibuprofen with the highest risk of stroke followed by diclofenac. Diclofenac and lumiracoxib were associated with the highest risk of cardiovascular death. Naproxen is viewed as being least harmful for cardiovascular safety but this advantage should be weighed against gastrointestinal toxicity (Trelle et al. 2011).

Opioid analgesics

Opioids are the first-line treatment for pain that follows major surgery (Macintyre and Jarvis 1996) and can also be prescribed for cancer and non-cancer-related chronic pain. Opioid doses need to be titrated carefully to achieve pain relief to suit each individual patient while minimizing any unwanted side-effects (McQuay et al. 1997).

A number of opioids are used for controlling pain following surgery. These include morphine, diamorphine, fentanyl and oxycodone. The most common routes of opioid administration are intravenous, epidural, subcutaneous, intramuscular or oral.

Evidence for the concept of opioid rotation when patients have intolerable opioid-related side-effects originates from cancer pain studies (Quigley 2004) but it may be a useful strategy to consider in the management of acute pain as well.

Opioids for mild-to-moderate pain

TRAMADOL

It has been suggested that despite progress in pain management, chronic non-cancer pain (CNCP) still represents a clinical challenge (Coluzzi and Mattia 2007). The efficacy and safety profile of tramadol make it suitable as a long-term treatment in a variety of CNCP conditions (Coluzzi and Mattia 2007). In recent studies tramadol has also been recognized as being efficacious in the management of chronic cancer pain of moderate severity (Davis et al. 2005).

It is uncertain whether tramadol is more effective than other opioids for mild-to-moderate neuropathic pain; one report suggests a reduction in allodynia (pain from stimuli which are not normally painful) (Sindrup and Jensen 1999, Twycross and Wilcock 2001). Nurses should be aware that circumstantial reports suggest that tramadol lowers seizure threshold, and therefore care needs to be taken in those patients who have a history of epilepsy, as well as any other medications that may contribute to the lowering of the seizure threshold, for example tricyclic antidepressants and selective serotonin reuptake inhibitors (SSRIs) (Twycross and Wilcock 2001). Few patients with severe pain will achieve a satisfactory level of pain control with tramadol. It is available in immediate and modified-release preparations.

Tramadol has been shown to be an effective analgesic for post-operative pain (McQuay and Moore 1998, Reicin et al. 2001). Although tramadol does have some side-effects, which include nausea and dizziness, it is free of NSAID side-effects and causes less constipation than codeine preparations and opioids (Bamigbade and Langford 1998). The combination of tramadol with paracetamol is more effective than either of the two components administered alone (McQuay and Edwards 2003).

CODEINE PHOSPHATE

Codeine is metabolized by the hepatic cytochrome CYP2D6 to morphine. Approximately 7% of Caucasians and 1–3% of the Asian population are poor CYP2D6 metabolizers and therefore do not experience effective analgesia with codeine.

Codeine is available in tablet and syrup formulations. Doses of 30–60 mg po qds are generally prescribed to a maximum of 240 mg/24 h. It is also available in combination preparations with a non-opioid. The combination preparations are available in varying strengths of codeine and paracetamol, including co-codamol 8 mg/500 mg, 15 mg/500 mg and 30 mg/500 mg.

Opioids for the management of chronic non-cancer pain

Opioids are being used increasingly to treat persistent pain. They have a well-established role in the management of acute pain and for those with cancer and palliative care needs. There is evidence from research that opioids can be helpful in the short and medium term in providing symptomatic pain relief from other non-cancer pain conditions (British Pain Society 2010). Opioids are prescribed to reduce pain intensity. Rarely is pain completely relieved by opioids alone (British Pain Society 2010). In approximately 80% of cases patients will experience at least one adverse side-effect from opioids. Opioids should be given careful consideration before they are commenced and patients should be informed that the effects of long-term use of opioids is unknown in terms of effects on endocrine and immune function (British Pain Society 2010). When opioid therapy is commenced, a plan to review the patient in terms of opioid effects must be in place. From a palliative care perspective, there is new guidance available from NICE to support safe prescribing of opioids (NICE 2012).

MORPHINE

A large amount of information and research is available concerning morphine and therefore it tends to be the first-line opioid (of choice). It is available in oral, rectal, parenteral and intraspinal preparations.

All strong opioids require careful titration from an expert practitioner. Where possible, modified-release preparations should be used at regular intervals in the management of persistent pain (British Pain Society 2010). For patients who are requiring in excess of 120–180 mg of morphine or equivalent, advice from a pain specialist should be sought. Patients should be informed of potential side-effects such as constipation, nausea and increased sleepiness, in order to allay any fear. The patient should also be told that nausea and drowsiness are transitory and normally improve within 48 hours, but that constipation can be an ongoing problem and it is recommended that a laxative should be prescribed when the opioid is started. The most effective laxative for this group of patients is a combination of both a softening and a stimulating laxative (Davis et al. 2005).

Patients often have many concerns about commencing strong drugs such as morphine. Fears frequently centre around addiction and abuse (Cherny 2010). Time should be taken to reassure patients and their families and provide verbal and written information (NICE 2012).

Although morphine is still considered to be the opioid drug of choice for moderate-to-severe pain (Hanks et al. 2004), alternative opioids allow the practitioner to carefully assess the patient on an individual basis and select the most appropriate one to use.

DUROGESIC (FENTANYL)

Fentanyl is a strong opioid, available in a patch, which is recommended in patients who have stable pain requirements. Transdermal patches are available in doses of 12, 25, 50, 75 or 100 micrograms per hour. It is reported to have an improved side-effect profile in comparison to morphine in relation to constipation, although some patients experience nausea and mild drowsiness (BMA/Royal Pharmaceutical Society of Great Britain 2008). Use of the patch has increased because it frees the patient from taking tablets.

Changing of the patch is recommended every 3 days but in some circumstances patients may require a dosing interval of 2 days. The patch should be applied to skin that is free from excess hair and any form of irritation and should not be applied to irradiated areas. It is advisable to change the location on the body to avoid an adverse skin reaction. Occasionally difficulties arise relating to the titration of the patch as each patch is equivalent to a range of morphine (Table 8.4).

METHADONE

Methadone is a synthetic opioid developed more than 40 years ago (Riley 2006). It is available in oral, rectal and parenteral preparations. There has been some reluctance amongst professionals to use methadone, which arose from the difficulties experienced in titrating the drug due to its long half-life (15 hours) that caused accumulation to occur, especially in the elderly (Gannon 1997). There are different methods of achieving effective titration (Gannon 1997); for example, one regimen is to calculate one-tenth of the total daily dose of morphine (maximum starting dose must not exceed 30 mg). Administer the methadone to the patient on an as-required basis but not within 3 hours of the last fixed dose. The total dose required over a 24-hour period is calculated after 5–6 days, divided and given as a two or three times daily regimen and this avoids the build-up of methadone within the body (Morley and Makin 1998). Titration is recommended in a hospital setting to ensure accurate administration. This can be difficult for patients because they have to experience pain before they are administered a dose of methadone in the titration period.

Methadone can be a cheap, effective alternative to morphine if titration is supervised by the specialist pain or palliative care team (Gardner-Nix 1996).

It is particularly useful in patients with renal failure. Morphine is excreted via the kidneys and, if renal failure occurs, this may lead to the patient experiencing severe drowsiness as a result of accumulation of morphine metabolites (Gannon 1997). Methadone is lipid soluble and is metabolized mainly in the liver. About half of the drug and its metabolites are excreted by the intestines and half by the kidneys. Methadone should be used with the advice of a pain specialist.

Table 8.4 **Recommended conversion rate guide from oral morphine to 72-hour fentanyl patch**

Morphine dose in 24 hours (mg)	Fentanyl TTS (μg/h)
30	12
60	25
120	50
180	75
240	100

TTS, transdermal therapeutic system.

OXYCODONE

Oxycodone is available as an immediate or modified-release preparation and titration should occur in the same way as morphine. Oxycodone is a useful alternative to morphine (Riley 2006). It has similar properties and can be administered orally, rectally and parenterally. Oxycodone has similar side-effects and is usually given 4–6 hourly. It has an analgesic potency 1.5–2.0 times higher than morphine. It has similar side-effects to morphine, although oxycodone has been found to cause less nausea (Heiskanen and Kalso 1997) and significantly less itchiness (Mucci-LoRusso et al. 1998).

A study by Riley (2012) identified that on a population level there is no difference between morphine and oxycodone in terms of analgesia efficacy and tolerability.

TARGINACT

This drug is a combination of modified-release oxycodone and naloxone. The aim of this combination is to prevent the potential negative effects on bowel function. It is suggested that approximately 97% of the naloxone is eliminated by first-pass metabolism in the healthy liver, preventing it from significantly affecting analgesic effects (Vondrackova et al. 2008).

TAPENTADOL

Tapentadol is a centrally acting opioid analgesic supported by evidence for the management of acute and severe chronic pain (Wild et al. 2010). It is available in oral preparations in immediate- and modified-release forms. The conversion factor for tapentadol from oral morphine is 2.5:1. Therefore 10 mg oral morphine is equivalent to 25 mg of tapentadol. Side-effects associated with tapentadol are similar to other opioids, including dizziness, headaches, somnolence, nausea and constipation.

DIAMORPHINE

Diamorphine is used parenterally in a syringe pump or PCA pump for the control of moderate-to-severe pain when patients are unable to take the oral form of morphine. It is calculated by dividing the total daily dose of oral morphine by three. Breakthrough doses are calculated by dividing the 24-hour dose of diamorphine by six and administering on an as-required basis (Fallon et al. 2010).

BUPRENORPHINE

Buprenorphine is an alternative strong opioid available in patch form. The patch has similar advantages to fentanyl but does not contain a reservoir of the drug. Instead, it is contained in a matrix form with effective levels of the drug being reached within 24 hours. Titration is recommended with an alternative opioid initially and then transfer to the patch when stable requirements have been reached. A lower dose patch (Butrans) is available in strengths of 5, 10 and 20 μg/h that should be worn continuously by the patient for 7 days. The higher dose patch (Transtec) of 35, 52.5 and 70 μg/h is now licensed to be used up to 96 hours or twice weekly for patient convenience. Conversion is based on the chart supplied by the pharmaceutical company which demonstrates equivalent doses. Buprenorphine is also available as a sublingual tablet, which is titrated from 200 to 800 μg 6 hourly. Conversion is based on multiplying the total daily dose of buprenorphine by 100 to give the total daily dose of morphine (i.e. 200 μg buprenorphine/8-hourly = 600 μg buprenorphine/24 hours = 60 mg morphine/24 hours) (Budd 2002).

Transmucosal opioids such as fentanyl citrate (Actiq), Abstral, Effentora and intranasal preparations such as Pecfent are licensed to be used for the treatment of cancer breakthrough pain. There are some circumstances when these agents are used off licence but they should always be used under the guidance of a specialist.

ORAL TRANSMUCOSAL FENTANYL CITRATE (ACTIQ)

Licensed for the management of breakthrough pain in patients who are already on an established maintenance dose of opioid for cancer pain, oral transmucosal fentanyl citrate (OTFC) is a lozenge which is rubbed against the oral mucosa on the side of the cheek which leads to the lozenge being dissolved by the saliva. The advantage of OTFC is its fast onset via the buccal mucosa (5–15 minutes) and its short duration (up to 2 hours). It is available in a range of doses (200–1600 μg) but there is no direct relation between the baseline analgesia and the breakthrough dose. Titration can be difficult and lengthy as the recommended starting dose is 200 μg with titration upwards (Portenoy et al. 1999). It is recommended that the lozenge be removed from the mouth if the pain subsides before it has completely dissolved. The lozenge should not be reused but should be dissolved under running hot water.

FENTANYL BUCCAL TABLET (EFFENTORA)

This is a licensed medication for breakthrough pain in adults with cancer who are already receiving a maintenance opioid for chronic cancer. Patients receiving maintenance opioid therapy are those who are taking at least 60 mg of oral morphine daily, at least 25 μg of transdermal fentanyl per hour, at least 30 mg of oxycodone daily, at least 8 mg of oral hydromorphone daily or an equi-analgesic dose of another opioid for a week or longer. This buccal tablet is available in 100, 200, 400, 600 and 800 μg. It is placed on the oral mucosa above the third upper molar which leads to the tablet being dissolved by the saliva. It usually takes 15–25 minutes for the tablet to dissolve. It is recommended that if the tablet has not completely dissolved within 30 minutes then the remainder of the tablet should be swallowed with water as it is thought that the tablet will then only be likely to consist of inactive substances rather than active fentanyl (Darwish et al. 2007).

Abstral is an oral transmucosal delivery formulation of fentanyl citrate, indicated for the management of breakthrough pain in patients using opioid therapy for chronic cancer pain (Rauch et al. 2009). The tablet is administered sublingually and it rapidly disintegrates, ensuring the fentanyl dissolves quickly. Abstral is available in six dosing strengths: 100, 200, 300, 400, 600 and 800 μg fentanyl citrate.

Adjuvant drugs (co-analgesics)

Most chronic pain contains elements of neuropathic pain. Patients with nociceptive pain are likely to gain some benefit from conventional medications such as NSAIDs but these drugs come with a strong side-effect profile. Individuals with neuropathic pain are likely to gain some relief from co-analgesics such as tricyclic antidepressants (e.g. amitriptyline and nortriptyline) and anticonvulsant drugs (e.g. gabapentin and pregabalin) (Mackintosh and Elson 2008).

The WHO analgesic ladder recommends the use of these drugs in combination with non-opioids, opioids for mild-to-moderate pain and opioids for moderate-to-severe pain (see Figure 8.13).

Nitrous oxide (Entonox)

Inhaled nitrous oxide provides analgesia that is short acting and works quickly. It has a special role in managing pain associated with procedures such as wound dressings, drain removal and in acute trauma (see section on 'Entonox administration' below for further details).

Local anaesthetics

In addition to epidural analgesia, local anaesthetics may be used to block individual or groups of peripheral nerves during surgical procedures and to infiltrate surgical wounds at the end of an operation (Carroll and Bowsher 1993). Occasionally these techniques may be used to extend the duration of post-operative analgesia beyond the finite period that a single injection technique provides (Macintyre et al. 2010). Techniques include regular intermittent bolus doses or continuous infusions of local anaesthetic.

A topical preparation (patch) containing local anaesthetic is also available to manage acute or chronic neuropathic pain in areas of intact skin with hypersensitivity.

Cannabis

Studies are currently examining the potential benefits of using cannabis for the management of chronic conditions, for example multiple sclerosis and cancer. There is some evidence for relief of spasticity and neuropathic pain and for improvement in sleep (Lynch and Campbell 2011). Further studies in pain and on long-term treatment risks and benefits are needed.

Anaesthetic interventions for managing complex cancer-related pain

Sometimes it is difficult to attain and maintain adequate pain control without significant side-effects and it is in situations such as this that anaesthetic interventions may be of benefit.

Effective control can be achieved by epidural or intrathecal (spinal) infusions:

- as single injections for simple nerve blocks, or
- regional nerve blocks which target individual nerves, plexi or ganglia (Hicks and Simpson 2004).

Examples include managing pelvic pain and post-radiation brachial plexopathy.

These interventions can be useful but careful consideration and assessment must take place to ensure that any potential side-effects are discussed with the patient (anaesthetic interventions may severely limit the patient's activities) and that future planning is addressed with the patient and family as an epidural/intrathecal infusion may limit discharge options for the patient who is dying.

Education of patient

Opioids and driving

In the UK patients who are prescribed opioids are permitted to drive. The British Pain Society has suggested under certain circumstances that patients who are taking opioids should not drive. These circumstances include:

- The condition for which they are being treated has physical consequences that might impair their driving ability.
- They feel unfit to drive.
- They have just started opioid treatment.
- The dose of opioid has been recently adjusted upwards or downwards (as withdrawal of opioids can also have an impact on driving).
- They have consumed alcohol or drugs that can produce an additive effect.

The Driving and Vehicle Licensing Agency (DVLA) is the only legal body that can advise a patient about their right to hold a driving licence. Patients starting opioids should be advised to inform the DVLA that they are now taking opioids and prescribers should document that this advice has been given (British Pain Society 2010).

COMPLICATIONS

The use of opioids in renal failure

Renal failure can cause significant and dangerous side-effects due to the accumulation of the drug. A systematic review in patients with cancer pain has concluded that fentanyl, alfentanil and methadone, with caveats, are the medications likely to cause least harm in patients with renal impairment when used appropriately (King et al. 2011). Basic guidelines for pain management in renal failure include the following.

- Reduce analgesia dose and/or dose frequency (6-hourly instead of 4-hourly).
- Select a more appropriate drug (not renally excreted).
- Avoid modified-release preparations.
- Seek advice from a specialist pain/palliative care team and/or pharmacist (Farrell and Rich 2000).

Non-pharmacological methods of managing pain

Optimal pain control is more likely to be achieved by combining non-pharmacological with pharmacological techniques. Despite the lack of research evidence to support the effectiveness of many non-pharmacological techniques, their benefits to patients and families should not be underestimated.

Psychological interventions

A number of simple psychological interventions can improve a patient's pain control by:

- reducing anxiety, stress and muscle tension
- distraction (distraction plays a role in pain management by pushing awareness of pain out of central cognition)
- increasing control and pain-coping mechanisms
- improving general well-being.

Some simple interventions include the following.

Creating trusting therapeutic relationships

By creating trusting relationships with patients, nurses are instrumental in reducing anxiety and helping patients to cope with pain. Nurses may underestimate the benefits and comfort they bring by staying with a patient who is experiencing pain (Mann and Carr 2006). Nurses can help to create a trusting relationship by:

- listening to the patient
- believing the patient's pain experience (Seers 1996)
- acting as a patient advocate
- providing patients with appropriate physical and emotional support.

The use of gentle humour

Pasero and McCaffery (1998) suggest that many patients find gentle humour an effective way of coping with pain. Humour may be particularly helpful prior to a painful procedure as it can have a lasting effect. In the clinical setting, humorous tapes, books and videos can be made available for patient use.

Information/education

Patient information/education can make all the difference between effective and ineffective pain relief. Information/education helps to reduce anxiety (Macintyre and Schug 2007, Taylor 2001) and enables patients to make informed decisions about their care. Patients should be given specific information about why pain control is important, what to expect in terms of pain relief, how they can participate in their management and what to do if pain is not controlled. Some caution is required, however, because not all patients respond positively to the same level of information. Patients with high levels of anxiety may find that detailed information can increase their anxiety and influence their pain control. New NICE guidance on the safe prescribing of opioids suggests that all patients who start on opioids should be offered written information to support them (NICE 2012).

Relaxation

Whilst scientific evidence for the effectiveness of relaxation techniques is limited (Carroll and Seers 1998, Seers and Carroll 1998), a number of studies have shown benefits for patients experiencing pain (Good et al. 1999, Lang et al. 2000, Sloman et al. 1994). Payne (1995) describes several relaxation techniques ranging from simple breathing techniques to progressive muscle relaxation and more complex techniques. One simple relaxation technique script that has been adapted for use at the Royal Marsden Hospital is outlined in Box 8.14. This technique can be taught to patients and used during painful procedures or at times when the patient feels anxious or stressed. Patients should be encouraged to practise the technique to gain mastery.

> **Learning Activity 8.4**
>
> **Learning in practice: Pain management and relaxation**
>
> Box 8.14 provides a simple relaxation technique that you can try yourself at home or in the classroom. For best results, ask a friend/colleague to work with you: one of you finds a comfortable and relaxing position and listens to the instructions, while the other reads through the steps outlined in the script.
>
> - After you have finished, discuss how the procedure made you feel.
> - Would you recommend this technique to patients who are in pain?

Music

The use of music in the healthcare setting can also provide relaxation and distraction from pain (Beck 1991, Good 1996, Heiser et al. 1997). Setting up a library of music (e.g. easy listening, classical) and having personal listening devices available for patient use is a simple way to provide patients with relaxing music. Vaajoki et al. (2012) reported significantly lower pain intensity and pain distress in bedrest on the second post-operative day in a music group compared with a control group after elective abdominal surgery.

Art

Art therapies can assist the patient in moving the focus of attention away from the physical sensation of pain (Bullington et al. 2005, Pavlek 2008). The skills of an art therapist are required to ensure the successful use of this intervention.

> **Learning Activity 8.5**
>
> **Learning in practice: Pain management**
>
> Think of a patient who you cared for recently who was in pain.
>
> - How was their pain being managed?
> - What pharmacological interventions were being used?
> - What non-pharmacological interventions were being used?
> - Based on your reading within this chapter, can you think of any other strategies that might have helped to manage their pain?

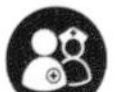

Box 8.14 **Simple relaxation technique script**

Relaxation technique script

Please note that breathing rate during this technique should be normal for the patient in their present condition.

1 Loosen any tight clothing and position yourself comfortably, either lying or sitting. Have your arms and legs uncrossed. Ensure your back and head are well supported.
2 Allow both your hands to rest on your abdomen, one on top of the other. It may be helpful to place a pillow on your lap for your hands to rest on.
3 Gently allow your eyes to close. Breathe normally in and out through your nose if you find this comfortable.
4 As you breathe in, be aware of your abdomen rising gently under your hands (do not force this movement).
5 As you breathe out, be aware of your abdomen relaxing under your hands.
6 Let your shoulders relax and drop down.
7 Let your jaw relax.
8 Now keep your attention softly focused on the rise and fall of your abdomen as this movement follows each breath.
9 Repeat steps 4–8 for between 3 and 5 minutes or longer if appropriate.

During the exercise

As you become aware of any thoughts that arise, let them go and just bring your attention back to the rise and fall of the abdomen. If you are still having difficulty focusing on the technique, try saying the following phrases: 'I am relaxed' or 'I feel calm'.

To finish the exercise

Now slowly become aware of your surroundings, stretch out your fingers and toes, gently open your eyes and come back to the room.

Physical interventions

In addition to psychological interventions, a number of physical interventions can be helpful in reducing pain.

Comfort measures

Simple comfort measures such as positioning pillows and bedlinen (such as supporting a painful limb) (Mann and Carr 2006) can help the patient feel more relaxed and improve patient comfort and pain control. Other comfort measures include ensuring that interruptions and noise are minimized to promote rest and ensuring the ambient temperature is comfortable.

Exercise

Both passive and active physical exercises may benefit patients by increasing range of motion (Feine and Lund 1997), preventing joint stiffness and muscle wasting which may further compound pain problems. Exercise should always be tailored to the patient's tolerance and stamina. A simple exercise regimen which is practised regularly and supervised by a therapist can help patients feel better and more in control as well as having benefits in terms of pain relief. It can increase mobility and flexibility whilst restoring confidence and challenging fear avoidance behaviour (Mann and Carr 2006).

Rest

In addition to exercise, teaching patients to rest comfortably in any position when in pain is a meaningful action and the base from which a person can learn to move more easily (O'Connor and Webb 2002). A person with a terminal illness may experience restriction of movement and neuromuscular pain with increased tension. For these patients, learning to rest and letting go of any tension can be helpful.

Transcutaneous electrical nerve stimulation

Transcutaneous electrical nerve stimulation (TENS) (Figure 8.14) is thought to work by sending a weak electrical current through the skin to stimulate the sensory nerve endings. Depending on the stimulation parameters used, TENS is thought to modulate pain impulses by closing the gate to pain transmission within the spinal cord by stimulating the release of natural pain-relieving chemicals in the brain and spinal cord (King 1999).

Evidence for the use of TENS is variable. Johnson and Martinson (2007) reported significant decreases in pain at rest and on movement in a meta-analysis of 38 studies on TENS and peripheral nerve stimulation for chronic musculoskeletal pain. The evidence for TENS for post-operative pain is often negative, but this may be due to how the studies are conducted.

Heat therapies

For decades superficial heat therapy has been used to relieve a variety of muscular and joint pains, including arthritis, back pain and period pain. There is much anecdotal and some scientific evidence to support the usefulness of heat as an adjunct to other pain treatments (French et al. 2006).

Heat works by:

- stimulating thermoreceptors in the skin and deeper tissues, thereby reducing the sensitivity to pain by closing the gating system in the spinal cord
- reducing muscle spasm
- reducing the viscosity of synovial fluid which alleviates painful stiffness during movement and increases joint range (Carr and Mann 2000).

In the home environment, people use a variety of different methods for applying heat therapies, such as warm baths, hot water bottles, wheat-based heat packs and electrical heating pads. In the hospital setting, caution is required with this equipment as it does not reach health and safety standards (no even and regular temperature distribution) and there have been incidences of serious burns (Barillo et al. 2000). Carr and Mann (2000) note that heat therapy should not be used immediately following tissue damage as it will increase swelling. The Medicines and Healthcare Products Regulatory Agency (MHRA 2005) has documented evidence of burns caused by using heat patches or packs and therefore urges caution in their use and also recommends regular checking of skin throughout therapy.

Figure 8.14 **TENS machine.**

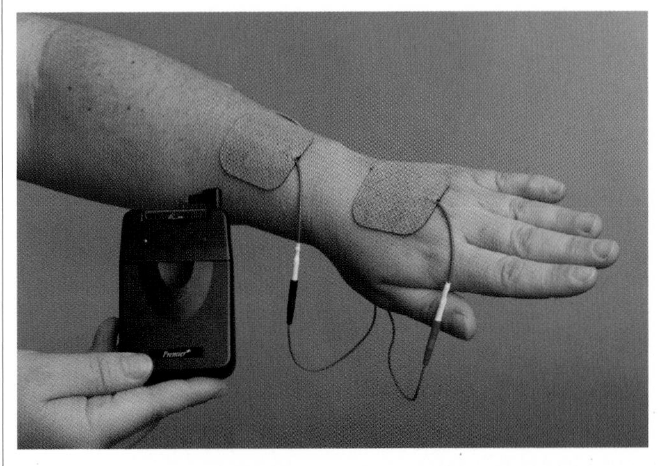

Cold therapies

Cold therapies can also be used to stimulate nerves and modulate pain (Carr and Mann 2000). Cold may be particularly valuable following an acute bruising injury where it can help to reduce inflammation and limit further damage. Cold can be applied in the form of crushed ice or gel-filled cold packs which should be wrapped in a towel to protect the skin from an ice burn.

End-of-life care

DEFINITION

There is considerable ambiguity surrounding the terms end-of-life care, palliative care and terminal care and they are often used interchangeably but are not synonymous.

Palliative care

Palliative care is the active, total care of the patient whose disease is not responsive to curative treatment. Control of pain, of other symptoms and of social, psychological and spiritual problems is paramount. Palliative care is interdisciplinary in its approach and encompasses the patient, the family and the community in its scope. Palliative care affirms life and regards dying as a normal process: it neither hastens nor postpones death (European Association for Palliative Care 2014).

Recent advances in healthcare mean that many people now live with advanced, incurable illness for many years. This has been acknowledged by the WHO which reviewed its definition of palliative care to advise that palliative care is 'applicable from early in the course of illness in conjunction with other therapies which aim to prolong life' (WHO 2002).

End-of-life care (EOLC)

A component of palliative care has been defined as care that helps all those with advanced, progressive, incurable conditions to live as well as possible until they die. It enables the supportive and palliative care needs of both patient and family to be identified and met throughout the last phase of life and into bereavement. By definition, EOLC encompasses the holistic assessment and management of physical care, pain and other symptoms which includes the provision of psychological, social, financial, spiritual and practical support for both the patient and their family/carers in their place of choice, during the last year of life and includes care given after bereavement (National Council for Palliative Care 2008).

Terminal care

Care that is given during the terminal phase. This is an ill-defined period of irreversible decline that signifies imminent death. This is usually a period of several days but may be as short as a few hours; occasionally this can be as long as a couple of weeks (Maltoni and Amadori 2001).

The term 'families and carers' is used throughout this chapter though it is acknowledged that not all family are carers and not all carers are family.

ANATOMY AND PHYSIOLOGY

In the days and hours leading up to an expected death, many physiological changes present as signs and symptoms that represent the closing down of the body before death. These can be alarming if not understood (Field et al. 1997). It is important for healthcare professionals to have an understanding of this process so that they can provide information and reassurance for patients and families. The following are common.

- Decreased social interaction – sleeping more.
- A decreasing level of consciousness leading eventually to coma, except in those few patients who remain awake until a few minutes before they die.
- Decreased food and fluid intake – no hunger or thirst.
- Changes in elimination – reduced urine output and bowel motions, occasional incontinence.
- A weaker pulse (but regular unless previously arrhythmic).
- A gradual drop in blood pressure, though at this stage it should not be routinely taken. It is important that healthcare professionals review the continued need for all interventions and discontinue any that are no longer felt to be conferring benefit to the patient (Ellershaw and Murphy 2011).
- Shallower, slower breathing, which varies in depth, often in a Cheyne–Stokes pattern.
- Cooling and clamminess of the skin from the periphery inwards.
- Cyanosis of the skin on the extremities and around the mouth.

The breathing will ultimately stop, followed several minutes later by cessation of the heart (Harlos 2010).

RELATED THEORY

Enabling people to die in comfort and with dignity is hugely important for the patient, their families and carers and is a core function of the NHS (NEoLCP 2011). There is evidence to indicate that the final elements of care not only have an impact at the time but also on the subsequent bereavement process (King's Fund 2008). *The End of Life Care Strategy* (DH 2008) is considered a blueprint for improving the care of all dying patients regardless of their diagnosis. Care for those approaching the end of life is often challenging and emotionally demanding but, if staff have the necessary knowledge, skills and attitudes, it can be one of the most important and rewarding areas of care (NEoLCP 2010).

End-of-life care has come to the forefront of international government health policies, including *The End of Life Care Strategy* (DH 2008) and *Quality Markers and Measures for End of Life Care* (DH 2009). The four countries of the UK have advocated numerous initiatives to enhance EOLC in the public and private sectors, integrated EOLC pathways being one example (Watts 2012). *The End of Life Care Strategy* (DH 2008) set guidance aimed at improving care and choices for all people regardless of their diagnosis and place of care. The principal aims are to improve the quality of care for those approaching the end of their life and to enable greater choices and control about their place of care and death. The strategy, which focuses on the role of health and social care, states that high-quality EOLC should be available wherever the person may be: at home, in a care home, in hospital, in a hospice or elsewhere (DH 2008).

The National End of Life Care Programme (NEoLCP 2010) was developed to implement the strategy. The programme advocates the following core principles for delivery of EOLC.

- Treat individuals with dignity and respect.
- Provide information and support to families and carers.
- Recognize and respect an individual's spiritual and religious needs.
- Provide effective pain and symptom management.
- Provide care after death.
- Ensure care is person centred and integrated.
- Provide a safe, comfortable environment for care.

Early identification that a patient is dying is a key element in quality EOLC. A major challenge for all staff is knowing how and when to open up a discussion with individuals, their relatives and others involved within their care, about what they wish for as they near the end of their life. Nurses are ideally placed to identify the various clinical triggers that indicate when someone could be in their last year of life, thus enabling and facilitating effective care planning. Agreement needs to be reached by the MDT caring for the individual and there should be negotiation as to which clinician is best placed to communicate this to the patient and their family/carers. It is important that healthcare professionals recognize that sometimes the individual and their families and carers may struggle to consider the future and therefore conversations and care should be guided and planned sensitively and appropriately (NEoLCP 2011).

This planned approach can lead to improved outcomes in terms of both patient care and best use of NHS resources. Early discussion enables the patient to have more control over their care and should result in the more frequent use of advance care planning (NEoLCP 2011).

EVIDENCE-BASED APPROACHES

Palliative care is a relatively new specialty in nursing and medicine; its services operate in different ways and vary in funding (voluntary or NHS), team composition, staff to patient ratio, out of hours care, and treatment regimens used. Palliative care's evidence base is comparatively small and, consequently, applying an evidence-based approach is not always easy. Higginson (1999) points out that an absence of evidence does not mean that a service or treatment is not effective, just that we have not validated its efficacy.

Outcomes such as quality of care and quality of life measures, including quality of death and the best resolution of the bereavement process, are extremely hard to determine, especially when patients are frail and ill. Thus, many studies exclude quality of life as an outcome variable or include only patients who can complete questionnaires. The challenge is to ensure that those aspects of care that are hard to measure do not become a lower priority than aspects, such as survival or function, that are easy to measure (Higginson 1999). However, in order to promote greater use of clinical protocols, best practice guidelines within services and guidance on the most effective models of care, more research evidence is undoubtedly needed.

Evidence suggests that those patients and carers who have had the opportunity to discuss EOLC about 3 months before death:

- are significantly less likely to receive inappropriate aggressive medical treatment
- have significantly reduced levels of depression
- have significantly better adjustment post bereavement (Shipman et al. 2008).

Care before death

Recognition of the dying phase

Care of the dying patient starts with a recognition from the multiprofessional team that the terminal phase has begun. This has been cited as perhaps the single most important factor in enabling the achievement of all the factors associated with a 'good death' (Faull and Nyatanga 2012).

It has been suggested that the following characteristics are central to a good death from medical, nursing and patient perspectives.

- Control.
- Comfort.
- Closure.
- Trust in healthcare providers.
- Recognition of impending death.
- An honouring of personal beliefs and values (Kehl 2006).

Evidence suggests that the dying phase can be difficult to identify. A study by Veerbeek et al. (2008) showed that of 489 deaths in several settings, the dying phase was only identified on the day of death for 50% of patients. The study also found that recognition of the dying phase decreased the chance of the patient having diagnostic interventions (57% versus 39%); 88% of patients in the study had received therapeutic interventions during the dying phase. Barriers to recognizing dying included a reluctance by healthcare professionals to make a diagnosis of dying; 'prognostic paralysis' has been described, whereby clinicians of patients with uncertain illness trajectories prevaricate when considering end-of-life issues (Stewart and McMurray 2002). Health professionals are often concerned that discussions about prognosis will cause distress and damage hope, and that there may be insufficient time to have such discussions. These same concerns are often voiced by patients and families (Maguire and Pitceathley 2002).

In an attempt to overcome these barriers, four basic criteria for recognizing the terminal phase are widely acknowledged. The presence of two or more of the following, commonly preceded by a progressive period of decline and where no other reversible cause is present, is said to denote the terminal phase of life.

- The patient is unable to get out of bed.
- The patient is semi-comatose.
- The patient is only able to take sips of fluid.
- The patient is no longer able to take tablets.

Nursing care during this period does not simply represent a continuation of previously given care, nor, necessarily, the complete cessation of all 'active treatment' measures which may previously have been undertaken. As with all aspects of nursing care, assessment of the individual patient and their family will help to determine the appropriate next steps, which can vary greatly from person to person. It is important that family members and carers of people approaching the end of life are involved in the provision of care. They need therefore to be closely involved in decision making with the recognition that they have their own needs (DH 2008).

Preferred priorities of care and death

Enabling patients to be cared for and to die in a place of their choice is a central tenet to the delivery of good-quality EoLC, and is an important aspect of meeting the psychosocial needs of patients and their relatives in the last days of life (DH 2008). NICE (2004b) guidelines recognized the importance of addressing patients' needs and preferences. They encourage sharing of information and good communication and documentation of patients' and carers' choice of care. They allow multidisciplinary teams and other services to plan and reduce inappropriate admissions and interventions, and help patients to prepare for the future and think about their values and beliefs. The *Preferred Priorities for Care* (PPC) document is designed to help people with advance care planning and enable them to prepare for the future. It gives them an opportunity to think about, talk about and write down their preferences and priorities for care at the end of life (NEoLCP 2011).

More recently, preferred place of care and death in place of choice have been used in the Commissioning for Quality and Innovation payment framework (NEoLCP 2010) which is seen as a lever for service improvement in many acute settings.

Nurses play a key role in assessing the patient's and carer's complex needs relating to preferred place of care and death. It is possible that carers may become tired or ill and informal carers may need more support to understand the complexity of looking after dying patients (Hudson 2005). Often these communications are extremely sensitive and need to be facilitated by an objective outsider who is able to voice the fears and concerns of all those involved. All resources should therefore be discussed and explored, especially for those who have no family or friends, or live in a deprived area where hospital admission is highly likely (Welch et al. 2010).

In communal settings, where possible, single room accommodation should be offered to patients and families or carers. This can provide a feeling of homeliness, allows dying people to rest, gives them privacy and enables them to have family to stay for extended periods without intruding on others (Waller et al. 2008). Nurses should be mindful that some dying patients do not wish to have a single room which they see as isolating. This too should be respected. There is evidence that although the witnessing of a death can be distressing, if this is well managed the process can be comforting for other patients (Payne et al. 1996).

Advance care planning

Advance care planning refers to 'the process by which patients, together with their families and healthcare practitioners, consider their values and goals and articulate their preferences for future care' (Tulsky 2005, p.360). Comprehensive advance care planning (ACP) can help to avoid certain courses of action such as inappropriate readmission to hospital. Ahearn et al. (2013) performed a retrospective study of 100 randomly selected notes which revealed that preferred place of death was not discussed with 92% of patients. The study also found in 10 patients that if ACP had occurred prior to acute decline, a better alternative to acute hospital admission could have been considered, thus allowing patients with a poor prognosis to die in their normal place of residence or a hospice.

Advance decisions to refuse treatment (ADRT)

These allow people who are 18+ years to make a legal decision to refuse, in advance, a proposed treatment or the continuation of that treatment, if at the relevant time the person lacks the capacity to consent to it. ADRTs can only be made by those who are deemed to have the mental capacity to do so, and allow only for the refusal of treatments – they cannot enforce the provision of specified treatments in the same circumstances (DH 2012).

Advance decisions to refuse treatment must be made in writing, be signed and witnessed, and must expressly state that the decision stands even if the person's life is at risk (DH 2012). They can be withdrawn verbally or in writing and are not considered valid if the person has conferred Lasting Power of Attorney on another person. Equally they can be invalidated if the person has done anything which is clearly inconsistent with the original advance decision, for example any change in religious faith.

The Mental Capacity Act (2005) contains statutory guidance about ADRTs. If ADRTs comply with all the tests set out in the Mental Capacity Act, they will be legally binding, so must be respected as if the person who had made the advance decision had capacity and refused the treatment at the time the decision was required. Please refer to the Mental Capacity Act (2005) for comprehensive information relating to ADRTs and Chapter 4: Communication.

Discharging patients for end-of-life care at home or nursing home

For individuals who wish to be discharged to their home or a care home, access to specialist palliative care and 24/7 advice and support are vital (NEoLCP 2011). Proactive working and a complex combination of services across many different settings are crucial; prior to discharge, nurses should ensure that appropriate referrals are made to specialists within the team who will work in partnership with primary and community care services to facilitate the patient's safe discharge.

Patients who are being discharged from hospital for EOLC at home will have their care delivered by a variety of multidisciplinary and multiagency teams, including GP practices, local care homes, pharmacies, hospices, ambulance services, local hospitals and local authority and voluntary sector support services whose aim should be to work together to meet the needs of the patient and their families and carers and ensure a rapid and seamless discharge (NEoLC 2012). Nurses must communicate effectively with other members of the health and social care teams, sharing with them the information necessary to provide the patient with safe, effective and timely care.

This move, between differing health and social care settings, at this very emotional time, can cause great anxiety for patients, their family and carers. It is imperative that nurses give reassurance and clear and concise information relating to responsibility for care and supply all necessary contact details (NEoLC 2012).

For care home and home settings, it is essential that the GP is notified immediately of any patient who is being discharged for EOLC. This will enable them to make arrangements to review the patient as soon as possible; it is crucial that the GP reviews the person regularly and at least every 14 days, both from a care point of view and in order that a Medical Certificate of Cause of Death (MCCD) can be appropriately issued without involving the coroner. The community nurses and hospice teams must be contacted and issued with all the necessary paperwork and information relating to the patient's urgent discharge. Any anticipatory drugs should be prescribed.

The End of Life Care Strategy (DH 2008) identified the need to improve co-ordination of care, recognizing that people at the end of life frequently received care from many different organizations. The subsequent national development of locality registers (now known as electronic palliative care co-ordination systems) was identified as a mechanism for enabling co-ordination between health and social care professionals involved in a patient's care. One such record, 'Co-ordinate my Care', has shown that in areas where these records are used, the successful achievement of preferred place of death has increased for those patients who have expressed a preference (Read 2012). Patients who are being discharged for EOLC at home should, where possible, be consented for the appropriate local electronic record in order to ensure that their wishes are adhered to.

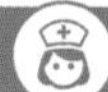 Learning Activity 8.6

Scenario: Discharging patients for end-of-life care at home

You have been asked to start arranging the discharge of a patient who is moving from hospital to home for end-of-life care.

1 Who needs to be informed of the discharge?
2 What other arrangements need to be put in place?

See the end of the chapter for the answers.

LEGAL AND PROFESSIONAL ISSUES

Next of kin

Despite the widespread use of the term 'next of kin' (NOK), it is not clearly defined by law (Advisory Services Alliance 2010) and should not be confused with the 'nearest relative', a legal term used in mental health (Mental Capacity Act 2005). The NOK has no legal liabilities and no rights to medical notes or personal possessions (Dimond 2004). Healthcare staff should respect the patient's wishes when identifying who is next of kin and who should be contacted in the event of their death: this could be a partner, relative or friend (Connecting for Health 2011).

Given the wide variety of relationships and family structures that can exist, it can be easy to make incorrect assumptions about the roles people have (DH 2005b). It is important that the ward or department establishes and documents at the earliest moment possible who is the NOK, who should be informed in the event of a death and who has permission to take any property away, visit, sit with the deceased or make decisions for them. If the deceased person was living in a care home but died in hospital, the care home should be informed because the staff may be aware of the patient's wishes and NOK details.

Documentation should contain not only the address and telephone number of the next of kin but also their relationship to the patient. If possible, a second contact person should also be recorded. These details should be confirmed with the patient if possible rather than transcribed from previous documentation.

In the event of the patient's condition deteriorating, it is vital that the person(s) identified by the patient as the NOK are informed. Nursing staff should also establish whether the NOK wishes to be contacted during the night and document this in the patient's notes.

If the NOK is not present at the time of death, the hospital will have to inform them that the death has occurred. In some cases of sudden death the police will inform the next of kin. Telling someone that a relative or friend has died has to be done with care and sensitivity, and all staff need to have some form of training to allow them to carry out this role sensitively and confidently. It may include being involved in a supportive conversation which may have to be continued later if time is restricted. Wherever possible, hospitals need to respond to the needs of the next of kin at the time they are informed of the death. This can involve phone conversations, making arrangements for the next of kin or others to come to the hospital, and even contacting other people on their behalf (DH 2005b).

In the event of no NOK being identified by the patient, healthcare staff should notify those identified in their local policy who will be responsible for registering the death at the town hall and liaising with the appropriate funeral directors to organize a contract funeral, if necessary. Contract funerals are organized by the local borough. Under Section 46 of the Public Health (Control of Diseases) Act 1984, the council has a statutory obligation to carry out the funeral arrangements of a person who dies within the local area where there is no one else willing or able to deal with the funeral arrangements, for whatever reason.

Hospital staff and volunteers do not have right of entry into the home of the deceased (even if they have the key). Nor do they have the right to go through the deceased's papers in order to identify a friend or relative who could help. In line with partnership working, NHS staff should consult the local protocols with other relevant agencies such as the police and Social Services who may be able to help in identifying relatives or others with responsibility (DH 2005b).

Marriages at the end of life

On occasion, critically or terminally ill patients may request assistance in arranging a marriage or civil partnership in the hospital. For patients too ill to be moved to a place registered for the ceremony (i.e. a register office or place of worship), it is possible to request a ceremony within a hospital or at the bedside.

The hospital chaplain or other religious official and the relevant manager will provide assistance in making necessary arrangements for patients who need a marriage/civil partnership ceremony within the hospital.

Where the parties to a marriage wish this to occur by any non-Church of England ceremony or where a civil marriage/civil partnership is required, the registrar must perform this under licence. The intended spouse/partner of the patient must give notice of the marriage/civil partnership personally to the superintendent registrar.

If the couple wish to be married according to the rites of the Church of England, they should be advised to approach the Church of England chaplain, or the vicar or rector of the parish in which the patient resides and then apply for a special licence to the appropriate registrar for their locality.

In all circumstances the registrar will need a letter, signed by a registered medical practitioner, stating that the patient is too ill to be moved and is not expected to recover. The letter will also confirm that the patient has capacity and does understand the nature and purpose of the marriage/civil partnership ceremony.

The registrar will also need a letter giving permission for the marriage/civil partnership to take place on hospital grounds.

Notice of the intended marriage/civil partnership must also be given to the ward sister/charge nurse so that she/he can adequately accommodate a celebration if desired by the patient and future spouse.

Last will and testament

There are times when a patient may wish to make a will in hospital and some may not be able to complete this process independently. Healthcare staff must ensure that a doctor has reviewed the patient to assess that he/she has capacity to make decisions (Mental Capacity Act 2005) and to record this in the patient's medical notes.

Where possible, wills should be drawn up professionally and patients should be encouraged to seek the assistance of a solicitor, particularly if this concerns complex property or financial matters. Patients may ask nurses to sign a will for them. The Royal College of Nursing (RCN 2013) states that though there is nothing in law preventing a nurse from witnessing a will, it advises against the signing of legal documents as this could lead to involvement in legal cases should there be a later dispute. It is therefore more appropriate for someone who is independent of the patient to undertake this task. This is endorsed by the Nursing and Midwifery Council, who remind nurses of the importance of maintaining clear professional boundaries and being impartial at all times (NMC 2015). All healthcare professionals should consult their hospital's local policy relating to the signing of last wills or any other legal documents.

Rarely, there may be circumstances where a healthcare professional (HCP) is the only person who can realistically witness a signature. This may be when the patient has no apparent relatives or friends, is living remotely from others or is terminally ill (though not mentally incompetent) and there is some urgency for a witness. In these exceptional circumstances, it is acceptable for nurses to witness the signature, although there is no obligation to do so unless local policy demands it. In all cases, the nurse should record the witnessing of the signature in the patient's notes as well as a record of why the HCP was needed to be the signatory witness (RCN 2013).

Most hospitals have will templates available for use. Equally, a patient may choose to draft his or her own will. Both are valid but, where at all possible, the patient should be strongly encouraged to seek a solicitor's advice.

Organ donation

Organ donation is an important consideration at the end of life. Current law is an opt-in system for donation, so express wishes must be made by patients or families (next of kin). Wherever possible, assess the dying person's wishes regarding organ, tissue and body donation and document this in a way that is consistent across organizations and accessible at the time of death (NICE 2011). Patients who have previously expressed a wish to donate (or carry a donor card), or whose family has expressed such a wish, might need specific preparation. Further information can be found at www.organdonation.nhs.uk/.

Euthanasia and assisted suicide

Euthanasia is the act of deliberately, by act or omission, ending a person's life to relieve suffering. For example, a doctor who gives a patient with terminal cancer an overdose of muscle relaxants to end their life would be considered to have carried out euthanasia. In the UK, euthanasia is against the law and carries a maximum penalty of life imprisonment.

Assisted suicide is the act of deliberately assisting or encouraging another person to commit, or attempt to commit, suicide. If a relative of a person with a terminal illness were to obtain powerful sedatives, knowing that the person intended to take an overdose of sedatives to kill themselves, they would be assisting suicide (DH 2013a).

Both euthanasia and assisted suicide are illegal in the UK despite current campaigns to change the law. Nurses must not therefore participate in either process. They should, however, be aware that those patients who approach healthcare professionals with a request for assisted suicide or euthanasia will be doing so from a position of significant vulnerability and must be treated with respect, care and compassion. Commonly, these requests stem from a fear of pain, indignity and dependence and it is imperative to ensure that patients are offered adequate opportunities to express these fears (Dowler 2011). Nurses have a duty of care to ensure that patients' concerns are communicated to the MDT in order that the appropriate specialist physical, psychosocial and spiritual support is offered to minimize their distress.

Artificial hydration

The patient has the right to refuse artificial hydration and those who are unable to communicate their wishes retain this right through advance refusal. Discussions with the patient or relatives and carers may result in the negotiation of a plan of care whereby artificial hydration is commenced for an agreed period, on the understanding that this will be discontinued if it is causing distress to the patient. The appropriateness of artificial hydration will depend on regular assessment of the intervention.

This subject requires skilled and experienced communication (see Chapter 4: Communication).

PRE-PROCEDURAL CONSIDERATIONS

Communication

Excellent communication is paramount in all areas of nursing practice but more so when dealing with dying patients and their relatives. If patients and their relatives and carers are to make educated end-of-life decisions, they need to have nurses who can engage and have open, honest and unambiguous dialogue (NNCG 2011). Nurses must have the confidence to raise the issue of planning for future care and death as well as responding to patients and families that raise these issues themselves (Henry and Wilson 2012). When it is recognized that the patient is dying, it is important that agreement is reached between medical and nursing teams, patients and their families about clinical decisions (NCCG 2011). This may include decisions relating to EOLC pathways, cardiopulmonary resuscitation or whether treatment ceilings are required. If an implanted cardiac device is *in situ* it is important to assess whether it should be left in place, as it may affect the dying phase. Pacing therapy is not normally discontinued but the deactivation of implantable cardiac defibrillators needs to be considered (British Heart Foundation 2007).

Fallowfield (2005) warns that healthcare professionals tend to underestimate patients' desire for information and advises that individualized assessment is necessary to clarify the information needs of patients, relatives and carers. It is vital that nurses remember that they are the patient's advocate; they need to ensure that individuals have sufficient space and time to reflect and discuss their concerns. Nurses must also remember that the patient and their families and carers may struggle to consider the future; conversations and care should therefore be guided sensitively. Communication is influenced by patients' and families' cultural and spiritual beliefs, which will also affect patients' information needs at the end of life. Nurses are more closely involved with patients and therefore ideally placed to establish their feelings and preferences concerning end-of-life wishes. These may include who they wish to be present at the time of their death or how they wish families and carers to be informed of their death. Ensuring that healthcare professionals at all levels have the skills to communicate with and care for the dying is critical to the success of improving EOLC (DH 2008). Please see Chapter 4: Communication for further information relating to communication skills.

Prognosis

Prognostication is an uncertain art and often only when wise after the event can these judgements be verified (GMC 2010). Over the past 20 years there has been a major shift in attitudes regarding disclosure of information to patients; more recently the culture is for complete disclosure. However, healthcare professionals should always be mindful of the individual needs of patients, families and carers and sensitively establish the amount of disclosure a patient and family wishes.

Guidance suggests that someone is approaching the end of life when they are likely to die within the next 12 months (Murray et al. 2005), whether from advanced, progressive, incurable conditions or general frailty and co-existing conditions; they may be at risk of dying from a sudden acute crisis in their existing condition or life-threatening acute conditions caused by sudden catastrophic events.

Those close to a patient who is at the end of life stage may want or need information about the patient's diagnosis and about the likely progression of the condition or disease. This will help them set goals and priorities and help them provide care, as well as enabling them to recognize and respond to changes in the patient's condition. If a patient has capacity to make decisions, you should check that they agree to you sharing this information (Watson et al. 2009). If a patient lacks capacity to make a decision about sharing information, it is reasonable to assume that, unless they indicate otherwise, they would want those closest to them to be kept informed of relevant information about their care.

Watson et al. (2009) assert that prognostication is not just about passing on clinical details and predictions of disease progression; it also involves assessing the following.

- What does the patient actually want to know? Too much information can be as harmful as inadequate information.
- How is the patient dealing with the information that is being given?
- How can the patient be helped to deal with the implications of the news?

To discuss prognostication without regard for the implications of those facts is to increase the risk of dysfunctional communication taking place.

Discussions surrounding prognosis should be undertaken by professionals confident in advanced communication skills and with the appropriate experience to offer an approximation on the grounds of their clinical knowledge and experience. Following communication about prognosis, advice and support should be offered to those who are finding the situation emotionally challenging. Sources of support may include patient and carer support and advocacy services, counselling and chaplaincy services. It is important that support is also offered to healthcare professionals (GMC 2010).

The principles of breaking bad news should be adhered to in undertaking discussions about prognosis.

Principles of care for dying patients

End-of-life care pathways were intended to exemplify a high standard of care through the terminal phase of palliative care into bereavement. The Liverpool Care Pathway for the Dying Patient (Ellershaw et al. 1997), commonly shortened to LCP, was developed by the Royal Liverpool University Hospital and the Marie Curie Hospice in Liverpool as a model of best practice in end-of-life-care (O'Hara 2011). It incorporated 'gold standard' care associated with the hospice setting into mainstream healthcare and was welcomed as a means of enabling professionals of all specialties to provide the best possible multidisciplinary care for their patients as they enter the terminal phase. The LCP was endorsed by successive national policy frameworks (DH 2003a), the *End of Life Care Strategy* (DH 2008), *Quality Markers and Measures for End of Life Care* (DH 2009), General Medical Council guidance (GMC 2010) and the NICE quality standard for EOLC for adults (NICE 2011).

However, EOLC pathways were criticized for reducing care of the dying to a flow diagram and a tick box exercise that did not improve patient care (Kelly 2003). Allen (2010, p.48) contests that EOLC pathways have transformed and changed into a 'hybrid ensemble' of clinical and management agendas.

Following substantial criticism of the LCP in the media and elsewhere, the government requested an independent review of its use. A panel lead by Baroness Julia Neuberger consulted professional bodies and reviewed relevant literature. They also consulted members of the public who described their personal experiences around usage of the LCP.

Following the consultation, a report entitled *More Care, Less Pathway: A Review of the Liverpool Care Pathway* was produced (DH 2013a). The review panel noted that before the introduction of the LCP into hospitals, the care that patients received at the end of life was variable, with many examples of poor care. They fully acknowledged the valuable contribution that approaches like the LCP have made in improving the timeliness and quality of clinical decisions in the care of dying patients, and urged that the overall findings of the review did not result in clinicians defaulting back to treating dying patients as though they are always curable for fear of censure. The review panel stated that, used correctly, the LCP could provide a model of good practice for dying patients. However, the evidence examined showed that the LCP had not always been used appropriately and had come to be seen as a generic protocol, intended to be applicable for all patients in the last hours or days of their lives, and that this was the wrong approach. The panel therefore recommended that the LCP be replaced by 'an end of life care plan for each patient backed up by condition-specific good practice guidance' (DH 2013a, p.47).

The importance of individually tailored care for those in the terminal phase of their lives, and their relatives, cannot be overemphasized. No framework, pathway or care plan is a substitute for careful assessment, information giving, listening, referral and skilled intervention. Each person will require slightly different care in one way or another and, as with all areas of nursing care, assumptions should never be made solely on the basis of previous preferences, sociocultural or religious stereotypes.

However, some principles and interventions, whilst not to be applied without bearing in mind the individual's needs, are important and should be routinely considered, even if not undertaken for each patient. These principles should reflect the ethos of palliative care and integrate the physical, psychological, social and spiritual aspects of care which are at no time more important than in the terminal phase of life (Watts 2013).

Guidance on many different aspects of terminal care, including comfort measures, the anticipatory prescription of medicines, the discontinuation of inappropriate interventions (including resuscitation) and care of the relatives and carers (both before and after the death of the patient), should be included in these principles of care.

Pharmacological support

Pharmacological symptom management can improve the quality of life of patients with a severe life-limiting illness. Depending on a person's position on the disease trajectory and their goals of care, drugs, including chemotherapy, may be prescribed to actively treat disease, prevent, reduce or eliminate symptoms or slow the disease process. A patient approaching the terminal phase may choose to have antibiotics to treat their symptomatic urinary tract infection but may decline to have antibiotics to treat a recurring episode of severe pneumonia (Clary and Lawson 2009). Palliative care, with its gradual shift in transition from curative and life-prolonging treatment toward palliative quality of life treatments, can relieve significant medical burdens and maintain a patient's dignity and comfort.

Symptoms such as pain, dyspnoea, nausea and vomiting should be treated proactively according to local regimens. Tumour-related bowel obstruction where surgery is not appropriate can be managed medically, also adhering to local policy. Normalizing the environment for patients may prevent delirium but pharmacological intervention may be needed as per local guidelines (Clary and Lawson 2009). Excessive respiratory secretions, which may lead to the phenomenon of the 'death rattle', can be a very distressing symptom for families and relatives and needs sensitive explanation and reassurance that this is unlikely to be distressing the patient and the reasons for the management of choice which may be pharmacologically but can also include non-pharmacological measures such as positioning the patient.

Any intervention should be consistent with the patient's preferences and goals, especially in the context of palliative care. If investigations or tests cannot possibly lead to a change in the patient's management, the investigation or test is not indicated. Currow et al. (2013) report that 20% of people take at least eight medications at the time of referral to a specialist palliative service, adding that many people admitted to palliative care services had an increase in prescribed medications as death approached, with reductions in long-term medications often surpassed by initiation of drugs for symptom management. Acknowledging that patients' rights to adequate medication are not lessened because they have a shorter prognosis, they point out that frail and vulnerable patients have diminished capacity for withstanding adverse drug reactions which increase the risk of iatrogenic harm. There is, therefore, a greater responsibility on those prescribing medication to palliative patients to optimize all medications, balancing benefit and risk, monitoring and adjusting for each individual in the context of a changing clinical picture (Currow et al. 2013).

Many medications for chronic conditions are continued in spite of changes in a person's prognosis that may render the initial intentions unnecessary or inappropriate. Changes in body composition and eating habits may affect blood glucose levels, requiring adjustment of diabetes management such as frequency and targets of monitoring and appropriateness of medication indication and dosage. Cessation of long-term medications often occurs as a result of suspected adverse drug reaction or loss of the oral route of administration rather than planned care. However, cessation of long-term medications without careful discussion with patients or their families carries the potential for both physiological and psychological harm (Clary and Lawson 2009). It can be extremely difficult for patients or families who for a lifetime have monitored blood glucose levels to suddenly let go of this practice.

At all times there should be clear discussion with patients and their families relating to the goals of treatment as well as specific time lines for reviewing these and if necessary discontinuing them; this is especially important when considering fluids, nutritional supplements and oxygen. It should also be pointed out to patients and their families that if symptoms, such as those previously mentioned, have not been an issue earlier in their trajectory then these may not necessarily be a problem at the end of life. Equally, they should be reassured that discontinuing medications or treatments does not mean a discontinuation of care, which will be delivered with competence and compassion right to the end of life. This reassurance alongside good management of physical symptoms allows patients and loved ones the space to work out unfinished emotional, psychological and spiritual issues and, thereby, the opportunity to find affirmation at life's end (Clary and Lawson 2009).

A patient's compliance relating to medication may be affected by concern about addiction, side-effects or incorrectly thinking that if pain killers are taken 'too soon' they will be without sufficient analgesia 'when pain gets worse'. As a result, people with severe symptoms may not use medicines even when effective management is available. This is particularly pertinent to opioids. Involving pharmacists to counsel patients can have a positive influence and improve patient outcomes. Team-based multidisciplinary care is considered integral to palliative care because of the complex biomedical and psychosocial needs of palliative care patients. Similar to palliative care, optimizing medication outcomes should have a multidisciplinary approach. Pharmacists are well placed to promote proactive review of pharmacotherapy. The can provide advice for other healthcare professionals and also facilitate discussion with patients to reset therapeutic goals to ensure they understand the reasons for, and are happy with, any proposed changes (Clary and Lawson 2009).

Non-pharmacological support

Research has indicated that non-pharmacological approaches to physical and psychological symptoms may be of benefit to EOLC patients (Booth et al. 2011). Non-pharmacological measures can help to empower patients at a time when the majority of their symptom management is prescriptive. There is a body of literature concerning the non-pharmacological management of breathlessness (Booth et al. 2011, Corner et al. 1996). This model advocates the involvement of the multidisciplinary team to draw on all resources available, e.g. using the physiotherapist to give advice on breathing exercises and the occupational therapist to teach relaxation techniques.

Florence Nightingale (1859) wrote of the effect that the environment had on health, highlighting the negative effects of factors such as noise, lack of air, light and sleep. Booth et al. (2011) also advocate assessment of the environment, acknowledging the benefits of a bright well-ventilated room with the positioning of a fan to reduce the sensation of breathlessness for patients. This multidisciplinary model should not be limited to the care of breathlessness and should be considered for all aspects of patient care for optimum outcomes.

The essence of non-pharmacological interventions is both holistic and heuristic (Taylor 2007). Nurses, who often spend most time with patients during EOLC, are often best placed to assist patients with non-pharmacological interventions. The element of reassurance or 'presence' is very important: knowing when to touch or not to touch a patient or relative, when to simply sit quietly with the patient or draw up a chair for a deeply anxious relative. Nursing routines, performed in a calm reassuring manner, bring normality to interactions, providing a sense of safety and security. These fundamental aspects of care are often extremely simple but are not always evident to those that do not have experience or specialist skills in relation to caring for EOLC patients. Specific non-pharmacological techniques such as relaxation techniques, counselling and music therapy are discussed in other chapters in this book.

Physical care

Physical discomfort can be one of the greatest concerns as patients with a terminal illness anticipate dying. NICE (2004b) guidelines advise that patients expect to be offered optimal symptom management at the end of life and recommend that this should be achieved in all healthcare settings, particularly in the community where effective well-managed symptom management can reduce unnecessary hospital admissions.

There should be a holistic assessment of the patient's needs followed by comprehensive care planning and regular review of symptoms. It is absolutely essential that the patient is central to the process of assessment and planning at all times (NEoLCP 2010). Nurses should be competent to build on this assessment in a dynamic, sensitive, consistent manner and observe and record subtle changes (NEoLCP 2011). They must be aware of the significance and governance risks involved when assessments are not comprehensive. This will often involve consideration of changes of equipment to keep the patient comfortable. Ensuring a pressure-relieving mattress is made available for patients either in their own home or in hospital is of paramount importance in order to ensure that pressure area care is maintained. However, many patients do not like the pressure-relieving mattress and will not wish to have this. In this situation the nurse's role is to advise the patient and their relative of the risk involved without alarming them unduly. Switching to a 24-hour syringe pump for patients who are unable to swallow medication must be considered alongside the patient's feelings of being attached to a pump that may limit their mobility in the home. All discussions should be documented clearly and contemporaneously.

Communication with other members of the multidisciplinary team can be an excellent resource when assessing the patient's need; the expertise of the patient's key worker, occupational therapist or social worker is often invaluable. Use of assessment tools such as the Pepsi-Cola aide memoire and the distress thermometer can also aid assessment (NEoLCP 2011).

Meeting the physical needs of patients at the end of life is aimed at providing as much comfort as possible. The change from curing to caring means providing comfort with the least invasive procedures, and maintaining privacy and dignity becomes paramount. If these physical needs are controlled to a manageable level, patients and their families and carers will be able to focus on maintaining hope, reaffirming important connections and attaining a sense of completion.

Table 8.5 lists some common physical symptoms present during the terminal phase of life and any management changes specific to the patient who is dying. Pain, sickness, nausea and respiratory tract secretions have been cited as the four most common symptoms (Ellershaw et al. 2010). Information relating to these and many of the other symptoms experienced in the terminal phase, including mouth care, nutrition and elimination, is discussed in relevant chapters of this book.

Psychosocial care

Ongoing psychosocial assessment, support and care of the patient and their relatives are extremely important as death approaches. Research has shown that improving psychosocial interventions alleviates distress for EOLC patients (Lloyd-Williams 2003). However, provision may need to be adjusted according to the changing needs of the patient – many will experience increasing anxiety and distress, increased feelings of social isolation and, alongside this, a decrease in physical energy available to them for dealing with these concerns. Relatives will naturally be distressed by the deterioration of the patient and may exhibit signs of grief even before death occurs. Nurses should ensure that, wherever possible, the physical environment is conducive to patients and relatives being able to express their thoughts and emotions, and that appropriately trained staff are available to listen and support them.

Alleviating distress when patients no longer feel connected with the world and are angry that their body has failed them can be challenging for healthcare professionals. Patients may find it difficult to discuss threats to their personhood and it is only through effective communication and interpersonal skills that nurses can address these issues (Lloyd-Williams 2003).

Evidence suggests that real change in EOLC will only happen if patients are allowed to prepare for and face death by expressing fears, hopes and desires (Neuberger 2004). Some managemen strategies prevent this; for example, medication to alleviate anxiety may also block fear. As a result, the source of fear or anxiety will not be understood and the cause will not be addressed. Patients have reasons to be afraid and allowing them to express their anxiety is crucial (Cannaerts et al. 2004).

The importance of psychosocial care should never be underestimated and psychological management should be considered just as important as physical management across primary, acute and tertiary care (Lloyd-Williams 2003). All healthcare professionals need to understand and recognize patients with complex psychosocial needs and be able to make comprehensive assessments of the distressing issues that patients may face. Nurses should be aware of their own limitations in this area and seek the support of specialists when needed.

Psychological, social and spiritual factors may exacerbate physical suffering. For instance, depression amplifies pain and other somatic symptoms. When physical, psychological and spiritual sources of distress are inseparably intermixed, causing 'total pain syndrome', a fully integrated clinical approach that addresses the multiple dimensions of suffering is required (Lloyd-Williams 2003).

Spiritual and religious care

Considerable energy and debate continue to be devoted to defining and exploring the concept of spirituality and its relationship to religion (NEoLCP 2011). Spiritual care has risen in visibility in health services over the last two decades, from a position where it was equated with religious care and regarded as the sole province of chaplains to one where a broad concept of spirituality is employed and spiritual care is recognized as having relevance for all sectors and to lie potentially within the remit of all health

Table 8.5 **Guidelines for symptom control**

Symptom	Management changes
Pain (see Chapter 9: Respiratory care)	Good assessment is a necessary precondition for effective pain management (Cherny 2010) Levels of pain may increase, decrease or remain stable. Analgesics may need to be rationalized and/or administered via a different route (e.g. subcutaneous syringe pump) as the patient may no longer be able to swallow Levels of consciousness, lucidity and respiratory rate will all be commonly altered during the terminal phase. It is important to bear this in mind when assessing the effects and side-effects of analgesic medications Some discomfort can be caused by immobility and pressure on the skin. If appropriate (i.e. if it will not cause patient or relative distress), the patient should be moved to a pressure-relieving mattress. Otherwise regular skin care should be carried out as tolerated (see Chapter 5: Elimination for further information)
Nausea/vomiting	Nausea and vomiting may increase, decrease or remain stable. Comprehensive assessment is paramount. In light of assessment reverse the reversible. Consider the complications of the disease process as well as side-effects of drugs (Faull and Woof 2002) Antiemetics may need to be rationalized and/or administered via a different route (e.g. subcutaneous syringe pump) as the patient may no longer be able to swallow Because the insertion of a nasogastric tube is considered a fairly invasive and uncomfortable procedure, it is unlikely to be appropriate for the management of nausea and vomiting in the terminal care setting. Those nasogastric tubes already *in situ* should remain unless causing distress to the patient Injectable hyoscine hydrobromide (Buscopan) or octreotide should be considered to dry gastric secretions in those patients with mechanical vomiting secondary to bowel obstruction
Respiratory secretions	'Noisy', 'bubbly' breathing or 'death rattle' in the terminal phase of life affects approximately 50% of dying patients and is the result of fluid pooling in the hypopharynx. Non-pharmacological methods should be used alongside medication. These can include distraction techniques, relaxation therapy and a hand-held fan. A multidisciplinary team approach with the physiotherapist, occupational therapist and palliative care team is often needed (Robinson and English 2010) Changing the position of the patient in the bed may reduce the noisiness of breathing. It is important to reassure family that the patient is not drowning or choking, and is unlikely to be distressed by the symptom themselves Antimuscarinic (hyoscine butylbromide) or anticholinergic (glycopyrronium or hyoscine hydrobromide) drugs are often used in this setting and can be administered subcutaneously via a syringe pump
Agitation/restlessness	Confusion, delirium, agitation and restlessness are all terms used to describe patient distress in the last 48 hours of life. The symptom is fairly common with up to 88% of patients experiencing symptoms in the last days or hours of life (Lawlor et al. 2000). Careful assessment should include consideration of any precipitating factors including medications, reversible metabolic causes, constipation, urinary retention, hypoxia, withdrawal from drugs or alcohol, uncontrolled symptoms and existential distress Clear, concise communication, continuity of carers if possible, the presence of familiar objects and people and a safe immediate environment can all be helpful nursing interventions Where the cause of the symptoms cannot be established or cannot be reversed, anxiolytics, antipsychotics or sedation may need to be considered. This may need to be discussed with relatives instead of the patient. It is important that the nurse is present for these conversations in order to facilitate reassurance of the relatives throughout
Breathlessness	Breathlessness may be a new symptom in the terminal phase or may worsen from its pre-existing state. Careful assessment is important as this symptom will usually involve physiological, psychological and environmental factors Low-dose opioids and anxiolytics can be of use for breathlessness, though as with other medications, the route of administration may need to be altered. Nebulized bronchodilators and oxygen may also be of benefit. Where the symptom is causing severe distress and is intractable, sedation may need to be considered in discussion with the patient and relatives (Booth 2006) Relaxation exercises, open windows or electric fans and massage may also be of benefit if the patient can tolerate these
Constipation	The focus of care with regard to constipation should remain on patient comfort. Oral laxatives are inappropriate if the patient cannot swallow and rectal interventions should only be undertaken if the patient is clearly distressed by this symptom

and social care workers. However, this perceptual shift has not necessarily occurred at the level of practice and there is anecdotal and other evidence of continuing uncertainty and ambiguity over how, when and where spiritual need should be addressed.

The (UK) Standards for Hospice and Palliative Care Chaplaincy affirm that assessment of spiritual and religious need should be available to all patients and carers, including those of no faith. Spiritual needs are defined as exploring the individual's sense of meaning and purpose in life; exploring attitudes, beliefs, ideas, values and concerns around life and death issues; affirming life and worth by encouraging reminiscence about the past; exploring the individual's hopes and fears regarding the present and future for themselves and their families/carers; exploring the 'why' questions in relation to life, death and suffering.

Each patient and their relatives should have the opportunity to express, in advance, any religous, cultural or practical needs they may have for the time of death or afterwards, particularly regarding urgent release for burial or cremation. This can be done as part of the advance care planning process or it can be completed nearer the point of death (NNCG 2011). It is important to try to discuss these with the patient, as even where relatives share a common faith, there may be differences in the way each person practises. It is vital that assumptions are not made on the basis of a previously disclosed religious preference; for example, not all Catholic believers will want to be given the sacrament of the sick. Further information about religious/cultural perspectives and practices is given in Table 8.6.

POST-PROCEDURAL CONSIDERATIONS

Nursing care does not end when the death of the patient occurs; it extends beyond death to provide care for the deceased person and support to their family and carers (NNCG 2011). This physical care given by nurses following death in hospitals has been traditionally referred to as 'last offices'. However, this chapter will refer to 'care after death', a term more appropriate in our multicultural society (NNCG 2011).

Care after death (last offices)

DEFINITION

'Care after death' has historically been referred to as 'last offices', a term related to the Latin *officium*, meaning service or duty which was associated with the military. This term also had religious connotations from its association with 'last rites', a Christian sacrament and prayer administered to the dying (Quested and Rudge 2003). It is used to refer to the final act performed on a person's body. Last offices, sometimes referred to as 'laying out', was the term for the nursing care given to a deceased patient which demonstrates continued respect for the patient as an individual (NMC 2015). More recently, there has been a move away from the term 'last offices' and its link with the military and religious association with 'last rites', to the terminology of 'care after death'. This move is appropriate for a variety of reasons. The term 'last offices' only applies to the physical care of the deceased body. 'Care after death' is a broader term that better reflects a multicultural society and also embraces all the differing nursing tasks involved, including the ongoing support of the family and carers (NNCG 2011).

Even though they have died, patients are still referred to as patients or people throughout this section.

RELATED THEORY

Death threatens the orderly continuation of social life, according to Seale (1998). Care after death can mark the social transition of the person and the biological death of the patient, and begins the process of handing over care to the family and funeral director. This care can be considered as an important act in the rite of passage in moving the deceased person into the world of the dead (van Gennep 1972) and is a procedure that people in all cultures recognize.

Care after death is the final act a nurse will carry out for the patient and remains associated with ritual (Pattison 2008a,b). Nursing care for a patient who has died has historical roots dating back to the 19th century (Wolf 1988). However, contemporary nursing practice has moved away from the ritualistic practices of cleansing, plugging, packing and tying the patient's orifices to prevent the leakage of body fluids to encompass much more than simply dealing with a dead body (Pattison 2008a,b, Pearce 1963). Consideration now has to be given to legal issues surrounding death, the removal (or non-removal) of equipment, washing and grooming, and ensuring correct identification of the patient (Costello 2004). The *End of Life Care Strategy* (DH 2008) emphasizes care after a patient has died, and in particular it points to the value of integrated care pathways in managing administrative and psychosocial care. This corresponds to a good death theory where being treated with dignity is an underlying premise (Kehl 2006, Smith 2000), and good death encompasses all stages of dying and death (NNCG 2011, Pattison 2008a,b). This principle, therefore, continues after death.

Carrying out such an intimate act that in many cultures would be carried out only by certain family or community members requires careful consideration by nurses and adequate preparation of procedures. This should include family members where possible. Since 60.6% of all men and women who die in England and Wales will die in an institution (hospice, hospital, care home) (ONS 2009), it is predominantly nurses who carry out after-death care, prior to patients being moved to mortuaries or undertakers. Quested and Rudge (2003) suggested that this aspect of care is largely invisible to other healthcare workers.

EVIDENCE-BASED APPROACHES

Care after death has its nursing foundation in traditional cultures although it is a nursing routine which does not have a large amount of research-based evidence (Cooke 2000). For nurses, this care should be seen as a privilege and treated with the utmost sensitivity. There is only one chance to get it right so it is imperative that nurses ensure the wishes of the family and carers are, where possible, adhered to. New guidance has been developed to assist nurses with this complex aspect of care (NNCG 2011). This new guidance encourages nurses to honour the integrity of the person who has died and places the deceased and their carers at the 'focus of the care whilst continuing to balance the legal and coronial system and the health and safety of staff' (NNCG 2011).

Care after death can have symbolic meaning for nurses, often providing a sense of closure. It can be a fulfilling experience as it is the final demonstration of respectful, sensitive care given to a patient (Nearney 1998) and also the family (Speck 1992). Philpin (2002) advises that there has been a move away from practice that is considered unscientific; however, care after death is a time when nurses must be mindful and show respect for patients' rituals and cultures as well as insight into the symbolic meanings that patients and their families hold dear. This can be a major source of comfort and structure for the patients and families at this traumatic time (Neuberger 2004, Wolf 1988).

It should be noted that many parts of the nursing procedures relating to care after death are based on general principles of infection prevention and control, and safe working. Care of the patient who has died must therefore take into account health and safety guidelines to ensure families, healthcare workers, mortuary staff and undertakers are not put at risk (HSAC 2003). This chapter incorporates this guidance with broader national guidance where appropriate. It aims to ensure that patients who have died are treated with respect and dignity even after death, that legalities are adhered to and that appropriate infection prevention and control measures are taken. *Patients Who Die in Hospital* (DH 2005b) and *What to Do After a Death* (DH 2006b) provide information for families and carers and focus on procedures around the legalities of organizing funerals.

Table 8.6 **Cultural and religious considerations in the care of the dying patient and their care after death**

	Beliefs about death	Cultural or religious routines	Preparing the body	Post-mortem/ transplantation	Specific burial requirements	For further information contact
Baha'i	Baha'is have a great respect for life, believing each person has a soul that comes into being at conception. During the lifetime the spiritual attributes are acquired for the next stage of existence that follows death	The body is to be treated with great respect as it is considered to be the vehicle of the soul. Friends and relatives will say the prayers for the dead	The body is to be washed and wrapped in plain cotton or silk. A special ring will be placed on the finger of the patient and is not to be removed	Organ donation is considered praiseworthy	Embalming and cremation are forbidden. The burial should take place no more than an hour's journey from the place of death	UK Bahai: www.bahai.org.uk
Buddhism	Death viewed as very important as it is a time of transition before rebirth as the person moves towards Nirvana – the freedom from suffering, death and rebirth	There is no one specific ritual but a state of calm is necessary. An example may be: • A monk may be called to recite prayers/ lead meditation • The family wanting the body to remain in one place for up to 7 days for the rebirth to take place. (It is recognized this is not possible in a healthcare setting)	At all times the body should be treated with greatest care and respect. When washing has taken place the body should be wrapped in a plain white sheet	No objections	Prefer cremation as symbol of impermanence of the body	Buddhist Hospice Trust: www. buddhisthospice. org.uk
Christianity/ Anglican / Church of England	God's forgiveness is available to all who ask because of the selfless/sinless death of Jesus Christ on the cross. As Christ was resurrected, death has been overcome and eternal life is a gift from God available to all who believe and seek forgiveness	Priest or minister may attend to say prayers. Primarily to support relatives and friends	No specific requests		No preference	Hospital Chaplaincies Council: www.nhs-chaplaincy-spiritualcare.org.uk
Nonconformist/ Free Church		Prayers may be offered but these will be informal in most situations	No specific requests			
Roman Catholicism		Priest requested to recite prayers for the dying and then prayers for the dead	A religious icon such as a crucifix or rosary may accompany the patient's body	No objections	Burial has in the past been preferred	

(continued)

Table 8.6 **Cultural and religious considerations in the care of the dying patient and their care after death** ***(continued)***

	Beliefs about death	Cultural or religious routines	Preparing the body	Post-mortem/ transplantation	Specific burial requirements	For further information contact
Church of Jesus Christ of Latter Day Saints (Mormon Church)	Earthly life is viewed as a test to see if individuals are fit to return to God on death. Death is viewed as a temporary separation from loved ones		The body should be washed and dressed in a shroud. Some may wear a religious undergarment which must remain in place after the patient has died	No religious objection	Burial preferred	Church of Jesus Christ of Latter Day Saints: www .ldschurch.org
Christian Scientist		There are no specific rituals associated with death	Females only to touch female body	This is generally not supported unless there is a legal requirement for it	Prefer cremation	For details of local Christian Science Church: www.christianscience .org.uk
Hinduism	Hindus believe that all human beings have a soul that passes through successive cycles of birth and rebirth. It is believed that eventually the soul will be purified and join the cosmic consciousness	Last rites include: Tying a thread around the neck or wrist to bless the dying person Sprinkling holy water from the Ganges on them Placing a sacred Tulsi leaf in their mouth If possible, placing the person on a sheet or mat on the floor to symbolize closeness to Mother Earth, freedom from physical constraints and the easing of the soul's departure	Close family members led by the eldest son usually wash the body. They may be distressed if a non-Hindu touches the body so gloves should be worn. A female must only be touched by a female and a male by a male. The body should be covered by a plain white sheet. All religious objects should remain in place	Only if absolutely necessary. If a post-mortem does take place, the organs must be returned to the body	Cremation within 24 hours of death arranged by the eldest son	National Council of Hindu Temples: www .hinducounciluk.org
Islam	Death is a mark of transition from one state of being to another. Muslims are encouraged to accept death as part of the will of Allah	The time before death is important for extending forgiveness to family and friends. The Koran is recited until the point of death	The body should be turned to the right (Quibla; Mecca) if this hasn't happened before the patient dies. The relatives will close the eyes and bandage the lower jaw so the mouth doesn't gape. Flex the joints of the arms and legs to stop them becoming rigid. A complete cleansing (Ghusal) will then take place performed by the relatives (this may take place after the body has been removed from the ward). The body will be wrapped in a Caffan. If there isn't one available, a sheet will do. A female must be handled by female nursing staff and a male by male staff. Maintaining modesty and dignity is essential	This is not acceptable, primarily because it will delay burial but also because the person may still be able to perceive pain	Burial will take place as quickly as possible	Muslim Council of Great Britain: www.mcb.org.uk/ downloads/Death-Bereavement.pdf

	Beliefs about death	Cultural or religious routines	Preparing the body	Post-mortem/ transplantation	Specific burial requirements	For further information contact
Jehovah's Witness	When a person dies their existence stops for ever	There are no special rituals or practices to perform	No special requirements are to be observed		Funeral must be modest and dignified	
Judaism		Orthodox Jews don't permit the touching or moving of a dying person. Following death, the rabbi will be requested to perform Last Rites. It is important somebody stays with the body until a member of Jewish Burial Society or family member arrives The family may want to keep watch with the body to pray even if it is in the mortuary	The body will receive the ritual washing Taharah performed by either trained members of the synagogue or the Jewish Burial Society. If the rabbi cannot be contacted, essential procedures can be performed by healthcare staff. Close eyes and mouth. All catheters and drains and the fluid in them must be left as they are considered part of the body. Open wounds must be covered. The body must be laid flat with hands open and arms parallel to the body. DON'T wash the body. Traditionally the body is covered by a plain white sheet with the feet facing the door	This is not permitted by Orthodox Jews except where the law requires it. Reform Jews permit it on the grounds of the furthering of medical knowledge	Orthodox Jews Cremation is permitted for non-Orthodox Jews	Burial Society of the United Synagogue: www.theus.org.uk 020 8343 3456 Office of the Chief Rabbi (Orthodox): www.chiefrabbi.org Union of Liberal and Progressive Synagogues: : www .liberaljudaism.org Montagu Centre, 21 Maple Street, London W1T 4BE.
Sikhism	Life after death is a continuous cycle of rebirth: the person's soul is their essence	Prior to the death comfort may be derived from reciting verses from the holy book (Guru Granth Sahib)	The relatives may wish to prepare the body but this shouldn't be assumed. The five Ks should be left on the body. 1 Kesh – uncut hair symbolic of sanctity and a love of nature 2 Kangha – a wooden comb symbolizing cleanliness 3 Kara – a steel band worn on the right wrist symbolic of strength and restraint 4 Kirpan – a sword or dagger symbolizing the readiness to fight against injustice 5 Kacha – unisex undershorts symbolizing morality The body must be touched only by staff of the same sex. The eyes and mouth must be closed, the face straight and clean	No objections	Cremation	Sikh Educational and Cultural Association: 01474 332356

Source: Adapted from Hollins (2009) and other sources.

Indications

- When a patient's death has been verified and documented.
- For adult patients who have died in hospital or in a hospice.

Contraindications

When to consult for further guidance before undertaking procedures.

- If a patient who has died is indicated for a post-mortem.
- If a patient who has died is a candidate for organ donation.

LEGAL AND PROFESSIONAL ISSUES

Nurses should be aware of the legal requirements for care of patients after death as it is essential that correct procedures are followed (Green and Green 2006). It is particularly important that nurses are aware of deaths that require referral to the coroner (discussed later) as this will facilitate the correct personal care and enable nurses to prepare the family for both a potential delay in the processing of the MCCD and also the possibility of a post-mortem examination (NNCG 2011).

Guidance relating to vulnerable adults is available (MCA 2005). If after death safeguarding issues are raised, it is important to follow the local policy and ensure that concerns are communicated with relevant agencies such as Social Services, police and coroner.

Every effort should be made to accommodate the wishes of the patient's relatives (Neuberger 2004). The UK is an increasingly multicultural and multifaith society which presents a challenge to nurses who need to be aware of the many different religious and cultural rituals that may accompany the death of a patient. There are notable cultural variations within and between people of different faiths, ethnic backgrounds and national origins. This may affect approaches to death and dying (Neuberger 2004). This needs to be remembered when administering care after death in order to avoid presumptions. While those who have settled in a society with a dominant faith or culture other than their own might appear to increasingly adopt that dominant culture, they may choose to retain their different practices at times of birth, marriage or death (Neuberger 1999). Approaches to death and dying also reveal as much about the attitude of society as a whole as they do about individuals within that society (Field et al. 1997).

Practices relating to care after death will vary depending on the patient's cultural background and religious practices (Nearney 1998). Table 8.6 provides a guide to cultural and religious variations in attitudes to death and how individuals may wish to be treated. This information is not designed to be a 'fact file' (Gilliat-Ray 2001, Gunaratnam 1997, Smaje and Field 1997) of information on culture and religion that seeks to give concrete information. Such a 'fact file' would not be appropriate as we need to be aware that whilst death and death-related beliefs, rituals and traditions can vary widely among each cultural group, within any given group there may be varying degrees of observance of these issues (Green and Green 2006), from orthodox to agnostic and atheist. Categorizing individuals into groups with clearly defined norms can lead to a lack of understanding of the complexities of religious and cultural practice and can depersonalize care for individuals and their families (Neuberger 1999, Smaje and Field 1997).

Expected deaths may be very different from those where a patient has died suddenly or unexpectedly (Docherty 2000). In certain cases the patient's death may need to be referred to the coroner or medical examiner for further investigation and possible post-mortem (DH 2003b). If those caring for the deceased are unsure about this then the person in charge of the patient's care should be consulted before care after death has commenced. If the death is going to be referred to the coroner, advice must be sought before interfering with anything that might be relevant to establishing the cause of death.

PRE-PROCEDURAL CONSIDERATIONS

Before undertaking care after death, several other events must take place.

Verification and certification of death

Death should be confirmed or verified by appropriate healthcare staff. The process of verifying death is not in itself a statutory process and can be performed by nurses as well as doctors (Academy of Medical Royal Colleges 2008). The NMC states that nurses may confirm death has occurred provided there is an explicit policy or protocol to allow such action and provided that the death is expected (NMC 2015). Nurses and other healthcare professionals must therefore be aware of local guidance, which should be in line with national guidance, regarding the criteria for verifying death. It is good practice for verification to occur as soon as possible.

The professional verifying the death is responsible for confirming the identity of the deceased person (where known) using the terminology of 'identified to me as'. This requires name, date of birth, address and NHS number (if known) (NNCG 2011). Details of the date and time death occurred should be documented in the notes and/or care pathway documentation along with the name and contact details of the responsible practitioner. Any relevant devices (such as cardiac defibrillators) should also be recorded as well as the verifier's own name and contact details in the nursing, medical or ambulance documentation (NNCG 2011). The certifying medical practitioner has overall responsibility for identifying and communicating the presence of any implanted devices or radioactive substances. They are also responsible for identifying the appropriate person to deactivate and remove implants, to liaise with the appropriate medical physics department regarding radioactive treatments and advise mortuary staff and funeral directors. If relatives have any concerns about the death, these should also be documented.

Unexpected deaths must be confirmed by a medical doctor (and usually a senior medical doctor). Confirmation of death must be recorded in the medical and nursing notes and care pathway documentation if necessary. If the death is suspicious or unexplained, a special forensic post-mortem may be required and means the family and carers can only view the body with agreement from the police and coroner. In many instances the restrictions will be minimal but, if the death is thought to be suspicious, it is important that forensic evidence is not contaminated; there should therefore be no removal of indwelling devices or other such equipment from the patient (NNCG 2011).

A registered medical doctor who has attended the deceased person during their last illness is required to give a MCCD (Home Office 1971). It is good practice to ensure that when the death need not be referred to the coroner, the MCCD is issued within 1 working day so burial or cremation arrangements can commence (NNCG 2011). The certificate requires the doctor to state on which date he/she last saw the deceased alive and whether or not he/she has seen the body after death (this may mean the certificate is completed by a different doctor from the one who confirmed death). Out-of-hours medical examiners (ME) can now certify death where there is a cultural/religious requirement to bury, cremate or repatriate patients quickly (DH 2008). The ME can also certify for reportable deaths where a post-mortem is not deemed necessary (DH 2008). The ME is an independent health professional who determines the need for coroner referral.

Burial and cremation

For those who need a burial within 24 hours, this remains at the discretion of the local births and deaths registrar in each council and depends on the individual opening hours and on-call facilities. Local hospital policy should outline procedures for out-of-hours death registration, and certification and burial is usually easier to accommodate than cremation within 24 hours.

Repatriation to another country needs further documentation, alongside the death certification and registration documents. This varies according to the country to which the person is being repatriated. Only a coroner or ME is authorized to permit the body to be moved out of England or Wales. A *Form of notice to a coroner of intention to remove a body out of England* (Form 104) is required which can be obtained from coroners or registrars. This form needs to be given to the coroner along with any certificate for burial or cremation already issued. The coroner's office will acknowledge receipt of notice and inform the family when repatriation can occur. Coroner authorization normally takes up to four working days so that necessary enquiries can be made. In urgent situations, this can sometimes be expedited and the coroner's office and relevant High Commission will have further information relating to this. In terms of infection control, different levels of packing of body orifices may be required by different countries. Those involved with repatriation must be informed if there is a risk of cross-infection (HSAC 2003). Funeral directors will assist with transportation issues.

Referral to a coroner
If the patient's death is to be referred to a coroner or ME, this will affect how their body is prepared. The need for referral to a coroner or ME needs to be ascertained with the person verifying the death (DH 2008). Preparation in this situation differs according to how the patient died. Broadly, two types of death are referred to the coroner:

- those from a list of cases where the coroner must be informed (which includes deaths within 24 hours of an operation, for example)
- cases where the treating doctor is unable to certify the cause of death (Home Office 2002, HTA 2006).

The DH website at www.dh.gov.uk gives more information about when to refer to the coroner or ME and when post-mortems are indicated.

Requirement for a post-mortem
Post-mortems can affect preparation after death, depending on whether this is a coroner's post-mortem (sometimes referred to as a legal post-mortem because it cannot be refused) or a post-mortem requested by the consultant doctor in charge to answer a specific query on the cause of death (also referred to as a hospital or non-legal post-mortem). A coroner's post-mortem might require specific preparation but the coroner or ME will advise on this and should be contacted as soon as possible after death to ascertain any specific issues. Individual hospitals, institutions and NHS trusts should provide further guidance on these issues. If the patient is to be referred to the coroner, cap off catheters and ensure there is no possibility of leakage. Do not remove any invasive devices until this has been discussed with the coroner (HTA 2006).

If the patient is *not* to be referred to the coroner, invasive and non-invasive attachments, such as central venous access catheters, peripheral venous access cannulas, Swan–Ganz catheters, tracheal tubes (tracheostomy/endotracheal) and drains, can all be removed.

If a post-mortem is necessary, the patient's family or carers may have questions that need to be sensitively answered. The DH (2003b) has published a simple guide to what actually takes place at a post-mortem.

Organ donation
Consider if the patient was a candidate for organ or tissue donation. Patients who previously expressed a wish to be a donor (or carry a donor card), or whose family has expressed such a wish, might need specific preparation. If an individual's wishes regarding organ and tissue donation were not formally recorded before death, consent can be sought from a nominated representative or someone else in a qualifying relationship, if they believe the deceased wanted to donate. Whole-body donation can only be agreed by individuals themselves and not by anybody else after death (HTA 2011). Advice on consent is available from NHS Blood and Transplant (NHSBT) specialist nurses organ donation (SN-OD) who are based in acute trusts or by contacting NHSBT directly (www.uktransplant.org.uk/ukt).

Infectious patients
The practitioner who verified the death is responsible for ascertaining whether the person had a known or suspected infection and whether this is notifiable. The Health and Safety Executive has issued guidelines on the handling of bodies with infections and nurses, doctors and other healthcare professionals should be aware of related local infection control policies and reporting responsibilities (HSE 2003). It is vital that processes are in place to protect confidentiality, which continues after death, but this does not prevent the use of sensible rules to safeguard the health and safety of all those who may care for the deceased.

Families and carers should also be supported in adhering to infection prevention and control procedures if they wish to assist in personal care after the death of an infectious patient. There are a few, very rare, exceptions where it is not possible for families to participate.

- If the patient has had any of the following infections prior to death: typhus, severe acute respiratory syndrome, yellow fever, anthrax, plague, rabies and smallpox. Assistance with care after death or viewing is not permitted because of the high risk of transmission of these infections (Healing et al. 1995).
- If the patient was exposed to radiation. Patients may have been treated with radioactive material as therapy or may have been exposed to it in accidental circumstances. Always seek expert radiation protection advice before beginning care after death in such cases.

If the patient was infectious, it needs to be established whether it is a notifiable infection, for example hepatitis B, C or tuberculosis, or non-notifiable (Healing et al. 1995, HPA 2010, HSAC 2003). There are additional requirements for patients with blood-borne infections, therefore the senior nurse on duty should be consulted and the local infection control policy adhered to. In the UK, notifiable infections must be reported via a local authority 'proper officer' and this is the attending doctor's duty. Infection prevention and control contacts in local trusts or services can provide more help and guidance around notification. Placing the patient who has died in a body bag is advised for all notifiable diseases and a number of non-notifiable infectious diseases (i.e. HIV, transmissible spongiform encephalopathies, e.g. Creutzfeldt–Jakob disease). A label identifying the infection must also be attached to the patient's body. Specific guidance is outlined in the procedure.

Certain extra precautions are required when handling a patient who has died from an infectious disease. However, the deceased will pose no greater threat of infection than when they were alive. It is assumed that staff will have practised universal precautions when caring for all patients, and this practice must be continued when caring for the deceased patient (HSAC 2003).

Porters, mortuary staff, undertakers and those involved with the care of patients who have died must also be informed if there is a danger of infection (HSAC 2003).

Patient and family considerations
Some families and carers may wish to assist with personal care after death, and within certain cultures it may be unacceptable for anyone other than a family member or religious leader to wash the patient (Green and Green 2006). It may also be required for somebody of the same sex as the patient to undertake the personal care after death (Neuberger 2004). Families and carers should be supported and encouraged to participate if possible as this may help to facilitate the grieving process. If children are involved, nurses should be mindful of their needs and should consider the physical environment. Adults may require guidance on how best to convey the news of a deceased relative to children (NNCG 2011).

Spiritual needs
Spiritual needs relating to preparation of the patient who has died can be diverse . The patient's previous wishes should be

established where possible and should always take precedence (Pattison 2008a,b). If not previously documented, try to determine patients' previous wishes from family or carers. The patient's last will and testament might have instruction on this, or an advance decisions or advance care plans might have information. Families, carers or members of the patient's community or faith may wish to participate in the care after death. If this is the case, they must be adequately prepared for this with careful and sensitive explanation of the procedure to be undertaken. Families may request other items to accompany the patient who has died to the mortuary and funeral home. This might be an item of sentimental value, for instance, or an item of jewellery and this should be discussed with the NOK and documented and witnessed in accordance with local policy.

Certain religious artefacts must never be removed from the patient, even after death, for example the five Ks in Sikhism (Kesh – uncut hair, Kangha – the wooden comb which fixes uncut hair into a bun, Kara – an iron, steel or gold bracelet worn on the right wrist, Kirpan – a symbolic sword worn under clothing in a cloth sheath or as a brooch or pendant, and Kacha – undergarments) (Neuberger 2004).

The information given above and in Table 8.6 is for guidance only. Families may require all, part or none of these actions to be carried out. The information has been adapted from Hollins (2009), Speck (1992), Pattison (2008a, 2008b), Neuberger (2004) and Green and Green (2006).

Regardless of the faith that the patient's record states they hold, wishes relating to care after death may differ from the conventions of their stated faith. Sensitive discussion is needed by nurses to establish what is wanted at this time. If patients are of a faith not listed above or hold no religious beliefs, ask the relatives to outline the patient's previously expressed wishes, if any, or establish the family's wishes. Furthermore, the patient may be non-denominational and/or the family members may be multidenominational so all possibilities must be taken into account.

Additional considerations

It is important to inform other patients, particularly if the person has died in an area where other people are present (such as a bay or open ward), and might know the patient. Residents in communal settings, such as care homes and prisons, have often built significant relationships with other residents and members of staff (Moss et al. 2002). It is important to consider how to address their needs within the boundaries of patient confidentiality. If the person has died in an environment where other people may be distressed by the death then sensitively inform them that the patient has died, being careful not to provide information about the cause and reason for death (NNCG 2011). Senior staff should offer guidance in the event of uncertainty about how to deal with the situation.

Finally, carry out all personal care after death in accordance with safe manual handling guidance and where possible within 2–4 hours of death. This is because rigor mortis can occur relatively soon after death, and this time is shortened in warmer environments (Berry and Griffie 2006). It is best practice to do this with two people, one of whom needs to be a registered nurse or a suitably trained person (NNCG 2011).

Learning Activity 8.7

Learning in practice: Care after death

Within your clinical area, find out what the local policy is for caring for patients after death.

- As a student nurse, consider what aspects of this process you are able to be involved in.
- Having read this section, what significant thing have you learnt that will help you if you are caring for a patient after death?

Procedure guideline 8.12 **Personal care after death**

Essential equipment

- Disposable plastic apron
- Disposable plastic gloves
- Bowl of warm water, soap, patient's own toilet articles
- Disposable wash cloths and two towels
- Disposable razor or patient's own electric, comb and equipment for nail care, a razor if there is a request for the patient to be shaved (see notes re shaving below)
- Equipment for mouth care, including equipment for cleaning dentures
- Identification labels ×2 or as defined in local policy
- Documents required by law and by organization/institution policy, e.g. notification of death forms
- Shroud or patient's personal clothing: night-dress, pyjamas, clothes previously requested by patient, or clothes which comply with deceased patient/family/cultural wishes
- Body bag if required (if there is actual or potential leakage of bodily fluids and/or if there is infectious disease)
- Labels for the patient's body defining the nature of the infection/disease (HSAC 2003)
- Gauze, tape, dressings and bandages if wounds, puncture sites or intravenous/arterial devices
- Plastic bags for clinical and domestic (household) waste
- Laundry skip and appropriate bags for soiled linen
- Clean bedlinen
- Record books for property and valuables
- Bags for the patient's personal possessions
- Disposable or washable receptacle for collecting urine if appropriate
- Sharps bin if appropriate

Optional equipment

- Caps/spigots for urinary catheters (if catheters are to be left *in situ*)
- Goggles
- Full gowns
- 3M masks (if highly infectious) (HSAC 2003)
- Petroleum jelly
- Suction equipment and absorbent pads (where there is the potential for leakage)
- Card or envelope to offer lock of hair as appropriate (Pattison 2008a)

Pre-procedure

Action	Rationale
1 Apply gloves and apron, gowns/masks/goggles if the patient is infectious.	Personal protective equipment (PPE) must be worn when performing personal care after death, and is used to both protect yourself and all of your patients from the risks of cross-infection (HSAC 2003, **C**; Loveday et al. 2014, **C**; RCN 2005, **C**).
2 If the patient is on a pressure-relieving mattress or device, consult the manufacturer's instructions before switching off.	If the mattress deflates too quickly it may cause a manual handling challenge to the nurses carrying out personal care after death. **E**
3 Lay the patient on his/her back with the assistance of additional nurses and straighten any limbs as far as possible (adhering to your own organization's manual handling policy). If it is not possible to lay the body flat due to a medical condition then inform the mortuary or relevant staff and the funeral director.	To maintain the patient's privacy and dignity (NMC 2015, **C**) and for future nursing care of the body. Stiff, flexed limbs can be difficult to fit easily into a mortuary trolley, mortuary fridge or coffin and can cause additional distress to any carers who wish to view the body. However, if the patient's body cannot be straightened, force should not be used as this can be corrected by the funeral director (Green and Green 2006, **E**).
4 Remove all but one pillow. Close the mouth and support the jaw by placing a pillow or rolled-up towel on the chest or underneath the jaw. Do not bind the patient's jaw with bandages. Some people have deformed jaws that will never close – notify the funeral director if this is the case.	To avoid leaving pressure marks on the face which can be difficult to remove.
5 Remove any mechanical aids such as syringe drivers, heel pads, etc. Apply gauze and tape to syringe driver/IV sites and document disposal of medication (adhering to your own organization's disposal of medication policy). Consider leaving prosthetics *in situ* as appropriate (e.g. limb, dental or breast prosthetics).	
6 Close the patient's eyes by applying light pressure to the eyelids for 30 seconds. If this is unsuccessful then explain sensitively to the family/carers that the funeral director will resolve the issue. If corneal or eye donation is to take place, close the eyes with gauze moistened with normal saline.	To maintain the patient's dignity (NMC 2015, **C**) and for aesthetic reasons. Closure of the eyelids will also provide tissue protection in case of corneal donation (Green and Green 2006, **E**).
7 Do not tie the penis. Spigot any urinary catheters. Pads and pants can be used to absorb any leakage of fluid from the urethra, vagina or rectum.	
8 Leakages from the oral cavity, vagina and bowel can be contained by the use of suctioning, drainage and incontinence pads respectively. Patients who do continue to have leakages from their orifices after death should be placed in a body bag following personal care after death. The packing of orifices can cause damage to the patient's body and should only be done by professionals who have received specialist training. It might be helpful to manage self-limiting leakages with absorbent pads and gently rolling the patient who has died to aid drainage of potential leakages.	Leaking orifices pose a health hazard to staff coming into contact with the patient's body (Green and Green 2006, **E**; HSAC 2003, **C**). Ensuring that the patient's body is clean will demonstrate continued respect for the patient's dignity (NMC 2015, **C**). The packing of orifices is considered unnecessary, as it increases the rate of bacterial growth that can occur when these areas of the patient's body are not allowed to drain naturally (Berry and Griffie 2006, **E**). However, there are certain situations where it is necessary (in severe leakage or where repatriation is required). A body bag is also necessary in these cases.
9 Exuding wounds or unhealed surgical scars should be covered with a clean absorbent dressing and secured with an occlusive dressing (e.g. Tegaderm). Stitches and clips should be left intact. Consider leaving intact recent surgical dressings for wounds that could potentially leak, e.g. large amputation wounds.	The dressing will absorb any leakage from the wound site (Naylor et al. 2001, **R2b**).
10 Stomas should be covered with a clean bag. Reinforcement of the dressing should be sufficient.	Open wounds and stomas pose a health hazard to staff coming into contact with the body (RCN 2005, **C**). Disturbing recent large surgical dressings may encourage seepage and leakage (Travis 2002, **E**).

(continued)

Procedure guideline 8.12 Personal care after death *(continued)*

Action	Rationale
11 a Remove drainage tubes, unless otherwise stated. b Record the tubes and devices that have been removed and those that have been left *in situ*. Open drainage sites need to be sealed with an occlusive dressing (e.g. Tegaderm). c Mortuary staff or appropriate healthcare staff should determine with the funeral director collecting the body their capacity to remove lines, drains, indwelling catheters, etc. If they are unable to remove these then the mortuary staff or those designated should attend to this before releasing the body. When a family collects the deceased all lines, drains and indwelling catheters should be removed.	Open drainage sites pose a health hazard to staff coming into contact with the patient's body (RCN 2005, **C**). When a death is being referred to the coroner or ME or for post-mortem, all lines, devices and tubes should be left in place (Green and Green 2006, **E**). The funeral director may need to ensure same-day burial and the family may wish to bathe and dress the body (NNCG 2011, **C**).
12 Wash the patient, unless requested not to do so for religious/cultural reasons or carer's preference. It is best to let the funeral directors shave the body if necessary. If the family/carers request that the body is shaved, sensitively discuss the consequences and document this in the notes. If shaving is to be carried out, apply water-based emollient cream to the face first. Be aware that some faith groups prohibit shaving.	For hygenic and aesthetic reasons. As a mark of respect and point of closure in the relationship between nurse and patient (Cooke 2000, **E**). Shaving the body whilst still warm can cause bruising and marking which only appears days later (NNCG 2011, **C**).
13 It may be important to family and carers to assist with washing, thereby continuing to provide the care given in the period before death. Prepare them sensitively for changes to the body after death and be aware of manual handling and infection control issues.	It is an expression of respect and affection, part of the process of adjusting to loss and expressing grief (Berry and Griffie 2006, **E**).
14 Mouth and teeth should be cleaned with foam sticks or a toothbrush. Insert clean dentures if the patient normally used them. Apply petroleum jelly to the lips and perioral area.	Teeth and mouth are cleaned for hygienic and aesthetic reasons (Cooke 2000, **E**) and to remove debris. Petroleum jelly can prevent skin excoriation or corrosion if stomach contents aspirate.
15 Remove all jewellery (in the presence of another nurse) unless requested by the patient's family to do otherwise. Jewellery remaining on the patient should be documented on the notification of death form. Record the jewellery and other valuables in the patient's property book and store the items according to local policy. Avoid the use of the names of precious metals or gems when describing jewellery to prevent potential later confusion. Instead, use terms such as 'yellow metal' or 'red stone'. Rings left on the patient's body should be secured with tape, if loose. Be aware of religious ornaments that need to remain with the deceased.	To meet with legal requirements, cultural practices and relatives' wishes (Green and Green 2006, **E**).
16 Dress the patient appropriately (use of shrouds is common practice in many hospitals), or as the family's wish before they are transferred from the ward. The body should never be transferrred naked or released to a funeral director from an organization without a mortuary. Be aware that soiling can occur. In community settings the community nurse may offer to do this, or the family may want to do it themselves, in which case they should be advised sensitively on the potential for soiling.	Honouring the rituals and cultures of patients' families and carers can be a major souce of comfort and structure at what for some is an extrememly traumatic time (Wolf 1988, **E**). For family and carers viewing the patient's body or religious or cultural reasons and to meet families' or carers' wishes (Green and Green 2006, **E**).
17 Ensure a correct hospital or organizational patient identification label is attached to the patient's wrist and attach a further label to one ankle. As a minimum, this should identify their name, date of birth, address, ward (if an inpatient) and ideally their NHS number. Complete any documents such as notification of death cards. Copies of such cards are usually required (refer to hospital policy for details). Tape one securely to clothing or shroud.	

18 Provided no leakage is expected and there is no infectious diseases present, the body can be then transferred to the body store or mortuary as per local policy which may use a body bag or else the body is wrapped in a sheet. If leakage is expected or if the patient was infectious, a body bag should be used. If the leakage is continuous, place it on absorbent pads in the body bag and advise the mortuary or funeral director.	To avoid actual or potential leakage of fluid, whether infection is present or not, as this poses a health hazard to all those who come into contact with the deceased patient. The sheet will absorb excess fluid (HSAC 2003, **C**).
If a sheet is used, do not tape too tightly.	This can cause disfigurement.
19 Tape the second notification of death card to the outside of the body bag.	For ease of identification of the patient's body in the mortuary (Green and Green 2006, **E**).
20 Request the portering staff to remove the patient's body from the ward and transport to the mortuary. In hospital settings, it is best practice for porters to take the body from the ward to the mortuary within 1 hour of request so it can be refrigerated within 4 hours of death. This ensures that tissue donation can take place (if requested).	To avoid decomposition which occurs rapidly, particularly in hot weather and in overheated rooms. Many pathogenic organisms survive for some time after death and so decomposition of the patient's body may pose a health and safety hazard for those handling it (Cooke 2000, **E**). Autolysis and growth of bacteria are delayed if the patient's body is cooled.
21 The privacy and dignity of the deceased on transfer from the place of death are paramount. The body should be placed in an appropriate container to avoid causing distress to others and bed areas that will be passed should be screened off as the body is removed.	To avoid causing unnecessary distress to other patients, relatives and staff.
22 Remove gloves and apron. Dispose of equipment according to local policy and wash hands.	To minimize risk of cross-infection and contamination (RCN 2005, **C**).
23 Record all details and actions within the nursing documentation.	To record the time of death, names of those present, and names of those informed (NMC 2010, **C**).
24 Transfer property and patient records to the appropriate administrative department.	The administrative department cannot begin to process the formalities such as the death certificate or the collection of property by the next of kin until the required documents are in its possession (Green and Green 2006, **E**).

Problem-solving table 8.2 **Prevention and resolution (Procedure guideline 8.12)**

Problem	Cause	Prevention	Action
Relatives not present at the time of the patient's death.	Possible unexpected death; uncontactable family.	Preparation of family for event of death where appropriate.	Inform the relatives as soon as possible of the death. Consider also that they may want to view the patient's body before personal care after death has been completed.
Relatives or next of kin not contactable by telephone or by the general practitioner.	Out of date or missing contact information.	Ensure next of kin contact information is documented and up to date.	If within the UK, local police will go to next of kin's house. If abroad, the British Embassy will assist.
Death occurring within 24 hours of an operation.	n/a	In relation to documentation, ensure information around circumstance of death is documented and handed over to relevant healthcare staff.	All tubes and/or drains must be left in position. Spigot or cap off any cannulas or catheters. Treat stomas as open wounds. Leave any endotracheal or tracheostomy tubes in place. Machinery can be disconnected (discuss with coroner) but settings must be left alone. Post-mortem examination will be required to establish the cause of death. Any tubes, drains, etc. may have been a major factor contributing to the death.
Unexpected death.	n/a	As above.	As above. Post-mortem examination of the patient's body will be required to establish the cause of death.
Unknown cause of death.	n/a	As above.	As above.

(continued)

Problem-solving table 8.2 **Prevention and resolution (Procedure guideline 8.12)** ***(continued)***

Problem	Cause	Prevention	Action
Patient brought into hospital who is already deceased.	n/a	Not preventable but, where possible, ensure patients' families are prepared for all eventualities, particularly if palliative care patients whose death is expected, and that family know who to call and what to do in the event of death.	As above, unless patient is seen by a medical practitioner within 14 days before death. In this instance the attending medical officer may complete the death certificate if he/she is clear as to the cause of death.
Patient who dies after receiving systemic radioactive iodine.	There is a potential risk of exposure to radiation (IPEM 2002).	Radiation protection should be undertaken according to local policy.	Ensure those in contact with the patient's body are aware and pregnant nurses should not be involved in care for these patients. For further information refer to local policy for radiation protection.
Patient who dies after insertion of gold grains, colloidal radioactive solution, caesium needles, caesium applicators, iridium wires or iridium hair pins.	There is a potential risk of exposure to radiation (IPEM 2002).	Radiation protection should be undertaken according to local policy when removing wires. Physicist may remove radioactive wires/ needles, etc. themselves, depending on source.	Inform the physics department as well as appropriate medical staff. Once a doctor has verified death, the sources are removed and placed in a lead container. A Geiger counter is used to check that all sources have been removed. This reduces the radiation risk when completing these procedures. Record the time and date of removal of the sources. Ensure those in contact with the patient's body are aware and pregnant nurses should not carry out nursing care for these patients. For further information refer to local policy for radiation protection.
Patient and/or relative wishes to donate organs/tissues for transplantation.	n/a	Discussion around transplantation should occur with families/NOK wherever appropriate (as deemed by clinical team). Exceptions apply.	As stated in the Human Tissue Act 1961, patients with malignancies can only donate corneas and heart valves (and more recently tracheas). Contact local transplant co-ordinator as soon as a decision is made to donate organs/tissue and before care after death is attempted. Obtain verbal and written consent from the next of kin, as per local policy. Prepare patient who has died as per transplant co-ordinator's instructions. For further guidance see www.organdonation.nhs.uk/.
Patient to be moved straight from ward to undertakers.	n/a	n/a	Contact senior nurse for hospital. Contact local register office as release of Certificate for Burial or Cremation ('green' document) needs to be obtained. Liaise with chosen funeral directors and the deceased's family. Perform personal care as per religious/cultural/family wishes. Obtain written authority for removal of person by the funeral directors, from the next of kin. Document all actions and proceedings (Travis 2002).
Relatives want to see the person who has died after removal from the ward.	n/a	n/a	Inform the mortuary staff in order to allow time for them to prepare the body. Occasionally nurses might be required to undertake this in institutions where there are no mortuary staff. The patient's body will normally be placed in the hospital viewing room. Ask relatives if they wish for a chaplain or other religious leader or appropriate person to accompany them. As required, religious artefacts should be removed from or added to the viewing room. The nurse should check that the patient's body and environment are presentable before accompanying the relatives into the viewing room. The relatives may want to be alone with the deceased but the nurse should wait outside in order that support may be provided should the relatives become distressed. After the relatives have left, the nurse should contact the portering service who will return the deceased patient to the mortuary.

POST-PROCEDURAL CONSIDERATIONS

Immediate care

Since there is a time limit to how long a patient should remain in the heat of a ward (there could potentially be early onset of rigor mortis), the senior nurse will have to exercise discretion over when to send the patient to the mortuary. This will vary according to family circumstances (there could be a short delay in a relative travelling to the ward/area) and to the ward situation (side rooms are obviously easier for the family/other patients). As a general rule, 1–2 hours would be considered the upper limit for a patient to remain in the ward area, after care after death has been completed.

Viewing the patient

Families may wish to view the patient in a viewing room. Again, it is important to ensure that the patient is in a presentable state before taking the family to see them.

Bereavement support

The bereaved family may find it difficult to comprehend the death of their family member and it can take great sensitivity and skill to support them at this time. Explaining all procedures as fully as possible can help understanding for the practices at the end of life. Offering bereavement care services may be useful to families for that difficult period immediately after death and in the future. National services such as CRUSE (www.cruse.org.uk) can be useful if local services aren't known. There may be extreme distress; this is a difficult situation to handle and other family members are likely to be of most comfort and support at this point. The family member may wish for their GP to be contacted.

Maintain a high degree of sensitivity when outlining the process after a patient has died since families frequently have to attend the hospital in the very near future to collect the documentation for registering the death.

Education of patient and relevant others

Helping the family to understand procedures after death is the role of many people in hospital but primarily this will fall upon those who first meet with the family after their relative has died. The Home Office leaflet *What to Do after a Death* can help families.

If the family suggest that they feel the death was unnatural or even that it was interfered with, we have a responsibility to explore these feelings and even outline their legal entitlement to a post-mortem.

- Prepare the family for what they might see.
- Invite the family into the bed space/room.
- Accompany family but respect their need for privacy should they require it.
- Anticipate questions.
- Offer the family the opportunity to discuss care (at that time or in the future).
- Offer to contact relatives on behalf of the family.
- Advise about the bereavement support services that can be accessed. Arrange an appointment with facilities.
- Provide them with a point of contact with the hospital.

Some families may wish for a memento of the patient, such as a lock of hair. Try to anticipate and accommodate these wishes as much as possible.

Support of nursing staff and others

End-of-life care has been described as challenging, complex and emotionally demanding but, if staff have the necessary knowledge, skills and attitudes, it can be one of the most important and rewarding areas of care (DH 2008, Poncet et al. 2007). Providing EOLC can expose staff to risks of emotional burnout or post-traumatic stress (Mealer et al. 2007). To prevent this, a supportive and nurturing environment for all those who provide EOLC is necessary. Pattison (2011) agrees, stating that the practical and emotional support needed by staff cannot be overestimated. She advises that this can be provided by mentorship and clinical supervision as well as staff counselling but warns that consideration needs to be given to workload and skill mix to enable this to take place. This support should extend to doctors and all members of the multidisciplinary team because the emotional implications of dealing with EOLC affect all (Ho et al. 2011).

The palliative care team can be a useful resource in providing informal teaching and educational support for staff relating to EOLC issues. This is often achieved by joint patient care or meetings with family members. This experiential learning can be valuable especially for junior team members who may have more confidence to ask questions on a one-to-one basis.

Learning for practice

After studying this chapter, list five key points you have learnt about patient comfort that you will be able to apply to your clinical practice.

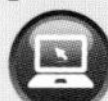
For further learning exercises visit **www.royalmarsdenmanual.com/student**.

Now Test Yourself

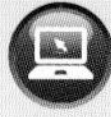
This section provides a range of exercises/activities to further test your learning. For additional exercises visit **www.royalmarsdenmanual.com/student**.

What have you learnt?

1 Which layer of the skin contains blood and lymph vessels, sweat and sebaceous glands?

A Epidermis
B Dermis
C Subcutaneous layer
D All of the above

2 What factors can influence the appearance of the skin?

3 Using a hot water bottle in bed may cause foot ulceration.

A True
B False

4 A clean technique should be used for all eye care procedures.
- A True
- B False – for vulnerable exposed eyes or to reduce the risk of infection, an aseptic technique may be required

5 What is xerostomia?
- A Dry mouth
- B Taste changes
- C Ulcerated mouth
- D All of the above

6 Which of the following is no longer a recommended method of mouthcare?
- A Chlorhexidine solution and foam sticks
- B Sodium bicarbonate
- C Normal saline mouthwash
- D Glycerine and lemon swabs

7 In pain assessment, a useful mnemonic is 'SOCRATES'. What does it stand for?

8 List at least four non-pharmacological methods of managing pain.

9 'The active, total care of the patient whose disease is not responsive to curative treatment' defines which term?
- A End of life care
- B Palliative care
- C Terminal care
- D All of the above

10 Which of the following IS NOT one of the four basic criteria that denote the terminal phase of life?
- A The patient is semi-comatose
- B The patient is unable to get out of bed
- C The patient is unable to verbally communicate
- D The patient is only able to take sips of fluid
- E The patient is no longer able to take tablets

See the end of the chapter for the answers.

Key points

- Hygiene is a highly personal matter determined by individual values and practices. It involves care of the skin, hair, nails, teeth, oral and nasal cavities, eyes, ears and perineal-genital areas (Berman et al. 2010).
- Evidence has shown that the knowledge and attitudes of caregivers are integral to the effective delivery of oral care. The mouth should be assessed as part of the initial nursing assessment and should be reassessed regularly thereafter.
- A range of factors can influence the nature and expression of pain and can be associated with the patient, the nurse or the clinical environment. Pain can have many dimensions including physical, psychological, spiritual and sociocultural.
- It is important for healthcare professionals to have an understanding of the process of dying so that they can provide information and reassurance for patients and families.
- The importance of individually tailored care for those in the terminal phase of their lives, and their relatives, cannot be overemphasized. No framework, pathway or care plan is a substitute for careful assessment, information giving, listening, referral and skilled intervention.

Websites

For further information about organ donation, contact the following website or your local transplant co-ordinator: www.organdonation.nhs.uk/
For further information about bereavement and bereavement advice:
Cruse Bereavement Care: www.cruse.org.uk
For advice following a death:
Citizens Advice Bureau: www.citizensadvice.org.uk
Some useful references for further reading around religious/spiritual practices:
Hospital Chaplaincies Council:
www.nhs-chaplaincy-spiritualcare.org.uk
Bahai: www.bahai.org.uk
Buddhist Hospice Trust: www.buddhisthospice.org.uk
Hindu Council UK: www.hinducounciluk.org
Jainism: www.jainism.org
Jehovah's Witness: www.jw.org
Judaism: www.bbc.co.uk/religion/religions/judaism
Sikhism: www.bbc.co.uk/religion/religions/sikhism
Rastafarianism: www.rastafarian.net
Zoroastrianism (Parsee): www.bbc.co.uk/religion/religions/zoroastrian

REFERENCES

Abbey, J., Piller, N., De Bellis, A., et al. (2004) The Abbey pain scale: a 1-minute numerical indicator for people with end-stage dementia. *International Journal of Palliative Nursing*, 10(1), 6–13.

Abidia, R.F. (2007) Oral care in the intensive care unit: a review. *Journal of Contemporary Dental Practice*, 8(1), 1–8.

Academy of Medical Royal Colleges (2008) *A Code of Practice for the Diagnosis and Confirmation of Death*. London: Academy of Medical Royal Colleges. Available at: www.aomrc.org.uk/doc_view/42-a-code-of-practice-for-the-diagnosis-and-confirmation-of-death

Advisory Services Alliance (2010) Available at: www.advicenow.org.uk/livingtogether accessed 22/7/2014

Ahearn, D.J., Nidh, N., Kallat, A., et al. (2013) Offering older hospitalised patients the choice to die in their preferred place. *Postgraduate Medical Journal*, 89, 20–24.

Alexander, M., Fawcett, J. & Runciman, P. (2007) *Nursing Practice: Hospital and Home*, 3rd edn. London: Churchill Livingstone.

Allen, D. (2010) Care pathways: some social scientific observations on the field. *International Journal of Care Pathways*, 14, 47–51.

Anderson, K.O. & Cleeland, C.S. (2003) The assessment of cancer pain. In: Bruera, E. & Portenoy, R.K. (eds) *Cancer Pain: Assessment and Management*. Cambridge: Cambridge University Press, pp.51–66.

Audit Commission for Local Authorities and the National Health Service in England and Wales (1997) *Anaesthesia Under Examination: The Efficiency and Effectiveness of Anaesthesia and Pain Relief Services in England and Wales.* Abingdon: Audit Commission Publications.

Aung, T. & Mulley, G.P. (2002) Removal of ear wax. *BMJ*, 325(7354), 27.

Bamigbade, T.A. & Langford, R.M. (1998) Tramadol hydrochloride: an overview of current use. *Hospital Medicine*, 59(5), 373–376.

Barillo, D.J., Coffey, E.C., Shirani, K.Z. & Goodwin, C.W. (2000) Burns caused by medical therapy. *Journal of Burn Care & Rehabilitation*, 21(3), 269–273.

Beacroft, M. & Dodd, K. (2010) Pain in people with learning disabilities in residential settings – the need for change. *British Journal of Learning Disabilities*, 38(3), 201–209.

Beck, S. (1991) The therapeutic use of music for cancer-related pain. *Oncology Nursing Forum*, 18(8), 1327–1337.

Beck, S. (2004) Mucositis. In: Yarbro, C.H., Frogge, M.H. & Goodman, M. (eds) *Cancer Symptom Management*, 3rd edn. Sudbury, MA: Jones and Bartlett, pp. 276–292.

Bennett, M. (2001) The LANSS Pain Scale: the Leeds assessment of neuropathic symptoms and signs. *Pain*, 92(1–2), 147–157.

Berchier, C.E., Slot, D.E., Haps, S. & van der Weijden, G.A. (2008) The efficacy of dental floss in addition to a toothbrush on plaque and parameters of gingival inflammation: a systematic review. *International Journal of Dental Hygiene*, 6, 265–279.

Berman, A., Snyder, S., Kozier, B. & Erb, G. (2010) *Kozier and Erb's Fundamentals of Nursing: Concepts, Process and Practice*, 8th edn. Upper Saddle River, NJ: Prentice Hall.

Berry, A.M., Davidson, P.M., Masters, J. & Rolls, K. (2007) Systematic literature review of oral hygiene practices for intensive care patients receiving mechanical ventilation. *American Journal of Critical Care*, 16(6), 552–562.

Berry, P. & Griffie, J. (2006) Planning for the actual death. In: Ferrell, B.R. & Coyle, N. (eds) *Textbook of Palliative Nursing*, 2nd edn. Oxford: Oxford University Press, pp.561–577.

Bissett, S. & Preshaw, P. (2011) Guide to providing mouth care for older people. *Nursing Older People*, 23(10), 14–21.

BNF (2014) *British National Formulary 67.* London: Pharmaceutical Press.

Booth, S. (2006) Palliative care for intractable breathlessness in cancer. *European Journal of Cancer Care*, 15, 303–314.

Booth, S., Moffat, C., Burkin, J., Galbraith, S. & Bausewein, C. (2011) Non-pharmacological interventions for breathlessness. *Current Opinion in Supportive and Palliative Care*, 5(2), 77–86.

Bourne, N. (2008) Managing acute pain in opioid tolerant patients. *Journal of Perioperative Practice*, 18(11), 498–503.

Bouza, C., Saz, Z., Munoz, A. & Amate, J.M. (2005) Efficacy of advanced dressings in the treatment of pressure ulcers: a systematic review. *Journal of Wound Care*, 14(5), 193–199.

Boyd-Monk, H. (2005) Bringing common eye emergencies into focus. *Nursing*, 35(12), 46–51.

Bristol-Myers Squibb (2012) *Perfalgan, Dosing Tool.* Uxbridge: Bristol-Myers Squibb Pharmaceuticals.

British Heart Foundation (2007) *Implantable Cardioverter Defibrillators in Patients who are Reaching the End of Life.* London: British Heart Foundation.

British Pain Society (2008) *FAQs.* London: British Pain Society. Available at: www.britishpainsociety.org/media_faq.htm

British Pain Society (2010) *Opioids for Persistent Pain: Good Practice.* London: British Pain Society.

British Pain Society and Royal College of Physicians (2004) *A Practical Guide to the Provision of Chronic Pain Services for Adults in Primary Care.* London: British Pain Society and Royal College of Physicians.

Bryant, R. & Rolstad, B. (2001) Examining threats to skin integrity. *Ostomy Wound Management*, 47(6), 18–27.

Budd, K. (2002) *Evidence-based Medicine in Practice. Buprenorphine: A Review.* Newmarket: Haywood Medical.

Bullington, J., Sjostrom-Flanagan, C., Nordemar, K. & Nordemar, R. (2005) From pain through chaos to new meaning: two case studies. *The Arts in Psychotherapy*, 32(4), 261–274.

Burns, S. & Day, T. (2012) A return to the basics: Interventional Patient Hygiene (A call for papers). *Intensive and Critical Care Nursing*, 28(5), 193–196.

Burr, S. & Penzer, R. (2005) Promoting skin health. *Nursing Standard*, 19(36), 57–65.

Cannaerts, N., Dierckx de Casterle, B. & Grypdonck, M. (2004) Palliative care, care for life: a study of the specificity of residential palliative care. *Qualitative Health Research*, 14(6), 816–835.

Carpenito-Moyet, L.J. & Ovid Technologies (2012) Oral mucous membrane. In: Carpenito-Moyet, L.J. (ed) *Nursing Diagnosis: Application to Clinical Practice*, 14th edn. Philadelphia: Lippincott Williams & Wilkins, pp.490–495.

Carr, E. (2007) Barriers to effective pain management. *Journal of Perioperative Practice*, 17(5), 200–203, 206–208.

Carr, E. & Mann, E.M. (2000) Recognising the barriers to effective pain relief. In: *Pain: Creative Approaches to Effective Management.* Basingstoke: Palgrave Macmillan, pp.109–129.

Carroll, D. & Bowsher, D. (1993) *Pain: Management and Nursing Care.* Oxford Butterworth-Heinemann.

Carroll, D. & Seers, K. (1998) Relaxation for the relief of chronic pain: a systematic review. *Journal of Advanced Nursing*, 27(3), 476–487.

Castledine, G. (2005) The 'Been There, Done That' attitude. *British Journal of Nursing*, 14(20), 1103.

Chalmers, J. & Pearson, A. (2005) Oral hygiene care for residents with dementia: a literature review. *Journal of Advanced Nursing*, 52(4), 410–419.

Chalmers, J.M, King, P.L., Spencer, A.J., Wright, F.A. & Carter, K.D. (2005) The oral health assessment tool – validity and reliability. *Australian Dental Journal*, 50(3), 91–199.

Chapman S. (2012) Cancer pain part 2: assessment and management. *Nursing Standard*, 26(48), 44–49.

Cherny, N.I. (2010) Pain assessment and cancer pain syndromes. In: Doyle, D., Cherny, N.I., Christakis, N.A., Fallon, M., Kasasa, S. & Portenoy, R.K. (eds) *Oxford Textbook of Palliative Medicine*, 4th edn. Oxford: Oxford University Press, pp.599–625.

Chumbley, G.M., Hall, G.M. & Salmon, P. (2002) Patient-controlled analgesia: what information does the patient want? *Journal of Advanced Nursing*, 39(5), 459–471.

Clarkson, J.E., Worthington, H.V. & Eden, T.O. (2007) Interventions for treating oral mucositis for patients with cancer receiving treatment. *Cochrane Database of Systematic Reviews*, 2, CD001973.

Clary, P.L. & Lawson, P. (2009) Pharmacologic pearls for end-of-life care. *American Family Physician*, 79(12), 1059–1065.

Clay, M. (2000) Oral health in older people. *Nursing Older People*, 12(7), 21–26.

Collins, F. & Hampton, S. (2003) The cost-effective use of BagBath: a new concept in patient hygiene. *British Journal of Nursing*, 12(16), 984, 986–990.

Coluzzi, F. & Mattia, C. (2007) Chronic non-cancer pain: focus on once-daily tramadol formulations. *Therapeutics and Clinical Risk Management*, 3(5), 819–829.

Connecting for Health (2011) *Advisory Service Alliance Living Together Next of Kin.* Available at: http://connectingforhealth.nhs.uk

Cooke, H. (2000) *A Practical Guide to Holistic Care at the End of Life.* Oxford: Butterworth Heinemann.

Cooley, C. (2002) Oral health: basic or essential care? *Cancer Nursing Practice*, 1(3), 33–39.

Corner, J., Plant, H., A'Hern, R. & Bailey, C. (1996) Non-pharmacological intervention for breathlessness in lung cancer. *Palliative Medicine*, 10(4), 299–305.

Costello, J. (2004) *Nursing the Dying Patient: Caring in Different Contexts.* Basingstoke: Palgrave Macmillan.

Cox, F. (2010) Basic principles of pain management: assessment and intervention. *Nursing Standard*, 25(1), 36–39.

Cunningham, C. & Gould, D. (1998) Eyecare for the sedated patient undergoing mechanical ventilation: the use of evidence-based care. *International Journal of Nursing Studies*, 35(1–2), 32–40.

Currow, D.C., Agar, M. & Abernethy, A.P. (2013) Hospital can be the actively chosen place for death. *Journal of Clinical Oncology*, 31, 651–652.

Cutler, C.J. & Davis, N. (2005) Improving oral care in patients receiving mechanical ventilation. *American Journal of Critical Care*, 14, 389–394.

Dahlin, C. (2004) Oral complications at the end of life. *American Journal of Nursing*, 104(7), 40–47.

Darwish, M., Kirby, M. & Giang, J.D. (2007) Effect of buccal dwell time on the pharmacokinetic profile of fentanyl buccal tablet. *Expert Opinion in Pharmacotherapy*, 8, 2011–2016.

Davies, A. (2000) A comparison of artificial saliva and chewing gum in the management of xerostomia in patients with advanced cancer. *Palliative Medicine*, 14, 197–203.

Davies, A. (2005a) Oral assessment. In: Davies, A. & Finlay, I. (eds) *Oral Care in Advanced Disease.* Oxford: Oxford University Press, pp.7–19.

Davies, A. (2005b) Salivary gland dysfunction. In: Davies, A. & Finlay, I. (eds) *Oral Care in Advanced Disease.* Oxford: Oxford University Press, pp.97–113.

Davis, B.D. & McVicker, A. (2000) Issues in effective pain control: from assessment to management. *International Journal of Palliative Nursing*, 6(4), 162–169.

Davis, M.P., Glare, P. & Hardy, J. (2005) *Opioids in Cancer Pain.* Oxford: Oxford University Press.

DH (1984) *Public Health (Control of Diseases).* London: HMSO.

DH (2001) *The Essence of Care: Patient Focussed Benchmarking for Healthcare Professionals.* London: HMSO.

DH (2003a) *The Essence of Care: Patient-Focused Benchmarking for Health Care Practitioners.* London: Stationery Office. Available at: www.dh.gov.uk/prod_consum_dh/groups/dh_digitalassets/@dh/@en/documents/digitalasset/dh_4127915.pdf (archived)

DH (2003b) *A Simple Guide to Post Mortem Examination Procedure.* London: HMSO.

DH (2005a) *Choosing Better Oral Health: An Oral Health Plan for England.* London: Department of Health. Available at: www.dh.gov.uk/prod_consum_dh/groups/dh_digitalassets/@dh/@en/documents/digitalasset/dh_4123253.pdf (archived)

DH (2005b) *Patients Who Die in Hospital.* London: Department of Health.

DH (2006a) *About Dignity in Care.* London: Department of Health. Available at: http://webarchive.nationalarchives.gov.uk/+/www.dh.gov.uk/en/SocialCare/Socialcarereform/Dignityincare/DH_4134922

DH (2006b) *What to Do After a Death.* London: Department of Health.

DH (2008) *End of Life Care Strategy: Promoting High Quality Care for All Adults at the End of Life.* Department of Health, London.

DH (2009) *End of Life Care Strategy: Quality Markers and Measures for End of Life Care.* London: Department of Health.

DH (2012) *End of Life Care Strategy: Fourth Annual Report.* London: Department of Health. Available at: www.gov.uk/government/uploads/system/uploads/attachment_data/file/136486/End-of-Life-Care-Strategy-Fourth-Annual-report-web-version-v2.pdf

DH (2013a) *Independent Review of the Liverpool Care Pathway – More Care, Less Pathway: A Review of the Liverpool Care Pathway.* London: Department of Health. Available at: www.gov.uk/government/uploads/system/uploads/attachment_data/file/212450/Liverpool_Care_Pathway.pdf

DH (2013b) *Water Systems: Health Technical Memorandum 04-01: Addendum. Pseudomonas Aeruginosa – Advice for Augmented Care Units.* London: Department of Health. Available at: www.gov.uk/government/uploads/system/uploads/attachment_data/file/140105/Health_Technical_Memorandum_04-01_Addendum.pdf

Diabetes UK (2012) *Putting Feet First: Diabetes UK Position on Preventing Amputations and Improving Foot Care for People with Diabetes.* Available at: tinyurl.com/b6nfl7o

Dickinson, L. & Porter, H. (2006) Oral care. In: Grundy, M. (ed) *Nursing in Haematological Oncology*, 2nd edn. Philadelphia: Baillière Tindall, pp.371–385.

Dimond, B. (2004) Health and safety considerations following the death of a patient. *British Journal of Nursing*, 13(11), 675–676.

Dingwall, P. (2010) *Personal Hygiene Care.* Oxford: John Wiley & Sons.

Disorbio, J.M., Bruns, D. & Barolat, G. (2006) Assessment and treatment of chronic pain. A physician's guide to a biopsychosocial approach. *Practical Pain Management*, March 2006. Available at: www.healthpsych.com/articles/biopsychosocial_tx.pdf

Docherty, B. (2000) Care of the dying patient. *Professional Nurse*, 15(12), 752.

Dowler, C. (2011) Nurses must not 'ignore' patients' requests for assisted suicide, RCN advises. *Nursing Times*, 20 October 2011. Available at: www.nursingtimes.net/nursing-practice/clinical-zones/end-of-life-and-palliative-care/nurses-must-not-ignore-patients-requests-for-assisted-suicide-rcn-advises/5036758.article#

Downey, L., & Lloyd, H. (2008) Bed bathing patients in hospital. *Nursing Standard*, 22(34), 35–40.

Doyle, S. & Dalton, C. (2008) Developing clinical guidelines on promoting oral health: an action research approach. *Learning Disability Practice*, 11(2), 12–15.

Drayer, R.A., Henderson, J. & Reidenberg, M. (1999) Barriers to better pain control in hospitalized patients. *Journal of Pain and Symptom Management*, 17(6), 434–440.

Drury, P. & Gatling, W. (2005) *Diabetes: Your Questions Answered.* London: Churchill Livingstone.

Duffin, C. (2008) Brushing up on oral hygiene. *Nursing Older People*, 20(2), 14–16.

Duffy, B. (2008) Managing chemical eye injuries.*Emergency Nurse*, 16(1) 25–30.

Eilers, J., Berger, A.M. & Petersen, M.C. (1988) Development, testing, and application of the oral assessment guide. *Oncology Nursing Forum*, 15(3), 325–330.

Eisenberg, E., Marinangeli, F., Birkhahn, J., Paladini, A. & Varrassi, G. (2005) Time to modify the WHO analgesic ladder? *Pain Clinical Updates*, 13, 1–4.

Ellershaw, J. & Murphy, S. (2011) What is the Liverpool Care Pathway for the Dying Patient (LCP)? In: Ellershaw, J. & Wilkinson, S. (eds) *Care of the Dying: A Pathway to Excellence*, 2nd edn. Oxford: Oxford University Press.

Ellershaw, J.E., Dewar, S. & Murphy, D. (2010) Achieving a good death for all. *BMJ*, 341, c4861. Available at: www.bmj.com/341/bmj.c4861full?sid=f197eb5bba77

Ellershaw, J., Foster, A., Murphy, D., Shea, T. & Overill, S. (1997) Developing an integrated care pathway for the dying patient. *European Journal of Palliative Care* 4(6), 203–207.

Ersser, S.J., Getliffe, K., Voegeli, D. & Regan, S. (2005) A critical review of the inter-relationship between skin vulnerability and urinary incontinence and related nursing intervention. *International Journal of Nursing Studies*, 42(7), 823–835.

European Association for Palliative Care (EAPC) (2014) Available at: www.eapcnet.eu/corporate/about the EAPC/definition and aims.aspx

Fallon, M., Cherny, N.I. & Hanks, G. (2010) Opioid analgesia therapy. In: Doyle, D., Cherny, N.I., Christakis, N.A., Fallon, M., Kasasa, S. & Portenoy, R.K. (eds) *Oxford Textbook of Palliative Medicine*, 4th edn. Oxford: Oxford University Press, pp.599–625.

Fallowfield, L. (2005) Communication with the patient and family. In: Doyle, D., Hanks, G., Cherny, N. & Calman, K. (eds) *Oxford Textbook of Palliative Medicine*, 3rd edn. Oxford: Oxford University Press.

Farrell, A. & Rich, A. (2000) Analgesic use in patients with renal failure. *European Journal of Palliative Care*, 7(6), 201–205.

Faull, C. & Nyatanga, B. (2012) Terminal care and dying. In: Faull, C. (ed) *Handbook of Palliative Care*, 3rd edn. Oxford: John Wiley & Sons, pp.295–322.

Faull, C. & Woof, R. (2002) *Palliative Care.* Oxford: Oxford University Press.

Feine, J.S. & Lund, J.P. (1997) An assessment of the efficacy of physical therapy and physical modalities for the control of chronic musculoskeletal pain. *Pain*, 71(1), 5–23.

Field, D., Hockley, J. & Small, N. (1997) *Death, Gender and Ethnicity.* London: Routledge.

Fink, R. & Gates, R. (2006) Pain assessment. In: Ferrell, B.R. & Coyle, N. (eds) *Textbook of Palliative Nursing*, 2nd edn. Oxford: Oxford University Press.

Finlay, I. & Davies, A. (2005) Fungal infections. In: Davies, A. & Finlay, I. (eds) *Oral Care in Advanced Disease.* Oxford: Oxford University Press, pp.55–71.

Fitzpatrick, J. (2000) Oral health needs of dependent older people: responsibilities of nurses and care staff. *Journal of Advanced Nursing*, 32(6), 1325–1332.

Forrester, J.V. (2002) *The Eye: Basic Sciences in Practice*, 2nd edn. Edinburgh: W.B. Saunders.

Fraise, A.P. & Bradley, T. (eds) (2009) *Ayliffe's Control of Healthcare-Associated Infection: A Practical Handbook*, 5th edn. London: Hodder Arnold.

Frazer, C.A., Frazer, R.Q. & Byron, R.J. (2009) Prevent infections with good denture care. *Nursing*, August 2009, 50–53.

French, S.D., Cameron, M., Walker, B.F., Reggars, J.W. & Esterman, A.J. (2006) Superficial heat or cold for low back pain. *Cochrane Database of Systematic Reviews*, 1, CD004750.

Gannon, C. (1997) Clinical management. The use of methadone in the care of the dying. *European Journal of Palliative Care*, 4(5), 152–159.

Gardner-Nix, J.S. (1996) Oral methadone for managing chronic nonmalignant pain. *Journal of Pain and Symptom Management*, 11(5), 321–328.

Geraghty, M. (2005) Nursing the unconscious patient. *Nursing Standard*, 20(1), 54–64.

Gilliat-Ray, S. (2001) Sociological perspectives on the pastoral care of minority faiths in hospital. In: Orchard, H. (ed) *Spirituality in Health Care Contexts.* London: Jessica Kingsley Publishers, pp.135–146.

GMC (2010) *Treatment and Care Towards the End of Life: Good Practice in Decision Making.* London: General Medical Council.

Godfrey, H. (2005) Understanding pain, part 1: physiology of pain. *British Journal of Nursing*, 14(16), 846–852.

Gooch, J. (1989) Skin hygiene. *Professional Nurse*, 5(1), 13–18.

Good, M. (1996) Effects of relaxation and music on postoperative pain: a review. *Journal of Advanced Nursing*, 24(5), 905–914.

Good, M., Stanton-Hicks, M., Grass, J.A., et al. (1999) Relief of postoperative pain with jaw relaxation, music and their combination. *Pain*, 81(1–2), 163–172.

Goodman, M. & Wickham, R. (2005) Endocrine malignancies. In: Yarbro, C., Goodman, M. & Frogge, M.H. (eds) *Cancer Nursing: Principles and Practice*, 6th edn. Sudbury, MA: Jones and Bartlett, pp.1215–1243.

Gould, D. (1994) Helping the patient with personal hygiene. *Nursing Standard*, 8(34), 30–32.

Grap, M.J., Munro, C.L., Ashtiani, B. & Bryant, S. (2003) Oral care interventions in critical care: frequency and documentation. *American Journal of Critical Care*, 12(2), 113–118.

Green, J. & Green, M. (2006) *Dealing with Death: A Handbook of Practices, Procedures and Law*, 2nd edn. Suffolk: Jessica Kingsley Publishers.

Griffiths, J., Jones, V., Leeman, I., et al. (2000) *Oral Health Care for People with Mental Health Problems Guidelines and Recommendations*: Gosforth: British Society for Disability and Oral Health.

Gunaratnam, Y. (1997) Culture is not enough: a critique of multiculturalism in palliative care. In: Field, D., Hockley, J. & Small, N. (eds) *Death, Gender and Ethnicity*. London: Routledge, pp.166–186.

Hahn, M. & Jones, A. (2000) *Head and Neck Nursing*. London: Churchill Livingstone.

Hanks, G., Cherny, N. & Fallon, M. (2004) Opioid analgesic therapy. In: Doyle, D. (ed) *Oxford Textbook of Palliative Medicine*, 3rd edn. Oxford: Oxford University Press, pp.316–342.

Harkin, H. (2005) A nurse-led ear care clinic: sharing knowledge and improving patient care. *British Journal of Nursing*, 14(5), 250–254.

Harkin, H. (2008) *Guidance Document in Ear Care*. Available at: www.earcarecentre.com/Health Professionals/Protocols

Harkin, H. & Kelleher, C. (2011) Caring for older adults with hearing loss. *Nursing Older People*, 23(9), 22–28.

Harlos M. (2010) *When Death is Near*. Winnipeg, MB: Canadian Virtual Hospice. www.virtualhospice.ca/en_US/Main+Site+Navigation/Home/Topics/Topics/Final+Days/When+Death+Is+Near.aspx.

Harmer, M. & Davies, K.A. (1998) The effect of education, assessment and a standardised prescription on postoperative pain management. The value of clinical audit in the establishment of acute pain services. *Anaesthesia*, 53(5), 424–430.

Healing, T.D., Hoffman, P.N. & Young, S.E. (1995) The infection hazards of human cadavers. *Communicable Disease Report*, 5(5), R61–R68.

Heiser, R.M., Chiles, K., Fudge, M. & Gray, S.E. (1997) The use of music during the immediate postoperative recovery period. *AORN Journal*, 65(4), 777–778, 781–785.

Heiskanen, T. & Kalso, E. (1997) Controlled-release oxycodone and morphine in cancer related pain. *Pain*, 73(1), 37–45.

Henry, C. & Wilson, J. (2012) Personal care at the end of life and after death. *Nursing Times*, 108. Available at: www.nursingtimes.net/Journals/2012/05/08/h/i/z/120805-Innov-endoflife.pdf

Hicks, F. & Simpson, K.H. (2004) Regional nerve blocks. In Hicks, F. & Simpson, K.H. (eds) *Nerve Blocks in Palliative Care*. Oxford: Oxford University Press, pp.53–55.

Higginson, I.J. (1998) Can professionals improve their assessments? *Journal of Pain and Symptom Management*, 15(3), 149–150.

Higginson, I.J. (1999) Evidence based palliative care: there is some evidence and there needs to be more. *BMJ*, 319(7208), 462–463.

Hitz Lindenmüller, I. & Lambrecht, J.T. (2011) Oral Care. *Topical Applications and the Mucosa*, 40, 107–115.

Ho, L.A., Englelberg, R.A., Curtis, J.R. et al. (2011) Comparing clinician ratings of the quality of palliative care in the intensive care unit. *Critical Care Medicine*, 39(5), 975–983.

Hobbs, G.J. & Hodgkinson, V. (2003) Assessment, measurement, history and examination. In: Rowbotham, D.J. & Macintyre, P.E. (eds) *Acute Pain*. London: Arnold, pp.93–112.

Hollins, S. (2009) *Religions, Cultures and Healthcare*, 2nd edn. Oxford: Radcliffe Publishing.

Holloway, S. & Jones, V. (2005) The importance of skin care and assessment. *British Journal of Nursing*, 14(22), 1172–1176.

Holman, C., Roberts, S. & Nicol, M. (2005) Promoting oral hygiene. *Nursing Older People*, 16(10), 37–38.

Holt, P. (2013) Assessment and management of patients with diabetic foot ulcers. *Nursing Standard*, 27(7), 49–55.

Home Office (1971) *Report of the Committee on Death Certification and Coroners*. CMND 4810. London: HMSO.

Home Office (2002) *When Sudden Death Occurs: Coroners and Inquests*. www.nnuh.nhs.uk/docs%5Cleafl ets%5C90.pdf.

HPA (2010) *Mortality Guidelines Management of Infection Control Associated with Human Cadavers*. London: Health Protection Agency. Available at: www.hpa.org.uk/topics/infectiousDiseases/InfectionsAZ/Mortality/Guidelines/

HSAC (2003) *Safe Working and the Prevention of Infection in the Mortuary and Post-Mortem Room*. London: Health and Safety Advisory Committee. Available at: www.hse.gov.uk/pubns/priced/mortuary-infection.pdf

HSE (2003) *Infection at Work: Controlling the Risks: A Guide for Employers and the Self-Employed on Identifying, Assessing and Controlling the Risks of Infection in the Workplace*. London: Health and Safety Executive, HMSO.

HTA (2006) *Code of Practice – Consent*. London: Human Tissue Authority. Available at: www.hta.gov.uk

HTA (2011) *How to Donate your Body (Body & Brain Donation Information Pack)*, Human Tissue Act, 2004. London: Human Tissue Authority. Available at: www.hta.gov.uk/bodyorganandtissuedonation/howtodonateyourbody.cfm

Hudson, P. (2005) A psycho-educational intervention for family caregivers of patients receiving palliative care: a randomised controlled trial. *Journal of Pain and Symptom Management*, 30(4), 329–341.

Huskinson, W. & Lloyd, H. (2009) Oral health in hospitalised patients: assessment and hygiene. *Nursing Standard*, 23(36), 43–47.

Husseini, A., Slot, D.E. & van der Weijden, G.A. (2008) The efficacy of oral irrigation in addition to a toothbrush on plaque and the clinical parameters of periodontal inflammation: a review. *International Journal of Dental Hygiene*, 6, 304–314.

Idvall, E., Hamrin, E., Sjostrom, B. & Unosson, M. (2002) Patient and nurse assessment of quality of care in postoperative pain management. *Quality and Safety in Health Care*, 11(4), 327–334.

IASP (1994) *IASP Pain Terminology*. Available at: www.iasp-pain.org/taxonomy

IASP (1996) Classification of chronic pain. *Pain*, 3(Suppl), 51–226.

IPEM (2002) *Medical and Dental Guidance Notes. A Good Practice Guide on All Aspects of Ionising Radiation Protection in the Clinical Environment*. York: Institute of Physics and Engineering in Medicine.

Jacobs, C. (2008) Ear irrigation. *Primary Health Care*, 18(7), 36–39.

Johnson, D., Lineweaver, L. & Maze, L. (2009) Patients' bath basins as potential sources of infection: a multicenter sampling study. *American Journal Critical Care*, 18(1), 31–40.

Johnson, M. & Martinson, M. (2007) Efficacy of electrical nerve stimulation for chronic musculoskeletal pain: a meta-analysis of randomized controlled trials. *Pain*, 130(1), 157–165.

Jones, C.V. (1998) The importance of oral hygiene in nutritional support. *British Journal of Nursing*, 7(2), 74–83.

Joseph, J. & Clifton, S.D. (2013) Nurses' knowledge of pressure ulcer risk assessment. *Nursing Standard*, 27(33), 54, 56, 58–60.

Kayser-Jones, J., Bird, W.F., Paul, S.M., et al. (1995) An instrument to assess the oral health status of nursing home residents. *Gerontologist*, 35(6), 814–824.

Kehl, K.A. (2006) Moving towards peace: an analysis of the concept of a good death. *American Journal of Hospice Palliative Care*, 23(4), 277–286.

Kelly, D. (2003) A commentary on 'An integrated care pathway for the last two days of life'. *International Journal of Palliative Nursing*, 9(1), 39.

King, A. (1999) *King's Guide to TENS for Health Professionals: A Health Professionals' Guide to Transcutaneous Electrical Nerve Stimulation for the Treatment of Pain*. London: King's Medical.

King, S., Forbes, K., Hanks, G.W., Ferro, C.J. & Chambers, E.J. (2011) A systematic review of the use of opioid medication for those with moderate to severe cancer pain and renal impairment: a European Palliative Care Research Collaborative opioid guidelines project. *Palliative Medicine*, 25(5), 525–552.

King's Fund (2008) *Improving Environments for Care at End of Life*. London: King's Fund.

Kitson, A. (1994) Post-operative pain management: a literature review. *Journal of Clinical Nursing*, 3(1), 7–18.

Kozier, B., Erb, G., Berman, A., Snyder, S. & Lake, R. (2008) Hygiene. In: Kozier, B., Harvey, S. & Morgan-Samuel, H. (eds) *Fundamentals of Nursing: Concepts, Process and Practice*. London: Pearson Education Ltd.

Kraszewski, S. (2008) Safe and effective ear irrigation. *Nursing Standard*, 22(43), 45–48.

Krishnasamy, M. (2008) Pain. In: Corner, J. & Bailey, C.D. (eds) *Cancer Nursing: Care in Context*, 2nd edn. Oxford: Blackwell Publishing, pp.449–461.

Kuckelkorn, R., Schrage, N., Keller, G. & Redbrake, C. (2002) Emergency treatment of chemical and thermal eye burns. *Acta Ophthalmologica Scandinavica*, 80(1), 4–10.

Lang, E.V., Benotsch, E.G., Fick, L.J., et al. (2000) Adjunctive non-pharmacological analgesia for invasive medical procedures: a randomised trial. *Lancet*, 355(9214), 1486–1490.

Larson, L., Ciliberti, T. & Chantler, C. (2004) Comparison of traditional and disposable bed baths in critically ill patients. *American Journal of Critical Care*, 13(3), 235–241.

Lawler, K. (1997) Pain assessment. *Professional Nurse*, 13(1 Suppl), S5–S8.

Lawlor, P.G., Gagnon, B., Mancini, I.L., et al. (2000) Occurrence, causes, and outcome of delirium in patients with advanced cancer. *Archives of Internal Medicine*, 160(6), 786–794.

Lee, A. (2006) The angle and aqueous. In: Marsden, J. (ed) *Ophthalmic Care*. Chichester: John Wiley & Sons, pp.420–460.

Lewis, N.L. & Williams, J.E. (2005) Acute pain management in patients receiving opioids for chronic and cancer pain. *Continuing Education in Anaesthesia and Critical Care Pain*, 5(4), 127–129.

Li, X., Kolltveit, K.M., Tronstad, L. & Olsen, I. (2000) Systemic disease caused by oral infection. *Clinical Microbiology Reviews*, 13(4), 547–558.

Lloyd-Williams, M. (2003) *Psychosocial Issues in Palliative Care*. Oxford: Oxford University Press.

Lockhart, J.S. & Resick, L.K. (2006) Anatomy and physiology. In: Clarke, L.K. & Dropkin, M.J. (eds) *Head and Neck Cancer*. Pittsburgh, PA: Oncology Nursing Society.

Lokich, J.J. & Moore, C. (1984) Chemotherapy-associated palmar-plantar erythrodysesthesia syndrome. *Annals of Internal Medicine*, 101(6), 798–799.

Loveday, H.P., Wilson, J.A., Pratt, R.J., et al. (2014) epic3: national evidence-based guidelines for preventing healthcare-associated infections in NHS hospitals in England . *Journal of Hospital Infection*, 86 (Suppl 1), S1–70 .

Loveman, E. & Gale, A. (2000) Factors influencing nurses' inferences about patient pain. *British Journal of Nursing*, 9(6), 334–337.

Lynch, M.E. & Campbell, F. (2011) Cannabinoids for treatment of chronic non-cancer pain; a systematic review of randomized trials. *British Journal of Clinical Pharmacology*, 72(5), 735–744.

Macintyre, P.E. (2001) Safety and efficacy of patient-controlled analgesia. *British Journal of Anaesthesia*, 87(1), 36–46.

Macintyre, P.E. & Jarvis, D.A. (1996) Age is the best predictor of postoperative morphine requirements. *Pain*, 64(2), 357–364.

Macintyre, P.E. & Schug, S.A. (2007) *Acute Pain Management: A Practical Guide*, 3rd edn. Edinburgh: Elsevier Saunders.

Macintyre, P.E., Schug, S.A., Scott, D.A., et al. (2010) *Acute Pain Management: Scientific Evidence*, 3rd edn. Melbourne: ANZCA and FPM.

Mackintosh, C. & Elson, S. (2008) Chronic pain: clinical features, assessment and treatment. *Nursing Standard*, 23(95), 48–56.

Maguire, P. & Pitceathly, C. (2002) Key communication skills and how to acquire them. *BMJ*, 325, 697–700.

Maher, K. (2004) Xerostomia. In: Yarbro, C., Frogge, M.H. & Goodman, M. (eds) *Cancer Symptom Management*, 3rd edn. Sudbury, MA: Jones and Bartlett.

Malkin, B. (2009) The important of patients' oral health and nurses' role in assessing and maintaining it. *Nursing Times*, 105(17), 19–23.

Malkin, B. & Berridge, P. (2009) Guidance on maintaining personal hygiene in nail care. *Nursing Standard*, 23(41), 35–38.

Maltoni, M. & Amadori, D. (2001) Palliative medicine and medical oncology. *Annals of Oncology*, 12, 443–451.

Mann, E. (2008) Neuropathic pain: could nurses become more involved? *British Journal of Nursing*, 17 (19), 1208–1213.

Mann, E. & Carr, E. (2006) *Pain Management*. Oxford: Blackwell Publishing.

Marchaim, D., Taylor, A. & Hayakawa, Y. (2011) Hospital bath basins are frequently contaminated with multidrug resistant human pathogens. *American Journal of Infection Control*, 40(6), 562–564.

Marieb, E. (2001) *Human Anatomy and Physiology*, 5th edn. Boston, MA: Benjamin Cummings.

Marsden, J. (2006) The care of patients presenting with acute problems. In: Marsden, J. (ed) *Ophthalmic Care*. Chichester: Whurr, pp.209–252.

Marsden, J. (2007) *An Evidence Base for Opthalmic Nursing Practice*. Chichester: John Wiley & Sons.

Massa, J. (2010) Improving efficiency, reducing infection and enhancing experience. *British Journal of Nursing*, 19(22), 1408–1414.

McAuliffe, L., Nay, R., O'Donnell, M. & Fetherstonhaugh, D. (2008) Pain assessment in older people with dementia: literature review. *Journal of Advanced Nursing*, 65(1), 2–10.

McCaffery, M. & Beebe, A. (1989) Perspectives on pain. In: McCaffery, M. & Beebe, A. (eds) *Pain: Clinical Manual for Nursing Practice*. St Louis, MO: Mosby, pp.1–5.

McCaffery, M. & Ferrell, B.R. (1997) Nurses' knowledge of pain assessment and management: how much progress have we made? *Journal of Pain and Symptom Management*, 14(3), 175–188.

McCaffery, M. & Pasero, C. (1999) *Pain Clinical Manual*, 2nd edn. St Louis, MO: Mosby.

McCaffery, M. & Robinson, E.S. (2002) Your patient is in pain – here's how you respond. *Nursing*, 32(10), 36–45.

McCaffrey, R. (1968) *Nursing Practice Theories Relating to Cognition, Bodily Pain and Man-Environment Interactions*. Los Angeles, CA: University of California Los Angeles.

McCaffrey, R. (2000) *Nursing Management of the Patient with Pain*, 3rd edn. Philadelphia: Lippincott Williams & Wilkins.

McLoughlin, C. (2005) A guide to wash creams. *Professional Nurse*, 20(6), 46–47.

McQuay, H.J. & Edwards, J. (2003) Meta-analysis of single dose oral tramadol plus acetaminophen in acute postoperative pain. *European Journal of Anaesthesiology*, 28(Suppl), 19–22.

McQuay, H.J. & Moore, R.A. (1998) Oral tramadol versus placebo, codeine and combination analgesics. In: McQuay, H.J. & Moore, R.A. (eds) *An Evidence-Based Resource for Pain Relief*. Oxford: Oxford University Press, pp.138–146.

McQuay, H.J., Moore, A. & Justins, D. (1997) Treating acute pain in hospital. *BMJ*, 314(7093), 1531–1535.

Mealer, M.L., Berg, A.S., Rothbaum, B. & Moss, M. (2007). Increased prevalence of post-traumatic stress disorder symptoms in critical care nurses. *American Journal of Respiratory Critical Care Medicine*, 175, 693–697.

Meechan, J. (2005) Oral pain. In: Davies, A. & Finlay, I. (eds) *Oral Care in Advanced Disease*. Oxford: Oxford University Press, pp.133–143.

Mehta, V. & Langford, R.M. (2006) Acute pain management for opioid dependent patients. *Anaesthesia*, 61(3), 269–276.

Melzack, R. (1975) The McGill Pain Questionnaire: major properties and scoring methods. *Pain*, 1(3), 277–299.

MHRA (2005) *Medical Device Alert Ref. MDA/2005/027. Heat patches or heat packs intended for pain relief.* London: Medicines and Healthcare Products Regulatory Agency.

Milligan, S., McGill, M., Sweeney, M.P. & Malarkey, C. (2001) Oral care for people with advanced cancer: an evidence-based protocol. *International Journal of Palliative Nursing*, 7(9), 418–426.

Moakes, H. (2012) An overview of foot ulceration in older people with diabetes. *Nursing Older People*, 24(7), 14–19.

Morley, J.S. & Makin, M.K. (1998) The use of methadone in cancer pain poorly responsive to other opioids. *Pain Reviews*, 5(1), 51–59.

Moss, M.S., Braunschweig, H. & Rubinstein, R.L. (2002). Terminal care for nursing home residents with dementia. *Alzheimer's Care Quarterly*, 3, 233–246.

Mucci-LoRusso, P., Berman, B.S., Silberstein, P.T., et al. (1998) Controlled-release oxycodone compared with controlled-release morphine in the treatment of cancer pain: a randomized, double-blind, parallel-group study. *European Journal of Pain*, 2(3), 239–249.

Munro, C.L. & Grap, M.J. (2004) Oral health and care in the intensive care unit: state of the science. *American Journal of Critical Care*, 13(1), 25–33.

Murray, SA, Boyd, K. & Sheikh, A. (2005) Palliative care in chronic illness: we need to move from prognostic paralysis to active total care. *BMJ*, 330, 611–612.

Narayan, M. (2010) Culture's effects on pain assessment and management. *American Journal of Nursing*, 110(4), 38–47.

National Council for Palliative Care (2008) *Palliative Care Explained*. Available at: www.ncpc.org.uk/palliative-care-explained

Naylor, W., Laverty, D. & Mallett, J. (2001) *The Royal Marsden Hospital Handbook of Wound Management in Cancer Care*. Oxford: Blackwell Science.

Nearney, L. (1998) Last offices, part 1. *Nursing Times*, 94(26), Insert.

Neuberger, J. (1999) Cultural issues in palliative care. In: Doyle, D., Hanks, G. & MacDonald, N. (eds) *Oxford Textbook of Palliative Medicine*. Oxford: Oxford University Press, pp.777–780.

Neuberger, J. (2004) *Caring for People of Different Faiths*. Abingdon: Radcliffe Medical Press.

NHSQIS (2004) *Working with Dependent Older People to Achieve Good Oral Health*. Edinburgh: NHS Quality Improvement Scotland.

NHS Choices (2013) *Euthanasia and Assisted Suicide*. Available at: www.nhs.uk/Conditions/Euthanasiaandassistedsuicide/Pages/Introduction.aspx

NHS NEoLCP (2010) *Route to Success: the Key Contribution of Nursing to End of Life Care*. Available at: www.endoflifecareforadults.nhs.uk (archived)

NHS NEoLCP (2011) *The Route to Success in End of Life Care – Achieving Quality in Acute Hospitals*. Available at: www.ncpc.org.uk/publication/transforming-end-life-care-acute-hospitals-route-success-%E2%80%98how-to%E2%80%99-guide

NHS NEoLCP (2012) Preferred Priorities for Care (PPC). Available at: www.nhsiq.nhs.uk/resource-search/publications/eolc-ppc.aspx

NICE (2004a) *Type 2 Diabetes: Prevention and Management of Foot Problems, CG10*. London: National Institute for Health and Clinical Excellence. Available at: www.nice.org.uk/guidance/CG10

NICE (2004b) *Improving Supportive and Palliative Care for Adults with Cancer: The Manual*. London: National Institute for Health and Clinical Excellence.

NICE (2008) *Type 2 Diabetes: The Management of Type 2 Diabetes, CG 66*. London: National Institute for Clinical Excellence. Available at: www.nice.org.uk/guidance/CG66

NICE (2011) *Organ Donation for Transplantation: Improving Donor Identification and Consent Rates for Deceased Organ Donation, CG135*. London: National Institute for Health and Clinical Excellence. Available at: www.nice.org.uk/guidance/CG135

NICE (2012) *Opioids in Palliative Care: Safe and Effective Prescribing of Strong Opioids for Pain in Palliative Care of Adults, CG140*. London: National Institute for Health and Clinical Excellence. Available at: www.nice.org.uk/guidance/CG140

Nicholas, M., Molloy, A., Tonkin, L. & Beeston, L. (2003) *Manage your Pain: Practical and Positive Ways of Adapting to Persistent Pain*. London: Souvenir Press Limited.

Ni Thuathail, A. & Welford, C. (2011) Pain assessment tools for older people with cognitive impairment. *Nursing Standard*, 26(6), 39–46.
Nigam, Y. & Knight, J. (2008) Exploring the anatomy and physiology of ageing. Part 6 – the eye and ear. *Nursing Times*, 104(36), 22–23.
Nightingale, F. (1859) *Notes on Nursing – What It Is and What It Is Not.* London: Churchill Livingstone.
NMC (2010) *Record Keeping: Guidance for Nurses and Midwives.* London: Nursing and Midwifery Council. Available at: http://tinyurl.com/9w9eqoy
NMC (2013) *Consent.* London: Nursing and Midwifery Council. Available at: www.nmc-uk.org/Nurses-and-midwives/Advice-by-topic/A/Advice/Consent
NMC (2015) *The Code: Standards of Conduct, Performance and Ethics for Nurses and Midwives.* London: Nursing and Midwifery Council. Available at: http://tinyurl.com/q9gwpgm
NNCG (2011) *National Nurse Consultant Group. Guidance for staff responsible for care after death.* London: National End of Life Care Programme.
O'Connor, M. & Webb, R. (2002) Learning to rest when in pain. *European Journal of Palliative Care*, 9(2), 68–72.
O'Hara, T. (2011) Nurses' views on using the Liverpool Care Pathway in an acute hospital setting. *International Journal of Palliative Nursing*, 17(5), 239–244.
Olver, J. & Cassidy, L. (2005) *Ophthalmology at a Glance.* Oxford: Blackwell Science.
ONS (2009) *Mortality Statistics: Deaths Registered in 2008.* London: OPSI.
Orenius, T., Koskela,.T., Koho, P., et al. (2013) Anxiety and depression are independent predictors of quality of life of patients with chronic musculoskeletal pain. *Journal of Health Psychology*, 18(2) 167–175.
Pargeon, K.L. & Hailey, B.J. (1999) Barriers to effective cancer pain management: a review of the literature. *Journal of Pain and Symptom Management*, 18(5), 358–368.
Parker, L. (2004) Infection control: maintaining the personal hygiene of patients and staff. *British Journal of Nursing*, 13(4), 474–478.
Pasero, C.L. & McCaffery, M. (1998) Is laughter the best medicine? *American Journal of Nursing*, 98(12), 12.
Pattison, N. (2008a) Care of patients who have died. *Nursing Standard*, 22(28), 42–48.
Pattison, N. (2008b) Caring for patients after death. *Nursing Standard*, 22(51), 48–56.
Pattison, N. (2011) End of life in critical care: an emphasis on care. *Nursing in Critical Care*, 16(3), 113–115.
Pavlek, M. (2008) Paining out: an integrative pain therapy model. *Clinical Social Work Journal*, 36(4) 385–393.
Payne, R.A. (1995) *Relaxation Techniques: A Practical Handbook for the Health Care Professional.* Edinburgh: Churchill Livingstone.
Payne, S., Hillier, R., Evans, L. & Roberts, T. (1996) Impact of witnessing death on hospice patients. *Social Science and Medicine*, 43(12), 1785–1794.
Pearce, E. (1963) *A General Textbook of Nursing.* London: Faber and Faber.
Pearson, L.S. & Hutton, J.L. (2002) A controlled trial to compare the ability of foam swabs and toothbrushes to remove dental plaque. *Journal of Advanced Nursing*, 39(5), 480–489.
Peate, I., Nair, M., Wild, K. (2014) *Nursing Practice: Knowledge and Care.* Oxford: John Wiley & Sons.
Pegram, A., Bloomfield, J. & Jones, A. (2007) Clinical skills: bed bathing and personal hygiene needs of patients. *British Journal of Nursing*, 16(6), 356–358.
Penzer, R. & Finch, M. (2001) Promoting healthy skin in older people. *Nursing Standard*, 15(34), 46–52.
Perkins, F.M. & Kehlet, H. (2000) Chronic pain as an outcome of surgery. A review of predictive factors. *Anesthesiology*, 93(4), 1123–1133.
Philips, L. & Buttery, J. (2009) Exploring pressure ulcer prevalence and preventative care. *Nursing Times*, 16, 105.
Philpin, S. (2002) Rituals and nursing: a critical commentary. *Journal of Advanced Nursing*, 38(2), 144–151.
Poncet, M.C., Toullic, P., Papazian, L. et al. (2007) Burnout syndrome in critical care nursing staff. *American Journal of Respiratory Critical Care Medicine*, 175, 698–704.
Portenoy, R.K., Payne, R., Coluzzi, P., et al. (1999) Oral transmucosal fentanyl citrate (OTFC) for the treatment of breakthrough pain in cancer patients: a controlled dose titration study. *Pain*, 79(2–3), 303–312.
Potter, P.A. & Perry, A.G. (2003) *Basic Nursing: Essentials for Practice*, 5th edn. St Louis, MO: Mosby.
Power, M., Wigglesworth, N., Donaldson, E., Chadwick, P. & Goldman, D. (2010) Reducing C. difficile infection in acute care by using an improvement collaborative. *BMJ*, 34, 351.
Pullen, R.L. Jr. (2006) Spin control: caring for a patient with inner ear disease. *Nursing*, 36(5), 48–51.
Quested, B. & Rudge, T. (2003) Nursing care of dead bodies: a discursive analysis of last offices. *Journal of Advanced Nursing*, 41(6), 553–560.
Quigley, C. (2004) Opioid switching to improve pain relief and drug tolerability. *Cochrane Database of Systematic Reviews*, 3, CD004847.
Quinn, B., Potting, C.M.J., Stone, R. et al. (2008) Guidelines for the assessment of oral mucositis in adult chemotherapy, radiotherapy and haematopoietic stem cell transplant patients. *European Journal of Cancer*, 44, 61–72.
Raiman, J. (1986) Coping with pain. Pain relief – a two-way process. *Nursing Times*, 82(15), 24–28.
Rauch, R.L., Tark, M., Reyes, E., et al. (2009) Efficacy and long term tolerability of sublingual fentanyl oral disintegrating tablet in the treatment of breakthrough cancer pain. *Current Medical Research and Opinion*, 25(12), 2877–2885.
RCN (2005) *Good Practice in Infection Prevention and Control: Guidance for Nursing Staff.* London: Royal College of Nursing.
RCN (2010) *Accountability and Delegation: What You Need to Know.* London: Royal College of Nursing.
RCN (2013) *Acting as a Witness – Signing Legal Documents in the Course of Your Employment.* London: Royal College of Nursing. Available at: www.rcn.org.uk/support/rcn_direct_online_advice/a-z2/acting_as_a_witness
Read, C. (2012) A kinder system: how technology is helping many more patients die where they want to – at home. Available at: www.hsj.co.uk/Journals/2012/12/05/b/x/m/INNOVATIONSUPP_121206.pdf
Ready, L. & Edwards, W. (1992) *Management of Acute Pain: A Practical Guide.* Seattle, WA: IASP Publications.
Reicin, A., Brown, J., Jove, M., et al. (2001) Efficacy of single-dose and multidose rofecoxib in the treatment of post-orthopedic surgery pain. *American Journal of Orthopedics*, 30(1), 40–48.
Richardson, M. (2007) Hearing and balance: the outer and middle ear. *Nursing Times*, 103(38), 24–25.
Riley, J. (2006) An overview of opioids in palliative care. *European Journal of Palliative Care*, 13(6), 230–233.
Riley, J. (2012) Conference Paper presentation: Morphine or oxycodone for cancer pain? A randomized controlled trial comparing response to first-line opioid and clinical efficacy of opioid switching. Norway: European Association of Palliative Care Research.
Roberts, J. (2001) Oral assessment and intervention. *Nursing Older People*, 13(7), 14–16.
Roberts, P. & Holdich, P. (2012) Fungal infections of the foot in people with diabetes. *Journal of Community Nursing*, 26(2) 2–6.
Robinson, D. & English, A. (2010) Physiotherapy in palliative care. In: Doyle, D., Cherny, N.I., Christakis, N.A., Fallon, M., Kasasa, S. & Portenoy, R.K. (eds) *Oxford Textbook of Palliative Medicine*, 4th edn. Oxford: Oxford University Press.
Robinson, P., Deacon, S.A., Deer, C., et al. (2005) Manual versus powered toothbrushing for oral health. *Cochrane Database of Systematic Reviews*, 2, CD002281.
Rodrigues, Z. (2009) Irrigation of the eye after alkaline and acidic burns.*Emergency Nurse*, 17(8), 26–29.
Romsing, J., Moiniche, S. & Dahl, J.B. (2002) Rectal and parenteral paracetamol, and paracetamol in combination with NSAIDs, for postoperative analgesia. *British Journal of Anaesthesia*, 88(2), 215–226.
Rowbotham, D.J. (2000) Non-steroidal anti-inflammatory drugs and paracetamol. In: Rowbotham, D.J. (ed) *Chronic Pain.* London: Martin Dunitz, pp.19–26.
Royal College of Anaesthetists (2006) Section 1 Key issues in developing new materials. In: Lack, J.A., Rollin, A.M., Thoms, G., White, L. & Williamson, C. (eds) *Raising the Standard: Information for Patients*, 2nd edn. London: Royal College of Anaesthetists, pp.14–29.
Royal College of Physicians (2005) *Cannabis and Cannabis-Based Medicines: Potential Benefits and Risks to Health.* Report of a Working Party. London: Royal College of Physicians.
Royal College of Physicians, British Geriatric Society and British Pain Society (2007) *The Assessment of Pain in Older People: National Guidelines.* London: Royal College of Physicians.
Sarin, J., Balasubramaniam, R., Corcoran, A.M., Laudenbach, J.M. & Stoopler, E.T. (2008) Reducing the risk of aspiration pneumonia among elderly patients in long-term care facilities through oral health interventions. *Journal of the American Medical Directors Association*, 9(2), 128–135.
Schiff, L. (2001) Market choices: hair-washing systems. Available at: www.modernmedicine.com/modern-medicine/news/market-choices-hair-washing-systems?page=full
Schug, S.A. & Chong, C. (2009) Pain management after ambulatory surgery. *Current Opinion in Anaesthesiology*, 22(6), 738–743.

Schug, S.A. & Torrie, J.J. (1993) Safety assessment of postoperative pain management by an acute pain service. *Pain*, 55(3), 387–391.

Scott, I.E. (1994) Effectiveness of documented assessment of postoperative pain. *British Journal of Nursing*, 3(10), 494–501.

Seale, C. (1998) *Constructing Death: The Sociology of Dying and Bereavement*. Cambridge: Cambridge University Press.

Seers, K. (1996) The patients' experiences of their chronic nonmalignant pain. *Journal of Advanced Nursing*, 24(6), 1160–1168.

Seers, K. & Carroll, D. (1998) Relaxation techniques for acute pain management: a systematic review. *Journal of Advanced Nursing*, 27(3), 466–475.

Shaw, M.E. (2006) Examination of the eye. In: Marsden, J. (ed) *Ophthalmic Care*. Chichester: Wiley, pp.66–84.

Sheppard, C.M. & Brenner, P.S. (2000) The effects of bathing and skin care practices on skin quality and satisfaction with an innovative product. *Journal of Gerontological Nursing*, 26(10), 36–45.

Sherman, D.W., Matzo, M.L., Paice, J.A., et al. (2004) Learning pain assessment and management: a goal of the End-of-Life Nursing Education Consortium. *Journal of Continuing Education in Nursing*, 35(3), 107–120.

Shipman, C., Gysels, M., White, P., et al. (2008) Making a difference improving generalist end of life care: national consultation with practitioners, commissioners, academics, and service user groups. *BMJ*, 337, a1720.

Sidebotham, D., Dijkhuizen, M.R. & Schug, S.A. (1997) The safety and utilization of patient-controlled analgesia. *Journal of Pain and Symptom Management*, 14(4), 202–209.

Simpson, K.H. (2008) Chronic non-cancer pain. In: Dickman, A. & Simpson, K.H. (eds) *Chronic Pain*. Oxford: Oxford University Press.

Sindrup, S.H. & Jensen, T.S. (1999) Efficacy of pharmacological treatments of neuropathic pain: an update and effect related to mechanism of drug action. *Pain*, 83(3), 389–400.

Sloman, R., Brown, P., Aldana, E. & Chee, E. (1994) The use of relaxation for the promotion of comfort and pain relief in persons with advanced cancer. *Contemporary Nurse*, 3(1), 6–12.

Smaje, C. & Field, D. (1997) Absent minorities? Ethnicity and the use of palliative care services. In: Field, D., Hockley, J. & Small, N. (eds) *Death, Gender and Ethnicity*. London: Routledge, pp.142–165.

Smith, R. (2000) A good death. An important aim for health services and for us all. *BMJ*, 320, 129–130.

Smoker, A. (1999) Skin care in old age. *Nursing Standard*, 13(48), 47–53.

Sonis, S.T., Elting, L.S., Keefe, D., et al. (2004) Perspectives on cancer therapy-induced mucosal injury. *Cancer*, 100(S9), 1995–2024.

Southern, H. (2007) Oral care in cancer nursing: nurses' knowledge and education. *Journal of Advanced Nursing*, 57(6), 631–638.

Speck, P. (1992) Care after death. *Nursing Times*, 88(6), 20.

Stannard. C.F. & Booth, S. (2004) Clinical pharmacology. In: Stannard, C.F. & Booth, S. (eds) *Churchill's Pocket Book of Pain*, 2nd edn. London: Elsevier Churchill Livingstone.

Stewart, S. & McMurray, J.J. (2002) Palliative care for heart failure. *BMJ*, 330, 611–612.

Stiefel, K.A., Damron, S., Sowers, N.J. & Velez, L. (2000) Improving oral hygiene for the seriously ill patient: implementing research-based practice. *Medsurg Nursing*, 9(1), 40–46.

Stockton, L. & Flynn, M. (2009) Sitting and pressure ulcers. 1: Risk factors, self-repositioning and other interventions. *Nursing Times*, 105(24), 12–14.

Stollery, R., Shaw, M.E. & Lee, A. (2005) *Ophthalmic Nursing*, 3rd edn. Oxford: Blackwell Publishing.

Sweeney, P. (2005) Oral hygiene. In: Davies, A. & Finlay, I. (eds) *Oral Care in Advanced Disease*. Oxford: Oxford University Press, pp.23–35.

Tan, G., Jensen, M.P., Thornby, J.I. & Shanti, B.F. (2004) Validation of the Brief Pain Inventory for chronic nonmalignant pain. *Journal of Pain*, 5(2), 1331–1337.

Taylor, H. (2001) The importance of providing good patient information. *Professional Nurse*, 17(1), 34–36.

Taylor, J. (2007) The non-pharmacological management of breathlessness. *End of Life Care* 1, 20–27. Available at: www.Endoflifecare.co.uk/journal/0101_breathlessness.pdf

Tortora, G.J. & Derrickson, B.H (2011) *Principles of Anatomy and Physiology*, 13th edn. Hoboken, NJ: John Wiley & Sons.

Travis, S. (2002) *Procedure for the Care of Patients Who Die in Hospital*. London: Royal Marsden NHS Foundation Trust.

Trelle, S., Reichenbach S., Wandel S., et al. (2011) Cardiovascular safety of non steroidal anti inflammatory drugs: network meta analysis. *BMJ*, 342, c7086.

Tulsky, J.A. (2005) Beyond advance directives: importance of communication skills at the end of life. *JAMA*, 294(3), 359–365.

Turk, D.C. & Okifuji, A. (1999) Assessment of patients' reporting of pain: an integrated perspective. *Lancet*, 353(9166), 1784–1788.

Twycross R. & Wilcock, A. (2001) Pain relief. In: *Symptom Management in Advanced Cancer*, 3rd edn. Abingdon: Radcliffe Medical Press.

Twycross, R., Harcourt, J. & Bergl, S. (1996) A survey of pain in patients with advanced cancer. *Journal of Pain and Symptom Management*, 12(5), 273–282.

Tye, T. & Gell-Walker, V. (2000) Patient-controlled analgesia. *Nursing Times*, 96(25), 38–39.

Vaajoki, A., Pietilä, A.M., Kankkunen, P. & Vehviläinen-Julkunen, K. (2012) Effects of listening to music on pain intensity and pain distress after surgery: an intervention. *Journal of Clinical Nursing*, 21(5–6), 708–717.

Van den Beuken-van Everdingen, M.H.J., de Rijke, J.M., Kessels, A.G., Schouten, H.C., van Kleef, M. & Patijin, J. (2007). Prevalence of pain in patients with cancer: a systematic review of the past 40 years. *Annals of Oncology*, 18(9), 1437–1449.

Van Gennep, A. (1972) *The Rites of Passage*. Chicago: Chicago University Press.

Veerbeek, L., van Zuylen, L., Swart, S.J., et al. (2008) The effect of the Liverpool Care Pathway for the dying: a multi-centre study. *Palliative Medicine*, 22(2), 145–151.

Voegeli, D. (2008) Care or harm: exploring essential components in skin care regimens. *British Journal of Nursing*, 17(1), 24–30.

Vondrackova, D., Leyendecker, P., Meissner, W. et al. (2008) Analgesic efficacy and safety of oxycodone in combination with naloxone as prolonged release tablets in patients with moderate to severe chronic pain. *Journal of Pain*, 9(12), 1144–1154.

Walker, S.M., Macintyre, P.E., Visser, E. & Scott, D. (2006) Acute pain management: current best evidence provides guide for improved practice. *Pain Medicine*, 7(1), 3–5.

Walker, V., Dicks, B. & Webb, P. (1987) Pain assessment charts in the management of chronic cancer pain. *Palliative Medicine*, 1(2), 111–116.

Waller, S., Deward, S., Masterson, A. & Hedley, F. (2008) *Improving Environments for Care at End of Life: Lessons from Eight Pilot Sites*. London: King's Fund, pp.1–54.

Watkinson, S. & Seewoodhary, R. (2007) Common conditions and practical considerations in eye care. *Nursing Standard*, 21(44), 42–47.

Watson, M., Lucas, C., Hoy, A. & Wells, J. (2009) *The Oxford Handbook of Palliative Care*, 2nd edn. Oxford: Oxford University Press.

Watts, T. (2012) End-of-life care pathways as tools to promote and support a good death; a critical commentary. *European Journal of Cancer Care*, 21(1), 20–30.

Watts, T. (2013) End-of-life care pathways and nursing: a literature review. *Journal of Nursing Management*, 21, 47–57.

Welch, A., Harrison, D.A., Hutchings, A. & Rowan, K. (2010) The association between deprivation and hospital mortality for admissions to critical care units in England. *Journal of Critical Care*, 25(3), 382–390.

Wheatley, R.G., Schug, S.A. & Watson, D. (2001) Safety and efficacy of postoperative epidural analgesia. *British Journal of Anaesthesia*, 87 (1), 47–61.

WHO (1979) *Handbook for Reporting Results of Cancer Treatment*, Vol. 48. Geneva: World Health Organization, pp.15–22.

WHO (1996) *Cancer Pain Relief*, 2nd edn (with a guide to opioid availability). Geneva: World Health Organization.

WHO (2002) *WHO Definition of Palliative Care*. Geneva: World Health Organization. Available at: www.who.int/cancer/palliative/en

WHO (2012) *Oral Health Fact Sheet No. 318, April 2012*. Geneva: World Health Organization. Available at: www.who.int/mediacentre/factsheets/fs318/en/

Wild, J.E., Grond, S., Kuperwasser, B., et al. (2010) Long-term safety and tolerability of tapentadol extended release for the management of chronic low back pain or osteoarthritis pain. *Pain Practice*, 10(5), 416–427.

Williamson, A. & Hoggart, B. (2005) Pain: a review of three commonly used pain rating scales. *Journal of Clinical Nursing*, 14(7), 798–804.

Wilson, D. (2006) Giving patients a choice of what to wear in hospital. *Nursing Times*, 102(20), 29–31.

Wolf, Z. (1988) *Nurses' Work: The Sacred and the Profane*. Philadelphia: University of Pennsylvania Press.

Wood, A. (2004) Mouth care and ritualistic practice. *Cancer Nursing Practice*, 3(4), 34–39.

Woodrow, P. (2006) *Intensive Care Nursing: A Framework for Practice*, 2nd edn. London: Routledge.

Worthington, H.V., Clarkson, J.E. & Eden, T.O. (2007) Interventions for preventing oral mucositis for patients with cancer receiving treatment. *Cochrane Database of Systematic Reviews*, 4, CD000978.

Answers

Learning Activity 8.1 Scenario: Bathing a patient

You have been asked to wash a 78-year-old male patient with limited mobility.
What factors should you take into account when considering how to meet his hygiene needs?

- Discuss his usual preferences for washing.
- Gain consent.
- Explain all stages of the procedure.
- Ensure privacy and dignity.
- Consider mobility and washing aids (shower chair, bath hoist, etc.).

Learning Activity 8.3 Case study: Pain

James is a 37-year-old man who was admitted to your ward having had knee surgery this morning following an injury he sustained playing football a couple of months ago. It is now early evening; he is using patient-controlled analgesia (PCA), containing morphine, in order to control his pain, and is also receiving regular doses of oral paracetamol and diclofenac (a non-steroidal anti-inflammatory).

James has said he has some pain. The nurse you are working with has asked you to assess James' pain.

1 What tool would you use to do this?
   - For example: numerical rating scale 0–10.

2 What else would you want to find out about his pain?
   - Location, duration, type (e.g. stabbing, dull ache), precipitating/alleviating factors.

3 What pharmacological interventions may be appropriate?
   - Review his oral and patient-controlled analgesia. Is the PCA working effectively? Has he had all of his oral analgesia as prescribed?

4 What non-pharmacological interventions may be appropriate?
   - For example: information and reassurance, comfort measures (positioning, pillow), relaxation, music, distraction, TV.

Learning Activity 8.6 Scenario: Discharging patients for end-of-life care at home

You have been asked to start arranging the discharge of a patient who is moving from hospital to home for end-of-life care.

1 Who needs to be informed of the discharge?
   - Family/carers, GP, community nurses, hospice teams, voluntary care support services (if appropriate).

2 What other arrangements need to be put in place?
   - Anticipatory drugs prescribed, patient consent for local electronic palliative care coordination system (where possible), equipment such as a bed, oxygen and incontinence aids, as appropriate.

Now Test Yourself What have you learnt?

1 Which layer of the skin contains blood and lymph vessels, sweat and sebaceous glands?
   A Epidermis
   B Dermis
   C Subcutaneous layer
   D All of the above

2 What factors can influence the appearance of the skin?
   - Nutrition and hydration
   - Incontinence
   - Age
   - Health
   - Mobility
   - Treatments
   - Concurrent conditions

3 Using a hot water bottle in bed may cause foot ulceration.
   A True
   B False

4 A clean technique should be used for all eye care procedures.
   A True
   B False – for vulnerable exposed eyes or to reduce the risk of infection, an aseptic technique may be required

5 What is xerostomia?
   A Dry mouth
   B Taste changes
   C Ulcerated mouth
   D All of the above

6 Which of the following is no longer a recommended method of mouthcare?
   A Chlorhexidine solution and foam sticks
   B Sodium bicarbonate
   C Normal saline mouthwash
   D Glycerine and lemon swabs

7 In pain assessment, a useful mnemonic is 'SOCRATES'. What does it stand for?
   S – severity: none, mild, moderate, severe
   O – onset: when and how did it start?
   C – characteristic: is it shooting, burning, aching – ask the patient to describe it
   R – radiation: does it radiate anywhere else?
   A – additional factors: what makes it better?
   T – time: is it there all the time, is there a time of day when it is worse?
   E – exacerbating factors: what makes it worse?
   S – site: where is the pain?

8 List at least four non-pharmacological methods of managing pain.
   - For example: information/education, music, art, comfort measures, exercise, heat, cold

9 'The active, total care of the patient whose disease is not responsive to curative treatment' defines which term?
   A End of life care
   B Palliative care
   C Terminal care
   D All of the above

10 Which of the following IS NOT one of the four basic criteria that denote the terminal phase of life?
   A The patient is semi-comatose
   B The patient is unable to get out of bed
   C The patient is unable to verbally communicate
   D The patient is only able to take sips of fluid
   E The patient is no longer able to take tablets

Respiratory care

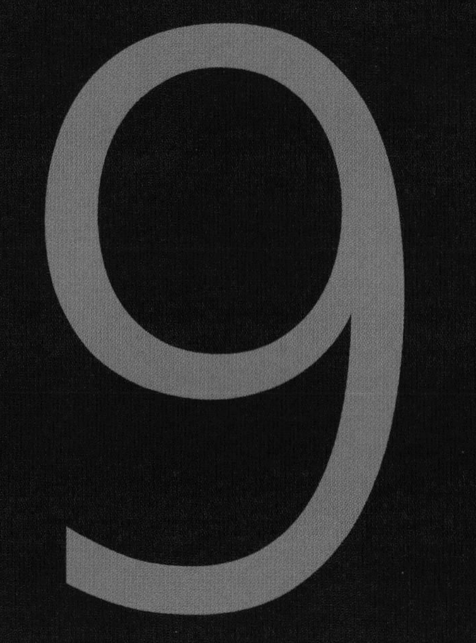

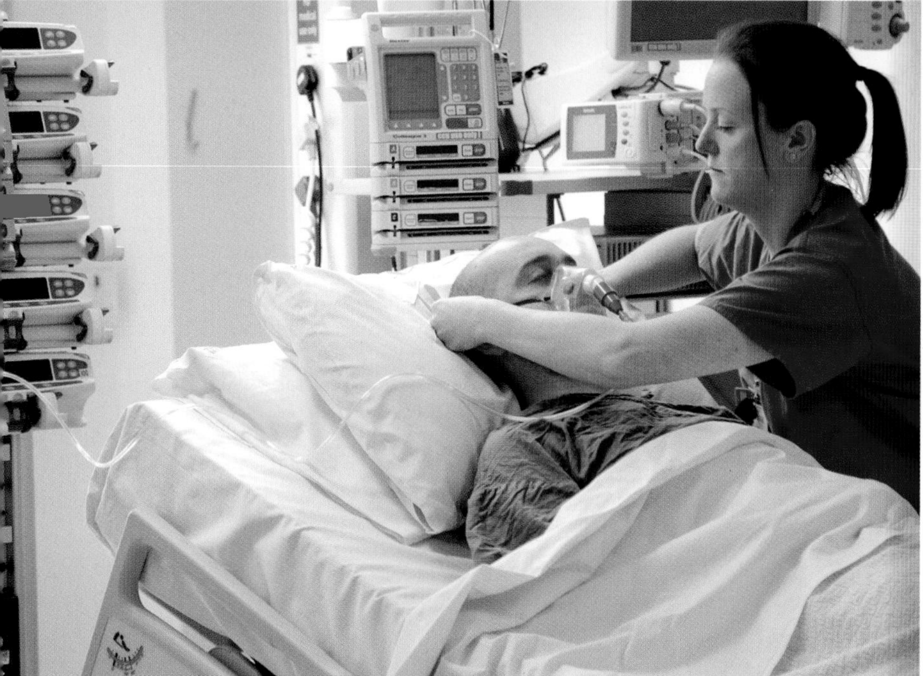

By reading this chapter and undertaking the learning activities within it, you should be able to:

1. Gain insight and understanding into the nursing management and assessment of patients with respiratory problems.
2. Understand the principles of administering oxygen therapy.
3. Demonstrate an understanding of safe management of tracheostomies.
4. Identify appropriate opportunities to discuss smoking cessation with patients.
5. Understand the principles of cardiorespiratory resuscitation.

Procedure guidelines

The Royal Marsden Manual of Clinical Nursing Procedures: Student Edition, Ninth Edition. Edited by Lisa Dougherty, Sara Lister and Alexandra West-Oram

Overview

This chapter explains the nursing management and assessment of patients with respiratory problems. Administration of oxygen therapy, managing patients with chest drains and tracheostomies, counselling patients regarding smoking cessation and performing cardiopulmonary resuscitation (CPR) will be discussed.

Respiratory therapy

DEFINITION

The principle of respiratory therapy is the application of pharmacological and non-pharmacological means to improve breathing and therefore gaseous exchange. This will include an assessment of the cause of the impaired breathing, reversal of causes where possible and therapies to optimize respiratory function (Shelledy and Mikles 2002).

ANATOMY AND PHYSIOLOGY

See also Chapter 11: Observations.

The respiratory system is a complex system that is responsible for the efficient exchange of the respiratory gases, primarily oxygen and carbon dioxide. The respiratory system is responsible for ensuring a continuous optimum supply of oxygen to the tissues and the elimination of carbon dioxide during expiration. Four separate functions are necessary to achieve optimal respiration (Marieb et al. 2012).

1. *Pulmonary ventilation*: adequate breathing and movement of air in and out of the lungs, ensuring a fresh supply of oxygen to the alveoli.
2. *External respiration*: ensuring adequate gas exchange, oxygen uptake and carbon dioxide unloading between the blood and the alveoli of the lungs.
3. *Transport of respiratory gases*: moving oxygen and carbon dioxide between the lungs and the body tissues. Transport is affected by the cardiovascular system and uses the blood as a carrying mechanism.
4. *Cellular respiration*: oxygen delivery and carbon dioxide uptake between the systemic blood and tissue cells.

The respiratory system is composed of the following structures.

- The two respiratory centres in the medulla oblongata and pons of the brain.
- The nose, mouth and connecting airways.
- The trachea, main bronchus, bronchioles and alveoli.
- The respiratory muscles: the diaphragm and the intercostal muscles.
- The respiratory nerves: the subphrenic nerve and the intercostal nerves.
- The bone structure of the thorax: the ribs, vertebrae and sternum.
- The lung parenchyma.
- The pleura (Urden et al. 2006).

Alteration, damage or blockage to any of the structures listed above may result in either respiratory impairment or respiratory failure. It is essential when considering respiratory function to remember the close association and dependence between the cardiovascular, neurological, musculoskeletal and respiratory systems (Marieb et al. 2012).

Tissue oxygenation

All the cells of the body require a continuous supply of oxygen to ensure growth and repair of tissues and optimum metabolism. Oxygen is drawn into the body through the nose and mouth; it then travels down the trachea and into the smaller airways and alveoli of the lungs. Once it has reached the alveoli, oxygen in solution is able to transfer into the network of capillaries and from there travels via the venous network to all cells of the body. This tissue oxygenation is known as cellular oxygenation. Low oxygen levels are called hypoxia. In low oxygen conditions, anaerobic cellular oxygenation will occur, generating the waste product lactic acid. If the low oxygen state is allowed to continue, lactic acid will accumulate, leading to a metabolic acidosis and cell death (Berne 2004, Bersten et al. 2009, Guyton and Hall 2006, Hess 2000, Jenkins and Tortora 2013, Kumar and Clark 2009, Marieb et al. 2012, Pierson 2000, West 2008).

There are three components to oxygenation: oxygen uptake, oxygen transportation and oxygen utilization. *Oxygen uptake* is the process of extracting oxygen from the environment. *Oxygen transportation* is the mechanism by which the uptake of oxygen results in the delivery of oxygen to the cells. *Oxygen utilization* is the metabolic need for molecular oxygen by the cells of the body (Jenkins and Tortora 2013, Marieb et al. 2012).

In order for oxygenation to take place there needs to be an adequate cardiac output.

Oxygen uptake

The air that we breathe in during normal conditions from the atmosphere is composed of the following gases:

- oxygen 21%
- carbon dioxide 0.03%
- nitrogen 79%
- rare gases 0.003%.

Inspired air at sea level has a total atmospheric pressure of 760 mmHg. According to Dalton's Law, where there is a mixture of gases, each gas exerts its own pressure as if there were no other gases present. The pressure of an individual gas in a mixture is called the partial pressure and is denoted as P, which is then followed by the type of gas, so that the partial pressure of oxygen is written PO_2 (Tortora and Derrickson 2011).

- Oxygen 0.21 × 760 = 159 mmHg (21 kPa)
- Carbon dioxide 0.03 × 760 = 22.8 mmHg (3.0 kPa)
- Nitrogen 0.79 × 760 = 600 mmHg (80 kPa)

The partial pressure of gases controls the movement of oxygen and carbon dioxide through the body between the atmosphere and the lungs, the lungs and the blood and finally the blood and the cells.

Gaseous exchange

Movement of gases is by diffusion. Diffusion is the movement of gas molecules from an area of relatively high partial pressure to one of lower partial pressure (Jenkins and Tortora 2013).

Diffusion of oxygen takes place from the alveolus into the pulmonary capillaries and movement of carbon dioxide from the capillary into the alveolus. From the alveolus, the oxygen diffuses from the capillaries into the tissues and mitochondria of the cells (Figure 9.1).

The alveolar oxygen partial pressure must be higher than the arterial oxygen partial pressure in order to push the oxygen through the alveolar membrane into the interstitial spaces and from there into the pulmonary capillaries.

As inspired air enters the respiratory tract, it encounters water vapour present in the upper airways which warms and humidifies it. Water vapour exerts its own partial pressure of 47 mmHg. The partial pressure of the water vapour must be subtracted from the total atmospheric pressure to give a corrected atmospheric pressure and partial pressure of each gas (Marieb et al. 2012).

- Corrected total atmospheric pressure 760 – 47 = 713 mmHg
- Oxygen 0.21 × 713 = 150 mmHg (20 kPa)
- Carbon dioxide 0.03 × 713 = 21 mmHg (2.8 kPa)

Figure 9.1 Gas movement in the body is facilitated by partial pressure differences. Top of figure illustrates pressure gradients that facilitate oxygen and carbon dioxide exchange in the lungs. Bottom of figure shows pressure gradients that facilitate gas movements from systemic capillaries to tissues.

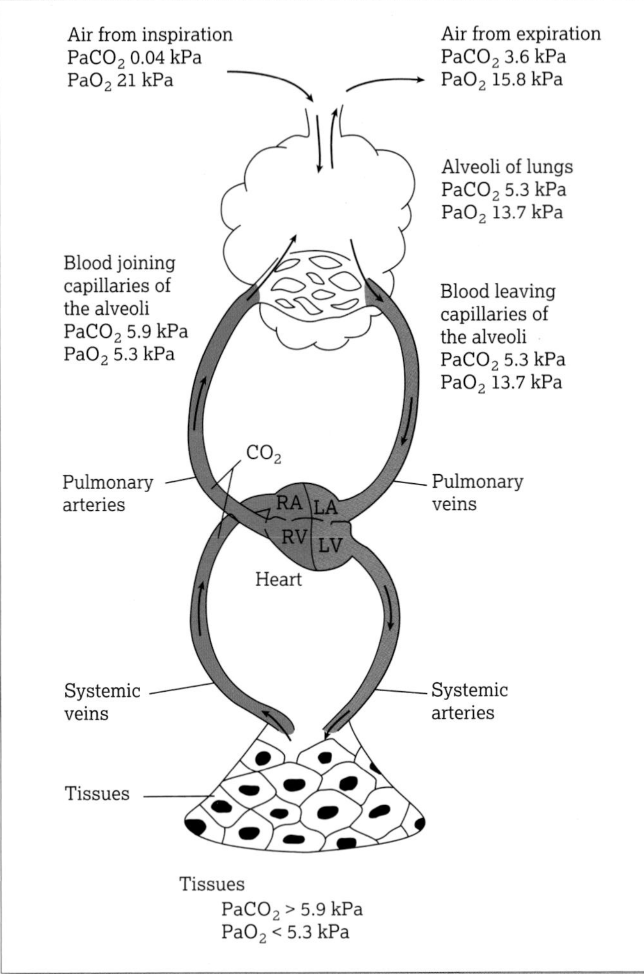

Figure 9.2 Oxyhaemoglobin dissociation curve. With a PaO_2 of 8 kPa and more, saturations will remain high (flat portion of curve). NB: The middle red line is the normal position of the curve.

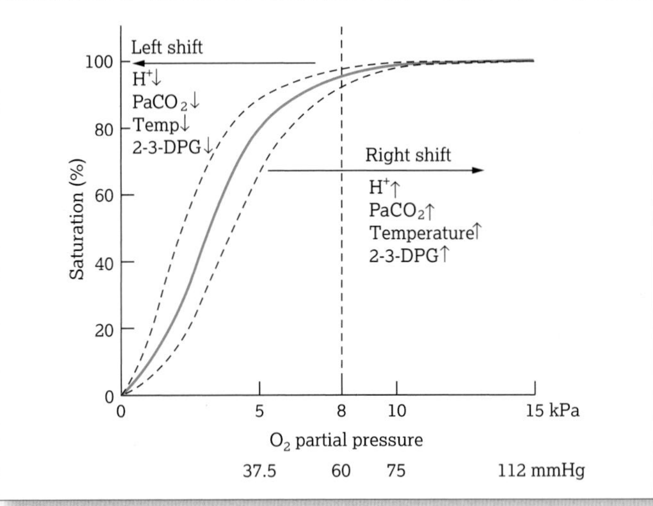

As oxygen continues to pass down the respiratory tract to the alveolus, it encounters carbon dioxide leaving the respiratory tract which also exerts a partial pressure, equal to 40 mmHg. This in turn must be subtracted to determine the correct values. Oxygen has a corrected value of 150 – 40 = 110–100 mmHg (14.6–13.3 kPa).

Oxygen transportation

Oxygen is carried in the blood in two ways.

- *Dissolved in the plasma (serum)*: only 2–3% is carried in this way as oxygen is not very soluble (Ahrens and Tucker 1999, Marieb et al. 2012). This is measured as the PaO_2. There is 0.003 mL of blood for each 1 mmHg partial pressure oxygen. At 100 mmHg partial pressure, only 0.3 mL of oxygen would be carried per 100 mL of plasma.
- *Bound to haemoglobin in the red blood cells*: 95–98% of oxygen is carried in this way and is measured as the percentage of oxygen saturated (SaO_2). Each gram of haemoglobin can carry 1.34 mL of oxygen per 100 mL blood.

Haemoglobin is composed of haem (iron) and globulin (protein). Each haemoglobin molecule has four binding sites, each able to carry one molecule of oxygen. A haemoglobin molecule is said to be fully saturated with oxygen when all four haem sites are attached to oxygen. When fewer than four are attached, the haemoglobin is said to be partially saturated.

The bond between haemoglobin and oxygen is affected by various physiological factors that shift the oxygen dissociation curve to the right or left (Figure 9.2) (Jenkins and Tortora 2013, Marieb et al. 2012).

OXYHAEMOGLOBIN CURVE SHIFT TO THE RIGHT

When a shift occurs to the right, there is reduced binding of oxygen to haemoglobin and oxygen is given up more easily to the tissues. The saturation will be lower (Pierson 2000).

Factors that cause the curve to shift to the right are an increase in:

- body temperature due to infection, sepsis
- hydrogen ion content (acidaemia), known as the Bohr effect, due to infection, sepsis or other shock conditions
- carbon dioxide due to sepsis, pulmonary disease, postoperatively
- 2-3-DPG (an enzyme found in the red blood cells that affects haemoglobin and oxygen binding).

OXYHAEMOGLOBIN CURVE SHIFT TO THE LEFT

When a shift occurs to the left, there is an increase in the binding of oxygen to the haemoglobin, oxygen is given up less easily to the tissues and cellular hypoxia can occur (Pierson 2000).

Factors that cause the curve to shift to the left are a decrease in:

- body temperature due to exposure, near drowning, trauma
- hydrogen ion content (alkalaemia)
- carbon dioxide
- 2-3-DPG.

Oxygen utilization

The relationship between the PaO_2 and the SaO_2 is represented as the oxygen dissociation curve. Oxygen uptake in the lungs is shown by the upper flat part of the curve. When the PaO_2 is between 8.0 and 13.3 kPa (60–100 mmHg), the haemoglobin is 90% or more saturated with oxygen. At this point of the curve, large changes in the PaO_2 lead to small changes in the SaO_2 of haemoglobin, because the haemoglobin is almost completely saturated. Release of oxygen to the tissues is shown by the lower part of the curve. There is easy removal of oxygen from the haemoglobin for use by the cells. It is at this part of the curve that small changes in the PaO_2 cause major changes in the SaO_2. This is important clinically (Guyton and Hall 2006, Hess 2000).

A patient's oxygen level must be kept at 8.5 kPa or above (60 mmHg). Below this level, desaturation can occur at a rapid rate, resulting in tissue hypoxia and cell death (Marieb et al. 2012).

Oxygen consumption

At rest, the normal oxygen consumption is approximately 200–250 mL/min. As the available oxygen per minute in a normal man is about 700 mL, this means there is an oxygen reserve of 450–500 mL/min. Factors that increase the consumption of oxygen include fever, sepsis, shivering, restlessness and increased metabolism (Bersten et al. 2009). It is difficult to say at which absolute level oxygen therapy is necessary, as each situation should be judged by the requirements for oxygen and the availability of oxygen. Therefore, all the above information needs to be taken into account together with the measurement of the arterial blood gases.

Generally, additional oxygen will be required when the PaO_2 has fallen to 8.5 kPa (60 mmHg) or less (Bersten et al. 2009).

Carbon dioxide excretion

The second function of the respiratory system is to excrete carbonic acid from the lungs during expiration. The normal level of carbon dioxide in the blood is 3.5–5.3 kPa. Carbon dioxide has a direct effect on the respiratory centre in the brain. As the carbon dioxide level rises and diffuses from the blood into the cerebrospinal fluid (CSF), it is hydrated and carbonic acid is formed. The acid then dissociates and hydrogen ions are liberated and as there are no proteins in the CSF to buffer the hydrogen ions, the pH of the CSF falls, which excites the central chemoreceptors and the respiratory rate is increased (Marieb et al. 2012).

EVIDENCE-BASED APPROACHES

Respiratory assessment

Once information about the person's past medical history has been obtained, one of the most reliable and important assessments is to closely observe and talk to the patient. During this time a patient's smoking status should be ascertained and, if appropriate, their smoking habits and the benefits of stopping should be discussed. For smoking cessation, brief interventions typically take about 5–10 minutes and may include one or more of the following.

- Simple opportunistic advice to stop.
- Assessment of patient's desire to stop.
- Offer of pharmacotherapy and/or behavioural support.
- Provision of self-help material and referral to more intensive support such as the NHS Stop Smoking services (NICE 2006).

Normal respiration is effortless and almost unconscious and the person can eat, drink and speak in full sentences without appearing breathless. Essential first steps in respiratory assessment are therefore to observe the person's breathing for the following.

- Ease and comfort.
- Rate.
- Pattern.
- Position the patient has adopted; for example, does the patient need to sit at 90° upright to breathe effectively?
- Rate and ease of breathing during speaking or movement.
- General colour and appearance: is there any evidence of greyness, cyanosis, pallor, sweating?
- Additional audible breath sounds: wheezing or stridor? (O'Driscoll et al. 2008)

Having rapidly made this assessment, other essential assessments are a chest X-ray and arterial blood gas, and a computed tomography (CT) scan or ventilation/perfusion (V/Q) scan may also be necessary (see Chapter 10: Interpreting diagnostic tests).

Having made a comprehensive assessment, the immediate cause of respiratory insufficiency should be corrected where possible. It is important to recognize that this may result from interruption to any part of respiration; for example, the patient may be in severe pain and appropriate pain management may improve their respiratory function, or conversely an opioid overdose may result in decreased or absent respiration and the antidote to the opioid will then need to be given. There may be a mechanical obstruction to respiration, such as an infective obstruction like epiglottitis, and the treatment is therefore directed at treating the infection whilst also oxygenating the patient (O'Driscoll et al. 2008).

Respiratory therapy therefore covers a wide area and will include any manipulation or management of alteration to any part of the respiratory tree. It may include pharmacological management including pain management, antidotes to drug toxicity, support and guidance on smoking cessation, antimicrobials for infections of the respiratory tract, respiratory stimulants, surgery to repair a ruptured diaphragm or to manage trauma, the insertion of a tracheostomy or chest drains, or a thoracoabdominal shunt for superior vena cava obstruction. Finally, positioning and physiotherapy play a major role in improving respiratory function (O'Driscoll et al. 2008).

Any person who is unable to maintain tissue oxygenation will need to receive supplemental oxygen until they are able to manage again on room air. This oxygen may be delivered in different ways depending on the severity of the condition and the level of hypoxia (Morton and Fontaine 2009).

Learning Activity 9.1 Case study: Respiratory assessment and smoking cessation

Ella Smith is a 29-year-old woman who was admitted to your unit overnight for observation following an acute exacerbation of her asthma. This is the second time in 6 weeks she has been admitted for this reason.

1 You need to assess her respiratory status; what else should you be observing for?

She is a smoker and on her previous admission was advised that she should try to stop smoking as this was a likely trigger for her asthma. She managed to stop for 4 weeks but started again one week ago when she was on a girls' night out and all her friends were smoking. She tells you that she usually smokes 5–10 cigarettes a day.

2 What would be your first step in encouraging her to stop smoking?
3 What other forms of support may she benefit from?

See the end of the chapter for the answers.

Oxygen therapy

DEFINITION

Oxygen therapy is the administration of oxygen at concentrations greater than that in ambient air with the intention of treating or preventing the symptoms and manifestations of hypoxia.

EVIDENCE-BASED APPROACHES

Rationale

Indications

- Respiratory failure, of which there are two types (Marieb et al. 2012, O'Driscoll et al. 2008, Tortora and Derrickson 2011).
  - *Type 1*, referred to as hypoxaemic respiratory failure (failure to oxygenate the tissues). The PaO_2 is <8 kPa (60 mmHg) while the carbon dioxide (PCO_2) is normal or low. Common causes include infectious conditions, pneumonia, pulmonary oedema and adult respiratory distress syndrome.
  - *Type 2*, referred to as hypercapnic (raised carbon dioxide) or respiratory pump failure. Alveolar ventilation is insufficient to excrete carbon dioxide accompanied by hypoxaemia (deficiency of oxygen in the arterial blood). The PCO_2 is >6 kPa (45 mmHg). Common causes include chronic obstructive pulmonary disease (COPD), chest wall deformities, drug overdose and chest injury (Kayner 2012).
- Acute myocardial infarction.
- Cardiac failure.
- Shock – haemorrhagic, bacteraemic and cardiogenic.
- Conditions in which there is a reduced ability to transport oxygen, for example anaemia.
- During anaesthesia.
- Post-operatively.
- Sleep apnoea.
- Severe pain.
- Asthma.
- Pulmonary embolus.
- Conditions that affect the neuromuscular control of breathing such as muscular dystrophy, Guillain–Barré.
- Severe trauma affecting the diaphragm, ribs, lungs or trachea.
- Tension pneumothorax.
- Pleural effusion (Kayner 2012).

Causes of respiratory failure are shown in Box 9.1.

Contraindications

No specific contraindications to oxygen therapy exist, but the following precautions or possible contraindications need to be considered.

- With increased PaO_2 ventilatory depression may occur in spontaneously breathing patients with elevated $PaCO_2$.
- With high flow of fractional inspired oxygen (FiO_2), absorption atelectasis, oxygen toxicity and/or depression of ciliary and/or leucocytic function may occur.
- Supplemental oxygen should be administered with caution to patients suffering from paraquat poisoning and those receiving bleomycin.
- During laser bronchoscopy, minimal levels of supplemental oxygen should be used to avoid intratracheal ignition.
- Fire hazard is increased in the presence of increased oxygen concentrations.
- Bacterial contamination associated with certain nebulization and humidification systems is a possible hazard (Fischer 2006).

Anticipated patient outcomes

Outcome is determined by clinical and physiological assessment to establish adequacy of the patient response to oxygen therapy. It should be geared towards achieving desired oxygen saturations with the least FiO_2 setting (O'Driscoll et al. 2008).

LEGAL AND PROFESSIONAL ISSUES

Competencies

Nursing staff must be trained to adequately administer oxygen therapy and their competency should be assessed. They should check and document that a device is being used appropriately and the flow is as prescribed and appropriate for the patient's needs. Nursing and physiotherapy staff may assess patients, initiate and monitor oxygen delivery systems within the prescribed parameters, except in emergencies when oxygen should be given first and documented later (NPSA 2009).

Governance

Clinical governance leads in local hospitals and organizations should audit current practice and develop local policies and evidence-based guidelines to ensure that:

- oxygen is administered and prescribed according to national guidelines (NPSA 2009)
- all equipment used, such as humidification, continuous positive airway pressure (CPAP), Optiflow, chest drains and CPR equipment, is regularly checked for safety and staff are adequately trained to use and troubleshoot when problems occur.

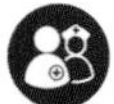

Box 9.1 **Causes of respiratory failure**

Common causes of type 1 respiratory failure (hypoxaemic) include the following:

- COPD
- Pneumonia
- Pulmonary oedema
- Pulmonary fibrosis
- Asthma
- Pneumothorax
- Pulmonary embolism
- Pulmonary arterial hypertension
- Pneumoconiosis
- Granulomatous lung diseases
- Cyanotic congenital heart disease
- Bronchiectasis
- Acute respiratory distress syndrome (ARDS)
- Fat embolism syndrome
- Kyphoscoliosis
- Obesity

Common causes of type 2 respiratory failure (hypercapnic) include the following:

- COPD
- Severe asthma
- Drug overdose
- Poisonings
- Myasthenia gravis
- Polyneuropathy
- Poliomyelitis
- Primary muscle disorders
- Porphyria
- Cervical cordotomy
- Head and cervical cord injury
- Primary alveolar hypoventilation
- Obesity-hypoventilation syndrome
- Pulmonary oedema
- ARDS
- Myxoedema
- Tetanus (Kayner 2012)

COPD, chronic obstructive pulmonary disease.

Risk management

The use of medical equipment relating to oxygen therapy will be monitored as identified within the local hospital medical equipment policies. All incident reports relating to oxygen therapy and supportive respiratory equipment as stated in this chapter should be reviewed by local risk management committees in order to identify themes and trends and propose appropriate risk reduction measures to prevent reoccurrence and improve patient safety (BTS 2008, MHRA 2010, NPSA 2008, 2009).

PRE-PROCEDURAL CONSIDERATIONS

Before commencing oxygen therapy, it is essential that it should be prescribed as can seen by the example prescription in Box 9.2. This should be in the form of parameters, for example 28–40% of oxygen to keep saturations (sats) >92%. This will allow nursing staff to alter the oxygen setting to achieve the target saturations without requiring a change to the prescription on each occasion, as well as individualizing treatment to meet the patient's needs. The only exception to this situation is during immediate management of critical illness or emergency situations when oxygen should be given without being formally prescribed (O'Driscoll et al. 2008).

Regular pulse oximetry monitoring must be available in all clinical environments where oxygen may be administered. Oxygen therapy will need to be adjusted to achieve target saturations rather than giving a fixed dose to all patients with the same disease. Nurses can make these adjustments without requiring a change to the prescription on each occasion. Most oxygen therapy will be from nasal cannulas rather than masks and will not be given to patients who are not hypoxaemic (except during critical illness) (O'Driscoll et al. 2008).

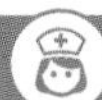
Learning Activity 9.2

Scenario: Administering oxygen

You are looking after a 78-year-old gentleman overnight whose oxygen saturations have dropped to 85%. The nurse in charge has asked you to give him some oxygen.

What would you do?

See the end of the chapter for the answers.

Equipment

Oxygen is an odourless, tasteless, colourless, transparent gas that is slightly heavier than air. Oxygen supports combustion so there is always a danger of fire when oxygen is being used. The following safety measures should be remembered.

- Oil or grease around oxygen connections should be avoided.
- Alcohol, ether and other inflammable liquids should be used with caution in the vicinity of oxygen.
- No electrical device must be used in or near an oxygen tent.
- Oxygen cylinders should be kept secure in an upright position and away from heat.

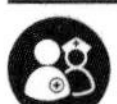
Box 9.2 **Example of oxygen section for hospital prescription charts**

Drug: OXYGEN	Date administered
Circle target oxygen saturation	06
88–92% 94–98% Other________	10
Starting device/flow rate ________	14
PRN/continuous (refer to local O_2 guideline)	18
Tick here if saturation not indicated ☐	22
Date and signature	
Print name	

Table 9.1 **Fixed performance mask oxygen flow rates**

Oxygen flow rate (L/min)	% Oxygen delivered
2	24
6	31
8	35
10	40
15	60

- There must be no smoking in the vicinity of oxygen.
- A fire extinguisher should be readily available.
- Care should be taken with high concentrations of oxygen when using the defibrillator in a cardiorespiratory arrest or during elective cardioversion.

All oxygen delivery systems should be checked at least once per day. Care should be taken to avoid interruption of oxygen therapy in situations including ambulation or transport for procedures (O'Driscoll et al. 2008).

Oxygen delivery

Any oxygen delivery system will include these basic components.

- *Oxygen supply*, from either a piped supply or a portable cylinder. All medical gas cylinders have to conform to a standardized colour coding: oxygen cylinders are black with a white shoulder and are labelled 'Oxygen' or 'O_2'. Since 2004, small portable oxygen cylinders have been in use: these are totally white and are a C-size cylinder.
- A *reduction gauge*: to reduce the pressure to atmospheric pressure.
- *Flowmeter*: a device that controls the flow of oxygen in litres per minute.
- *Tubing*: disposable tubing of varying diameter and length.
- *Mechanism for delivery*: a mask or nasal cannulas (Table 9.1).
- *Humidifier*: to warm and moisten the oxygen before administration.
- *Water trap* if humidifier in use (O'Driscoll et al. 2008).

Nasal cannulas

Nasal cannulas (Figure 9.3) consist of two plastic prongs that are inserted inside the anterior nares and supported on a light frame. Advantages to the patient are that they may seem less

Figure 9.3 **Nasal cannulas.**

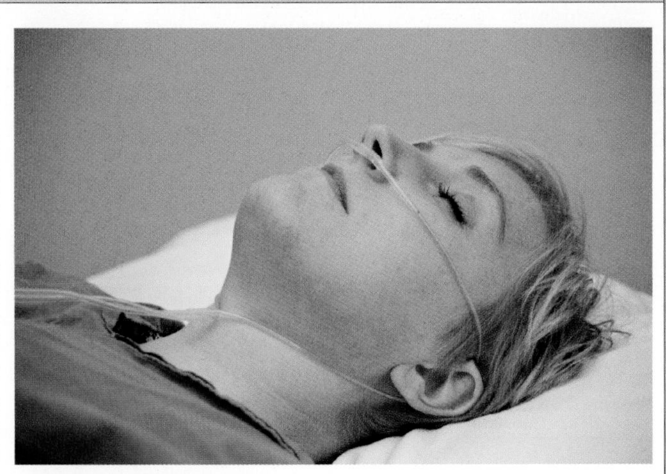

Table 9.2 **Oxygen flow rates for nasal cannulas**

Oxygen flow rate (L/min)	% Oxygen delivered
1	24
2	28
3	32
4	36
5	40
6	44

Table 9.3 **Approximate oxygen concentration related to flow rates of semi-rigid masks**

Oxygen flow rate (L/min)	% Oxygen delivered
2	24
4	35
6	50
8	55
10	60
12	65
15	70

claustrophobic and do not interfere with eating, drinking and communication (Fell and Boehm 1998). Nasal cannulas provide an alternative to a mask, but can be used only where the patient requires a low percentage of oxygen and are usually used with flow rates of 1–4 litres of oxygen per minute and provide approximately 28–35% oxygen (Table 9.2). They cannot be attached satisfactorily to an external humidification device but in many cases the oxygen will be humidified as it passes through the nasal passages into the trachea (Marieb et al. 2012). They are generally well tolerated and are useful post-operatively or where the patient requires minimal support and are also used in the chronic setting where a patient at home requires long-term oxygen therapy.

Simple semi-rigid plastic masks

Simple semi-rigid plastic masks (Figure 9.4) are low-flow (5–10 L/min) masks which entrain the air from the atmosphere and therefore are able to deliver a variable oxygen percentage (anything from 40% to 60%). Oxygen concentrations vary depending on the flow rate and the patient's breathing pattern (Table 9.3). Large discrepancies between the delivered FiO_2 and the actual amount received by the patient will occur, dependent on the patient's rate and depth of breathing (O'Driscoll et al. 2008). These masks are useful for patients who need a higher percentage of oxygen temporarily whilst the cause of their hypoxia is treated. This type of mask may be worn for hours or several days, but should be used in conjunction with a humidifier if used for more than 12 hours).

Note that if the oxygen flow on this mask is less than 5 L/min, increased resistance to breathing occurs, causing a possible build-up of CO_2 within the mask, resulting in rebreathing (O'Driscoll et al. 2008).

If the patient requires 60% oxygen or more, expert help should be sought as the patient may require more invasive respiratory support (NICE 2007).

Non-rebreathing mask (high-concentration reservoir mask)

Non-rebreathing masks (Figure 9.5) are similar to the simple semi-rigid plastic masks with the addition of a reservoir bag, which allows the oxygen to be delivered at concentrations between 60% and 90% when used at flow rates of 10–15 L/min (O'Driscoll et al. 2008). Oxygen flows into the bag and mask during inhalation and the valve prevents expired air from flowing back into the bag.

Note that if the oxygen flow is too low, the carbon dioxide can accumulate in the reservoir bag and fail to meet the patient's requirements, resulting in an increase in carbon dioxide (Pierce 1995). This device should only be used in the presence of expert nursing and medical support and usually during emergency intervention or before more invasive ventilatory therapy is instituted.

Fixed performance masks or high-flow masks (Venturi-type masks)

Venturi-type oxygen masks deliver high-flow oxygen via a Venturi adaptor (Figure 9.6). The adaptors are colour coded according to

Figure 9.4 **Simple semi-rigid plastic mask.**

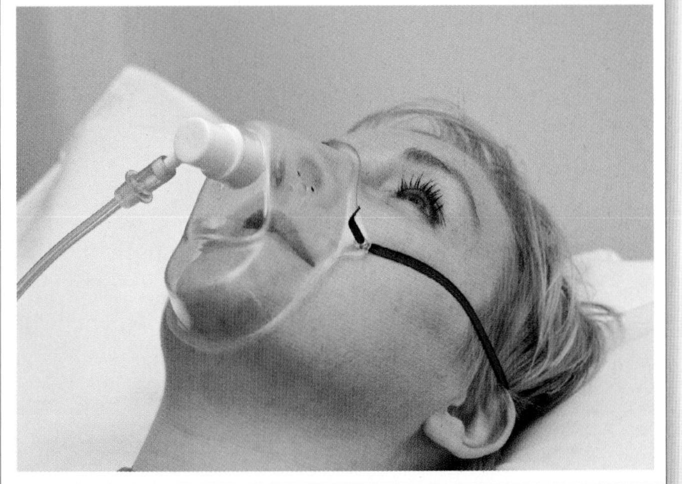

Figure 9.5 **Non-rebreathing mask.**

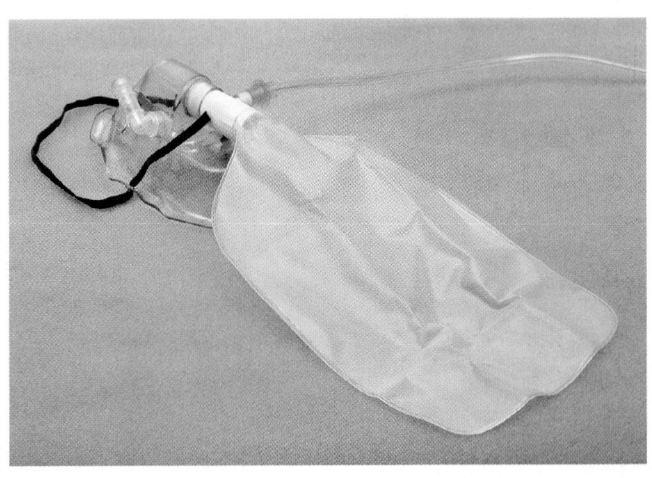

Figure 9.6 Venturi barrels.

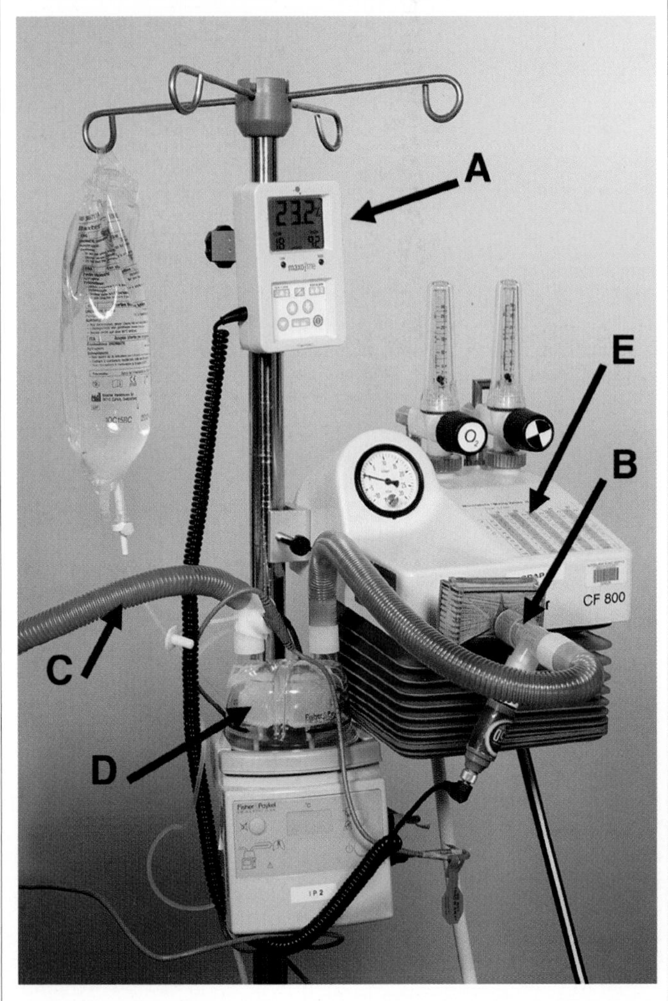

Figure 9.7 (a) Oxygen analyser. (b) T-piece. (c) Oxygen (elephant) tubing. (d) Warm bath humidifier. (e) Flow generator oxygen and air Drager bellows.

the percentage of oxygen they deliver with different oxygen flow rates. Venturi masks are available in the following concentrations: 24%, 28%, 35%, 40% and 60%. Venturi masks with 24% and 28% are suited to those at risk of CO_2 retention (O'Driscoll et al. 2008).

Tracheostomy mask

Tracheostomy masks perform in a similar way to the simple semi-rigid plastic facemask (see Figure 9.4). The mask is placed over the tracheostomy tube or stoma.

T-piece circuit

The T-piece circuit is a simple, large-bore, non-rebreathing circuit which is attached directly to an endotracheal or tracheostomy tube (Figure 9.7b). Humidified oxygen is delivered through one part of the T and expired gases leave through the other part. This device may be used as part of the weaning process when a patient has been ventilated previously by a mechanical ventilator (Bersten et al. 2009).

Assessment and recording tools

All patients should be assessed and monitored using a *track and trigger system* (e.g. National Early Warning Score – NEWS) (NICE 2007, RCP 2012). Observations for respiratory rate, pulse oximetry and oxygen saturation alongside oxygen delivery system, heart rate and blood pressure need to be recorded on observation charts (Box 9.3).

Arterial blood gas (ABG) analysis should be measured as soon as possible in all critically ill patients and situations involving hypoxaemic patients, and is part of the essential assessment in patients who may develop carbon dioxide retention (type 2 respiratory failure) (NICE 2007, O'Driscoll et al. 2008). ABG (see Chapter 10: Interpreting diagnostic tests) should be measured with the administered inspired oxygen concentration noted at the time of arterial blood sampling. This should be repeated in accordance with the patient' clinical response to treatment (O'Driscoll et al. 2008).

Box 9.3 **Codes for recording oxygen delivery on observation chart**

A Air (not requiring oxygen, or weaning or on PRN oxygen)
N Nasal cannula
SM Simple mask
V24 Venturi 24%
V28 Venturi 28%
V35 Venturi 35%
V40 Venturi 40%
V60 Venturi 60%
H28 Humidified oxygen 28% (also H35, H40, H60 for humidified oxygen at 35%, 40%, 60%)
RM Reservoir mask/non-rebreathe mask
TM Tracheostomy mask
CP CPAP system
NIV Non-invasive system
Other device: specify__________

Learning Activity 9.3

Learning in practice: Assessment and recording tools

In your clinical area, find out what track and trigger system is used for patient assessement and monitoring of vital signs (e.g. National Early Warning Score – NEWS).

- What vital signs does it include?
- How easy do you find the tool to use?
- If you assess a patient and one of your observations is outside normal limits, how do you know this from the tool? Does it indicate what you should do in such cases?

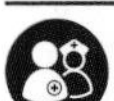

Pharmacological support
Oxygen cylinders and equipment may be ordered from the pharmacy whilst other medical equipment comes from external sources via stores and needs to be ordered before stocks run out to ensure ready availability in the event of an emergency. Nebulizers and broncholitic agents may improve respiratory status.

Domiciliary oxygen and portable oxygen

Some patients are so disabled by chronic respiratory disease that they require continual supplementary oxygen at home. Low-flow oxygen given over a period of time improves the prognosis of some patients (Benditt 2000, O'Driscoll et al. 2008).

Long-term oxygen may be prescribed for treatment of COPD, cystic fibrosis, interstitial lung disease, neuromuscular and skeletal disorders, pulmonary hypertension and palliation in lung cancer. It may be provided in the form of cylinders. The problem with this is that the cylinders need changing frequently. Oxygen condensers (concentrators) are far more economical than cylinders. A condenser consists of a compressor powered by electricity. The condenser works by drawing in room air that is passed through a bacterial filter and a sieve bed. The sieve bed contains zeolite which has an affinity for nitrogen and when under pressure works by removing nitrogen and other gases, concentrating oxygen and delivering it through a meter at the front of the compressor (O'Driscoll et al. 2008).

The oxygen can be delivered to the patient by nasal cannulas or mask (Esmond 2001).

Specific patient preparations
Oxygen delivery to the patient should be explained, including what equipment is to be used (such as a mask or nasal cannula) and the importance of keeping the apparatus in place. The patient should know about the flammability of oxygen and the dangers of any naked flames/lit cigarettes in their immediate vicinity. The nurse should instruct the patient to notify him or her of increasing distress, air hunger, nausea, anxiety, dry nasal passages or 'sore throat' (due to drying) (O'Driscoll et al. 2008).

Procedure guideline 9.1 **Oxygen therapy**

Essential equipment
- Piped/wall oxygen and medical air
- Oxygen flow meter/regulator
- Oxygen cylinders for transport of patients
- Ambu-bag for emergencies
- Nasal cannulas
- Selection of oxygen masks
- Oxygen tubing, varying lengths and types
- Oxygen analysers

Optional equipment
- Non-invasive equipment in non-critical care areas (essential within critical care environments)
- High-flow O_2 and medical air mixers for use in HDU setting
- Humidification equipment
- Cold water bubble humidifiers

Medicinal products
- Asthma inhalers or nebulizers
- Oxygen as prescribed for patient
- Nicotine patches to aid smoking cessation

Pre-procedure

Action	Rationale
1 Assess the patient's condition and level of oxygen therapy required, e.g. facemask, humidified oxygenation, nasal cannulas.	To ensure that the appropriate method for delivery of oxygen is chosen to suit the patient's condition (O'Driscoll et al. 2008, **C**).
2 Ensure an oxygen prescription is in place with clear target oxygen saturations for O_2 therapy titration. See Box 9.2.	Medical oxygen is a drug. National guidelines and clinical governance require that the intentions of the clinician who initiates oxygen therapy should be communicated clearly to the person who actually administers oxygen to the patient and an accurate record must be kept of exactly what has been given to the patient (O'Driscoll et al. 2008, **C**).
3 Explain to the patient why they require oxygen therapy and the benefits and problems thereof.	To minimize apprehension and anxiety and improve understanding of treatment. **E**
4 Attach oxygen tubing to the port on the wall oxygen or cylinder (and not to the medical air port).	To ensure proper oxygen delivery and prevent hypoxia if connected to medical air port (NPSA 2007, **C**).

Procedure

Action	Rationale
5 Set oxygen flowmeter to required setting (L/min) and check oxygen is flowing through system by using fingertips.	To ensure system is working properly. **E**

(continued)

Procedure guideline 9.1 Oxygen therapy *(continued)*

Action	Rationale
6 *Either: Apply a nasal cannula* by gently placing the nasal prongs of the cannula into the patient's nostrils, draping the tubing over the patient's ears and sliding the fit connector up under the chin to hold the tubing securely in place.	To ensure the mask or cannula is applied correctly to enable the patient to receive the oxygen. **E**
Or:	
Apply an oxygen mask by placing the mask over the patient's mouth and nose, then pull the elastic strap over the head and adjust the strap on both sides to secure the mask in a position that seals it against the face.	To ensure patient comfort. **E**
Post-procedure	
7 Check that the patient is comfortable.	To ensure patient comfort. **E**
8 Record that oxygen therapy has been commenced, time and flow rate.	To maintain accurate records (NMC 2010, **C**).
9 Provide continued reassurance to patient and opportunity to ask questions.	To minimize apprehension and anxiety and improve understanding of treatment. **E**

Problem-solving table 9.1 Prevention and resolution (Procedure guideline 9.1)

Problem	Cause	Prevention	Suggested action
Inability to maintain an airway.	Position of patient.	Provide pillows to support patient. Elevate head of bed. Demonstrate to patient orthopnoeic position.	Position patient preferably sitting up at an angle of greater than 45°.
	Airway secretions.	Provide sputum pot for expectoration. Saline nebulizers if prescribed to loosen secretions.	Encourage patient to cough and expectorate if able or remove secretions by suction if patient unable to do so.
Inability to maintain adequate oxygenation.	Inadequate oxygen delivery, patient's condition deteriorating. More breathless. Oxygen saturation decreased. Deteriorating blood gases.	Increased frequency and recording of cardiovascular observations and respiration rate. Attach pulse oximeter. Use of NEWS scoring.	Assess level of oxygen support required by assessing previous medical history and current respiratory assessment. Increase oxygen delivery using the lowest percentage of oxygen to achieve the individual goal for the patient.
Dry mouth.	Oxygen therapy can lead to a dry mouth.	Provide regular mouthcare or artificial saliva if prescribed.	Add humidification to the circuit (see Procedure guideline 9.2: Humidification for respiratory therapy). Give regular mouthcare.
Nasal cannula or mask discomfort.	Position or use of cannula and oxygen mask.	Use appropriate size mask.	Ensure correct placement and that the patient is comfortable. Cut off tip of cannulas that protrude into nares to a comfortable length.
Intolerance of oxygen therapy.	Fear and anxiety. Confusion. Hypoxia.	Explain need for therapy and benefit it will have. Allow patients to express their fears/concerns. Encourage relatives/carers to stay with patient.	Assess patient for change. Ensure continual reassurance given to patient. Ensure patient remains orientated to the environment and oxygen device. If intolerant of mask, nasal cannulas may be tolerated. If hypoxic, oxygen may need to be increased.

Problem	Cause	Prevention	Suggested action
Inability to communicate.	Mask makes communication difficult; patient may not hear carer and nurse may not hear patient.	Provide patient with non-verbal means of communication, either pen and paper or symbol board.	Assist patient to move around bed area if not able to go far. Mobilize patient with portable oxygen cylinder if appropriate.
Inability to maintain personal hygiene.	Immobility. On bedrest. Mask restricting independence.	Provide patient with hygiene wipes or offer assistance if unable to meet own hygiene needs.	Provide reassurance for patient to remain independent where able. Allow them to carry out their own hygiene if able or help patient with hygiene if not.
Inability to maintain safe environment.	Detachment of oxygen from flowmeter. Kinked or looped oxygen tubing. Mask removed by patient.	Pulse oximeter with audible alarm.	Ensure oxygen attached to flowmeter. Check patient regularly. Ensure no kinks or loops arise. Ensure patient is attached to oxygen.

POST-PROCEDURAL CONSIDERATIONS

Immediate care

Explain the reasons for oxygen therapy and the benefits of keeping the device in place until further review. Allow opportunities to express discomfort. Document what percentage of oxygen was commenced and the patient's related observations, and continue to monitor the patient's respiratory status as frequently as necessary.

Ongoing care

For patients requiring oxygen therapy for more than 24 hours or when the patient reports discomfort due to dryness, humidification should be commenced to protect airway defences (Dysart et al. 2009, Ward and Park 2000) as well as for the general comfort of the patient.

Encouraging patients to sit out in chairs rather than lying or even sitting up in bed will help prevent atelectasis and aid removal of secretions. Ensuring that post-operative patients have effective pain relief will allow for early ambulation, as well as deep breathing and other basic exercises which will help prevent post-operative atelectasis or possible chest infections (Shelledy and Mikles 2002).

Accurate and frequent monitoring of vital signs and recording of observations as well as oxygen concentration and flow rates administered to the patient in conjunction with a track and trigger scoring system (e.g. NEWS) allow for early identification and referral of patients at risk of deterioration (NICE 2007, RCP 2012).

Weaning from oxygen therapy

Titrate or reduce oxygen therapy dose if the patient is clinically stable and the oxygen saturation has been in the upper zone of the target range for some time (usually 4–8 hours). Observe the patient 5 minutes after lowering the dose of oxygen therapy and document. Discontinue oxygen therapy once the patient is clinically stable on the lowest dose oxygen and the target saturations are maintained within the desired range on two consecutive observations or as per written protocol of timed oxygen. Post-operative patients may require oxygen administration whilst on intravenous opiate, patient-controlled analgesia (BTS 2008).

Documentation

Baseline vital signs and oxygen flow rates or concentrations administered as well as the patient's response to therapy must be recorded on the patient's observation chart (NICE 2007). All patients on oxygen therapy should have an added score of 2 documented on NEWS scording on the vital signs observation chart (RCP 2012).

Education of patient and relevant others

Patients should be educated regarding the necessity of keeping their oxygen masks on, and ambulatory patients must recommence oxygen with the help of nurses after mobilizing.

Before sending a patient home on oxygen, healthcare providers must be sure the patient and family members understand the dangers of smoking in an oxygen-enriched environment. An increased amount of oxygen in the environment increases the speed at which things burn once a fire starts. Oxygen can saturate clothing, fabric, hair, beards and anything in the area. Even flame-retardant clothing can burn when the oxygen content increases. It is important to keep all flames and heat sources away from oxygen containers and oxygen systems. Patients should be advised never to smoke or light a match while using oxygen or allow others in the same room to do so. Patients should also be advised not to smoke in bed. Every home should have at least one working smoke detector on every level and near all bedrooms. As many people on home oxygen therapy have limited mobility, home sprinkler systems can add an extra layer of protection (www.gov.uk/firekills). They also need to inform their home and car insurers that oxygen therapy will be used, as well as the local Fire Brigade. They should be reassured that a full written package of training on safe use and storage of equipment will be provided by the contractor supplying their home oxygen.

COMPLICATIONS

Carbon dioxide narcosis

Carbon dioxide is the chemical that most directly influences respiration by its effect on the efficiency of alveolar ventilation. The normal partial pressure of carbon dioxide in the blood is 4.0–6.0 kPa (30–45 mmHg). When this level rises, the pH of the CSF drops which in turn causes excitation of the central chemoreceptors, and hyperventilation occurs (Marieb et al. 2012).

In people who always retain carbon dioxide and are therefore usually hypercapnic because of chronic pulmonary disease such as chronic bronchitis, the chemoreceptors are no longer sensitive to a raised level of carbon dioxide. In these cases the falling PaO_2 becomes the principal respiratory stimulus (the hypoxic drive) (Marieb et al. 2012). Therefore, if a high level of supplementary oxygen was delivered to such patients in non-emergency situations, severe respiratory depression would ensue and ultimately unconsciousness and death. The Resuscitation Council UK and British Thoracic Society advise the administration of high-flow oxygen during an acute respiratory distress or arrest situation. Start with 15 litres of oxygen per minute and wean down to the flow rate required to maintain adequate peripheral saturations of 94–98% (O'Driscoll et al. 2008).

Oxygen toxicity
Pulmonary toxicity following prolonged higher percentages of oxygen therapy is recognized clinically, but there is still much to be learnt about the condition. The degree of injury is related to the length of time and percentage of oxygen to which the individual is exposed. The pattern is one of decreasing lung compliance as a result of a sequence of events, tracheal bronchial inflammation, haemorrhagic interstitial and intra-alveolar oedema, leading ultimately to fibrosis (Winslow 2013).

Where possible, long periods (i.e. 24 hours or more) of oxygen therapy above 50% should be avoided (Winslow 2013).

Retrolental fibroplasia
Retrolental fibroplasia is a disease affecting premature babies who weigh under 1200 g (about 28 weeks' gestation) if they are exposed to high concentrations of oxygen within the first 3–4 weeks of life. It appears that the oxygen stimulates immature blood vessels in the eye to vasoconstrict and obliterate, which results in neovascularization, accompanied by haemorrhage, fibrosis and then retinal detachment and blindness (Bersten et al. 2009, Pierce 1995).

Humidification

DEFINITION
Humidity is the amount of water vapour present in a gas. The terms used to define humidity are absolute humidity, maximum capacity and relative humidity. *Absolute humidity* is the mass of water vapour that a given volume of gas can carry at a set temperature. When a gas is at its *maximum capacity*, it is said to be fully saturated. *Relative humidity* is the ratio of the absolute humidity to the maximum capacity. The warmer the gas, the more vapour it can hold but if the temperature of the gas falls, water held as vapour will condense out of the gas into the surrounding atmosphere (Khan and O'Driscoll 2004, O'Driscoll et al. 2008).

ANATOMY AND PHYSIOLOGY
The respiratory tract is lined with ciliated epithelial cells that secrete mucus. Each cell has about 200 hair-like structures known as cilia, whose role is to remove unwanted mucus and secretions. Less than optimal humidification results in the reduction of adequate ciliary activity and can lead to squamous epithelial changes, dehydration with thickening of secretions, atelectasis and heat loss (Jenkins and Tortora 2013).

The provision of humidification and heat can improve patient tolerance of oxygen therapy and minimize symptoms of dryness. It also reduces the metabolic cost of gas conditioning and, through adequate gas flow, improves lung and airway mechanics (Chanques et al. 2009, Lenglet et al. 2012).

RELATED THEORY
Normal room air has an approximate temperature of 22°C with a relative humidity of 50% and a water content of 10 mgH_2O. For effective gas exchange to occur in the lungs, the air would need to be at a temperature of 37°C with 100% humidity and a water content of 44 mgH_2O per litre by the time it reaches the bifurcation in the trachea, which is referred to as the isothermic point. When the temperature falls below 37°C and humidity falls below 100%, several changes take place in the airways. The mucus that collects in the airways thickens and movement of the cilia is reduced. If there is no improvement, the mucus will become thicker and immobile; the cilia will also lose their mobility so clearance of all secretions will stop and infection can set in (Marieb et al. 2012).

If there is a continuing lack of humidity further damage occurs. The cilia can break off, causing damage to the mucosal lining of the respiratory tract. The isothermic point of saturation moves from the bifurcation of the trachea to a lower point in the lungs, resulting in further damage which can lead to collapse of the alveoli, decrease in lung function and hypoxaemia (Jenkins and Tortora 2013, O'Driscoll et al. 2008).

EVIDENCE-BASED APPROACHES
Many devices can be used to supply humidification; the best of these will fulfil the following requirements.

- The inspired gas must be delivered to the trachea at a room temperature of 32–36°C with 100% humidity and should have a water content of 33–43 g/m^3 (Bersten et al. 2009).
- The set temperature should remain constant; humidification and temperature should not be affected by large ranges of flow.
- The device should have a safety and alarm system to guard against overheating, overhydration and electric shocks.
- It is important that the appliance should not increase resistance or affect the compliance of respiration.
- It is essential that whichever device is selected, wide-bore tubing (elephant tubing) is used to allow efficient formation of water vapour (BTS 2008) (see Figure 9.7c).

Rationale
Inhalation of oxygen, which is a dry gas, used during respiratory therapy can cause evaporation of water from the respiratory tract and damage of the mucosal lining if humidification is not provided. In patients who are intubated or have a tracheostomy, the natural pathway of humidification is bypassed (Branson and Gentile 2010).

Indications

- Used for mechanical ventilation and non-invasive ventilation such as CPAP/non-invasive positive end-expiration (NIPEE).

Contraindications

- There are no contraindications to humidification, though the device chosen will depend upon type of oxygen therapy, tenacity of secretions and the patient's clinical condition (i.e. mechanical ventilation, self-ventilating at home, etc.).
- Humidification should not be used for patients requiring open system (mask) ventilation when 'droplet contact' isolation precautions are required.

Anticipated patient outcomes
The provision of adequate humidification of gases enabling clearance of secretions, a reduction in the tenacity of secretions and improved gas exchange. The patient's airway is to remain patent at all times.

PRE-PROCEDURAL CONSIDERATIONS

Equipment

Heat and moisture exchanger (HME)
During ventilatory humidification an HME performs the function of the nose and pharynx in conditioning the inspired air. It works passively by retaining heat and moisture from the expired air and returns it to the patient in the next inspired breath (Chiumello et al. 2004, Restrepo and Walsh 2012). HMEs may contain a bacterial filter and consist of spun, pleated, highly thermal conductive material (Figure 9.8). A type of HME known as an artificial or 'Swedish' nose (Figure 9.9) can be used in a self-ventilating patient with a tracheostomy who is being weaned from oxygen. It can also be used in ventilated patients, inserted between the patient's airway and the ventilator circuit.

Figure 9.8 Heat and moisture exchanger (HME).

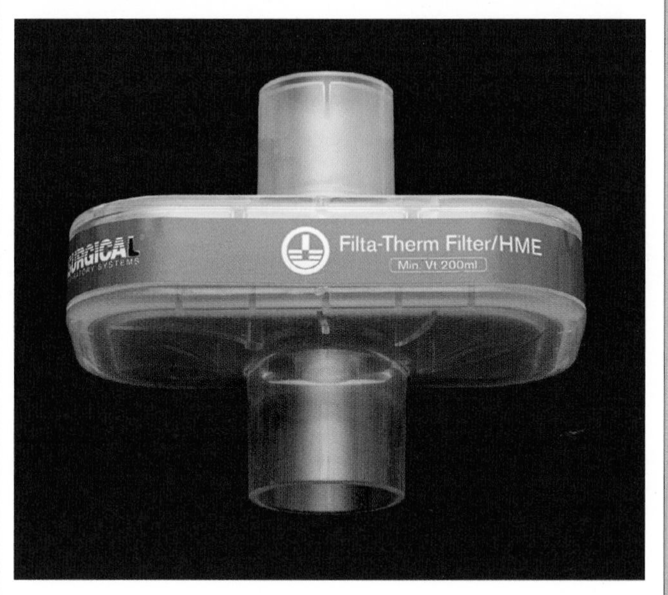

Figure 9.9 Swedish nose.

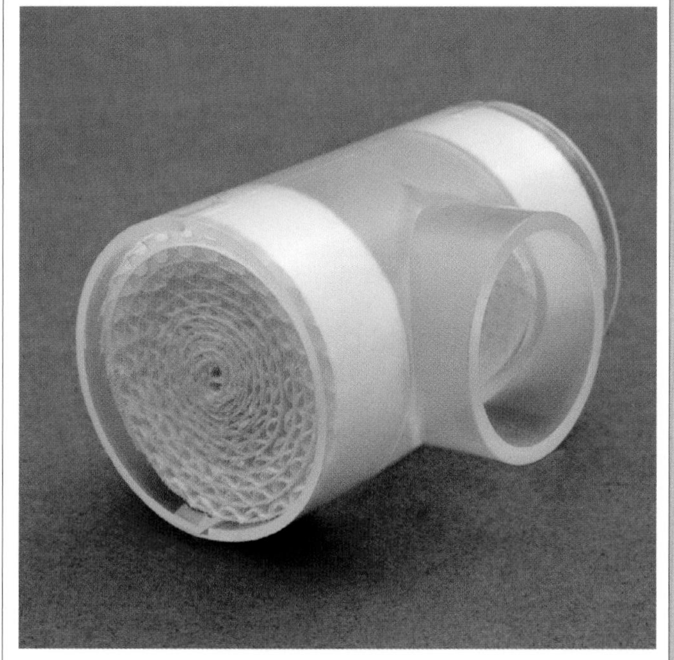

Cold water bubble humidifier

This device (Figure 9.10) delivers partially humidified oxygen at about 50% relative humidity. Gas is either forced across or bubbled through water at room temperature. This method is not advised as it is inefficient (Bersten et al. 2009).

Water humidification chamber

With these devices, inspired gas is forced over, or through, a heated reservoir of water (water humidification chamber)

Figure 9.10 Cold water bubble humidifier.

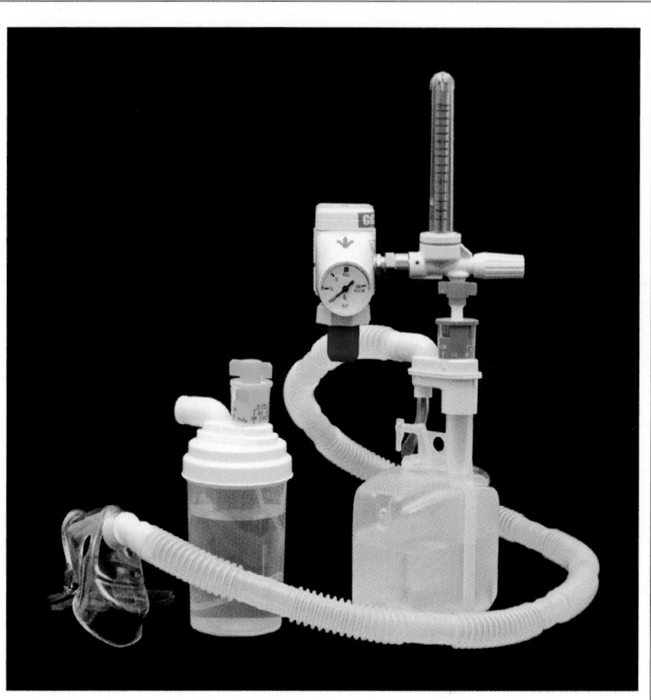

(see Figure 9.7d). To achieve an adequate humidity for the patient, the water bath must reach a set temperature. The gas will then cool as it moves down the breathing circuit to the patient, and a relative humidity of 100% will be reached. Hot water bath humidifiers are therefore very efficient and useful for humidification for immobile patients, particularly if they are receiving mechanical ventilatory support. However, they have three main disadvantages.

- Danger of overheating and causing damage to the trachea.
- Their efficiency can alter with changes in gas flow rate, surface area and the water temperature.
- Condensation can form collections of contaminated water in the oxygen delivery tubes and can wash colonized biofilm from the inner lumen of the tracheal tube towards the patient (Mackenzie 2008).

Aerosol generators

These devices are not governed by temperature but provide microdroplets of water suspended in the gas (Bersten et al. 2009). The gas provided through aerosol devices can be very highly saturated with water. There are three main types of aerosol humidifier.

- Gas-drive nebulizer
- Mechanical (spinning disc) nebulizer
- Ultrasonic nebulizer

These devices are useful for the spontaneously breathing patient with chronic chest disease.

Procedure guideline 9.2 **Humidification for respiratory therapy**

Various humidifiers exist. Select the system most appropriate for the patient.

Essential equipment

- Water humidification chamber (see Figure 9.7d)
- Heating equipment
- Oxygen (elephant) tubing (see Figure 9.7c)
- Oxygen analyser (see Figure 9.7a)
- Sterile H_2O bottle or bag depending on type of humidifier used

Pre-procedure

Action	Rationale
1 Discuss with the patient's doctor the choice of system to be used.	To ensure the most appropriate device is selected to meet the patient's needs. **E**
2 Explain to the patient the reason for use of the humidifier and how it works.	To enable the patient to understand what is happening and to be able to tolerate the humidification. **E**

Procedure

Action	Rationale
3 Prepare the device to be used (although some circuits are ready prepared with humidifier).	To ensure the circuit is in working condition and patent to oxygen flow. **E**
(a) Prepare humidifier and circuit. (b) Attach humidifier/wide-bore oxygen tubing; ensure minimal length of tubing, water trap and mask.	Connecting all equipment to oxygen and mask and ensuring all connections are secure. **E** To reduce dead space from excess tubing. **E**
4 Once the circuit is set up, run the system to check it is functioning correctly and the circuit is intact and check oxygen delivered through the oxygen analyser.	To ensure that oxygen is being delivered through the circuit as set. **E** To ensure the system is humidifying the oxygen and that no leaks exist, which causes suboptimal oxygen delivery to the patient (BTS 2008, **C**; Intersurgical 2009, **C**; MDA 2000, **C**).
5 If the hot water system is in use, check it is running within recommended temperature range and attach to patient.	To ensure no damage to the patient's lungs if temperature above range. **E**
6 Check water is present in water source of system; do not allow to run dry.	To aid adequate delivery of humidity to the patient and prevent damage to the humidifier. **E**
7 Position the circuit tubing below the patient.	To ensure collection of humidity in the circuit is able to drain into the water trap or circuit rather than into the patient. **E**
8 Ask the patient if they find the humidification comfortable.	To ensure patient comfort. **E**

Post-procedure

Action	Rationale
9 Monitor the running of the system.	To ensure the system is functioning adequately and delivering humidity (MDA 2000, **C**).
10 Reassure the patient as they may find the system noisy and the excessive moisture in the circuit difficult to cope with.	To allow patient to adjust to the feel of the mask, preventing anxiety and panic at the initial increase of work of breathing (Moser and Chung 2003, **E**).
11 Assess the tenacity of secretions on a regular basis, and document all findings.	To assess how effective the choice of humidification device has been. **E**. This will enable the same care to be continued or an alternative method to be evaluated. Documentation is imperative to the multidisciplinary approach to allow for ongoing best practice (Woodrow 2002, **E**).
12 Change the humidification and circuit on a weekly basis, and document.	To prevent contamination of equipment and minimize the risk of infection (Demers 2002, **E**).

Problem-solving table 9.2 **Prevention and resolution (Procedure guideline 9.2)**

Problem	Cause	Prevention	Suggested action
Potential blockage of humidifier.	Kinking of oxygen tubing or secretions in humidification filter.	Change filter 4–6 hourly or more frequently for patients with copious secretions. Administer 0.9% sodium chloride nebulizers if prescribed to loosen secretions. Check tubing not kinked underneath the patient.	Encourage patient to cough and expectorate if able or remove secretions by suction if patient unable to do so. Ensure tubing is not too long which would allow kinking.

COMPLICATIONS
Possible contamination of water in humidification if the tubing collects water and it is reintroduced into the humidification chamber. This chamber provides the perfect environment for contaminants to grow as it is moist and warm (Demers 2002).

High-flow oxygen therapy

DEFINITION
High-flow oxygen therapy (HFOT) (Figure 9.11) is the provision of high-flow, heated and humidified oxygen therapy to the patient through a wide-bore nasal cannula, facemask, tracheostomy mask or tracheostomy tube (Waugh and Granger 2004).

EVIDENCE-BASED APPROACHES
High-flow oxygen therapy allows the accurate delivery of oxygen therapy of up to 100% FiO_2 at a flow rate of up to 60 L/min (system dependent), previously unfeasible via conventional methods of oxygenation (15 L via a non-rebreathable facemask and 6 L via a nasal cannula) (O'Driscoll et al. 2008). Higher flow rates are of particular benefit for patients with hypoxaemic respiratory failure who have greater inspiratory flow requirements. HFOT can meet or exceed the patient's demand, minimizing the risk of air dilution and the inaccurate delivery of oxygen (Masclans and Roca 2012, Sztrymf et al. 2012). Invariably, oxygenation and work of breathing improve (Roca et al. 2010).

High-flow oxygen therapy emulates the temperature and humidity of a healthy adult lung (37°C and 44 mg/L H_2O), optimizing mucociliary clearance by preserving the function of the ciliated mucosa, reducing the risk of respiratory tract infections and ensuring good oxygenation and ventilation. HFOT also reduces dryness of the upper airway mucosa (Cuquemelle et al. 2012).

Although research on the effects of HFOT is limited, several studies have shown that high-flow nasal therapy helps to flush out the anatomical dead space, increasing the alveolar ventilation over minute ventilation. It also provides low levels of positive end-expiratory airway pressure which aid alveolar recruitment and reduce atelectasis formation (Dysart et al. 2009, Groves and Tobin 2007, Masclans and Roca 2012, Parke et al. 2007).

The nasal cannula allows the patient to communicate freely and does not interfere with daily activities such as speaking, eating and drinking, thereby increasing patient compliance (Roca et al. 2010, Tiruvoipati et al. 2010).

High-flow oxygen therapy can be used as a step between conventional oxygen therapy, non-invasive ventilation or mechanical ventilation, allowing the patient to receive level 2 care on the ward setting and possibly prevent admission to the intensive therapy unit (ITU) (Sztrymf et al. 2011). It can also help to wean patients off non-invasive or mechanical ventilation, facilitating earlier discharge from the ITU back to the ward.

Figure 9.11 **High-flow Optiflow circuit.**

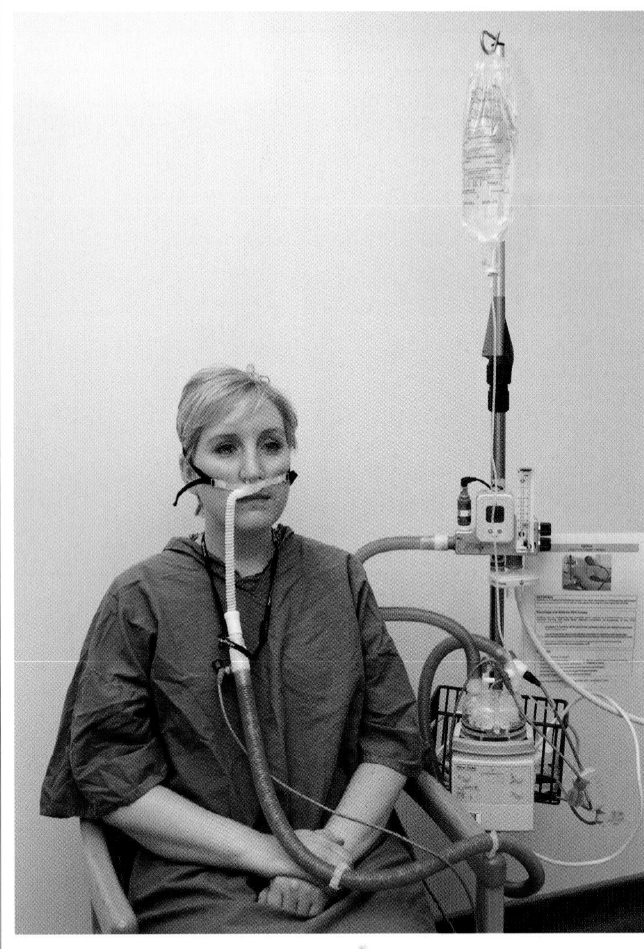

Indications

- Mild-to-moderate hypoxaemic respiratory failure.
- Difficulty clearing secretions.
- Respiratory wean.
- Symptomatic breathlessness (Hui et al. 2013, Ritchie et al. 2011, Sztrymf et al. 2011).

Contraindications

There are no documented absolute contraindications but relative contraindications may include:

- upper gastrointestinal or head and neck surgery and cancers
- obstructed nasopharynx
- haemoptysis or uncontrolled oral or nasal bleeding
- deranged clotting.

Procedure guideline 9.3 **High-flow oxygen therapy**

Essential equipment

- Oxygen supply
- Drip stand
- Air/O_2 blender
- Oxygen analyser (see Figure 9.7a)
- Heating equipment
- Water humidification chamber (see Figure 9.7d)
- Breathing circuit
- High-flow oxygen nasal cannula, mask or tracheostomy attachment
- HME/bacterial filter (see Figure 9.9)
- Bag of sterile water (see Figure 9.11)

(continued)

Procedure guideline 9.3 High-flow oxygen therapy *(continued)*

Pre-procedure

Action	Rationale
1 Assess the patient using patient assessment, vital signs and ABG measurements to decide whether HFOT is indicated.	To determine if patient is hypoxaemic (O'Driscoll et al. 2008,**C**).
2 Explain the principles of HFOT to the patient and family and gain consent.	To increase patient knowledge, minimize anxiety, gain consent and aid patient compliance (NMC 2013, **C**).
3 Obtain and document patient's observations prior to commencing HFOT: (a) Respiratory rate (b) SpO_2 (c) Heart rate (d) Blood pressure (e) Temperature (f) EWS/NEWS	To provide baseline observations prior to commencing oxygen therapy. **E**
4 Ensure patient is sitting upright and in a comfortable position.	To promote comfort and aid lung expansion and breathing (O'Driscoll et al. 2008, **C**).

Procedure

Action	Rationale
5 Set up HFOT as per manufacturer's instructions and attach sterile water bag to water humidification chamber (see Figure 9.11).	Adhering to manufacturer's guidelines ensures the safe and correct use of equipment. **E**
6 Turn on water humidifier and allow it to reach minimum temperature (37°C).	To warm the water in the chamber. **E**
7 Calibrate oxygen analyser (see Figure 9.7a) to room air (21%).	To ensure an accurate reading of the oxygen concentration which is to be delivered. **E**
8 Set desired flow rate and oxygen concentration.	To enable the delivery of blended air and oxygen at a high flow. **E**
9 Place the nasal cannula, facemask or tracheostomy attachment onto the patient and tighten the straps.	To ensure the fit is snug and comfortable. Uncomfortable devices will result in poor patient compliance. **E**
10 Monitor vital signs and EWS/NEWS for first 5 minutes after therapy is started.	To detect any deterioration in the patient's condition (O'Driscoll et al. 2008, **C**).
11 Document the indication for HFOT, the patient's vital signs, the target oxygen saturation and the set FiO_2 and flow rate.	Aim for saturations of 95% for most acutely unwell patients, and 88–92% for those at risk of hypercapnic respiratory failure (O'Driscoll et al. 2008, **C**). To maintain accurate records (NMC 2010, **C**) and ensure continuity of care.

Post-procedure

Action	Rationale
12 Continue to monitor and document vital signs and EWS/NEWS at least 4 hourly or more frequently if unstable.	To monitor for signs of deterioration (O'Driscoll et al. 2008, **C**).
13 Escalate any problems regarding equipment or patient to an appropriate member of staff (e.g. senior nursing staff, critical care outreach team, medical staff or physiotherapists).	To ensure equipment is working properly. **E** To prevent patient deterioration (NICE 2007, **C**).
14 Monitor patient's response to HFOT and wean flow or oxygen as per senior nursing/medical staff advice.	To reduce oxygen as per patient's requirements (O'Driscoll et al. 2008, **C**).
15 Check equipment regularly (e.g. 4 hourly) to ensure the correct flow and oxygen concentration are being administered.	To ensure patient is not being over- or underoxygenated. **E**
16 Check tubing regularly to ensure it is free from trapped water. If found, lift tubing and drain water back into the water humidification chamber.	Trapped water will result in poor delivery of the oxygen therapy. **E**
17 Replace bag of sterile water approximately every 12 hours or as required so that the water humidification chamber does not dry out.	Drying out will cause an increase in the temperature of unhumidified air/oxygen being delivered which may damage the patient's airway. **E** Drying out of the water chamber may damage equipment. **E**

Problem-solving table 9.3 **Prevention and resolution (Procedure guideline 9.3)**

Problem	Cause	Prevention	Action
The oxygen analyser shows fluctuating oxygen concentrations.	The oxygen was turned on before the flow during the initial set-up. The tubing is logged with water.	Turn on the flow first, and then increase the oxygen to get the desired oxygen concentration. Check the tubing regularly.	Hold tubing upright to allow any logged water to flow back into the water chamber.
The patient is unable to tolerate the high flow of air/oxygen.		Explain the rationale for the high flow to the patient as this may aid compliance.	Reduce flow but continue to monitor vital signs, in particular SpO_2, respiratory rate and work of breathing.
The patient complains that the air/oxygen is too warm.		Explain to the patient that the air/oxygen will be warm, as this may aid compliance.	Change the humidifier setting from invasive mode to non-invasive mode but only if absolutely necessary as the invasive mode ensures optimal temperature and humidity.
The humidifier temperature alarms sounds.	The patient has removed the nasal cannula or mask and the HFOT system has been left on. The temperature/flow probes are not pushed into the circuit properly or have become disconnected. The bag of sterile water has run out.	Turn the HFOT system and humidifier off when not in use.	Check all fittings and connections. Replace the bag of sterile water.

Tracheostomy and laryngectomy care

DEFINITION

A tracheostomy is the surgical creation of an opening (stoma) in the anterior wall of the trachea to facilitate ventilation; this opening is usually maintained by the use of a tracheostomy tube (Figure 9.12a). The opening is commonly made at the level of the second or third cartilaginous ring (McGrath et al. 2012). When a total laryngectomy (the surgical removal of the larynx) is performed, a permanent stoma is formed by stitching the end of the trachea to the skin of the neck (McGrath et al. 2012).

ANATOMY AND PHYSIOLOGY

Figure 9.12a shows the anatomy of the neck. The larynx, situated at the top of the trachea, houses the vocal cords and is the point of transition between the upper and lower airways (Epstein 2009). It is made up of nine cartilage segments, the largest of which is called the thyroid cartilage. Inferior to this is the cricoid cartilage which attaches to the large cylindrical tube/elastic structure known as the trachea. This is usually approximately 11 cm long and is made up of rigid cartilage anteriorly and a posterior membranous portion (Epstein 2009). The trachea then divides at the carina to form the right and left mainstem bronchi of the lungs.

RELATED THEORY

The exact location of the stoma will be determined on an individual basis according to the patient's neck and rationale for tracheostomy. Low stomas (i.e. beyond the third tracheal ring) increase the risk of bleeding from the brachiocephalic trunk, and a tracheostomy that is too close to the cricoid has an increased risk of subglottic stenosis, a condition that is difficult to treat (De Leyn et al. 2007).

EVIDENCE-BASED APPROACHES

Rationale

Indications for a tracheostomy

- The patient has an obstructed upper airway, for example by a foreign object or oedema of the soft tissues.
- The patient is likely to need prolonged artificial ventilation – the tracheostomy reduces the risk of tissue damage and work of breathing by shortening the dead space, therefore promoting the weaning process from artificial ventilation.
- The patient is unable to independently maintain their airway, i.e. those with reduced consciousness levels may be unable to maintain a patent airway or protect from aspiration.
- The patient's bronchial secretions cannot be cleared due to poor cough effort and the patient is therefore at risk of aspiration.
- The patient is undergoing upper airway surgery.
- The patient has undergone a laryngectomy – the stoma will be permanent (McGrath et al. 2012).

Contraindications

The only absolute contraindications for tracheostomy are severe localized sepsis/skin infection, uncontrollable coagulopathy (ICS 2008) or prior major neck surgery which completely obscures the anatomy (De Leyn et al. 2007).

Types of tracheostomy

A *temporary tracheostomy* usually refers to a stoma formed as an elective procedure at the time of major surgery (such as a total glossectomy) (Prior and Russell 2004) (see Figure 9.12b), although percutaneous techniques, performed by the bedside in intensive care units, are becoming commonplace (ICS 2008).

A *permanent tracheostomy* is the creation of a tracheostomy usually following a total laryngectomy (Prior and Russell 2004)

Figure 9.12 (a) Anatomy of the head and neck. (b) Temporary tracheostomy. (c) Permanent tracheostomy.

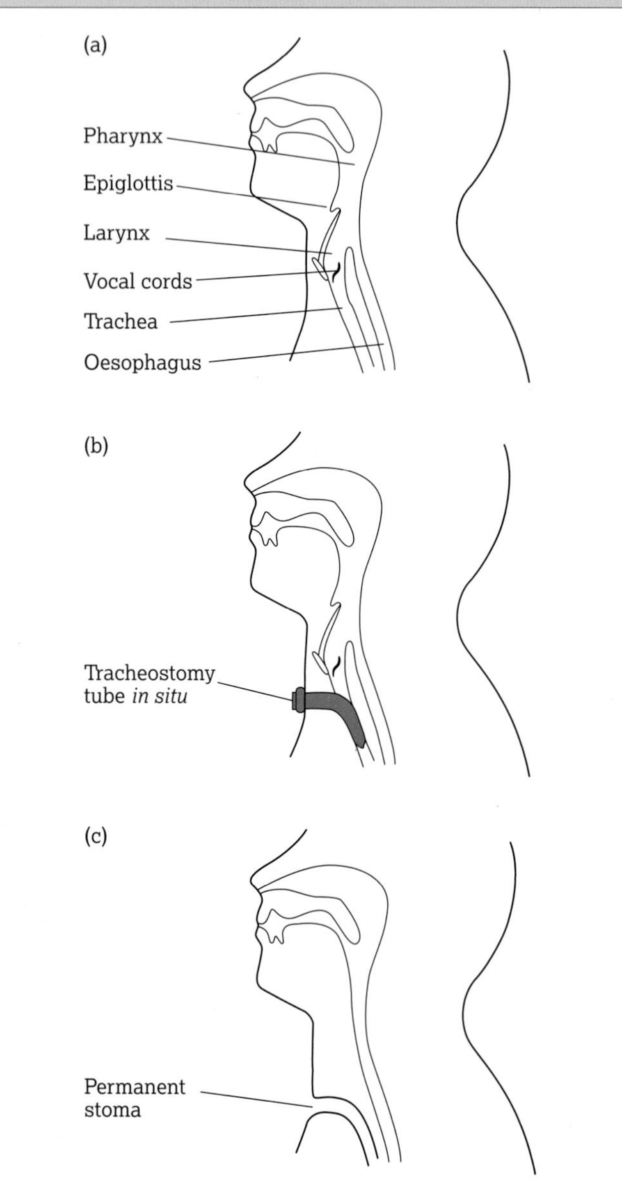

(see Figure 9.12c). The larynx is removed and the trachea is sutured in position to form a permanent stoma, known as a laryngectomy stoma (Clotworthy 2006a). The patient will breathe through this stoma for the remainder of their life. As a result, there is no connection between the nasal passages and the trachea (Edgtton-Winn and Wright 2005).

Percutaneous tracheostomy

The percutaneous method most commonly used is known as percutaneous dilational tracheostomy (PDT) (De Leyn et al. 2007), enabling the pretracheal tissues to be incised under local anaesthesia. A sheath is inserted into the trachea between the cricoid and the first tracheal ring or between the first and second rings. The trachea is progressively dilated with a series of conical dilators, which are slipped over a guidewire, ready for a tracheostomy tube to be inserted. Now frequently performed in the critical care setting as an early intervention post initiation of mechanical ventilation, the procedure takes less time and requires fewer resources, such as theatres and surgeons, resulting in fewer costs, than a surgical tracheostomy (Patel and Matta 2004). Another potential benefit of percutaneous tracheostomy is more rapid stomal closure and smaller scar formation once the tracheostomy tube has been removed (Patel and Matta 2004).

Surgical tracheostomy

Elective surgical tracheostomy is ideally performed in the operating theatre under general anaesthetic, although it can be performed under local anaesthetic (De Leyn et al. 2007). A horizontal incision is made halfway between the sternal notch and the cricoid cartilage (Price 2004). The strap muscles are divided and the thyroid isthmus is retracted/divided, enabling the trachea to be exposed and the tracheal cartilages to be counted. The tracheostomy should be sited over the second and third or third and fourth tracheal cartilages (Price 2004).

LEGAL AND PROFESSIONAL ISSUES

Competencies

The most common problems associated with tracheostomy, in both general wards and critical care, are related to obstruction or displacement (ICS 2008). All hospitals or community settings should have a procedure for managing such situations and all staff involved in the care of the patient must be both aware of the procedure and appropriately trained in either managing the situation or supporting additional staff. At all times, if there is any doubt about the appropriate care that needs to be given, or the management of a situation, call for more senior or emergency help, according to local policy, as soon as possible.

Having emergency equipment readily available is paramount at all times for all types of altered airways (see 'Pre-procedural considerations' for equipment required). All staff caring for the patient should also know the type of tube in place at any one time; this and details of all care provided should be clearly documented.

Managing difficult situations with a tracheostomy is stressful for both the patient and staff, so prevention is always better than cure. All procedures should be undertaken only after approved training, supervised practice and competency assessment, and carried out in accordance with local policies and protocols.

Risk management

The standards within each hospital should be based upon evidence and recommendations from the following sources.

- Intensive Care Society
- St George's Hospital Tracheostomy Guidelines
- National Tracheostomy Safety Project
- Difficult Airway Society
- Fourth National Audit Project (NAP 4)

PRE-PROCEDURAL CONSIDERATIONS

Equipment

The following should always be at the bedside, during transfers or accessible if the patient is self-caring or ambulant.

- Operational oxygen with tracheostomy mask and non-rebreathe mask available.
- Operational suction, checked each shift, with a selection of suction catheters present, including Yankauer suction catheters.
- Sterile water (Serra 2000) can be used to help clear suction tubing of secretions after suctioning has been performed.
- Non-powdered latex-free gloves, aprons and eye protection (Day et al. 2002).
- Two spare cuffed tracheostomy tubes, one the same size as the patient is wearing, the other a size smaller, in case of an emergency tracheostomy tube change (Serra 2000, Tamburri 2000).
- One 10 mL syringe to inflate cuff.

Figure 9.13 Tracheal dilator.

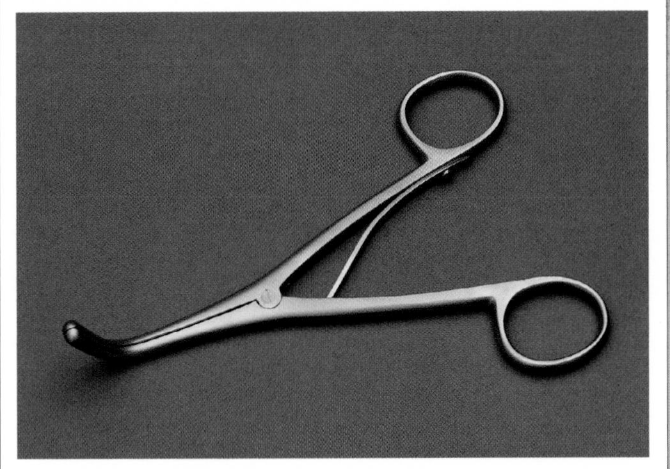

Figure 9.14 Cuff pressure manometer.

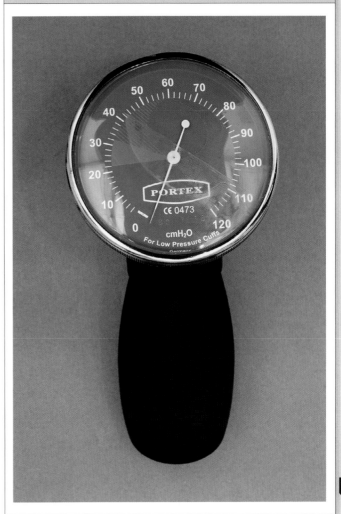

- Tracheal dilators (ICS 2008) (Figure 9.13).
- Spare soft neck ties or tape.
- Suture cutter and lubricating gel.
- Cuff pressure manometer (Serra 2000) (Figure 9.14).
- Readily available resuscitation equipment (ICS 2008) including bag valve mask.
- Tracheostomy tube holder and dressing.
- Catheter mount and tracheostomy disconnection wedge.

It can be useful to have the above equipment in a small 'tracheostomy box' that can remain by the patient's bedside or move with the patient during transfer.

When caring for the patient who has undergone a total laryngectomy, the equipment listed above should always be by the bedside, and in addition the following equipment is recommended.

- Tilley's forceps: these are angled forceps that can be used to remove crusts or plugs of mucus from in and around the stoma.
- Pen torch (or access to a light source).
- Micropore or Elastoplast tape for those patients with a tracheo-oesophageal puncture, to ensure that the catheter keeping the puncture patent is secured firmly with tape or a suture.

Similar to the 'tracheostomy box', it may be useful to have a 'laryngectomy box' readily available by the bedside and for transfers.

Tracheostomy tubes

Tracheostomy tubes are made of either metal or plastic, and therefore vary considerably in rigidity, durability and kink resistance (ICS 2008). Most tubes manufactured now are dual-cannula tracheostomies and are inherently safer and most commonly preferred, particularly for use in acute settings. The outer tube maintains the patency of the airway while the inner tube, which fits snugly inside the outer tube, can be removed for cleaning without disturbing the stoma site. The major advantage of an inner cannula is that it allows immediate relief of life-threatening airway obstruction in the event of blockage of a tracheostomy tube with clots or tenacious secretions. Disposable inner tubes are now available; these single-use items are quicker to use (McGrath et al. 2012) and minimize cross-infection as no cleaning is required.

The majority of tracheostomy tubes are manufactured from plastics of varying types, some of which become softer at body temperature (e.g. polyvinyl chloride construction). Some also have a high-volume, low-pressure cuff which distributes the pressure evenly on the tracheal wall and aims to minimize the risk of tracheal ulceration, necrosis and/or stenosis at the cuff site (ICS 2008, Russell 2004). The cuff when inflated provides a seal between the tube and tracheal wall, enabling effective ventilation and protection of the lower respiratory tract against aspiration (Russell 2004).

Most tubes are sized according to their internal diameter in millimetres, varying also in their length and shape. The size and style of the tube chosen will depend upon the size of the trachea and the needs of the individual patient (Bond et al. 2003, Lewarski 2005, Serra 2000). It is essential that all staff caring for a patient with a tracheostomy know the type of tube in place at any one time, and that this information is readily available and clearly documented in the patient's notes (ICS 2008).

A selection of tube types and commonly seen tubes is described below.

CUFFED TRACHEOSTOMY TUBES

Portex Blue Line and Portex Blue Line Ultra cuffed tracheostomy tubes

These are single-use tracheostomy tubes constructed of siliconized polyvinyl chloride with an introducer and inflatable cuff of 'high-volume/low-pressure' design (Figure 9.15). They are softer and more pliable and are often used when percutaneous tracheostomy is performed in the critical care setting. The cuff

Figure 9.15 **Portex cuffed tube.**

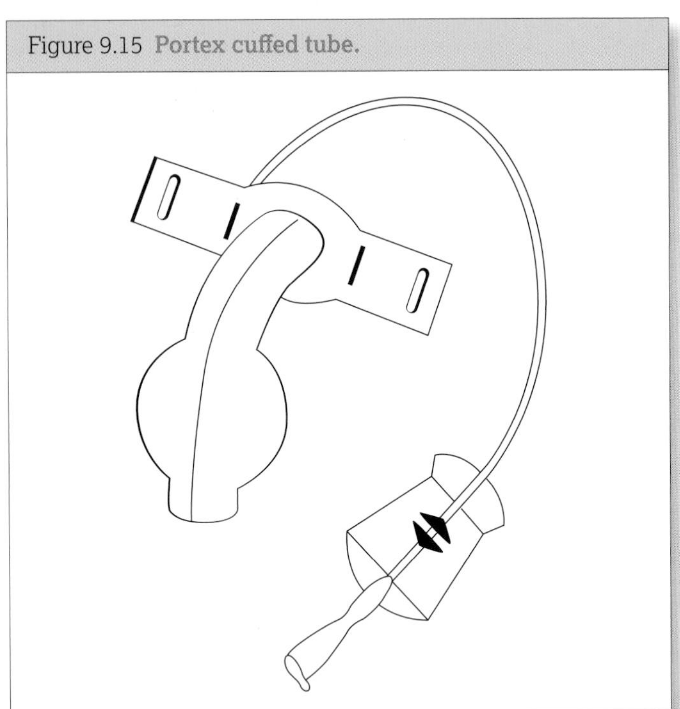

pressure should be monitored regularly. Once the stoma is well-formed, after about 7–10 days, and depending on the patient's specific weaning needs, the Portex tube may be replaced by a more suitable, sturdier tube such as a Shiley tube (Hess 2005).

Shiley cuffed tracheostomy tube

This is a plastic tube with an introducer and one inner tube (Figure 9.16a). The inner tube has the universal 15 mm extension at its upper aspect to facilitate connection to other equipment. The outer tube has an inflatable cuff to give an airtight seal and facilitate ventilation and prevention of aspiration. Shiley tubes are often used in the immediate post-operative phase, that is, at 24–72 hours. As with all cuffed tracheostomies, the internal cuff pressure should not exceed 25 cmH_2O (ICS 2008) and should be monitored on a regular basis. The cuff should be deflated to remove the tube (to prevent mucosal damage and allow the tube to be removed safely) when the patient is eating and drinking, or when a speaking valve or decannulation plug is *in situ* (ICS 2008). Failure to deflate the cuff when a speaking valve or plug is in place will result in complete occlusion of the patient's airway.

CUFFLESS TRACHEOSTOMY TUBES

Shiley cuffless tracheostomy tube

This is a plastic tube with an introducer and two inner tubes (see Figure 9.16b). One inner tube has an extension known as a 15 mm

Figure 9.16 **(a) Shiley cuffed tube. (b) Shiley plain tube. (c) Shiley plain fenestrated tube. (d) Shiley cuffed fenestrated tube.**

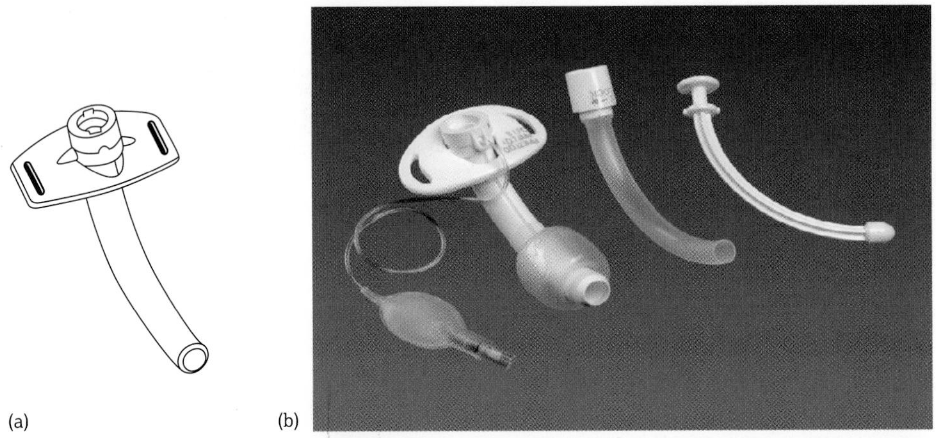

(a) (b)

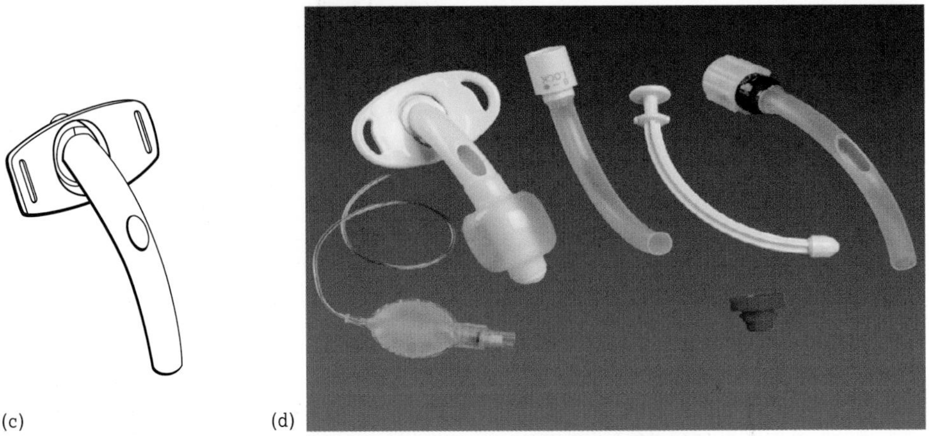

(c) (d)

hub or adaptor at its upper aspect. The majority of tracheostomy tubes used in the hospital setting have the universally sized 15 mm hub to allow attachment to speaking valves and other equipment (Russell 2004). The other tube has no 15 mm hub extension and is less obtrusive and suitable for those patients not requiring attachment to other equipment (Russell 2004).

A cuffless Shiley tube is usually used for the following reasons.

- To keep the tracheostomy tract patent if the patient is going to have further surgery.
- In place of a metal tracheostomy tube if the patient is going to have radiotherapy to the neck area (Prior and Russell 2004). Keeping the metal tube *in situ* during radiotherapy can cause reactions due to interference of the metal with the radiotherapy beam and leads to an increased dose being given to the underlying stoma and surrounding skin (Prior and Russell 2004).
- For a laryngectomy patient who has a benign or malignant stenosis of the trachea and requires a longer tube than the regular length laryngectomy tube to keep the stenosis patent.

FENESTRATED TRACHEOSTOMY TUBES

Shiley fenestrated cuffless tube

The Shiley fenestrated cuffless tube (see Figure 9.16c) is a plastic tube with an introducer and three inner tubes. One inner tube has no hub jutting out, is less obtrusive and is suitable for those patients not requiring attachment to other equipment (Russell 2004). The other two inner tubes have the universal 15 mm extension at the upper aspect to facilitate connection to other apparatus, and one of these (with a green coloured hub) also has a fenestration midway down the tube (the clear or white hubbed inner has no fenestrations down the side and sits flush with the outer tube). This is to encourage the passage of air and secretions into the oral and nasal passages. It is useful when attempting to encourage a return to normal function following long-term use of a temporary tracheostomy, for example enabling the patient to communicate verbally. Fenestrated tubes are not recommended for use following percutaneous tracheostomy or when patients are requiring mechanical ventilation due to a risk of surgical emphysema (ICS 2008).

A fenestrated tube is the most suitable for phonation and weaning. A cap (known as a decannulation plug) is placed onto the tube, occluding the artificial airway. This enables air flow through as well as around the tracheostomy tube, allowing the patient to breathe via the oral and nasal passages again. The cap can be left *in situ* for certain periods of time until the patient can tolerate the tube occluded continuously for an uninterrupted period of time. The Intensive Care Society (ICS 2008) states that this period of time should be a *minimum of 4 hours* uninterrupted, though common practice is 24 hours in ward environments. Once this has occurred, removal of the entire tube, known as decannulation, can be considered (Harkin 2004, Serra 2000). The decannulation procedure should ideally take place in the morning, during normal working hours, to ensure that a specialist assessment can be sought if the patient requires tracheostomy tube reinsertion (Harkin 2004).

Shiley fenestrated cuffed tube

This tube is very similar to the cuffless fenestrated tube although it has an outer cuff to facilitate ventilation and protect against aspiration, and only two inner tubes (see Figure 9.16d). Both inner tubes have the universal 15 mm extension at the upper aspect to facilitate connection to other apparatus, and one of these (with a green coloured hub) also has a fenestration midway down the tube. The outer tube also has a fenestration in the middle of the cannula, again to encourage a return to normal function. The fenestrated tube can also be occluded with a cap, to assess the patient's oral and nasal airway, first ensuring that the *cuff has been completely deflated* and that the fenestrated inner tube is *in situ*. This tube is particularly useful for weaning patients who require both periods of cuff inflation (to protect the airway) and cuff deflation (to enable a speaking valve to be used) (Russell 2004).

Figure 9.17 Kapitex Tracheotwist cuffed fenestrated tube.

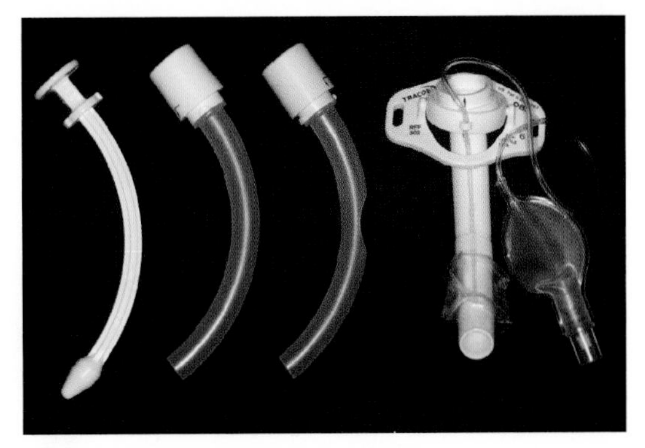

SPECIALIST FUNCTION TUBES

Kapitex Tracheotwist fenestrated tube

This is a plastic tube with an introducer and two inner tubes (Figure 9.17). One of these inner tubes has an extension at its upper end to facilitate connection to other apparatus. The other inner tube has a fenestration midway down the tube, while the outer tube also has a fenestration consisting of a series of small holes. This helps to reduce the risk of granulation tissue growing through the fenestration. The neck plate or flange moves in a vertical and horizontal direction, enabling the plate to move as the patient moves. An inner tube with integrated speaking valve can be ordered separately.

Portex Blue Line Ultra 'Suctionaid' (Figure 9.18) and Tracheotwist 306 tracheostomy tubes

These are specialist tracheostomy tubes that have a facility for aspiration of subglottic secretions. They are mostly used for the prevention of ventilator-associated pneumonia (VAP) in critically ill patients, although they are now also indicated for patients with conditions such as bulbar palsy who are unable to effectively clear secretions accumulating above the tracheostomy tube. Suction should not be applied continuously due to the risk of laryngeal injury (ICS 2008).

Figure 9.18 Portex Blue-Line Suctionaid tracheostomy tube.

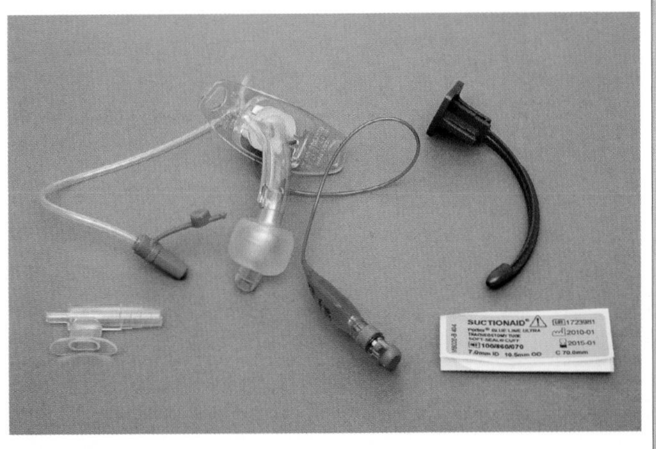

Figure 9.19 (a) Jackson silver tube. (b) Negus silver tube.

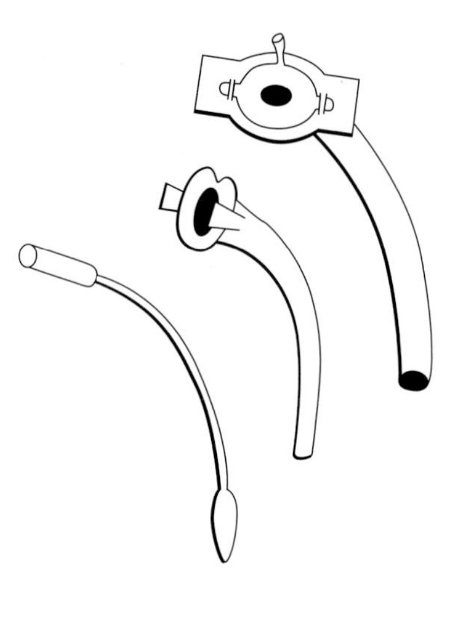

(a)

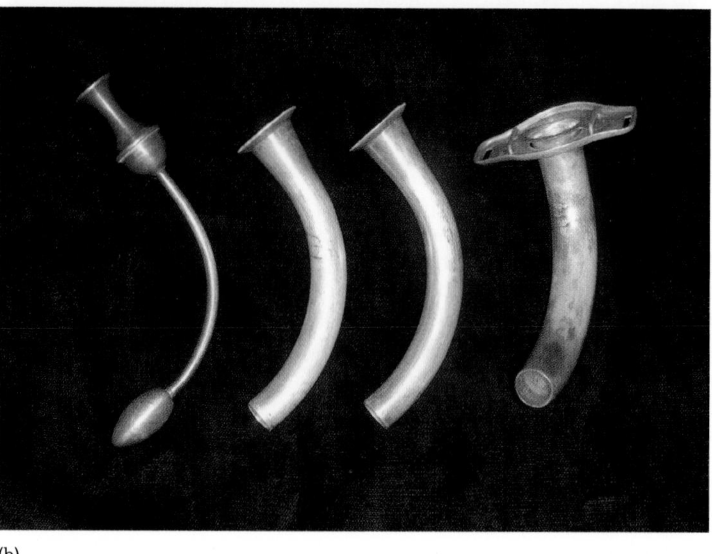

(b)

METAL TUBES

Jackson silver tracheostomy tube

This is a silver tube with an introducer and inner tube (Figure 9.19a). The inner tube is locked in position by a small catch on the outer tube and may be removed and cleaned as necessary without disturbing the outer tube.

Negus silver tracheostomy tube

This is a silver tracheostomy tube with an introducer and a choice of inner tubes, with and without speaking valves (Figure 9.19b). The outer tube does not have a safety catch so the inner tube can at times be coughed out inadvertently.

Learning Activity 9.4

Learning in practice: Tracheostomy and laryngectomy care

If you are working in a clinical area that cares for patients with tracheostomies or permanent laryngectomies, find out what the local procedures are for the care of such patients.

- What emergency equipment should be available?
- Ask the nurse in charge if you can carry out a short audit/check of one or two patients with a tracheostomy/laryngectomy. Do they have the correct emergency equipment available?
- Compare your findings to the list of recommended emergency equipment in this chapter. Are there any differences? Discuss your findings with your mentor/supervising nurse.

Additional tracheostomy supplies

SPEAKING VALVES

These are plastic devices with two-way valves that fit onto the 15 mm hub of the fenestrated inner tube. Distinction should be made between open and closed position valves.

- The open position speaking valve (e.g. Rusch valve) (Figure 9.20) is open by default and closes with positive pressure (expiration) which diverts air through the upper airways past the vocal cords, thus allowing production of a voice.
- The closed position speaking valve (e.g. Passy Muir valve) (Figure 9.21) is closed by default and requires negative pressure (i.e. the patient's inspiratory effort) to open. Once expiration starts, it closes, causing air to be diverted as described above. This type of valve can be used in ventilator circuits, always with cuff deflation, for patients who are mechanically ventilated.

If a non-fenestrated cuffed tube is in place, the cuff should always be deflated before a speaking valve is fitted as the patient will not be able to exhale (Clotworthy 2006b). Ordinarily, practitioners will also consider changing a non-fenestrated tube for a fenestrated tube (double lumen, with fenestrated inner tube). This will allow air to be diverted through the fenestrations of the tube in addition to air already diverted around the tube to the

Figure 9.20 Rusch speaking valve.

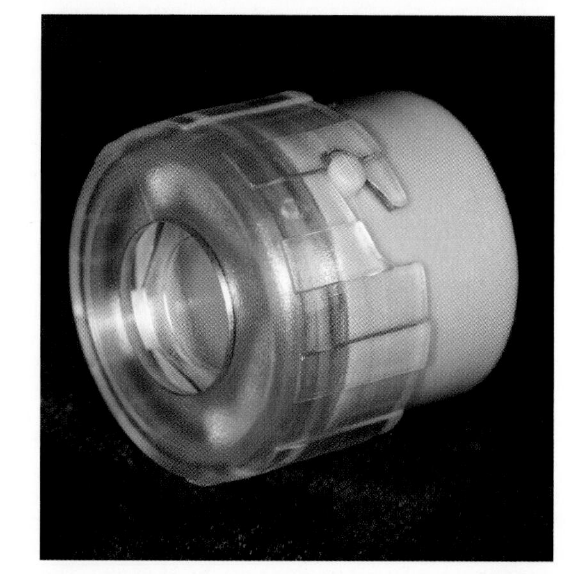

Figure 9.21 Passy Muir valve.

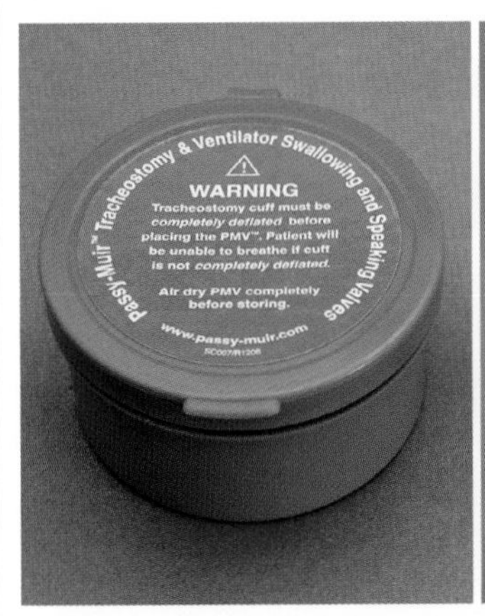

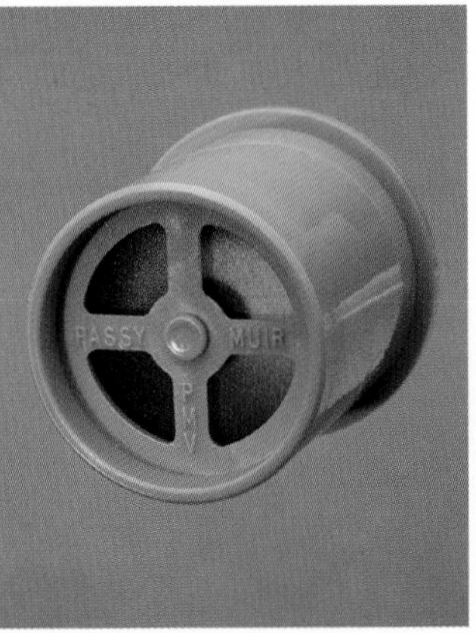

Figure 9.22 Decannulation plug.

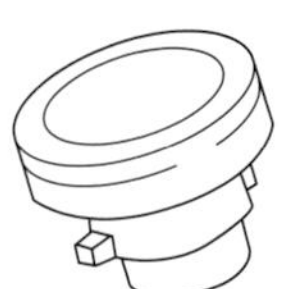

upper airways. If a non-fenestrated tube is in place, depending on the size of the tracheostomy tube and the diameter of the patient's trachea, sufficient air may not be diverted past the cuff. This will result in pressure building up because the patient will not be able to breathe out and the valve will not be tolerated. In this case a complete outer tube change to a fenestrated tube will be necessary.

However, anecdotal evidence from practice (often in critical care environments) would suggest that in some instances, cuff deflation alone (without changing a non-fenestrated tube for a fenestrated tube) may be sufficient to allow air diversion past the cuff through the upper airways as described above. It is important that each individual case is considered carefully and that practitioners weigh up the potential discomfort and distress a complete tracheostomy tube change may cause against the potential risks of fitting a speaking valve on a non-fenestrated tube. It is therefore imperative that, when a speaking valve is used for the first time, the patient is carefully monitored for any signs of respiratory distress. If the patient experiences difficulty in breathing, an inability to vocalize or they begin to sound wheezy or stridulous, the speaking valve should be removed immediately and the patient reassessed (ICS 2008).

DECANNULATION PLUG

This is a small plastic plug which fits into the outer fenestrated tube (Figure 9.22). It is used to encourage patients to divert air around the tube and into the nose and mouth before removal of the tracheostomy tube as described previously. Alternatively, a small plastic plug (Kapitex) or a blind hub (Shiley) can be fitted into or over the inner fenestrated tube. This is particularly useful for patients who are still producing tenacious secretions as the plug or hub can be removed to enable the inner tube to be cleaned (Harkin 2004).

Laryngectomy tubes

Patients who have undergone a total laryngectomy may require a cuffed tracheostomy tube for the first 24–48 hours. The tube stents the often oedematous stoma and the inflated cuff prevents blood-stained secretions from entering the lungs. During the immediate post-operative phase, the decision on whether a tube is required and which type is made by the surgeon (Clotworthy 2006a). For those patients with no tube in place, the nurse must be extremely vigilant, assessing the bare stoma frequently to ensure that it is not at risk of stenosis. A stenosed stoma will restrict the patient's breathing, hinder the removal of secretions and prevent the insertion of a cuffed tube in an emergency situation. Stoma size should be sufficiently large, ideally 20–25 mm in diameter (Rhys Evans et al. 2003), in order to insert a size 6 or above Shiley tracheostomy tube or equivalent. In the longer term, many patients no longer require a tube of any type.

COLLEDGE SILVER LARYNGECTOMY TUBE

This is a silver laryngectomy tube with an introducer (Figure 9.23a). It is often used to dilate a laryngectomy stoma which has stenosed. These tubes can be cleaned, autoclaved and reused.

SHILEY LARYNGECTOMY TUBE

This is a plastic tube with an introducer and inner tube (Figure 9.23b). The inner tube has the universal 15 mm hub enabling attachment to other equipment. It is shorter in length than a tracheostomy tube, thereby conforming to the slightly shorter trachea in the patient who has undergone a total laryngectomy. The inner tube may be removed and cleaned frequently without disturbing the outer tube. It is sometimes worn post-operatively while the stoma is healing to help facilitate a 'neater' shaped stoma.

SHAW SILVER LARYNGECTOMY TUBE

This is a silver laryngectomy tube with an introducer and an inner tube beyond both lower and upper aspects of the outer tube. Thus pressure dressings may be secured without occluding the stoma. The silver catch on the outer tube keeps the inner tube in position (Figure 9.23c).

Stoma button

This is a soft silastic 'button' (Figure 9.23d). It may be used in place of a laryngectomy tube. It is very light and comfortable to wear and can be used in conjunction with a Blom–Singer speaking valve. In order to facilitate the use of the Blom–Singer speaking valve, a diamond shape is cut out of the silastic (see Chapter 4: Communication, for specific information on surgical voice restoration).

Silastic laryngectomy tube

This is a slightly opaque silastic tube which is longer in length in comparison to the stoma button. It is available in 36 and 55 mm lengths and in a variety of different sizes (Figure 9.23e). It is most suitable for patients who experience a degree of stenosis further down the trachea (see Chapter 4: Communication, for further information).

Specific patient preparation

Care of the patient with a tracheostomy requires a multidisciplinary approach. Patients may have issues with pain and discomfort, swallowing, speech, mobility and general care. Speech and language therapists will play a pivotal role in the assessment and management of the patient's impaired swallowing and speech. Specialized physiotherapists are skilled in mobilization rehabilitation (see Chapter 6: Moving and positioning), humidification techniques and general care for tracheostomies. Patients may have difficulty with an altered body image and need psychological support not only from the team closely involved in their care but also potentially from a formal psychological support team. Other key support teams include rehabilitation teams (for

Figure 9.23 **(a) Colledge silver tube. (b) Shiley laryngectomy tube. (c) Shaw laryngectomy tube. (d) Stoma button. (e) Laryngectomy tube.**

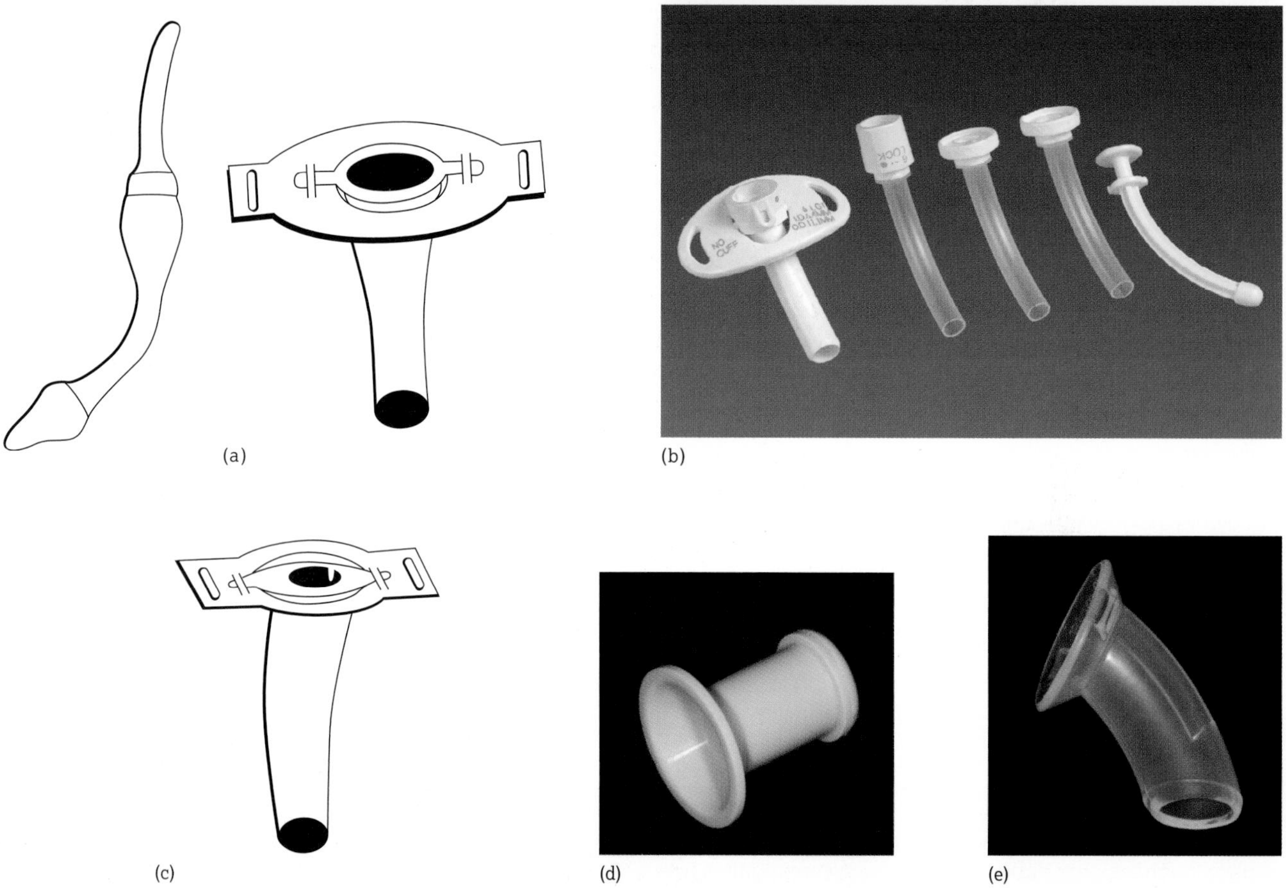

(a) (b)

(c) (d) (e)

rehabilitation, relaxation and occupational therapy), critical care outreach teams (particularly for newly formed stomas in the ward environment and/or the deteriorating patient with airway difficulties), anaesthetists in the event of an airway emergency, discharge co-ordinators and community teams for patients with airways who are going home.

Humidification

Humidification may be required initially while a new stoma adapts to the outside environment. It can be provided for patients requiring low-rate (1–5 L/min) oxygen therapy by using a disposable nebulizer set with sterile 0.9% sodium chloride (approximately 5 mL), attached to the oxygen supply and setting the gas rate for the liquid to form into humidification droplets. The nebulizer is administered using a specific tracheostomy mask (Figure 9.24) rather than via the nose and mouth, as is usual practice. Local policy will determine frequency which may need to be every 4–6 hours or more frequently in patients with more tenacious secretions. 0.9% sodium chloride nebulizers can also be given using air instead of oxygen if the patient is not on oxygen therapy. Patients requiring continual high concentrations of oxygen (≥28%) require humidification via a heated circuit where possible or a cold water Venturi humidified system at all other times (see Figure 9.7, Figure 9.10). Patients no longer requiring oxygen therapy can receive humidification in the form of a HME and a patient with a laryngectomy stoma can effectively humidify using laryngeal stoma protectors that combine protection along with humidification, for example Laryngofoam, Buchanan bib, Romet (McGrath et al. 2012).

Humidification of a tracheostomy is important to prevent drying of the airway which impairs mucus and cilia function, resulting in thickened airway secretions. Devices such as HME filters or a Trachphone (Figure 9.25), which also has an integral speaking valve and oxygen port, may be used for tracheostomy patients (McGrath et al. 2012).

Figure 9.24 **Tracheostomy mask.**

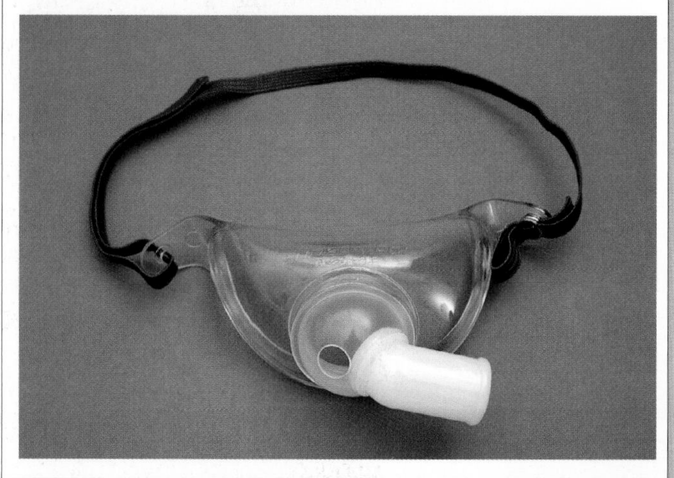

Figure 9.25 Trachphone.

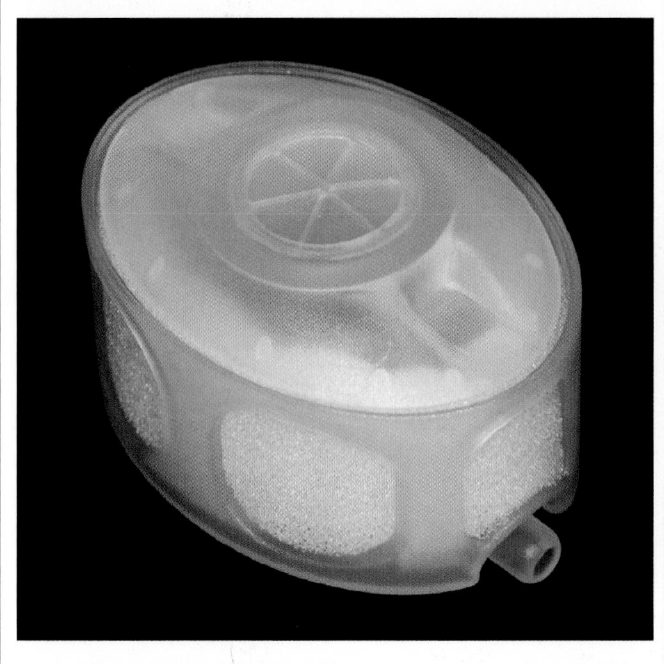

Education

Patient education is paramount to providing quality care. In the initial post-operative/post-procedural phase, this may be purely to aid comfort and relaxation, explaining and stressing the rationale and importance of suctioning, positioning and how to strengthen cough. This will involve a multidisciplinary approach with all members of the team educating, supporting and providing comfort throughout all interventions.

For patients with long-term tracheostomy needs, early education is vital. Supporting an individual with a tracheostomy of any type requires an understanding of the impact the tracheostomy tube has on the patient's airway and knowing how to manage potential complications (Serra 2000). In order to support and teach the patient and/or their carer, staff must confirm whether the tube serves as the primary airway (i.e. a permanent stoma) or if the patient has a functioning upper airway (Bowers and Scase 2007, McGrath et al. 2012).

Patient education will come from various sources but primarily the clinical nurse specialists, nursing staff, physiotherapists and community nursing teams will play pivotal roles. Education will be both practical (i.e. through demonstration with their own tracheostomy, possibly utilizing mirrors) or through the use of posters and pictures. Practical tracheal suctioning on a specialized mannequin and examining the tracheostomy tubes can also be beneficial (McGrath et al. 2012).

Tracheostomy: dressing change

EVIDENCE-BASED APPROACHES

A tracheostomy is a surgical opening into the trachea and hence a potential route of infection, so the area should be kept clean. Tracheostomies can also cause damage to the surrounding tissues through pressure and the presence of irritant secretions (McGrath et al. 2012), necessitating regular inspection and appropriate care of the area to prevent tissue damage and wound breakdown. Changing the dressing will ensure that the surrounding skin remains clean, dry and free from irritation and infection (Edgtton-Winn & Wright 2005).

Rationale

Indications

In some patients, dressing may not be indicated as it creates an ideal environment for bacterial colonization (Higgins 2009). Secretions from the stoma can also cause excoriation around the site. The decision to dress a tracheostomy should be based on clinical need, although a thorough assessment of the stoma is indicated for all patients with altered airways (i.e. tracheostomy or laryngectomy). The dressing around the tracheostomy tube can be renewed without removing the tube, which should be done twice a day or more frequently if necessary (Serra 2000).

Contraindications

Occasionally a surgical team may request that the original dressing remain intact for a period of time, usually 24–48 hours. There may be an increased risk of bleeding associated with the stoma formation and in this instance the dressing should not be changed until consultation with the surgeon has occurred.

Principles of care

Changing the tracheostomy dressing always requires two people (McGrath et al. 2012): one to secure the tracheostomy and the other to assess and dress the stoma site. When assessing the wound, if infection is suspected, that is, the area is reddened, excoriated, painful, discoloured or exudate is present, a microbiology swab should be sent for culture (Higgins 2009, ICS 2008, McGrath et al. 2012).

The stoma should be cleaned thoroughly with 0.9% sodium chloride and an appropriate dressing applied where indicated. This should be a foam dressing, usually manufactured with a cross-shaped incision to fit around the tracheostomy tube (McGrath et al. 2012). For those patients with secretions that tend to accumulate around the stoma, a specialized barrier product can be used to prevent the skin becoming red and excoriated (Hampton 1998).

Stoma sutures (secured to the flange of the tracheostomy tube) are removed on day 7 (day 7–10 if the tracheostomy has been inserted using a percutaneous technique). If the patient has previously received external beam radiotherapy to the neck, stoma sutures are removed on day 10.

Procedure guideline 9.4 **Tracheostomy: dressing change**

This procedures requires two nurses: one to hold the tracheostomy in place and the other to change the dressing.

Essential equipment

- Sterile dressing pack
- Tracheostomy dressing or keyhole dressing
- Cleaning solution, such as 0.9% sodium chloride
- Tracheostomy securing tapes
- Bactericidal alcohol handrub

Medicinal products

- Review a possible need for analgesia

(continued)

Procedure guideline 9.4 Tracheostomy: dressing change *(continued)*

Pre-procedure

Action	Rationale
1 Explain and discuss the procedure with the patient.	To ensure that the patient understands the procedure and gives their valid consent (NMC 2013, **C**).
2 Screen the bed or cubicle.	To ensure the patient's privacy. **E**
3 Wash hands using bactericidal soap and water or bactericidal alcohol handrub, and prepare the dressing tray or trolley.	To minimize the risk of infection (Fraise and Bradley 2009, **E**).
4 Perform the procedure using aseptic technique, i.e. apply apron and gloves.	To minimize the risk of infection. **E**
Procedure	
5 Remove the soiled dressing from around the tube, clean around the stoma with 0.9% sodium chloride using low-linting gauze.	To reduce the risk of dressing fragments entering the altered airway (Russell 2005, **E**) and to remove secretions and any crusts.
6 Replace with a tracheostomy dressing or a comfortable foam-backed keyhole dressing (**Action figure 6**).	To ensure the patient's comfort. **E** To avoid pressure from the tube (Scase 2004, **E**).
7 Renew tracheostomy tapes, checking that 1–2 fingers can be placed between the tapes and neck.	To secure the tube. **E** To ensure that the tapes are not too tight (Scase 2004, **E**; Woodrow 2002, **E**) or too loose, thus decreasing the chance of necrosis caused by excessive pressure from the tapes (Serra 2000, **E**).
Post-procedure	
8 Monitor patient closely for changes in respiratory rate and pattern of breathing, pulse, dyspnoea.	Any procedure to the tracheostomy if not managed correctly may lead to possible dislodgement of tube or secretions, leading to respiratory deterioration or distress. **E**

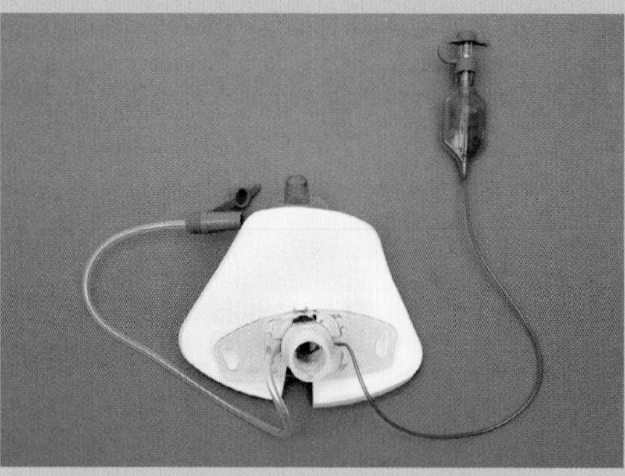

Action Figure 6 Sterile tracheostomy keyhole dressing.

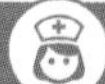

Learning Activity 9.5

Scenario: Tracheostomy dressing change

You have been asked to prepare the equipment required to change the tracheostomy dressing for one of your patients. It is now day 5 following his neck operation, which included the formation of a temporary tracheostomy.

1 Is this a procedure you can do on your own?
2 Make a list of the equipment required.
3 How should you prepare the patient for the procedure?

See the end of the chapter for the answers.

Tracheostomy: suctioning

EVIDENCE-BASED APPROACHES

Rationale

An effective cough requires closure of the glottis, then reopening of the glottis once an adequate intrathoracic pressure is achieved. When a tracheostomy is *in situ*, the mechanism of closing the glottis is compromised, so the patient's ability to remove secretions is reduced as they are unable to generate the high flows required for coughing. In addition to this, the natural mechanisms of warming and humidifying the gases are lost, altering the consistency of secretions. Secretions become thick and dry, inhibiting mucociliary transport (Higgins 2009), leading to a potential blocking of the tracheostomy tube. Tracheal suction is an essential component of managing secretions, maintaining respiratory function and a patent airway.

Indications

The use of routine suctioning should be avoided and careful assessment of the patient's respiratory function should be carried out instead. Inspection, auscultation, percussion and palpation will help to determine the following (Hough 2001, Pryor and Prasad 2008).

- The patient's ability to clear their own secretions.
- Location of any secretions.
- Whether these secretions could be reached by the catheter.
- How detrimental these secretions might be for the patient.

The presence of prominent audible secretions, visible secretions, decreased oxygenation or diminished breath sounds during the assessment would indicate a need for suction (Ireton 2007).

Contraindications

Tracheal suction is an essential component of care for all patients with artificial airways. Most contraindications are relative to the patient's risk of developing adverse reactions or worsening clinical condition as a result of the procedure. Hence choosing to not suction in order to avoid a potential side-effect may sometimes be more harmful to the patient.

However, despite its necessity, suction may be painful and distressing to the patient and can also be complicated by hypoxaemia, bradycardia and cardiovascular compromise (particularly in patients with autonomic dysfunction such as spinal injuries), alveolar collapse, tracheal mucosal damage, bleeding and the introduction of infection (Higgins 2009, ICS 2008).

Principles of care

Infection risk

Universal precautions must be used at all times when suctioning; this includes wearing aprons, gloves and eye protection. Both the caregiver and patient are at risk of infection when suctioning is performed and, in order to minimize this, examination gloves should be worn and an aseptic technique should be used, decontaminating hands with an alcohol handrub before and after the suction procedure (DH 2005). Suction catheters are for single use only and should be disposed of after each suction.

Suction should be performed using aseptic techniques, with the patient upright and in a neutral head alignment.

Method of suctioning

Shallow suctioning, where the catheter is inserted to a premeasured depth not beyond the distal end of the tracheostomy tube, is preferred to deep suctioning, in which the suction catheter is inserted until resistance is met. Deep suctioning should be avoided as it is associated with increased risks of mucosal damage, inflammation (De Leyn et al. 2007) and bleeding, subsequently increasing the risk of airway occlusion. Always suction with the inner tube *in situ* and change to a non-fenestrated inner tube before the procedure. The instillation of 0.9% sodium chloride to 'aid' suctioning is not recommended (Celik and Kanan 2006, ICS 2008). Suction should always be performed with the inner tube *in situ*, and if necessary changed to a non-fenestrated inner tube. The suction catheter should have a diameter no greater than half the internal diameter of the tracheostomy tube; for example, suction catheter size = 2 × (tracheostomy size – 2).

The lowest possible vacuum should be applied to minimize atelectasis. Pre-oxygenation may be necessary in those with high O_2 requirements. The catheter should be inserted approximately 10–15 cm, depending on the length of the tracheostomy tube, before applying suction and slowly withdrawing the catheter. Suction should be applied for a maximum of 10 seconds. The application of 0.9% sodium chloride to 'loosen' or 'aid' suctioning is not recommended (ICS 2011, McGrath et al. 2012).

Any difficulty in passing the suction catheter should lead to the consideration that the tube is blocked or misplaced and requires immediate attention (ICS 2011).

Anticipated patient outcomes

Suctioning can cause distress, is uncomfortable and is associated with airway changes and cardiovascular instability, and should therefore only be performed when indicated and not at fixed intervals. Frequency should be determined on an individual patient basis and suctioning should aim to clear airway secretions when the patient is not able to, ensuring airway patency and patient safety at all times.

Equipment

Suction catheter size and suction pressure

Choosing the correct suction catheter size depends on the size of the tracheostomy tube. As a guide, the diameter of the suction catheter should not exceed one-half of the internal diameter of the tracheostomy tube (Griggs 1998, Hough 2001).

The following formula can be used to determine the correct size catheter.

$$\text{Suction catheter size (Fg)} = 2 \times (\text{size of tracheostomy tube} - 2)$$

$$\text{For example: 8.00mm ID tube}: 2 \times (8 - 2) = 12\ \text{Fg (ICS 2008)}$$

The incorrect choice of catheter, poor technique and the use of an excessively high suction pressure may all lead to mucosal trauma. The lowest possible vacuum pressure should be used, ≤100–120 mmHg (13–16 kPa) to minimize atelectasis (ICS 2008) and mucosal damage.

PRE-PROCEDURAL CONSIDERATIONS

Within a critical care setting, a closed-circuit suction system is an alternative method to the open suction system for patients being mechanically ventilated. This closed system has the catheter sealed in a protective plastic sleeve, which is connected permanently into a standard ventilator circuit, thus preventing the catheter becoming contaminated (Figure 9.26). This also reduces the number of times the patient is disconnected from the ventilator, avoiding further hypoxia and cross-infection. Patients who are immunosuppressed, actively infectious patients or those who require high levels of PEEP may in particular benefit from a closed unit (Billau 2004).

Figure 9.26 **Components of a closed-circuit catheter. The control valve locks the vacuum on or off. The catheter is protected inside an airtight sleeve. A T-piece connects the device to the tracheal tube. The irrigation port allows saline instillation for irrigating the patient's airway or for cleaning the catheter.**

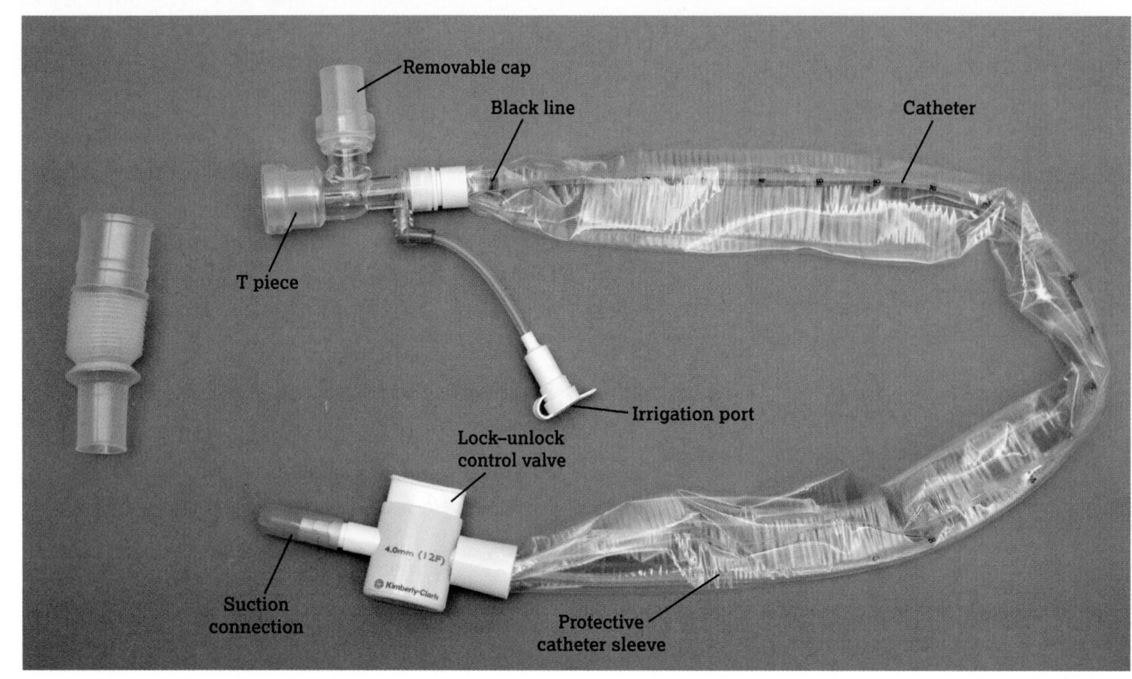

Procedure guideline 9.5 **Tracheostomy: suctioning a patient**

Essential equipment

- Suction source (wall or portable), collection container and tubing, changed every 24 hours to prevent growth of bacteria (Billau 2004)
- Disposable plastic apron
- Eye protection, for example goggles
- Bactericidal alcohol handrub
- Sterile suction catheters (assorted sizes according to tube size)
- A selection of non-sterile, powder-free, clean boxed gloves
- Sterile bottled water (labelled 'suction' with opening date), changed every 24 hours to prevent the growth of bacteria (Billau 2004)

Pre-procedure

Action	Rationale
1 If secretions are tenacious, consider using, as prescribed, 2 hourly or more frequently 0.9% sterile sodium chloride nebulizers or other mucolytic agents such as nebulized acetylcysteine.	Suctioning may not be as effective if the secretions become too tenacious or dry. Anecdotal evidence through practice suggests that frequent 0.9% sterile sodium chloride or acetylcysteine nebulizers may assist in loosening dry and thick secretions. **E**
2 Explain procedure to patient and ensure upright position if possible. If the patient is able to perform their own suction, self-suction should be taught. This is not appropriate in critical care settings.	To obtain the patient's co-operation and to help them relax. **E** The procedure is unpleasant and can be frightening for the patient (Billau 2004, **E**). Reassurance is vital. **E** Self-control of the patient's suction is preferable with long-term stomas, if the patient is able to manage it. **E**
3 If a patient has a fenestrated outer tube, ensure that a plain inner tube is *in situ*, rather than a fenestrated inner tube (Russell 2005).	Suction via a fenestrated inner tube allows a catheter to pass through the fenestration and cause trauma to the tracheal wall (Billau 2004, **E**).

Procedure	
4 Wash hands with bactericidal soap and water or bactericidal alcohol handrub, and put on a disposable plastic apron, disposable gloves and eye protection.	To minimize the risk of cross-infection. **E** Gloves minimize the risk of infection transfer to the catheter or from the sputum to the nurse's hands (Fraise and Bradley 2009, **E**). Some patients may accidentally cough directly ahead at the nurse; standing to one side with tissues at the patient's tracheostomy minimizes this risk. **E**
5 If patient is oxygen dependent, hyperoxygenate for a period of 3 minutes.	To minimize the risk of acute hypoxia (Billau 2004, **E**).
6 Ensure that the suction pressure is set to the appropriate level.	Recommended suction pressure is ≤100–120 mmHg (13–16 kPa) to minimize atelectasis (ICS 2008, **C**).
7 Select the correct size catheter. As a guide, the diameter of the suction catheter should not exceed one-half of the internal diameter of the tracheostomy tube (Griggs 1998, Hough 2001). The following formula can be used to determine the correct size catheter: Suction catheter size (Fg) = 2 × (size of tracheostomy tube – 2) For example: 8.00 mm ID tube: 2 × (8 – 2) = 12 Fg (ICS 2008).	This ensures that hypoxia does not occur while suctioning: the larger the volume, the greater the bore of the tube. **E** Incorrect choice of catheter size can cause mucosal damage. **E** A tube with too small a diameter may not be able to remove thick secretions. **E**
8 Open the end of the suction catheter pack and use the pack to attach the catheter to the suction tubing. Keep the rest of the catheter in the sterile packet. Use an aseptic technique throughout.	To reduce the risk of transferring infection from hands to the catheter and to keep the catheter as clean as possible. **E**
9 An additional clean, disposable glove can be used on the dominant hand at this stage.	To facilitate easy disposal of the suction catheter after suction. **E**
10 Remove the catheter from the sleeve and introduce the catheter to about one-third of its length or approximately 10–15 cm (ICS 2008) or until the patient coughs. If resistance is felt, withdraw catheter approximately 1 cm before applying suction by placing the thumb over the suction port control and slowly withdraw the remainder of the catheter (McGrath et al. 2012).	Gentleness is essential; damage to the tracheal mucosa can lead to trauma and respiratory infection. **E** The catheter should go no further than the carina to prevent trauma (McGrath et al. 2012, **E**). The catheter is inserted with the suction off to reduce the risk of trauma (McGrath et al. 2012, **E**).
11 Do not suction the patient for more than 10 seconds (ICS 2008).	Prolonged suctioning may result in acute hypoxia, cardiac arrhythmias (Day et al. 2002, **E**), mucosal trauma, infection and the patient experiencing a feeling of choking.
12 Wrap catheter around dominant hand, then pull back glove over soiled catheter, thus containing catheter in glove, then discard.	Catheters are used only once to reduce the risk of introducing infection. **E**
13 If the patient is oxygen dependent, reapply oxygen immediately.	To prevent hypoxia. **E**
14 Rinse the suction tubing by dipping its end into the sterile water bottle and applying suction until the solution has rinsed the tubing through.	To loosen secretions that have adhered to the inside of the tube. **E**
15 If the patient requires further suction, repeat the above actions using new gloves and a new catheter. Allow the patient sufficient time to recover between each suction, particularly if oxygen saturation is low or if patient coughs several times during the procedure. The patient should be observed throughout the procedure.	To ensure general condition is stable (Billau 2004, **E**).
16 Repeat the suction until the airway is clear. No more than three suction passes should be made during any one suction episode (Day 2000, Glass and Grap 1995) unless in emergency such as tube occlusion (Nelson 1999).	To minimize the risk of hypoxaemia (Day 2000, **E**).
Post-procedure	
17 Where appropriate, reconnect the patient to oxygen within 10 seconds post suctioning.	To minimize the risk of hypoxaemia (Day 2000, **E**).
18 Observe patient's respiratory rate and pattern, oxygen saturations, heart rate and work of breathing closely over the following 15 minutes. Observe for signs of bleeding.	Suctioning can be complicated by hypoxaemia, bradycardia, tracheal mucosal damage and bleeding (ICS 2008, **C**).

COMPLICATIONS

Hypoxia

The act of suctioning reduces vital lung volume from the lungs and upper airways. Each suctioning procedure should last no longer than 10 seconds to decrease the risk of trauma, hypoxia and other side-effects (ICS 2008). Ventilator disconnection or removal of the oxygen supply will also add to the risk of hypoxia prior to suctioning. Within a critical care setting, this risk can be avoided by hyperoxygenating the lungs with 100% oxygen, either manually or via a ventilator (Glass and Grap 1995, Hough 2001), which should be considered for all patients with high oxygen requirements.

Cardiac arrhythmias

Arrhythmias may be brought about by the onset of hypoxaemia or a vagal reflex instigated by tracheal stimulation by the catheter (MacIntyre and Branson 2009).

Raised intracranial pressure

This may occur if the suction catheter causes excessive tracheal stimulation and results in coughing and an increase in the patient's intrathoracic pressure, both of which compromise cerebral venous drainage (Pryor and Prasad 2008).

Problem-solving table 9.4 **Prevention and resolution (Procedure guidelines 9.4 and 9.5)**

Problem	Cause	Prevention	Suggested action
Profuse tracheal secretions.	Local reaction to tracheostomy tube.	Maintain euvolaemia with adequate and not excessive hydration. Hyoscine can be considered by clinicians to aid in the reduction of excessive secretions following the immediate post-operative phase when excessive secretions are common.	Suction frequently, for example every 1–2 hours, or on clinical need.
Lumen of tracheostomy tube occluded.	Tenacious mucus in tube.	Frequent suction as required and regular inner tube changes. Humidify airways. Encourage coughing to clear secretions from within the tube.	Change the inner tube. Use 0.9% sodium chloride nebulizers, HMEs and suction. Continue to change the inner tube regularly, for example 1–3 hourly.
	Dried blood and mucus in the tube, especially in the post-operative period.	As above.	Provide humidification (see Procedure guideline 9.2). Humidification, administering air if there is no need for oxygen.
Tracheostomy tube dislodged accidentally.	Tapes/ties not secured adequately. Tracheostomy tube not secured adequately by staff during moving and handling of patient.	Ensure tapes secure at all times with 1–2 finger spaces maximum between skin and tapes/ties. Educate patient and staff about safe mobilization of patients with tracheostomy.	Insert spare tube. This should be clean and ready at the bedside (Serra 2000). *Note:* tracheal dilators must be kept at the bedside aof patients with tracheostomies (Serra 2000).
Infection.	Nature of surgery and condition of patient often predispose to infection.	Ensure dressings are changed when soiled and universal infection precautions are adhered to.	Encourage the patient to cough up secretions and/or suction regularly. Change the tube and clean the stoma area frequently, for example 4 hourly. Protect permanent stomas with a bib or gauze. Following result of sputum specimen, commence appropriate antibiotics as needed.

POST-PROCEDURAL CONSIDERATIONS

Documentation

All interventions and care given should be clearly documented in the patient's notes once performed. It is essential that all staff caring for a patient with a tracheostomy know the type of tube in place at any one time, and that this information is readily available and clearly documented in the patient's notes (ICS 2008). As discussed, the use of care plans and bundles may aid in standardizing documentation of patients with a tracheostomy, though this should comply with local policy at all times.

COMPLICATIONS

The main complications associated with tracheostomies are blockage, dislodgement of tracheostomy tube and bleeding at tracheostomy site or inside trachea due to suction injury or coagulopathy, usually presenting with respiratory difficulty. A systematic approach should be adopted and the situation given urgent attention (Box 9.4). When all types of tracheostomies are considered, the likelihood that an airway stoma encountered in an emergency situation is a laryngectomy is between 1 in 20 and 1 in 30. A patient with a tracheostomy is more likely to come to harm by not having oxygen applied to the face if confusion

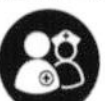 Box 9.4 **Tracheostomy emergency**

- DONT PANIC!
- Call for help – senior medical and nursing staff.
- Reassure patient.
- Assess patency of airway and breathing – is the patient breathing via the nose or mouth? Check oxygen saturations.
- If the airway is not patent it must be cleared immediately ONLY by those with appropriate airway and tracheostomy management experience.
- Multiple attempts to reinsert the tracheostomy should not be made.
- If in doubt, remove the tracheostomy tube and allow the patient to breathe through the mouth/nose (cover the stoma site).
- Apply oxygen masks over both sites of air entry.

Source: Adapted from ICS (2011).

surrounds the nature of the stoma; the default emergency action is therefore to apply oxygen to the face and the stoma for all neck breathers when there is any doubt as to the nature of a stoma. Any oxygen applied to the upper airway can be removed in the case of a laryngectomy once this has been confirmed to be the case. Ventilation via laryngectomy stomas can be achieved using paediatric facemasks or laryngeal masks applied to the anterior neck (RCUK 2012).

The National Tracheostomy Safety Project has published distinct guidelines for management of emergencies for patients with either a tracheostomy (Figure 9.27) or laryngectomy (Figure 9.28), with both carrying a clear message emphasizing the need for oxygenation of the patient and the need to call for help early. It also designed 'the green algorithm' for emergency tracheostomy management with a patent upper airway (RCUK 2012).

Cardiopulmonary resuscitation

DEFINITION

Cardiopulmonary resuscitation is an emergency procedure such as cardiac compressions and ventilation, which are performed in an effort to manually preserve cardiac output and oxygenation to ensure intact brain function until further measures are taken to return spontaneous blood circulation and breathing in a person in cardiac arrest (RCUK 2010a, 2010b).

ANATOMY AND PHYSIOLOGY

The heart

The heart is made up of four chambers: two upper atria and two lower ventricles (see Figure 11.5). The right atrium receives deoxygenated blood via the venous circulation. From the right atrium, blood flows into the right ventricle which pumps it into the lungs via the pulmonary arteries. Carbon dioxide is released and oxygen is absorbed. This blood is oxygenated and returns to the heart via the pulmonary veins that empty into the left atrium. The blood then passes into the left ventricle which pumps it into the aorta and arterial circulation (Waugh and Grant 2010).

The atrioventricular septum completely separates the right and left sides of the heart. From shortly after birth, the two sides of the heart never directly communicate. Blood travels from right side to left side via the lungs only. However, the chambers themselves work together. The two atria contract simultaneously and the two ventricles contract simultaneously (Waugh and Grant 2010).

To prevent backflow of blood, the heart has valves. The atrioventricular (AV) valves are between the atria and ventricles. The right AV valve between the right atrium and right ventricle is also called the tricuspid valve because it consists of three cusps. The left AV valve between the left atrium and ventricle is called the bicuspid as it has two cusps. Both arteries that emerge from the heart have a valve to prevent blood from flowing back into the heart – the semi-lunar (SL) valves. The pulmonary SL valve lies where the pulmonary trunk leaves the right ventricle and the aortic SL valve is situated at the opening between the aorta and left ventricle. The valves open and close in response to pressure changes as the heart contracts and relaxes (Jenkins and Tortora 2013, Moran 2010).

Cardiac conduction system

This pathway is made up of the:

- sinoatrial (SA) node
- AV node
- bundle of His
- left and right bundle branches
- Purkinje fibres.

The SA node is the natural pacemaker of the heart. It releases electrical stimuli at a regular rate, which will vary depending on whether the body is at rest or in action. As each stimulus passes through the myocardial cells of the atria, it creates a wave of contraction which spreads rapidly through both atria (Jenkins and Tortora 2013).

The rapidity of atrial contraction is such that around 100 million myocardial cells contract in less than one-third of a second; this is so fast it appears instantaneous.

When the electrical stimulus from the SA node reaches the AV node, it is delayed briefly so that the contracting atria have enough time to pump all the blood into the ventricles. Once the atria are empty of blood, the valves between the atria and ventricles close. At this point the atria begin to refill and the electrical stimulus passes through the AV node, through the bundle of His, along the left and right bundle branches and the Purkinje fibres. In this way all the cells in the ventricles receive an electrical stimulus causing them to contract (Becker 2007).

Around 400 million myocardial cells that make up the ventricles contract in less than one-third of a second. As the ventricles contract, the right ventricle pumps blood to the lungs where carbon dioxide is released and oxygen is absorbed, whilst the left ventricle pumps blood into the aorta from where it passes into the coronary and arterial circulation.

At this point the ventricles are empty, the atria are full and the valves between them are closed. The SA node is about to release another electrical stimulus and the process is about to repeat itself. However, there is a third section to this process. The SA node and AV node contain only one stimulus. Therefore every time the nodes release a stimulus, they must recharge before they can do it again (Jenkins and Tortora 2013).

In the heart, the SA node recharges whilst the atria are refilling, and the AV node recharges when the ventricles are refilling. This means there is no need for a pause in heart function. Again, this process takes less than one-third of a second. (The times given for the three different stages are based on a heart rate of 60 beats per minute, or 1 beat per second.)

The term used for the release of an electrical stimulus is 'depolarization' and the term for recharging is 'repolarization'.

So, the three stages of a single heart beat are:

- atrial depolarization
- ventricular depolarization
- atrial and ventricular repolarization (Jenkins and Tortora 2013, Moran 2010).

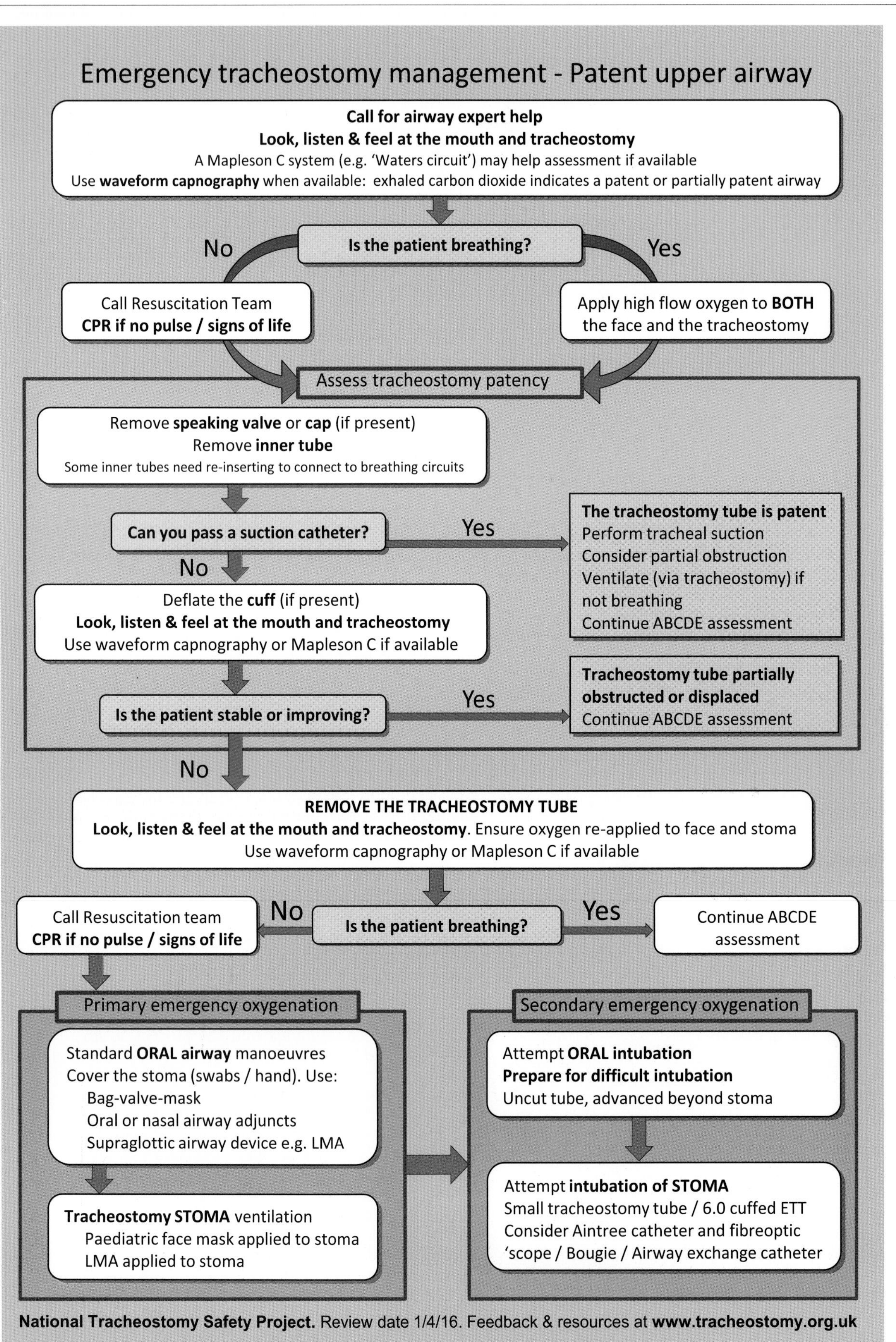

Figure 9.27 Emergency tracheostomy guidelines. Source: Reproduced with permission from the National Tracheostomy Safety Project (www.tracheostomy.org.uk).

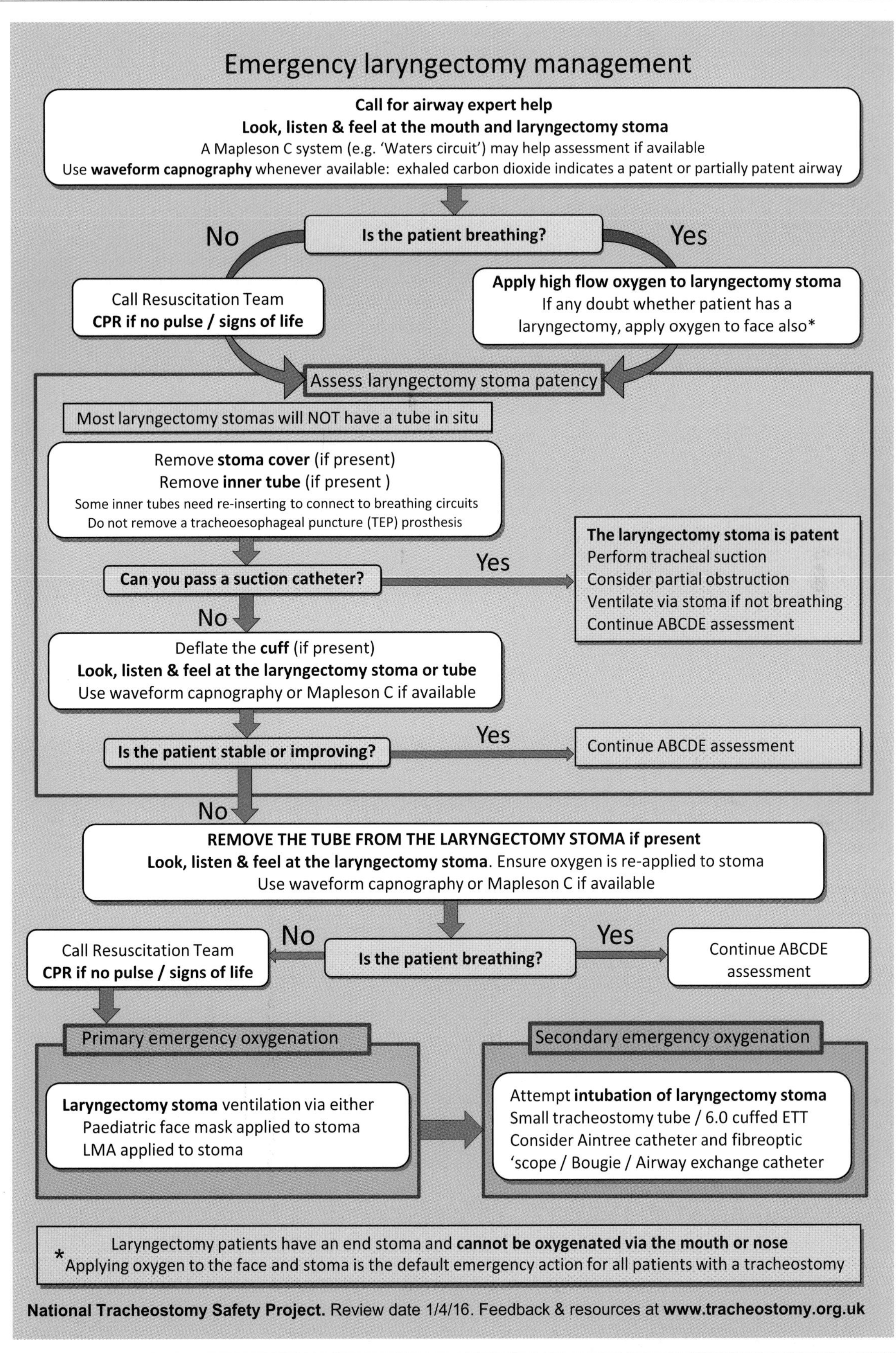

Figure 9.28 Emergency laryngectomy guidelines. Source: Reproduced with permission from the National Tracheostomy Safety Project (www.tracheostomy.org.uk).

RELATED THEORY

Cardiac arrest implies a sudden interruption of cardiac output. It may be reversible with appropriate treatment (Handley 2004, RCUK 2010a, 2010b). The patient will collapse, lose consciousness, stop breathing and will be pulseless (Jevon 2001, Paradis 2007).

The four arrhythmias that cause cardiac arrest are:

- asystole
- ventricular fibrillation (VF)
- pulseless ventricular tachycardia (VT)
- pulseless electrical activity (PEA).

For the purposes of resuscitation guidelines, these rhythms are divided into two groups by their treatment:

- VF and pulseless VT, which require defibrillation
- non-VF/VT, which do not require defibrillation (RCUK 2010b).

Resuscitation is the emergency treatment of any condition in which the brain fails to receive enough oxygen.

Potentially reversible causes of a cardiopulmonary arrest

During cardiac arrest, potential causes or aggravating factors for which specific treatment exists should be considered. For ease of memory, there are eight common causes of arrest, four of which begin with the letter H and four with the letter T.

- Hypoxia
- Hypovolaemia
- Hypo-/hyperkalaemia/metabolic
- Hypothermia
- Thrombosis – coronary or pulmonary
- Tamponade – cardiac
- Toxins
- Tension pneumothorax (RCUK 2010a, 2010b)

Hypoxia

There are many reasons why a patient may become severely hypoxic, the most common being the following.

- Acute respiratory failure (O'Driscoll et al. 2008)
- Airway difficulties (RCUK 2012)
- Acute lung injury (O'Driscoll et al. 2008)
- Severe anaemia
- Neuromuscular disorders

For healthy cell metabolism, the body requires a constant supply of oxygen. When this is interrupted for more than 3 minutes in most situations (except when there is severe hypothermia), cell death occurs, followed by lactic acidosis and very rapidly a cardiorespiratory arrest. The risk of hypoxia is minimized by ensuring that the patient's lungs are ventilated adequately with 100% oxygen (RCUK 2010b).

Hypovolaemia

Hypovolaemia in adults that results in PEA is usually due to severe blood loss. While it is not the nurse's role to make a medical diagnosis, they may be aware of significant factors in the history of a patient that may have led to PEA.

The most common causes of severe blood loss are:

- trauma
- surgical procedure
- gastrointestinal mucosa erosion
- oesophageal varices
- peripheral vessel erosion (by tumour usually)
- clotting abnormality.

Note: Blood loss, although usually overt, can be covert such as a gastrointestinal bleed which may only become apparent when the patient collapses.

The treatment for hypovolaemia is identifying and stopping the source of fluid or blood loss, and replacing the circulating volume with the appropriate fluid. Fluid resuscitation is normally started with a crystalloid, for example 0.9% sodium chloride, and/or colloid, for example Gelofusine (depending on local protocols); there is no evidence that colloids are more effective than crystalloids. Blood is likely to be required rapidly if the blood loss exceeds 1500–2000 mL in an adult (Perel et al. 2007, RCUK 2010b).

Hypo-/hyperkalaemia and other metabolic disorders

Because potassium is so closely linked with muscle and nerve excitation, any imbalance will affect both the nervous conduction and the muscular working of the heart. Therefore a severe rise or fall in potassium can cause arrest arrhythmias. The causes of hypokalaemia are:

- gastrointestinal fluid losses
- urinary fluid loss
- drugs that affect cellular potassium, for example antifungal agents such as amphotericin.

The immediate treatment for hypokalaemia that has resulted in an arrest is to give concentrated infusions of potassium while carefully monitoring the serial potassium measurements. Most ICU/accident and emergency (A&E) departments and coronary care units (CCUs) will have an arterial blood gas analyser that enables the potassium to be measured in 1 minute.

The patients who are most at risk of hyperkalaemia are those with renal failure or Addison's disease (Weisberg 2008). The immediate treatment for hyperkalaemia is to give intravenous calcium. This has the effect of protecting the myocardium during the cardiac arrest. If the patient is successfully resuscitated, it will be essential to monitor their serum potassium and, if it remains high, to commence therapy to lower or remove the potassium (RCUK 2010a, 2010b).

Hypothermia

Hypothermia should be suspected in any submersion or immersion injury. During a prolonged resuscitation attempt, a patient who was normothermic at the onset of cardiac arrest may become hypothermic (RCUK 2010b). A low-reading thermometer should be used if available. Resuscitation in the presence of hypothermia may be prolonged.

Thrombosis – coronary or pulmonary

The most common cause of thromboembolic or mechanical circulatory obstruction is a massive pulmonary embolus. Options for definitive treatment include thrombolysis or, if available, cardiopulmonary bypass and operative removal of the clot (RCUK 2010b).

Tamponade

This is where there is an acute effusion of fluid in the pericardial space and as it enlarges, the heart is splinted and finally cannot beat. The fluid is usually blood but can be malignant or infected fluid (Dolan and Preston 2006). The most common cause for a sudden tamponade is trauma. The immediate treatment is the insertion of a catheter or surgical drainage of the fluid (Harper 2010). After drainage, the cause of the tamponade should be sought and corrected where possible, for example with appropriate antibiotic therapy for a bacterial aetiology or surgical repair of a myocardial laceration (Harper 2010).

Toxicity: poisoning and drug intoxication

Poisoning rarely leads to cardiac arrest but it is a leading cause of death in patients less than 40 years old. Self-poisoning with therapeutic or recreational drugs is the main reason for hospital admission (RCUK 2010b). There are few specific therapeutic measures for poisons that are useful in the immediate situation. The emphasis must be on intensive supportive therapy, with correction of hypoxia, acid/base balance and electrolyte disorders. Specialist help can be obtained by telephoning one of the regional National Poisons Information Service Centres (RCUK 2010b).

Tension pneumothorax

A tension pneumothorax is the sudden collapse of a lung, usually under pressure, which results in a severe change in intrathoracic pressure and cessation of the heart as a pump (Bersten et al. 2009). The most common causes are:

- trauma
- acute lung injury
- mechanical ventilation of the newborn.

The immediate treatment is the insertion of a large-bore cannula into the second intercostal space at the midclavicular line of the affected side (RCUK 2010b). Arrangements should be made for the insertion of a formal chest tube and underwater seal drain.

EVIDENCE-BASED APPROACHES

Sudden death as a result of cardiac arrest is responsible for 60% of ischaemic heart disease deaths across Europe (RCUK 2010b). Survival to hospital discharge is cited as 10.7% of all types of cardiac arrest with survival being higher (21.2%) in ventricular fibrillation arrests (RCUK 2010b).

Changes to adult basic life support (BLS) guidelines have been made to reflect the importance of performing high-quality chest compressions. The rescuer should reduce the number and duration of pauses during chest compressions (RCUK 2010b).

Cardiopulmonary resuscitation guidelines in the UK are researched and implemented by the Resuscitation Council UK, and BLS and advanced life support (ALS) guidelines are changed according to their recommendations. The duration of collapse is frequently difficult to estimate accurately, so CPR should be given before attempted defibrillation outside hospital, unless the arrest is witnessed by a healthcare professional or an automated external defibrillator (AED) is being used (RCUK 2010b).

In contrast, there is no evidence to support or refute the use of CPR before defibrillation for in-hospital cardiac arrest. For this reason, after in-hospital VF/VT cardiac arrest, a shock should be given as soon as possible (RCUK 2010b). Continuing good-quality CPR may improve the amplitude and frequency of fine VF and improve the chance of successful defibrillation to a perfusing rhythm, as fine VF is difficult to distinguish from asystole and very unlikely to be shocked successfully (Eftestol et al. 2002, RCUK 2010a).

Rationale

The basic technique involves a rapid simple assessment of the patient followed by BLS resuscitation. The first international consensus evidence-based guidelines on resuscitation were published in 2000 (AHA/ILCOR 2000, Shuster et al. 2010). These guidelines were reviewed in 2004/05 by the International Liaison Committee on Resuscitation and published in 2005 (AHA/ILCOR 2000). These internationally agreed guidelines based on research and audit now form the basis for the European resuscitation guidelines (Baskett et al. 2005) as well as the UK resuscitation guidelines (RCUK 2010b).

Changes to Resuscitation Council UK guidelines suggest that the rescuer should not stop to check the patient or discontinue CPR unless the person starts to show signs of regaining consciousness, such as coughing, opening eyes, speaking or moving purposefully, and starts to breathe normally (RCUK 2010b).

Indications

- The patient is unconscious, has absent or agonal (gasping) respirations and has no pulse (Perkins et al. 2005). Other clinical features such as pupil size, cyanosis and pallor are unreliable and so the practitioner should not waste time looking for them (Skinner and Vincent 1997).

Contraindications

- Do not attempt cardiopulmonary resuscitation orders (DNACPR).
- If the environment is going to place the rescuer at risk, do not attempt resuscitation until the environment is secured.

DO NOT ATTEMPT CARDIOPULMONARY RESUSCITATION

Survival after in-hospital cardiac arrest is still only in the region of 10–20% depending on numerous factors, such as initial cardiac ECG rhythm, co-morbidities, age, performance status, reason for hospital admission and cause of cardiac arrest (Meaney et al. 2010, NCEPOD 2012). In an attempt to reduce the number of futile resuscitation attempts, many hospitals and organizations have introduced formal DNACPR policies, which can be applied to individual patients in specific circumstances. Healthcare professionals must be able to show that their decisions relating to CPR are compatible with the Human Rights Act 1998 implemented on 2 October 2000 (e.g. the right to life, the right to be free from inhuman or degrading treatment and freedom of expression) (BMA 2000, 2007, BMA et al. 2002). The following guidelines are based on those provided in a joint statement by the British Medical Association (BMA), the Royal College of Nursing (RCN) and the Resuscitation Council UK (BMA 2007). (*Note*: Where no decision has been made and the express wishes of the patient are unknown, CPR should be performed without delay.) Each hospital should audit all CPR attempts and assess what proportion of patients should have had a DNACPR decision in place prior to the arrest and should not have undergone CPR, rather than have the decision made after the first arrest. This will improve patient care by avoiding undignified and potentially harmful CPR attempts during the dying process (NCEPOD 2012).

- Sensitive advance discussion between experienced medical/nursing staff and patients regarding attempting CPR should be encouraged but not forced. Neither patients, nor those close to them, can demand treatment that is clinically inappropriate. If the healthcare team believes that CPR will not restart the heart and breathing, this should be explained to the patient in a sensitive way. (*Note:* In England, Wales and Northern Ireland, no person is legally entitled to give consent to medical treatment on behalf of another adult.) Information about CPR needs to be realistic. Written information explaining CPR should be available for patients and those close to them to read. The BMA, in liaison with the Resuscitation Council UK, RCN and Age Concern England, has published an information leaflet that may help patients and families to discuss DNAR with medical and nursing staff (BMA 2007).
- Patients are entitled to refuse CPR even when there is a reasonable chance of success (Mental Capacity Act 2005).
- Some patients may ask that no DNACPR order be made. Patients cannot demand treatment which the healthcare team judges to be inappropriate, but all efforts should be made to accommodate their wishes and preferences.
- An advance DNACPR order should only be made after consideration of the likely clinical outcome, the patient's wishes and their human rights. It should be considered on an individual patient basis where:
  - attempting CPR will not start the patient's heart and breathing
  - there is no benefit in restarting the patient's heart and breathing

– the expected benefit is outweighed by the burdens (RCUK 2010b).

- The overall responsibility for decisions about CPR and DNACPR orders rests with the consultant in charge of the patient's care. Issues should, however, be discussed with other members of the healthcare team, the patient and people close to the patient where appropriate.
- There are exceptional cases where resuscitation discussions with a patient may be inappropriate, for example where senior members of the medical and nursing team consider that CPR would be futile and that such a discussion would cause the patient unnecessary distress and anguish. This could apply to patients in the terminal phase of their illness.
- The most senior members of the medical and nursing team available should clearly document any decisions made about CPR in the patient's medical and nursing notes. The decision should be dated and the reasons for it given. This information must be communicated to all other relevant healthcare professionals (NCEPOD 2012). Unless it is against the wishes of the patient, their family should also be informed.
- The DNACPR order should be reviewed on each admission or in light of changes in the patient's condition (BMA et al. 2002).
- Finally, it should be noted that a DNACPR order applies only to CPR and should not reduce the standard of medical or nursing care (NCEPOD 2012).

Figure 9.29 **Initial verbal assessment.**

Principles of care

Failure of the circulation for 3–4 minutes will lead to irreversible cerebral damage (Docherty and Hall 2002). BLS acts to slow down the deterioration of the brain and the heart until defibrillation and/or ALS can be provided (RCUK 2010b).

Assessment

There are two stages of assessment.

- An immediate assessment by the rescuer to ensure that CPR may safely proceed (i.e. checking there is no immediate danger to the rescuer from any hazard, for example electrical power supply).
- Assessment by the rescuer of the likelihood of injury sustained by the patient, particularly injury to the cervical spine. Although there may be no external evidence of injury, the immediate situation may provide the necessary evidence. For example, trauma to the cervical spine should be suspected in an accelerating/decelerating injury such as a road traffic accident with a motorbike travelling at speed.

Once these two aspects have been assessed, the patient's level of consciousness should be checked by gently shaking his shoulders and asking loudly if he is all right (Figure 9.29). If there is no response, the rescuer should commence the BLS assessment (Figure 9.30) immediately.

Note: If the arrest is witnessed or monitored and a defibrillator is not immediately to hand, a single precordial thump should be administered. If delivered within 30 seconds after cardiac arrest, a sharp blow with a closed fist on the patient's sternum may convert VF back to a perfusing rhythm (RCUK 2010b).

Defibrillation

Defibrillation causes a simultaneous depolarization of the myocardium and aims to restore normal rhythm to the heart. This is the definitive treatment for VF and pulseless VT. It has been suggested that about 60% of adults who collapse because of non-traumatic cardiac arrest are found to be in VF when first attached to a monitor (Nolan et al. 2010). In hospital, cardiac arrest is more likely to present as non-VF/VT, in other words asystole or PEA. Early defibrillation is a vital link in the chain of survival and developments in public access defibrillation and first responder defibrillation by ward nurses in hospitals are focusing firmly on this link. Delay in defibrillation decreases the chances of success,

Figure 9.30 **Basic life support algorithm. Source: Reproduced with permission from the Resuscitation Council (resus.org.uk).**

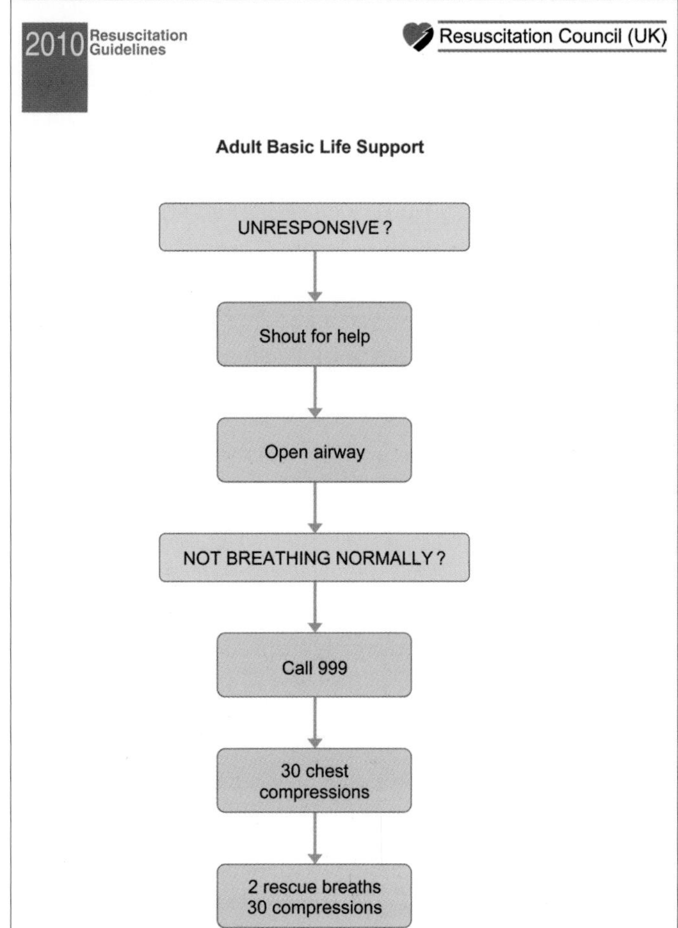
2010 Resuscitation Guidelines
Resuscitation Council (UK)
Adult Basic Life Support
UNRESPONSIVE ?
Shout for help
Open airway
NOT BREATHING NORMALLY ?
Call 999
30 chest compressions
2 rescue breaths 30 compressions

in the absence of bystander CPR, by 10–12% each minute (Nolan et al. 2010).

Nurses are often first on the scene at a cardiac arrest, highlighting the obvious need for nurse-led defibrillation at ward level. While not all nurses are trained in defibrillation, they should understand why it is necessary and how it is done and be able to assist in an emergency (Austin and Snow 2000). Resuscitation guidelines suggest asking for an AED, if one is available, as it can be used safely and effectively without previous training (RCUK 2010b). The aim of an effective defibrillation strategy is to reduce the pre-shock pause to less than 5 seconds by planning ahead and continuing cardiac compressions during charging, and using a very brief safety check (RCUK 2010b).

Method of basic life support

Basic life support is sometimes known as the 'ABC'.

Airway

The rescuer should look in the mouth and remove any visible obstruction (leave well-fitting dentures in place). The most likely obstruction in an unconscious person is the tongue. The head tilt/chin lift manoeuvre (Figure 9.31), which removes the tongue from occluding the oropharynx, is an effective method of opening an airway and relieving obstruction in 80% of patients (Simmons 2002).

Note: If there is any suspicion of cervical spine injury, establish a clear upper airway by performing a jaw thrust or chin lift with manual in-line stabilization.

Breathing

Keeping the airway open, the rescuer should look, listen and feel for breathing (more than an occasional gasp or weak attempts at breathing) for up to 10 seconds. If the patient is breathing, they should be turned into the recovery position (Figure 9.32). If the adult patient is not breathing and there is no suspicion of trauma or drowning, an immediate call for the cardiac arrest team should be made. It should be noted that in 40% of cases a person who has arrested still has agonal (gasping) respirations and these can be mistaken for normal breaths (Hauff et al. 2003).

Artificial ventilation must then be commenced and maintained. If there are no aids to ventilation available then direct mouth-to-mouth ventilation should be used. There have been isolated reports of infections such as tuberculosis (TB) and severe acute respiratory syndrome (SARS) following mouth-to-mouth ventilation but never transmission of HIV (RCUK 2010a). There is no evidence to quantify the degree of risk to the rescuer by performing mouth-to-mouth ventilation but, as it is widely acknowledged that some people are reluctant in spite of the lack of evidence, an allowance has been made for them to only perform chest compressions (RCUK 2010b). The recommended length for each breath is now 1 second (RCUK 2010b).

Figure 9.31 **Head tilt/chin lift manoeuvre.**

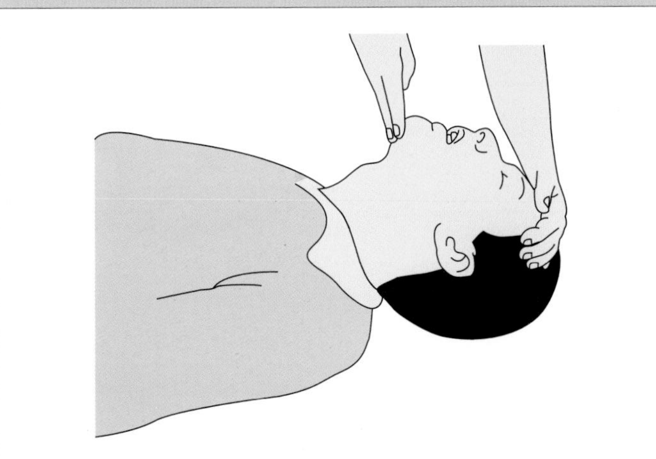

Figure 9.32 **The recovery position.**

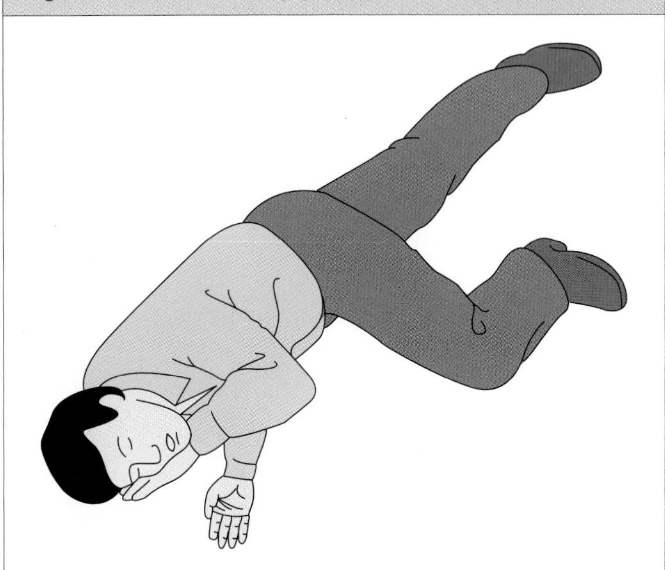

When cardiac arrest occurs in hospital, the Resuscitation Council recommends the use of adjuncts such as the pocket mask or the bag mask unit. These can be used to avoid direct person-to-person contact and some devices may reduce the risk of cross-infection between patient and rescuer (RCUK 2010b). In 2005, in recognition of the concern about providing mouth-to-mouth resuscitation, the guidelines changed and the BLS algorithm now starts with chest compressions and then proceeds to two breaths (RCUK 2010b).

One of the most easily learnt aids is the 'mouth-to-facemask' method (Figure 9.33) in which a ventilation mask with a one-way valve and an oxygen attachment port is used. The mask directs the patient's exhaled air and any fluid away from the rescuer and the oxygen port allows attachment of oxygen with enrichment up to 45%.

If the operator is skilled in airway management, a bag valve mask may be used. When the bag is attached to oxygen, high levels, of up to 85%, can be obtained. However, it should be emphasized that to manipulate the head tilt and hold on a facemask while squeezing a bag is a procedure that requires considerable skill and practice and is most safely achieved by two people, one holding the mask and one squeezing the bag (RCUK 2010b) (Figure 9.34).

The most effective method of airway management is to use an endotracheal tube, thus enabling the application of 100% oxygen (RCUK 2010b, Robertson et al. 1998). This method of airway management is included in the ALS algorithm.

Circulation

Circulation is assessed by looking for any signs of movement, including swallowing or breathing. If trained to do so, a check should also be made for the carotid pulse (Figure 9.35) for up to 10 seconds. If no circulation is detected, it must be maintained by compressions. The correct place to compress is in the centre of the lower half of the sternum (Figure 9.36). The rescuer should position themselves vertically above the patient with arms straight and elbows locked. The sternum should be pressed down to depress it by 5–6 cm. This should be repeated at a rate of about 100–120 times a minute. After 30 compressions, two rescue breaths are given, continuing compressions and rescue breaths in a ratio of 30:2 (RCUK 2010b). There is evidence that chest

Figure 9.33 Mask with one-way valve over patient's nose and mouth and rescuer giving breath.

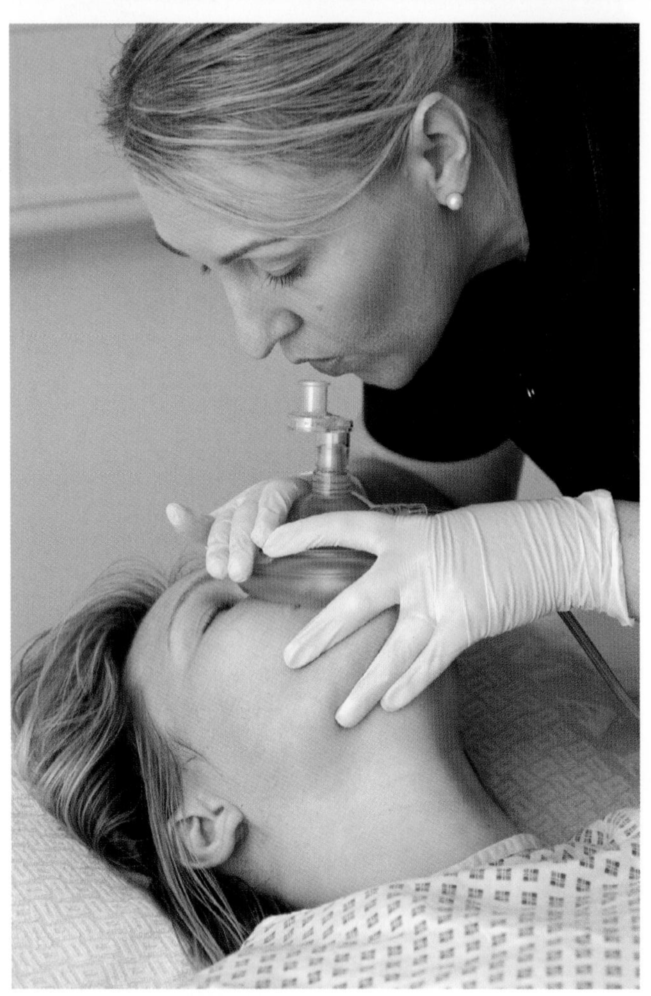

Figure 9.35 Carotid pulse check.

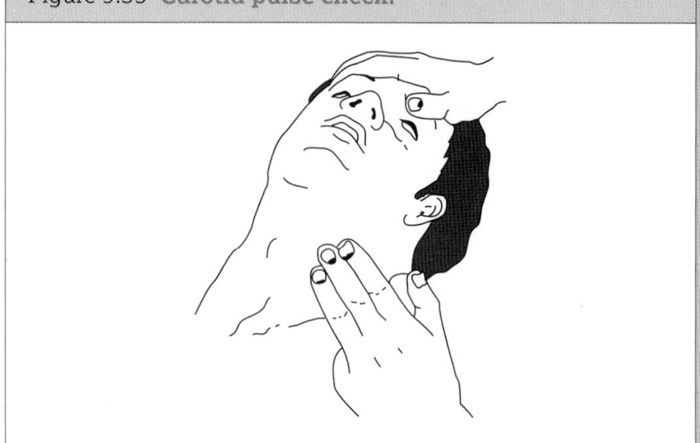

compressions are often interrupted and that this is associated with a reduction in the chance of survival. New adult ALS guidelines (RCUK 2010b) suggest an increased emphasis on the importance of minimal interruption in high-quality chest compressions throughout any ALS intervention; therefore, chest compressions are now continued while a defibrillator is charging, which will minimize the pre-shock pause. It is therefore imperative that interruptions to chest compressions are minimized by effective co-ordination between rescuers (Eftestol et al. 2002, RCUK 2010b, van Alem et al. 2003).

LEGAL AND PROFESSIONAL ISSUES

All members of the healthcare professions who attempt resuscitation will be expected to employ the highest professional standards of care, in line with their level of training. In general, there are two means by which the risk of personal liability may be minimized. The first is by good practice and the second is by taking out adequate indemnity insurance (NMC 2015, RCUK 2010a). To ensure best practice, make sure that regular updates for BLS and if appropriate ALS training are maintained.

The Resuscitation Council UK guidelines state that if rescuers are not able, or are unwilling, to give rescue breaths, they should give chest compressions alone (RCUK 2010b).

Whenever CPR is carried out (outside the hospital setting), particularly on an unknown victim, there is some risk of cross-infection, associated particularly with giving rescue breaths.

Figure 9.34 Two people using Ambu-bag and mask.

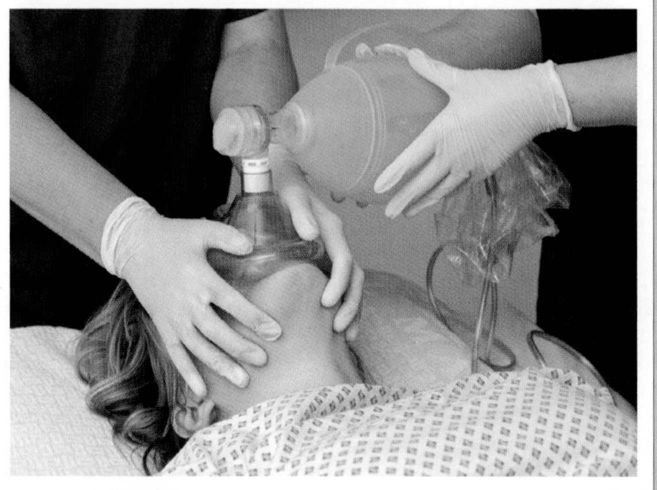

Figure 9.36 Correct positioning of hands for external compressions.

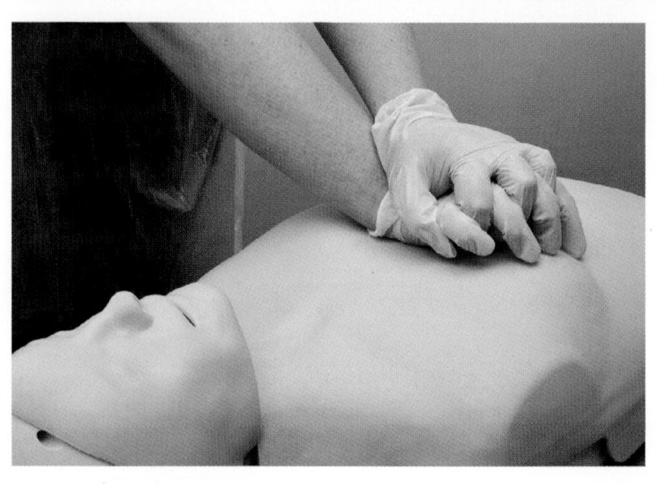

Normally, this risk is very small and has to be set against the inevitability that a person in cardiac arrest will die if no assistance is given.

Competencies

Cardiopulmonary resuscitation standards and training

The Resuscitation Council UK (RCUK), formed in 1981, aims to promote the education of lay and professional personnel in the most effective methods of resuscitation appropriate to their needs. In its report *CPR Guidance for Clinical Practice and Training in Hospitals* (Resuscitation Council 2004), the Council made a number of recommendations relating to the provision of a resuscitation service in hospital.

- *Resuscitation committee*: this should comprise medical and nursing staff who advise on the role and composition of the cardiac arrest team, resuscitation equipment and resuscitation training equipment.
- *Resuscitation training officer* (RTO), who should be responsible for training in resuscitation, equipment maintenance and the auditing of resuscitation/clinical trials.
- *Resuscitation training*: hospital staff should receive at least annual resuscitation training appropriate to their level and role. Medical and nursing staff should receive basic resuscitation training and should be encouraged to recognize patients who are at risk of having a cardiac arrest and call for appropriate help early. This is the most effective method of improving outcome (Jevon 2002). All medical staff should have advanced resuscitation training and senior nurses and doctors working in acute specialities (CCU, ITU, A&E) should hold a valid RCUK ALS certificate.
- *Cardiac arrest team*: each hospital should have a team of approximately five people including a minimum of two doctors (physician and anaesthetist), an ALS-trained nurse, the RTO and a porter when possible. Clear procedures should be available for calling the cardiac arrest team. The Resuscitation Council has recommended the development of a medical emergency team which recognizes patients at risk of having a cardiac arrest and initiates the most appropriate clinical intervention to prevent it (Jevon 2002). Track and trigger systems and NEWS (NICE 2007, RCP 2012) alert nurses to when a patient is deteriorating so that they can initiate interventions and early referral to critical care outreach teams or medical emergency teams (DH 2000, NICE 2007, RCP 2012). Hospital staff are often trained in BLS techniques (see Figure 9.30) that are more appropriate for the single lay rescuer in an out-of-hospital environment. These new guidelines are aimed primarily at healthcare professionals who are first to respond to an in-hospital cardiac arrest (Figure 9.37). Some of the guidelines are also applicable to healthcare professionals in other clinical settings (Resuscitation Council 2004).

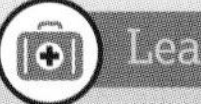

Learning Activity 9.6

Learning in practice: Cardiac arrest

Thinking about your clinical area:

- Do you know the procedure in the event of a cardiac arrest?
- What number do you call for the cardiac arrest/medical emergency team?
- Find out who is included within the medical emergency team and is likely to respond in the event of a cardiac arrest in your area.
- Do you know where the cardiac arrest equipment is?
- Look through the equipment and drugs with your mentor/supervising nurse. Do you know what all the equipment is for?

Figure 9.37 **In-hospital resuscitation algorithm. CPR, cardiopulmonary resuscitation; IV, intravenous. Source: Resuscitation Council (2010b). Reproduced with permission from the Resuscitation Council (resus.org.uk).**

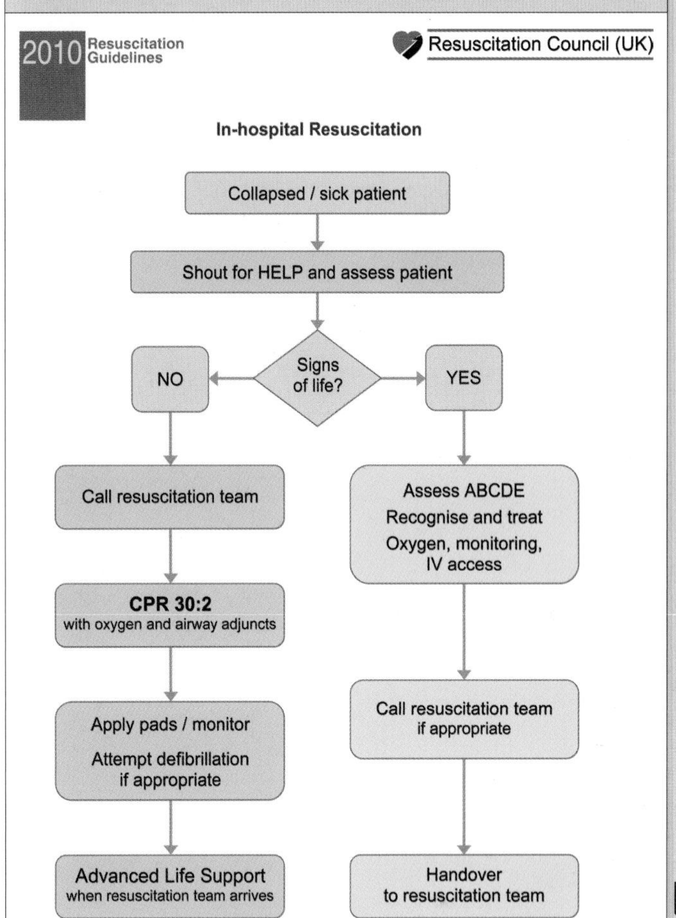

PRE-PROCEDURAL CONSIDERATIONS

Equipment

All hospital wards and appropriate departments, for example theatre, computed tomography (CT) scanning, should have a standardized cardiac arrest trolley or box. Resuscitation equipment should be checked on a daily basis (RCUK 2010b) by the staff on the wards or clinical areas responsible for it, and a record of this check should be maintained. Defibrillators should also be standardized. The use of AEDs or shock advisory defibrillators (Colquhoun 2008) is recommended to reduce mortality from cardiac arrests related to ischaemic heart disease (Jevon 2002). The RCUK recommends that defibrillation should be a basic skill requirement of all nurses (Colquhoun 2008, RCUK 2010a).

Training should be provided in the use of AEDs but if there is no trained individual present when a cardiac arrest occurs, the RCUK advises that an untrained individual should attempt AED defibrillation. The administration of a defibrillatory shock should not be delayed by waiting for more highly trained personnel to arrive. The same principle should apply to individuals whose period of qualification has expired (RCUK 2010b).

Placement of self-adhesive electrodes (defibrillation pads)

The right electrode should be placed to the right of the sternum below the clavicle and the left paddle vertically in the

Figure 9.38 **Placement of defibrillation pads attached to defibrillator on patient's chest.**

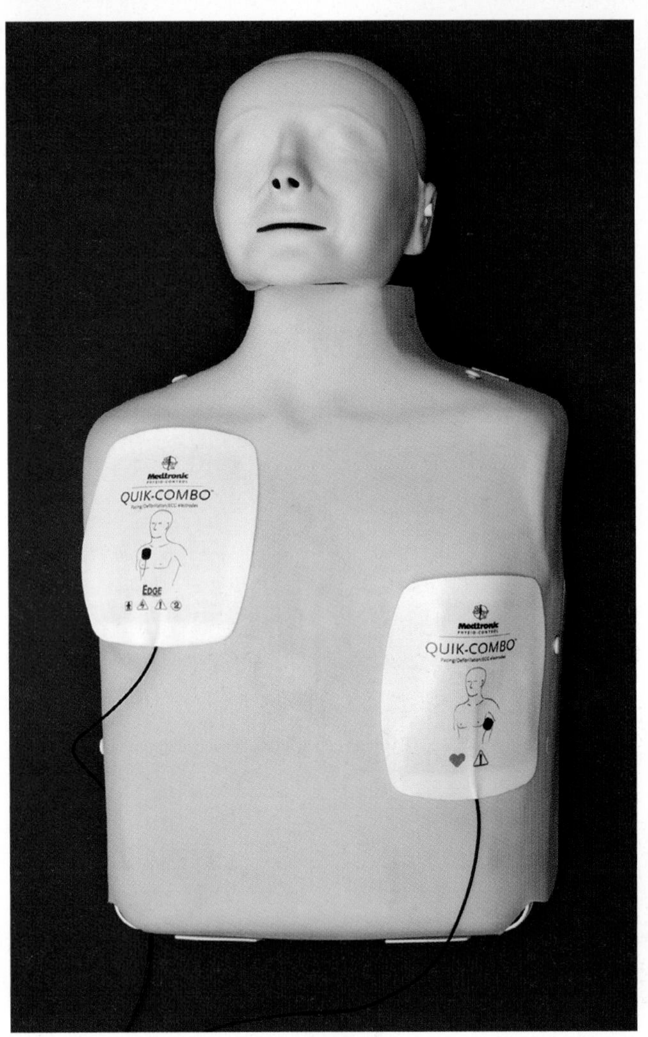

Figure 9.39 **Pocket mask with oxygen port.**

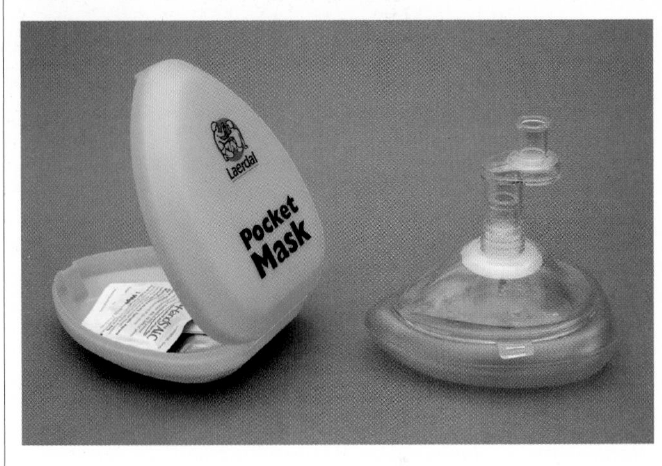

midaxillary line approximately level with the position V6 used in electrocardiogram (ECG) monitoring (Figure 9.38).

Safe defibrillation practice

Defibrillation in an environment where high flows of oxygen are present could represent a danger to patients and rescuers. It is therefore essential to ensure that oxygen tubing and equipment are moved away from the chest when defibrillation is performed. Using adhesive electrodes to deliver the shock as opposed to paddles may also minimize the danger (RCUK 2010b).

A *pocket mask with oxygen port* (Figure 9.39) may be used as an adjunct to administer mouth-to-mask ventilation for a patient with respiratory arrest. The patient should be in the supine position with the head in the sniffing position (head tilt, chin lift – see Figure 9.31). Apply the mask to the patient's face using the thumbs of both hands. Lift the jaw into the mask with the remaining fingers by exerting pressure behind the angles of the jaw (jaw thrust). Blow through the inspiratory valve and watch the chest rise. Stop inflation and allow the chest to fall before blowing in the second breath.

A *self-inflating resuscitation bag* with oxygen reservoir (Nolan et al. 2010) and tubing (Figure 9.40) may be used to administer high inspired oxygen concentrations to a patient and can be connected to a facemask, laryngeal mask or tracheal mask. As the bag is squeezed, the contents are delivered to the patient's lungs and, on release, the expired gas is diverted to the atmosphere via a one-way valve and the bag then refills automatically via an inlet at the opposite end. Used alone, the bag-valve apparatus ventilates the patient's lungs with ambient air only (FiO_2: 0.21), which can be increased to around 45% by attaching oxygen tubing and increasing the flow to 5–6 L/min directly to the bag adjacent to the air intake. If a reservoir system is attached and the oxygen flow is increased to 10 L/min, an inspired oxygen concentration of approximately 85% can be achieved (RCUK 2010b).

An *oropharyngeal airway* is a curved plastic tube, flanged and reinforced at the oral end with a flattened shape to ensure that it fits neatly between the tongue and the hard palate (Nolan et al. 2010). It is used to overcome backward tongue displacement in an unconscious patient. Oropharngeal airways come in sizes 2, 3 and 4, for small, medium and large adults respectively. The right size is chosen by measuring the oropharyngeal airway from the patient's incisors to the angle of the jaw/mandible, as indicated in Figure 9.41a.

Figure 9.40 **Self-inflating resuscitation bag with oxygen reservoir.**

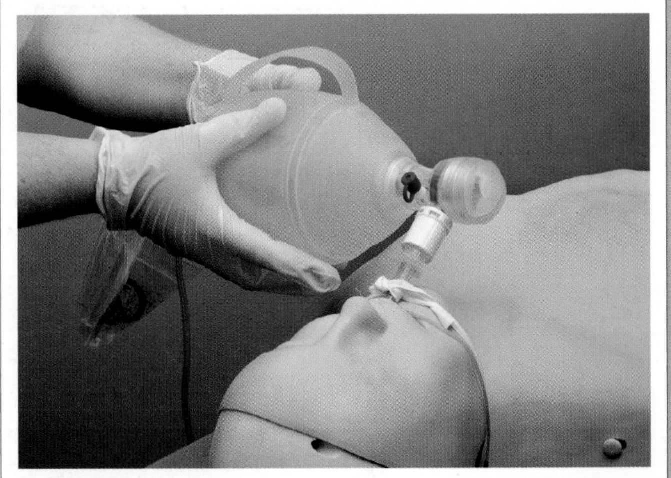

Figure 9.41 (a) Measure the Guedel airway from the corner of the mouth to the angle of the jaw. (b) Insert the airway in an upside-down position to the junction of the hard and soft palate. (c) Rotate the airway 180° once you have reached the junction of the hard and soft palate. (d) Insert the airway until it lies in the oropharynx.

(a) (b) (c) (d)

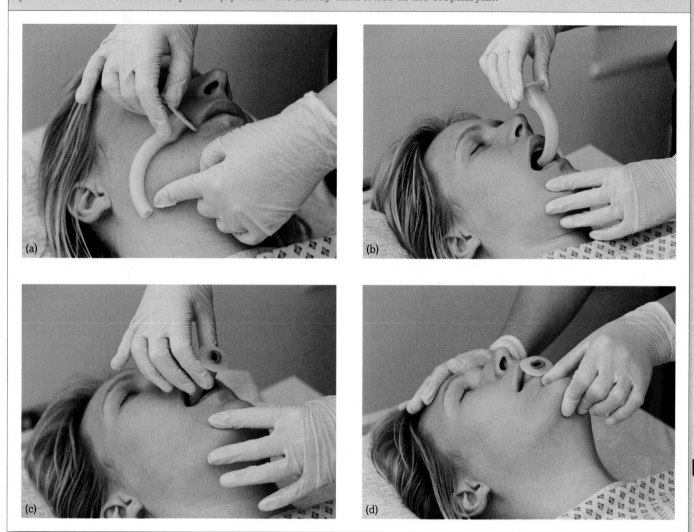

The technique for insertion of an oropharyngeal airway in the unconscious patient is as follows.

- Open the patient's mouth and ensure, by looking into the mouth, that there is no foreign material that may be pushed into the larynx.
- Insert the airway into the mouth in the 'upside-down' position as far as the junction of the hard and soft palate and then rotate the airway through 180° (see Figure 9.41). Then insert the airway until it lies in the oropharynx. This rotation technique minimizes the chance of pushing the tongue backwards and downwards which would further obstruct the airway (RCUK 2010b).

Use of the incorrect size oropharyngeal airway may result in trauma, laryngospasm and/or worsening of the airway obstruction.

Suction equipment such as a wide-bore suction end (Yankauer sucker – Figure 9.42) should be used to remove liquid (blood, saliva and gastric contents) from the upper airway. This is done best under direct vision during intubation but should not result in any delay in achieving a definitive airway. If tracheal suction

Figure 9.42 Yankauer sucker.

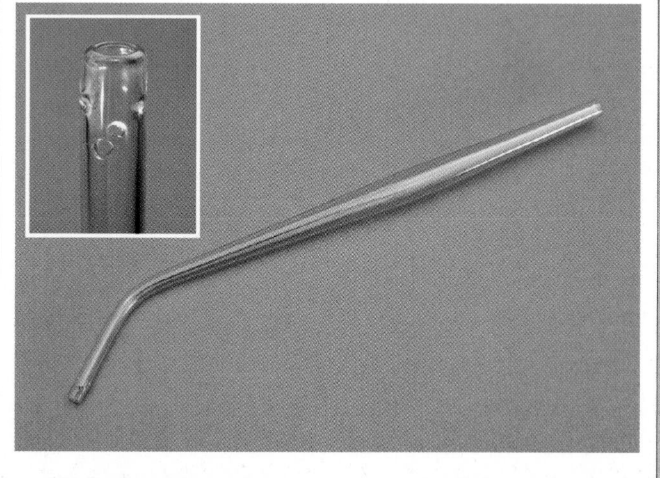

Figure 9.43 **Endotracheal/tracheostomy suction catheter.**

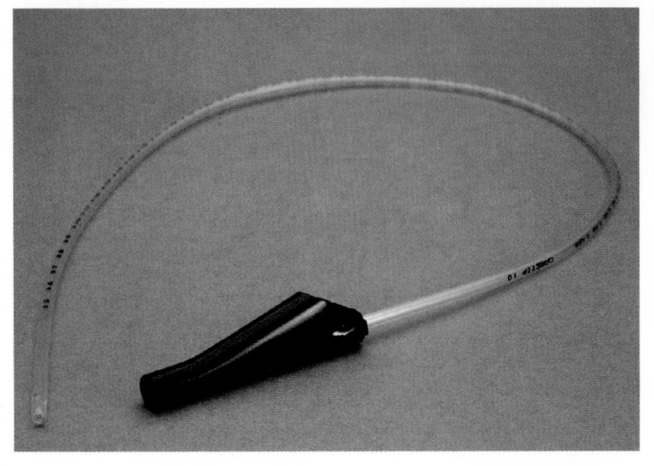

is necessary, it should be as brief as possible and preceded and followed by ventilation with 100% oxygen.

Endotracheal suction catheters (Figure 9.43) are used to clear secretions from endotracheal or tracheostomy tubes or laryngeal airway masks (Hallstrom et al. 2000, RCUK 2010b).

A *laryngeal mask airway* (LMA) (size 4) or Combitube (small) consists of a wide-bore tube with an elliptical inflated cuff designed to seal around the laryngeal opening. It is easier to ventilate a patient using bag-valve-LMA ventilation than using bag-valve-facemask ventilation, because of difficulty in ensuring no air leak on the facemask, especially if there is only one person available to ventilate the patient. The LMA is a reliable and safe device and has a high success rate, after a short period of training (Figure 9.44) (Hallstrom et al. 2000, RCUK 2010b).

A *McGill forceps* (Figure 9.45) is a curved forceps which can be used by the anaesthetist for a difficult intubation and to help introduce an endotracheal tube during intubation (Figure 9.46). Tracheal intubation is considered to be superior to other advanced techniques of airway management because the airway is reliably isolated from foreign material in the oropharynx (Hallstrom et al. 2000). Extensive training and regular practice are required to acquire and maintain the skills of intubation, and endotracheal tubes (oral, cuffed, sizes 6, 7 and 8) are kept

Figure 9.45 **McGill forceps.**

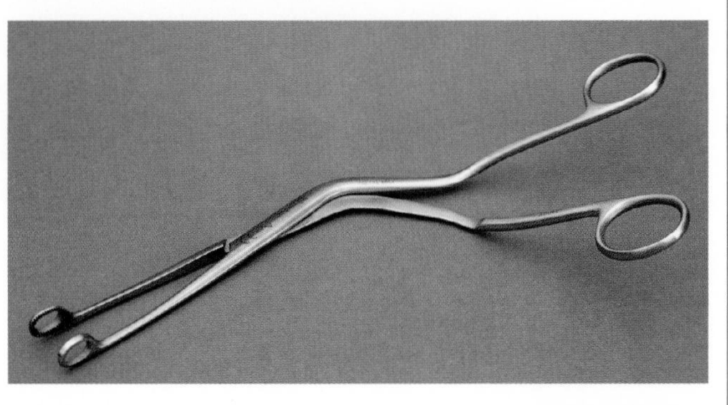

on emergency trolleys and should be sized according to the patient's size and gender.

An *introducer* such as a gum elastic bougie (Figure 9.47) or a semi-rigid stylet is a useful aid to intubation. Water-soluble lubricating jelly is used prior to intubation or insertion of the LMA or nasopharyngeal airway to aid smooth insertion.

A *laryngoscope* (Figure 9.48) with both curved Macintosh and long blades is used by the anaesthetist to visualize the vocal cords prior to intubation. It consists of a handle with either rechargeable or removable batteries and a light source, which needs to be checked regularly, as well as just before use, and in case of malfunction spare batteries and light sources need to be available (RCUK 2010b).

Assessment and recording tools

Decisions relating to CPR ideally should have been documented prior to a cardiac arrest. Every hospital should have a 'do not attempt resuscitation' (DNAR) policy based on national guidelines (BMA et al. 2002, Jevon 2001).

During and after a cardiac arrest, all resuscitation attempts should be documented for auditing purposes, ideally using a nationally recognized template such as the Utstein template (recommended for use by the RCUK). If these recommendations are implemented, standards in resuscitation and resuscitation training should improve (Jevon 2002).

Figure 9.44 **Laryngeal mask airway.**

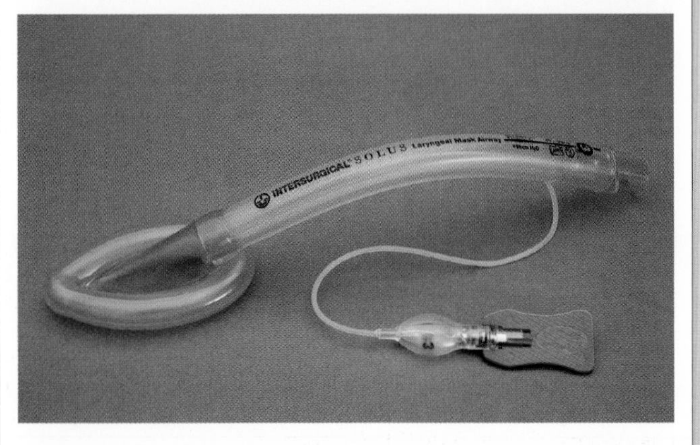

Figure 9.46 **Endotracheal tubes.**

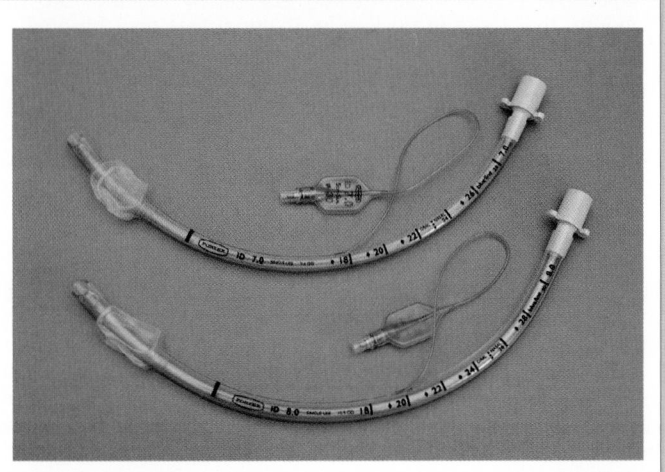

Figure 9.47 Bougie.

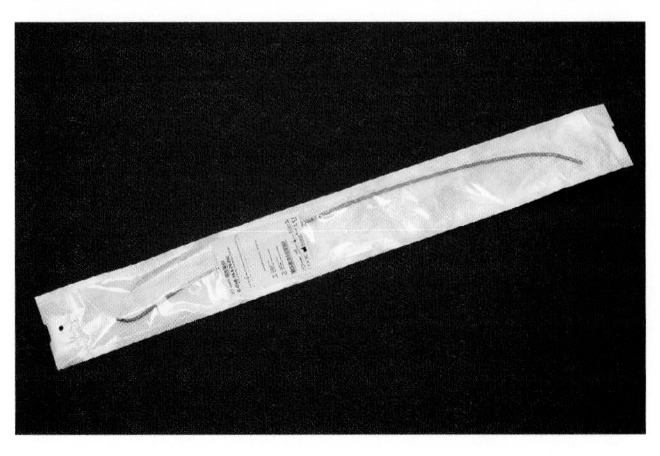

Pharmacological support

Only a few drugs are indicated during the immediate management of a cardiac arrest and there is only limited scientific evidence supporting their use. Drugs should be considered only after a sequence of shocks has been delivered (if indicated) and chest compressions and ventilation started (RCUK 2010b). Central venous access is optimum as it allows for drugs to be delivered rapidly. However, this is dependent on the skills available. If a peripheral intravenous cannula is already in place, it should be used first (RCUK 2010b). It is also possible to administer drugs using the intraosseous route, which is used commonly in the resuscitation of children.

The drugs used in the treatment of cardiac arrest are as follows.

- *Adrenaline* 1 mg (10 mL of a 1:10,000 solution) given intravenously. The main purpose of adrenaline is to utilize its inotropic effect to maintain coronary and cerebral perfusion during a prolonged resuscitation attempt. It is the first drug used in cardiac arrest of any aetiology. Adrenaline is included in the ALS universal algorithm (Figure 9.49), 1 mg to be given every 3–5 minutes (Nolan et al. 2010).

Figure 9.48 Laryngoscope handle and blade.

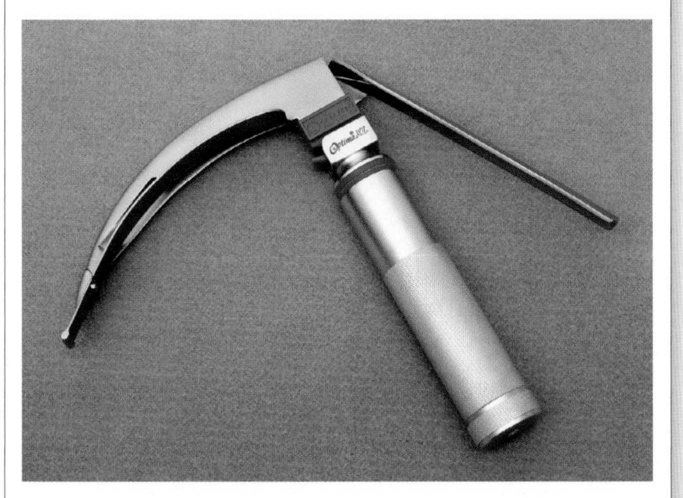

Figure 9.49 The advanced life support algorithm for the management of cardiac arrest in adults. CPR, cardiopulmonary resuscitation; ECG, electrocardiogram, PEA, pulseless electrical activity; VF, ventricular fibrillation; VT, ventricular tachycardia. Source: Resuscitation Council (2010b). Reproduced with permission from the Resuscitation Council (resus.org.uk).

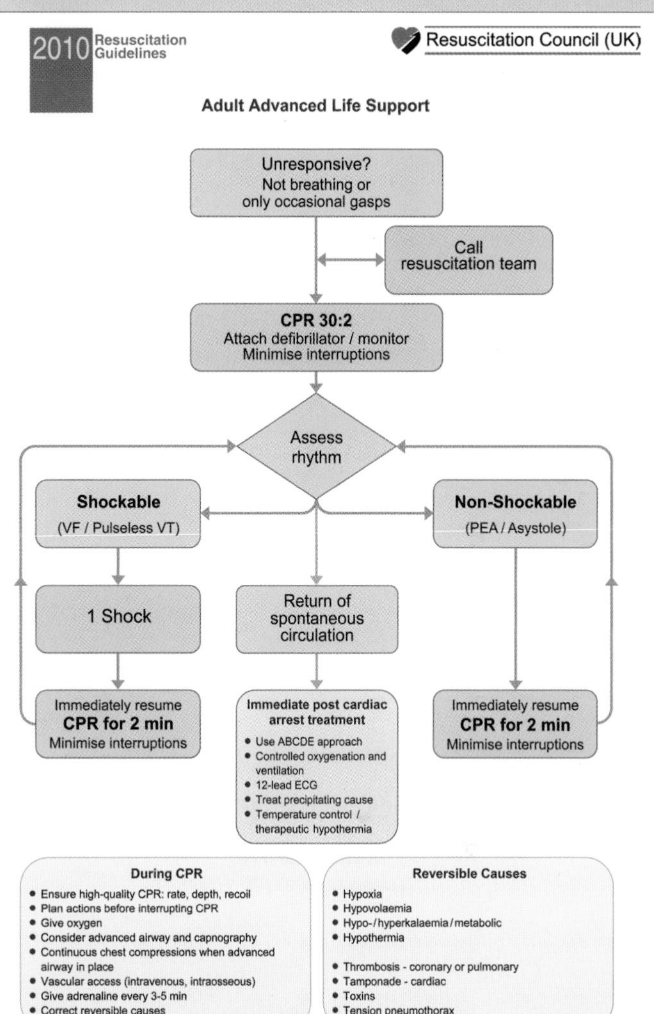

- *Atropine* is no longer recommended routinely in patients with asystole or PEA, since the 2010 RCUK guidelines update (RCUK 2010b).
- *Amiodarone* (300 mg in 20 mL) should be considered in VF or pulseless VT. It increases the duration of the action potential in the atrial and ventricular myocardium; thus the QT interval is prolonged. In refractory VT or VF following recovery from cardiac arrest, a further 300 mg may be given followed by an infusion of 900 mg over 24 hours (RCUK 2010b). *Note*: Lidocaine can still be considered if amiodarone is not available (RCUK 2010b).
- *Calcium chloride* (10 mL of 10%) is only given during resuscitation when specifically indicated; that is, for the treatment of PEA caused by hyperkalaemia, hypocalcaemia or overdose of calcium channel-blocking drugs (RCUK 2010b). Although it plays a vital role in the cellular mechanisms underlying myocardial contraction, there are few data supporting any beneficial action for calcium following most cases of cardiac arrest (RCUK 2010b).

- *Sodium bicarbonate* 8.4% is only used in prolonged cardiac arrest or according to serial blood gas analyses. Potential adverse effects of excessive sodium bicarbonate administration include hypokalaemia, exacerbation of respiratory acidosis and increased affinity of haemoglobin for oxygen. The high concentration of sodium can also exacerbate cerebral oedema. Other adverse effects are increased cardiac irritability and impaired myocardial performance. Sodium bicarbonate is usually given in 25–50 mmol aliquots and repeated as necessary. It can also be given in the special circumstances of tricyclic overdose or hyperkalaemia (Winser 2001).
- *Magnesium sulphate*: magnesium (4–8 mmol of 50%) should be given in cardiac arrest where there is a suspicion of hypomagnesaemia as this may precipitate refractory VF/VT (Nolan et al. 2010). It is important to recognize torsades de pointes. Many of these patients are hypomagnesaemic and/or hypokalaemic and part of effective treatment (prevention of recurrent episodes) will be giving intravenous magnesium and correction of any other electrolyte abnormality. The normal value for magnesium is 0.8–1.2 mmol/L (Nolan et al. 2010).

Use pre-filled syringes (mini-jets) whenever possible for speed and ease of use (Figure 9.50). Drugs should be considered only after chest compressions and ventilation have been started and, where indicated, defibrillation attempted.

Learning Activity 9.7 Case study: Cardiac arrest

Mrs Grange is a 69-year-old woman who has had recent extensive gynaecological surgery. During the shift handover this morning, you were told that she had not been feeling herself overnight and that she was slightly tachycardic with lower than normal blood pressure. You have been asked to keep a close eye on her with regular hourly observations. You go to her bed to carry out your next set of observations and as you approach her you find her on her bed and she appears pale and slightly slumped to one side on her pillows. You go up to Mrs Grange and touch her arm but she does not respond.

1 What should you do next?
2 One of the healthcare assistants comes to help you. What should you ask him to do?
3 You now know that Mrs Grange is not breathing and has no pulse. One of the qualified nurses comes to help you and the healthcare assistant brings the cardiac arrest trolley. What do you do next?
4 What should you be prepared to do once the cardiac arrest team arrive?
5 What may be the possible causes for her cardiac arrest?

See the end of the chapter for the answers.

Figure 9.50 **(a) Mini-jet vial and administration chamber with Luer-Lok connector. (b) Remove caps from both mini-jet vials and administration chamber. (c) Screw mini-jet vial into administration chamber. (d) Push vial gently to ensure that medication can be administered and connect Luer-Lok to intravenous device and inject entire contents, followed by 0.9% sodium chloride flush.**

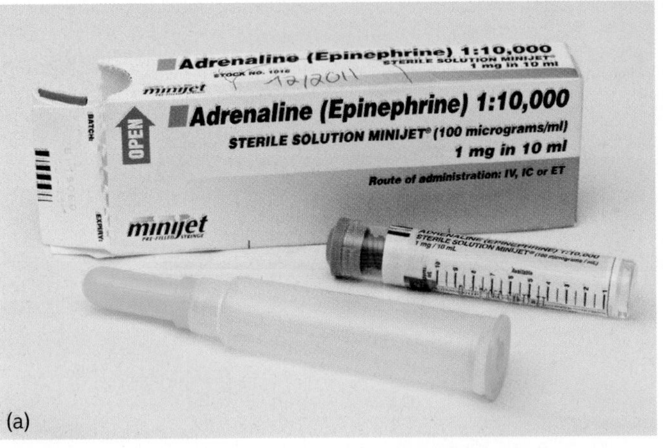

(a)

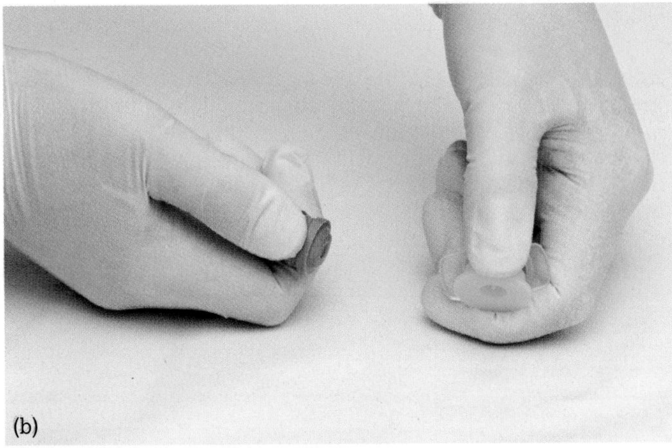
(b)

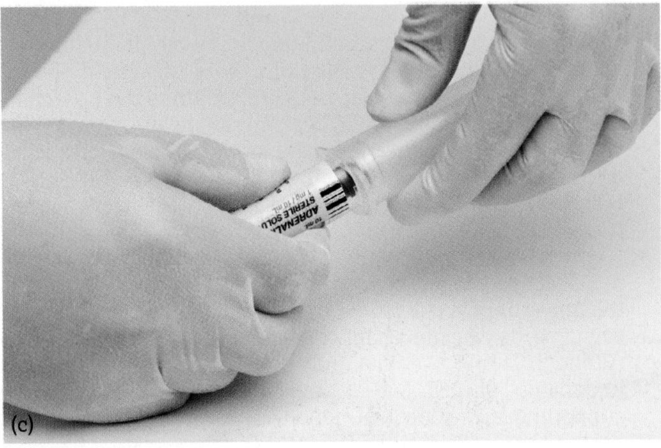
(c)

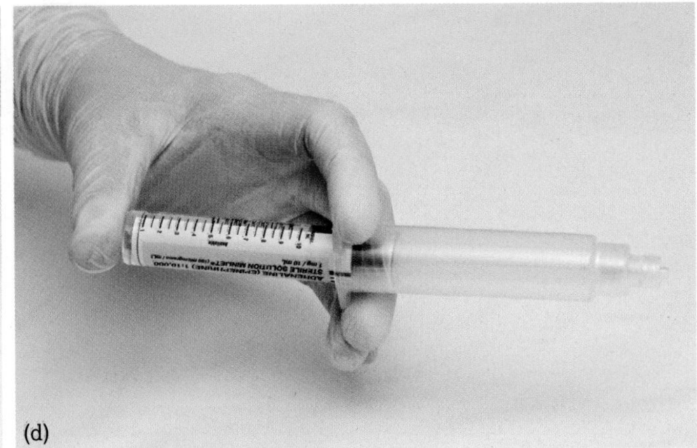
(d)

Specific patient preparation

Education

NEWS (National Early Warning Score) (RCP 2012) is a track and trigger system which alerts nurses to when a patient is deteriorating in order to initiate interventions and early referral to critical care outreach teams (DH 2000, NICE 2007, RCP 2012). This is the most effective method of improving outcome (Jevon 2002). All medical staff should have advanced resuscitation training and senior nurses and doctors working in acute specialties (CCU, ITU, A&E) should hold a valid RCUK ALS certificate.

The importance of prevention of cardiac arrest cannot be highlighted enough. Using a structured communication tool, such as Situation, Background, Assessment, Recommendation (SBAR) (Christie and Robinson 2009, NHS Institute for Innovation and Improvement 2011, RCP 2012), may help to identify patients at risk in a timely manner (RCUK 2010b).

Procedure guideline 9.6 Cardiopulmonary resuscitation

Essential equipment

Airway management

- Pocket masks with oxygen port
- Self-inflating resuscitation bag with oxygen reservoir and tubing
- Clear facemasks in sizes 4, 5 and 6
- Oropharyngeal airways in sizes 2, 3 and 4
- Yankauer suckers × 2
- Endotracheal suction catheters × 10
- Laryngeal mask airway (size 4) or Combitube (small)
- McGill forceps
- Endotracheal tubes: oral, cuffed, sizes 6, 7 and 8
- Gum elastic bougie
- Lubricating jelly
- Laryngoscopes × 2: normal and long blades
- Spare laryngoscope bulbs and batteries
- 1 inch ribbon gauze/tape
- Scissors
- Syringe: 20 mL
- Clear oxygen mask with reservoir bag
- Oxygen cylinders × 2 (if no wall oxygen)
- Cylinder key

Circulation equipment

- Intravenous cannulas: 18 gauge × 3, 14 gauge × 3
- Hypodermic needles: 21 gauge × 10
- Syringes: 2 mL × 6, 5 mL × 6, 10 mL × 6, 20 mL × 6
- Cannula securement dressings and tapes × 4
- Seldinger wire central venous catheter kits × 2
- 12 gauge non-Seldinger central venous catheter × 2
- Intravenous administration sets × 3
- 0.9% sodium chloride: 1000 mL bags × 2

Optional equipment

- Extra ECG electrodes
- Extra defibrillation gel pads unless using fast patch electrodes
- Clock
- Gloves/goggles/aprons
- A sliding sheet or similar device should be available for safe handling

Medicinal products

Immediately available pre-filled syringes of:

- Amiodarone: 300 mg × 1
- Adrenaline: 1 mg (1:10,000) × 4

Other readily available drugs used in CPR

- Epinephrine (adrenaline): 1 mg (1:10,000) × 4
- Sodium bicarbonate 8.4%: 50 mL × 1
- Calcium chloride 10%: 10 mL × 2
- Lidocaine: 100 mg × 2
- 0.9% sodium chloride: 10 mL ampoules × 10
- Naloxone: 400 g × 2
- Epinephrine/adrenaline 1:1000 × 2
- Amiodarone: 150 mg × 4
- Magnesium sulphate 50% solution: 2 g (4 mL) × 1
- Potassium chloride 40 mmol × 1
- Adenosine: 6 mg × 10
- Hydrocortisone: 200 mg × 1
- Glucose 10%: 500 mL × 1

Pre-procedure

Action	Rationale
1 Note time of arrest, if witnessed.	Lack of cerebral perfusion for approximately 3–4 minutes can lead to irreversible brain damage (RCUK 2010b, **C**).

Procedure

Action	Rationale
2 Give patient precordial thump only in witnessed collapse and in cardiac monitored arrest if defibrillator not immediately available.	This may restore cardiac rhythm, which will give a cardiac output. **E** Single precordial thump has low success rate for cardioversion of shockable rhythm (Haman et al. 2009, **E**).
3 Summon help. If a second nurse is available, they can call for the cardiac arrest team, bring emergency equipment and screen off the area.	Maintain patient's privacy and dignity. CPR is more effective with two rescuers. One is responsible for inflating the lungs and the other for chest compressions. Continue until medical help arrives (RCUK 2010b, **C**).
4 Lie patient flat on a firm surface/bed. If on a chair, lower the patient to the floor, ensuring that the head is supported.	Effective external cardiac massage can be performed only on a hard surface (RCUK 2010b, **C**).

(continued)

Procedure guideline 9.6 Cardiopulmonary resuscitation *(continued)*

Action	Rationale
5 If patient is in bed, remove bed head and ensure adequate space between back of bed and wall.	To allow easy access to patient's head in order to facilitate intubation. **E**
6 Ensure a clear airway. If cervical spine injury is excluded, extend, not hyperextend, the neck (thus lifting the tongue off the posterior wall of the pharynx). This is best achieved by lifting the chin forwards with the finger and thumb of one hand while pressing the forehead backwards with the heel of the other hand (see Figure 9.31). If this fails to establish an airway, there may be obstruction by a foreign body. Try to remove the obstruction if visible. Insert oropharyngeal Guedel airway if you have appropriate training. See Figure 9.41.	To establish and maintain airway, thus facilitating ventilation (RCUK 2010b, **C**).
Do not remove well-fitted dentures.	They help to create a mouth-to-mask seal during ventilation. **E**
7 Place the heel of one hand in the centre of the sternum and place the other on top, ensuring that the hands are located between the middle and the lower half of the sternum. Ensure that only the heel of the dominant hand is touching the sternum.	To ensure accuracy of external cardiac compression and reduced delay in commencing cardiac compressions (RCUK 2010b, **C**).
Place the other hand on top, straighten the elbows and make sure shoulders are directly over the patient's chest.	
The sternum should be depressed sharply by 5–6 cm. The cardiac compressions should be forceful, and sustained at a rate of 100–120 per minute.	This produces a cardiac output by applying direct downward force and compression (Smith 2000, **R3**).
8 Apply facemask with Ambu-bag over nose and mouth. Compress bag in a rhythmical fashion: the bag should be attached to an oxygen source, 12–15 litres. In order to deliver +85% oxygen, a reservoir may be attached to the Ambu-bag. However, if oxygen is not immediately available, the Ambu-bag will deliver ambient air.	Room air contains only 21% oxygen. In shock, a low cardiac output, together with ventilation/perfusion mismatch, results in severe hypoxaemia. The importance of providing a high oxygen gradient from mouth to vital cells cannot be exaggerated and so oxygen should be added during CPR as soon as it is available (80–100% is desirable) (Simmons 2002, **R3**).
9 Maintain cardiac compression and ventilation at a ratio of 30:2. This rate can be achieved effectively by counting out loud 'one and two and', and so on. There should be a slight pause to ensure that the delivered breath is sufficient to cause the patient's chest to rise. This must continue until cardiac output returns and the patient has a palpable blood pressure.	Counting aloud will ensure co-ordination of ventilation and compression ratio. To maintain circulation and oxygenation, thus reducing risk of damage to vital organs. **E**
10 When the cardiac arrest team arrives, it will assume responsibility for the arrest in liaison with the ward staff.	To ensure an effective expert team co-ordinates the resuscitation (RCUK 2010b, **C**).
11 Attach patient to ECG monitor using three electrodes or defibrillation patches/paddles.	To obtain adequate ECG signal. Accurate recording of cardiac rhythm will determine the appropriate treatment to be initiated. **E**
Intubation in CPR	
12 Continue to ventilate and oxygenate the patient before intubation.	The risks of cardiac arrhythmias due to hypoxia are decreased (RCUK 2010b, **C**).
13 Equipment for intubation should be checked before handing to appropriate medical/nursing staff. (a) Suction equipment is operational. (b) The cuff of the endotracheal tube inflates and deflates. (c) The endotracheal tube is well lubricated. (d) That catheter mount with swivel connector is ready for use.	To ensure all equipment is working prior to use. **E**
14 During intubation, the anaesthetist may request cricoid pressure. This involves compressing the oesophagus between the cricoid ring and the sixth cervical vertebra.	To prevent the risk of regurgitation of gastric contents and the consequent risk of pulmonary aspiration (RCUK 2010b, **C**).
15 Recommence ventilation and oxygenation once intubation is completed.	Intubation should interrupt resuscitation only for a maximum of 16 seconds to prevent the occurrence of cerebral anoxia (Handley et al. 1997, **R3**).

Action	Rationale
16 Once the patient's trachea has been intubated, chest compressions, at a rate of 100–120 per minute, should continue uninterrupted (except for defibrillation and pulse check when indicated) and ventilation should continue at approximately 12 breaths per minute. Compression should continue while the defibrillator is charging.	Uninterrupted compression results in a substantially higher mean coronary perfusion pressure. A pause in chest compressions allows the coronary perfusion pressure to fall. On resuming compressions, there is some delay before the original coronary perfusion pressure is restored (RCUK 2010b, **C**). Reducing the pre-shock pause improves time of compression which has a more favourable outcome for the patient (Deakin et al. 2010, **C**).
Intravenous access in CPR	
17 Venous access must be established through a large vein as soon as possible.	To administer emergency cardiac drugs and fluid replacement (RCUK 2010b, **C**).
18 Asepsis should be maintained throughout.	To prevent local and/or systemic infection (Fraise and Bradley 2009, **E**).
19 The correct rate of infusion is required.	To ensure maximum drug and/or solution effectiveness. **E**
20 Accurate recording of the administration of solutions infused and drugs added is essential.	To maintain accurate records, provide a point of reference in the event of queries and prevent any duplication of treatment (NMC 2010, **C**).
Defibrillation	
21 Apply pads/paddles to chest. It may be necessary to shave the chest.	To ensure the pads/paddles are applied correctly and make adequate contact which enhances electrical contact (van Alem et al. 2003, **E**).
22 Remove oxygen source at least 1 metre from patient unless intubated.	To reduce the risk of sparks igniting the oxygen source (Nolan et al. 2005, **E**).
23 The person delivering the shock must ask all members of the resuscitation team to stand clear of the patient.	To ensure that none of the resuscitation team are in contact with the patient or the bed as they may also receive the shock (Perkins and Lockey 2008, **E**).
24 Deliver a single shock to treat VF/pulseless VT.	To terminate pulseless VT, VF and restart the heart by depolarizing its electrical conduction system and delivering brief measured electrical shocks to the chest wall or the heart muscle itself (Eftestol et al. 2002, **E**; Wik et al. 2003, **R1**).
Post-procedure	
25 Check patient by assessing airway, breathing, circulation, blood pressure and urine output.	To ensure a clear airway, adequate oxygenation and ventilation and aim to maintain normal sinus rhythm and a cardiac output adequate for perfusion of vital organs. To ensure adequacy of ventilation and oxygenation (Perkins and Lockey 2008, **E**).
26 Check arterial blood gases.	To ensure rapid correction of acid/base balance, potassium, glucose and haemoglobin results as an ABG result is available much quicker than laboratory blood results (RCUK 2010b, **C**).
27 Check full blood count, clotting and biochemistry.	To exclude anaemia as a contributor to myocardial ischaemia. A clotting disorder may have contributed to a major haemorrhage. Replacement stored blood for transfusion has fewer clotting factors and the patient may require replacement of clotting factors usually in the form of fresh frozen plasma. **E** To assess renal function and electrolyte balance (K^+, Mg^{2+} and Ca^{2+}). To ensure normoglycaemia. To commence serial cardiac enzyme assay (Nolan et al. 2005, **C**; RCUK 2010b, **C**).
28 Monitor patient's cardiac rhythm and record 12-lead ECG.	Normal sinus rhythm is required for optimum cardiac function (RCUK 2010b, **C**). An assessment of whether cardiac arrest has been associated with a myocardial infarction should be made, as the patient may be suitable for coronary angioplasty or thrombolytic therapy (Nolan et al. 2005, **C**).
29 A chest X-ray should be taken.	To establish correct position of tracheal tube, gastric tube and central venous catheter. To exclude left ventricular failure, pulmonary aspiration and pneumothorax. To establish size and shape of heart (Nolan et al. 2006, **C**).
30 Continue respiratory therapy aiming for SaO_2 94–98% for adults.	Hypoxia and hypercarbia both increase the likelihood of a further cardiac arrest (RCUK 2010b, **C**).

(continued)

Procedure guideline 9.6 Cardiopulmonary resuscitation *(continued)*

Action	Rationale
31 Assess patient's level of consciousness. This can be done by use of the Glasgow Coma Scale. Although this is intended primarily for head injury, it is clinically relevant. It contains five levels of consciousness. (a) Conscious and alert (b) Drowsy but responsive to verbal commands (c) Unconscious but responsive to minimal painful stimuli (d) Unconscious and responsive to deep painful stimuli (e) Unconscious and unresponsive.	Once a heart has been resuscitated to a stable rhythm and cardiac output, the organ that influences an individual's survival most significantly is the brain. Initial assessment and regular monitoring will alert the nurse to any changes in function (RCUK 2010b, **C**).
32 The patient should be stable prior to any transfer and nursed in the appropriate position, that is semi-Fowler or the recovery position. Avoid nursing supine as this physiologically hinders cardiac output and respiration, unless clinically indicated for patients with acute head or spinal cord injury. Careful explanation and reassurance are vital at all times, particularly if the patient is conscious and aware.	Transferring a patient post arrest may pose risks because of changes in their haemodynamic status. This is due to movement of the trolley – inertia, changes in environment and/or changing equipment, which may impact negatively on the patient's physiological status (Shirley and Bion 2004, **E**). Nursing a patient in semi-Fowler's position ensures good air entry and reduces risks of aspiration for patients not contraindicated for head of bed to be elevated (Tablan et al. 2004, **C**).

Problem-solving table 9.5 Prevention and resolution (Procedure guideline 9.6)

Problem	Cause	Prevention	Suggested action
Defibrillator not working.	Battery pack not charged.	Ensure defibrillator is plugged into the mains so battery can recharge.	Check defibrillator when doing emergency trolley checks as per hospital policy.
No trace when ECG dots or pads are on patient.	ECG dots or pads dry. Test plug connected to lead.	Change ECG dots/pads as they can dry out. Ensure that the test plug is not attached.	Check expiry dates of ECG dots/pads when checking emergency trolley/equipment. After emergency trolley checks, ensure that the test plug is no longer attached.
Staff unable to use defibrillator.	Not had training.	Mandatory yearly BLS training for staff who will be present during CPR, and ALS every 3 years for staff who work in specialized areas, for example critical care. Standardize equipment throughout the hospital.	Find a member of staff who is trained in using defibrillator. AED defibrillators should be available as they can be used by people without previous training.
Laryngoscope light not working.	Laryngoscope handle not charged.	Ensure that the laryngoscope handle is charged using rechargeable batteries or new batteries inserted. Change laryngoscope light.	Check laryngoscope when doing resuscitation equipment checks as per hospital policy. If using rechargeable batteries, ensure laryngoscope handle is docked. Have spare batteries if not using rechargeable. Have spare light bulbs/spare disposable laryngoscope blades on the emergency trolley.
Portable suction not working.	Battery pack not charged. Incorrectly connected tubing.	Ensure that suction unit is plugged in so battery can charge. Check that tubing correctly connected.	Check portable suction is on charge and tubing correctly connected when checking resuscitation equipment as per hospital policy.
Emergency drugs missing/expired.	Trolley not checked. Equipment removed without being replaced.	Have a checklist of the emergency drugs that need to be on the resuscitation trolley.	Check drugs and expiry dates when checking resuscitation equipment and resuscitation trolley as per hospital policy and lock trolley for safekeeping of drugs.
Equipment missing off resuscitation trolley.	Removal of equipment without replacing or returning it.	Have a checklist of all equipment needed on resuscitation trolley.	Check resuscitation trolley list as per hospital policy. Replace any missing or expired equipment. Seal/lock trolley after checks/use. Educate all staff not to remove equipment from trolley other than in a cardiac arrest.

POST-PROCEDURAL CONSIDERATIONS

Immediate care

Following stabilization of the patient post cardiac or respiratory arrest, consideration should be given to moving them to an appropriate critical care or high-dependency environment. All established monitoring should continue during transfer and the patient should be transferred by individuals capable of monitoring the patient and responding appropriately to any change in their condition, including a further cardiac arrest. A critical care outreach service or designated transfer team, if available, may contribute to the care of the patient during stabilization and transfer (Nolan et al. 2006, RCUK 2010b, Shirley and Bion 2004).

Ongoing care

The patient's haemodynamic status should be continually monitored post resuscitation, as well as observing their level of consciousness, respiration rate and if possible urine output. Monitor blood glucose levels in adults with sustained return of spontaneous circulation (ROSC) after cardiac arrest. Maintaining blood glucose values >10 mmol/L, they should be treated in an HDU/ICU environment, but hypoglycaemia must be avoided (RCUK 2010b). Documentation of physiological parameters needs to continue and any change in haemodynamic status needs to be reported to the medical team or senior nursing staff attending to the patient prior to transfer to the CCU or HDU.

The Intensive Care Society (UK) has published guidelines for the transport of the critically ill adult (www.ics.ac.uk). These outline the requirements for equipment and personnel when transferring critically ill patients (Nolan et al. 2006, RCUK 2006, Sandroni et al. 2007, Shirley and Bion 2004).

Careful explanation and reassurance must be given to the patient before transfer, particularly if the patient is conscious and aware. The patient's relatives will require considerable support and will need to be kept informed of the transfer of their relative and to where. It is important that if the family were not present during the arrest, the appropriate member of the medical team contacts the next of kin and informs them of the arrest and its outcome. If the patient has survived, the next of kin/family will need to know that the patient has been moved to a more appropriate environment for continued monitoring.

Note: Whether the resuscitation attempt was successful or not, the pastoral needs of all those associated with the arrest should not be forgotten (RCUK 2010b, Sandroni et al. 2007).

Documentation

Good record keeping is an integral part of nursing practice, and is essential to the provision of safe and effective care (NMC 2010). There must be documentary evidence of how decisions relating to the patient were made. Accurate recording of the administration of solutions infused and drugs added is essential. All resuscitation attempts should be audited, ideally using a nationally recognized template such as the Utstein template (recommended by the RCUK 2010b). Hospitals should collect data regarding cardiac arrest for the National Cardiac Arrest Audit (NCAA) (RCUK 2010b).

Education of patient and relevant others

Prevention of cardiac arrest is the most important factor for survival. Education of the patient and relevant others needs to start at first contact with healthcare professionals regarding lifestyle changes, diet, exercise, smoking cessation, and regular check-ups to treat or control any underlying causes such as hypertension and diabetes.

COMPLICATIONS

Some possible complications may arise from cardiopulmonary resuscitation.

- Gastric distension due to bagging too forcefully and/or too quickly, causing air to enter the stomach. A nasogastric tube should be inserted as soon as the airway is secure, to help prevent and manage gastric distension which may cause vomiting and possible aspiration into the lungs.
- Fractured ribs, sternum, punctured lungs can occur as a result of chest compressions. The correct placement of hands during chest compression is vital in helping to prevent fracturing of ribs and sternum.
- Transmission of disease through mouth-to-mouth ventilation. The use of a pocket resuscitation mask with a one-way valve will prevent the transmission of infection from bodily fluids during ventilation (DH 2007).

Learning for practice

After studying this chapter, list five key points you have learnt about respiratory care that you will be able to apply to your clinical practice.

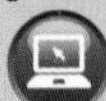
For further learning exercises visit **www.royalmarsdenmanual.com/student**.

Now Test Yourself

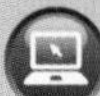
This section provides a range of exercises/activities to further test your learning. For additional exercises visit **www.royalmarsdenmanual.com/student**.

What have you learnt?

1 There are four functions necessary to achieve optimal respiration, one of which is cellular respiration. Which of the following definitions best describes cellular respiration?

A Adequate breathing and movement of air in and out of the lungs, ensuring a fresh supply of oxygen to the alveoli

B Adequate gas exchange, oxygen uptake and carbon dioxide unloading between the blood and the alveoli of the lungs

C The movement of oxygen and carbon dioxide between the lungs and the body tissues

D Oxygen delivery and carbon dioxide uptake between the systemic blood and tissue cells

2 What percentage of the air we breathe is made up of oxygen?
A 16%
B 21%
C 26%
D 31%

3 In an emergency, oxygen can be administered by a nurse without a prescription and documented later
A True
B False

4 Which of the following oxygen masks is able to deliver between 60–90% oxygen when delivered at a flow rate of 10–15 L/min?
A Simple semi-rigid plastic masks
B Venturi high flow mask
C Nasal cannulas
D Non-rebreathing mask

5 What are the benefits of administering humidified oxygen?

6 Most tracheostomy tubes consist of an outer and inner tube. What are the two main reasons for having the inner tube?

7 When considering the conduction system of the heart, which of the following is considered the natural pacemaker of the heart?
A Sinoatrial (SA) node
B AV node
C Bundle of His
D Purkinje fibres

8 In the event of a cardiac arrest, which are the two rhythms that require defibrillation?
A Asystole and PEA
B PEA and VF
C PEA and pulseless VT
D VF and pulseless VT

9 What are the eight common causes of cardiac arrest? Can you list the four Hs and four Ts?

10 Which is the first drug to be used in cardiac arrest of any aetiology?
A Adrenaline
B Amiodarone
C Atropine
D Calcium chloride

See the end of the chapter for the answers.

Key points

- An understanding of respiratory physiology and oxygen transportation and utilization is fundamental to respiratory assessment and the provision of effective respiratory care.
- Nursing and physiotherapy staff may assess patients, initiate and monitor oxygen delivery systems within the prescribed parameters, except in emergencies when oxygen should be given first and documented later (NPSA 2009).
- All patients should be assessed and monitored using a *track and trigger system*, e.g. NEWS (National Early Warning Score) (NICE 2007, RCP 2012).
- In general wards and critical care, the most frequent problems with tracheostomies relate to obstruction or displacement. All hospitals and community settings should have a procedure for managing such situations and all staff involved in the care of the patient must be both aware of the procedure and appropriately trained.
- Cardiac arrest implies a sudden interruption of cardiac output. It may be reversible with appropriate treatment (Handley 2004, RCUK 2010b). All members of the healthcare professions who attempt resuscitation will be expected to employ the highest professional standard of care, in line with their level of training.

REFERENCES

AHA/ILCOR (2000) Guidelines 2000 for CPR and emergency care: an international consensus on science. *Resuscitation*, 46(1), 73–92, 109–114.

Ahrens, T. & Tucker, K. (1999) Pulse oximetry. *Critical Care Nursing Clinics of North America*, 11(1), 87–98.

Austin, R. & Snow, A. (2000) Defibrillation. In: Cheller, A. (ed) *Resuscitation: A Guide for Nurses*. London: Harcourt, pp.141–157.

Baskett, P.J., Nolan, J.P., Handley, A., Soar, J., Biarent, D. & Richmond, S. (2005) European Resuscitation Council guidelines for resuscitation 2005. Section 9. Principles of training in resuscitation. *Resuscitation*, 67(Suppl 1), S181–189.

Becker, D. (2007) Cardiac anatomy and physiology and assessment. In: Kaplow,R. & Hardin, S.R. (eds) *Critical Care Nursing: Synergy for Optimal Outcomes*. Sudbury, MA: Jones and Bartlett, pp.121–138.

Benditt, J.O. (2000) Adverse effects of low-flow oxygen therapy. *Respiratory Care*, 45(1), 54–61.

Berne, R.M. (2004) *Physiology*, 5th edn. St Louis, MO: Mosby.

Bersten, A.D., Soni, N. & Oh, T.E. (2009) *Oh's Intensive Care Manual*, 6th edn. Oxford: Butterworth-Heinemann.

Billau, C. (2004) Suctioning. In: Russell, C. & Matta, B.F. (eds) *Tracheostomy: A Multiprofessional Handbook*. Cambridge: Cambridge University Press, pp.157–172.

Bjorling, G. (2007) *Long-Term Tracheostomy: Outcome, Cannula Care and Material Wear*. Stockholm: Karolinska Institute.

BMA (2000) *The Impact of the Human Rights Act on Medical Decision-Making*. London: British Medical Association.

BMA (2007) *Withholding or Withdrawing Life-Prolonging Medical Treatment*, 3rd edn. London: Blackwell Publishing.

BMA, RCN, Resuscitation Council (UK) & Age Concern (2002) *Decisions Relating to Cardiopulmonary Resuscitation: Model Information Leaflet*. London: British Medical Association.

Bond, P., Grant, F., Coltart, L. & Elder, F. (2003) Best practice in the care of patients with a tracheostomy. *Nursing Times*, 99(30), 24–25.

Bowers, B. & Scase, C. (2007) Tracheostomy: facilitating successful discharge from hospital to home. *British Journal of Nursing*, 16(8), 476–479.

Branson, R.D. & Gentile, A. (2010) Is humidification always necessary during noninvasive ventilation in the hospital? *Respiratory Care*, 55(2), 209–216.

BTS (2008) *BTS Guideline for Emergency Oxygen Use in Adult Patients.* London: British Thoracic Society. Available at: www.brit-thoracic.org.uk/document-library/clinical-information/oxygen/emergency-oxygen-use-in-adult-patients-guideline/emergency-oxygen-use-in-adult-patients-guideline/

Celik, S.A. & Kanan, N. (2006) A current conflict: use of isotonic sodium chloride solution on endotracheal suctioning in critically ill patients. *Dimensions of Critical Care Nursing*, 25(1), 11–14.

Chanques, G., Constantin, J-M., Sauter, M., et al. (2009) Discomfort associated with underhumidified high-flow oxygen therapy in critically ill patients. *Intensive Care Medicine*, 35, 996–1003.

Chiumello, D., Pelosi, P., Park, G., et al. (2004) In vitro and in vivo evaluation of a new active heat moisture exchanger. *Critical Care*, 8(5), 281–288.

Christie, P. & Robinson, H. (2009) Using a communication framework at handover to boost patient outcomes. *Nursing Times*, 105(47), 13–15.

Clotworthy, N. (2006a) Post-operative care of the patient following a laryngectomy. In: *Guidelines for the Care of Patients with Tracheostomy Tubes.* London: St George's Healthcare NHS Trust, pp.15–16.

Clotworthy, N. (2006b) Tracheostomy tubes. In: *Guidelines for the Care of Patients with Tracheostomy Tubes.* London: St George's Healthcare NHS Trust, pp.9–14.

Colquhoun, M.C. (2008) A national scheme for public access defibrillation in England and Wales: Early results. *Resuscitation*, 78(3), 275–280.

Cuquemelle, E., Pham, T., Papon, J-F., Louis, B., Danin, P-E. & Brochard, L. (2012) Heated and humidified high-flow oxygen therapy reduces discomfort during hypoxemic respiratory failure. *Respiratory Care*, 57(10), 1571–1577.

Day, T. (2000) Tracheal suctioning: when, why and how. *Nursing Times*, 96(20), 13–15.

Day, T., Farnell, S. & Wilson-Barnett, J. (2002) Suctioning: a review of current research recommendations. *Intensive Care Nursing*, 18(2), 79–89.

Deakin, C.D., Nolan, J.P., Sunde, K. & Koster, R.W. (2010) European Resuscitation Council Guidelines for Resuscitation 2010 Section 3. Electrical therapies: automated external defibrillators, defibrillation, cardioversion and pacing. *Resuscitation*, 81(10), 1293–1304.

De Leyn, P., Bedert, L., Delcroix, M., et al. (2007) Tracheotomy: clinical review and guidelines. *European Journal of Cardiothoracic Surgery*, 32(3), 412–421.

Demers, R.R. (2002) Bacterial/viral filtration. Let the breather beware! *Chest*, 120, 1377–1389.

DH (2000) *Comprehensive Critical Care: A Review of Adult Critical Care Services.* London: Department of Health.

DH (2005) *Hazardous Waste (England) Regulations.* London: Department of Health.

DH (2007) *Pandemic Influenza: Guidance for Infection Control in Hospitals and Primary Care Settings.* London: Department of Health.

Docherty, B. & Hall, S. (2002) Basic life support and AED. *Professional Nurse*, 17(12), 705–706.

Dolan, S. & Preston, N.J. (2006) Malignant effusions. In: Kearney, N. & Richardson, A. (eds) *Nursing Patients with Cancer: Principles and Practice.* Edinburgh: Elsevier Churchill Livingstone, pp.619–632.

Dysart, K., Miller, T.L., Wolfson, M.R. & Shaffer, T.H. (2009) Research in high-flow therapy: mechanisms of action. *Respiratory Medicine*, 103(10), 1400–1405.

Edgtton-Winn, M. & Wright, K. (2005) Tracheostomy: a guide to nursing care. *Australian Nursing Journal*, 13(5), 17–20.

Eftestol, T., Sunde, K. & Steen, P.A. (2002) Effects of interrupting precordial compressions on the calculated probability of defibrillation success during out-of-hospital cardiac arrest. *Circulation*, 105(19), 2270–2273.

Epstein, O. (2009) *Pocket Guide to Clinical Examination*, 4th edn. Edinburgh: Mosby.

Esmond, G. (2001) *Respiratory Nursing.* London: Baillière Tindall.

Fell, H. & Boehm, M. (1998) Easing the discomfort of oxygen therapy. *Nursing Times*, 94(38), 56–58.

Fischer, R. (2006) Oxygen delivery device can also deliver infections. *Nursing*, 36(7), 18.

Fraise, A.P. & Bradley, T. (eds) (2009) *Ayliffe's Control of Healthcare-Associated Infection: A Practical Handbook*, 5th edn. London: Hodder Arnold.

Glass, C.A. & Grap, M.J. (1995) Ten tips for safer suctioning. *American Journal of Nursing*, 95(5), 51–53.

Griggs, A. (1998) Tracheostomy: suctioning and humidification. *Nursing Standard*, 13(2), 49–53.

Groves, N. & Tobin, A. (2007) Nasal high-flow therapy delivers low-level positive airway pressure. *Australian Critical Care*, 20, 126–131.

Guyton, A.C. & Hall, J.E. (2006) *Textbook of Medical Physiology*, 11th edn. Philadelphia: Elsevier Saunders.

Hallstrom, A., Cobb, L., Johnson, E. & Copass, M. (2000) Cardiopulmonary resuscitation by chest compression alone or with mouth-to-mouth ventilation. *New England Journal of Medicine*, 342, 1546–1553.

Haman, L., Parizek, P. & Vojacek, J. (2009) Precordial thump efficacy in termination of induced ventricular arrhythmias. *Resuscitation*, 80, 14–16.

Hampton, S. (1998) Film subjects win the day. *Nursing Times*, 94(24), 80–82.

Handley, A.J. (2004) Basic life support. In: Colquhoun, M., Handley, A. & Evans, T. (eds) *ABC of Resuscitation*, 4th edn. London: BMJ Books, pp.1–4.

Handley, A.J., Becker, L.B., Allen, M., van Drenth, A., Kramer, E.B. & Montgomery, W.H. (1997) Single rescuer adult basic life support. An advisory statement from the Basic Life Support Working Group of the International Liaison Committee on Resuscitation (ILCOR). *Resuscitation*, 34(2), 101–108.

Harkin, H. (2004) *Decannulation.* In: Russell, C. & Matta, B.F. (eds) *Tracheostomy: A Multiprofessional Handbook.* Cambridge: Cambridge University Press, pp.255–268.

Harper, R.J. (2010) Pericardiocentesis. In: Roberts, J.R. & Hedges, J.R. (eds). *Clinical Procedures in Emergency Medicine*, 5th edn. Philadelphia: Saunders Elsevier, pp. 287–307.

Hauff, S.R., Rea, T.D., Culley, L.L., et al. (2003) Factors impeding dispatcher-assisted telephone cardiopulmonary resuscitation. *Annals of Emergency Medicine*, 42(6), 731–737.

Hess, D. (2000) Detection and monitoring of hypoxemia and oxygen therapy. *Respiratory Care*, 45(1), 65–80.

Hess, D.R. (2005) Tracheostomy tubes and related appliances. *Respiratory Care*, 50(4), 497–510.

Higgins, D. (2009) Basic nursing principles of caring for patients with a tracheostomy. *Nursing Times*, 105(3), 14–15.

Hough, A. (2001) *Physiotherapy in Respiratory Care: An Evidence-Based Approach to Respiratory and Cardiac Management*, 3rd edn. Cheltenham: Nelson Thornes.

Hui, D., Morgado, M., Chisholm, G., et al. (2013) High-flow oxygen and bilevel positive airway pressure for persistent dyspnoea in patients with advanced cancer: A phase II randomised trial. *Journal of Pain and Symptom Management*, 46(4), 463–473.

ICS (2008) *Standards for the Care of Adult Patients with a Temporary Tracheostomy.* Intensive Care Society: Standards and Guidelines. London: Intensive Care Society.

ICS (2011) *Standards for the Care of Adult Patients with a Temporary Tracheostomy.* Intensive Care Society: Standards and Guidelines. London: Intensive Care Society.

Intersurgical (2009) Complete Respiratory Systems. Available at: http://media.intersurgical.com/global/documents/info_sheets/Humidification.pdf

Ireton, J. (2007) Tracheostomy suction: a protocol for practice. *Paediatric Nursing*, 19(10), 14–18.

Jenkins, G. & Tortora, G.J. (2013) *Anatomy and Physiology: From Science to Life*, 3rd edn. Hoboken, NJ: John Wiley & Sons.

Jevon, P. (2001) Cardiopulmonary resuscitation. Initial assessment. *Nursing Times*, 97(41), 41–42.

Jevon, P. (2002) Resuscitation in hospital: Resuscitation Council (UK) recommendations. *Nursing Standard*, 16(33), 41–44.

Kayner, A.M. (2012) Respiratory failure. Available at: http://emedicine.medscape.com/article/167981-overview

Khan, S.Y. & O'Driscoll, B.R. (2004) Is nebulized saline a placebo in COPD? *BMC Pulmonary Medicine*, 30(4), 9.

Kumar, P.J. & Clark, M.L. (2009) *Kumar and Clark's Clinical Medicine*, 7th edn. Edinburgh: Saunders/Elsevier.

Lenglet, H., Sztrymf, B., Leroy, C., Brun, P., Dreyfuss, D. & Ricard, J-D. (2012) Humidified high-flow nasal oxygen during respiratory failure in the emergency department: feasibility and efficacy. *Respiratory Care*, 57(11), 1873–1878.

Lewarski, J.S. (2005) Long-term care of the patient with a tracheostomy. *Respiratory Care*, 50(4), 534–537.

MacIntyre, N.R. & Branson, R.D. (2009) *Mechanical Ventilation*, 2nd edn. St Louis, MO: Saunders Elsevier.

Mackenzie, I. (2008) *Core Topics in Mechanical Ventilation*. Cambridge: Cambridge University Press.

Marieb, E.N., Hoehn, K. & Hutchinson, M. (2012) *Human Anatomy and Physiology*, 9th edn. San Francisco, CA: Pearson Benjamin Cummings.

Masclans, J.R. & Roca, O. (2012) High-flow oxygen therapy in acute respiratory failure. *Clinical Pulmonary Medicine*. 19(3), 127–130.

McGrath, B., Bates, L., Atkinson, D. & Moore, J. (2012) Anaesthesia: multidisciplinary guidelines for the management of tracheostomy and laryngectomy airway emergencies. *Journal of the Association of Anaesthetists of Great Britain and Ireland*, 67, 1025–1041.

MDA (2000) *Continuous Positive Airway Pressure (CPAP) Circuits: Risk of Misassembly*. Available at: www.mhra.gov.uk/Safetyinformation/Safetywarningsalertsandrecalls/MedicalDeviceAlerts/Safetynotices/CON008853

Meaney, P.A., Nadkami, V.M., Kern, K.B., Indik, J.H., Haperin, H.R. & Berg, R.A. (2010) Rhythms and outcomes of adult in-hospital cardiac arrest. *Critical Care Medicine*, 38, 101–108.

MHRA (2010) All chest drains when used with high-flow, low-vacuum suction systems (wall mounted). Available at: www.mhra.gov.uk/home/groups/dts-bs/documents/medicaldevicealert/con081898.pdf

Moran, G. (2010) *A Beginner's Guide to Normal Heart Function, Sinus Rhythm and Common Cardiac Arrhythmias*. Nottingham: Division of Nursing, University of Nottingham. Available at: www.nottingham.ac.uk/nursing/practice/resources/cardiology/introduction/index.php

Morton, P.G. & Fontaine, D.K. (2009) *Critical Care Nursing: A Holistic Approach*, 9th edn. Philadelphia: Lippincott Williams & Wilkins.

Moser, D.K. & Chung, M.L. (2003) Critical care nursing practice regarding patient anxiety assessment and management. *Intensive Care and Critical Care Nursing*, 19(5), 275–288.

NCEPOD (2012) Time to intervene. A review of patients who underwent pulmonary resuscitation as a result of an in-hospital cardiopulmonary arrest. London: National Confidential Enquiry into Patient Outcome and Death. Available at: www.ncepod.org.uk

Nelson, L. (1999) Points of friction. *Nursing Times*, 95(34), 72–75.

NHS Institute for Innovation and Improvement (2011) Available at: www.institute.nhs.uk/quality_and_service_improvement_tools/quality_and_service_improvement_tools/sbar_-_situation_-_background_-_assessment_-_recommendation.html

NICE (2006) *Brief Interventions and Referral for Smoking Cessation in Primary Care and Other Settings*. London: National Institute for Health and Clinical Excellence.

NICE (2007) *Acutely Ill Patients in Hospital: Recognition of and Response to Acute Illness in Adults in Hospital*. London: National Institute for Health and Clinical Excellence. Available at: www.nice.org.uk/guidance/CG50

NMC (2010) *Record Keeping: Guidance for Nurses and Midwives*. London: Nursing and Midwifery Council. Available at: http://tinyurl.com/9w9eqoy

NMC (2013) *Consent*. London: Nursing and Midwifery Council. Available at: www.nmc-uk.org/Nurses-and-midwives/Advice-by-topic/A/Advice/Consent/

NMC (2015) *The Code: Standards of Conduct, Performance and Ethics for Nurses and Midwives*. London: Nursing and Midwifery Council.

Nolan, J.P., Deakin, C.D., Soar, J., Bottiger, B.W. & Smith, G. (2005) European Resuscitation Council Guidelines for Resuscitation 2005 Section 4. Adult advanced life support. *Resuscitation*, 67(Suppl 1), S39–86.

Nolan, J.P., Soar, J., Lockey, A., et al. (2006) *Advanced Life Support*, 5th edn. London: Resuscitation Council (UK).

Nolan, J.P., Soar, J, Zideman, D.A., et al. (2010) European Resuscitation Council Guidelines for Resuscitation 2010 Section 1. Executive summary. *Resuscitation*, 81, 1219–1276.

NPSA (2007) *The Fifth Report from the Patient Safety Observatory. Safety Care for the Acutely Ill Patient: Learning from Incidents*. London: National Patient Safety Agency. Available at: www.nrls.npsa.nhs.uk/resources/?entryid45=59828

NPSA (2008) *Chest Drains. Rapid Response Report: Risks Associated with the Insertion of Chest Drains*. London: National Patient Safety Agency.

NPSA (2009) *Rapid Response Report NPSA/2009/RRR006: Oxygen Safety in Hospitals*. London: National Patient Safety Agency.

O'Driscoll, B.R., Howard, L.S., Davison, A.G. & British Thoracic Society (2008) BTS guideline for emergency oxygen use in adult patients. *Thorax*, 63(Suppl 6), 1–73.

Paradis, N. (2007) *Cardiac: The Science and Practice of Resuscitation Medicine*, 2nd edn. Cambridge: Cambridge University Press, pp.3–26.

Parke, R., Eccleston, M., McGuiness, S., Korner, S. & Gerard, C. (2007) High-flow humidified nasal oxygen therapy (F&P OptiflowTM) delivers low-level positive pressure in a study of 15 post-operative cardiac patients. Available at: http://www.aaic.net.au/document/?D=2007670

Patel, J. & Matta, B. (2004) Percutaneous dilatational tracheostomy. In: Russell, C. & Matta, B.F. (eds) *Tracheostomy: A Multiprofessional Handbook*. Cambridge: Cambridge University Press, pp.59–68.

Perel, P., Roberts, I. & Pearson, M. (2007) Colloids versus crystalloids for fluid resuscitation in critically ill patients. *Cochrane Database of Systematic Reviews*, 4, CD000567.

Perkins, G.D. & Lockey, A.S. (2008) Defibrillation – safety versus efficacy. *Resuscitation*, 79, 1–3.

Perkins, G.D., Stephenson, B., Hulme, J. & Monsieurs, K.G. (2005) Birmingham assessment of breathing study (BABS). *Resuscitation*, 64(1), 109–113.

Pierce, L.N. (1995) *Guide to Mechanical Ventilation and Intensive Respiratory Care*. Philadelphia: W.B. Saunders.

Pierson, D.J. (2000) Pathophysiology and clinical effects of chronic hypoxia. *Respiratory Care*, 45(1), 39–51.

Price, T. (2004) Surgical tracheostomy. In: Russell, C. & Matta, B.F. (eds) *Tracheostomy: A Multiprofessional Handbook*. Cambridge: Cambridge University Press, pp.35–58.

Prior, T. & Russell, S. (2004) Tracheostomy and head & neck cancer. In: Russell, C. & Matta, B.F. (eds) *Tracheostomy: A Multiprofessional Handbook*. Cambridge: Cambridge University Press, pp.269–283.

Pryor, J.A. & Prasad, S.A. (2008) *Physiotherapy for Respiratory and Cardiac Problems: Adults and Paediatrics*, 4th edn. Edinburgh: Churchill Livingstone Elsevier.

RCP (2012) *National Early Warning Score: Standardising the Assessment of Acute Illness and Severity in the NHS. Report of a Working Party*. London: Royal College of Physicians.

RCUK (2010a) *Legal Status of Those Who Attempt Resuscitation*. London: Resuscitation Council.

RCUK (2010b) *Resuscitation Guidelines October 2010*. London: Resuscitation Council.

RCUK (2012) *The National Tracheostomy Safety Project – The Emergency Management of Tracheostomies and Laryngectomies*. London: Resuscitation Council.

Restrepo, R.D. & Walsh, B.K. (2012) humidification during invasive and noninvasive mechanical ventilation. *Respiratory Care*, 57 (5), 782–788.

Resuscitation Council (2004) *CPR Guidance for Clinical Practice and Training in Hospitals*. London: Resuscitation Council. Available at: www.resus.org.uk/pages/standard.pdf

Rhys Evans, P.H., Montgomery, P.Q. & Gullane, P.J. (2003) *Principles and Practice of Head and Neck Oncology*. London: Dunitz.

Ritchie, J.E., Williams, A.B., Gerard, C. & Hockey, H. (2011) Evaluation of a humidified nasal high-flow oxygen system, using oxygraphy, capnography and measurement of upper airway pressures. *Anaesthesia and Intensive Care*, 39(6), 1103–1110.

Robertson, C., Steen, P., Adgey, J., et al. (1998) The 1998 European Resuscitation Council Guidelines for adult advanced life support. *Resuscitation*, 37(2), 81–90.

Roca, O., Riera, J., Torres, F. & Masclans, J.R. (2010) High-flow oxygen therapy in acute respiratory failure. *Respiratory Care*, 55(4), 408–413.

Russell, C. (2004) Tracheostomy tubes. In: Russell, C. & Matta, B.F. (eds) *Tracheostomy: A Multiprofessional Handbook*. Cambridge: Cambridge University, pp.85–114.

Russell, C. (2005) Providing the nurse with a guide to tracheostomy care and management. *British Journal of Nursing*, 14(8), 428–433.

Sandroni, C., Nolan, J., Cavallaro, F. & Antonelli, M. (2007) In-hospital cardiac arrest: incidence, prognosis and possible measures to improve survival. *Intensive Care Medicine*, 33, 237–245.

Scase, C. (2004) Wound care. In: Russell, C. & Matta, B.F. (eds) *Tracheostomy: A Multiprofessional Handbook*. Cambridge: Cambridge University Press, pp.173–186.

Serra, A. (2000) Tracheostomy care. *Nursing Standard*, 14(42), 45–52.

Shelledy, D.C. & Mikles, S.P. (2002) Patient assessment and respiratory care plan development. In: Mishoe, S.C. & Welch, M.A. (eds) *Critical Thinking in Respiratory Care: A Problem-Based Learning Approach*. New York: McGraw-Hill, pp.181–234.

Shirley, P.J. & Bion, J.F. (2004) Intra-hospital transport of critically ill patients: minimising risk. *Intensive Care Medicine*, 30, 1505–1510.

Shuster, M., Billi, J.E., Bossaert, L., et al. (2010) International consensus on cardiopulmonary resuscitation and emergency cardiovascular care science with treatment recommendations. Part 4: Conflict of interest management before, during and after the 2010 International Consensus Conference on Cardiopulmonary Resuscitation and Emergency Cardiovascular Care Science with Treatment Recommendations. *Resuscitation*, 81, e41–e47.

Simmons, R. (2002) The airway at risk. In: Colquhoun, M., Handley, A. & Evans, T. (eds) *ABC of Resuscitation*, 5th edn. London: BMJ Books, pp.25–31.

Simpson, G., Vincent, S. & Ferns, J. (2012) Spontaneous tension pneumothorax: what is it and does it exist? *Internal Medicine Journal*, 42(10), 1157–1160.

Skinner, D.V. & Vincent, R. (1997) *Cardiopulmonary Resuscitation*, 2nd edn. Oxford: Oxford University Press.

Smith, D. (2000) Basic life support. In: Cheller, A. (ed) *Resuscitation: A Guide for Nurses*. London: Harcourt, pp.65–80.

Sztrymf, B. Messika, J., Bertrand, F., et al. (2011) Beneficial effects of humidified high flow nasal oxygen in critical care patients: a prospective study. *Intensive Care Medicine*, 37, 1780–1786.

Sztrymf, B., Messika, J., Mayot, T., Lenglet, H., Dreyfuss, D. & Ricard, J. (2012) Impact of high-flow nasal oxygen on intensive care unit patients with acute respiratory failure: a prospective observational study. *Journal of Critical Care*, 27, 324e9–324e13.

Tablan, O.C., Anderson, L.J., Besser, R., et al. (2004) CDC Healthcare Infection Control Practices Advisory Committee. Guidelines for preventing health care-associated pneumonia, 2003: recommendations of CDC and the Healthcare Infection Control Practices Advisory Committee. *Morbidity and Mortality Weekly Report*, 53(RR-3), 1–36.

Tamburri, L.M. (2000) Care of the patient with a tracheostomy. *Orthopaedic Nursing*, 19(2), 49–58.

Tiruvoipati, R., Lewis, D., Haji, K. & Botha, J. (2010) High-flow nasal oxygen vs high-flow face mask: a randomised crossover trial in extubated patients. *Journal of Critical Care*, 25, 463–468.

Tortora, G.J. & Derrickson, B. (2011) *Principles of Anatomy & Physiology*, 13th edn. Hoboken, NJ: John Wiley & Sons.

Urden, L.D., Stacy, K.M. & Lough, M.E. (2006) *Thelan's Critical Care Nursing: Diagnosis and Management*, 5th edn. St Louis, MO: Mosby/Elsevier.

Van Alem, A.P., Sanou, B.T. & Koster, R.W. (2003) Interruption of cardiopulmonary resuscitation with the use of the automated external defibrillator in out-of-hospital cardiac arrest. *Annals of Emergency Medicine*, 42(4), 449–457.

Ward, B. & Park, G.R. (2000) Humidification of inspired gases in the critically ill. *Clinical Intensive Care*, 11(4), 169–176.

Waugh, A. & Grant, A. (2010) *Ross and Wilson's Anatomy and Physiology in Health and Illness*. Edinburgh: Churchill Livingstone Elsevier, pp.77–129.

Waugh, J.B. & Granger, W.M. (2004) An evaluation of two new devices for nasal high-flow gas therapy. *Respiratory Care*, 49(8), 902–906.

Weisberg, L.S. (2008) Management of severe hyperkalaemia. *Critical Care Medicine*, 36(12), 3246–3251.

West, J.B. (2008) *Pulmonary Pathophysiology: The Essentials*, 7th edn. Philadelphia: Wolters Kluwer/Lippincott Williams and Wilkins.

Wik, L., Hansen, T.B., Fylling, F., et al. (2003) Delaying defibrillation to give basic cardiopulmonary resuscitation to patients with out-of-hospital ventricular fibrillation: a randomized trial. *JAMA*, 289(11), 1389–1395.

Winser, H. (2001) An evidence base for adult resuscitation. *Professional Nurse*, 16(7), 1210–1213.

Winslow, R.M. (2013) Oxygen is the poison. *Transfusion*, 53(2), 424–437.

Woodrow, P. (2002) Managing patients with a tracheostomy in acute care. *Nursing Standard*, 16(44), 39–46.

Answers

Learning Activity 9.1 Case study: Respiratory assessment and smoking cessation

Ella Smith is a 29-year-old woman who was admitted to your unit overnight for observation following an acute exacerbation of her asthma. This is the second time in 6 weeks she has been admitted for this reason.

1 You need to assess her respiratory status; what else should you be observing for?
- Ease and comfort of breathing, rate, pattern, her position, rate and ease of breathing when speaking or moving, her colour and appearance, any audible breath sounds.

She is a smoker and on her previous admission was advised that she should try to stop smoking as this was a likely trigger for her asthma. She managed to stop for 4 weeks but started again one week ago when she was on a girls' night out and all her friends were smoking. She tells you that she usually smokes 5–10 cigarettes a day.

2 What would be your first step in encouraging her to stop smoking?
- Assess her desire to stop smoking.
- Have a discussion about the benefits of stopping smoking.

3 What other forms of support may she benefit from?
- In consultation with other members of the nursing and multidisciplinary team, suggest pharmacotherapy and behavioural support.
- Provide any available self-help material and potentially refer her to more intensive support such as the NHS Stop Smoking services http://www.nhs.uk/smokefree.

Learning Activity 9.2 Scenario: Administering oxygen

You are looking after a 78-year-old gentleman overnight whose oxygen saturations have dropped to 85%. The nurse in charge has asked you to give him some oxygen.

What would you do?
- Inform and discuss what you are going to do with the patient.
- Find out at what rate to administer the oxygen and with which device.

- Check whether oxygen has been prescribed and, if so, whether the required rate is within the prescribed parameters.
- If not prescribed, discuss with the nurse in charge/medical team whether this constitutes an emergency situation where oxygen can be administered first and formally prescribed later.
- Commence oxygen administration as directed.
- Continue to monitor oxygen saturations and other vital signs (including respiratory rate).
- Document all decisions and ensure this is countersigned by your supervising nurse.

Learning Activity 9.5 **Scenario: Tracheostomy dressing change**

You have been asked to prepare the equipment required to change the tracheostomy dressing for one of your patients. It is now day 5 following his neck operation, which included the formation of a temporary tracheostomy.

1 Is this a procedure you can do on your own?
- No, it requires two nurses, one to hold the tracheostomy in place, the other to change the dressing.

2 Make a list of the equipment required.
- Sterile dressing pack, tracheostomy/keyhole dressing, 0.9% sodium chloride cleaning solution, tracheostomy securing tapes, alcohol handrub.

3 How should you prepare the patient for the procedure?
- Explain and discuss the procedure with the patient.
- Review whether any additional analgesia is required in advance of the procedure.

Learning Activity 9.6 **Case study: Cardiac arrest**

Mrs Grange is a 69-year-old woman who has had recent extensive gynaecological surgery. During the shift handover this morning, you were told that she had not been feeling herself overnight and that she was slightly tachycardic with lower than normal blood pressure. You have been asked to keep a close eye on her with regular hourly observations. You go to her bed to carry out your next set of observations and as you approach her you find her on her bed and she appears pale and slightly slumped to one side on her pillows. You go up to Mrs Grange and touch her arm but she does not respond.

1 What should you do next?
- Shout for help.
- Check the surrounding area to make sure it is safe, no slip/trip hazards, no wires/electric cables in the way.
- Check level of consciousness by gently shaking shoulders saying, Are you alright?
- Use ABC to check airway – breathing – circulation.

2 One of the healthcare assistants comes to help you. What should you ask him to do?
- Call the cardiac arrest team, get another nurse to come and help and bring the cardiac arrest trolley.

3 You now know that Mrs Grange is not breathing and has no pulse. One of the qualified nurses comes to help you and the healthcare assistant brings the cardiac arrest trolley. What do you do next?
- Along with the other nurse you commence 30 chest compressions followed by two rescue breaths using the Ambu-bag.

4 What should you be prepared to do once the cardiac arrest team arrive?
- Continue to help as directed by the team and your nursing colleagues. This may include reassuring other patients in the immediate ward area.

5 What may be the possible causes for her cardiac arrest?
- The most likely causes may include hypovolaemia, thrombosis, metabolic causes.

Now Test Yourself **What have you learnt?**

1 There are four functions necessary to achieve optimal respiration, one of which is cellular respiration. Which of the following definitions best describes cellular respiration?
   A Adequate breathing and movement of air in and out of the lungs, ensuring a fresh supply of oxygen to the alveoli
   B Adequate gas exchange, oxygen uptake and carbon dioxide unloading between the blood and the alveoli of the lungs
   C The movement of oxygen and carbon dioxide between the lungs and the body tissues
   D Oxygen delivery and carbon dioxide uptake between the systemic blood and tissue cells

2 What percentage of the air we breathe is made up of oxygen?
   A 16%
   B 21%
   C 26%
   D 31%

3 In an emergency, oxygen can be administered by a nurse without a prescription and documented later.
   A True
   B False

4 Which of the following oxygen masks is able to deliver between 60–90% oxygen when delivered at a flow rate of 10–15 L/min?
   A Simple semi-rigid plastic masks
   B Venturi high flow mask
   C Nasal cannulas
   D Non-rebreathing mask

5 What are the benefits of administering humidified oxygen?
- Maintains effective ciliary activity, helping to ensure the effective removal of mucus and secretions from the respiratory tract.
- Minimises symptoms of dryness.
- Improves patient tolerance of oxygen therapy.
- Improves lung and airway mechanics.

6 Most tracheostomy tubes consist of an outer and inner tube. What are the two main reasons for having the inner tube?
- It can be removed for cleaning without disturbing the stoma site.
- Allows immediate relief of life-threatening airway obstruction in the event of a blockage with clots or secretions.

7 When considering the conduction system of the heart, which of the following is considered the natural pacemaker of the heart?
   A Sinoatrial (SA) node
   B AV node
   C Bundle of His
   D Purkinje fibres

8 In the event of a cardiac arrest, which are the two rhythms that require defibrillation?
A Asystole and PEA
B PEA and VF
C PEA and pulseless VT
D VF and pulseless VT

9 What are the eight common causes of cardiac arrest? Can you list the four Hs and four Ts?
- Hypoxia, Hypovolaemia, Hypo/hyperkalaemia, Hypothermia
- Thrombosis, Tamponade, Toxins, Tension pneumothorax

10 Which is the first drug to be used in cardiac arrest of any aetiology?
A Adrenaline
B Amiodarone
C Atropine
D Calcium chloride

Part Three
Supporting the patient through the diagnostic process

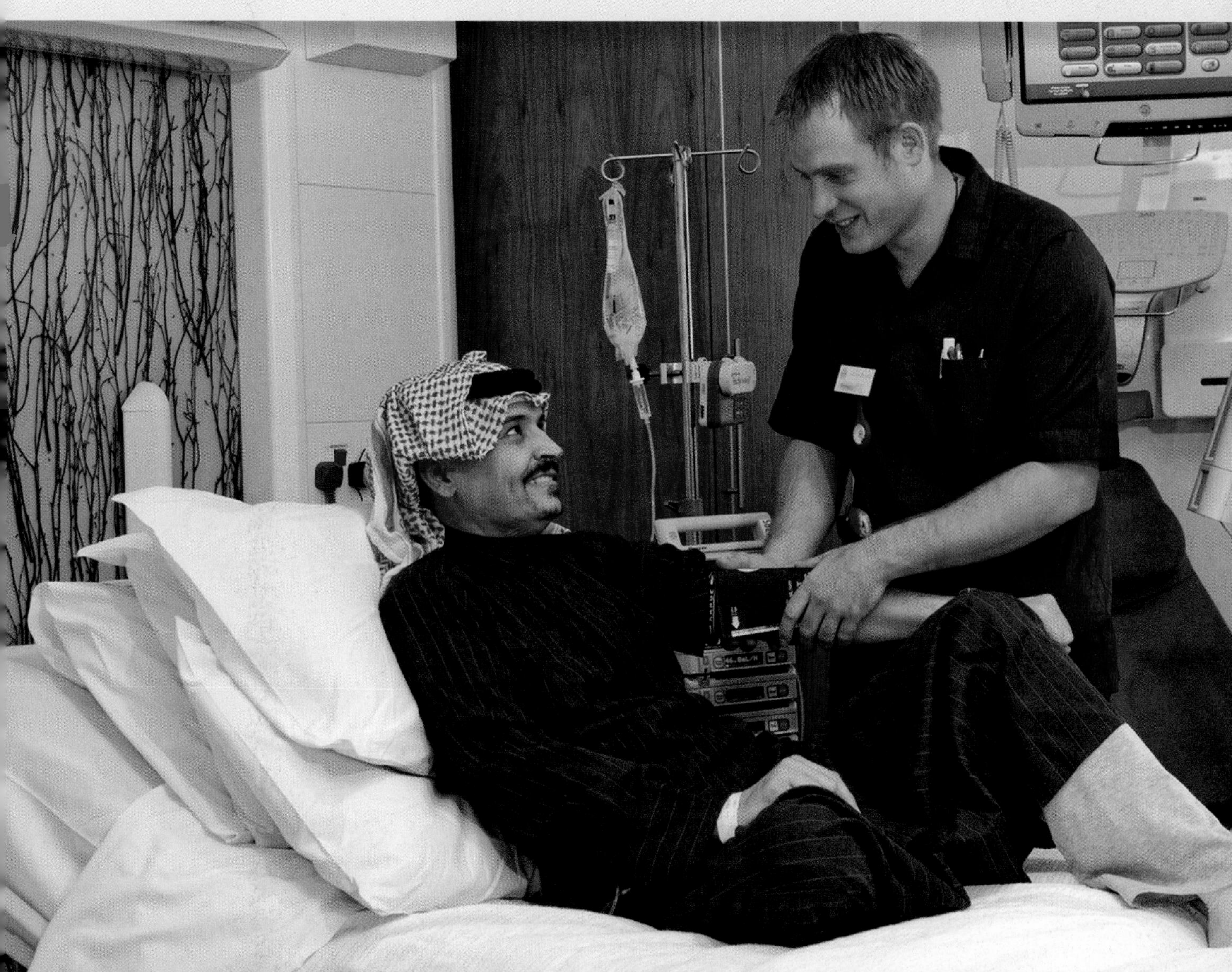

Interpreting diagnostic tests

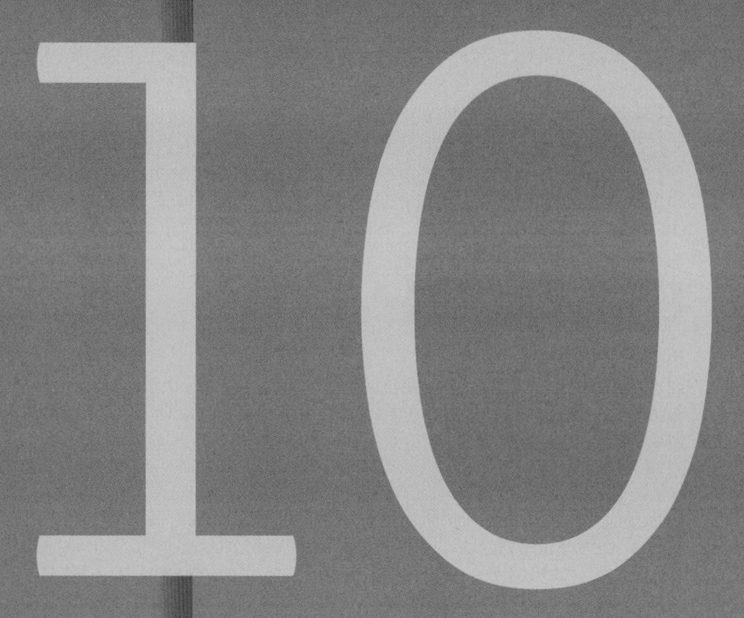

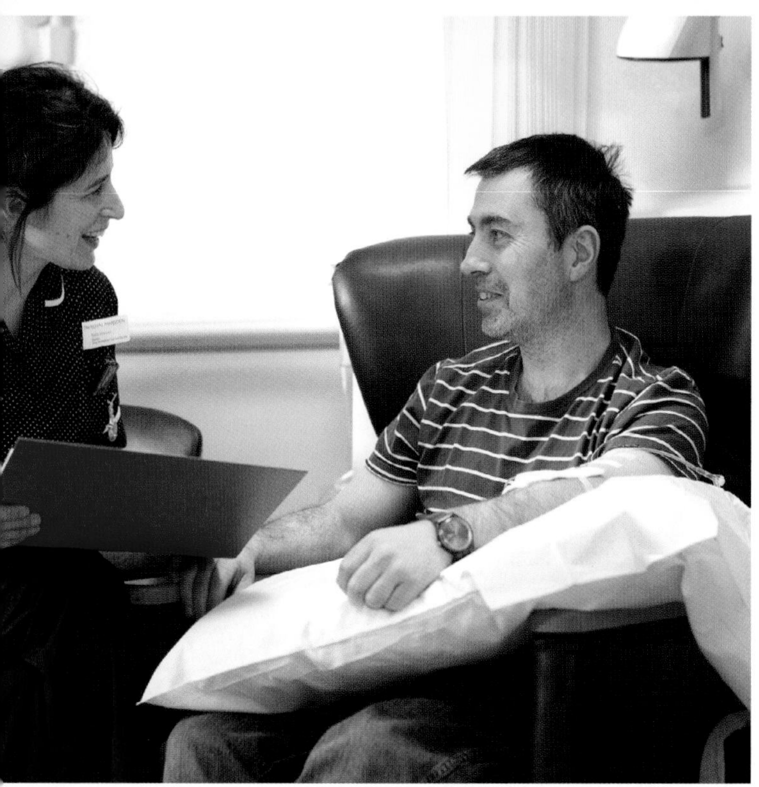

By reading this chapter and undertaking the learning activities within it, you should be able to:

1. Identify the importance of the nursing role in instigating, participating and assisting in diagnostic tests and specimen collection.
2. Demonstrate an understanding of the rationale for common diagnostic tests encountered in clinical practice.
3. Demonstrate an understanding of the clinical procedures for common diagnostic tests and associated infection control precautions.

Procedure guidelines

The Royal Marsden Manual of Clinical Nursing Procedures: Student Edition, Ninth Edition. Edited by Lisa Dougherty, Sara Lister and Alexandra West-Oram

Overview

In clinical practice nursing staff are required to instigate, participate or assist in diagnostic tets and the collection of body fluids and/or specimens for varying purposes. This chapter will discuss common diagnostic tests encountered in clinical practice.

Diagnostic tests

DEFINITION

A diagnostic test is a procedure that is used to aid in the detection and or diagnosis of disease (Chernecky and Berger 2013, Higgins 2013).

RELATED THEORY

Diagnostic tests are undertaken to aid in diagnosis and treatment of various conditions. The tests are used to identify diseases from their characteristics, signs and symptoms and to identify changes or abnormalities. Diagnostic tests include blood sampling from a vein or from central venous access devices to determine the haematological and biochemical status of patients, lumbar puncture for diagnostic and treatment purposes, liver biopsy, semen collection and cervical swabbing. Depending on the clinical picture, radiological investigations such as X-ray, computed tomography (CT) or magnetic resonance imaging (MRI) may be required. Other more invasive diagnostic procedures such as endoscopy may also be required.

EVIDENCE-BASED APPROACHES

Rationale

Diagnostic tests are essential in the healthcare setting but their selection and use must be considered carefully. The overuse of diagnostic tests is a contributor to needless healthcare costs, hence it is essential that healthcare providers and professionals ensure that the tests used are of adequate benefit to the patient's health (Qaseem et al. 2012). This leads to poor quality services and continuing financial pressure on departments and organizations (Korenstein et al. 2012). For example, a faecal sample from a patient who also has a history of recent travel would be investigated for organisms not normally looked for in a specimen from a patient without such a history. The sensitivity of the organism to a range of antimicrobials can then be tested to decide on the most appropriate and effective mode of treatment (Higgins 2013). Diagnostic tests may include the collection of samples or procedures that assist in the diagnosis and treatment of a patient's condition.

Successful laboratory diagnosis depends upon the collection of specimens at the appropriate time, using the correct technique and equipment, and transporting them to the designated laboratory safely without delay (Box 10.1). For this to be achieved, it is essential that there is good liaison between medical, nursing, portering and laboratory staff (Mims 2004).

Box 10.1 **Good practice in specimen collection**

- Appropriate to the patient's clinical presentation.
- Collected at the right time.
- Collected in a way that minimizes the risk of contamination.
- Collected in a manner that minimizes the health and safety risk to all staff handling the sample.
- Collected using the correct technique, with the correct equipment and in the correct container.
- Documented clearly, informatively and accurately on the request forms.
- Stored/transported appropriately.

Source: Higgins (2008b). Reproduced with permission from EMAP Publishing Ltd.

Indications

Conducting a diagnostic test or collecting a specimen is often the first crucial step in determining diagnosis and subsequent mode of treatment for patients with suspected infections or to aid in the diagnosis of specific conditions. In other aspects the collection or test may help determine variation from normal values such as blood sampling or endoscopic findings.

Principles of care

Nursing staff play a key role within the diagnostic testing process because they often identify the need for diagnostic and/or microbiological investigations, initiate the collection of specimens and assume responsibility for timely and safe transportation to the laboratory (Higgins 2013). Specimen collection is often the first crucial step in investigations that define the nature of the disease, determine a diagnosis and therefore the mode of treatment.

Methods of investigation

Initial examination

The initial assessment of the patient will determine the potential diagnostic tests or samples that are required. Dependent on how the patient progresses, their clinical history and/or symptom progression will determine the need for further diagnostic tests. For example, specimens will be initially examined for clinical variables such as odour, appearance, consistency and turbidity. Foul-smelling, purulent material is suggestive of anaerobic bacteria, cloudy cerebrospinal fluid (CSF) or urine suggests the presence of neutrophils, stool may contain blood or mucus and parasites such as roundworms or tapeworms which are visible to the naked eye (Gould and Brooker 2008).

Direct microscopy

The majority of specimens will then undergo direct microscopic investigation which is valuable as an early indication of the causative organism. High magnification is required to visualize viruses, which are then identified according to their characteristic shapes (Gould and Brooker 2008). Certain parasitic protozoa, such as those causing malaria, are identified by direct microscopy which necessitates the specimen being delivered to the laboratory as quickly as possible whilst the protozoa are mobile and therefore visible (Higgins 2013). In combination with clinical presentations, this may be enough to initiate or change targeted treatments until a more definitive diagnosis is reached (Weston 2008).

Gram staining

Gram staining is a process by which staining substances are added to a sample to differentiate the type of organisms present. Cells with differing properties stain differently in relation to the structure of their cell wall (Mims 2004).

Gram staining allows for the differentiation between Gram-positive bacteria (e.g. *Staphylococcus aureus*), which stain purple, and Gram-negative bacteria (e.g. *Escherichia coli*), which stain pink when viewed under the microscope. This can be used to guide the choice of antimicrobial therapy until other investigation methods can provide a definitive identification of pathogenic micro-organisms (Mims 2004).

Culture

Depending upon the type of specimen sent to the laboratory and the suspected causative organism, a liquid or solid medium will be selected to enable further identification. Clinical specimens are inoculated onto agar plates or into nutrient broth, then incubated for a certain period of time and observed for growth (Weston 2008). Different species or strains have different growth rates; for example, *Pseudomonas* and *Clostridium* multiply in approximately 10 minutes, *Escherichia coli* has a growth rate of 8 hours whilst

Mycobacterium tuberculosis takes 18–24 hours to grow (Weston 2008). Growth of bacteria is seen as colonies on the culture media and the size, colour and shape vary according to the type of bacteria identified (Gould and Brooker 2008).

Fungal organisms grow in the same type of media as those used for bacteria, although they generally require an incubation period of 24–48 hours (Higgins 2013). Pathogenic fungi can also be grown on special mycological media, upon which they grow better with less risk of bacterial overgrowth (Mims 2004). Fungi are identified by their characteristic appearance on the surface of the agar and microscopic appearance (Gould and Brooker 2008). The presence of fungi, such as *Candida albicans*, is sometimes difficult to interpret because they are commonly present in the upper respiratory, alimentary and female genital tracts, and on the skin of healthy people. However, in patients who are immunocompromised this fungus can lead to systemic disease (Garber 2001).

Viruses cannot be cultured outside living cells, although cells grown in nutrient material can be used to culture certain viruses. Their identification is indicated by the characteristic way in which they change the shape of the cell (Gould and Brooker 2008).

Antibiotic sensitivity

Once the pathogenic organism has been identified, it is vital to establish which antibiotics it is sensitive to so the appropriate therapy can be prescribed (Gould and Brooker 2008). The bacteria are inoculated onto a solid media plate and paper discs impregnated with different antibiotics are placed over them and incubated. If the bacteria are sensitive to a particular antibiotic, their growth is inhibited, resulting in a clear zone around the disc.

Serology

Serology is useful in identifying viral infections and bacterial infections with difficult culture organisms and is based upon the host's immunological reaction. Detection of antigens or antibodies in serum, which are activated in response to infection, may suggest that the patient is, or has been, infected (Higgins 2013).

Despite the disadvantage of the test being performed retrospectively, antibody testing is the main method for diagnosing viral infections (Mims 2004). Two serum tests are collected, once at the beginning of the illness and again at 10–14 days, and compared for changes in antibody content. A raised content suggests that the patient's infection is current (Mims 2004).

Histology

Histology is the study of cells and tissues within the body. It also studies how the tissues are arranged to form organs. The histological focus is on the structure of individual cells and how they are arranged to form the individual organs. The types of tissues that are recognized are epithelial, connective, muscular and nervous (Junqueira and Carneiro 2005).

The tissues are examined under a light microscope where light passes through the tissue components after they have been stained. As most tissues are colourless, they are stained with dyes to enable visualization. An alternative is the electron microscope in which the cells and tissue can be viewed at magnifications of about 120,000 times (Junqueira and Carneiro 2005).

LEGAL AND PROFESSIONAL ISSUES

An organization providing diagnostic services must have clear identifiable policies and procedures. Bidirectional communication must be open between the department, organizational board and national bodies to ensure appropriate care is delivered. Monitoring processess must be in place to identify potential clinical or organizational risks and have a clear reporting mechanism.

Competencies

In accordance with the NMC's *The Code: Standards of Conduct, Performance and Ethics* (NMC 2015), the collection of specimens should be undertaken by professionals who are competent and feel confident that they have the knowledge, skill and understanding to do so, following a period of appropriate training and assessment. For microbiological sampling, this will include knowledge and understanding of the collection, handling and transportation of samples to optimize quality and minimize contamination and inadvertent subversion of the specimen, all of which may have subsequent implications for patient treatment and care.

Consent

It is therefore essential that healthcare practitioners gain consent before beginning any treatment or care; this includes the collection of samples or conducting a diagnostic test (NMC 2013). Consent is continuous throughout any patient episode and the practitioner must ensure that the patient is kept informed at every stage (Marsden 2007). For specimen collection this includes:

- informing the patient of the reason for specimen collection
- what the procedure will involve
- ascertaining their level of understanding (especially if they need to be directly involved in the sampling technique)
- how long the results may take to be processed
- how the results will be made available
- information about the implications this may have for their care.

Risk management

New research and evidence continue to be produced. It is essential that any risk or change in practice is communicated to clinicians. Alerts from the Medicines and Healthcare Products Regulatory Agency (MHRA) and changes in practice should be acted upon. Several agencies such as the Health Protection Agency (HPA) also contribute new guidance and best practice using the the latest available evidence.

Accurate record keeping and documentation

Good record keeping is an integral part of nursing practice, and it is essential to the provision of safe and effective care (NMC 2010). Accurate, specific and timely documentation of specimen collection or diagnostic tests should be recorded in the patient notes, care plan or designated record charts/forms such as a microbiological flow chart that details when a specimen was collected, results of analysis, sensitivities or resistance to antimicrobials and changes/modifications to treatment. It is also important to ensure that electronic records are up to date. This assists in the communication and dissemination of information between members of the interprofessional healthcare team.

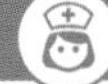
Learning Activity 10.1

Scenario: Gaining consent

You have been asked to take a sputum sample from a patient with a productive cough.

Before undertaking this procedure what information should you give to the patient in order to gain their verbal consent?

See the end of the chapter for the answers.

PRE-PROCEDURAL CONSIDERATIONS

Equipment

There is a variety of equipment/tools designed for the collection of specimens such as sterile pots, swabs and other receptacles (Figure 10.1, Figure 10.2, Figure 10.3, Figure 10.4). Advice should be sought from the microbiology department about the best type of container for the required investigation (Higgins 2013).

Figure 10.1 **Sputum pot.**

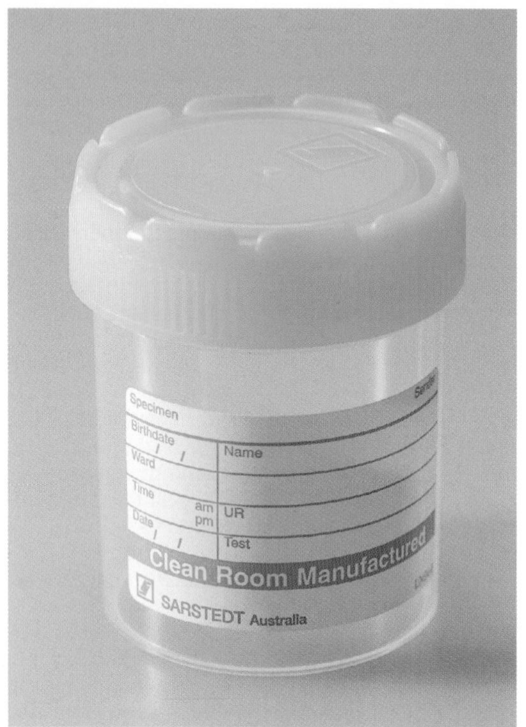

It is essential that the specimen and its transport container are appropriate for the type of organism being investigated; for example, bacterial swabs contain a transport medium that is incompatible with viral specimen analysis. Failure to utilize the correct collection method leads to inaccurate results so it is vital that an adequate quantity of material is obtained to allow complete microbiological examination.

Figure 10.2 **Various stool pots.**

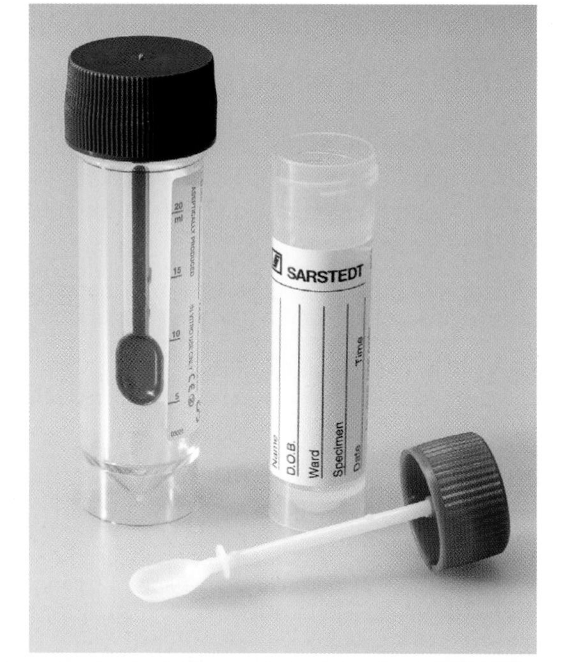

Figure 10.3 **Urine pot.**

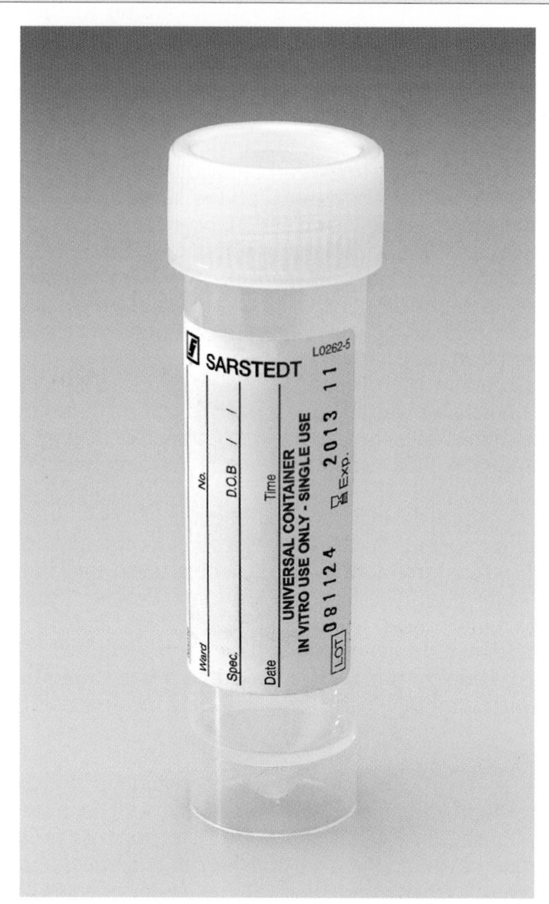

Equipment used for transportation

Within healthcare institutions, specimens should be transported in deep-sided trays that are not used for any other purpose, and are disinfected weekly and whenever contaminated (HSE 2003), or robust, leak-proof containers that conform to 'Biological Substances, Category B – UN3373' regulations (HSE 2005). Specimens that need to be moved outside the hospital must be transported using a triple-packaging system (HSE 2005). This consists of a watertight, leak-proof, absorbent primary container, a durable, watertight, leak-proof secondary container and an outer container that complies with 'Biological Substances,

Figure 10.4 **Variety of swabs.**

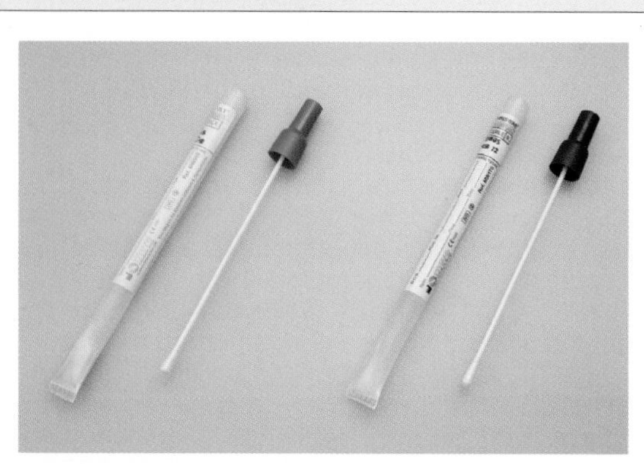

Category B – UN 3373' standards (Pankhurst and Coulter 2009). A box for transportation is essential and should carry a warning label for hazardous material. It must be made of smooth impervious material, such as plastic or metal, which will retain liquid and can be easily disinfected and cleaned in the event of a spillage (HSE 2003).

Handling specimens

Specimens should be obtained using safe techniques and practices, and practitioners should be aware of the potential physical and infection hazards associated with the collection of diagnostic specimens within the healthcare environment. Standard (universal) infection control precautions should be adopted by healthcare workers who have direct contact or exposure to the blood, bodily fluids, secretions and excretions of patients (European Biosafety Network 2010, Gould and Brooker 2008). In addition to personal protection, the person collecting the specimen should also be mindful of the collective health and safety of other people involved in the handling of samples. Every health authority must ensure that medical, nursing, phlebotomy, portering and any other staff involved in handling specimens are trained to do so (RCN 2012).

In relation to specimen collection, standard (universal) infection control precautions should include the following (Tilmouth and Tilmouth 2009).

- Hand hygiene.
- The use of personal protection equipment (PPE).
- Safe sharps management.
- Safe handling, storage and transportation of specimens.
- Waste management.
- Clean environment management.
- Personal and collective management of exposure to body fluids and blood.

Selection of PPE should be based upon an assessment of risk of exposure to body fluids. As minimum precautions, gloves and aprons should be worn when handling all body fluids. Protective face wear (e.g. goggles, masks and visors) should be worn during any procedure where there is risk of blood, bodily fluid, secretions or excretions splashing into the eyes or face (Gould 2002, RCN 2012).

Specimens should be placed in a double, self-sealing bag with one compartment containing the specimen and the other containing the request form. The specimen container used should be appropriate for the purpose and the lid should be securely closed immediately to avoid spillage and contamination. The specimen should not be overfilled and not be externally contaminated by the contents. Any accidental spillages must be cleaned up immediately by staff wearing appropriate protective equipment (HSE 2003, RCN 2012).

If a specimen is suspected or known to present an infectious hazard, particularly Hazard Group 3 pathogens (such as hepatitis B or C virus, HIV, *Mycobacterium tuberculosis*), this must be clearly indicated with a 'danger of infection' label on the specimen and the request form to enable those handling the specimen to take appropriate precautions (HSE 2003).

Specimens from patients who have recently been treated with toxic therapy such as gene therapy, cytotoxic drugs, radioactivity or active metabolites need to be handled with caution. Local guidelines on the labelling, bagging and transportation of such samples to the laboratory should be followed. For example, in the case of gene therapy, the specimen must be labelled with a 'biohazard' label, double bagged and transported to the laboratory in a secure box with a fastenable lid.

Selecting specimens

Selecting a specimen that is representative of the disease process is critical to the ability of the laboratory to provide information that is accurate, significant and clinically relevant. Incorrect specimen selection or technique can be life threatening to patients (Wegerhoff 2006). Specimens should only be taken when there are clinical signs of infection (or in the case of specific swabs, such as skin or nasal swabs, as part of an infection screening regimen). Signs of infection such as fever should trigger a careful clinical assessment to ensure that unnecessary tests are avoided and the most useful laboratory samples are obtained to identify therapeutic options (Gould and Brooker 2008). Specimens may also be collected for other diagnostic procedures such as cervical smears, semen collection and lumbar puncture. Tissue sampling may also be indicated during endoscopy or biopsies.

Wherever possible, specimens should be collected before patients are commenced on any treatment such as antibiotics or antiseptics. Treatment with antibiotics before the causative organism has been identified may inhibit its growth, so that it is not easily detected during analysis, yielding a misleading false negative (Weston 2008). If, however, the patient is already receiving such treatment, this must be clearly indicated on the requisition form.

Assessment and recording tools

Request forms

The form should include as much information as possible as this allows the laboratory or department conducting the investigation to select the most appropriate equipment and/or media for examination (Weston 2008).

Request forms should include the following information.

- Patient's name, date of birth, ward and/or department.
- Hospital number.
- Investigation required so as to avoid indiscriminate specimen analysis which wastes time and money.
- Date and time of specimen collection.
- Type and site of specimen. This should specify the actual anatomical site, such as 'abdominal wound', as this allows the laboratory to differentiate the target and non-target pathogens and assess the significance of results based upon the flora normally associated with that site (Wegerhoff 2006).
- Diagnosis and relevant clinical information which can help in the interpretation of a sample (Higgins 2013).
- Relevant signs and symptoms.
- Relevant history, for example recent foreign travel.
- Present or recent antimicrobial therapy.
- Whether the patient is immunocompromised as these patients are highly susceptible to opportunistic infections and non-pathogenic organisms (Weston 2008).
- Consultant's name.
- Name and contact details of the doctor requesting the investigation, as it may be necessary to telephone the result before the report is dispatched.
- If a high-risk specimen, it should be labelled with a 'danger of infection' label (HSE 2003).

Communication

For certain specimens that have specific collection techniques or require prompt processing, communication with the laboratory before the sample collection and/or providing information that a sample is being sent to the laboratory can improve efficiency of processing and accuracy of results. Where a diagnostic test is to be undertaken, it is essential that the patient is prepared appropriately with consideration of fasting times, the cessation of certain medications and post-procedural care. A patient information leaflet explaining the test can be given to prepare the patient. Communication with the department where the test will be conducted is essential.

Collecting specimens

The production of high-quality, accurate results which are clinically useful is very much dependent upon the quality of the specimen collection (Higgins 2013, Wegerhoff 2006). The greater the quantity of material sent for laboratory examination, the greater the chance of isolating a causative organism.

Specimens should be taken as soon as possible after the manifestation of clinical signs and symptoms. The timing of specimen collection is especially important during the acute phase of viral infections. Many viral illnesses have a prodromal phase where multiplication and shedding of the virus are usually at their peak and when the patient is most infective (Mims 2004). This is often before the onset of clinical illness and has often ceased by about day 5 from the onset of symptoms. At this stage, the patient's immune response against the virus has already been mounted and may therefore affect organism isolation (Winter 2005).

Specimens are readily contaminated by poor technique and analysis of such specimens could lead to adverse outcomes such as misdiagnosis, misleading results, extended length of stay, inappropriate therapy or potentially disastrous consequences for the patient (Wegerhoff 2006). Therefore, a clean technique must be used to avoid inadvertent contamination of the site of the sample or the specimen itself. Specimens should also be collected in sterile containers with close-fitting lids.

POST-PROCEDURAL CONSIDERATIONS

Labelling specimens

Prompt microbiological analysis is only possible if specimens and their accompanying request forms are sent with specific, accurate and complete patient information. Incorrectly labelled or unlabelled specimens will be discarded (HSE 2003).

Samples should include the following information.

- Patient's name, date of birth, ward and/or department.
- Hospital number.
- Date and time of specimen collection.
- Type and site of specimen. This should specify the actual anatomical site such as 'abdominal wound' as this allows the laboratory to differentiate the target and non-target pathogens and assess the significance of results based upon the flora normally associated with that site (Wegerhoff 2006).
- If a high-risk specimen, it should be labelled with a 'danger of infection' label (HSE 2003).

Transporting specimens

An awareness of the type of organism being investigated and their growth requirements gives the healthcare professional an insight into the correct collection, storage and transportation methods (Table 10.1). Most micro-organisms are also extremely susceptible to environmental fluctuations such as pH, temperature, ultraviolet rays and oxidizing agents (Gould and Brooker 2008). Incorrect or prolonged storage or transportation may result in the organism not surviving before cultures can be made (Gill et al. 2005). Delays in transporting a specimen to the laboratory can compromise the specimen's integrity, leading to false-negative or -positive results, because the sample is no longer representative of the disease process (Higgins 2013).

The sooner a specimen arrives in the laboratory, the greater the chance of organisms being identified. Some pathogens do not survive once they have left the host, whilst normal body flora within the sample may proliferate and overgrow, inhibiting or killing the pathogen (Weston 2008).

If delays are anticipated, samples need to be stored appropriately, depending on the nature of the specimen, until they can be processed. For example, blood cultures need to be incubated at 37°C, whereas swabs must be either refrigerated or kept at ambient temperature, depending on the site from which they were taken.

The transport of clinical specimens must conform to health and safety legislation and regulations, and there are more specific guidelines on the labelling, transport and reception of specimens within clinical laboratories and similar facilities (HSE 2003).

Table 10.1 **Types of organisms**

Organism	Definition
Aerobic	Aerobic bacteria will only grow in the presence of oxygen
Anaerobic	Anaerobic bacteria prefer an atmosphere of reduced oxygen, such as deep in wound bed tissue, and facultative anaerobes can grow in either the presence or absence of oxygen
Bacteria	Bacteria are unicellular organisms that multiply and die very rapidly, especially once removed from their optimum environment
Virus	Viruses are intracellular parasites that hijack the genetic material of the host cell, and are therefore unable to multiply outside living cells

Source: Adapted from Gould and Brooker (2008), Higgins (2013), Winter (2005).

Learning Activity 10.2

Learning in practice: Specimen handling and collection

Within your clinical area, make sure that you are familiar with the various containers used for specimen collection.

- Ask your mentor/supervising nurse to go through the forms that should be completed for different specimens.
- Familiarize yourself with the process for specimen storage and collection. Where do the samples go when they are ready for collection? Who collects them? Where is the laboratory?
- If you haven't already been, ask if you can arrange a visit to the laboratory to see how the specimens are processed.

Blood: obtaining samples from a peripheral vein (venepuncture)

DEFINITION

Venepuncture is the procedure of entering a vein with a needle (Weller 2009).

ANATOMY AND PHYSIOLOGY

The superficial veins of the upper limb are most commonly chosen for venepuncture. These veins are numerous and accessible, ensuring that the procedure can be performed safely and with minimum discomfort (McCall and Tankersley 2012). In adults, veins located on the dorsal portion of the foot may be selected but there is an increased risk of complications, especially if the patient has diabetes or a history of vascular/coagulation disorders (Hoeltke 2013). Therefore, veins in the lower limbs should be avoided where possible.

Vein choice

The veins commonly used for venepuncture are those found in the antecubital fossa because they are sizeable veins capable of providing copious and repeated blood specimens (Weinstein and Plumer 2007). However, the venous anatomy

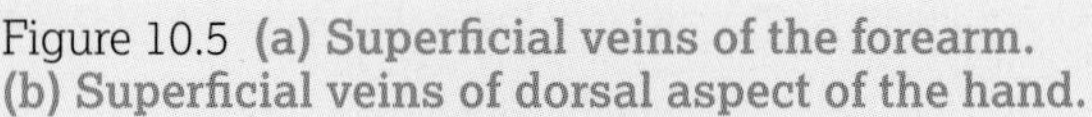

Figure 10.5 **(a) Superficial veins of the forearm. (b) Superficial veins of dorsal aspect of the hand.**

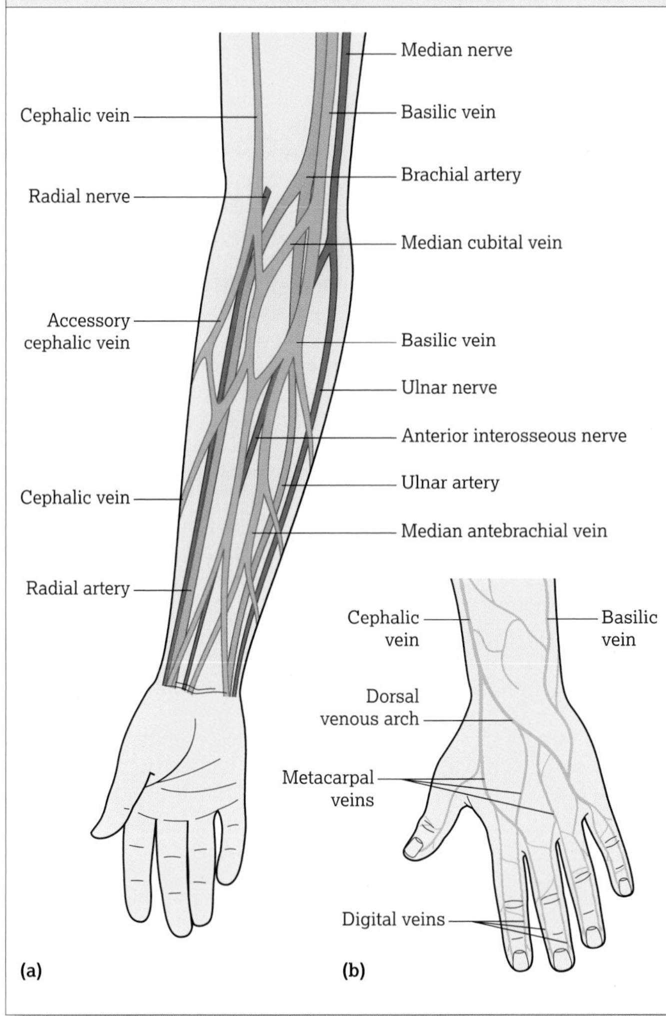

of each individual may differ. The main veins of choice are the (Figure 10.5):

- median cubital veins
- cephalic vein
- basilic vein
- metacarpal veins (used only when the others are not accessible).

Median cubital vein
The median cubital vein may not always be visible, but its size and location make it easy to palpate. It is also well supported by subcutaneous tissue, which prevents it from rolling under the needle (Hoeltke 2013).

Cephalic vein
On the lateral aspect of the wrist, the cephalic vein rises from the dorsal veins and flows upwards along the radial border of the forearm as the median cephalic, crossing the antecubital fossa as the median cubital vein. Care must be taken to avoid accidental arterial puncture, as this vein crosses the brachial artery. It is also in close proximity to the radial nerve (Dougherty 2008, Jenkins and Tortora 2013).

Basilic vein
The basilic vein, which has its origins in the ulnar border of the hand and forearm (Marieb and Hoehn 2010), is often overlooked as a site for venepuncture. It may well be prominent but is not well supported by subcutaneous tissue, making it roll easily, which can result in difficult venepuncture. Owing to its position, a haematoma may occur if the patient flexes the arm on removal of the needle, as this squeezes blood from the vein into the surrounding tissues (McCall and Tankersley 2012, Weinstein and Plumer 2007). Care must also be taken to avoid accidental puncture of the median nerve and brachial artery (Garza and Becan-McBride 2013).

Metacarpal veins
The metacarpal veins are easily visualized and palpated. However, the use of these veins may not be suitable in the elderly because skin turgor and subcutaneous tissue are diminished which makes the veins more difficult to anchor (McCall and Tankersley 2012, Weinstein and Plumer 2007).

Layers of the vein
Veins consist of three layers: the tunica intima, the tunica media and the tunica adventitia.

Tunica intima
The tunica intima is a smooth endothelial lining, which allows the passage of blood cells. If it becomes damaged, the lining may become roughened, leading to an increased risk of thrombus formation (Jenkins and Tortora 2013, Weinstein and Plumer 2007). Within this layer are folds of endothelium called valves, which keep blood moving towards the heart by preventing backflow. Valves are present in larger vessels and at points of branching and are seen as noticeable bulges in the veins (Jenkins and Tortora 2013). However, when suction is applied during venepuncture, the valve can compress and close the lumen of the vein, thus preventing the withdrawal of blood (Weinstein and Plumer 2007). Therefore, if detected, venepuncture should be performed above the valve in order to facilitate collection of the sample (Weinstein and Plumer 2007).

Tunica media
The tunica media, the middle layer of the vein wall, is composed of muscular tissue and nerve fibres, both vasoconstrictors and vasodilators, which can stimulate the vein to contract or relax. This layer is not as strong or stiff as an artery and therefore veins can distend or collapse as the pressure rises or falls (Jenkins and Tortora 2013, Waugh and Grant 2010, Weinstein and Plumer 2007). Stimulation of this layer by a change in temperature, mechanical or chemical stimulation can produce venous spasm, which can make a venepuncture more difficult.

Tunica adventitia
The tunica adventitia is the outer layer and consists of connective tissue, which surrounds and supports the vessel (Jenkins and Tortora 2013).

Arteries tend to be placed more deeply than veins and can be distinguished by the thicker walls, which do not collapse, the presence of a pulse and the bright red blood. It should be noted that aberrant arteries may be present; these are arteries located superficially in an unusual place (Jenkins and Tortora 2013, Weinstein and Plumer 2007).

Choosing a vein
The choice of vein must be that which is best for the individual patient. The most prominent vein is not necessarily the most suitable vein for venepuncture (Weinstein and Plumer 2007). There are two stages to locating a vein:

1 visual inspection
2 palpation.

Visual inspection
Visual inspection is the scrutiny of the veins in both arms and is essential prior to choosing a vein. Veins adjacent to foci of

infection, bruising and phlebitis should not be considered, owing to the risk of causing more local tissue damage or systemic infection (Dougherty 2008). An oedematous limb should be avoided as there is danger of stasis of lymph, predisposing to complications such as phlebitis and cellulitis with increased risk of causing tissue damage from the torniquet application (Hoeltke 2013, Smith 1998). Areas of previous venepuncture should be avoided as a build-up of scar tissue can cause difficulty in accessing the vein and can result in pain due to repeated trauma (Hoeltke 2013).

Palpation

Palpation is an important assessment technique, as it determines the location and condition of the vein, distinguishes veins from arteries and tendons, identifies the presence of valves and detects deeper veins (Dougherty 2008). The nurse should always use the same fingers for palpation as this will increase sensitivity and the ability of the nurse to know what they are feeling. The less dominant hand should be used for palpation so that in the event of a missed vein, the nurse can repalpate and realign the needle (Hoeltke 2013). The thumb should not be used as it is not as sensitive and has a pulse, which may lead to confusion in distinguishing veins from arteries in the patient (Weinstein and Plumer 2007).

Thrombosed veins feel hard and cord-like, and should be avoided along with tortuous, sclerosed, fibrosed, inflamed or fragile veins, which may be unable to accommodate the device to be used and will result in pain and repeated venepunctures (Dougherty 2008). Use of veins which cross over joints or bony prominences and those with little skin or subcutaneous cover, for example the inner aspect of the wrist, will also subject the patient to more discomfort (Dougherty 2008). Therefore, preference should be given to a vessel that is unused, easily detected by inspection and palpation, patent and healthy. These veins feel soft and bouncy and will refill when depressed (Weinstein and Plumer 2007).

EVIDENCE-BASED APPROACHES

Rationale

Indications

Venepuncture is carried out for two reasons:

- to obtain a blood sample for diagnostic purposes
- to monitor levels of blood components and a patient's condition (Garza and Becan-McBride 2013).

Contraindications (to using certain veins/areas)

- Previous surgery to an affected limb with axillary lymph node clearance.
- Lymphoedema on a particular limb.
- Amputation, fracture and cerebrovascular accident affecting limb.

Methods of improving venous access

- *Application of a tourniquet*: this promotes venous distension. The tourniquet should be tight enough to impede venous return but not restrict arterial flow. It should be placed about 7–8 cm above the venepuncture site. It may be more comfortable for the patient to position it over a sleeve or paper towel to prevent pinching the skin. The tourniquet should not be left on for longer than 1 minute as this may result in haemoconcentration, or pooling of the blood or haemolysis leading to inaccurate blood results (Hoeltke 2013, Saleem et al. 2009).
- The patient may be asked to clench the fist and encourage venous distension but should avoid 'pumping' as this action may affect certain blood results, for example potassium where cell damage releases potassium (Ernst 2005, Garza and Becan-McBride 2013).
- Lowering the arm below heart level also increases blood supply to the veins.
- Light tapping of the vein may be useful but can be painful and may result in the formation of a haematoma in patients with fragile veins, for example thrombocytopenic patients (Dougherty 2008).
- The use of heat in the form of a warm pack or by immersing the arm in a bowl of warm water for 10 minutes helps to encourage venodilation and venous filling (Lenhardt et al. 2002).
- Ointment or patches containing small amounts of glyceryl trinitrate have been used to improve local vasodilation to aid venepuncture (Weinstein and Plumer 2007).

Methods for insertion

Asepsis is vital when performing a venepuncture as the skin is breached and a foreign device is introduced into a sterile circulatory system. The two major sources of microbial contamination are:

- cross-infection from practitioner to patient
- skin flora of the patient.

Good handwashing and drying techniques are essential on the part of the nurse or healthcare professional and gloves should be changed between patients (see Chapter 3: Infection prevention and control).

To remove the risk presented by the patient's skin flora, firm and prolonged rubbing with an alcohol-based solution, such as chlorhexidine 0.5% in 70% alcohol, is advised (RCN 2010). This cleaning should continue for about 30 seconds, although some authors state a minimum of 1 minute or longer (Weinstein and Plumer 2007). The area that has been cleaned should then be allowed to dry to: (i) facilitate coagulation of the organisms, thus ensuring disinfection, and (ii) prevent a stinging pain on insertion of the needle due to the alcohol on the end of the needle. The skin must not be touched or the vein repalpated prior to venepuncture (McCall and Tankersley 2012).

LEGAL AND PROFESSIONAL ISSUES

Venepuncture is one of the most commonly performed invasive procedures in the NHS and is now routinely undertaken by nurses. In order to perform venepuncture safely, the nurse must have basic knowledge of the following.

- The relevant anatomy and physiology.
- The criteria for choosing both the vein and device to use.
- The potential problems which may be encountered, how to prevent them and necessary interventions.
- The health and safety/risk management of the procedure, as well as the correct disposal of equipment (RCN 2010).

Certain principles, such as adherence to an aseptic technique, must be applied throughout (see Chapter 3: Infection prevention and control). The circulation is a closed sterile system and a venepuncture, however quickly completed, is a breach of this system, providing a means of entry for bacteria.

Nurses must be aware of the physical and psychological comfort of the patient (Hoeltke 2013). They must appreciate the value of adequate explanation and simple measures to prevent the complications of venepuncture, such as haematoma formation, when it is neither a natural nor acceptable consequence of the procedure (Hoeltke 2013).

Risk management

The number of litigation cases within the healthcare environment has increased in recent years (Garza and Becan-McBride 2013). It is therefore vital that nurses receive accredited and appropriate training, supervision and assessment by an experienced member of staff (RCN 2010). The nurse is then accountable and responsible for ensuring that skills and competence are maintained and knowledge is kept up to date, in order to fulfil the criteria set out in *The Code* (NMC 2015).

PRE-PROCEDURAL CONSIDERATIONS

Safety of the practitioner

It is recommended that well-fitting gloves are worn during any procedure that involves handling blood and body fluids, particularly venepuncture and cannulation (ICNA 2003, NHS Employers 2007, RCN 2010). This is to prevent contamination of the practitioner from potential blood spills. Whilst it is recognized that gloves will not prevent a needlestick injury, the wiping effect of a glove on a needle may reduce the volume of blood to which the hand is exposed, thereby reducing the volume inoculated and the risk of infection (ICNA 2003, Mitchell Higgs 2002, NAO 2003). However, there is no substitute for good technique and practitioners must always work carefully when performing venepuncture.

A range of safety devices is now available for venepuncture which can reduce the risk of occupational percutaneous injuries amongst healthcare workers, in particular vacuum blood collection systems (CDCP 1997). New regulations require the use of safer sharps systems that incorporate protective mechanisms such as safety shields or covers. Where practical, all conventional devices are to be replaced (HSE 2013). Used needles should always be discarded directly into an approved sharps container, without being resheathed (Garza and Becan-McBride 2013, RCN 2010). Specimens from patients with known or suspected infections such as hepatitis or HIV should have a biohazard label attached. The accompanying request forms should be kept separately from the specimen to avoid contamination (HSE 2003). All other non-sharp disposables should be placed in a universal clinical waste bag.

Equipment

Tourniquets

There are several types of tourniquet available. A good-quality, buckle closure, single hand release type is most effective but the choice will depend on availability and operator. Consideration should be given to the type of material and the ability to decontaminate the tourniquet. Fabric tourniquets that cannot be cleaned are not recommended (Golder et al. 2000, RCN 2010). Disposable tourniquets are available for single use and should be discarded immediately after use, especially where there is potential for microbial cross-contamination (RCN 2010, Warekois et al. 2007). A blood pressure cuff can be applied instead of a tourniquet as it will apply pressure over a wider area and make the veins more prominent. The cuff should be inflated halfway between the diastolic and systolic reading. The need for disposable cuffs should also be considered where cross-contamination may occur.

Needles

The intravenous devices commonly used to perform a venepuncture for blood sampling are a straight steel needle and a steel winged infusion device. The optimum gauge to use is 21 swg (standard wire gauge), which measures internal diameter: the smaller the gauge size, the larger the diameter. This enables blood to be withdrawn at a reasonable speed without undue discomfort to the patient or possible damage to the blood cells (McCall and Tankersley 2012).

Vacuum systems

A vacuum system consists of a plastic holder which contains or is attached to a double-ended needle or adaptor (Figure 10.6). It is important to use the correct Luer adaptor to ensure a good connection and avoid blood leakage (Garza and Becan-McBride 2013). The blood tube is vacuumed in order to ensure that the exact amount of blood required is withdrawn when the tube is pushed into the holder. Filling ceases once the tube is full, which removes the need for decanting blood and also reduces blood wastage. The system can also be attached to winged infusion devices (Dougherty 2008).

Figure 10.6 **A vacuumed collection system: two blood culture bottles, Vacutainer holder and Vacutainer 'butterfly'.**

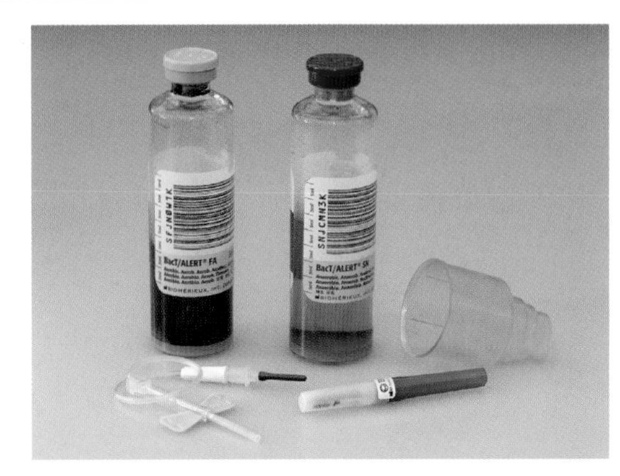

A number of vacuum systems can be used for taking blood samples. These are simple to use and cost-effective. The manufacturer's instructions should be followed. Vacuum systems reduce the risk of healthcare workers being contaminated, because they offer a completely closed system during the process of blood withdrawal and there is no necessity to decant blood into bottles (Dougherty 2008). This makes them the safest method for collecting blood samples.

Blood collection tubes are available in various sizes and have different coloured tops dependent on the type of additives. The colour coding of the tops is generally universal but may vary depending on manufacturer. Local policy must be referred to in order to select the correct tubes for specific tests (Table 10.2). Blood tubes should be used in a sequence referred to as the 'order of draw' to minimize the transferring of additives. The correct volume of blood should be collected into each tube to prevent erroneous results. The expiry dates on the tubes should also be monitored regularly.

Equipment available will depend on local policy (Table 10.3), but with increasing concern about the possibility of contamination to the practitioner, blood collection systems with integrated safety devices are now readily available and should be used for all procedures (HSE 2013, RCN 2010). However, the nurse must always select the device after assessing the condition and accessibility of the vein.

Pharmacological support

It is important to remember that patients may fear venepuncture and in some cases suffer from needle phobia. The use of topical local anaesthetic cream may be beneficial for anxious patients or for venepuncture in children (Weinstein and Plumer 2007).

Non-pharmacological support

Patient anxiety about the procedure may result in vasoconstriction. The nurse's manner and approach will also have a direct bearing on the patient's experience (Garza and Becan-McBride 2013). Approaching the patient with a confident manner and giving adequate explanation of the procedure may reduce anxiety. Careful preparation and an unhurried approach will help to relax the patient and this in turn will increase vasodilation (Dougherty 2008, Weinstein and Plumer 2007).

Table 10.2 **Blood collection tubes**

Tube	Additive	Specimen	Determinations	Instructions
Blood culture	Culture medium and anticoagulant	Whole blood	Aerobic followed by anaerobic – use aerobic bottle only if not enough blood for both bottles	
Light blue	Sodium citrate	Plasma	PT, INR, APTT, D-dimers, fibrinogen, thrombophilia screen (4 light blue + 1 EDTA tube), lupus (3 light blue tubes)	Fill tube completely and invert tube gently 3–4 times
Red	No additive	Serum	Antibiotic levels, steroid hormones, B_{12}	Do not need to invert tube
Gold	Clot activator and serum separator	Serum	Routine chemistry, lipids, thyroid (TFT), drug levels including lithium, proteins, supply additional tube for troponin I levels	Invert 5–6 times
Green	Sodium or lithium heparin and plasma separator	Plasma	Plasma determinations in chemistry	Invert 8–10 times
Lavender	EDTA	Whole blood	FBC, sickle screen, haemoglobin, electrophoresis, red cell folate, malaria, lead, mercury, thalassaemia, PTH, ESR	Invert 8–10 times
Pink	EDTA	Whole blood	Antibody and group screen	Invert 8–10 times
Grey	Sodium fluoride & (K) oxalate	Plasma	Alcohol, glucose, lactate	Invert 8–10 times
Royal blue	Heparin or EDTA or nothing	Plasma or serum	Trace elements, manganese, zinc, whole blood	Invert 8–10 times

Source: Dojcinovska (2011). Reproduced with permission from John Wiley & Sons.
APTT, activated partial thromboplastin time; EDTA, ethylenediamine tetra-acetic acid; ESR, erythrocyte sedimentation rate; FBC, full blood count; INR, international normalized ratio; PTH, parathyroid hormone; PTT, partial thromboplastin time; TFT, thyroid function test.

Table 10.3 **Choice of intravenous device**

Device	Gauge	Advantages	Disadvantages	Use
Needle	21	Cheaper than winged infusion devices. Easy to use with large veins	Rigid. Difficult to manipulate with smaller veins in less conventional sites. May cause more discomfort. Venous access only confirmed when sample tube attached	In large, accessible veins in the antecubital fossa. When small quantities of blood are to be drawn
Winged infusion device with safety feature	21	Flexible due to small needle shaft. Easy to manipulate and insert at any site. Increases the success rate of venepuncture and causes less discomfort (Hefler et al. 2004). Usually shows a 'flashback' of blood to indicate a successful venepuncture	More expensive than steel needles. The 12–30 cm length of tubing on the device may be caught and dislodge the needle	Veins in sites other than the antecubital fossa. When quantities of blood greater than 20 mL are required from any site
	23	Flexible due to small needle shaft. Easy to manipulate and insert at any site. Causes less discomfort. Smaller swg and therefore useful with fragile veins	More expensive than steel needles, plus there can be damage to cells which can cause inaccurate measurements in certain blood samples, for example potassium	Small veins in more painful sites, for example inner aspect of the wrist, especially if measurements are related to plasma and not cellular components

swg, standard wire gauge.

Specific patient preparation

- Injury, disease or treatment, for example amputation, fracture and cerebrovascular accident, may prevent the use of a limb for venepuncture, thereby reducing the venous access. Use of a limb may be contraindicated because of an operation on one side of the body, for example mastectomy and axillary node dissection, as this can lead to impairment of lymphatic drainage, which can influence venous flow regardless of whether there is obvious lymphoedema (Cole 2006, Berreth 2010, Hoeltke 2013).
- The age and weight of the patient will also influence choice. Young children have short fine veins and the elderly have prominent but fragile veins. Care must be taken with fragile veins and the largest vein should be chosen along with the smallest gauge device to reduce the amount of trauma to the vessel (Weinstein and Plumer 2007). Malnourished patients will often present with friable veins (Dougherty 2008).
- If the patient is in shock or dehydrated there will be poor superficial peripheral access. It may be necessary to take blood after the patient is rehydrated as this will promote venous filling and blood will be obtained more easily (Dougherty 2008).
- Medications can influence the choice of vein in that patients on anticoagulants or steroids or those who are thrombocytopenic tend to have more fragile veins and will be at greater risk of bruising both during venepuncture and on removal of the needle. Therefore choice may be limited by areas of bruising present or the inability to access the vessel without causing bruising (Dougherty 2008).
- The temperature of the environment will influence venous dilation. If the patient is cold, no veins may be evident on first inspection. Application of heat, for example in the form of a warm compress or soaking the arm in warm water, will increase the size and visibility of the veins, thus increasing the likelihood of a successful first attempt (Lenhardt et al. 2002, Weinstein and Plumer 2007).
- Venepuncture itself may cause the vein to collapse or go into a spasm. This will produce discomfort and a reduction in blood flow. Careful preparation and choice of vein will reduce the likelihood of this and stroking the vein or applying heat will help resolve it (Dougherty 2008).
- Involving patients in the choice of vein, even if it is simply to choose the non-dominant arm, can increase a feeling of control which in turn helps to relieve anxiety (Hudak 1986, Morris 2011).
- The environment is also another important consideration. In the inpatient and outpatient settings, lighting, ventilation, privacy and position must be checked and optimized where possible. This will ensure that the patient and the operator are both comfortable. Having adequate lighting is also beneficial as it illuminates the procedure, ensuring the operator has a good view of the vein and equipment (Dougherty 2008).

Procedure guideline 10.1 Venepuncture

Essential equipment

- Clean tray or receiver
- Tourniquet or sphygmomanometer and cuff
- 21 swg multiple sample safety needle or 21/23 swg winged safety infusion device and multiple sample Luer adaptor
- Plastic tube holder, standard
- Appropriate vacuumed specimen tubes
- Swab saturated with chlorhexidine in 70% alcohol, or isopropyl alcohol 70%
- Low-linting gauze swabs
- Sterile adhesive plaster or hypoallergenic tape
- Specimen request forms
- Non-sterile, well-fitting gloves
- Plastic apron (optional)
- Sharps bin

Pre-procedure

Action	Rationale
1 Approach the patient in a confident manner and explain and discuss the procedure with the patient.	To ensure that the patient understands the procedure and gives their valid consent (NMC 2013, **C**).
2 Allow the patient to ask questions and discuss any problems which have arisen previously.	Anxiety results in vasoconstriction; therefore, a patient who is relaxed will have dilated veins, making access easier. **E**
3 Consult the patient as to any preferences and problems that may have been experienced at previous venepunctures. Check if they have any allergies.	To involve the patient in the treatment. To acquaint the nurse fully with the patient's previous venous history and identify any changes in clinical status, for example mastectomy, as both may influence vein choice (Dougherty 2008, **E**). To prevent allergic reactions, for example to latex or chlorhexidine (McCall and Tankersley 2012, **E**; MHRA 2012, **C**).
4 Check that the identity of the patient matches the details on the request form by asking for their full name and date of birth and checking their identification bracelet (where appropriate). If the patient is unable to communicate then check the identity band for full name, date of birth and hospital number. Clarity may need to be gained with a relative/carer or registered nurse/doctor to whom the patient is known.	To ensure the sample is taken from the correct patient (NPSA 2007a, **C**; RCN 2010, **C**).
5 Assemble the equipment necessary for venepuncture.	To ensure that time is not wasted and that the procedure goes smoothly without unnecessary interruptions. **E**

(continued)

Procedure guideline 10.1 Venepuncture *(continued)*

Action	Rationale
6 Carefully wash hands using bactericidal soap and water or bactericidal alcohol handrub, and dry before commencement.	To minimize risk of infection (DH 2010, **C**; Fraise and Bradley 2009, **E**).
7 Check hands for any visibly broken skin, and cover with a waterproof dressing.	To minimize the risk of contamination to the practitioner (DH 2010, **C**; Fraise and Bradley 2009, **E**).
8 Check all packaging before opening and preparing the equipment on the chosen clean receptacle.	To maintain asepsis throughout and check that no equipment is damaged. **E**
Procedure	
9 Take all the equipment to the patient, exhibiting a confident manner.	To help the patient feel more at ease with the procedure. **E**
10 Support the chosen limb on a pillow.	To ensure the patient's comfort and facilitate venous access. **E**
11 Apply a tourniquet to the upper arm on the chosen side, making sure it does not obstruct arterial flow. If the radial pulse cannot be palpated then the tourniquet is too tight (Weinstein and Plumer 2007). The position of the tourniquet may be varied; for example, if a vein in the hand is to be used it may be placed on the forearm. A sphygmomanometer cuff may be used as an alternative.	To dilate the veins by obstructing the venous return (Dougherty 2008, **E**). To increase the prominence of the veins. **E** To promote blood flow and therefore distend the veins (Lenhardt et al. 2002, **R3**).
12 If the tourniquet does not improve venous access, the following methods can be used. *Either:* The arm may be placed in a dependent position. The patient may be asked to clench their fist. *Or:* The veins may be tapped gently or stroked. *Or:* Remove the tourniquet and apply moist heat, for example a warm compress, soak limb in warm water or, with prescription, apply glyceryl trinitrate ointment/patch (Weinstein and Plumer 2007).	To improve venous access (Dougherty 2008, **E**).
13 Select the vein by careful palpation to determine size, depth and condition (**Action figure 13**).	To prevent inadvertent insertion of the needle into other anatomical structures (Witt 2011, **E**).
14 Release the tourniquet.	To ensure patient comfort. **E**
15 Select the device, based on vein size, site and volume of blood to be taken. Use a 23 swg winged infusion device for small veins, metacarpal or feet veins.	To reduce damage or trauma to the vein and prevent haemolysis (Dougherty 2008, **E**; RCN 2010, **C**).
16 Wash hands with bactericidal soap and water or bactericidal alcohol handrub.	To maintain asepsis and minimize the risk of infection (DH 2010, **C**; Fraise and Bradley 2009, **E**).
17 Reapply the tourniquet.	To dilate the veins by obstructing the venous return (Dougherty 2008, **E**).
18 Put on gloves.	To prevent possible contamination of the practitioner (NHS Employers 2007, **C**).
19 Clean the patient's skin carefully for 30 seconds using an appropriate preparation, for example chlorhexidine in 70% alcohol, and allow to dry. Do not repalpate or touch the skin (**Action figure 19**).	To maintain asepsis and minimize the risk of infection (DH 2010, **C**; Fraise and Bradley 2009, **E**). To prevent pain on insertion (Dougherty 2008, **E**; Fraise and Bradley 2009, **E**; RCN 2010, **C**).
20 Remove the cover from the needle and inspect the device carefully.	To detect faulty equipment, for example bent or barbed needles. If these are present place them in a safe container, record batch details and return to manufacturer (MHRA 2005, **C**; RCN 2010, **C**).
21 Anchor the vein by applying manual traction on the skin a few centimetres below the proposed insertion site (**Action figure 21**).	To immobilize the vein. To provide countertension to the vein which will facilitate a smoother needle entry (Dougherty 2008, **E**).

Action	Rationale
22 Insert the needle smoothly at an angle of approximately 30°. However, the angle will depend on size and depth of the vein (see **Action figure 21**).	To facilitate a successful, pain-free venepuncture. **E**
23 Reduce the angle of descent of the needle as soon as a flashback of blood is seen in the tubing of a winged infusion device or when puncture of the vein wall is felt.	To prevent advancing too far through vein wall and causing damage to the vessel (Dougherty 2008, **E**).
24 Slightly advance the needle into the vein, if possible.	To stabilize the device within the vein and prevent it becoming dislodged during withdrawal of blood. **E**
25 Do not exert any pressure on the needle.	To prevent a puncture occurring through the vein wall. **E**
26 Withdraw the required amount of blood using a vacuumed blood collection system (**Action figure 26**). Collect blood samples in the following order: • blood culture • coagulation • serum tube with or without clot activator or gel separator (glass, non-additive tubes can be filled before the coagulation tube) • additive tubes such as: (a) gel separator tubes (may contain clot activator or heparin) (b) heparin tubes (c) EDTA • all other tubes (Garza and Becan-McBride 2013).	To minimize the risk of transferring additives from one tube to another and bacterial contamination of blood cultures (manufacturer's guidelines, **C**).
27 Release the tourniquet. In some instances this may be necessary at the beginning of sampling as inaccurate measurements may be caused by haemostasis, for example when taking blood to assess calcium levels.	To decrease the pressure within the vein. **E**
28 Remove tube from plastic tube holder.	To prevent blood spillage caused by vacuum in the tube (Campbell et al. 1999, **E**).
29 Place a low-linting swab over the puncture point.	To apply pressure. **E**
30 Remove the needle, but do not apply pressure until the needle has been fully removed.	To prevent pain on removal and damage to the intima of the vein. **E**
31 Activate safety device and then discard the needle immediately in sharps bin.	To reduce the risk of accidental needlestick injury (HSE 2013, **C**).
32 Apply digital pressure directly over the puncture site. Pressure should be applied until bleeding has ceased; approximately 1 minute or longer may be required if current disease or treatment interferes with clotting mechanisms.	To stop leakage and haematoma formation. To preserve vein by preventing bruising or haematoma formation. **E**
33 The patient may apply pressure with a finger but should be discouraged from bending the arm if a vein in the antecubital fossa is used.	To prevent leakage and haematoma formation (Morris 2011, **E**).
34 Gently invert the tube at least six times.	To prevent damage to blood cells and to mix with additives (manufacturer's guidelines, **C**).
35 Label the bottles with the relevant details at the patient's side.	To ensure that the specimens from the right patient are delivered to the laboratory, the requested tests are performed and the results returned to the correct patient's records (NMC 2010, **C**; NPSA 2007a, **C**).
Post-procedure	
36 Inspect the puncture point before applying a dressing.	To check that the puncture point has sealed. **E**
37 Confirm whether the patient is allergic to adhesive plaster.	To prevent an allergic skin reaction. **E**
38 Apply an adhesive plaster or alternative dressing.	To cover the puncture and prevent leakage or contamination. **E**
39 Ensure that the patient is comfortable.	To ascertain whether patient wishes to rest before leaving (if an outpatient) or whether any other measures need to be taken. **E**
40 Remove gloves and discard waste, making sure it is placed in the correct containers, for example sharps into a designated receptacle.	To ensure safe disposal and avoid laceration or other injury of staff (DH 2006a, **C**; Fraise and Bradley 2009, **E**). To prevent reuse of equipment (MDA 2000, **C**).

(continued)

Procedure guideline 10.1 Venepuncture *(continued)*

Action	Rationale
41 Follow hospital procedure for collection and transportation of specimens to the laboratory.	To make sure that specimens reach their intended destination. **E**
42 Document the procedure in the patient's records if taken whilst an inpatient.	To ensure timely and accurate record keeping (NMC 2010, **C**).

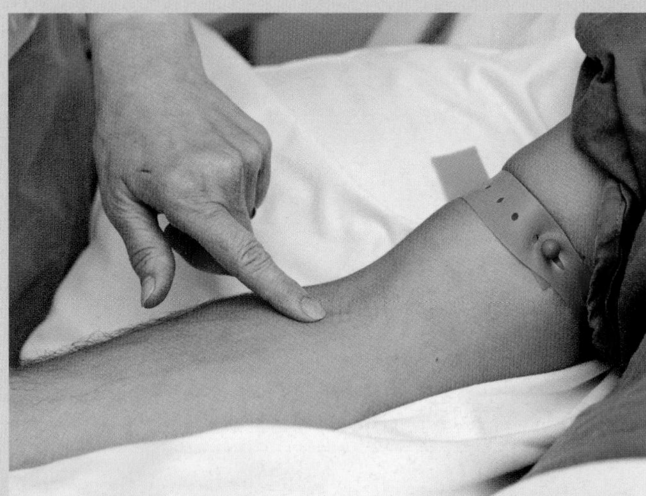

Action Figure 13 Palpating the vein.

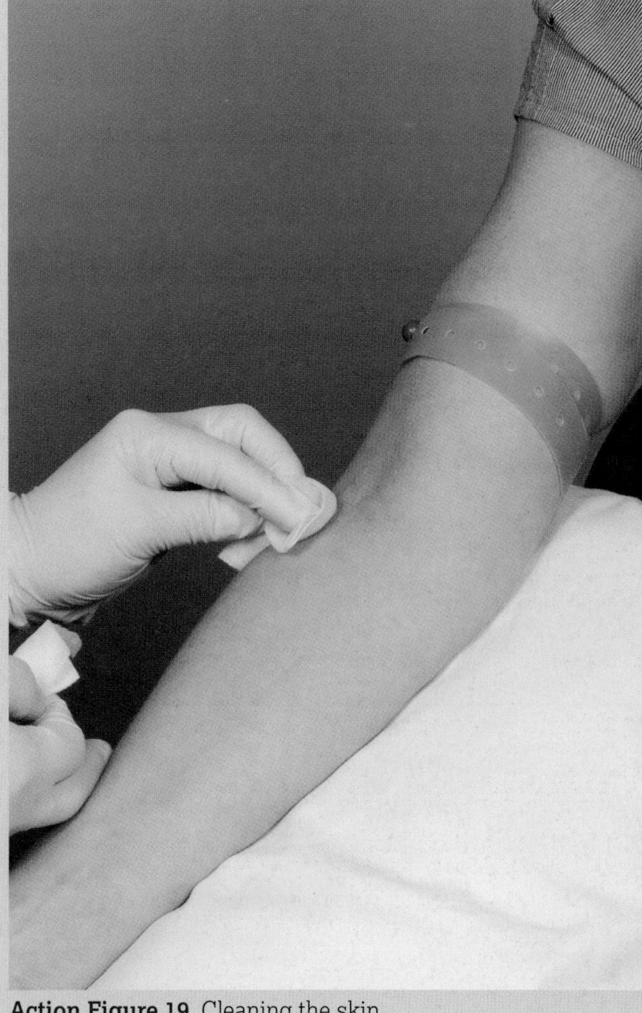

Action Figure 19 Cleaning the skin.

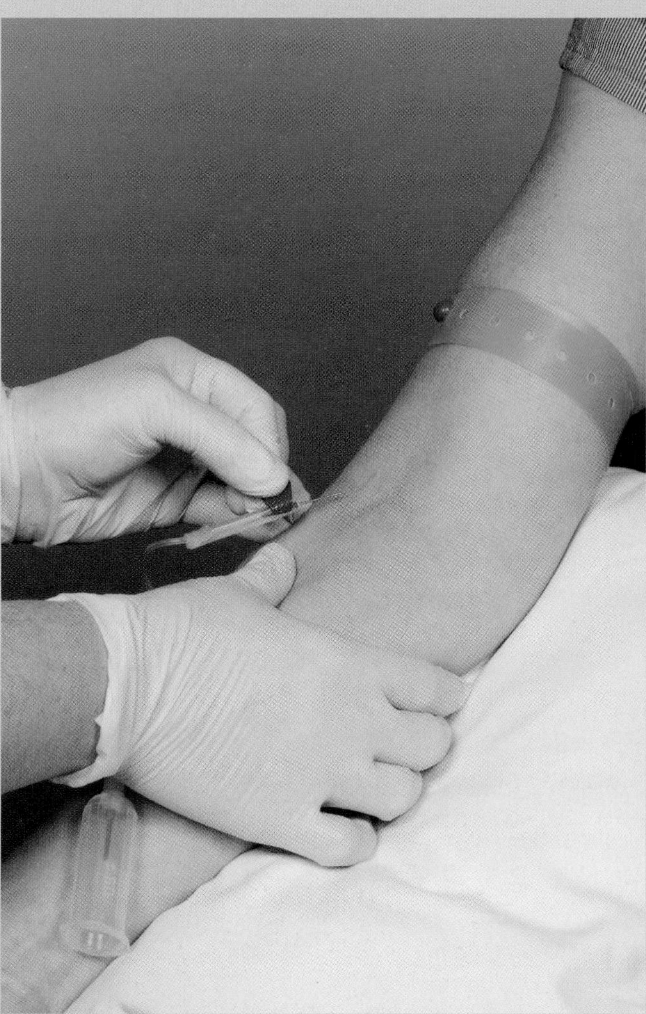

Action Figure 21 Anchoring the skin.

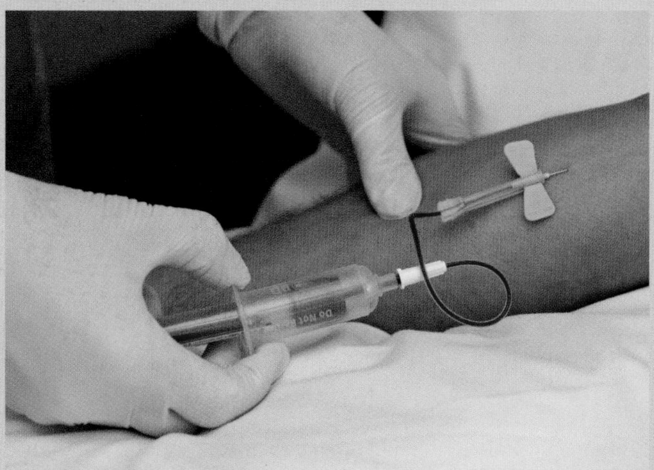

Action Figure 26 Attach sample bottle to holder.

Problem-solving table 10.1 Prevention and resolution (Procedure guideline 10.1)

Problem	Cause	Prevention	Suggested action
Pain.	Use of vein in sensitive area (e.g. wrist).	Avoid using veins in sensitive areas wherever possible. Use local anaesthetic cream.	Complete procedure as quickly as possible.
Anxiety.	Previous trauma.	Minimize the risk of a traumatic venepuncture. Use all methods available to ensure successful venepuncture.	Approach patient in a calm and confident manner. Listen to the patient's fears and explain what the procedure involves. Offer patient opportunity to lie down. Suggest use of local anaesthetic cream (Lavery and Ingram 2005).
	Fear of needles.		All of the above and perhaps referral to a psychologist if fear is of phobic proportions.
Limited venous access.	Repeated use of same veins.	Use alternative sites if possible.	Do not attempt the procedure unless experienced.
	Peripheral shutdown.	Ensure the room is not cold.	Put patient's arm in warm water. Apply glycerol trinitrate patch.
	Dehydration.		May be necessary to rehydrate patient prior to venepuncture.
	Hardened veins (due to scarring and thrombosis).		Do not use these veins as venepuncture will be unsuccessful.
	Poor technique/choice of vein or device.	Ensure correct device and technique are used.	
Needle inoculation of or contamination to practitioner.	Unsafe practice. Incorrect disposal of sharps.	Maintain safe practice. Activate safety device. Ensure sharps are disposed of. immediately and safely.	Follow accident procedure for sharps injury, for example make site bleed and apply a waterproof dressing. Report and document. An injection of hepatitis B immunoglobulin or triple therapy may be required.
Accidental blood spillage.	Damaged/faulty equipment.	Check equipment prior to use.	Report within hospital and/or MHRA.
	Reverse vacuum.	Use vacuumed plastic blood collection system. Remove blood tube from plastic tube holder before removing needle.	Ensure blood is handled and transported correctly.
Missed vein.	Inadequate anchoring. Poor vein selection. Wrong positioning. Lack of concentration. Poor lighting.	Ensure that only properly trained staff perform venepuncture or that those who are training are supervised. Ensure the environment is well lit.	Repalpate, withdraw the needle slightly and realign it, providing the patient is not feeling any discomfort. Ensure all learners are supervised. If the patient is feeling pain, then the needle should be removed immediately.
	Difficult venous access.		Ask experienced colleague to perform the procedure.
Spurt of blood on entry.	Bevel tip of needle enters the vein before entire bevel is under the skin; usually occurs when the vein is very superficial.		Reassure the patient. Wipe blood away on removal of needle.
Blood stops flowing.	Through puncture: needle inserted too far.	Correct angle.	Draw back the needle, but if bruising is evident, then remove the needle immediately and apply pressure.
	Contact with valves.	Palpate to locate.	Withdraw needle slightly to move tip away from valve.
	Venous spasm.	Results from mechanical irritation and cannot be prevented.	Gently massage above the vein or apply heat.
	Vein collapse.	Use veins with large lumen. Use a smaller device.	Release tourniquet, allow veins to refill and retighten tourniquet.
	Small vein.	Avoid use of small veins wherever possible.	May require another venepuncture.
	Poor blood flow.	Use veins with large lumens.	Apply heat above vein.

POST-PROCEDURAL CONSIDERATIONS

Immediate care

It is important to ensure that the needle is removed correctly on completion of blood sampling and that the risk of haematoma formation is minimized. Pressure should be applied as the needle is removed from the skin. If pressure is applied too early, it causes the tip of the needle to drag along the intima of the vein, resulting in sharp pain and damage to the lining of the vessel (McCall and Tankersley 2012).

The practitioner should ensure that firm pressure is maintained until bleeding has stopped. The patient should also be instructed to keep their arm straight and not bend it as this also increases the risk of bruising (Moini 2013). A longer period of pressure may be necessary where the patient's blood may take longer to clot, for example if the patient is receiving anticoagulants or is thrombocytopenic. The practitioner may choose to apply the tourniquet over the venepuncture site to ensure even and constant pressure on the area (Dougherty 2008). Alternatively, they can elevate the arm slightly above the heart to decrease venous pressure (McCall and Tankersley 2012).

The practitioner should inspect the site carefully for bleeding or bruising before applying a dressing to the site, and the patient leaving the department. If bruising has occurred, the patient should be informed of why this has happened and given instructions for what to do to reduce the bruising and any associated pain.

COMPLICATIONS

Complications that may occur when venepuncture is performed include arterial puncture, nerve injury, haematoma, fainting and infection. Careful assessment and preparation will minimize the risks but if they occur then appropriate action should be taken immediately.

Arterial puncture

To prevent an arterial puncture, careful assessment of vein selection is necessary. The nurse should palpate the vessel prior to needle insertion to confirm the absence of a pulse; the angle of insertion should be less than 40° and in the event of a missed vein, blind probing should be avoided (McCall and Tankersley 2012).

An arterial puncture can be identified by bright red blood, rapid blood flow and pain. The needle should be removed immediately and pressure applied for 5 minutes by the nurse. A pressure dressing should be applied and the patient should receive verbal and written advice to follow in the event of increased pain, swelling or loss of sensation. No tourniquet or blood pressure cuff should be reapplied to the arm for 24 hours. The incident should be documented in the patient's notes (Dougherty 2008).

Nerve injury

Careful vein selection and needle insertion should minimize the risk of nerve injury. The angle of insertion should be less than 40° and blind probing should be avoided (Morris 2011). In the event of a nerve injury, the patient may complain of a sharp shooting pain, burning or electric shock sensation that radiates down the arm and they may experience numbness/tingling in the fingers. The needle should be removed immediately to prevent further nerve damage (McCall and Tankerlsey 2012). The patient should receive verbal and written advice to follow if the pain/numbness continues for more than a few hours. The incident should be documented in the patient's notes (Dougherty 2008).

Haematoma

Haematoma formation is the most common complication of venepuncture (McCall and Tankersley 2012). A haematoma develops when blood leaks from the vein into the surrounding tissues. It may be caused by the needle penetrating completely through the vein wall, the needle only being partially inserted, or insufficient pressure on the site when the needle is removed. If a haematoma develops, the needle should be removed immediately and pressure applied. In the event of a large haematoma developing, the nurse can apply an ice pack to relieve pain and swelling. The application of Hirudoid cream, which is used for the treatment of superficial thrombophlebitis, or arnica cream may be beneficial (BNF 2014).

The patient should receive verbal and written advice as a haematoma may lead to a compression injury to the nerve (Morris 2011). The incident should be documented in the patient's notes (Dougherty 2008).

Fainting

Fainting may occur during or immediately following venepuncture. The patient may complain of feeling light-headed and appear pale and sweaty. Loss of consciousness may occur suddenly so the nurse should be vigilant throughout the procedure and routinely confirm with the patient that they do not feel unwell or faint. In the event of the patient feeling faint, the nurse should remove the device immediately, apply pressure to the site and encourage the patient to lower the head and breathe deeply. The application of a cold compress to the forehead and increased ventilation (open a window if clinically acceptable) may help to make the patient more comfortable. If the patient suffers a loss of consciousness, the nurse should call for assistance and ensure the patient's safety until they recover. The patient should not be allowed to leave the department until fully recovered and be advised not to drive for at least 30 minutes (Garza and Becan-McBride 2013, McCall and Tankersley 2012). The incident should be documented in the patient's notes and the patient advised to inform staff on future occasions.

Infection

Infection at the venepuncture site is a rare occurrence (McCall and Tankersley 2012). Aseptic technique should be maintained with careful attention to hand washing and skin preparation. The venepuncture site should not be repalpated after cleaning and the site should be covered for 15–20 minutes after the procedure. Infection at the venepuncture site should be reported to a doctor as antibiotics may be required (Hart 2008).

Blood tests

EVIDENCE-BASED APPROACHES

Rationale

Blood tests are routinely collected to:

- define baseline results
- confirm disease
- monitor disease
- regulate therapy/treatment.

It is important that the correct blood tube is used for each test. The blood tubes contain special additives relevant to the type of test required, usually indicated by the colour of the tube top. The practitioner should ensure that the correct tube is selected by referring to local hospital guidelines. Correct 'order of draw' should be followed to avoid transferring additive from one tube to another when filling (Garza and Becan-McBride 2013).

Numerous blood tests are available. Blood samples are sent to various departments within the laboratory, such as haematology, biochemistry and microbiology. Brief outlines of some routine tests are given below. Please refer to specialist reference texts for more detail.

Haematology

The full blood count (FBC) is the most commonly requested blood test (Higgins 2013). The FBC involves monitoring the levels of red blood cells (erythrocytes), white blood cells (leucocytes) and platelets (thrombocytes). Variations to normal values can indicate anaemia, infection and thrombocytopenia (Table 10.4).

Table 10.4 **Haematology**

Test	Reference range	Functions/additional information
Red blood cells	Men: $4.5–6.5 \times 10^{12}$/L Women: $3.9–5.6 \times 10^{12}$/L	The main function of the RBC is the transport of oxygen and carbon dioxide
Haemoglobin	Men: 135–175 g/L Women: 115–155 g/L	Haemoglobin (Hb) is a protein pigment found within the RBC which carries the oxygen. Anaemia (deficiency in the number of RBCs or Hb content) may occur for many reasons. Changes to cell production, deficient dietary intake or blood loss may be relevant and need to be investigated further
White blood cells	Men: $3.7–9.5 \times 10^{9}$/L Women: $3.9–11.1 \times 10^{9}$/L	The function of the WBC is defence against infection There are different kinds of WBC: neutrophils, lymphocytes, monocytes, eosinophils and basophils Leucopenia is a WBC count lower than 3.7 and is usually associated with the use of cytotoxic drugs Leucocytosis (high levels of neutrophils and lymphocytes) occurs as the body's normal response to infection and after surgery Leukaemia involves an increased WBC count caused by changes in cell production in the bone marrow. The leukaemic cells enter the blood in increased numbers in an immature state
Platelets	Men: $150–400 \times 10^{9}$/L Women: $150–400 \times 10^{9}$/L	Clot formation occurs when platelets and the blood protein fibrin combine A patient may be thrombocytopenic (low platelet count) due to drugs/poor production or have a raised count (thrombocytosis) with infection or autoimmune disease
Coagulation/INR	INR range 2–3 (in some cases a range of 3–4.5 is acceptable)	Coagulation occurs to prevent excessive blood loss by the formation of a clot (thrombus). However, a clot that forms in an artery may block the vessel and cause an infarction or ischaemia which can be fatal (Blann 2007) Aspirin, warfarin and heparin are three drugs used for the prevention and/or treatment of thrombosis It is imperative that patients on warfarin therapy receive regular monitoring to ensure a balance of slowing the clot-forming process and maintaining the ability of the blood to clot (Blann 2007)

INR, international normalized ratio; RBC, red blood cell; WBC, white blood cell.

Group and save (blood transfusion)

All patients who require a blood transfusion need to have their blood type confirmed. It is essential that correct patient identification and accurate labelling are maintained. The sample will be screened to determine the ABO and Rh (Rhesus) type. All staff should receive formal documented training in blood transfusion practice (McClelland 2007). (See Chapter 7: Nutrition, fluid balance and blood transfusion.)

Biochemistry

Urea and electrolytes are the most common biochemistry tests requested (Table 10.5).

Liver function tests

There are numerous tests which are used to assess liver function. Additional tests include alkaline phosphatase (AP), gamma-glutamyl transpeptidase (GGT), aspartate aminotransferase (AST) and alanine aminotransferase (ALT).

Microbiology

Various types of sample may be sent to the microbiology laboratory for screening, for example microbiological drug assays. Blood tests sent to microbiology may include screening for hepatitis B, hepatitis C and HIV.

Blood cultures

DEFINITION

A blood culture is a specimen of blood obtained from a single venepuncture or CVAD for the purpose of detecting blood-borne organisms (bacteria or fungi) and their associated infections (Lee et al. 2007). Inoculation of an aerobic and an anaerobic sample of blood in two separate bottles comprises a set of blood cultures.

RELATED THEORY

Blood cultures are an essential part of the management of patients with serious blood-borne infections and are known as the gold standard investigation (HPA 2014a), enabling the identification of the causative pathogens, antimicrobial susceptibility and treatment guidance (Shore and Sandoe 2008). Bacteraemia and fungaemia are associated with high morbidity and mortality amongst hospitalized patients, particularly those with compromised host defences (Panceri et al. 2004). The accurate and timely detection of the organism and sensitivities has significant diagnostic and prognostic importance (HPA 2014a).

Micro-organisms may be present in the blood intermittently or continuously, depending upon the source of infection

Table 10.5 **Biochemistry**

Test	Reference range	Functions/additional information
Sodium	135–145 mmol/L	The main function of sodium is to maintain extracellular volume (water stored outside the cells), acid/base balance and the transmitting of nerve impulses Hypernatraemia (serum sodium >145 mmol/L) may be an indication of dehydration due to fluid loss from diarrhoea, excessive sweating, increased urinary output or a poor oral intake of fluid. An increased salt intake may also cause an elevation Hyponatraemia (serum sodium <135 mmol/L) may be indicated in fluid retention (oedema)
Potassium	3.5–5.2 mmol/L	Potassium plays a major role in nerve conduction, muscle function, acid/base balance and osmotic pressure. It has a direct effect on cardiac muscle, influencing cardiac output by helping to control the rate and force of each contraction The most common cause of hyperkalaemia (serum potassium >5.2 mmol/L) is chronic renal failure. The kidneys are unable to excrete potassium. The level may be elevated due to an increased intake of potassium supplements during treatment. Tissue cell destruction caused by trauma/cytotoxic therapy may cause a release of potassium from the cells and an elevation in the potassium plasma level. It may also be observed in untreated diabetic ketoacidosis Urgent treatment is required as hyperkalaemia may lead to changes in cardiac muscle contraction and cause subsequent cardiac arrest The main cause of hypokalaemia (serum potassium <3.5 mmol/L) is the loss of potassium via the kidneys during treatment with thiazide diuretics. Excessive/chronic diarrhoea may also cause a decreased potassium level
Urea	2.5–6.5 mmol/L	Urea is a waste product of metabolism that is transported to the kidneys and excreted as urine. Elevated levels of urea may indicate poor kidney function
Creatinine	55–105 μmol/L	Creatinine is a waste product of metabolism that is transported to the kidneys and excreted as urine. Elevated levels of creatinine may indicate poor kidney function
Calcium	2.20–2.60 mmol/L	Most of the calcium in the body is stored in the bone but ionized calcium, which circulates in the blood plasma, plays an important role in the transmission of nerve impulses and functioning of cardiac and skeletal muscle. It is also vital for blood coagulation High calcium levels (hypercalcaemia >2.6 mmol/L) can be due to hyperthyroidism, hyperparathyroidism or malignancy. Elevation in calcium levels may cause cardiac arrhythmia, potentially leading to cardiac arrest (Blann 2007) Tumour cells can cause excessive production of a protein called parathormone-related polypeptide (PTHrP) which causes a loss of calcium from the bone and an increase in the blood calcium levels. This is a major reason for hypercalcaemia in cancer patients (Higgins 2013) Hypocalcaemia (<2.20 mmol/L) is often associated with vitamin D deficiency due to inadequate intake or increased loss due to gastrointestinal disease. Mild hypocalcaemia may be symptomless but severe hypocalcaemia may cause increased neuromuscular excitability and cardiac arrhythmias. It is also a common feature of chronic renal failure (Higgins 2013)
C-reactive protein (CRP)	<10 mg/L	Elevation in the CRP level can be a useful indication of bacterial infection. CRP is monitored after surgery and for patients who have a high risk of infection. The CRP level can help monitor the severity of inflammation and assist in the diagnosis of conditions such as systemic lupus erythematosus (SLE), ulcerative colitis and Crohn's disease (Higgins 2013)
Albumin	35–50 g/L	Albumin is a protein found in blood plasma which assists in the transport of water-soluble substances and the maintenance of blood plasma volume
Bilirubin	(total) <17 μmol/L	Bilirubin is produced from the breakdown of haemoglobin; it is transported to the liver for excretion in bile. Elevated levels of bilirubin may cause jaundice

(HPA 2014a). In order to determine whether there is a bacteraemia (bacteria in the blood), the bacteria must be 'grown' or 'cultured'. The blood sample taken must be added to a culture medium (a liquid containing nutrients essential for bacterial growth). The blood cultures then need time in an appropriate environment for the bacteria (if any) to grow. This usually takes around 6–18 hours, but slow-growing species can take longer. If there is evidence of bacterial growth, this will then be stained and examined under a microscope to determine species and then tested for sensitivity (Higgins 2013).

EVIDENCE-BASED APPROACHES

Rationale

Indications

There are many signs and symptoms in the patient which may suggest bacteraemia but clinical judgement is required. The following indicators should be taken into account when assessing a patient for signs of bacteraemia or sepsis which would then indicate the need for blood culture sampling (Dellinger et al. 2013, HPA 2014a).

- Core temperature out of normal range (>38°C or <36°C)
- Focal signs of infection
- Abnormal heart rate (raised), blood pressure (low or raised) or respiratory rate (raised)
- Chills or rigors
- Raised or very low white blood cell count
- New or worsening confusion/altered levels of consciousness (Higgins 2013)

Coburn et al. (2012) suggest that an isolated fever or leucocytosis does not necessitate the collection of blood cultures, unless the patient is immunocompromised or endocarditis is suspected. Asai et al. (2012) also recognized the limitations of blood culture sampling in the terminally ill patient and do not recommend the routine use of this diagnositic tool for patients at the end of life. However, professional judgement will be required for each individual case.

Methods of blood culture specimen collection

In recognition of the importance of taking accurate blood cultures, there is now national guidance that implements procedure and policy to improve the quality of blood culture investigations and to reduce the risk of blood sample contamination (HPA 2014a). Contamination can come from a number of sources: the patient's skin, the equipment used to obtain the sample, the practitioner or the general environment (Murray and Masur 2012). Failure to use an aseptic technique or careful procedures when obtaining blood cultures can cause a 'false-positive' result which may lead to extensive diagnostic testing, excessive antibiotic use, prolonged hospitalization and artificially raised incidence rates (Dellinger et al. 2013).

In order to optimize the identification of causative organisms, the taking of a peripheral sample is recommended and two sets of cultures should be taken at separate times and from separate sites. This will help eliminate the possibility of a false positive (Myers and Reyes 2011).

The initial samples should be obtained directly from a peripheral vein and not from existing peripheral cannulas or immediately above a cannula site, and the femoral vein should be avoided for venepuncture because it is difficult to ensure adequate skin cleansing and disinfection (DH 2007b).

If the patient has an existing vascular access device (VAD) which has been *in situ* for more than 48 hours or is suspected as a source of infection, a sample should also be taken from the device by a qualified and competent nurse or other healthcare practitioner (Myers and Reyes 2011). If feasible, a set of cultures should be taken from each lumen of the VAD.

It is suggested that the blood cultures should be taken when the temperature is rising or as soon as possible following a spike in temperature as this is when the serum concentration of the bacteria is at its highest (Higgins 2013).

Blood cultures should be taken prior to commencing or changing antimicrobial therapy as antibiotics may delay or prevent bacterial growth, causing a falsely negative result (HPA 2014a). In accordance with the Surviving Sepsis Campaign 2012 (Dellinger et al. 2013), antimicrobial therapy should be started within the first hour of recognition of severe sepsis and blood cultures should be taken before antimicrobial therapy is initiated. This is essential to confirm infection and the responsible pathogens whilst not causing significant delay in antibiotic administration (Dellinger et al. 2013). If antibiotic therapy has already been commenced, blood cultures should ideally be taken immediately prior to the next dose, except in paediatric patients (DH 2007b).

LEGAL AND PROFESSIONAL ISSUES

Competencies

Blood cultures should be collected by practitioners who have been trained in the collection procedure and whose competence has been assessed (DH 2007b). Practitioners must be competent and feel confident that they have the knowledge, skill and understanding to undertake blood culture sampling for microbiological analysis (NMC 2015).

Risk management

Contamination of a blood sample can lead to false-positive results which may in turn lead to inappropriate antibiotic therapy. This also has cost and resource implications (HPA 2014a). Contamination can be avoided by correctly decontaminating the patient's skin, adequate hand hygiene and decontamination of the bottle tops prior to obtaining a sample (Aziz 2011).

False negatives can occur due to inadequate sample volumes resulting in incorrect blood to media ratios and the administration of antimicrobials prior to taking the samples. False negatives result in present bacteria going undetected and therefore potentially being missed or untreated which has clear consequences for the patient (HPA 2014a).

PRE-PROCEDURAL CONSIDERATIONS

Equipment

Most blood culture systems involve two different collection bottles. Both bottles contain a particular medium that provides an optimal environment for bacterial growth. One bottle contains oxygen in the space above the medium for aerobic or oxygen-requiring bacteria and the other is suitablefor anaerobic bacteria not requiring oxygen. The aerobic bottle should be filled first to avoid oxygen entering the anaerobic bottle (HPA 2014a).

The use of a needle to decant blood into the culture bottles is now largely redundant due to the wide use of closed, vacuumed blood collection systems (for example, the Bio-Merieux BacT/ALERT system which utilizes either a holder for venous access device sampling or a Luer adaptor safety winged device for peripheral sampling) (see Figure 10.6). This reduces the health and safety risk to the healthcare professional and the risk of culture contamination. Needle-free or safety systems should be used where possible (HSE 2013).

Volume of blood culture specimen collection

Care should be taken not to under- or overfill the bottles as it is difficult to accurately judge the sample volume with this method (Shore and Sandoe 2008). The volume of blood taken for a culture is also critical to ensure correct blood to liquid culture medium ratio. A false-negative result could occur if an insufficient volume is introduced or if too much blood is introduced, due to the culture medium in the bottles being diluted (Higgins 2013). The liquid culture medium is a mixture of nutrients that supports microbial growth and inhibits phagocytosis and lysozyme activity (Shore and Sandoe 2008). This helps to determine if there are pathogenic micro-organisms present in the blood. As there are a number of systems in use, the manufacturer's instructions should be followed as to the total volume required for each bottle. Adult patients with clinically significant bacteraemias often have a low number of colony-forming units per millilitre of blood and a minimum of 10 mL per culture bottle is recommended (Dellinger et al. 2013).

Pharmacological support

Skin preparation products

Poor aseptic technique and skin decontamination can cause contamination of a blood culture with the patient's own skin flora, such as coagulase-negative staphylococci (Weston 2008). A combination of 2% chlorhexidine gluconate in 70% isopropyl alcohol is recommended as being effective for skin antisepsis (DH 2010, Loveday et al. 2014, Madeo and Barlow 2008). Chlorhexidine gluconate maintains a persistent antimicrobial function by disrupting the cell membrane and precipitating their contents, whilst the isopropyl alcohol quickly destroys micro-organisms by denaturing cell proteins (Inwood 2007). In order to achieve reduction and inhibition of the micro-organisms living on the skin, gentle friction is required for 30 seconds and the solution should be allowed to dry to achieve good skin antisepsis and to expose the cracks and fissures of the skin to the solution (Loveday et al. 2014). The top of each blood culture collection bottle should also be cleaned with 2% chlorhexidine gluconate in 70% isopropyl alcohol (DH 2010, Higgins 2013).

Procedure guideline 10.2 **Blood cultures: peripheral (winged device collection method)**

Essential equipment

- Alcohol-based skin cleaning preparation (2% chlorhexidine in 70% isopropyl alcohol)
- Alcohol-based swab for blood culture bottle decontamination (2% chlorhexidine in 70% isopropyl alcohol)
- A set of blood culture bottles (anaerobic and aerobic)
- Vacuum-assisted collection system (some include a winged device for peripheral cultures)
- Non-sterile gloves
- Gauze swabs
- Appropriate document/form
- Clean tray or receiver
- Trolley

Pre-procedure

Action	Rationale
1 Explain and discuss the procedure with the patient.	To ensure the patient understands the procedure and gives valid consent (NMC 2013, **C**).
2 Wash hands with bactericidal soap and water, or decontaminate physically clean hands with alcohol-based handrub.	To reduce the risk of cross-infection and specimen contamination (DH 2010, **C**).
3 Clean any visible soiled skin on the patient with soap and water then dry.	To reduce the risk of contamination (DH 2010, **C**).

Procedure

Action	Rationale
4 Apply a disposable tourniquet and palpate to identify vein. Release tourniquet.	To improve venous access and choose appropriate vein (Witt 2011, **E**).
5 Clean skin with a 2% chlorhexidine in 70% isopropyl alcohol swab for 30 seconds and allow to dry for 30 seconds. Do not palpate site again after cleaning.	To enable adequate skin antisepsis and decontamination, and to prevent contamination from practitioner's fingers (DH 2010, **C**; Inwood 2007, **E**).
6 Remove flip-off caps from culture bottles and clean with second 2% chlorhexidine in 70% isopropyl alcohol swab and allow to dry.	To reduce the risk of environmental contamination causing false-positive results (DH 2010, **C**).
7 Wash and dry hands again or use alcohol handrub and apply non-sterile gloves (sterile gloves are not essential).	To decontaminate hands having been in contact with the patient's skin to palpate vein and to prevent cross-infection. **E**
8 Attach winged blood collection set into the appropriate vacuum holder for taking blood cultures.	To reduce risk of contamination and health and safety risk to practitioner (DH 2006a, **C**; DH 2010, **C**).
9 Reapply tourniquet.	To improve venous access (Dougherty 2008, **E**).
10 Remove sheath covering needle at wings and perform venepuncture.	To obtain blood samples. **E**
11 If blood is being taken for other tests, collect the blood culture first. Inoculate the aerobic culture first.	To reduce the risk of contamination of culture bottles after inoculating other blood bottles. **E**
12 Attach aerobic bottle first, hold upright and use bottle graduation lines to accurately gauge sample volumes (at least 10 mL in each bottle or as recommended by manufacturer). Remove bottle and replace with anaerobic bottle, take same volume and remove bottle.	To ensure anaerobic bottle does not become contaminated with oxygen from the sample (Myers and Reyes 2011, **E**).
13 Release tourniquet and remove winged device, apply pressure to the venepuncture site.	To prevent bleeding at the site (de Verteuil 2011, **E**).

Post-procedure	
14 Activate safety feature and discard winged collection set in sharps container.	To reduce risk of sharps injury (HSE 2013, **C**).
15 Remove gloves and wash/decontaminate hands.	To ensure correct clinical waste management and reduce risk of cross-infection (DH 2006a, **C**).
16 Apply appropriate dressing.	To cover the puncture site after checking the patient has no allergy to the dressing (de Verteuil 2011, **E**).
17 Label bottles with appropriate patient details while in the presence of the patient, ensuring the bar codes on the bottles are not covered or removed.	To ensure that the specimens from the right patient are delivered to the laboratory, the requested tests are performed and the results returned to the patient's records (NHSBT 2011, **C**; NHSBT 2012, **C**; NMC 2010, **C**; NPSA 2007a, **C**).
18 Complete microbiology request form (including relevant information such as indications, site and time of culture).	To maintain accurate records and provide accurate information for laboratory analysis (NMC 2010, **C**; Weston 2008, **E**).
19 Arrange prompt delivery to the microbiology laboratory to process immediately (or incubate at 37°C).	To increase the chance of accurate organism identification (Higgins 2013, **E**).
20 Document the procedure in the patient's records.	To ensure timely and accurate record keeping (NMC 2010, **C**).

POST-PROCEDURAL CONSIDERATIONS

Immediate care

Blood cultures should be dispatched to the laboratory for immediate processing. If cultures cannot be processed immediately, they should be incubated at 37°C in order for bacterial growth to begin and to prevent deterioration in pathogenic micro-organism yield (Higgins 2013).

Ongoing care

Decisions on commencing, changing or adding antimicrobial therapy may need to be considered depending upon the patient's condition and history. Drug-resistant micro-organisms have highlighted the need for prudent control of antibiotic prescribing and usage. It is estimated that up to 40% of patients with moderate-to-severe infections are given unnecessary or inappropriate antibiotics to treat the *in vitro* susceptibility of the pathogen that is subsequently cultured (Johannes 2008).

The possibility of false results should also be considered before commencing any therapy. A false negative may be due to disproportionate blood volume to culture medium, inadequate incubation time and/or antibiotic administration prior to taking the sample. If the results are positive, the possibility of contamination should be considered, especially if the bacterium is one that commonly causes contamination (Higgins 2013). Occasionally a blood culture will provide a positive result for *Staph. epidermidis* which is normally present on the skin and therefore can contaminate the sample due to poor technique (Higgins 2013). Decisions regarding appropriate choice of empirical therapy as well as the duration and dosage should be made in conjunction with advice from the microbiology team (Tacconelli 2009).

Antimicrobial drug assay

DEFINITION

Therapeutic drug monitoring of blood serum ensures that there are sufficient levels of particular antimicrobial drugs to be therapeutically effective, whilst avoiding potentially toxic excess that may lead to adverse effects (Thomson 2004, Walker and Whittlesea 2012).

RELATED THEORY

The majority of drugs used in clinical practice have a wide therapeutic window and quantitative analysis of serum levels is unnecessary. However, there are certain drugs that require monitoring of serum concentration levels due to their narrow therapeutic index where toxicity is associated with persistently high serum concentrations, whilst therapeutic failure can result from low concentrations (Egan et al. 2012, Thomson 2004). Swallow et al. (2012) describe the use of saliva for testing drug levels. They suggest this is a reliable alternative to blood sampling and has been found to be particularly useful for children and babies.

Examples of drugs that need monitoring in clinical practice include lithium, digoxin, theophylline, phenytoin, ciclosporin and certain antibiotics (Higgins 2013). This section will focus on aminoglycoside antibiotics, such as gentamicin and amikacin, and glycopeptide antibiotics such as vancomycin as these are the most commonly monitored antimicrobial assays.

These drugs are excreted almost entirely by glomerular filtration and are potentially nephrotoxic and ototoxic. When aminoglycosides or glycopeptides are used as single modes of treatment, renal toxicity is estimated to be 5–10%, although this can increase to as much as 30% if both are used synergistically (Pannu and Nadim 2008).

- Nephrotoxicity involves the proximal tubules that are capable of regeneration; therefore adverse effects may be reversible over time (Hadaway and Chamallas 2003, Huth et al. 2011).
- Ototoxicity causes damage within the neuroepithelial cells of the inner ear, which can cause cochlear damage and/or vestibular impairment. These cells cannot be regenerated so the effects are irreversible (Huth et al. 2011). Ototoxicity occurs in 0.5–3% of patients and is usually associated with very high serum concentrations of the drugs (Pagkalis et al. 2011, Sha 2005).

Aminoglycoside antibiotics

Aminoglycosides such as gentamicin and amikacin are potent antibiotics, which are mainly used against aerobic, gram-negative bacteria and are often used synergistically against certain gram-positive organisms (Hammet-Stabler and Johns 1998). Administering extended dosing (single daily dosing) of aminoglycosides has been found to be associated with fewer adverse events and, because of their rapid 'concentration-dependent' action, the rate and extent of bacterial cell death are increased (Owens and Shorr 2009, Pagkalis et al. 2011). The timing of serum sampling will be determined by the patient's clinical manifestations, particularly renal function. Generally, for gentamicin, the post-dose level should be lower than 12 mg/L and the trough level should be lower than 2 mg/L (Walker and Whittlesea 2012).

Glycopeptide antibiotics

Vancomycin is the glycopeptide antibiotic most widely used for the treatment of serious infections caused by gram-positive pathogens, such as those suspected to be meticillin resistant (Jones 2006). Glycopeptides exhibit 'time-dependent' effects, meaning that their effectiveness increases with the duration of time that the antibiotic serum concentration is above the minimum inhibitory concentration (MIC) of susceptible pathogens (Owens and Shorr 2009).

The use and monitoring of vancomycin have increased due to the emergence of meticillin-resistant *Staphylococcus aureus* (MRSA) but the emergence of vancomycin-resistant *Staphylococcus aureus* has further complicated its clinical use (Roberts et al. 2011).

Determination of serum blood levels of vancomycin depends on the frequency of administration. If given intermittently (usually twice-daily doses), trough levels should be taken at set times, immediately before the administration of the next bolus dose (Jones 2006). An alternative method of administration is the continuous infusion of vancomycin providing higher and more sustained serum levels which may enhance the effect (Kitzis and Goldstein 2006). If given intermittently, the trough level should be between 5 and 15 mg/L, whilst continuous infusions aim to maintain serum concentrations at between 15 and 25 mg/L.

EVIDENCE-BASED APPROACHES

Rationale

The main criterion for monitoring serum drug concentration is to ensure that there is enough drug given for efficacy whilst avoiding concentrations associated with a significant risk of toxicity (Roberts et al. 2011).

Indications

Accurate and timely monitoring of microbial assay levels is indicated in patients receiving intravenous aminoglycoside or glycopeptide antibiotics:

- to ensure optimum therapeutic range
- to minimize high serum levels which may cause adverse side-effects of the drugs (particular caution should be exercised in patients who have renal impairment) (Roberts et al. 2011).

Contraindications

The samples should not be taken if there has been insufficient time lapse between dose administration and sample collection.

Principles of care

The initial dosage regimen should be appropriate for the clinical condition being treated, the patient's clinical characteristics (age, weight, renal function and so on) and concomitant drug therapy (Thomson 2004). The timing of the sample and interpretation of the results of analysis need consideration in relation to the dose given and the timing of previous dose administration.

Serum samples can be taken at two different times: the peak or the trough. A peak sample is collected at the drug's highest therapeutic concentration within the dosing period. The post-dose peak level timing will vary depending on the drug; ordinarily this is 1 hour after the completion of an infusion, although in the case of vancomycin, which has a slow distribution phase, it is recommended that the sample is taken at least 1–2 hours after the infusion ends (Tobin et al. 2002, Walker and Whittlesea 2012).

Trough levels are measured just prior to the administration of the next dose, that is, at the lowest concentration in the dosing period (Tobin et al. 2002). Therefore, trough levels are more commonly used because the level is more representative of how the different variables such as drug absorption and renal function affect the concentration within a predetermined timeframe. The results can then be used to adjust dosages to achieve the optimal response with the minimal toxicity.

Abnormally elevated serum levels may be obtained if the samples are taken from a CVAD through which the drug has been administered. This is more likely when residual drugs remain in the catheter if it has not been flushed correctly following administration of the drug or the first 5–10 mL of blood has not been discarded (Himberger and Himberger 2001). If a multilumen CVAD is *in situ*, a different lumen from the one used to administer the drug should be used to obtain the blood specimen.

Procedure guideline 10.3 **Blood sampling: antimicrobial drug assay**

Essential equipment

- Appropriate blood sample bottles
- Vacuum-assisted blood collection system
- Non-sterile gloves and apron
- Clean tray or receiver
- Appropriate documentation/forms

Pre-procedure

Action	Rationale
1 Discuss indication for procedure with patient.	To ensure the patient understands the procedure and gives valid consent (NMC 2013, **C**).
2 Wash hands with bactericidal soap and water, or decontaminate physically clean hands with alcohol-based handrub. Apply gloves.	To reduce the risk of cross-infection and specimen contamination (Fraise and Bradley 2009, **E**).
Procedure	
3 For trough levels: following venepuncture (see Procedure guideline 10.1: Venepuncture), withdraw the volume of blood appropriate to the blood sample bottle using the vacuum-assisted collection system.	To ensure the correct volume of blood is obtained and to reduce the safety risk to the practitioner (DH 2006a, **C**; DH 2010, **C**).

4 Clearly label blood sample bottle and appropriate form with 'pre-drug administration blood'.	To ensure there is no confusion between the pre-drug and post-drug serum level specimens. **E**
5 Administer intravenous antibiotics as prescribed via the patient's established vascular access device.	To continue with patient's prescribed drug regimen. **E**
6 If peak level required: within an allotted time after administration, repeat step 3. Clearly label blood sample bottle and appropriate form with 'post-drug administration blood'.	To allow time for even distribution of the drug through the blood for peak blood levels to be achieved (Jones 2006, **E**).
Post-procedure	
8 Ensure microbiology request forms are completed correctly, including date, exact time and dosage of previously administered dose.	To maintain accurate records and provide accurate information for laboratory analysis (NMC 2010, **C**; Weston 2008, **E**).
9 Arrange prompt delivery to the microbiology laboratory.	To allow for prompt analysis and timely adjustments to patient's drug therapy regimen if indicated. **E**
10 Document the procedure in the patient's records.	To ensure timely and accurate record keeping (NMC 2010, **C**).

POST-PROCEDURAL CONSIDERATIONS

Ongoing care

Changes in dosage regimens will depend upon interpretation of the results by the microbiology, medical and nursing team. Notably, high serum drug levels should prompt the microbiology team to telephone a result through to the medical team in charge of the patient's care, especially if this warrants withholding subsequent doses of the drug. A low drug serum level would instigate an increase in the dosage of the drug (Roberts et al. 2011). Any changes to the drug regimen should be communicated and clearly documented on the patient's prescription.

Documentation

In accordance with the principles of good record keeping, the date and time of when a trough and/or peak drug assay level is sent to the laboratory should be documented clearly and promptly in the patient's notes, care plan and/or on the patient's drug chart (or antimicrobial flow charts as provided by the pharmacy department) (NMC 2010). This assists in communication and the dissemination of information between members of the interprofessional healthcare team.

Semen collection

DEFINITION

Human male semen is collected for a variety of reasons; this chapter focuses on two of these. First, to facilitate semen analysis in the investigation of infertility and second, to procure and preserve sperm prior to interventions that carry the risk of future infertility. The physiology of semen is described, as are the ethics and legislation guiding the collection and storage of male gametes; key methods of procurement are outlined and finally the biopsychosocial process of the most common method of semen collection (self-masturbation and collection) is explained.

ANATOMY AND PHYSIOLOGY

Two of the three key functions of the male reproductive system are to produce and deliver sperm to the female ova for fertilization; the third is to produce and secrete male sex hormones in order to maintain the male reproductive system (Jenkins and Tortora 2013, Mawhinney and Mariotti 2000).

Spermatogenesis takes place in the testes in a constant and continuous cycle throughout adult human male life. On average, 85 million sperm are made per testicle per day. Primary male germ cells are initially created in the outer wall of the germinal epithelium of the seminiferous tubules (Gilbert 2000). As the sperm cells mature, they move into the lumen of the tubule to begin a circuitous journey through the male reproductive system. On this journey, sperm cells are augmented with nutritional and biochemical supplements (Jeyendran 2003), resulting in a greyish-white viscous fluid (semen). Semen not only helps sperm to survive but also eases the transfer of sperm into the female reproductive tract and facilitates successful fertilization (Jenkins and Tortora 2013).

Components of normal semen

The volume of semen released per ejaculate varies between 2.3 mL and 4.99 mL. The average ejaculate is 3.4 mL.

- Fructose-rich fluid from the seminal vesicles (65–70%).
- Secretions from the prostate gland containing enzymes, citric acid, lipids and acid phosphatase (25–30%).
- 200–500 million sperm (2–5%).
- Secretions produced by the bulbourethral glands that aid the mobility of sperm in the vagina and cervix (1%) (Mandal 2010).

Semen is released during the two-phase process of ejaculation (Mulhall 2013). Controlled by the central nervous system, ejaculation occurs when there is friction on the genitalia or other forms of sexual stimulation leading to impulses that are sent via the spinal cord to the brain. Phase 1 occurs when the vas deferens contracts to squeeze the sperm toward the base of the penis through the prostate gland and into the urethra. The seminal vesicles release their part of the semen that combines with the sperm (Mulhall 2013).

Phase 2 is when the muscles at the base of the penis and urethra contract. This forces the semen out of the penis. At this phase, the bladder neck contracts to prevent the backflow of the semen into the urinary tract (retrograde ejaculation if this occurs). The final components of semen join together in the posterior urethra and mix only after ejaculation (Mulhall 2013).

EVIDENCE-BASED APPROACHES

Rationale

Semen collection may be required for diagnostic and/or therapeutic purposes (Gerris 1999). Common reasons to collect semen include:

- to investigate the cause of infertility (Gerris 1999)
- to assess the success of a vasectomy or vasectomy reversal (Dohle et al. 2012)

- cryopreservation of semen prior to treatments that may affect fertility, i.e. for cancer (NICE 2013, Royal College of Physicians 2007)
- prior to artificial insemination (Hammarberg et al. 2010)
- sperm donation (van den Broek et al. 2013).

Principles of care

Studies have shown that male infertility can cause extreme loss of self-esteem and impaired gender identity (Schmidt et al. 2005). There exists evidence on the importance of the relationship between body and mind in self-identity and perception (Greil et al. 2010) and that male infertility threatens the perception of masculinity (Gannon et al. 2004).

However, much of the infertility literature suggests that the focus has previously been on the female rather than male partner so best practice is now that couples (opposite sex or same sex) having difficulty conceiving should be seen together as decisions made in relation to investigations and treatment affect both partners (HFEA 2012). Access to evidence-based information should be made available to ensure informed decisions are made. Information can be given verbally and supplemented with written and/or audio-visual information (NICE 2013). The HFEA (2012) Code of Practice also recommends that three distinct types of counselling should be offered to both partners so they understand the implications and consequences of their actions in seeking treatment.

- Implication counselling – to understand the implications of proposed treatment.
- Support counselling – to give emotional support.
- Therapeutic counselling – to cope with the consequences of infertility (HFEA 2012).

For men and boys with cancer, semen collection as fertility preservation is common. Education and information should be given to inform their consent for cryopreservation. Practical issues of how sperm is collected, stored and managed in the event of death is essential prior to any cancer treatment (Pacey and Eiser 2011). Clinical judgement should be employed in the timing of this consultation, but doing so at the earliest opportunity is encouraged (Lee et al. 2006).

Whatever the reason for collecting semen, the donor should have adequate verbal and written information with time and counselling to consider the decision to collect and reflect on the consequences of donation and fully understand the process of how their semen will be collected.

Methods of semen collection

Masturbation

Collecting semen for sperm cryopreservation is generally obtained by masturbation. For many men, this may be an embarrassing or uncomfortable process (Williams 2010). It is critical that men understand how to collect semen and that they be offered a private and relaxing environment to do so.

For adolescent males, careful counselling, tactful and age-appropriate instructions are necessary, as these patients are at risk for emotional distress from this process (Crawshaw and Hale 2005). Parents should be included in discussions, although separate sessions with the adolescent are often useful. Unfortunately, no guidelines exist for the best approach to semen cryopreservation in the adolescent male, but individual institutional strategies are available (Leonard et al. 2004).

Electroejaculation

In some patients who have suffered a spinal cord injury, ejaculation by masturbation is not an option for sperm collection. In this case, the ejaculatory nerves can be electrically stimulated using a low-voltage rectal probe. This is usually sufficient to produce a semen ejaculate, although the quality of the ejaculate is often less using this method compared to masturbation (Brackett et al. 2010).

Microepididymal sperm aspiration

Microepididymal sperm aspiration (MESA) is a surgical procedure for collection of sperm when the ejaculatory tubes are blocked or have been interrupted by a previous vasectomy (Nudell 1998). A surgical incision is made into the outer covering of the testis and the epididymis is exposed; expanded areas of the epididymis likely to contain sperm are incised and the sperm extracted (Nudell 1998).

Percutaneous epididymal sperm aspiration

Percutaneous epididymal sperm aspiration (PESA) is a variant of MESA; rather than an incision, needle aspiration is used to extract sperm from the epididymis. PESA can be performed under local anaesthesia, but less sperm is often collected using this approach (Esteves et al. 2013). Both MESA and PESA yield enough sperm for use with assisted reproductive methods but not enough for a standard insemination (Esteves et al. 2013, Nudell 1998).

Testicular sperm extraction (TESE)

For men who produce extremely small numbers of sperm, recovery of sperm from the epididymis may not be successful (Dabaja and Schlegel 2012). Testicular extraction and possibly tissue biopsy may be the best option for collecting sperm suitable for assisted reproductive techniques (ART). The outer covering of the testicle is pulled back so that seminiferous tubules can be visualized. An enlarged tubule is cut to permit sperm to flow from the tubule, where it can be aspirated (Schlegel 1999). Testicular tissue can be dissected in a culture dish and the released sperm collected for ART (Dabaja and Schlegel 2012, Gerris 1999). Some men with permanent azoospermia after chemotherapy can be successfully treated by TESE-intracytoplasmic sperm injection (ICSI) (Meseguer et al. 2003).

Anticipated patient outcomes

It would be expected that a diagnosis and/or analysis of results in relation to fertility treatments would be available to patients after semen collection had taken place. Cryopreserved semen will give the patient the opportunity to conceive after treatment for fertility-damaging treatment such as chemotherapy and/or radiotherapy.

LEGAL AND PROFESSIONAL ISSUES

The 1990 Human Fertilisation and Embryology Act provided for the establishment of the Human Fertilisation and Embryology Authority (HFEA), the first statutory body of its type in the world. With the creation of the HFEA, the 1990 Act ensured the regulation, through licensing, of:

- the creation of human embryos outside the body and their use in treatment and research
- the use of donated gametes and embryos
- the storage of gametes and embryos.

The Act was radically amended in 2008 (Human Fertilisation and Embryology Act 2008) to ensure that the legislative framework was in line with radical technological, social and medical changes since its original publication. Amendments include:

- extending regulation to the creation and use of all embryos outside the human body, regardless of the processes used in their creation

- increasing the scope of legitimate embryo research activities, i.e. allowing hybrid embryos to be created for research purposes
- banning sex selection of offspring for non-medical reasons
- retention of a duty, when providing fertility treatment, to take account of the welfare of the child, but removal of the reference to 'the need for a father'
- recognizing same-sex couples as legal parents of children conceived through the use of donated sperm, eggs or embryos (Birk 2009).

Human Fertilisation and Embryology Authority

The HFEA is the independent regulator for the licensing and monitoring of fertility clinics and research involving human embryos in the UK. In accordance to the Human Fertilisation and Embryology Act (1990, 2008) and the European Union Tissues and Cells Directive (2004), the HFEA provides authoritative information for the public, in particular for people seeking treatment, donor-conceived people and donors. The HFEA also determines the policy framework for fertility issues, which are sometimes ethically and clinically complex.

European Union Tissues and Cells Directives

The European Union Tissues and Cells Directives, published in 2004 (EUTCD 2004), introduced common safety and quality standards for human tissues and cells across the European Union (EU). The purpose of the directive is to facilitate a safer and easier exchange of tissues and cells (including human eggs and sperm) between member states of the EU and to improve safety standards for European citizens.

Ethical considerations

Beyond the scientific processes in ART and cryopreservation, there are ethical considerations to consider in the collection, storage and use of semen (Gong et al. 2009). The legal ownership of sperm as unfertilized gametes varies from country to country (Pennings 2000). However, ethical principles must respect the interests and welfare of those who will be born as a result of semen collection as well as the health and welfare of the donor (Gong et al. 2009).

Consent

Counselling and gaining informed consent are an integral part of all patient activities. Prior to the collection of semen for any reason, it is essential that practitioners gain fully informed consent (NMC 2013). Consent is continuous throughout any patient episode and the practitioner must ensure that the patient is kept informed at every stage (Stuart and White 2012). For semen collection, this includes:

- informing the patient of the rationale for specimen collection
- what the procedure will involve
- ascertaining their level of understanding (especially if they need to be directly involved in the sampling technique)
- how long the results may take to be processed
- how the results will be made available
- information on how this may affect their care.

In the UK, if the donor is a child, i.e. under the age of 18 years, then the normal rules of gaining consent in this age group apply (Shaw 2001).

- When obtaining consent, the person gaining consent must establish whether the child is legally competent (has capacity) to give consent.
- All people aged 16 and over are presumed in law to have capacity unless there is evidence to the contrary.
- However, as with adults, it does not mean that all 16-year-olds have capacity, and competence must be assessed along the following lines.
  - Are they able to understand and retain the information pertinent to the decision about their care, i.e. the nature, purpose and possible consequences of undergoing and not undergoing the proposed investigations or treatment?
  - Are they able to use this information to consider whether or not they should consent to the intervention offered?
  - Are they able to communicate their wishes?

If the child is deemed not legally competent, consent will need to be obtained from someone with parental responsibility (Shaw 2001).

PRE-PROCEDURAL CONSIDERATIONS

Equipment

A sterile specimen container from the laboratory is required. Container lids must not be waxed cardboard or have plastic or rubber liners to maintain the quality of the sample. Contraceptive condoms are not suitable as the lubricants are spermicidal. Men who are unable to provide a sample on religious or moral grounds may use silastic condoms such as the seminal collection device (Brinsden 2005).

Recording tools

Labelling specimens

Prompt specimen analysis is only possible if specimens and their accompanying request forms are sent with specific, accurate and complete patient information. Incorrectly labelled or unlabelled specimens will be discarded (HSE 2003). The form should include as much information as possible as this allows the laboratory to select the most appropriate media inoculation for examination and result interpretation (Weston 2008). General labelling should be conducted accurately as discussed at the beginning of the chapter.

Specific patient preparation

It takes between 3 and 4 days for the sperm count to return to normal after ejaculation (Brinsden 2005, NCCWCH and NICE 2004) so patients should be advised that sexual intercourse or masturbation should not have taken place for 48 hours prior to semen collection. This will ensure that the semen will have an optimum count and motility (NCCWCH and NICE 2004). The patient should have ejaculated at least once between 48 hours and and 7 days before collection. The patient should also be screened for the use of medicines and/or herbal remedies which may impact on sperm production or motility, such as St John's wort which has a mutagenic effect on sperm cells (Chernecky and Berger 2013).

Education

Patients who are to be treated with ICSI should undergo appropriate investigations to determine the diagnosis and enable informed discussion prior to the procedure. This will prepare the patient/couple for the potential implications of treatment. Genetic counselling and testing should be offered to men who have a specific or suspected genetic defect in relation to their infertility (NCCWCH and NICE 2004).

Patients who are undergoing treatments that may lead to infertility should be offered independent counselling to prepare them to cope with the possible physical and psychological implications of the treatment and its side-effects prior to commencing treatment (NCCWCH and NICE 2004, Wo and Viswanathan 2009).

Procedure guideline 10.4 **Semen collection**

Essential equipment

- Private room
- Sterile specimen collection container supplied by laboratory
- Tissues

Pre-procedure

Action	Rationale
1 Explain and discuss the procedure with the patient, giving clear, comprehensive instructions explaining what should and should not be done. Ask when he last had sexual intercourse or masturbated.	To ensure the patient understands the procedure and gives valid consent (Brinsden 2005, **E**; NMC 2013, **C**). To ensure the sperm count will be at maximum levels (Brinsden 2005, **E**).
2 Ensure the patient has a private room.	To ensure privacy for the patient. **E**
Procedure	
3 Instruct the patient to only open the lid prior to ejaculation and replace it immediately after collection.	To minimize microbiological contamination (Brinsden 2005, **E**).
4 A fresh masturbated specimen must be collected in a sterile container.	To ensure optimum sample is obtained (Chernecky and Berger 2013, **E**).
Post-procedure	
5 Complete specimen form and label specimen container (including relevant information such as date and time of collection).	To maintain accurate records and provide accurate information for laboratory analysis (NMC 2010, **C**).
6 Specimens must be transported to the laboratory as quickly as possible, within 1 hour of collection, and analysed within 3 hours.	To ensure optimum sample is obtained (Brinsden 2005, **E**; Chernecky and Berger 2013, **E**).
7 The specimen must be kept at between 25°C and 37°C in a laboratory incubator.	To ensure optimum sample is obtained (Brinsden 2005, **E**).
8 Document the procedure in the patient's records.	To ensure timely and accurate record keeping (NMC 2010, **C**).

POST-PROCEDURAL CONSIDERATIONS

Immediate care

It is important that the patient has information to take away and has a contact number in case further questions arise. The patient should be informed when results are likely to be available and how they will be communicated (NICE 2013).

Ongoing care

Patients who are undergoing treatments that may lead to infertility should be offered independent counselling to help them cope with the possible physical and psychological implications of the treatment and its side-effects (NICE 2013).

Specimen collection: swab sampling

DEFINITION

Sterile swabs are commonly used in clinical practice to obtain samples of material from skin and mucous membranes. They are utilized to identify micro-organisms in suspected infection or as part of a screening programme to identify patients who may be carrying pathogens without displaying clinical signs or symptoms (Ferguson 2005). Swab cultures provide useful data to augment diagnostic and therapeutic decision making (Bonham 2009).

RELATED THEORY

Swabbing is aimed at quantitative or qualitative collection of bodily fluid or cutaneous material for the purpose of obtaining a specimen for microbiological analysis (Bowler et al. 2001, Kingsley 2001) and when properly performed, a swab is a simple, non-invasive and cost-effective method of culturing in clinical practice (Bonham 2009). Samples of infected material can be obtained from any accessible part of the body by using a sterile swab tipped with cotton wool or synthetic material (Hampson 2006).

Swabs for screening programmes

Meticillin-resistant *Staphylococcus aureus* is one of the most significant problematic organisms within healthcare (Weston 2008). Colonized and infected patients represent the most important reservoir of MRSA strains within hospitals (HPA 2014b). The transmission of MRSA and the risk of MRSA infection can only be effectively addressed if MRSA carriers are identified and treated to reduce this risk of transmission (DH 2006b). These screening control measures guide staff in the protection of patients from MRSA colonization and infection. Active screening of patients for MRSA carriage is performed based on a risk assessment approach to the use of isolation and cohorting facilities (Coia et al. 2006).

Obtaining swabs is a key component of an effective MRSA prevention programme and certain patient groups are deemed to be at higher risk of contracting serious MRSA infections: critical care, burns, transplantation, cardiothoracic surgery, orthopaedic surgery, trauma, vascular surgery and renal patients (Coia et al. 2006).

The normal habitat of *Staphylococcus aureus*, including MRSA, is human skin, particularly the anterior nares (nose), axilla (armpit) and perineum (groin) (DH 2006b). The essential site to sample is the anterior nares (nose) as this is the most common carriage site for MRSA and most patients positive at other sites have positive results from nose samples (DH 2006b). Other samples can be taken from the following sites: skin lesions and wounds, vascular access device sites and other skin breaks, tracheostomies, catheter specimens of urine (CSU) and sputum from patients with a productive cough (Coia et al. 2006). The microbiological request form should clearly indicate that the samples are for MRSA screening to ensure that correct laboratory techniques are used and to avoid potential waste of resources.

EVIDENCE-BASED APPROACHES

Rationale

Indications

Taking a swab is indicated:

- if there are clinical signs of infection which may manifest as symptoms such as pain, redness, inflammation, heat, pus and odour
- if a patient shows signs of systemic infection or has a pyrexia of unknown origin (PUO)
- as part of a screening programme.

Contraindications

- As routine use (unless part of a screening regimen).
- On chronic wounds which will be colonized with skin flora.

Principles of care

Although swabs are relatively simple to use, absorbency of infected material is variable and adequate material collection that is representative of pathogenic changes, for example to wounds, is often dependent upon correct sampling technique (Gould and Brooker 2008). Swab specimens should be collected using an aseptic technique with sterile swabs, with the principal aim of gathering as much material as possible from the site of infection/inflammation. Care should be taken to avoid contamination with anything other than sample material such as surrounding tissue, which will be contaminated with other pathogens such as skin flora (Weston 2008).

If an infected area is producing copious amounts of pus or exudate, a specimen should be aspirated using a sterile syringe because swabs tend to absorb excess overlying exudate, resulting in an inadequate specimen (Gilchrist 2000). If the area to be swabbed is relatively dry, for example nasal or skin swabs, the tip of the swab can be moistened with sterile 0.9% sodium chloride which makes it more absorbent and increases the survival of pathogens (Weston 2008).

Obtaining a swab should be considered in conjunction with a comprehensive nursing assessment. This could include observation of localized infection such as inflammation or discharge from a wound during a dressing change.

Practitioners should know what type of pathogenic micro-organisms they are testing, for example whether a bacterial or viral infection is suspected, as this will determine which swab is the most appropriate. Advice should be sought from the microbiology laboratory prior to taking a swab to ensure appropriate and resource-effective sampling or specimen collection. For example, whilst viruses cause the majority of throat infections, group A streptococcus is the main bacterial cause of sore throats and therefore, if suspected, a swab with bacterial transport medium would need to be used rather than one containing viral transport medium (HPA 2014c).

LEGAL AND PROFESSIONAL ISSUES

Competencies

Obtaining specimens for microbiological analysis is a key component in the patient's assessment and subsequent nursing care. Therefore, practitioners must be competent and feel confident that they have the knowledge, skill and understanding to obtain and correctly process samples for specimen collection (RCN 2012).

PRE-PROCEDURAL CONSIDERATIONS

Equipment

Commercially available transport media offer a cheap and effective method to enable the culture of both aerobic and anaerobic micro-organisms (Bowler et al. 2001). Wound swabbing most frequently involves the use of a cotton- or alginate-tipped swab (Bowler et al. 2001), although these have been found to inhibit the detection of certain bacteria (Faoagali 2010). Despite being more expensive, flocked nylon swabs now provide a sensitive collection method for culture, rapid, near patient testing and molecular detection of a variety of bacteria and viruses. This is because of their ability to absorb cells then release them effectively to increase the sensitivity of detection of infecting microbes (Faoagali 2010). If unsure, the practitioner should liaise with the microbiology laboratory to clarify which is the most suitable swab for a particular investigation or type of specimen. See Figure 10.4.

Specific patient preparation

It may be necessary to position the patient in order to obtain the required sample.

Procedure guideline 10.5 **Swab sampling: ear**

Essential equipment

- Non-sterile gloves
- Apron
- Sterile swab (with transport medium)
- Appropriate documentation/form

Pre-procedure

Action	Rationale
1 Explain and discuss the procedure with the patient.	To ensure the patient understands the procedure and gives valid consent (NMC 2013, **C**).
2 Wash hands with bactericidal soap and water, or decontaminate physically clean hands with alcohol-based handrub. Don apron and gloves.	To reduce the risk of cross-infection and specimen contamination (Fraise and Bradley 2009, **E**; RCN 2012, **C**).
3 Ensure no antibiotics or other therapeutic drops have been used in the aural region 3 hours before taking the swab.	To prevent collection of such therapeutic agents which may mask pathogenic organisms and invalidate the specimen (Hampson 2006, **E**).

(continued)

Procedure guideline 10.5 Swab sampling: ear *(continued)*

Procedure

Action	Rationale
4 Remove the swab from outer packaging and place at the entrance of the auditory meatus as shown in **Action figure 4**. Rotate gently once.	To avoid trauma to the ear and to collect secretions/suitable specimen material (Mims 2004, **E**).
Post-procedure	
5 Remove cap from plastic transport tube.	To avoid contamination of the swab and to maintain the viability of the sampled material during transportation (HPA 2014b, **C**).
6 Carefully place swab into plastic transport tube, ensuring it is fully immersed in the transport medium. Ensure cap is firmly secured.	To avoid contamination of the swab and to maintain the viability of the sampled material during transportation (Ferguson 2005, **E**).
7 Remove gloves and apron and wash/decontaminate hands.	To reduce risk of cross-infection (Loveday et al. 2014, **C**; Sax et al. 2007, **E**).
8 Complete microbiology request form (including relevant information such as exact site, nature of specimen and investigation required).	To maintain accurate records and provide accurate information for laboratory analysis (NMC 2010, **C**; Weston 2008, **E**).
9 Arrange prompt delivery to the microbiology laboratory or refrigerate at 4–8°C.	To achieve optimal conditions for analysis (HPA 2014b, **C**).
10 Document the procedure in the patient's records.	To ensure timely and accurate record keeping (NMC 2010, **C**).

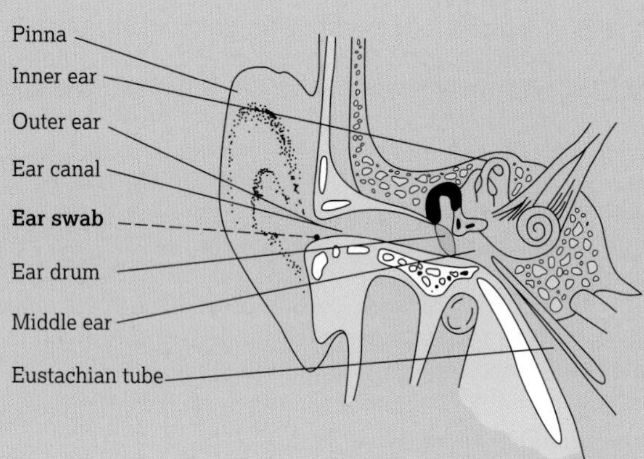

Action Figure 4 Area to be swabbed when sampling the outer ear.

Procedure guideline 10.6 Swab sampling: eye

Essential equipment

- Non-sterile gloves
- Apron
- Appropriate documentation/form
- Sterile bacterial or viral swab (with transport medium)

Pre-procedure

Action	Rationale
1 Explain and discuss the procedure with the patient.	To ensure the patient understands the procedure and gives valid consent (NMC 2013, **C**).
2 Seek advice from the microbiology laboratory as to the correct culture medium and swab required.	Different culture media and swabs are required for bacteria, viruses and chlamydia (Shaw et al. 2010, **E**).
3 Wash hands with bactericidal soap and water, or decontaminate physically clean hands with alcohol-based handrub. Don apron and gloves.	To reduce the risk of cross-infection and specimen contamination (Fraise and Bradley 2009, **E**; RCN 2012, **C**).

Procedure	
4 Remove swab from outer packaging.	To ensure collection of specimen material (Mims 2004, **E**).
5 Ask patient to look upwards.	To prevent corneal damage (Shaw et al. 2010, **E**).
6 Hold the swab parallel to the cornea and gently rub the conjunctiva in the lower eyelids from nasal side outwards.	To ensure that a swab of the correct site is taken and to avoid contamination by touching the eyelid (Shaw et al. 2010, **E**).
7 *If for chlamydia specimen:* apply slightly more pressure when swabbing.	To obtain as many organisms as possible from the follicles and to sweep organisms away from the lower punctum (Shaw et al. 2010, **E**).
8 If both eyes are to be swabbed, label swabs 'right' and 'left' accordingly.	To prevent the wrong swab being placed in the wrong culture medium (Shaw et al. 2010, **E**).
Post-procedure	
9 Remove cap from plastic transport tube.	To avoid contamination of the swab (HPA 2014b, **C**).
10 Carefully place swab into plastic transport tube, ensuring it is fully immersed in the transport medium. Ensure cap is firmly secured.	To avoid contamination of the swab and to maintain the viability of the sampled material during transportation (Ferguson 2005, **E**).
11 Remove gloves and apron and wash/decontaminate hands.	To reduce risk of cross-infection (Loveday et al. 2014, **C**; Sax et al. 2007, **E**).
12 Complete microbiology request form (including relevant information such as exact site, nature of specimen and investigation required).	To maintain accurate records and provide accurate information for laboratory analysis (NMC 2010, **C**; Weston 2008, **E**).
13 Arrange prompt delivery to the microbiology laboratory.	To achieve optimal conditions for analysis (HPA 2014b, **C**).
14 Document the procedure in the patient's records.	To ensure timely and accurate record keeping (NMC 2010, **C**).

Procedure guideline 10.7 **Swab sampling: nose**

Essential equipment

- Non- sterile gloves
- Apron
- Sterile bacterial or viral swab (with transport medium)

Optional equipment

- 0.9% sodium chloride
- Appropriate documentation/form

Pre-procedure

Action	Rationale
1 Explain and discuss the procedure with the patient.	To ensure the patient understands the procedure and gives valid consent (NMC 2013, **C**).
2 Wash hands with bactericidal soap and water, or decontaminate physically clean hands with alcohol-based handrub. Don apron and gloves.	To reduce the risk of cross-infection and specimen contamination (Fraise and Bradley 2009, **E**; RCN 2012, **C**).
Procedure	
3 Remove swab from outer packaging.	To ensure collection of specimen material (Mims 2004, **E**).
4 Ask patient to tilt head backwards.	To optimize visualization of area to be swabbed (Gould and Brooker 2008, **E**).
5 Moisten swab with sterile saline.	To prevent discomfort to the patient as the nasal mucosa is normally dry and organisms will adhere more easily to a moist swab (Hampson 2006, **E**).
6 Insert swab inside the anterior nares with the tip directed upwards and gently rotate (**Action figure 6**).	To ensure that an adequate specimen from the correct site is obtained and to avoid damage to the delicate epithelium (Gould and Brooker 2008, **E**).
7 Repeat the procedure with the same swab in the other nostril.	To optimize organism collection. **E**

(continued)

Procedure guideline 10.7 Swab sampling: nose *(continued)*

Post-procedure

Action	Rationale
8 Remove cap from plastic transport tube.	To avoid contamination of the swab (HPA 2014d, **C**).
9 Carefully place swab into plastic transport tube, ensuring it is fully immersed in the transport medium. Ensure cap is firmly secured.	To avoid contamination of the swab and to maintain the viability of the sampled material during transportation (Ferguson 2005, **E**).
10 Provide the patient with a tissue if required.	For patient comfort (Higgins 2013, **E**).
11 Remove gloves and apron and wash/decontaminate hands.	To reduce risk of cross-infection (Loveday et al. 2014, **C**; Sax et al. 2007, **E**).
12 Complete microbiology request form (including relevant information such as exact site, nature of specimen and investigation required).	To maintain accurate records and provide accurate information for laboratory analysis (NMC 2010, **C**; Weston 2008, **E**).
13 *If sample taken for screening:* state clearly on the microbiology request form, for example for MRSA screening.	To ensure only these organisms are being analysed, so the result will only indicate their presence or absence, and sensitivities (Weston 2008, **E**).
14 Arrange prompt delivery to the microbiology laboratory.	To achieve optimal conditions for analysis (HPA 2014d, **C**).
15 Document the procedure in the patient's records.	To ensure timely and accurate record keeping (NMC 2010, **C**).

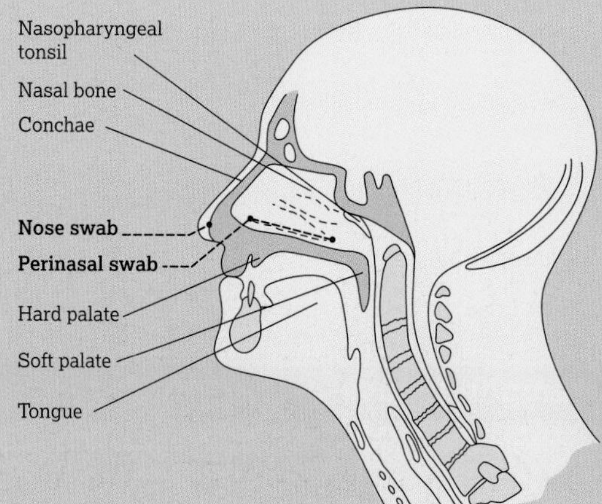

Action Figure 6 Area to be swabbed when sampling the nose.

Procedure guideline 10.8 Swab sampling: penis

Essential equipment

- Non-sterile gloves
- Apron
- Sterile bacterial or viral swab (with transport medium)
- Appropriate documentation/form

Pre-procedure

Action	Rationale
1 Explain and discuss the procedure with the patient.	To ensure the patient understands the procedure and gives valid consent (NMC 2013, **C**).
2 Wash hands with bactericidal soap and water, or decontaminate physically clean hands with alcohol-based handrub. Don apron and gloves.	To reduce the risk of cross-infection and specimen contamination (Fraise and Bradley 2009, **C**; RCN 2012, **C**).

Procedure

Action	Rationale
3 The patient should not have passed urine for at least 1 hour.	To ensure a representative sample from the area being swabbed (HPA 2014e, **C**).

4 Remove swab from outer packaging.	To ensure collection of specimen material (Mims 2004, **E**).
5 Retract prepuce.	To obtain maximum visibility of area to be swabbed (HPA 2014e **C**).
6 Pass the swab gently through the urethral meatus and rotate gently.	To collect a specimen of discharge or secretions (HPA 2014e, **C**).
Post-procedure	
7 Remove cap from plastic transport tube.	To avoid contamination of the swab (HPA 2014e, **C**).
8 Carefully place swab into plastic transport tube, ensuring it is fully immersed in the transport medium. Ensure cap is firmly secured.	To avoid contamination of the swab and to maintain viability of the sampled material during transportation (Ferguson 2005, **E**).
9 Remove gloves and apron and wash/decontaminate hands.	To reduce risk of cross-infection (Loveday et al. 2014, **C**; Sax et al. 2007, **E**).
10 Complete microbiology request form (including relevant information such as exact site, nature of specimen and investigation required).	To maintain accurate records and provide accurate information for laboratory analysis (NMC 2010, **C**; Weston 2008, **E**).
11 Arrange prompt delivery to the microbiology laboratory (within 4 hours).	To increase the chance of accurate organism identification and to ensure the best possible conditions for laboratory analysis (HPA 2014e, **C**).
12 Document the procedure in the patient's records.	To ensure timely and accurate record keeping (NMC 2010, **C**).

Procedure guideline 10.9 **Swab sampling: rectum**

Essential equipment

- Non-sterile gloves
- Apron
- Appropriate documentation/form
- Sterile bacterial or viral swab (with transport medium)

Pre-procedure

Action	Rationale
1 Explain and discuss the procedure with the patient.	To ensure the patient understands the procedure and gives valid consent (NMC 2013, **C**).
2 Ensure a suitable location in which to carry out the procedure.	To maintain patient privacy and dignity (Hampson 2006, **E**).
3 Wash hands with bactericidal soap and water, or decontaminate physically clean hands with alcohol-based handrub. Don apron and gloves.	To reduce the risk of cross-infection and specimen contamination (Fraise and Bradley 2009, **E**; RCN 2012, **C**).
Procedure	
4 Remove swab from outer packaging.	To ensure collection of specimen material (Mims 2004, **E**).
5 Pass the swab, with care, through the anus into the rectum and rotate gently.	To avoid trauma and to ensure that a rectal, not an anal, sample is obtained. **E**
6 *If specimen is for suspected threadworm:* take swab from the perianal area.	Threadworms lay their ova on the perianal skin (Hampson, 2006, **E**).
Post-procedure	
7 Remove cap from plastic transport tube.	To avoid contamination of the swab (HPA 2014b, **C**).
8 Carefully place swab into plastic transport tube, ensuring it is fully immersed in the transport medium. Ensure cap is firmly secured.	To avoid contamination of the swab and to maintain viability of the sampled material during transportation (Ferguson 2005, **E**).
9 Remove gloves and apron and wash/decontaminate hands.	To reduce risk of cross-infection (Loveday et al. 2014, **C**; Sax et al. 2007, **E**).

(continued)

Procedure guideline 10.9 Swab sampling: rectum *(continued)*

Action	Rationale
10 Complete microbiology request form (including relevant information such as exact site, nature of specimen and investigation required).	To maintain accurate records and provide accurate information for laboratory analysis (NMC 2010, **C**; Weston 2008, **E**).
11 Arrange prompt delivery to the microbiology laboratory.	To achieve optimal conditions for analysis (HPA 2014b, **C**).
12 Document the procedure in the patient's records.	To ensure timely and accurate record keeping (NMC 2010, **C**).

Procedure guideline 10.10 Swab sampling: skin

Essential equipment

- Non-sterile gloves
- Apron
- Appropriate documentation/form
- Sterile bacterial or viral swab (with transport medium)

Optional equipment

- Scalpel blade/U blade (for trained practitioners only)

Pre-procedure

Action	Rationale
1 Explain and discuss the procedure with the patient.	To ensure the patient understands the procedure and gives valid consent (NMC 2013, **C**).
2 Wash hands with bactericidal soap and water, or decontaminate physically clean hands with alcohol-based handrub. Don apron and gloves.	To reduce the risk of cross-infection and specimen contamination (Fraise and Bradley 2009, **E**; RCN 2012, **C**).
3 Remove swab from outer packaging.	To ensure collection of specimen material (Mims 2004, **E**).

Procedure

Action	Rationale
4 *For cutaneous sampling (for screening, for example groin)*: moisten swab with sterile saline and roll one swab along the area of skin along the inside of the thighs closest to the genitalia.	Organisms adhere more easily to a moist swab (Hampson 2006, **C**).
5 *For suspected fungal infection*: skin scrapings should be obtained. Take a scalpel blade and, with the affected area of skin stretched taut between two fingers, gently scrape the skin with a piece of dark paper underneath. Do not cause bleeding.	To identify superficial fungi that inhabit the outer layer of the skin (Mackie 2003, **E**). To visualize amount of sample and to allow easier transfer. **E**

Post-procedure

Action	Rationale
6 *Either*:	To avoid contamination of the swab (HPA 2014b, **C**).
For swab specimen: (a) Remove cap from plastic transport tube. (b) Carefully place swab into plastic transport tube, ensuring it is fully immersed in the transport medium. Ensure cap is firmly secured.	To avoid contamination of the swab and to maintain the viability of the sampled material during transportation (Ferguson 2005, **E**).
Or: *For skin scrapings:* (c) Transfer scrapings into sterile container.	To allow samples to be processed appropriately in the laboratory. **E**
7 Remove gloves and apron and wash/decontaminate hands.	To reduce risk of cross-infection (Loveday et al. 2014, **C**; Sax et al. 2007, **E**).
8 Complete microbiology request form (including relevant information such as exact site, nature of specimen and investigation required).	To maintain accurate records and provide accurate information for laboratory analysis (NMC 2010, **C**; Weston 2008, **E**).
9 Arrange prompt delivery to the microbiology laboratory (keep at room temperature).	To achieve optimal conditions for analysis (HPA 2014b, **C**).
10 Document the procedure in the patient's records.	To ensure timely and accurate record keeping (NMC 2010, **C**).

Procedure guideline 10.11 **Swab sampling: throat**

Essential equipment

- Non-sterile gloves
- Apron
- Sterile bacterial or viral swab (with transport medium)
- Light source
- Tongue spatula
- Appropriate documentation/form

Action	Rationale
Pre-procedure	
1 Explain and discuss the procedure with the patient.	To ensure the patient understands the procedure and gives valid consent (NMC 2013, **C**).
2 Wash hands with bactericidal soap and water, or decontaminate physically clean hands with alcohol-based handrub. Don apron and gloves.	To reduce the risk of cross-infection and specimen contamination (Fraise and Bradley 2009, **E**; RCN 2012, **C**).
3 Remove swab from outer packaging.	To ensure collection of specimen material (Mims 2004, **E**).
Procedure	
4 Ask patient to sit upright facing a strong light, tilt head backwards, open mouth and stick out tongue.	To ensure maximum visibility of the area to be swabbed and avoid contact with the oral mucosa (Gould and Brooker 2008, **E**).
5 Depress tongue with a spatula.	The procedure may cause the patient to gag. The spatula prevents the tongue moving to the roof of the mouth, which would contaminate the specimen (Hampson 2006, **E**).
6 Ask patient to say 'Ah'.	Assists with depression of the tongue and prevents patient from feeling the gag reflex (Keir et al. 2007, **E**).
7 Quickly but gently roll the swab over any area of exudate or inflammation or over the tonsils and posterior pharynx (**Action figure 7**).	To obtain the required sample (Weston 2008, **E**).
8 Carefully withdraw the swab, avoiding touching any other area of the mouth or tongue.	To prevent contamination of the specimen with the resident flora of the oropharynx (Weston 2008, **E**).
Post-procedure	
9 Remove cap from plastic transport tube.	To avoid contamination of the swab (HPA 2014b, **C**).
10 Carefully place swab into plastic transport tube, ensuring it is fully immersed in the transport medium. Ensure cap is firmly secured.	To avoid contamination of the swab and maintain the viability of the sampled material during transportation (Ferguson 2005, **E**).
11 Remove gloves and apron and wash/decontaminate hands.	To reduce risk of cross-infection (Loveday et al. 2014, **C**; Sax et al. 2007, **E**).
12 Complete microbiology request form (including relevant information such as exact site, nature of specimen and investigation required).	To maintain accurate records and provide accurate information for laboratory analysis (NMC 2010, **C**; Weston 2008, **E**).
13 Arrange prompt delivery to the microbiology laboratory.	To achieve optimal conditions for analysis (HPA 2014c, **C**).
14 Document the procedure in the patient's records.	To ensure timely and accurate record keeping (NMC 2010, **C**).

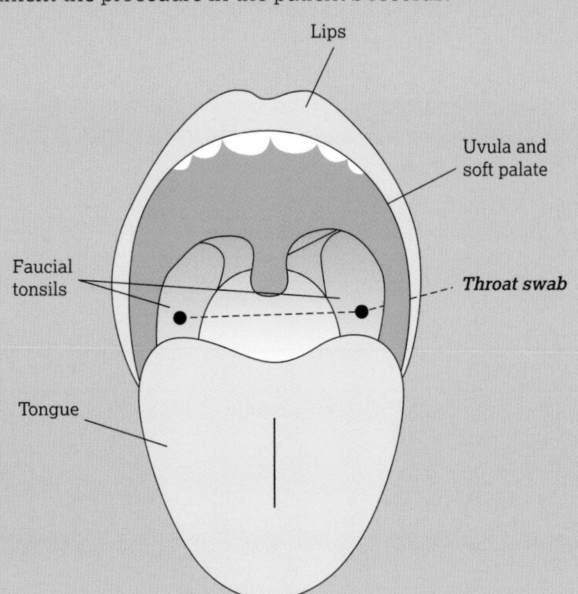

Action Figure 7 Area to be swabbed when sampling the throat.

Procedure guideline 10.12 **Swab sampling: vagina**

Essential equipment

- Non-sterile gloves
- Apron
- Sterile bacterial or viral swab (with transport medium)
- Appropriate documentation/form
- Light source
- Sterile speculum

Pre-procedure

Action	Rationale
1 Explain and discuss the procedure with the patient.	To ensure the patient understands the procedure and gives valid consent (NMC 2013, **C**).
2 Ensure a suitable location in which to carry out the procedure.	To maintain patient privacy and dignity and to help her to relax and be comfortable during procedure (Hampson 2006, **E**).
3 Wash hands with bactericidal soap and water, or decontaminate physically clean hands with alcohol-based handrub. Don apron and gloves.	To reduce the risk of cross-infection and specimen contamination (Fraise and Bradley 2009, **E**; RCN 2012, **C**).
4 Position the patient with her knees bent and legs apart. Adjust the light.	To be able to visualize the vulva and cervix. **E**
5 Remove swab from outer packaging.	To ensure collection of specimen material (Mims 2004, **E**).
Procedure	
6 Allow patient to resume a comfortable position.	To aid patient comfort. **E**
Post-procedure	
7 Remove cap from plastic transport tube.	To avoid contamination of the swab (HPA 2014b, **C**).
8 Carefully place swab into plastic transport tube, ensuring it is fully immersed in the transport medium. Ensure cap is firmly secured.	To avoid contamination of the swab and to maintain the viability of the sampled material during transportation (Ferguson 2005, **E**).
9 Remove gloves and apron and wash/decontaminate hands.	To reduce risk of cross-infection (Loveday et al. 2014, **C**; Sax et al. 2007, **E**).
10 Complete microbiology request form (including relevant information such as exact site, nature of specimen and investigation required).	To maintain accurate records and provide accurate information for laboratory analysis (NMC 2010, **C**; Weston 2008, **E**).
11 Arrange prompt delivery to the microbiology laboratory (within 4 hours).	To achieve optimal conditions for analysis (HPA 2014b, **C**).
12 Document the procedure in the patient's records.	To ensure timely and accurate record keeping (NMC 2010, **C**).

Procedure guideline 10.13 **Swab sampling: wound**

Essential equipment

- Non-sterile gloves
- Apron
- Sterile bacterial or viral swab (with transport medium)

Optional equipment

- 0.9% sodium chloride
- Appropriate documentation/form
- Dressing pack containing sterile gloves, cleansing solution and dressing (post sampling procedure)

Pre-procedure

Action	Rationale
1 Explain and discuss the procedure with the patient.	To ensure the patient understands the procedure and gives valid consent (NMC 2013, **C**).
2 Wash hands with bactericidal soap and water, or decontaminate physically clean hands with alcohol-based handrub. Don apron and gloves.	To reduce the risk of cross-infection and specimen contamination (Fraise and Bradley 2009, **E**; RCN 2012, **C**).
3 Remove current dressing, if applicable.	To expose wound in preparation for swabbing. **E**

4 Remove gloves and decontaminate hands. Open sterile dressing pack, decant sterile swab and don sterile gloves.	To reduce the risk of cross-infection (RCN 2012, **C**) and prepare equipment for sampling (Fraise and Bradley 2009, **E**).
5 Remove swab from outer packaging.	To ensure collection of specimen material (Mims 2004, **E**).
Procedure	
6 Rotate the swab tip over a 1 cm^2 area of viable tissue, at or near the centre of the wound for 5 seconds, applying enough pressure to express tissue fluid from the wound bed.	Expressed tissue fluids are likely to contain the true infecting organisms and less likely to contain surface contaminants (Kingsley 2003, **E**).
7 If the wound is dry, the tip of the swab should be moistened with 0.9% sodium chloride.	To make the swab more absorbent and to increase survival of pathogens present prior to culture (Weston 2008, **E**).
8 If pus is present, it should be aspirated using a sterile syringe and decanted into a sterile specimen pot.	To yield the optimum number of micro-organisms present within the wound (Weston 2008, **E**).
Post-procedure	
9 Remove cap from plastic transport tube.	To avoid contamination of the swab (HPA 2014b, **C**).
10 Carefully place swab into plastic transport tube, ensuring it is fully immersed in the transport medium. Ensure cap is firmly secured.	To avoid contamination of the swab and to maintain the viability of the sampled material during transportation (Ferguson 2005, **E**).
11 Redress the wound, if applicable, as per patient care plan.	To redress the wound. **E**
12 Remove gloves and apron, discard all clinical waste and wash/decontaminate hands.	To reduce risk of cross-infection (Loveday et al. 2014, **C**; Sax et al. 2007, **E**).
13 Complete microbiology request form (including relevant information such as exact site, nature of specimen and investigation required).	To maintain accurate records and provide accurate information for laboratory analysis (NMC 2010, **C**; Weston 2008, **E**).
14 Arrange prompt delivery to the microbiology laboratory (keep at room temperature).	To achieve optimal conditions for analysis (HPA 2014b, **C**).
15 Document the procedure in the patient's records.	To ensure timely and accurate record keeping (NMC 2010, **C**).

POST-PROCEDURAL CONSIDERATIONS

Immediate care

Commercially available transport media maintain the viability of both aerobic and anaerobic micro-organisms (Bowler et al. 2001). Specimens should be sent immediately to the laboratory or no later than 2 hours following collection (Bonham 2009). For specimens that cannot be transferred to the laboratory within 2 hours, storage at room temperature is considered to be appropriate for the maintenance of aerobic and anaerobic micro-organisms (Bowler et al. 2001). Advice should be sought from the microbiology laboratory if practitioners are unsure of the storage requirements for the sample.

Documentation

Relevant and detailed information such as clinical presentation, signs and symptoms of infection, and the site and nature of the swab should be indicated on the sample and microbiology request form (Ferguson 2005). This allows the microbiology laboratory to select the most appropriate processing technique and assist in differentiating organisms which would normally be expected at a particular site from those causing infection (Weston 2008).

In accordance with the principles of good record keeping, the date and time when a swab is sent to the laboratory should be documented clearly and promptly in the patient's notes and care plan (NMC 2010). This should be done alongside documentation of the clinical nursing assessment, particularly in relation to significant findings that have prompted the collection of the sample such as observation of inflammation or discharge at the site. This assists in communication and the dissemination of information between members of the interprofessional healthcare team.

Learning Activity 10.3 Case study: Swab sampling

Mr Wills is a 68-year-old man who has been admitted to hospital for IV antibiotics via his GP. Following surgery to his abdomen 3 weeks ago, he now has a dehisced laparotomy wound which is showing signs of infection (red, inflamed, producing pus). He has been admitted to your unit and, as part of his risk assessment, requires an MRSA screen.

1 Before carrying out the MRSA screen, what should you do to prepare Mr Wills?
2 Which is the most important area of the body to take a swab sample from when screening for MRSA?
3 What other areas of Mr Wills' body would you need to take swab samples from?
4 Once you have taken the swabs, what should you do with them in order to ensure they are ready for collection?

See the end of the chapter for the answers.

Specimen collection: urine sampling

DEFINITION

Urine samples are intended to identify any organisms causing infection within the urinary tract. Urinalysis is the tests that involve microbiological, chemical, microscopical and physical examination of the urine (Higgins 2013). Urinary tract infections (UTIs) result from the presence and multiplication of bacteria in one or more structures of the urinary tract with associated tissue invasion (HPA 2014h).

RELATED THEORY

Protection against infection is normally given by the constant flow of urine and regular bladder emptying, which prevent the colonization of micro-organisms (HPA 2014h). The urethra is colonized with naturally occurring flora but urine proximal to the distal urethra is normally sterile. As urine passes through the urethra, some of these micro-organisms are flushed through and normal urine will naturally contain a small number of bacteria. Therefore, the presence of bacteriuria is insignificant in the absence of clinical symptoms of an infection (Weston 2008).

Urinary tract infections account for up to 20% of all overall hospital-acquired infections. This is the second largest group of infections in the healthcare setting (HPA 2014h). The majority of the 20% are generally catheter-related infections with only 2–6% actual UTIs (HPA 2014h). UTIs in adults are common, particularly in women due to the short female urethra and its close proximity to the perineum, but age, sex and predisposing factors are other important considerations (HPA 2014h).

EVIDENCE-BASED APPROACHES

Rationale

Urine sample requests for Microscopy, Culture and Sensitivity (MC&S) constitute the largest single category of specimens examined in microbiological laboratories. The main value of urine culture is to identify bacteria and their sensitivity to antibiotics (Higgins 2013).

Urine sampling should be considered in combination with clinical assessment and urinalysis to avoid unnecessary sample processing which has time and cost implications for the microbiology laboratory (Simerville et al. 2005, Thomas 2008). A clinical assessment would involve examination of the odour, turbidity and colour, whether there are obvious signs of haematuria and pain particularly around the suprapubic area (Dulczak and Kirk 2005). Urinalysis may reveal a high pH, the presence of blood or positivity to leucocyte esterase (an enzyme released by white blood cells) or nitrite, all of which indicate a high probability of bacteriuria (Higgins 2013).

Indications

Obtaining a urine specimen is indicated:

- when there are clinical signs and symptoms to indicate an UTI
- if there are signs of a systemic infection or in patients with a PUO
- on development of new patient confusion as toxicity from infection can cause alterations in mental status or impairments in cognitive ability (Pellowe 2009).

Principles of care

Urine may be collected using a midstream urine (MSU) clean-catch technique or from a catheter using a sterile syringe to access the sample port (HPA 2014h). To minimize the contamination of a specimen by bacteria, which may be present on the skin, the perianal region or the external genital tract, good hand and genital hygiene should be encouraged. Therefore, patients should be encouraged to wash their hands prior to collecting a clean-catch midstream urine specimen and to clean around the urethral meatus prior to sample collection (Higgins 2013).

The principle for obtaining a midstream collection of urine is that any bacteria present in the urethra are washed away in the first portion of urine voided and therefore the specimen collected more accurately represents the urine in the bladder. A study conducted by Jackson et al. (2005) using a urinary collection device showed a reduction in contamination from different MSU techniques. However, a study in pregnant women found that there was no difference between MSU, clean-catch or morning samples with regard to potential contamination (Schneeberger et al. 2013).

Catheter-associated urinary tract infections (CAUTI)

The presence of a urinary catheter, and the duration of its insertion, are contributory factors in the development of a UTI. For every day the catheter remains *in situ*, the risk of bacteriuria is 5% so that 50% of patients catheterized for longer than 7–10 days will have bacteriuria (Pellowe 2009). Although often asymptomatic, 20–30% of patients with bacteriuria will develop a CAUTI and 1–4% will develop a bacteraemia, which has significant implications for patient morbidity, increased hospital stay and increased cost (HPA 2014h). Bacteriuria in patients who are catheterized for more than 30 days is up to 100%, although the patient may be asymptomatic (HPA 2014h).

In order to minimize CAUTIs, catheters should only be inserted where absolutely necessary and should not be placed for the management of urinary incontinence except in exceptional circumstances when all other management methods have been unsuccessful. Additional techniques such as closed catheter systems, antimicrobial coated catheters and routine catheter changes every 2–4 weeks should be considered to reduce the risks of a CAUTI (Hooton et al. 2010).

PRE-PROCEDURAL CONSIDERATIONS

Equipment

Specimen jars for urine collection must be sterile to ensure no contamination occurs which may lead to an incorrect diagnosis and treatment. The jars must close securely to prevent leakage of the sample and have a CE marking (HPA 2014h). See Figure 10.3.

Specific patient preparation

When collecting a MSU, the patient must pass a small amount of urine before collecting the specimen. This reduces the risk of contamination of the specimen with naturally occurring micro-organisms/flora within the urethra. Periurethral cleansing is recommended although the need for this has been questioned in both men and women as its effectiveness has been debated (HPA 2014h, Prandoni et al. 1996, Saint and Lipsky 1999).

Procedure guideline 10.14 **Urine sampling: midstream specimen of urine: male**

Essential equipment

- Cleaning solution (e.g. soap and water, 0.9% sodium chloride or disinfectant-free solution)
- Sterile specimen container (with wide opening)
- Non-sterile gloves
- Apron
- Appropriate documentation/forms

Pre-procedure

Action	Rationale
1 Discuss need and indication for procedure with patient.	To obtain valid consent (NMC 2013, **C**).
2 Fully explain the steps of the procedure.	The patient needs to fully understand the procedure in order to avoid inadvertent contamination of specimen and optimize the quality of the sample (Higgins 2013, **E**).
3 Ensure a suitable, private location.	To maintain patient privacy and dignity (Gilbert 2006, **E**).
Procedure	
4 Ask patient to wash hands with soap and water.	To reduce risk of cross-infection (Fraise and Bradley 2009, **E**).
5 *If practitioner's assistance required:* wash hands with bactericidal soap or decontaminate physically clean hands with alcohol rub and don apron.	To prevent cross-contamination (Fraise and Bradley 2009, **E**; RCN 2012, **C**).
6 Ask patient to retract the foreskin and clean the skin surrounding the urethral meatus with soap and water, 0.9% sodium chloride or a disinfectant-free solution.	To optimize general cleansing and minimize contamination of specimen with other organisms. **E** Disinfectant solutions may irritate the urethral mucous membrane (Higgins 2013, **E**).
7 Ask patient to begin voiding first stream of urine (approx. 15–30 mL) into a urinal, toilet or bedpan.	To commence the flow of urine and avoid contamination of specimen with naturally occurring micro-organisms/flora within the urethra (HPA 2014h, **C**).
8 Place the wide-necked sterile container into the urine stream without interrupting the flow.	To prevent contamination of specimen and ensure the collection of the midstream urine which most accurately represents the urine in the bladder (HPA 2014h, **C**).
9 Ask the patient to void his remaining urine into the urinal, toilet or bedpan.	For patient to comfortably continue passing urine (HPA 2014h, **C**).
10 Transfer specimen into sterile universal container.	For despatch to the laboratory (HPA 2014h, **C**).
11 Allow patient to wash hands.	To maintain personal hygiene. **E**
Post-procedure	
12 Label sample and complete microbiological request form including relevant clinical information, such as signs and symptoms of infection, antibiotic therapy.	To maintain accurate records and provide accurate information for laboratory analysis (NMC 2010, **C**; Weston 2008, **E**).
13 Dispatch sample to laboratory immediately (within 4 hours) or refrigerate at 4°C.	To ensure the best possible conditions for microbiological analysis and to prevent micro-organism proliferation (HPA 2014h, **C**).
14 Document the procedure in the patient's records.	To ensure timely and accurate record keeping (NMC 2010, **C**).

Procedure guideline 10.15 **Urine sampling: midstream specimen of urine: female**

Essential equipment

- Cleaning solution (e.g. soap and water, 0.9% sodium chloride or disinfectant-free solution)
- Sterile specimen container with wide opening (CE marked)
- Non-sterile gloves
- Appropriate documentation/forms
- Apron

Pre-procedure

Action	Rationale
1 Discuss need and indication for procedure with patient.	To obtain valid consent (NMC 2013, **C**).
2 Fully explain the steps of the procedure.	The patient needs to fully understand the procedure in order to avoid inadvertent contamination of specimen and optimize the quality of the sample (Higgins 2008a, **C**).
3 Ensure a suitable, private location.	To maintain patient privacy and dignity (Gilbert 2006, **E**).

(continued)

Procedure guideline 10.15 Urine sampling: midstream specimen of urine: female *(continued)*

Procedure

Action	Rationale
4 Ask patient to wash hands with soap and water.	To reduce risk of cross-infection (Fraise and Bradley 2009, **E**).
5 *If practitioner's assistance required:* wash hands with bactericidal soap or decontaminate physically clean hands with alcohol rub and don apron.	To prevent cross-contamination (Fraise and Bradley 2009, **E**; RCN 2012, **C**).
6 Ask patient to part the labia and clean the urethral meatus with soap and water, 0.9% sodium chloride or a disinfectant-free solution.	To optimize general cleansing and to minimize other organisms contaminating the specimen. **E** Disinfectant solutions may irritate the urethral mucous membrane (Higgins 2013, **E**).
7 Use a separate swab for each wipe and wipe downwards from front to back.	To prevent cross-infection and perianal contamination (Weston 2008, **E**).
8 Ask patient to begin voiding first stream of urine (approx. 15–30 mL) into a toilet or bedpan whilst separating the labia.	To commence the flow of urine and avoid contamination of specimen with naturally occurring micro-organisms/flora within the urethra (HPA 2014h, **C**).
9 Place the wide-necked sterile container into the urine stream without interrupting the flow.	To prevent contamination of specimen and to ensure the collection of the midstream of urine which most accurately represents the urine in the bladder (HPA 2014h, **C**).
10 Ask the patient to void her remaining urine into the toilet or bedpan.	For patient to comfortably continue passing urine (HPA 2014h, **C**).
11 Transfer specimen into sterile universal container.	For dispatch to the laboratory (HPA 2014h, **C**).
12 Allow patient to wash hands.	To maintain personal hygiene. **E**

Post-procedure

Action	Rationale
13 Label sample and complete microbiological request form including relevant clinical information, such as signs and symptoms of infection, antibiotic therapy.	To maintain accurate records and provide accurate information for laboratory analysis (NMC 2010, **C**; Weston 2008, **E**).
14 Dispatch sample to laboratory immediately (within 4 hours) or refrigerate at 4°C.	To ensure the best possible conditions for microbiological analysis and to prevent micro-organism proliferation (HPA 2014h, **C**).
15 Document the procedure in the patient's records.	To ensure timely and accurate record keeping (NMC 2010, **C**).

Procedure guideline 10.16 Urine sampling: catheter specimen of urine (CSU)

Essential equipment

- Sterile gloves
- Apron
- Syringe
- Non-traumatic clamps
- Appropriate documentation/forms
- Universal specimen container
- Alcohol-based swab

Optional equipment

- Non-sterile gloves

Pre-procedure

Action	Rationale
1 Explain and discuss the procedure with the patient.	To ensure the patient understands the procedure and gives valid consent (NMC 2013, **C**).
2 Ensure a suitable, private location.	To maintain patient privacy and dignity (Gilbert 2006, **E**).
3 Prepare equipment and place on sterile trolley.	To prepare equipment for use. **E**

Procedure

Action	Rationale
4 *If no urine visible in catheter tubing*: wash/decontaminate physically clean hands with alcohol rub, don apron and apply non-sterile gloves prior to manipulating the catheter tubing.	To minimize the risk of cross-infection (Pellowe 2009, **E**; RCN 2012, **C**).

5 Apply non-traumatic clamp a few centimetres distal to the sampling port.	To ensure sufficient sample has collected to allow for accurate sampling (Higgins 2013, **E**).
6 Wash hands with bactericidal soap and water, or decontaminate physically clean hands with alcohol rub and don gloves.	To prevent cross-contamination (Fraise and Bradley 2009, **E**; RCN 2012, **C**).
7 Wipe sampling port with 2% chlorhexidine in 70% isopropyl alcohol and allow drying for 30 seconds.	To decontaminate sampling port and prevent false-positive results (DH 2007a, **C**).
8 *If using needle and syringe:* using a sterile syringe and needle, insert needle into port at an angle of 45° and aspirate the required amount of urine, then withdraw needle. *Or in a needle-less system:* insert syringe firmly into centre sampling port (according to manufacturer's guidelines), aspirate the required amount of urine and remove syringe.	To enable safe inoculation of urine specimen and to minimize the risk of penetration of the wall of the catheter tubing (Hampson 2006, **E**). Reduces the risk of sharps injury (DH 2006a, **C**; European Biosafety Network 2010, **C**).
9 Transfer an adequate volume of the urine specimen (approx. 10 mL) into a sterile container immediately.	To avoid contamination and to allow for accurate microbiological processing (HPA 2014h, **C**).
10 Discard needle and syringe into sharps container.	To prevent the risk of needlestick injury. **E**
11 Wipe the sampling port with an alcohol wipe and allow to dry.	To reduce contamination of access port and to reduce risk of cross-infection (DH 2007a, **C**).
Post-procedure	
12 Unclamp catheter tubing.	To allow drainage to continue. **E**
13 Dispose of waste, remove apron and gloves and wash hands.	To ensure correct clinical waste management and reduce risk of cross-infection (DH 2006a, **C**).
14 Label sample and complete microbiological request form including relevant clinical information, such as signs and symptoms of infection, antibiotic therapy.	To maintain accurate records and provide accurate information for laboratory analysis (NMC 2010, **C**; Weston 2008, **E**).
15 Dispatch sample to laboratory immediately (within 4 hours) or refrigerate at 4°C.	To ensure the best possible conditions for microbiological analysis and to prevent micro-organism proliferation (HPA 2014h, **C**).
16 Document the procedure in the patient's records.	To ensure timely and accurate record keeping (NMC 2010, **C**).

Procedure guideline 10.17 **Urine sampling: sampling from an ileal conduit**

Essential equipment

- Sterile trolley
- Sterile dressing pack (with gloves)
- Urinary catheter (not larger than 14 Fr)
- Apron
- Universal specimen container
- Clean stoma appliance
- Appropriate documentation/forms
- Sterile water or 0.9% sodium chloride

Pre-procedure

Action	Rationale
1 Explain and discuss the procedure with the patient.	To ensure the patient understands the procedure and gives valid consent (NMC 2013, **C**).
2 Ensure a suitable, private location.	To maintain patient privacy and dignity (Gilbert 2006, **E**).
3 Ensure patient is in a comfortable position (sitting up, supported by pillows) and that stoma is easily accessible.	For patient comfort and to allow access to the stoma. **E**
4 Prepare equipment and place on sterile trolley.	To prepare equipment for use. **E**
Procedure	
5 Wash hands with bactericidal soap and water and dry or decontaminate physically clean hands with alcohol rub. Don non-sterile gloves.	To prevent cross-contamination (Fraise and Bradley 2009, **E**; RCN 2012, **C**).
6 Remove the appliance from stoma. Decontaminate hands, apply gloves and place sterile towel/pad under stoma.	To absorb any spillage from the stoma. **E**

(continued)

Procedure guideline 10.17 Urine sampling: sampling from an ileal conduit *(continued)*

Action	Rationale
7 Clean around the stoma with sterile water or 0.9% sodium chloride, from the centre outwards.	Cleaning of the area reduces the risk of introducing surface pathogens into the ileal conduit. **E**
8 Apply gentle skin traction to allow the stoma opening to be more visible.	To avoid catheter coming into contact with external surface of the stoma. **E**
9 Insert catheter tip gently into the stoma to a depth of 2.5–5 cm only.	Gentle handling reduces the risk of ileal perforation and is more comfortable for the patient. **E**
10 Allow approximately 10 mL of drain through into a sterile specimen container.	To avoid contamination and to allow for accurate microbiological processing (HPA 2014h, **C**).
11 Remove the catheter and discard.	As catheter is no longer required. **E**
12 Change gloves, attend to stoma and apply new stoma appliance.	To ensure patient comfort. **E**
Post-procedure	
13 Dispose of waste, remove apron and gloves and wash/ decontaminate hands.	To ensure correct clinical waste management and reduce risk of cross-infection (DH 2006a, **C**).
14 Label sample and complete microbiological request form including relevant clinical information, such as signs and symptoms of infection, antibiotic therapy.	To maintain accurate records and provide accurate information for laboratory analysis (NMC 2010, **C**; Weston 2008, **E**).
15 Dispatch sample to laboratory immediately (within 4 hours) or refrigerate at 4°C.	To ensure the best possible conditions for microbiological analysis and to prevent micro-organism proliferation (HPA 2014h, **C**).
16 Document the procedure in the patient's records.	To ensure timely and accurate record keeping (NMC 2010, **C**).

Procedure guideline 10.18 Urine sampling: 24-hour urine collection

Essential equipment

- Clean urine collection containers (e.g. wide-necked pot)
- Large urine containers with label attached for patient details
- Appropriate documentation/forms

Optional equipment

- Written patient instruction sheet

Pre-procedure

Action	Rationale
1 Discuss need and indication for procedure with patient.	To obtain valid consent (NMC 2013, **C**).
2 Fully explain the steps of the procedure, emphasizing the importance of not discarding any urine within the 24-hour period (provide written information if needed).	The patient needs to fully understand the procedure in order to avoid inadvertent contamination of specimen and optimize the quality of the sample. **E**
Procedure	
3 Ask patient to void urine and discard this specimen.	To establish the exact start time of the 24-hour period. **E**
4 All urine passed in the next 24 hours from this appointed time should be collected in a clean urine collection container.	To ensure the specimen is representative of the variables of altering body chemistry within the 24 hours (Thomson 2002, **E**).
5 *If catheter in situ:* completely empty catheter bag and hourly chamber (if applicable) or attach new catheter bag. Attach label indicating start time of 24-hour urine collection.	To clearly indicate to all practitioners the 24-hour collection period. **E**
6 If applicable, transfer urine from collection container into large specimen container.	To ensure specimen is collected in a suitable container for safe transportation to the laboratory. **E**
Post-procedure	
7 Label sample and complete request form.	To maintain accurate records and provide accurate information for laboratory analysis (NMC 2010, **C**; Weston 2008, **E**).
8 Dispatch sample to laboratory as soon as possible after completion of the 24-hour period.	To allow accurate laboratory processing and analysis (Higgins 2013, **E**).
9 Document the procedure in the patient's records.	To ensure timely and accurate record keeping (NMC 2010, **C**).

POST-PROCEDURAL CONSIDERATIONS

Immediate care

Urine is a very good culture medium so any bacteria present at the time of collection will continue to multiply in the specimen container. Rapid transport or special measures to ensure preservation of the sample are essential for laboratory diagnosis. The specimens should be transported and processed within 4 hours (HPA 2014h). Therefore, specimens should be processed immediately as delays of more than 2 hours at room temperature between collection and examination will yield unreliable results, suggesting falsely raised bacteriuria. If a delay was to occur the sample should be stored in a designated sample refrigerator (Higgins 2013).

Where delays in processing are unavoidable, specimens should be refrigerated at 4°C or a boric acid preservative, which holds the bacterial population steady for 48–96 hours, should be utilized. Facilities with semi-automated urine analysers should ensure that they have been validated and follow the manufacturer's and local guidance (HPA 2014h).

Specimen collection: faecal sampling

DEFINITION

Faecal specimens are primarily obtained for microbiological analysis to isolate and identify pathogenic bacterial, viral or parasitic organisms suspected of causing gastrointestinal infections or in patients with diarrhoea of potentially infectious aetiology (Higgins 2008b). Faecal specimens may also be obtained for other non-microbiological testing to detect the presence of other substances, such as occult blood or as part of the national screening programme for colorectal cancer (NHS BCSP 2008).

RELATED THEORY

There are a number of enteric pathogens normally present within the gastrointestinal (GI) tract, along with resident flora, that play an important role in digestion and in forming a protective, structural and metabolic barrier against the growth of potentially pathogenic bacteria (Kelly et al. 2005). Pathogenic agents that disrupt the balance within the GI tract manifest in symptoms such as prolonged diarrhoea, bloody diarrhoea, nausea, vomiting, abdominal pain and/or fever. Bacteria in faeces are representative of the bacteria present in the GI tract, so the culture of a faecal sample is necessary for identification of GI tract colonization (Lautenbach et al. 2005).

Laboratory investigations are requested for bacterial infections such as *Salmonella, Campylobacter, Helicobacter, Shigella, Escherichia coli* and *Clostridium difficile*, viral infections such as norovirus and rotavirus, and parasitic pathogens such as protozoa, tapeworms and amoebiasis (HPA 2014f, Weston 2008).

Diarrhoea can be defined as an unusual frequency of bowel actions with the passage of loose, unformed faeces and may be associated with other symptoms such as nausea, abdominal cramping, fever and malaise. It may be attributable to a variety of bacterial, viral or parasitic pathogens and may be associated with antibiotic use, food or travel-related agents (HPA 2014f, HPA 2014g). Prompt collection of a faecal sample for microbiological investigation is essential in determining the presence and identification of such agents.

Clostridium difficile

Clostridium difficile (C. diff) is recognized as a major healthcare-acquired infection causing diarrhoea associated with antibiotic use and environmental contamination globally. It is an anaerobic, gram-positive bacterium that produces spores that are resistant to many disinfectants and can survive in harsh environmental conditions for prolonged periods (Soyfoo and Shaw 2008). It has a significant impact upon patient morbidity and mortality and the signs and symptoms range from mild, self-limiting diarrhoea to severe, life-threatening conditions (HPA 2014f, Lessa et al. 2012). Those most at risk are older patients, immunocompromised patients and those who have had a recent course of antibiotics.

Antimicrobials, particularly broad-spectrum antibiotics, alter the normal gut flora, allowing *C. diff* to proliferate and become pathogenic in the absence of other organisms. This leads to the production of toxins that irritate and cause mucosal damage of the intestinal tract (Lessa et al. 2012).

The diagnosis of *C. diff* is through faecal sampling for culture and toxin analysis on patients who develop diarrhoea or who are admitted to healthcare institutions with unexplained diarrhoea. The control of antimicrobial drugs and improved infection control practices can limit or reduce the incidence of infection (HPA 2014f, Lessa et al. 2012). The use of faecal microbiota transplantation in the treatment of patients with recurrent infection has also shown positive results in the management of *C. diff* but this technique is not currently widely used and can be controversial (Kelly et al. 2012).

EVIDENCE-BASED APPROACHES

Rationale

Timely and accurate identification of patients with infective diarrhoea is crucial in individual management of colonization and within the context of effective infection control management. Obtaining the specimen provides important diagnostic information that can be used to decide how to manage the patient's condition and the mode of treatment (HPA 2014f, HPA 2014g). Prompt diagnosis can influence aspects of care such as isolation and cohort nursing of infected patients, infection control procedures, environmental decontamination and antibiotic prescribing (DH 2007b).

Indications

Collection of a faecal specimen is indicated:

- to identify an infective agent in the presence of chronic, persistent or extended periods of diarrhoea
- if patients are systemically unwell with symptoms of diarrhoea, nausea and vomiting, pain, abdominal cramps, weight loss and/or fever
- to investigate diarrhoea occurring after foreign travel
- to identify parasites, such as tapeworms (Pellatt 2007)
- to identify occult (hidden) blood if rectal bleeding is suspected (Pellatt 2007)
- in the presence of diarrhoea associated with prolonged antibiotic administration
- for symptomatic contacts of individuals with certain organisms (e.g. *E. coli* O157) where an infection can have serious clinical sequelae (HPA 2014f).

Contraindications

- As routine testing.
- In the absence of diarrhoea in suspected infective colonization.

Principles of care

A sample should be obtained as soon as possible after the onset of symptoms, ideally within the first 48 hours of illness, as the chance of successfully identifying a pathogen diminishes once the acute stage of the illness passes (Weston 2008). The specimen should be obtained using a clean technique in order to avoid inadvertent contamination (HPA 2014f).

PRE-PROCEDURAL CONSIDERATIONS

Assessment and recording tools

Collecting a faecal sample should be considered in conjunction with a comprehensive nursing assessment. This includes the observation of faeces for colour, presence of blood, consistency and odour (Pellatt 2007). The most widely used assessment tool is the Bristol Stool Chart (Lewis and Heaton 1997), which categorizes faeces into seven classifications (types) based upon the appearance and consistency. Samples sent to the microbiology laboratory for analysis of suspected *C. difficile* should be classified as Type 6/7 on the Bristol Stool Chart (HPA 2014g).

In addition to other associated symptomatology such as vomiting, fever, myalgia or abdominal pain, an accurate history should also include the onset, frequency and duration of diarrhoea, and other information such as history of foreign travel or potential food poisoning.

Procedure guideline 10.19 **Faecal sampling**

Essential equipment

- A clinically clean bedpan or disposable receiver
- Sterile specimen container (CE marked) (with integrated spoon) (see Figure 10.2)
- Non-sterile gloves
- Apron
- Appropriate documentation/forms

Pre-procedure

Action	Rationale
1 Discuss need and indication for procedure with patient.	To ensure the patient understands the procedure and gives valid consent (NMC 2013, **C**).
2 Wash hands with bactericidal soap and water, or decontaminate physically clean hands with alcohol-based handrub. Don apron and gloves.	To reduce the risk of cross-infection and specimen contamination (Fraise and Bradley 2009, **E**; RCN 2012, **C**).

Procedure

Action	Rationale
3 Ask patient to defaecate into a clinically clean bedpan or receiver.	To avoid unnecessary contamination from other organisms (Kyle 2007, **E**).
4 *If the patient has been incontinent:* a sample may be obtained from bedlinen or pads: try to avoid contamination with urine.	Urine would cause contamination of the sample (Higgins 2008b, **E**).
5 Using the integrated 'spoon', scoop enough faecal material to fill a third of the specimen container (or 10–15 mL of liquid stool).	To obtain a suitable amount of specimen for laboratory analysis. **E**
6 Apply specimen container lid securely.	To prevent risk of spillage. **E**

Post-procedure

Action	Rationale
7 Dispose of waste, remove apron and gloves, and wash hands with soap and water.	To reduce risk of cross-infection (DH 2006a, **C**). Soap and water must be used as alcohol-based handrubs are ineffective for *C. diff* (DH 2007b, **C**).
8 Examine the specimen for features such as colour, consistency and odour. Record observations in nursing notes/care plans.	To complete a comprehensive nursing assessment (Pellatt 2007, **C**).
9 *In cases of suspected tapeworms:* segments of tapeworm are easily seen in faeces and should be sent to the laboratory for identification.	Unless the head is dislodged, the tapeworm will continue to grow. Laboratory confirmation of the presence of the head is essential (Gould and Brooker 2008, **E**).
10 Label sample and complete microbiology request form (including relevant information such as onset and duration of diarrhoea, fever or recent foreign travel).	To maintain accurate records and provide accurate information for laboratory analysis (NMC 2010, **C**; Weston 2008, **E**).
11 Dispatch sample to the laboratory as soon as possible or refrigerate at 4–8°C and dispatch within 12 hours.	To increase the chance of accurate organism identification and to ensure the best possible conditions for laboratory analysis (Higgins 2013, **E**).
12 *In cases of suspected amoebic dysentery:* dispatch the sample to the laboratory immediately.	The parasite causing amoebiasis must be identified when mobile and survives for a short period only. Therefore, faeces should remain fresh and warm (Kyle 2007, **E**).
13 *In cases of prolonged diarrhoea, especially in the presence of a fever:* dispatch the sample to the laboratory immediately.	Due to the risk of *C. diff* and to ensure prompt diagnosis and initiation of appropriate infection control measures (DH 2007b, **C**).
14 Document the procedure in the patient's records.	To ensure timely and accurate record keeping (NMC 2010, **C**).

POST-PROCEDURAL CONSIDERATIONS

Immediate care

A faecal sample should be transported to the laboratory and processed as soon as possible because a number of important pathogens, such as *Shigella*, may not survive changes in pH and temperature once outside the body (HPA 2014f). If there is an anticipated delay in despatching the sample to the laboratory, it should be refrigerated at 4–8°C and processed within 12 hours (HPA 2014f).

Ongoing care

The result of specimen analysis will determine the patient's ongoing care. The involvement of the microbiology and infection control teams is essential to ensure prudent and safe treatment and nursing care. This should include:

- effective handwashing techniques to minimize the transmission of organisms
- implementation of Standard Precautions (gloves and aprons)
- nursing patients with unexpected or unexplained diarrhoea in isolation *or* cohorted with other infected patients (DH 2007b)
- thorough environmental decontamination (DH 2007b)
- prudent antibiotic prescribing (DH 2007a).

Education of patient and others

Patients should be provided with information and involved in their care as much as they choose to be (NMC 2015). Confirmation of an infection diagnosis should be relayed to patients and their families alongside information on management strategies (such as antibiotic therapy, the use of PPE, reasons for isolation and visiting restrictions). The provision of written information, such as leaflets, may also be useful.

Specimen collection: respiratory tract secretion sampling

DEFINITION

Obtaining a specimen from the respiratory tract is important in diagnosing illness, infections and conditions such as tuberculosis and lung cancer (Guest 2008). A sample can be obtained invasively or non-invasively and the correct technique will enable a representative sample to identify respiratory tract pathology and to guide treatment.

RELATED THEORY

Excessive respiratory secretions may be due to increased mucus production in cases of infection, impaired mucociliary transport or a weak cough reflex (Hess 2002). Lower airway secretions that are not cleared provide an ideal medium for bacterial growth. Suitable microbiological analysis in diagnosing infection will depend upon (HPA 2014i):

- the adequacy of lower respiratory tract specimens
- avoidance of contamination by upper respiratory tract and oral flora
- use of microscopic techniques and culture methods
- current and recent antimicrobial therapy.

EVIDENCE-BASED APPROACHES

Rationale

The main aim of sputum/secretion collection is to provide reliable information on the causative agent of bacterial, viral or fungal infection within the respiratory tract and its susceptibility to antibiotics for guiding treatment (Ioanas et al. 2001).

Indications

A respiratory tract secretion specimen is indicated:

- when there are clinical signs and symptoms of a respiratory tract infection, such as a productive cough, particularly with purulent secretions
- if there are signs of systemic infection or in patients with a PUO of >38°C (Perry 2007).

The presence of sputum, especially when discoloured, is commonly interpreted to represent the presence of bacterial infection and as an indication for antibiotic therapy. However, purulence primarily occurs when inflammatory cells or sloughed mucosal epithelial cells are present, and can result from either viral or bacterial infection (Johnson et al. 2008). One strategy for limiting or targeting antimicrobial prescribing is to send a respiratory tract specimen for microbiological analysis to either demonstrate that a substantial infection is not present or to identify an organism for which antimicrobial treatment is deemed necessary.

The accuracy of microbiological analysis can depend on the quality of the specimen obtained as well as the time taken for transportation and the method by which it is stored and transported (Perry 2007).

Methods of non-invasive and semi-invasive sampling

A sufficient quality of sputum will yield a representative sample and early morning sputum samples are preferred as they contain pooled overnight secretions in which pathogenic bacteria are more likely to be concentrated (Philomina 2009).

Obtaining a sputum sample

Sputum is a combination of mucus, inflammatory and epithelial cells, and degradation products from the lower respiratory tract (Dulak 2005). It is never free from organisms since material originating from the lower respiratory tract has to pass through the pharynx and the mouth, which have commensal populations of bacteria (Thomson 2002). However, it is important to ensure that material sent to the microbiology laboratory is of sputum rather than a saliva sample, which will contain squamous epithelial cells and be unrepresentative of the underlying pulmonary pathology.

Sputum produced as a result of infection is usually purulent and a good sample can yield a high bacterial load (Weston 2008). For patients who are self-ventilating, co-operative, able to cough, expectorate and follow commands, a sputum sample is a suitable collection method. In cases of suspected *Mycobacterium tuberculosis*, three sputum specimens are required as the release of the organism is intermittent, before the pathogenic organisms can be isolated (Damani 2012). See Figure 10.1 and Procedure guideline 10.20: Sputum sampling.

LEGAL AND PROFESSIONAL ISSUES

Competencies

Practitioners must be competent and feel confident that they have the knowledge, skill and understanding to undertake respiratory tract secretion sampling for microbiological analysis (NMC 2015). For more advanced skills of specimen collection such as suctioning, the practitioner should receive training and be assessed on their knowledge and understanding of the technique and potential adverse effects that may occur, such as hypoxia, cardiovascular instability and mucosal trauma (Thomson 2000).

PRE-PROCEDURAL CONSIDERATIONS

Pharmacological support

Adequate analgesia is a key consideration in ensuring that an effective sputum expectoration technique can be achieved. For example, pre-procedural analgesia should be given time to be effective, and wounds need to be supported to maximize inhalation and minimize pain (Guest 2008).

Nebulization of 0.9% sodium chloride and/or mucolytic agents, such as N-acetylcysteine, may need to be administered to help loosen tenacious secretions and to elicit an effective cough (Rajiv 2007).

Non-pharmacological support

Collaboration with the physiotherapy team may assist in obtaining a good-quality sample (Hess 2002). For sputum sampling, physiotherapeutic modalities implemented may include appropriate positioning, active cycle of breathing, deep breathing and effective coughing techniques (HPA 2014i).

Specific patient preparation

Patient position is important in optimizing secretion sampling. Patients should be sat upright or on the edge of the bed, if able, or in a high semi-Fowler position (head elevated to 30–45°) in bed supported by pillows (Dulak 2005).

The quality and quantity of secretion production and mucociliary clearance depend on systemic hydration. Patient hydration can boost sputum production to enable a good sample (Dulak 2005). This can be further enhanced with sufficient airway humidity and nebulization.

Procedure guideline 10.20 **Sputum sampling**

Essential equipment

- Universal container
- Apron
- Non-sterile gloves

Optional equipment

- Nebulizer
- Appropriate documentation/form
- Eye protection (e.g. goggles/visor)

Action	Rationale
Pre-procedure	
1 Explain and discuss the procedure with the patient.	To ensure the patient understands the procedure and gives valid consent (NMC 2013, **C**).
2 Fully explain the steps of the procedure.	The procedure requires the patient to fully understand and co-operate in order to optimize the quality of the sample (Dulak 2005, **E**).
3 Position patient upright in a chair or in a semi- or high Fowler position, supported as necessary with pillows.	For comfort and to facilitate optimum chest/lung expansion. **E**
4 *If secretions thick/tenacious or having difficulty clearing secretions:* administer nebulization therapy and/or enlist help of the physiotherapist.	To loosen secretions and assist in techniques that will optimize sputum sample collection (Hess 2002, **E**).
5 Wash hands with bactericidal soap/decontaminate physically clean hands with alcohol rub. Don apron, gloves and eye protection.	To reduce the risk of cross-infection or splash injury to practitioner and specimen collection (Damani 2012, **E**).
Procedure	
6 Ask patient to take three deep breaths in through their nose, exhale through pursed lips and then force a deep cough.	Deep breathing helps loosen secretions and a deep cough will ensure a lower respiratory tract sample is obtained (Dulak 2005, **E**).
7 Ask patient to expectorate into a clean container and secure lid.	To prevent contamination. **E**
Post-procedure	
8 Dispose of waste, remove apron, gloves and eye protection and wash/decontaminate hands.	To ensure correct clinical waste management and reduce the risk of cross-infection (DH 2006a, **C**).
9 Label sample and complete microbiology request form (including relevant information such as indication for sample and current/recent antimicrobial therapy).	To maintain accurate records and provide accurate information for laboratory analysis (NMC 2010, **C**; Weston 2008, **E**).
10 Dispatch to the laboratory as soon as possible within 4 hours.	To increase the chance of accurate organism identification (Higgins 2013, **E**).
11 Document the procedure in the patient's records.	To ensure timely and accurate record keeping (NMC 2010, **C**).

POST-PROCEDURAL CONSIDERATIONS

Immediate care

Many organisms responsible for infection of the lower respiratory tract do not survive well outside the host, so specimens should be dispatched to the laboratory immediately and processed within 2 hours (Gould and Brooker 2008). If there is an anticipated delay in despatching the sample to the laboratory, it should be refrigerated at 4–8°C and sent as soon as possible (HPA 2014i).

Documentation

The date and time when a sputum sample is sent to the laboratory should be documented clearly and promptly in the patient's notes and care plan (NMC 2010). This should be done alongside

Figure 10.7 **Endoscopy.** ***Source:*** **Reproduced with permission from the patient information website of Cancer Research UK (www.cancerresearchuk.org/cancerhelp).**

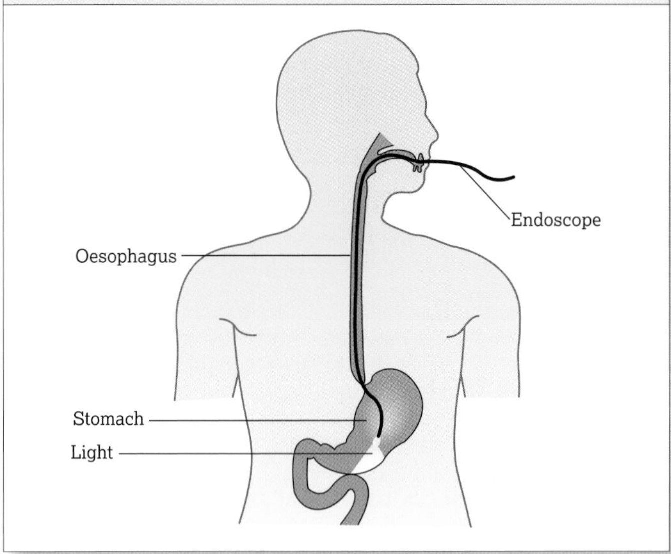

Figure 10.8 **Anatomy of the lower gastrointestinal tract. RUQ, right upper quadrant; LUQ, left upper quadrant; RLQ, right lower quadrant; LLQ, left lower quadrant.**

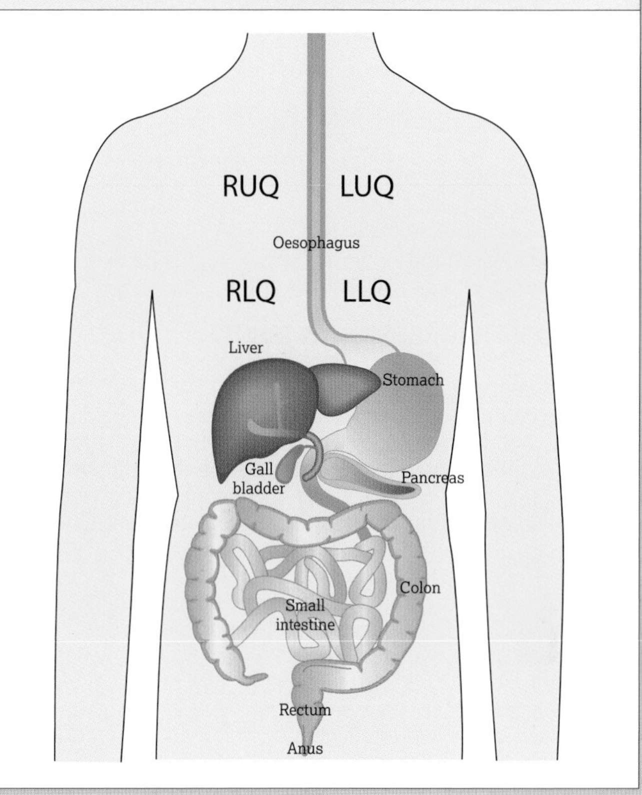

documentation in relation to significant findings that have prompted the collection of the sample, such as a description of the type and colour of sputum/secretions and method used to obtain the sample.

Endoscopic investigations

DEFINITION

Occasionally patients will be required to undergo further invasive diagnostic procedures such as an endoscopy. An endoscopy is the direct visual examination of the GI tract (Figure 10.7) which may include gastroscopy or colonoscopy. Endoscopy allows the practitioner to evaluate the appearance of the visualized mucosa for the purpose of diagnosis and therapeutic procedures (Smith and Watson 2005).

Gastroscopy

DEFINITION

A gastroscopy or oesophagogastroduodenoscopy (OGD) is a procedure in which a long flexible endoscope is passed through the mouth, allowing the doctor or nurse endoscopist to look directly at the mucosal lining of the oesophagus, stomach and proximal duodenum. The endoscope is generally less than 10 mm in diameter but a larger scope may be required for therapeutic procedures where suction channels are required (Smith and Watson 2005) (see Figure 10.7).

ANATOMY AND PHYSIOLOGY

See Figure 10.8.

Oesophagus

The oesophagus is a muscular thin-walled tube approximately 25 cm long and about 2 cm in diameter. It is located behind the trachea and in front of the vertebral column. It begins at the inferior end of the laryngopharynx and ends at the stomach. There are two sphincters within the oesophagus: the upper or hypopharyngeal sphincter and the lower gastro-oesophageal or cardiac sphincter. The upper moves food from the pharynx to the oesophagus and the lower the food passing into the stomach. The oesophagus has three layers, the mucosa, submucosa and the muscularis, with the innermost layer consisting of stratified squamous epithelium (Jenkins and Tortora 2013).

Stomach

The stomach connects the oesophagus and the small intestine or duodenum. It is a J-shaped dilated portion of the alimentary tract and one of its functions is a holding reservoir and mixing chamber. It is also located between the epigastric, umbilical and left hypochondriac regions of the abdomen. It is divided into four regions: the cardia, fundus, body and pyloric part. Distally, the pyloric sphincter is located between the stomach and the duodenum. The stomach has three muscle layers to allow for gastric motility to move the contents adequately whereas other parts of the alimentary tract only have two muscle layers (Jenkins and Tortora 2013).

Duodenum

The duodenum is part of the small intestine. It is approximately 25 cm long and 3.5 cm in diameter and is the shortest region. It begins at the pyloric sphincter of the stomach and joins the jejunum. Both the pancreas and the gallbladder release secretions into the duodenum (Jenkins and Tortora 2013).

EVIDENCE-BASED APPROACHES

Rationale

A gastroscopy is undertaken to investigate symptoms originating from the upper GI tract such as reflux and dysphagia. The doctor or nurse endoscopist uses direct vision to diagnose, sample and document changes in the upper GI tract.

Indications

- Dysphagia.
- Odynophagia.

- Achalasia.
- Unresponsive reflux disease.
- Gastric and peptic ulcers.
- Haematemesis and melaena.
- Suspected carcinoma.
- Oesophageal or gastric varices.
- Monitoring Barrett's oesophagus disease.

Contraindications

- Fractured base of skull.
- Metastatic adenocarcinoma.
- Some head/neck tumours.
- Thrombocytopenia.
- Symptoms that are functional in origin.

LEGAL AND PROFESSIONAL ISSUES

Nurse endoscopists

In some centres nurse endoscopists work alongside medical endoscopists undertaking endoscopy. In 1995, the British Society of Gastroenterology supported the development of non-medical endoscopists. The nurse endoscopist must work within their own professional boundaries and complement the medical endoscopist teams (BSG 2005, Smith and Watson 2005). It has also been shown that nurse endoscopists perform procedures at a high standard and adhere to international standards. Most patients also had no specific preference for doctor or nurse endoscopist and expressed high patient satisfaction (Tursi 2013, van Putten et al. 2012). It is essential that all practitioners are adequately trained in the administration of conscious sedation, and are aware of its side-effects and reversal agents. Conscious sedation is used to relax the patient, minimize pain during the procedure and improve procedural efficiency (Choi 2012). Clinical units must also limit the possibility of overdose, particularly with midazolam, as highlighted by the NPSA (2008).

Consent

It is essential that valid consent is obtained as previously discussed in this chapter prior to any investigation. This is important as conscious sedation may be utilized during this procedure.

Governance

It is a priority that an organization providing endscopic services has clear identifiable policies and procedures. Bidirectional communication must be open between the department, organizational board and national bodies to ensure that appropriate care is delivered. Monitoring processess must be in place to identify potential clinical or organizational risks and there must be a clear reporting mechanism.

Risk management

The organization must ensure that relevant policies and procedures are in place to reduce risk. Responding to national alerts and guidance is essential as well as implementing relevant evidence. In 2008, the NPSA issued an alert regarding the use of midazolam during conscious sedation. It was found that some patients were receiving an overdose of midazolam with a subsequent over-reliance on the use of flumazenil as a reversal agent.

PRE-PROCEDURAL CONSIDERATIONS

Equipment

To conduct a gastroscopy, a flexible side- or end-viewing endoscope is required. The endoscope allows visualization of the oesophagus, stomach and proximal duodenum (MacKay et al. 2010, Smith and Watson 2005). Access to resuscitation equipment is also essential if conscious sedation is going to be administered (BSG 2007).

Assessment and recording tools

A medical and nursing history and assessment must be undertaken to identify any care needs or concerns that may be significant, in particular the patient's current drug therapy, drug reactions or allergies, any organ dysfunctions such as cardiac and/or respiratory disease and previous or current illnesses. It is also important to be aware of any coagulopathies as samples of tissue or biopsy may need to be taken during the procedure. This can be pre-empted by reviewing blood results prior to the gastroscopy. A set of observations including temperature, pulse, blood pressure, respiration rate and oxygen saturations should also be taken to identify any pre-procedural abnormalities and provide a baseline. If the patient has diabetes, a blood glucose level should also be checked (BSG 2003, BSG 2007, MacKay et al. 2010, Smith and Watson 2005).

Pharmacological support

Prior to the procedure, a local anaesthetic spray may be used on the back of the throat. In some cases conscious sedation may be administered. This technique involves the administration of a benzodiazepine such as midazolam in small doses. Doses must be titrated for elderly patients or those with co-morbidities such as cardiac or renal failure (BNF 2014). Oxygen therapy should also be administered for patients at risk of hypoxia or those requiring sedation. Generally 2 litres per minute is adequate for most circumstances to maintain oxygen saturation levels and prevent hypoxaemia (BSG 2003, BSG 2007).

Specific patient preparation

The patient must fast for at least 4–8 hours prior to the gastroscopy to ensure that the stomach is relatively empty. Clear fluids may be taken up to 2 hours before, but local guidelines must be followed. This increases the visual field for the endoscopist and also minimizes the risk of aspiration if the patient vomits (Kang and Hyun 2013, Saied et al. 2012). If the patient has undergone previous gastric surgery, this fasting time may be longer, dependent on the type of surgery, to ensure gastric emptying (Ahn et al. 2013). The nurse can also assist by getting the patient to lie on their left side on the trolley (Smith and Watson 2005). If a sedative is used, it is essential that the patient is monitored with pulse oximetry and observed for any respiratory depression. Nursing staff can observe and record oxygen saturations and respiratory rate. ECG monitoring may only be required if a patient is at risk of cardiac instability during the procedure (BSG 2003).

POST-PROCEDURAL CONSIDERATIONS

Immediate care

Physiological monitoring must continue in the immediate recovery period. Supplemental oxygen and oxygen saturations may be required, especially if a sedative has been used. The patient should avoid drinking or eating for an hour after the use of the throat spray to minimize the risk of aspiration. Once stable, awake and reviewed by the team, the patient may be discharged or transferred to another department (BSG 2003, BSG 2007).

Ongoing care

It is recommended that patients who have been sedated with an intravenous benzodiazepine do not drive a car, operate machinery, sign legal documents or drink alcohol for 24 hours (BSG 2003). This is irrespective of whether their sedation has been reversed with flumazenil. The patient must be accompanied home if they have been given a sedative. The accompanying adult should stay with the patient for 12 hours at home if they live alone. It is important to remember that aspiration pneumonia may develop hours or days later and the patient should be informed to report any symptoms such as temperatures or breathing difficulty (BSG 2003, BSG 2007, Smith and Watson 2005).

Documentation
Any samples should be clearly documented with the appropriate forms as previously discussed in this chapter. All drugs administered, complications and/or findings should be documented.

COMPLICATIONS

Respiratory depression
If oversedation occurs, respiratory function will be affected. It is essential that close monitoring occurs during and after the procedure. A reversal agent may be required such as flumazenil for midazolam (BSG 2003, NPSA 2008, Smith and Watson 2005).

Perforation
Although rare, it is possible that perforation of the oesophagus, stomach or duodenum may occur. Further medical and/or surgical intervention will be required to manage this potential complication (Borgaonkar et al. 2012, Smith and Watson 2005).

Haemorrhage
Where biopsy samples have been taken, this may increase the risk of post-procedural bleeding. Further intervention may be required to stop the bleeding. Patients should be advised to seek medical assistance if there are signs of bleeding following discharge, which include the presence of fresh blood in the sputum and melaena (Chernecky and Berger 2013).

This will be dependent on the specific aetiology of the bleed, for example whether it is from varices when variceal band ligation may be required (Borgaonkar et al. 2012, SIGN 2008, Smith and Watson 2005).

Colonoscopy

DEFINITION
A colonoscopy is conducted by inserting a colonoscope through the anus into the colon. It provides information regarding the lower GI tract and allows a complete examination of the colon. The colonoscope is similar to the endoscope used in gastroscopy. Its length ranges from 1.2 to 1.8 metres. It is the most effective method of diagnosing rectal polyps and carcinoma (MacKay et al. 2010, Smith and Watson 2005, Swan 2005, Taylor et al. 2009).

ANATOMY AND PHYSIOLOGY
The large intestine is about 1.5 metres long. It begins at the ileum and ends at the anus. The four major structures are the caecum, colon, rectum and anal canal (Jenkins and Tortora 2013). See Figure 10.8.

Caecum
The caecum is about 6 cm long and opens from the ileum and ileocaecal valve (Jenkins and Tortora 2013).

Colon
The colon consists of three parts. The ascending colon runs from the caecum and joins the transverse colon and the hepatic flexure. The transverse colon is in front of the duodenum where it joins the descending colon at the splenic flexure. The descending colon travels down toward the middle of the abdomen where it joins the sigmoid colon which is S-shaped and becomes the rectum (Jenkins and Tortora 2013).

Rectum and anal canal
The rectum is approximately 20 cm long and is a dilated section of the colon. It joins the anal canal which is approximately 2–3 cm long (Jenkins and Tortora 2013).

EVIDENCE-BASED APPROACHES

Rationale
A colonoscopy is performed to investigate specific symptoms originating from the lower GI tract such as bleeding. The endoscopist uses direct vision to diagnose, sample and document changes in the lower GI tract (MacKay et al. 2010, Taylor et al. 2009).

Indications

- Screening of patients with family history of colon cancer, a serious but highly curable malignancy.
- Determining the presence of suspected polyps.
- Monitoring ulcerative colitis.
- Monitoring diverticulosis and diverticulitis.
- Active or occult lower gastrointestinal bleeding.
- Unexplained bleeding or faecal occult blood specifically in patients >50 years.
- Abdominal symptoms, such as pain or discomfort, particularly if associated with weight loss or anaemia.
- Chronic diarrhoea, constipation or a change in bowel habits.
- Surveillance of inflammatory bowel disease.
- Population screening for colorectal carcinoma.
- Palliative supportive treatments such as stent insertion.

Contraindications

- Upper gastrointestinal bleeding.
- Acute diarrhoea.
- Recent colon anastomosis.
- Toxic megacolon.
- Pregnancy (Chernecky and Berger 2013).

LEGAL AND PROFESSIONAL ISSUES

Competencies and consent
Competencies and consent will be the same as those discussed in the section on 'Gastroscopy', above.

Risk management
The NPSA (2009) highlighted the risks in relation to bowel preparation and actions required to minimize these. Harm to patients has occurred where oral bowel preparations were prescribed to those with definite contraindications; however, the majority of the incidents were related to the administration of the bowel preparations (56%) (Connor et al. 2012). The NPSA (2009) report identified that one death and 218 patient safety incidents resulting in moderate harm were related to the use of oral bowel preparations where contraindications were not considered or assessed.

PRE-PROCEDURAL CONSIDERATIONS

Equipment
A colonoscope is a flexible endoscope which generally uses fibreoptics to allow direct visualization of the rectum and colon (Chernecky and Berger 2013, MacKay et al. 2010, Smith and Watson 2005).

Pharmacological support
Bowel preparation agents, such as senna tablets and Citramag, are given to the patient to take 1 day before the colonoscopy to clear the bowel and minimize faecal contamination (Connor et al. 2012). A sedative and possibly an analgesic are usually administered before the procedure. This involves the administration of a benzodiazepine such as midazolam and an opioid such as fentanyl or pethidine which have been prescribed. Doses must be titrated for elderly patients or those with co-morbidities such as cardiac or renal failure. An antispasmodic may also be given. Oxygen therapy should also be administered during sedation. Generally 2 litres per minute is adequate for most circumstances to maintain oxygen saturation levels and prevent hypoxaemia (BSG 2003, BSG 2007, MacKay et al. 2010, Riley 2008, Swan 2005).

Specific patient preparation

A medical and nursing history and assessment must be undertaken to identify any care needs or concerns that may be significant. In particular, this should cover the patient's current drug therapy, drug reactions or allergies, any organ dysfunctions such as cardiac and/or respiratory disease, and previous or current illnesses. It is also important to be aware of any coagulopathies as samples of tissue or biopsy may need to be taken during the procedure. This can be pre-empted by reviewing blood results prior to the colonoscopy (Chernecky and Berger 2013).

To complete a successful colonoscopy, the bowel must be clean so that the physician can clearly view the colon. Most patients will require a bowel preparation. It is very important that the patient is given clear written instructions for bowel preparation well in advance of the procedure. Without proper preparation, the colonoscopy will not be successful and the test may have to be repeated. The patient must be individually assessed before being supplied the bowel preparation and the potential contraindications considered as below.

Contraindications to bowel preparation

- Gastrointestinal obstruction, perforation, ileus or gastric retention.
- Severe acute inflammatory bowel disease.
- Toxic megacolon.
- A reduction in consciousness level.
- Allergies or hypersensitivity to bowel preparation.
- The inability to swallow.
- Ileostomy (Connor et al. 2012).

The choice of bowel preparation must consider the advantages and disadvantages of each product, the tolerability, efficacy and possible side-effects. If the patient feels nauseated or vomits while taking the bowel preparation, they are advised to wait 30 minutes before drinking more fluid and start with small sips of solution. Some activity such as walking or a few cream crackers may help decrease the nausea (Connor et al. 2012, Smith and Watson 2005, Swan 2005).

Two days prior to the colonoscopy, specific light foods may be eaten, such as steamed white fish, and others avoided, such as high-fibre foods. On the day before the colonoscopy, breakfast from the approved food groups may be eaten while drinking plenty of clear fluids. The period of bowel cleansing generally should not be longer than 24 hours. On the day of the procedure, patients can drink tea/coffee with no milk 4 hours before and water up to 2 hours before. Some patients who are at risk of hypovolaemia and dehydration may need to be admitted to hospital for prehydration (Connor et al. 2012, MacKay et al. 2010, Smith and Watson 2005, Swan 2005).

A set of observations including temperature, pulse, blood pressure, respiration rate and oxygen saturations should also be taken to identify any pre-procedural abnormalities and provide a baseline. If the patient has diabetes, a blood glucose level should also be checked (BSG 2003, BSG 2007, Connor et al. 2012, Smith and Watson 2005).

Learning Activity 10.4

Scenario: Preparing a patient for a colonoscopy

A patient has called your unit from home and is asking you to explain what they need to do prior to coming in for their colonoscopy in 2 days time. They have been given some medication to take at home before being admitted, but don't understand what they are allowed to eat and until when.

Based on the evidence provided within this chapter, jot down some bullet points of what your advice would be to them around food and fluid intake.

See the end of the chapter for the answers.

POST-PROCEDURAL CONSIDERATIONS

Immediate care

Physiological monitoring and care post sedation should be the same as those for gastroscopy. However, larger doses of sedative and opioids may have been used so further observation is required. The patient may feel some cramping or a sensation of having gas, but this quickly passes on eating and drinking. Bloating and distension typically occur for about an hour after the examination until the air is expelled. Unless otherwise instructed, the patient may immediately resume a normal diet, but it is generally recommended that the patient waits until the day after the procedure to resume normal activities (BSG 2007, MacKay et al. 2010).

Ongoing care

If a biopsy was taken or a polyp was removed, the patient may notice light rectal bleeding for 1–2 days after the procedure; large amounts of bleeding, the passage of clots or abdominal pain should be reported immediately.

COMPLICATIONS

Polypectomy syndrome

When an endoscopic mucosal resection (EMR) or an endoscopic submucosal dissection (ESD) is conducted, a thermal injury to the bowel wall may occur. The patient may present with localized tenderness and pyrexia. Generally conservative management is adequate, but it is essential to monitor their condition as they may go on to develop a perforation (MacKay et al. 2010).

Perforation

During the procedure, the greatest risk or possible complication is bowel perforation; this may be apparent during the procedure but it can present 3–4 days after the procedure. This occurs in 1 in 1000 cases (MacKay et al. 2010, Smith and Watson 2005). If a snare polypectomy was conducted, the incidence of perforation is 0.1–0.3%. The incidence rises to 5% following an EMR (MacKay et al. 2010, Smith and Watson 2005). The nurse monitoring the patient after colonoscopy should be familiar with potential signs and symptoms such as unresolved abdominal pain, rigidity and/or bleeding. If a perforation occurs, surgical intervention is likely to be required (MacKay et al. 2010, Smith and Watson 2005, Suissa et al. 2012).

Haemorrhage

On average, haemorrhage occurs in 3 in 1000 procedures but the incidence and complication rates may be higher where a procedure involves a polypectomy. MacKay et al. (2010) state that the incidence post polypectomy should be <1% and 0.5–6.0% following EMR. The post-procedure monitoring by the nurse again includes observing for signs and symptoms of bleeding (MacKay et al. 2010, Smith and Watson 2005). Depending on the severity of the bleed, it may be managed conservatively or in haemodynamically unstable patients embolization may be required (MacKay et al. 2010, Suissa et al. 2012).

Cystoscopy

DEFINITION

Cystoscopy examines the inside of the urethra and bladder using a cystoscope and is one of the most widely used invasive urological investigations. It gives direct visualization of the urethra and bladder for both males and females but it is especially important in males as the urethra is much more complex (Fillingham and Douglas 2004, Rodgers et al. 2006).

ANATOMY AND PHYSIOLOGY

Urethra

The urethra extends from the external urethral orifice to the bladder (Jenkins and Tortora 2013).

Male urethra
The male urethra is approximately 20 cm long and provides a common pathway for urine, semen and reproductive organ secretions. The three parts of the male urethra are the prostatic urethra, membranous urethra and spongy or penile urethra. Originating at the urethral orifice of the bladder, the prostatic urethra passes through the prostate gland (Figure 10.9). The narrowest and shortest part of the urethra is the membranous urethra, originating from the prostate gland and extending to the bulb of the penis. The penile urethra ends at the urethral orifice (Jenkins and Tortora 2013).

Female urethra
The female urethra is located behind the symphysis pubis and opens at the external urethral orifice (Figure 10.10). It is approximately 4 cm long (Jenkins and Tortora 2013).

EVIDENCE-BASED APPROACHES

Rationale
A cystoscopy is undertaken to gain direct visualization of the urethra and the bladder to aid diagnosis of urological complications and diseases such as bladder cancer (Fillingham and Douglas 2004).

Indications

- Bladder dysfunction.
- Unexplained haematuria.
- Diagnosis of bladder cancer.
- Staging of bladder cancer.
- Obstruction or strictures.
- Dysuria.

Contraindications

- Confirmed urinary tract infection.

PRE-PROCEDURAL CONSIDERATIONS

Equipment
A cystoscope may be flexible or rigid. A rigid cystoscope is utilized in the operating theatre where the patient is anaesthetized. The flexible cystoscope can be used in the outpatient setting with local anaesthesia. The flexible cystoscope is useful for patients who require more regular examinations for follow-up after bladder cancer treatment (Fillingham and Douglas 2004).

Figure 10.9 **Cystoscopy for a man.** ***Source:*** **Reproduced with permission from the patient information website of Cancer Research UK (www.cancerresearchuk.org/cancerhelp).**

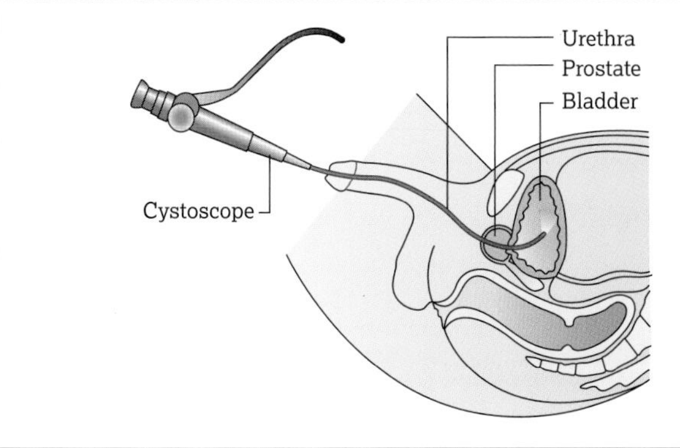

Figure 10.10 **Cystoscopy for a woman.** ***Source:*** **Reproduced with permission from the patient information website of Cancer Research UK (www.cancerresearchuk.org/cancerhelp).**

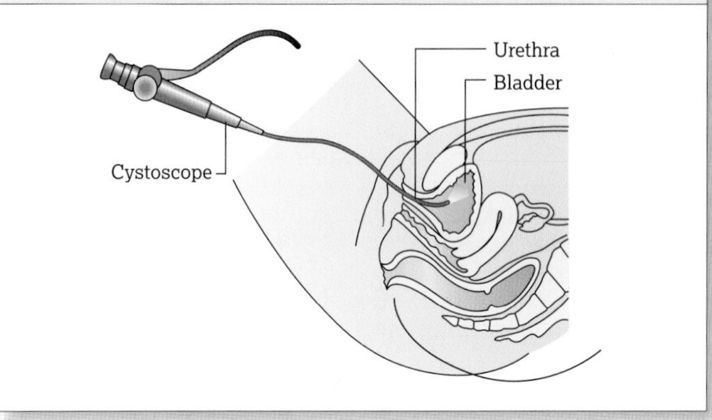

Specific patient preparation
It is essential that the patient does not have a UTI as the organism responsible for the infection may be spread into the bloodstream during the procedure. If the patient is having a general anaesthetic, they will have to fast prior to the procedure, dependent on anaesthetic instruction. Prior to the procedure, patients undergoing a local anaesthetic can usually eat and drink as normal and should empty their bladder prior to the procedure (Fillingham and Douglas 2004). It may be necessary for some patients to be treated with antibiotics before the procedure to reduce the risk of infection (AUA 2012).

POST-PROCEDURAL CONSIDERATIONS

Immediate care
Dependent on the type of procedure, recovery will vary. After a general anaesthetic, the patient will be recovered by recovery nursing staff. In the outpatient setting, physiological observations may be required. Nursing staff should monitor for signs of haematuria, infection, urinary retention and excessive pain in the abdomen or urethral area. It is also possible that the patient may experience bladder spasms which can be minimized with prescribed analgesics. Oral fluids should be encouraged (Chernecky and Berger 2013).

Ongoing care
It is common for the patient to experience some burning sensations whilst passing urine for a few days. It is advised that the patient drink plenty of water post procedure to flush the bladder and reduce the risk of infection. Any signs of excessive bleeding should be reported to the medical team (Chernecky and Berger 2013, Fillingham and Douglas 2004).

COMPLICATIONS

Infection
There is a risk of urinary infection in approximately 5% of cystoscopies performed. If an infection were to occur, relevant prescribed antimicrobial therapy may be required (Rodgers et al. 2006).

Liver biopsy

DEFINITION
Liver biopsy involves percutaneous puncture using a biopsy needle and removal of a small piece of the liver (Al Knawy and Shiffman 2007).

ANATOMY AND PHYSIOLOGY

The liver is the heaviest organ in the body. It weighs approximately 1.4 kg and is highly vascular. It is incompletely covered by a layer of peritoneum and enclosed in a thin inelastic capsule. There are two main lobes in the liver: the large right lobe and the smaller left lobe which is wedge shaped. The caudate and quadrate lobes are on the posterior surface and are continuations of the left lobe (Jenkins and Tortora 2013).

Functions of the liver

The liver has many functions including:

- *carbohydrate metabolism* and contributing to maintenance of blood glucose levels
- *lipid metabolism*
- *protein metabolism:* converting ammonia into urea
- *drug and hormone processing:* detoxifying the body
- *activation of vitamin D*
- *excretion of bilirubin*
- *phagocytosis* of some bacteria and aged blood cells
- *storage* of some vitamins, iron, copper and glycogen (Jenkins and Tortora 2013).

EVIDENCE-BASED APPROACHES

Rationale

A liver biopsy is an invaluable tool for diagnosing or monitoring conditions affecting the liver, such as cirrhosis, inflammation or hepatitis of various causes and some metabolic liver disorders. The risks, although small, must be weighed against the potential benefitss (Al Knawy and Shiffman 2007, Tannapfel et al. 2012).

Indications

- Diagnosis of cirrhosis.
- Diagnosis of cancer both primary and secondary.
- Miliary tuberculosis.
- Amyloidosis.
- Viral hepatitis for grading, staging and exclusion of co-morbidities.
- Diagnosis of autoimmune diseases affecting the liver.
- Grading and staging of chronic hepatitis B or C.

Contraindications

- An unco-operative or confused patient.
- Severe purpura.
- Coagulation defects.
- Prolonged clotting time.
- Increased bleeding time.
- Severe jaundice.
- Under 3 years of age.
- Current right lower lobe pneumonia.
- Current pleuritis (Al Knawy and Shiffman 2007, Tannapfel et al. 2012).

Methods of liver biopsy

There are a variety of methods for conducting a liver biopsy. A retrospective study by Manolakopoulos et al. (2007) found that the ultrasound-assisted approach was as safe as the ultrasound-guided approach and both obtained adequate samples. The ultrasound-guided technique is considered the standard (Tannapfel et al. 2012).

Percussion palpation approach

This method is also known as the blind approach where the liver is palpated in order to determine the position required for the liver biopsy.

Image-guided approach

Image guidance may be conducted using ultrasound, CT or MRI but the preferred method is ultrasound. The ultrasound method utilizes continuous ultrasound or site marking immediately prior to the procedure (Al Knawy and Shiffman 2007).

Ultrasound-assisted approach

The ultrasound is utilized immediately prior to the procedure and a mark is left on the skin indicating the puncture site. It is also known as the 'X marks the spot' technique. This technique has been shown to yield larger tissue samples, require fewer needle passes and have a decreased biopsy failure rate than the non-ultrasound-assisted approach (Di Teodoro et al. 2013).

Ultrasound-guided approach

The ultrasound is utilized throughout the procedure where the liver and biopsy needle are viewed in real time. This method is simple, reasonably fast, inexpensive and safer than other methods. In 1% of the cases significant complications have been reported with a mortality of 0.1% (Tannapfel et al. 2012).

Transjugular liver biopsy

When the percutaneous approach is contraindicated due to coagulopathy, vascular tumours, ascites or failed percutaneous attempts, the transjugular technique is indicated and is a safer approach (BSG 2004). The biopsy needle is inserted via the hepatic vein and this approach avoids the peritoneum and liver capsule (Keshava et al. 2008).

PRE-PROCEDURAL CONSIDERATIONS

Equipment

Aspiration or suction type needle

There are a few varieties of aspiration or suction type needles such as the Jamshidi, Klatskin and Menghini (Figure 10.11). The Menghini needle has a retaining device to minimize the risk of the sample being aspirated into the syringe and is the most commonly used. It is 6 cm long and approximately 1.4 mm wide.

Cutting type needles

The Tru-Cut and Vim-Silverman needle utilizes a cutting sheath to obtain the specimen. It is advanced approximately 2–3 cm into the liver and a sample of 1–2 cm with a diameter of 1 mm is collected. These needles are associated with a low failure rate but they also have a higher complication rate (Karamshi 2008).

Automated spring-loaded needle biopsy guns

Automated spring-loaded needle biopsy guns automatically trigger and insert the needle. These generally only require one

Figure 10.11 **Liver biopsy needles.**

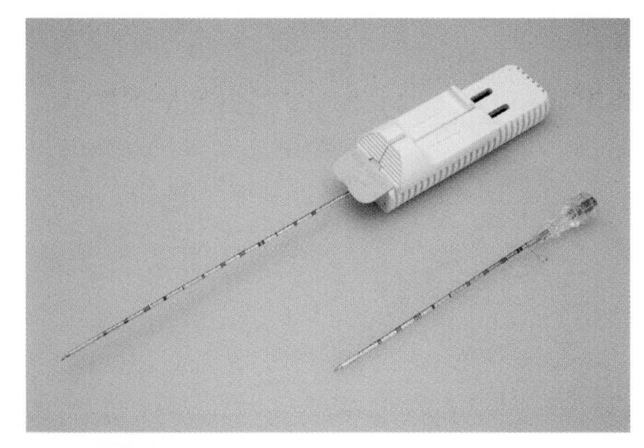

hand to operate, allowing the clinican to use the other hand for visual guidance such as the use of ultrasound (Karamshi 2008).

Pharmacological support
Medications should be reviewed by medical and nursing staff and arrangements made by the medical team for alternative anticoagulant and diabetic medication if necessary. A local anaesthetic such as lidocaine 2% is infiltrated into the area where the biopsy is to be taken. In some cases where the patient is extremely anxious, conscious sedation may be considered (Al Knawy and Shiffman 2007).

Specific patient preparation
Nursing staff should take a nursing history, reviewing social and medical history and determining allergy status. Up to 7 days prior to the procedure, the referring medical team must ensure that a full blood count, clotting screen and biochemistry have been taken. Nursing staff should review bloods as part of their pre-procedure assessment. If a patient is currently taking an anticoagulant such as warfarin, a clotting sample must be taken within 24 hours of the procedure.

A baseline set of physiological observations must be undertaken. If conscious sedation is used, the patient must be nil by mouth and they must have patent intravenous (IV) access (Royal College of Radiologists 2006). The patient is usually in the supine position with the right side as close to the edge of the bed as possible. The left side may be supported by a pillow. The patient's right hand is positioned under their head and their head turned to the left. Oxygen therapy may be required if there are pre-existing conditions or when conscious sedation is used. The patient may be asked to hold their breath at the end of expiration so nursing staff should explain this prior to the procedure (Karamshi 2008).

POST-PROCEDURAL CONSIDERATIONS

Immediate care
Immediately following the procedure, the patient must lie on their right side for 3 hours and remain on bedrest for a total of 6 hours. They may be able to go to the toilet after 3 hours. Physiological observations are required every 15 minutes for the first hour, every 30 minutes for the following 2 hours and then the frequency can be reviewed by the Registered Nurse (Chernecky and Berger 2013, Karamshi 2008). Any abnormality must be reported to the medical team immediately. The nurse should also observe the puncture site and abdomen for signs of bleeding and ensure that pain is adequately controlled. Pain is the most common problem reported by patients which can develop within 3 hours after the procedure, so recording the pain score and analgesia may be required. Severe pain must always be reported to the medical team as it may be an indicator of a bleed or bile leak (Karamshi 2008). The patient may also require emotional care throughout and after the procedure (Karamshi 2008).

Ongoing care/education
A post-procedure information sheet should be given to the patient identifying possible complications and instructions on what to do if any symptoms occur (Royal College of Radiologists 2006).

COMPLICATIONS

Haemorrhage
An inadvertent puncture of an intrahepatic or extrahepatic blood vessel can lead to haemorrhage manifesting within 4 hours. However, it is normal to lose approximately 5–10 mL of blood from the surface of the liver after the biopsy. Conservative management with blood products may be appropriate but surgical intervention may also be required to treat haemorrhage (Chernecky and Berger 2013, Karamshi 2008).

Peritonitis
An inadvertent puncture of the bile duct which consequently results in bile leaking into the peritoneal cavity can lead to peritonitis. Treatment may range from antimicrobial therapy to surgical and/or critical care intervention dependent on the severity (Chernecky and Berger 2013, Karamshi 2008).

Pneumothorax
An inadvertent puncture of the pleura can lead to a pneumothorax. If this occurs, urgent medical intervention is required. A formal chest drain may be necessary to relieve the pneumothorax (Chernecky and Berger 2013, Denzer et al. 2007).

Radiological investigations: X-ray

DEFINITION
An X-ray is a short-wavelength electromagnetic radiation that passes through matter and is used in diagnostic radiology and radiotherapy (Martin 2010).

EVIDENCE-BASED APPROACHES

Rationale
The general X-ray department performs a wide range of examinations, many of which require no patient preparation in advance and can often be performed on the day of the request. In accordance with the Ionizing Radiation Regulations (1999), to ensure radiation safety, there is a requirement for radiographers to justify, optimize and limit radiation dosage to a patient.

Indications
Diagnostic X-rays are performed to diagnose medical conditions such as damage to the skeletal structures and organ dysfunction, for example chest X-rays for respiratory complications.

Contraindications
The Ionizing Radiation (Medical Exposure) Regulations (2000) (Regulations 6 and 7) prohibit any medical exposure from being carried out which has not been justified and authorized, and provides an optimization process to ensure that doses arising from exposures are kept as low as reasonably practicable (ALARP).

In accordance with the *Medical and Dental Guidance Notes* (2002) for women known or likely to be pregnant, where the examination has been justified on the basis of clinical urgency and involves irradiation of the abdomen, operators must optimize the technique to minimize irradiation of the fetus (IPEM 2002). Radiography of areas remote from the fetus, for example chest, skull or hand, may be carried out safely at any time during pregnancy as long as good beam collimation and proper shielding equipment are used.

LEGAL AND PROFESSIONAL ISSUES
The Ionizing Radiation (Medical Exposure) Regulations (2000) set out the legal roles and responsibilities of all duty holders related to medical exposures to X-rays.

In accordance with the Ionizing Radiation (Medical Exposure) Regulations (IR(ME)R) (2000), the completed request form for a medical exposure must be clear and legible and the following information must be supplied.

- Unique patient identification – to include at least three identifiers from name, date of birth, hospital number or NHS number.
- Sufficient details of the clinical problem to allow the IR(ME)R practitioner to justify the medical exposure, and indication of examination thought to be appropriate.
- If applicable, information on the patient's possible pregnancy status.
- Signature uniquely identifying the referrer as it is important that the referrer is qualified to order an X-ray.

Blank request cards, pre-signed by a referrer, are a breach of the Regulations and any entries on the request form made by others should be checked and initialled by the referrer prior to signing the form.

Competencies

Non-medical 'referrers'

The IR(ME)R (2000) require employers to only accept requests for X-ray or nuclear medicine investigations from approved and authorized 'referrers'. When the referrer is not a trained medical doctor or dentist, the Regulations further require that the referrer has received appropriate information, instruction and training in radiation protection, and the scope and range of investigations for which they are authorized to request must be documented. All 'referrers' must be made aware of the appropriate referral criteria for such investigations as set down by each individual's organization in its IR(ME)R procedures and protocols.

Risk management

Radiation protection is based on the three principles of justification, optimization and limitation. The procedure must be justified and of net benfit to the patient. Optimization ensures that exposure to the patient, staff and public shall be as low as reasonably possible (ALARP). The limitation is essential to ensure that dose equivalent to staff and members of the public does not exceed the dose limits (IR(ME)R 2000).

PRE-PROCEDURAL CONSIDERATIONS

Pharmacological support

For some types of X-ray such as the barium swallow or enema, the patient is usually required to drink the contrast or have it administered via an enema, and a series of X-ray pictures is taken at various intervals. Afterwards the patient will be advised to drink plenty of fluids to clear their system of the contrast as quickly as possible (Chernecky and Berger 2013).

Specific patient preparation

The radiology department will inform the patient of any requirements prior to the booked procedure, such as being nil by mouth. For most examinations, the patient will be asked to remove some of their clothing and change into a hospital gown, to ensure that no artefacts (any feature in an image which misrepresents the object in the field of view) (McRobbie 2007) are caused in the area of clinical interest on the X-ray image. It is advisable for the patient not to wear jewellery at the time of the appointment as in most cases this will have to be removed, again to prevent the presence of artefacts on the image. For all X-rays the patient will be required to keep still to prevent any blurring of the images. Some procedures are performed on inspiration/ expiration, and the patient will be given the appropriate breathing instruction by the operator performing the procedure (Chernecky and Berger 2013).

Magnetic resonance imaging

DEFINITION

Magnetic resonance imaging provides cross-sectional images of the body. The patient lies inside the bore of a very strong magnet, typically 1.5 tesla, although 3 tesla scanners are becoming increasingly prevalent. Protons in the body's water molecules spin or 'precess' when exposed to such a strong magnetic field. Radio waves are transmitted into the patient at the same frequency at which the protons are precessing and the patient transmits a signal that is detected by a receiver coil (Chernecky and Berger 2013, Weishaupt et al. 2006). This signal contains specific information or 'weighting' about the individual tissues that can be mapped to form a two- or three-dimensional image (Weishaupt et al. 2006).

EVIDENCE-BASED APPROACHES

Rationale

Soft tissue structures such as the brain, spinal cord, musculoskeletal system, liver and pelvic structures are particularly well demonstrated using MRI. Although MRI is often targeted to particular areas of the body, it is also possible to scan the whole body with scan times ranging from 20 to 60 minutes. MRI is increasingly being used as a tool in radiotherapy treatment planning (Prestwich et al. 2012) and has begun to be used to guide interventional procedures, e.g. breast biopsies (O'Flynn et al. 2010). MRI does *not* use ionizing radiation and can therefore be used for repeated examinations. The magnetic field is always present so strict safety procedures are necessary to protect staff and patients (Shellock and Spinazzi 2008).

Indications

- Scanning of the brain to assess stroke, tumour, meningeal disease.
- Spinal pathology is particularly well demonstrated, including intervertebral disc pathology, tumour, infarction, spinal dysraphism, infection and degenerative diseases.
- Differentiation and characterization of benign versus malignant pathology in the liver.
- MRI is highly sensitive for imaging of the breast.
- MRI is the gold standard for assessment of pelvic malignancy and pelvic anatomy (Royal College of Radiologists 2012).

Contraindications

Patients with non-MRI-compatible implanted devices, such as cardiac pacemakers and cochlear implants, must not be scanned. Other implanted devices, for example stents, must be confirmed as MR safe prior to scanning.

Magnetic resonance imaging tends not to be used for acute trauma, for which CT is usually the preferred imaging modality, or for primary whole-body staging of malignancies, although a role for whole-body MRI is increasingly being proposed in some areas for non-oncological and oncological diagnostic purposes (Lambregts et al. 2011, Lin et al. 2012).

PRE-PROCEDURAL CONSIDERATIONS

Assessment and recording tools

A pre-MRI checklist is undertaken for all patients to identify risks from implanted devices which may be harmful to the patient or may severely degrade the image quality (Shellock and Spinazzi 2008).

Pharmacological support

The patient may require intravenous access for contrast injection, most often of a gadolinium-based contrast agent. This is used to enhance areas of suspected pathology, to define tumour bulk or to improve the efficacy of the scan by delineation or characterization of a pathological process (Runge et al. 2009). These contrast agents may be contraindicated in patients with poor renal function and therefore recent blood results to demonstrate adequate renal function will usually be required before contrast administration (Baert and Knauth 2009). It is also routine practice in some centres to administer antispasmodic agents prior to abdominal or pelvic scans to reduce bowel peristalsis and improve image quality. Claustrophobia can also be an issue and in some cases patients may require an oral sedative to relax them during the procedure. In severe claustrophobia or when scanning young children or individuals with learning difficulties, general anaesthetic may be necessary.

Non-pharmacological support

The scanner is very noisy so it is mandatory that patients are given ear protection during the scan. If the patient feels claustrophobic there are strategies to manage this, such as:

- adapting the patient's position
- changing the scanning technique
- using blindfolds or mirrors
- relaxation therapy (Chernecky and Berger 2013).

Specific patient preparation
Apart from safety checking, for most scans there is no preparation but for certain body scans the patient may have to abstain from food but may drink clear (non-caffeine) fluids to ensure their bladder does not fill too quickly, resulting in movement artefacts (Chernecky and Berger 2013).

Patients must be able to lie very still, usually lying on their back for significant time periods. Patient comfort is paramount so patients requiring pain relief should continue with pain medication as normal.

Computed tomography

DEFINITION
Computed tomography images are created when radiation passes through a patient and is absorbed in varying degrees by the body tissue. Multislice data are acquired as a three-dimensional block in a matter of seconds and digitally displayed in coronal, sagittal or axial planes (Fishman and Jeffrey 2004).

EVIDENCE-BASED APPROACHES

Rationale
Multislice CT has excellent image resolution and is used for diagnosis, staging and monitoring treatment response in the oncology setting, as well as being a research tool. Soft tissues as well as bone and lung anatomy are all seen well on CT scans. Routinely patients are given intravenous contrast medium which perfuses the body tissues and enhances the blood vessels and lesions (Husband and Reznek 2010).

Computed tomography does use radiation but protocols are optimized to give the best image with the lowest dose. Also, the number of body areas scanned and the intervals between scans are closely monitored in accordance with IR(ME)R regulations.

Indications
Computed tomography can image all parts of the body and is used for:

- pre-treatment staging
- interval scans to monitor treatment
- follow-up post treatment
- diagnosis and assessment of complications:
  - bowel obstructions and perforation
  - pulmonary embolism
  - stroke, cerebral bleeds
- perfusion CT (Chernecky and Berger 2013).

Contraindications

- Pregnancy: CT is not recommended unless clinical benefit outweighs radiation risk.
- Patients with poor renal function or those having iodine therapy may have CT without intravenous contrast.
- Previous CT within short timeframe unless clinically urgent.
- Patients who are unable to lie down in order to pass through the machine (Royal College of Radiologists 2010).

PRE-PROCEDURAL CONSIDERATIONS

Assessment and recording tools
Patients complete a questionnaire prior to CT in order to assess their suitability for CT and IV contrast. Intravenous contrast contains iodine, so patients with an iodine allergy, an allergy to shellfish or previous history of reaction to IV contrast should have a non-IV contrast CT.

Pharmacological support
The patient is cannulated for the intravenous injection of iodine-based contrast medium to enhance the blood vessels and bodily organs. During the injection it is normal for the patient to transiently feel warm over their whole body and to experience a metallic taste at the back of the throat, and some patients feel nauseous. CT examinations such as CT pulmonary angiograms demand contrast to flow at a fast rate and therefore a large-gauge cannula (20 G) is required. CT-compatible ports and PICCs may also be used (Thomsen et al. 2009).

Non-pharmacological support
Although CT is a fast imaging technique (5–20 seconds), some patients are very concerned about being claustrophobic during scanning but with kind careful explanation, most manage to be scanned.

Specific patient preparation
Patients are prepared for CT by drinking an oral contrast, usually water, which shows the digestive tract. This serves to hydrate the patient which is beneficial post IV contrast and also acts as a negative contrast agent in the digestive tract. Patients refrain from eating for 2 hours prior to CT in order to allow them to drink easily and to reduce nausea post IV contrast medium (Thomsen et al. 2009). IV access must be established prior to the CT scan to facilitate injection of the IV contrast. Radiopaque objects such as jewellery must be removed (Chernecky and Berger 2013).

Patients lie on the CT scan couch and pass through the doughnut-shaped machine. The examination is painless and the majority of patients tolerate the examinations well. Small children require general anaesthetic for CT (Thomsen et al. 2009). Emergency equipment must be available if IV contrast or a general anaesthetic is used (Chernecky and Berger 2013).

POST-PROCEDURAL CONSIDERATIONS

Immediate care
If any monitoring leads were moved prior to the CT, they should be replaced immediately. Some patients may experience side-effects which should be observed for after the administration of a contrast. These may include headache, nausea and vomiting. If an allergic reaction occurs this must be treated and the allergy status of the patient amended. The patient must then be informed that they have had an allergic reaction (Chernecky and Berger 2013).

Learning Activity 10.5

Learning in practice: Visiting the radiology department

In your clinical area, ask your mentor/supervising nurse if you can arrange a visit to the radiology department. You may wish to do this by following a patient who is going for an investigation such as an X-ray, CT or MRI scan.

- Find out what the difference is between these scanning techniques.
- What other investigations are carried out within the department?

Learning for practice

After studying this chapter, list four key points you have learnt about interpreting diagnostic tests that you will be able to apply to your clinical practice.

For further learning exercises visit **www.royalmarsdenmanual.com/student**.

Now Test Yourself

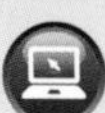

This section provides a range of exercises/activities to further test your learning. For additional exercises visit **www.royalmarsdenmanual.com/student**.

What have you learnt?

1 Gram staining is used to guide the choice of antimicrobial therapy.
- A True
- B False

2 What is histology?
- A A method for testing antibiotic sensitivity
- B The detection of antigens of antibodies within serum
- C The study of cells and tissues in the body
- D The use of a culture media to grow and identify bacteria from a specimen

3 In relation to specimen collection, what infection control precautions should be taken?
- A The use of personal protection equipment
- B Hand hygiene
- C Waste management
- D All of the above

4 In venepuncture, which vein(s) are used only when the others are not accessible?
- A Median cubital vein
- B Cephalic vein
- C Basilic vein
- D Metacarpal veins

5 Venepuncture does not require an aseptic technique.
- A True
- B False

6 What is the most common complication of venepuncture?
- A Nerve injury
- B Arterial puncture
- C Haematoma
- D Fainting

7 How many sputum samples are required in cases of suspected Mycobacterium tuberculosis?
- A 1
- B 2
- C 3
- D 4

8 How long should a patient fast for, prior to a gastroscopy, to ensure the stomach is relatively empty?
- A At least 2 hours
- B At least 4 hours
- C At least 6 hours
- D At least 8 hours

9 What is a cystoscopy?
- A Examination of cells under a microscope
- B An investigation examining a lump in the body
- C An investigation examining the bladder and urethra
- D An investigation examining the colon and rectum

10 Which of the following does not use ionizing radiation so can be used for repeated examinations?
- A X-ray
- B MRI scan
- C CT scan
- D None of the above, they all use ionizing radiation

See the end of the chapter for the answers.

Key points

- Diagnostic tests are undertaken to aid in the diagnosis and treatment of various conditions. The tests are used to identify diseases from their characteristics, signs and symptoms and to identify changes or abnormalities.
- Successful laboratory diagnosis depends upon the collection of specimens at the appropriate time, using the correct technique and equipment, and transporting them to the designated laboratory safely without delay.
- Nursing staff are in a unique position within the diagnostic testing process because they often identify the need for diagnostic and/or microbiological investigations, initiate the collection of specimens and assume responsibility for timely and safe transportation to the laboratory.
- Nurses play a key role in ensuring patients are appropriately prepared for, supported through and cared for after diagnostic investigations.

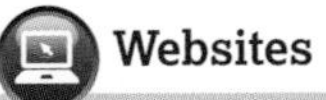
Websites

Diagnostic tests
www.library.wmuh.nhs.uk/pil/diagnostictests.htm

British Infertility Counselling Association
www.bica.net

Cancer Research UK
www.cancerhelp.org.uk

Infertility Network UK
www.infertilitynetworkuk.com

Human Fertilisation and Embryology Authority
www.hfea.gov.uk

Macmillan Cancer Support
www.macmillan.org.uk

NHS Cancer Screening Programme publications related to cervical screening
www.cancerscreening.nhs.uk/cervical

NHS Information Centre
www.ic.nhs.uk

REFERENCES

Ahn, J.I., Jung, H.Y., Bae, S.E., et al. (2013) Proper preparation to reduce endoscopic reexamination due to food residue after distal gastrectomy for gastric cancer. *Surgical Endoscopy*, 27(3), 910–917.

Al Knawy, B. & Shiffman, M. (2007) Percutaneous liver biopsy in clinical practice. *Liver International*, 27(9), 1166–1173.

Asai, A., Aoshima, M., Ohkui, Y., Otsuka, Y. & Kaneko, N. (2012) Should blood cultures be performed in terminally ill cancer patients? *Indian Journal of Palliative Care*, 18(1), 40–44.

AUA (2008) *Best Practice Policy Statement on Urological Surgery Antimicrobial Prophylaxis*. American Urological Assosciation. Available at: www.auanet.org/education/guidelines/antimicrobial-prophylaxis.cfm

Aziz, A.M. (2011) Audit of blood culture technique and documentation to improve practice. *British Journal of Nuring*, 20(8), 26–34.

Baert, A. & Knauth, M. (2009) *Contrast Media: Safety Issues and ESUR Guidelines*, 2nd rev. edn. Berlin: Springer.

Berreth, M. (2010) Minimizing the risk of lymphoedema: implications for the infusion nurse. *INS Newsline*, 32(3), 6–7.

Birk, D. (2009) *Human Fertilization and Embryology: The New Law*. London: Jordan Publishing.

Blann, A.D. (2007) *Routine Blood Results Explained*, 2nd edn. Keswick, Cumbria: M & K Update Ltd.

BNF (2014) *British National Formulary 67*. London: Pharmaceutical Press.

Bonham, P.A. (2009) Swab cultures for diagnosing wound infections: a literature review and clinical guideline. *Journal of Wound, Ostomy and Continence Nursing*, 36(4), 389–395.

Borgaonkar, M.R., Hookey, L., Hollingworth, R., et al. (2012) Indicators of safety compromise in gastrointestinal endoscopy. *Canadian Journal of Gastroenterology*, 26(2), 71–78.

Bowler, P.G., Duerden, B.I. & Armstrong, D.G. (2001) Wound microbiology and associated approaches to wound management. *Clinical Microbiology Reviews*, 14(2), 244–269.

Brackett, N., Lynne, C., Ibrahim, E., Ohl, D. & Sønksen, J. (2010) Treatment of infertility in men with spinal cord injury. *Nature Reviews: Urology*, 7(3), 162–172.

Brinsden, P.R. (2005) *Textbook of In Vitro Fertilization and Assisted Reproduction: The Bourn Hall Guide to Clinical and Laboratory Practice*, 3rd edn. London: Taylor & Francis.

BSG (2003) *Guidelines on Safety and Sedation During Endoscopic Procedures*. London: British Society of Gastroenterology. Available at: www.bsg.org.uk/clinical-guidelines/endoscopy/guidelines-on-safety-and-sedation-during-endoscopic-procedures.html

BSG (2004) *Guidelines on the Use of Liver Biopsy in Clinical Practice*. London: British Society of Gastroenterology. Available at: www.bsg.org.uk/pdf_word_docs/liver_biopsy.pdf

BSG (2005) *Non-Medical Endoscopists*. London: British Society of Gastroenterology. Available at: www.bsg.org.uk/pdf_word_docs/endo_%20nonmed.pdf

BSG (2007) *BSG Quality and Safety Indicators for Endoscopy*. London: British Society of Gastroenterology. Available at: www.thejag.org.uk/downloads%5CUnit%20Resources%5CBSG%20Quality%20and%20Safety%20Indicators.pdf.

Campbell, H., Carrington, M. & Limber, C. (1999) A practice guide to venepuncture and management of complications. *British Journal of Nursing*, 8(7), 426–431.

CDCP (1997) Evaluation of safety devices for preventing percutaneous injuries among health-care workers during phlebotomy procedures – Minneapolis-St Paul, New York City, and San Francisco, 1993–1995. *JAMA*, 277(6), 449–450.

Chernecky, C.C. & Berger, B.J. (2013) *Laboratory Tests and Diagnostic Procedures*, 6th edn. St Louis, MO: Elsevier.

Choi, C.H. (2012) Safety and prevention of complications in endoscopic sedation. *Digestive Diseases and Sciences*, 57, 1745–1747.

Coburn, B., Morris, A.M., Tomlinson, G. & Detsky, A.S. (2012) Does this adult with suspected bacteremia require blood cultures? *JAMA*, 300(5), 502–511.

Coia, J.E., Duckworth, G.J., Edwards, D.I., et al. (2006) Guidelines for the control and prevention of meticillin-resistant *Staphylococcus aureus* (MRSA) in healthcare facilities. *Journal of Hospital Infection*, 63 (Suppl 1), S1–44.

Cole, T. (2006) Risks and benefits of needle use in patients after axillary surgery. *British Journal of Nursing*, 15(18), 969–979.

Connor, A., Tolan, D., Hughes, S., Carr, N. & Tomson, C. (2012) Consensus guidelines for the safe prescription and administration of oral bowel-cleansing agents. Available at: https://www.rcr.ac.uk/docs/radiology/pdf/obca_12.pdf

Crawshaw, M. & Hale, J. (2005) Sperm storage and the adolescent male: a multi-disciplinary approach. *Human Fertility*, 8(3), 175–176.

Dabaja, A. & Schlegel, P. (2012) Microdissection testicular sperm extraction: an update. *Asian Journal of Andrology*, 15, 35–39.

Damani, N. (2012) *Manual of Infection Prevention and Control*, 3rd edn. Oxford: Oxford University Press.

de Verteuil, A. (2011) Procedures for venepuncture and cannulation. In: Phillips, S., Collins, M. & Dougherty, L. (eds) *Venepuncture and Cannulation*. Oxford: John Wiley & Sons.

Dellinger, R.P., Levy, M.M., Rhodes, A., et al. (2013) Surviving Sepsis Campaign: International Guidelines for Management of Severe Sepsis and Septic Shock: 2012. *Critical Care Medicine*, 41(2), 580–637.

Denzer, U., Arnoldy, A., Kanzler, S., et al. (2007) Prospective randomised comparison of minilaparoscopy and percutaneous liver biopsy: diagnosis of cirrhosis and complications. *Journal of Clinical Gastroenterology* 41(1), 103–110.

DH (2006a) *Safe Management of Healthcare Waste*. London: Department of Health.

DH (2006b) *Screening for Meticillin-Resistant Staphylococcus aureus (MRSA) Colonisation: A Strategy for NHS Trusts: Summary of Best Practice*. London: Department of Health. Available at: http://webarchive.nationalarchives.gov.uk/20130107105354/http://dh.gov.uk/prod_consum_dh/groups/dh_digitalassets/@dh/@en/documents/digitalasset/dh_078128.pdf

DH (2007a) *Saving Lives: Reducing Infection, Delivering Clean and Safe Health Care. High Impact Intervention No.6: Urinary Catheter Care Bundle*. London: Department of Health. Available at: http://webarchive.nationalarchives.gov.uk/20130107105354/http://dh.gov.uk/prod_consum_dh/groups/dh_digitalassets/@dh/@en/documents/digitalasset/dh_078125.pdf

DH (2007b) *Saving Lives: Reducing Infection, Delivering Clean and Safe Health Care: Taking Blood Cultures, Summary of Best Practice*. London:

Department of Health. Available at: http://webarchive.nationalarchives.gov.uk/20130107105354/http://dh.gov.uk/prod_consum_dh/groups/dh_digitalassets/@dh/@en/documents/digitalasset/dh_078118.pdf

DH (2010) *Clean Safe Care. High Impact Intervention. Taking Blood Cultures: A Summary of Best Practice*. London: Department of Health.

Di Teodoro, L.I., Pudhota, S.G., Vega K.J., et al. (2013) Ultrasound marking by gastroenterologists prior to percutaneous liver biopsy removes the need for a separate radiological evaluation. *Hepato-Gastroenterology*, 60, 821–824.

Dohle, G., Diemer, T., Kopa, Z., Krausz, C., Giwercman, A. & Jungwith, A. (2012) European Association guidelines on vasectomy. *European Urology*, 61, 159–163.

Dojcinovska, M. (2011) Selection of equipment. In: Phillips, S., Collins, M. & Dougherty, L. (eds) *Venepuncture and Cannulation*. Oxford: John Wiley & Sons.

Dougherty, L. (2008) Obtaining peripheral venous access. In: Dougherty, L. & Lamb, J. (eds) *Intravenous Therapy in Nursing Practice*, 2nd edn. Oxford: Blackwell Publishing, pp.225–270.

Dulak, S.B. (2005) Hands-on help: sputum sample collection. *RN*, 68(10), 24ac2.

Dulczak, S. & Kirk, J. (2005) Overview of the evaluation, diagnosis, and management of urinary tract infections in infants and children. *Urologic Nursing*, 25(3), 185–191.

Egan, S. Murphy, P.G., Fennell, J.P., et al. (2012) Using six sigma to improve once daily gentamicin dosing and therapeutic drug monitoring performance. *British Medical Journal Quality and Safety*, 21, 1042–1051.

Ernst, D.J. (2005) *Applied Phlebotomy*. Philadelphia: Lippincott Williams & Wilkins.

Esteves, S., Lee, W., David, B., Seol, B., Verza, S. & Agarwal, A. (2013) Reproductive potential of men with obstructive azoospermia undergoing percutaneous sperm retrieval and intracytoplasmic sperm injection according to the cause of obstruction. *Journal of Urology*, 189(1), 232–237.

European Biosafety Network (2010) *Prevention of Sharps Injuries in the Hospital and Healthcare Sector*. European Union. Available at: www.europeanbiosafetynetwork.eu/EU%20Sharps%20Injuries%20Implementation%20Guidance.pdf

European Union Tissues and Cells Directive (2004) *The European Parliament and The Council on Setting Standards of Quality and Safety for the Donation, Procurement, Testing, Processing, Preservation, Storage and Distribution of Human Tissues and Cells*. Brussels: European Parliament.

Faoagali, J. (2010) 'Swabs' then and now: cotton to flocked nylon. *Microbiology Australia*, September, 133–136.

Ferguson, A. (2005) Taking a swab. *Nursing Times*, 101(39), 26–27.

Fillingham, S. & Douglas, J. (2004) *Urological Nursing*, 3rd edn. Edinburgh: Baillière Tindall.

Fishman, E.K. & Jeffrey, R.B. (2004) *Multidetector CT: Principles, Techniques, and Clinical Applications*. Philadelphia: Lippincott Williams & Wilkins.

Fraise, A.P. & Bradley, T. (2009) *Ayliffe's Control of Healthcare-associated Infection: A Practical Handbook*, 5th edn. London: Hodder Arnold.

Gannon, K., Glover, L. & Able, P. (2004) Masculinity, infertility, stigma and media reports. *Social Science & Medicine*, 59(6), 1169–1175.

Garber, G. (2001) An overview of fungal infections. *Drugs*, 61(Suppl 1), 1–12.

Garza, D. & Becan-McBride, K. (2013) *Phlebotomy Simplified*, 2nd edn. Upper Saddle River, NJ: Pearson Education Inc.

Gerris, J. (1999) Methods of semen collection not based on masturbation or surgical sperm retrieval. *Human Reproduction Update*, 5, 211–225.

Gilbert, R. (2006) Taking a midstream specimen of urine. *Nursing Times*, 102(18), 22–23.

Gilbert, S. (2000) *Developmental Biology*, 6th edn. Sunderland, MA: Sinauer Associates.

Gilchrist, B. (2000) Taking a wound swab. *Nursing Times*, 96(4 Suppl), 2.

Gill, V., Fedorko, D. & Witebsky, F. (2005) The clinician and the microbiological laboratory. In: Mandell, G.L., Douglas, R.G., Bennett, J.E. & Dolin, R. (eds) *Mandell, Douglas, and Bennett's Principles and Practice of Infectious Diseases*, 6th edn. Philadelphia: Elsevier Churchill Livingstone.

Golder, M., Chan, C.L.H., O'Shea, S., Corbett, K., Chrystie, I.L. & French, G. (2000) Potential risk of cross-infection during peripheral-venous access by contamination of tourniquets. *Lancet*, 355(9197), 44.

Gong, D., Liu, Y.L., Zheng, Z., Tian, Y.F. & Li, Z. (2009) An overview on ethical issues about sperm donation. *Asian Journal of Andrology*, 11, 645–652.

Gould, D. (2002) Preventing cross-infection. *Nursing Times*, 98(46), 50–51.

Gould, D. & Brooker, C. (2008) *Infection Prevention and Control: Applied Microbiology for Healthcare*, 2nd edn. Basingstoke: Palgrave Macmillan.

Greil, A., Slausen-Blevens, K. & McQuillan, J. (2010) The experience of infertility: a review of recent literature. *Sociology of Health & Illness*, 32(1), 140–162.

Guest, J. (2008) Specimen collection. Part 5 – Obtaining a sputum sample. *Nursing Times*, 104(21), 26–27.

Hadaway, L. & Chamallas, S.N. (2003) Vancomycin: new perspectives on an old drug. *Journal of Infusion Nursing*, 26(5), 278–284.

Hammarberg, K., Baker, H. & Fisher, J. (2010) Men's experiences of infertility and infertility treatment 5 years after diagnosis of male factor infertility: a retrospective cohort study. *Human Reproduction*, 25(11), 2815–2820.

Hammett-Stabler, C.A. & Johns, T. (1998) Laboratory guidelines for monitoring of antimicrobial drugs. National Academy of Clinical Biochemistry. *Clinical Chemistry*, 44(5), 1129–1140.

Hampson, G.D. (2006) *Practice Nurse Handbook*, 5th edn. Oxford: Blackwell Publishing.

Hart, S. (2008) Infection control. In: Dougherty, L. & Lamb, J. (eds) *Intravenous Therapy in Nursing Practice*. Oxford: Blackwell.

Hefler, L., Grimm, C., Leodolter, S. & Tempfer, C. (2004) To butterfly or to needle: the pilot phase. *Annals of Internal Medicine*, 140(11), 935–936.

Hess, D.R. (2002) The evidence for secreting clearance techniques. *Cardiopulmonary Physical Therapy Journal*, 13(4), 7–21.

HFEA (2012) *Code of Practice*, 7th edn. London: Human Fertilisation and Embryology Authority. Available at: www.hfea.gov.uk

Higgins, C. (2013) *Understanding Laboratory Investigations for Nurses and Health Professionals*, 3rd edn. Oxford: Blackwell Publishing.

Higgins, D. (2008a) Specimen collection: obtaining a midstream specimen of urine. *Nursing Times*, 104(17), 26–27.

Higgins, D. (2008b) Specimen collection. Part 3 – collecting a stool specimen. *Nursing Times*, 104(19), 22–23.

Himberger, J.R. & Himberger, L.C. (2001) Accuracy of drawing blood through infusing intravenous lines. *Heart & Lung*, 30(1), 66–73.

Hoeltke, L.B. (2013) *The Complete Textbook of Phlebotomy*, 4th edn. Clifton Park, NY: Delmar Cengage Learning.

Hooton, T.M., Bradley, S.F., Cardens, D.D., et al. (2010) Diagnosis, prevention, and treatment of catheter-associated urinary tract infection in adults: 2009 International Clinical Practice Guidelines from the Infectious Diseases Society of America. *Infectious Diseases Society of America*, 50(5), 625–663.

HPA (2014a) *UK Standards for Microbiology Investigations: Investigation of Blood Cultures (for Organisms other than Mycobacterium species)*. London: Health Protection Agency.

HPA (2014b) *UK Standards for Microbiology Investigations: Investigation of Specimens for Screening for MRSA*. London: Health Protection Agency. Available at: www.hpa.org.uk/webc/hpawebfile/hpaweb_c/1317132861509

HPA (2014c) *UK Standards for Microbiology Investigations: Investigation of Throat Swabs*. Wales: Health Protection Agency. Available at: www.hpa.org.uk/webc/hpawebfile/hpaweb_c/1317132856329

HPA (2014d) *UK Standards for Microbiology Investigations: Investigation of Nose Swabs*. London: Health Protection Agency. Available at: www.hpa.org.uk/webc/hpawebfile/hpaweb_c/1317132855931

HPA (2014e) *UK Standards for Microbiology Investigations: Investigation of Genital Tract and Associated Specimens*. London: Health Protection Agency. Available at: www.hpa.org.uk/webc/hpawebfile/hpaweb_c/1317132861109

HPA (2014f) *UK Standards for Microbiology Investigations: Investigation of Faecal Specimens for Enteric Pathogens*. Wales: Health Protection Agency. Available at: www.hpa.org.uk/webc/hpawebfile/hpaweb_c/1317132856754

HPA (2014g) *UK Standards for Microbiology Investigations: Processing of Faeces for Clostridium difficile*. Wales: Health Protection Agency. Available at: http://www.hpa.org.uk/webc/hpawebfile/hpaweb_c/1317132856426

HPA (2014h) *Investigation of Urine: BSOP 41: Issue 7*. Wales: Health Protection Agency. Available at: www.hpa.org.uk/webc/hpawebfile/hpaweb_c/1317132858791

HPA (2014i) *Investigation for Bronchovascular Lavage, Sputum and Associated Specimens: BSOP57: Issue 2.3*. Wales: Health Protection Agency. Available at: www.hpa.org.uk/webc/hpawebfile/hpaweb_c/1317132860548

HSE (2003) *Safe Working and the Prevention of Infection in Clinical Laboratories and Similar Facilities*, 2nd edn. Sudbury: HSE Books.

HSE (2005) *Biological Agents: Managing the Risks in Laboratories and Healthcare Premises*. Sudbury: HSE Books.

HSE (2013) *Health and Safety (Sharp Instruments in Healthcare) Regulations 2013*. London: Health and Safety Executive.

Hudak, K. (1986) Compliance in IV therapy. *Journal of the Canadian Intravenous Nurses Association*, 2(3), 3–8.

Human Fertilisation and Embryology Act (1990) London: Stationery Office.

Human Fertilisation and Embryology Act. (2008) London: Stationery Office.

Husband, J.E. & Reznek, R.H. (2010) *Husband & Reznek's Imaging in Oncology*, 3rd edn. London: Informa Healthcare.

Huth, M.E., Ricci, A.J. & Cheng, A.G. (2011) Mechanisms of aminoglycoside ototoxicity and targets of hair cell protection. *International Journal of Otolaryngology*, 2011, 1–19.

ICNA (2003) *Reducing Sharps Injury and Prevention and Risk Management*. London: Infection Control Nurses Association.

Inwood, S. (2007) Skin antisepsis: using 2% chlorhexidine gluconate in 70% isopropyl alcohol. *British Journal of Nursing*, 16(22), 1390, 1392–1394.

Ioanas, M., Ferrer, R., Angrill, J., Ferrer, M. & Torres, A. (2001) Microbial investigation in ventilator-associated pneumonia. *European Respiratory Journal*, 17(4), 791–801.

Ionizing Radiation (Medical Exposure) Regulations (2000) SI 2000/1059. London: The Stationery Office. Available at: www.opsi.gov.uk/si/si2000/20001059.htm

Ionizing Radiations Regulations (1999) SI 1999/3232. London: Stationery Office. Available at: www.opsi.gov.uk/si/si1999/19993232.htm

IPEM (2002) *Medical and Dental Guidance Notes: A Good Practice Guide on All Aspects of Ionising Radiation Protection in the Clinical Environment*. York: Institute of Physics and Engineering in Medicine.

Jackson, S.R., Dryden, M., Gillett, P. Kearney, P. & Wetherall, R. (2005) A novel midstream urine-collection device reduces the contamination rates in urine cultures amongst women. *BJU International*, 96, 360–364.

Jenkins, G. & Tortora, G.J. (2013) *Anatomy and Physiology: From Science to Life*, 3rd edn. Hoboken, NJ: John Wiley & Sons.

Jeyendran, R. (2003) *Sperm Collection and Processing Methods – A Practical Guide*. Cambridge: Cambridge University Press.

Johannes, R.S. (2008) Epidemiology of early-onset bloodstream infection and implications for treatment. *American Journal of Infection Control*, 36(10), S171 e13–17.

Johnson, A.L, Hampson, D.F. & Hampson, N.B. (2008) Sputum color: potential implications for clinical practice. *Respiratory Care*, 53(4), 450–454.

Jones, R.N. (2006) Microbiological features of vancomycin in the 21st century: minimum inhibitory concentration creep, bactericidal/static activity, and applied breakpoints to predict clinical outcomes or detect resistant strains. *Clinical Infectious Diseases*, 42(Suppl 1), S13–24.

Junqueira, L.C. & Carmeiro, J. (2005) *Basic Histology: Text and Atlas*, 11th edn. London: McGraw-Hill Medical.

Kang, H. &. Hyun, J.J. (2013) Preparation and patient evaluation for safe gastrointestinal endoscopy. *Clinical Endoscopy*, 46(3), 212–218.

Karamshi, M. (2008) Performing a percutaneous liver biopsy in parenchymal liver diseases. *British Journal of Nursing*, 9(17), 746–752.

Keir, L., Wise, B., Krebs, C., et al. (2007) *Medical Assisting: Administrative and Clinical Competencies*, 6th edn. New York: Thomson Delmar Learning.

Kelly, C., de Leon, L. & Jasutkar, N. (2012) Fecal microbiota transplantation for relapsing *Clostridium difficile* infection in 26 patients: methodology and results. *Journal of Clinical Gastroenterology*, 46, 145–149.

Kelly, D., Conway, S. & Aminov, R. (2005) Commensal gut bacteria: mechanisms of immune modulation. *Trends in Immunology*, 26(6), 326–333.

Keshava, S., Mammen, T., Surendrababu, N.R.S. & Moses, V. (2008) Transjugular liver biopsy: what to do and what not to do. *Interventional Radiology Symposium*, 18(3), 245–248.

Kingsley, A. (2001) A proactive approach to wound infection. *Nursing Standard*, 15(30), 50–4, 56, 58.

Kingsley, A. (2003) Audit of wound swab sampling: why protocols could improve practice. *Professional Nurse*, 18 (6), 338–343.

Kitzis, M.D. & Goldstein, F.W. (2006) Monitoring of vancomycin serum levels for the treatment of staphylococcal infections. *Clinical Microbiology and Infection*, 12(1), 92–95.

Korenstein, D., Falk, R., Howell, E.A., Bishop, T. & Keyhani, S. (2012) Overuse of health care services in the United States: an understudied problem. *Archives of Internal Medicine*, 172(2), 171–178.

Kyle, G. (2007) Bowel care. Part 3 – obtaining a stool sample. *Nursing Times*, 103(44), 24–25.

Lambregts, D.M., Maas, M., Cappendijk, V.C., et al. (2011) Whole-body diffusion-weighted magnetic resonance imaging: current evidence in oncology and potential role in colorectal cancer staging. *European Journal of Cancer*, 47(14), 2107–2116.

Lautenbach, E., Harris, A.D., Perencevich, E.N., Nachamkin, I., Tolomeo, P. & Metlay, J.P. (2005) Test characteristics of perirectal and rectal swab compared to stool sample for detection of fluoroquinolone-resistant *Escherichia coli* in the gastrointestinal tract. *Antimicrobial Agents and Chemotherapy*, 49(2), 798–800.

Lavery, I. & Ingram, P. (2005) Venepuncture: best practice. *Nursing Standard*, 19(49), 55–65.

Lee, A., Mirrett, S., Reller, L.B. & Weinstein, M.P. (2007) Detection of bloodstream infections in adults: how many blood cultures are needed? *Journal of Clinical Microbiology*, 45(11), 3546–3548.

Lee, S., Schover, L., Partridge, A., et al. (2006) American Society of Clinical Oncology recommendations on fertility preservation in cancer patients. *Journal of Clinical Oncology*, 24(18), 2917–2931.

Lenhardt, R., Seybold, T., Kimberger, O., Stoiser, B. & Sessler, D.I. (2002) Local warming and insertion of peripheral venous cannulas: single blinded prospective randomised controlled trial and single blinded randomised crossover trial. *BMJ*, 325(7361), 409–410.

Leonard, M., Hammelef, K. & Smith, G. (2004) Fertility considerations, counseling, and semen cryopreservation for males prior to the initiation of cancer therapy. *Clinical Journal of Oncology Nursing*, 8(2), 127–131.

Lessa, F.C., Gould, C.V. & McDonald, L.C. (2012) Current status of *Clostridium difficile* infection epidemiology. *Clinical Infectious Diseases*, 55(2), S65–70.

Lewis, S.J. & Heaton, K.W. (1997) Stool form scale as a useful guide to intestinal transit time. *Scandinavian Journal of Gastroenterology*, 32(9), 920–924.

Lin, C., Luciani, A., Itti, E., et al. (2012) Whole-body diffusion magnetic resonance imaging in the assessment of lymphoma. *Cancer Imaging*, 12(2), 403-408.

Loveday, H., Wilson, J.A., Pratt, R.J., et al. (2014) epic 3: National Evidence-Based Guidelines for Preventing Healthcare-Associated Infections in NHS Hospitals in England. *Journal of Hospital Infection 86S1*, S1-S70. Available at: http://www.his.org.uk/files/3113/8693/4808/epic3_National_Evidence-Based_Guidelines_for_Preventing_HCAI_in_NHSE.pdf

MacKay, G.J., Dorrance, H.R., Molloy, R.G. & O'Dwyer, P.J. (2010) *Colorectal Surgery*. Oxford: Oxford University Press.

MacKie, R.M. (2003) *Clinical Dermatology*, 5th edn. Oxford: Oxford University Press.

Madeo, M. & Barlow, G. (2008) Reducing blood-culture contamination rates by the use of a 2% chlorhexidine solution applicator in acute admission units. *Journal of Hospital Infection*, 69(3), 307–309.

Mandal, A. (2010) *Semen Physiology*. Available at: www.news-medical.net/health/Semen-Physiology.aspx

Manolakopoulos, S., Triantos, C., Bethanis, S., et al. (2007) Ultrasound-guided liver biopsy in real life: comparison of same-day prebiopsy versus real-time ultrasound approach. *Journal of Gastroenterology and Hepatology*, 22(9), 1490–1493.

Marieb, E.N. & Hoehn, K. (2010) *Human Anatomy and Physiology*, 8th edn. San Francisco: Benjamin Cummings.

Marsden, J. (2007) *An Evidence Base for Ophthalmic Nursing Practice*. London: John Wiley & Sons.

Martin, E.A. (2010) *Concise Colour Medical Dictionary*, 5th edn. Oxford: Oxford University Press.

Mawhinney, M. & Mariotti, A. (2000) Physiology, pathology and pharmacology of the male reproductive system. *Periodontology*, 61(1), 232–251.

McCall, R.E. & Tankersley, C.M. (2012) *Phlebotomy Essentials*, 5th edn. Philadelphia: Lippincott Williams & Wilkins.

McClelland, D. (2007) *Handbook of Transfusion Medicine*, 4th edn. London: Stationery Office.

McRobbie, D.W. (2007) *MRI from Picture to Proton*, 2nd edn. Cambridge: Cambridge University Press.

MDA (2000) *Single-Use Medical Devices: Implications and Consequences of Reuse. Device Bulletin 2000, 04*. London: Department of Health.

Meseguer, M., Garrido, N., Remohí, J., et al. (2003) Testicular sperm extraction (TESE) and ICSI in patients with permanent azoospermia after chemotherapy. *Human Reproduction*, 18(6), 1281–1285.

MHRA (2005) *Reporting Adverse Incidents and Disseminating Medical Device Alerts*. London: Medicines and Healthcare Products Regulatory Agency.

MHRA (2012) *All Medical Devices and Medicinal Products Containing Chlorhexidine*. London: Medicines and Healthcare Products Regulatory Agency.

Mims, C.A. (2004) *Medical Microbiology*, 3rd edn. Edinburgh: Mosby.

Mitchell Higgs, N. (2002) Personal protective equipment – improving compliance. All Points Conference. London.

Moini, J (2013) *Phlebotomy Principles and Practice*. Burlington, MA: Jones and Bartlett Learning.

Morris, W. (2011) *Complications*. In: Phillips, S., Collins, M. & Dougherty, L. (eds) *Venepuncture and Cannulation*. Oxford: John Wiley & Sons, pp.175–222.

Mulhall, J. (2013) Physiology of ejaculation. In: Mulhall, J., Applegarth, L., Oates, R. & Schlegel, P. (eds) *Fertility Preservation in Male Cancer Patients*. Cambridge: Cambridge University Press.

Murray, P.R. & Masur, H. (2012) Current approaches to the diagnosis of bacterial fungal bloodstream infections in the ITU. *Critical Care Medicine*, 40(12), 3277–3282.

Myers, F.E. & Reyes, C. (2011) Blood cultures: 5 steps to doing it right. *Nursing*, March, 62–63.

NAO (2003) *A Safer Place to Work: Improving the Management of Health and Safety Risks to Staff in NHS Trusts*. London: Stationery Office. Available at: www.nao.org.uk/report/a-safer-place-to-work-improving-the-management-of-health-and-safety-risks-to-staff-in-nhs-trusts/

NCCWCH & NICE (2004) *Fertility: Assessment and Treatment for People with Fertility Problems*. London: RCOG Press. Available at: www.rcog.org.uk/womens-health/clinical-guidance/fertility-assessment-and-treatment-people-fertility-problems

NHS Bowel Screening Programme (BSCP) (2008) *Evidence Summary: Patient Information for the NHS Bowel Cancer Screening Programme*. Sheffield: NHS Cancer Screening Programmes.

NHSBT (2011) *Blood and Transplant Matters*. Watford: NHSBT.

NHSBT (2012) *Blood and Transplant Matters*. Watford: NHSBT.

NHSCSP (2013) *Achievable Standards, Benchmarks for Reporting, and Criteria for Evaluating Cervical Cytopathology*, 3rd edn. Sheffield: NHS Cancer Screening Programmes.

NHS Employers (2007) Needlestick injury. In: *The Healthy Workplaces Handbook*. London: NHS Employers.

NICE (2013) *Fertility: Assessment and Treatment for People with Fertility Problems*. London: National Institute for Health and Clinical Excellence.

NMC (2010) *Record Keeping: Guidance for Nurses and* Midwives. London: Nursing and Midwifery Council. Available at: www.nmc-uk.org/Documents/NMC-Publications/NMC-Record-Keeping-Guidance.pdf

NMC (2013) *Consent*. London: Nursing and Midwifery Council. Available at: www.nmc-uk.org/Nurses-and-midwives/Regulation-in-practice/Regulation-in-Practice-Topics/consent/

NMC (2015) *The Code: Standards of Conduct, Performance and Ethics for Nurses and Midwives*. London: Nursing and Midwifery Council. Available at: www.nmc-uk.org/Documents/Standards/The-code-A4-20100406.pdf

NPSA (2007a) *Standardising Wristbands Improves Patient Safety*. London: National Patient Safety Agency.

NPSA (2007b) *Promoting the Safer Use of Injectable Medicines*. London: National Patient Safety Agency.

NPSA (2008) *Reducing Risk of Overdose with Midazolam Injection in Adults*. London: National Patient Safety Agency.

NPSA (2009) *Reducing Risk of Harm from Oral Bowel Cleansing Solutions*. London: National Patient Safety Agency.

Nudell, D. (1998) The micro-epididymal sperm aspiration for sperm retrieval: a study of urological outcomes. *Human Reproduction*, 13(5), 1260–1265.

O'Flynn, E.A.M., Wilson, A.R.M. & Michell, M.J. (2010) Image-guided breast biopsy: state-of-the-art. *Clinical Radiology*, 65(4), 259–270.

Owens, R.C. Jr. & Shorr, A.F. (2009) Rational dosing of antimicrobial agents: pharmacokinetic and pharmacodynamic strategies. *American Journal of Health-System Pharmacy*, 66(12 Suppl 4), S23–30.

Pacey, A. & Eiser, C. (2011) Banking sperm is only the first of many decisions for men: what healthcare professionals and men need to know. *Human Fertility*, 14(4), 208–217.

Pagkalis, S., Mantadakis, E., Mavros, M.N., Ammari, C. & Falagas, M.E. (2011) Pharmacological considerations for the proper clinical use of aminoglycosides. *Drugs*, 71(17), 2277–2294.

Panceri, M.L., Vegni, F.E., Goglio, A., et al. (2004) Aetiology and prognosis of bacteraemia in Italy. *Epidemiology and Infection*, 132(4), 647–654.

Pankhurst, C. & Coulter, W. (2009) *Basic Guide to Infection Prevention and Control and Dentistry*. Oxford: John Wiley & Sons.

Pannu, N. & Nadim, M.K. (2008) An overview of drug-induced acute kidney injury. *Critical Care Medicine*, 36(4 Suppl), S216–223.

Pellatt, G.C. (2007) Clinical skills: bowel elimination and management of complications. *British Journal of Nursing*, 16(6), 351–355.

Pellowe, C. (2009) Using evidence-based guidelines to reduce catheter related urinary tract infections in England. *Journal of Infection Prevention*, 10(2), 44–49.

Pennings, G. (2000) What are the ownership rights for gametes and embryos? *Human Reproduction*, 15(5), 979–986.

Perry, C. (2007) *Infection Prevention and Control*. Oxford: Blackwell Publishing

Philomina, B. (2009) Role of respiratory samples in the diagnosis of lower respiratory tract infections. *Pulmonology*, 11(1), 12–14.

Prandoni, D., Boone, M.H., Larson, E., Blane, C.G. & Fitzpatrick, H. (1996) Assessment of urine collection technique for microbial culture. *American Journal of Infection Control*, 24(3), 219–221.

Prestwich, R.J., Sykes, J., Carey, B., et al. (2012) Improving target definition for head and neck radiotherapy: a place for magnetic resonance imaging and 18-fluoride fluorodeoxyglucose positron emission tomography? *Clinical Oncology*, 24(8), 577–589.

Qaseem, A., Alguire, P., Dallas, P., et al. (2012) Appropriate use of screening and diagnostic tests to foster high-value, cost-conscious care. *Annals of Internal Medicine*, 156(2), 147–149.

Rajiv, D. (2007) Inhalation therapy in invasive and non-invasive mechanical ventilation. *Current Opinion in Critical Care*, 13(1), 27–38.

RCN (2010) *Standards for Infusion Therapy*, 3rd edn. London: Royal College of Nursing.

RCN (2012) *Wipe It Out: Essential Practice for Infection Prevention and Control: Guidance for Nursing Staff*. London: Royal College of Nursing.

Riley, S. (2008) *Colonoscopic Polypectomy and Endoscopic Mucosal Resection: A Practical Guide*. London: British Society of Gastroenterology. Available at: www.bsg.org.uk/pdf_word_docs/polypectomy_08.pdf

Roberts, J., Norris, R., Paterson, D.L. & Martin, J.H. (2011) Therapeutic drug monitoring of antimicrobials. *British Journal of Clinical Pharmacology*, 73(1), 27–36.

Rodgers, M., Nixon, J., Hempel, S., et al. (2006) Diagnostic tests and algorithms used in the investigation of haematuria: systematic reviews and economic evaluation. *Health Technology Assessment*, 10(18). Available at: www.hta.ac.uk/1363

Royal College of Physicians, RCR & RCOG (2007) *The Effects of Cancer Treatment on Reproductive Functions: Guidance on Management*. London: Royal College of Physicians. Available at: www.rcog.org.uk/files/rcog-corp/uploaded-files/WPREffectCancerReproduction2007.pdf

Royal College of Radiologists (2006) *Recommendations for Cross Sectional Imaging in Cancer Management*. London: Royal College of Radiologists.

Royal College of Radiologists (2010) *Standards for Intravascular Contrast Agent Administration to Adult Patients*. London: Royal College of Radiologists.

Royal College of Radiologists (2012) *iRefer, Making the Best Use of Clinical Radiology*. London: Royal College of Radiologists.

Runge, V.M., Nitz, W.R. & Schmeets, S.H. (2009) *The Physics of Clinical MR Taught Through Images*, 2nd edn. New York: Thieme.

Saied, N., Chopra, A. & Agarwal, B. (2012) Parenteral erythromycin for potential use to empty retained gastric contents encountered during upper gastrointestinal endoscopic procedures. *Open Journal of Gastroenterology*, 2, 119–123.

Saint, S. & Lipsky, B.A. (1999) Preventing catheter-related bacteriuria. *Archives of Internal Medicine*, 159, 800–808.

Saleem, S., Mani, V., Chadwick, M.A., Creanor, S. & Ayling, R.M. (2009) A prospective study of causes of haemolysis during venepuncture: torniquet time should be kept to a minimum. *Annals of Clinical Biochemistry*, 46, 244–246.

Sax, H., Allegranzi, B., Uçkay, I., et al. (2007) 'My five moments for hand hygiene': a user-centred design approach to understand, train, monitor and report hand hygiene. *Journal of Hospital Infection*, 67 (1), 9–21.

Schlegel, P. (1999) Testicular sperm extraction: microdissection improves sperm yield with minimal tissue excision. *Human Reproduction*, 14(1), 131–135.

Schmidt, L., Christensen, U. & Holstein, B.E. (2005) The social epidemiology of coping with infertility. *Human Reproduction*, 20(4), 1044–1052.

Schneeberger, C., van den Heuvel, E.R., Erwich, J.J., et al. (2013) Contamination rates of three urine-sampling methods to assess bacteriuria in pregnant women. *Obstetrics and Gynecology*, 121, 299.

Sha, S. (2005) Physiological and molecular pathology of aminoglycoside ototoxicity. *Volta Review*, 105(3), 325–335.

Shaw, M. (2001) Competence and consent to treatment in children and adolescents. *Advances in Psychiatric Treatment*, 7, 150–159.

Shaw, M., Lee, A. & Stollery, A. (2010) *Ophthalmic Nursing*, 4th edn. Oxford: Blackwell Publishing.

Shellock, F.G. & Spinazzi, A. (2008) MRI safety update 2008: part 2, screening patients for MRI. *American Journal of Roentgenology*, 191(4), 1140–1149.

Shore, A. & Sandoe, J. (2008) Blood cultures. *BMJ*, 16(4), 324–325.

SIGN (2008) *Management of Acute Upper and Lower Gastrointestinal Bleeding: A National Guideline*. Edinburgh: NHS Quality Improvement Scotland. Available at: www.sign.ac.uk/pdf/sign105.pdf

Simerville, J.A., Maxted, W.C. & Pahira, J.J. (2005) Urinalysis: a comprehensive review. *American Family Physician*, 71(6), 1153–1162.

Smith, G.D. & Watson, R. (2005) *Gastrointestinal Nursing*. Oxford: Blackwell.

Smith, J. (1998) The practice of venepuncture in lymphoedema. *European Journal of Cancer Care*, 7(2), 97–99.

Soyfoo, R. & Shaw, K. (2008) How to cut *Clostridium difficile* infection. *Nursing Times*, 104(25), 42–44.

Stuart, M. & White, M. (2012) Consent. *Anaesthesia & Intensive Care Medicine*, 13(4), 141–144.

Suissa, A., Bentur, S., Lachter, J., et al. (2012) Outcome and complications of colonoscopy: a prospective multicenter study in northern Israel. *Diagnostic and Therapeutic Endoscopy*, 2012, 612542.

Swallow, V., Hughes, J., Roberts, D. & Webb, N. (2012) Assessing children's and parents' opinions on salivary sampling for therapeutic drug monitoring. *Nurse Researcher*, 19(3), 32–37.

Swan, E. (2005) *Colorectal Cancer*. London: Whurr.

Tacconelli, E. (2009) Antimicrobial use: risk driver of multidrug resistant microorganisms in healthcare settings. *Current Opinion in Infectious Diseases*, 22(4), 352–358.

Tannapfel, A., Dienes, H.P. & Lohse, A.W. (2012) The indications for liver biopsy. *Deutsches Arzteblatt International*, 109(27-28), 477–483.

Taylor, I., van Cutsem, E. & Garcia-Aguilar, J. (2009) *Colorectal Disease*, 3rd edn. Abingdon: Health Press.

Thomas, N. (2008) *Renal Nursing*, 3rd edn. Edinburgh: Baillière Tindall Elsevier.

Thomsen, H.S., Webb, J.A.W. & Aspelin, P. (eds) (2009) *Contrast Media: Safety Issues and ESUR Guidelines*, 2nd rev. edn. Berlin: Springer.

Thomson, A. (2004) Why do therapeutic drug monitoring? *Pharmaceutical Journal*, 273(7310), 153–155.

Thomson, L. (2000) Tracheal suctioning of adults with an artificial airway. *Best Practice*, 4(4), 1–7.

Thomson, R. (2002) Use of microbiology laboratory tests in the diagnosis of infectious disease. In: Tan, J.S. (ed.) *Expert Guide to Infectious Diseases*. Philadelphia: American College of Physicians, American Society of Internal Medicine.

Tilmouth, T. & Tilmouth, S. (2009) *Safe and Clean Care: Infection Prevention and Control for Health and Social Care Students*. London: Reflect Press.

Tobin, C.M., Darville, J.M., Thomson, A.H., et al. (2002) Vancomycin therapeutic drug monitoring: is there a consensus view? The results of a UK National External Quality Assessment Scheme (UK NEQAS) for Antibiotic Assays questionnaire. *Journal of Antimicrobial Chemotherapy*, 50(5), 713–718.

Tursi, A. (2013) Colonoscopy by nurse endoscopists: the right answer for the growing demand for colonoscopy in clinical practice? *Endoscopy*, 45(05), 408.

Van den Broek, U., Vandermeeren, M., Vanderschueren, D., Enzlin, P. & Demyttenaere, K. (2013) A systematic review of sperm donors: demographic characteristics, attitudes, motives and experiences of the process of sperm donation. *Human Reproduction Update*, 19(1), 37–51.

Van Putten, P.G., ter Borg, F., Adang, R.P., et al. (2012) Nurse endoscopists perform colonoscopies according to the international standard and with high patient satisfaction. *Endoscopy*, 44(12), 1127–1132.

Walker, R. & Whittlesea, C. (2012) *Clinical Pharmacy and Therapeutics*, 5th edn. London: Churchill Livingstone.

Warekois, R.S., Robinson, R. & Sommer, S.R. (2007) *Phlebotomy: Worktext and Procedures Manual*, 2nd edn. St Louis, MO: Elsevier Saunders.

Waugh, A. & Grant, A. (2010) *Ross and Wilson Anatomy and Physiology in Health and Illness*, 11th edn. Edinburgh: Churchill Livingstone.

Wegerhoff, F. (2006) It's a bug's life – specimen collection, transport, and viability. *Microbe*, 1, 180–184.

Weinstein, S. & Plumer, A.L. (2007) *Plumer's Principles & Practice of Intravenous Therapy*, 8th edn. Philadelphia: Lippincott Williams & Wilkins.

Weishaupt, D., Köchli, V.D. & Marincek, B. (2006) *How does MRI work? An Introduction to the Physics and Function of Magnetic Resonance Imaging*, 2nd edn. Berlin: Springer.

Weller, B.F. (2009) *Bailliere's Nurses' Dictionary*, 25th edn. Edinburgh: Elsevier.

Weston, D. (2008) *Infection Prevention and Control: Theory and Clinical Practice for Healthcare Professionals*. Oxford: John Wiley & Sons.

Williams, D. (2010) Sperm banking and the cancer patient. *Therapeutic Advances in Urology*, 2(1), 19–34.

Winter, G. (2005) It's probably a virus. *Practice Nurse*, 30(3), 26–28.

Witt, B. (2011) Vein selection. In: Phillips, S., Collins, M. & Dougherty, L. (eds) *Venepuncture and Cannulation*. Oxford: John Wiley & Sons, pp.91–107.

Wo, J.Y. & Viswanathan, A.N. (2009) Impact of radiotherapy on fertility, pregnancy, and neonatal outcomes in female cancer patients. *International Journal of Radiation Oncology, Biology, Physics*, 73(5), 1304–1312.

Answers

Learning Activity 10.1 Scenario: Gaining consent

You have been asked to take a sputum sample from a patient with a productive cough.

Before undertaking this procedure what information should you give to the patient in order to gain their verbal consent?

- Informing the patient of the rationale for specimen collection.
- What the procedure will involve (refer to Procedure guideline 10.20: Sputum sampling).
- Ascertaining their level of understanding.
- How long the results may take to be processed, how the results will be made available and the implications these results may have on their care.

Learning Activity 10.3 Case study: Swab sampling

Mr Wills is a 68-year-old man who has been admitted to hospital for IV antibiotics via his GP. Following surgery to his abdomen 3 weeks ago, he now has a dehisced laparotomy wound which is showing signs of infection (red, inflamed, producing pus). He has been admitted to your unit and, as part of his risk assessment, requires an MRSA screen.

1 Before carrying out the MRSA screen, what should you do to prepare Mr Wills?
  - Provide information about the procedure and why it is required.
  - Gain verbal consent prior to commencing the procedure.
  - As he has been in hospital recently, check his recent records for previous MRSA screening results.

2 Which is the most important area of the body to take a swab sample from when screening for MRSA?
  - The nose.

3 What other areas of Mr Wills' body would you need to take swab samples from?
  - Axilla.
  - Groin.
  - Abdominal wound.
  - Check whether he has any other broken areas of skin that should also be swabbed.

4 Once you have taken the swabs, what should you do with them in order to ensure they are ready for collection?
- Ensure there is a completed laboratory form.
- Ensure that each specimen swab is correctly labelled with the patient's full details.
- Ensure that specimens are placed in a plastic bag along with the laboratory form.
- Ensure that the specimen bag is placed in the designated collection box.

Learning Activity 10.4 Scenario: Preparing a patient for a colonoscopy

A patient has called your unit from home and is asking you to explain what they need to do prior to coming in for their colonoscopy in 2 days time. They have been given some medication to take at home before being admitted but don't understand what they are allowed to eat and until when.

Based on the evidence provided within this chapter, jot down some bullet points of what your advice would be to them around food and fluid intake.

- Two days prior to the colonoscopy, specific light foods may be eaten, such as steamed white fish, and others avoided, such as high-fibre foods.
- On the day before the colonoscopy, breakfast from the approved food groups may be eaten while drinking plenty of clear fluids. The period of bowel cleansing generally should not be longer than 24 hours.
- On the day of the procedure patients can drink tea/coffee with no milk 4 hours before, and water up to 2 hours before.

Now Test Yourself What have you learnt?

1 Gram staining is used to guide the choice of antimicrobial therapy.
A True
B False

2 What is histology?
A A method for testing antibiotic sensitivity
B The detection of antigens of antibodies within serum
C The study of cells and tissues in the body
D The use of a culture media to grow and identify bacteria from a specimen

3 In relation to specimen collection, what infection control precautions should be taken?
A The use of personal protection equipment
B Hand hygiene
C Waste management
D All of the above

4 In venepuncture, which vein(s) are used only when the others are not accessible?
A Median cubital vein
B Cephalic vein
C Basilic vein
D Metacarpal veins

5 Venepuncture does not require an aseptic technique.
A True
B False

6 What is the most common complication of venepuncture?
A Nerve injury
B Arterial puncture
C Haematoma
D Fainting

7 How many sputum samples are required in cases of suspected Mycobacterium tuberculosis?
A 1
B 2
C 3
D 4

8 How long should a patient fast for, prior to a gastroscopy, to ensure the stomach is relatively empty?
A At least 2 hours
B At least 4 hours (Always check local guidelines)
C At least 6 hours
D At least 8 hours

9 What is a cystoscopy?
A Examination of cells under a microscope
B An investigation examining a lump in the body
C An investigation examining the bladder and urethra
D An investigation examining the colon and rectum

10 Which of the following does not use ionizing radiation so can be used for repeated examinations?
A X-ray
B MRI scan
C CT scan
D None of the above, they all use ionizing radiation

Observations

11

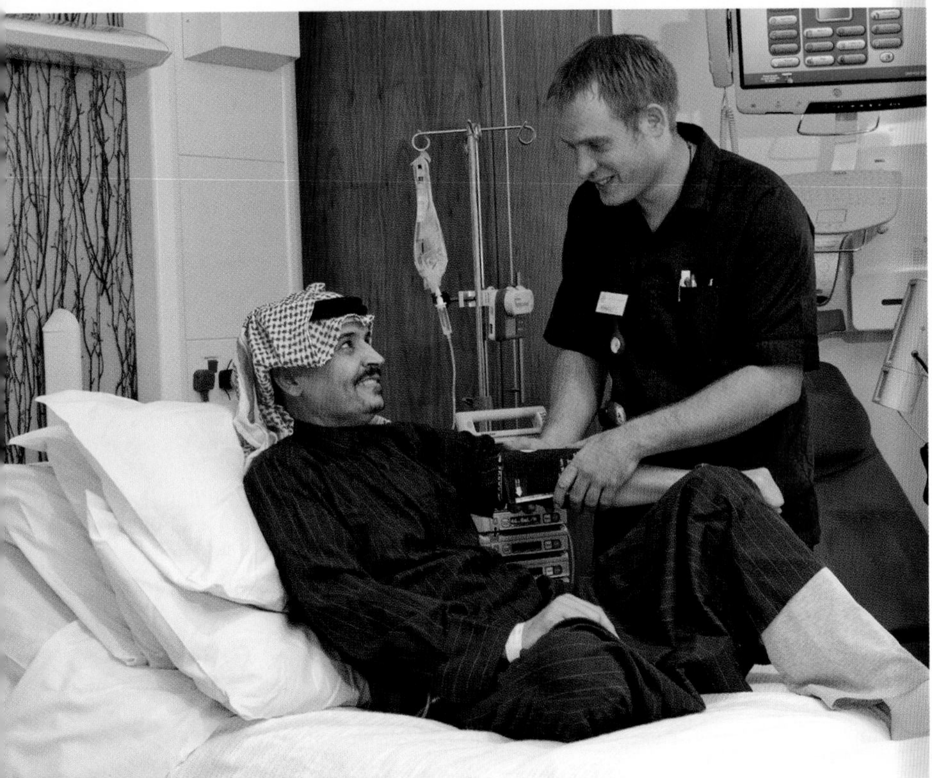

By reading this chapter and undertaking the learning activities within it, you should be able to:

1 Identify the need for a range of observations and how they inform the assessment process.
2 Demonstrate an understanding of the rationale, legal and professional issues for a range of key observations performed by nurses.
3 Demonstrate understanding of the procedure that should be undertaken for each observation and identify common problems that may arise.

Procedure guidelines

The Royal Marsden Manual of Clinical Nursing Procedures: Student Edition, Ninth Edition. Edited by Lisa Dougherty, Sara Lister and Alexandra West-Oram

Overview

The following observations will be discussed: pulse, blood pressure, respiration, peak flow, temperature, urinalysis, blood glucose, central venous pressure and neurological observations. For each observation discussed, we provide a definition, the rationale, legal and professional issues, procedural guidelines and a guide to problem solving.

Observations

DEFINITIONS

The term 'observation' refers to the physical assessment of a patient, including assessment of wounds, intravenous therapy, wound drains, pain and vital signs collection and specialized assessments such as neurological observations (Zietz and McCutcheon 2006). 'Vital signs' are traditionally used in the context of the collection of a cluster of physical measures, such as pulse, respiration, temperature and blood pressure, and more recently pulse oximetry.

EVIDENCE-BASED APPROACHES

Rationale

The taking of patient observations forms a fundamental part of the assessment process. The interpretation of the data from the assessment is vital in determining the level of care a patient requires, providing an intervention or treatment and preventing a patient deteriorating from an otherwise preventable cause (Wheatley 2006) (see Chapter 2: Assessment and discharge).

Indications

Observations are usually undertaken:

- to act as a baseline to help determine the patient's usual range (Bickley and Szilagyi 2009)
- to assist in recognizing if a patient's condition is deteriorating or indeed improving (Kisiel and Perkins 2006).

Principles of care

Adult patients in acute hospital settings should have:

- observations taken when they are admitted or initially assessed (including on transfer to a ward setting from critical care or transfer from one ward to another)
- a clearly documented plan which identifies which observations should be taken and how frequently subsequent observations should be done. This plan should take into consideration:
  - the diagnosis
  - plan for patient's treatment
  - any co-morbidities which may affect their health (NICE 2007a).

All patients in hospital should have their observations taken at least once every 12 hours, unless specified otherwise by senior staff (NICE 2007a).

Methods of measuring, recording and documenting observations

To assist with the identification of critically ill patients and those at risk of deterioration, physiological scoring systems were introduced (DH 2000, Wheatley 2006), referred to as 'track and trigger systems'. Examples include the National Early Warning System (NEWS) (RCP 2012) (Figure 11.1), medical emergency team (MET) scoring and patient-at-risk team (PART) score (DH 2001, Hodgetts et al. 2002). These scoring systems rely on nursing staff performing basic patient observations, that is, respiratory rate, heart rate, blood pressure, temperature and fluid balance (Wheatley 2006) and informing medical staff/critical outreach team of deviations from normal.

Data entry in terms of entering a patient's score can be recorded on:

- a paper medical record system
- a clinical documentation system with 'computers on wheels' workstation, or
- a clinical documentation system with a tablet PC/hand-held device affixed to the vital signs monitor.

Hand-held devices have been reported to contribute to the management of vulnerable patient groups. These devices have been shown to improve accuracy and timeliness in the recording of vital signs when the activity is delegated to non-registered healthcare support workers such as technicians (Wager et al. 2010). Hand-held computer methods have demonstrated speed and accuracy of charting when compared to the traditional pen/paper method where incorrect entries or omissions have been reported to occur (Prytherch et al. 2006).

Early warning systems help ward nurses to improve and focus their recognition of patients who may need further support and monitoring (DH 2000). As there are several track and trigger scoring systems in use, including locally adapted versions, it is important that time is taken to accurately calculate an individual patient's vital sign parameters in relation to the individual tool.

Currently no track and trigger system is validated for use across all diagnoses (Kyriacos et al. 2011). There is concern with the use of NEWS, in the assessment of patients with brain dysfunction, due to the use of 'alert, verbal, pain, unresponsive (AVPU)' components (Teasdale 2012). Within the field of haematology, emphasis is placed on the increase in referrals to critical outreach teams when using a system that has not been modified for a specific patient population (Teasdale 2012). It is also suggested that any track and trigger system should be used as an adjunct to identifying patients developing critical illness (Mulligan 2010). In order to avoid 'alarm fatigue', any early warning system escalation levels should be used in conjunction with clinical judgement and a holistic assessment rather than being relied on as an absolute measure of the patient's condition (Critical Care Stakeholders Forum and National Outreach Forum 2007).

Critical care outreach teams are now available in many hospitals following the recommendation of a review of the critical care services in England (DH 2000).Where such teams exist, they must be informed of any patients who are deteriorating or at risk of deteriorating, so that they can provide support to ward staff, assess the patient and avert critical care admissions (DH 2000).

A tool that assists with structuring and standardizing communication when reporting concern is the Situation-Background-Assessment-Recommendation (SBAR) tool (Figure 11.2). SBAR is an easy-to-remember, concrete mechanism useful for framing any conversation, especially critical ones, requiring a clinician's immediate attention and action. It gives an easy and focused way to set expectations for what will be communicated and how, between members of the team. This is essential for developing teamwork and fostering a culture of patient safety (Woodhall 2008). For an example of how to use the SBAR tool in clinical practice, refer to the Institute for Innovation and Improvement website (2008).

Anticipated patient outcomes

Physiological observations are extremely important in recognizing if a patient's condition is deteriorating or indeed improving (Kisiel and Perkins 2006).

LEGAL AND PROFESSIONAL ISSUES

Nurses are accountable and responsible for providing optimum care for their patients. The Nursing and Midwifery Council's (NMC) *The Code* provides the main source of professional accountability for nurses (NMC 2015). It is essential that nursing staff objectively examine the information gathered from assessments and observations, including the patient's baseline,

National Early Warning Score (NEWS)*

PHYSIOLOGICAL PARAMETERS	3	2	1	0	1	2	3
Respiration rate	≤8		9 – 11	12 – 20		21 – 24	≥25
Oxygen saturations	≤91	92 – 93	94 – 95	≥96			
Any supplemental oxygen		Yes		No			
Temperature	≤35.0		35.1 – 36.0	36.1 – 38.0	38.1 – 39.0	≥39.1	
Systolic BP	≤90	91 – 100	101 – 110	111 – 219			≥220
Heart rate	≤40		41 – 50	51 – 90	91 – 110	111 – 130	≥131
Level of consciousness				A			V, P, or U

*The NEWS initiative flowed from the Royal College of Physicians' NEWS Development and Implementation Group (NEWSDIG) report, and was jointly developed and funded in collaboration with the Royal College of Physicians, Royal College of Nursing, National Outreach Forum and NHS Training for Innovation

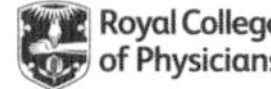

NHS
Training for Innovation

Figure 11.1 **NEWS – National Early Warning Scoring System (Royal College of Physicians 2012). In some settings, patients will have an impaired level of consciousness as a consequence of sedation, e.g. following surgical procedures. Thus, the assessment of consciousness level and the necessity to escalate care should be considered in the time-limited context of the appropriateness of the consciousness level in relation to recent sedation. For patients with known hypercapneic respiratory failure due to chronic obstructive pulmonary disease (COPD), recommended British Thoracic Society target saturations of 88–92% should be used. These patients will still 'score' if their oxygen saturations are below 92 unless the score is 'reset' by a competent clinical decision maker and patient-specific target oxygen saturations are prescribed and documented on the patient's chart and in the clinical notes. All supplemental oxygen, when administered, must be prescribed.** ***Reproducing this chart:*** **please note that this chart must be reproduced in colour, and should not be modified or amended.** ***Source:*** **Reproduced with permission from the Royal College of Physicians. National Early Warning Score (NEWS): Standardising the assessment of acute illness severity in the NHS. Report of a working party. London: RCP, 2012. Copyright © 2012 Royal College of Physicians.**

as well as any information previously recorded (Crouch and Meurier 2005).

For nurses' own professional accountability and for the achievement of safe, effective and proficient care of the patient, it is essential that nurses are able to discuss (using physiological rationale) the potential reasons for the observations they have recorded (Kisiel and Perkins 2006). Professional accountability demands more than nurses just undertaking observations. It is about nurses being able to interpret them and then to take appropriate action (Kisiel and Perkins 2006).

Observations should be taken by staff who have undergone the appropriate training regarding the procedure, not only so that they are able to perform the procedure correctly and accurately but also, crucially, so they are able to act on and understand the clinical relevance of the results (NICE 2007a). The degree of training should be suitable to the level of care that the practitioner is providing and the equipment they are using (NICE 2007a). However, all staff should have competencies in relation to measuring, monitoring, interpretation and when to respond promptly (NICE 2007a).

PRE-PROCEDURAL CONSIDERATIONS

Equipment

All practitioners need to be aware of the strengths and limitations of the devices they are using and need to have adequate training on the use of all equipment. They must ensure that the devices are validated, checked, maintained and recalibrated regularly according to the manufacturer's instructions (NICE 2011a). In addition to this, the device should only be used as the manufacturer intends; the user needs to know how it works normally, be able to use it effectively and safely (MHRA 2006).

Prior to the procedure, check when the device was last serviced. All devices, manual or automated, are only accurate if they are working and used correctly. Most trusts have the devices checked annually and the date documented on the device and staff should check this and report when it is due for servicing (Woodrow 2004).

Pulse (heart rate)

DEFINITION

The pulse is a pressure wave that is transmitted through the arterial tree with each heart beat following the alternating expansion and recoil of arteries during each cardiac cycle (Marieb and Hoehn 2010). A pulse is strongest in the arteries closest to the heart, becomes weaker in the arterioles and disappears in the capillaries altogether (Tortora and Derrickson 2011). A pulse can be palpated in any artery that lies close to the surface of the body. The radial artery at the wrist is easily accessible and therefore the radial pulse is frequently used, but there are several other clinically important arterial pulse points, such as the carotid,

Royal Marsden NHS Foundation Trust
SBAR report to Doctor or Outreach Nurse about a critical situation
Hospital Number: Date: Time:

Situation
I am calling about <patient name and location>. Consultant:
The patient's resuscitation status is For Resus? Not for Resus?
The problem I am calling about is__________________________.
The patient was admitted with__________________________.
I have informed__________________________the Nurse in Charge.
☐ I am afraid the patient is going to arrest.
I have just assessed the patient personally:
Observations are: BP_____, Pulse_____, Respirations_____and temperature_____.
Blood Glusose___mmol/l, Potassium____mmol/l, Magnesium____mmol/l.
Pain = Site / Duration Epidural Y/N or PCA Y/N
I am concerned about the:
Observation in the red or yellow bands on the observation chart
☐ Blood pressure because it is ☐ over 150 systolic or ☐ less than 100 systolic or
☐ 30 mmHg below usual
☐ Pulse because it is ☐ over 110 or ☐ less than 50
☐ Respiration because it is ☐ less than 9 or ☐ over 21
☐ Temperature because it is ☐ less than 36°C or over 38°C
☐ Conscious level / general condition is deteriorating
☐ Urine output is less than 0.5ml/kg/hr
☐ Oxygenation
☐ The MEWS is______________.

Background
The patient's mental status is:
☐ Alert and orientated to person, place and time
☐ Confused and ☐ cooperative or ☐ non-cooperative
☐ Agitated
☐ Lethargic but conversant and able to swallow
☐ Drowsy and not talking clearly and possibly not able to swallow
☐ Comatose ☐ Eyes closed ☐ Not responding to stimulation.
The skin is:
☐ Warm and dry
☐ Pale / Clammy
☐ Sweaty
☐ Extremities are cold
☐ Extremities are warm
The patient ☐ is not or ☐ is on oxygen.
☐ The patient has been on____(l/min) or (%) oxygen for____minutes (hours)
☐ The oximeter is reading____%
☐ The oximeter does not detect a good pulse and is giving erratic readings
The patient has ☐ no access ☐ a peripheral cannula ☐ a CVAD.

Assessment
☐ I think the problem is__________________________.
☐ I don't know what the problem is but the patient is deteriorating.
☐ The patient has fallen in the ward

Recommendation
☐ Patient to be seen within the next 30 minutes
☐ Patient to be seen now
☐ Would like approval of my course of action which is_______________.
Are any tests needed:
☐ Do you need any tests?__________________________.
If a change in treatment is ordered then ask:
☐ How often do you want the observations done?
☐ If the patient does not get better when would you want us to call again?

Call initiated by Nurse:__________________To:__________________.

Figure 11.2 **Situation-Background-Assessment-Recommendation (SBAR) tool.**

femoral and brachial plexus (Marieb and Hoehn 2010, Tortora and Derrickson 2011) (Figure 11.3).

ANATOMY AND PHYSIOLOGY

In health, the arterial pulse is one of the measurements used to assess the effects of activity, postural changes and emotions on the heart rate. In ill health, the pulse can be used to assess the effects of disease, treatments and response to therapy. Each time the heart beats, it pushes blood through the arteries. The pumping action of the heart causes the walls of the arteries to expand and distend, causing a wave-like sensation which can then be felt as the pulse (Marieb and Hoehn 2010).

The pulse is measured by lightly compressing the artery against firm tissue and counting the number of beats in a minute. The pulse is palpated to note the following:

- rate
- rhythm
- amplitude.

Rate

A person's pulse rate can be influenced by several factors including age, gender, exercise, pyrexia, medications, hypovolaemia, stress, positioning, pathology, hormones and electrolytes (Field

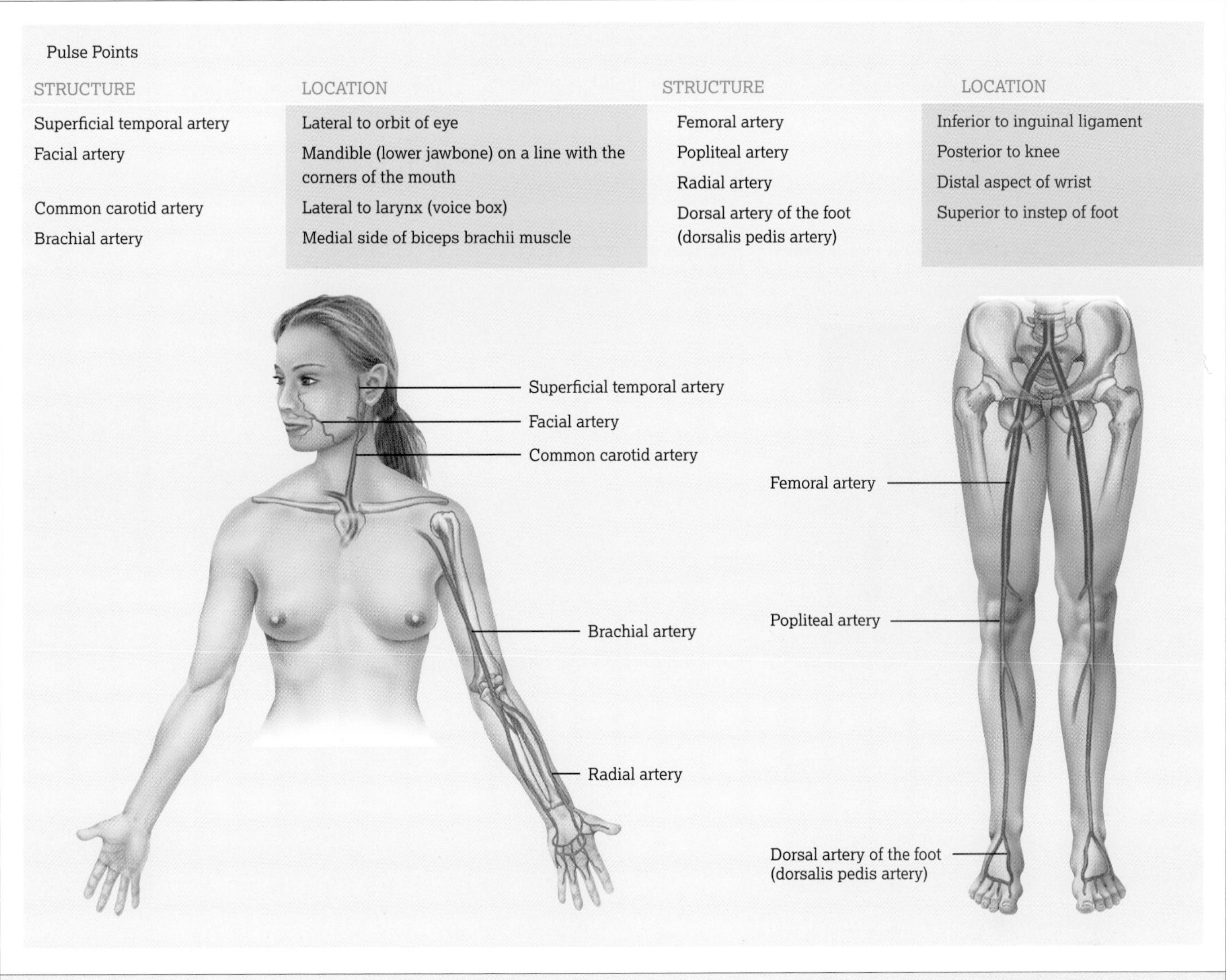

Pulse Points

STRUCTURE	LOCATION	STRUCTURE	LOCATION
Superficial temporal artery	Lateral to orbit of eye	Femoral artery	Inferior to inguinal ligament
Facial artery	Mandible (lower jawbone) on a line with the corners of the mouth	Popliteal artery	Posterior to knee
Common carotid artery	Lateral to larynx (voice box)	Radial artery	Distal aspect of wrist
Brachial artery	Medial side of biceps brachii muscle	Dorsal artery of the foot (dorsalis pedis artery)	Superior to instep of foot

Figure 11.3 **Pulse points.** ***Source:*** **Tortora and Derrickson (2011). Reproduced with permission from John Wiley & Sons.**

2008, Kozier et al. 2008). The approximate range is illustrated in Table 11.1.

The pulse may vary depending on posture. For example, the pulse of a healthy man may be around 66 beats per minute when he is lying down; this increases to 70 beats per minute when sitting up and 80 beats per minute when he suddenly stands (Marieb and Hoehn 2010).

The pulse rate of an individual with a healthy heart tends to be relatively constant. However, when blood volume drops suddenly or when the heart has been weakened by disease, the stroke volume declines and cardiac output is maintained only by increasing the rate of the heart beat.

Cardiac output (CO) is the amount of blood pumped out by each ventricle in 1 minute. It is the product of heart rate (HR) and stroke volume (SV). Stroke volume is defined as the volume of blood pumped out by one ventricle with each beat. Using normal resting values for HR (75 beats/minute) and SV (70 mL/beat), the average adult cardiac output can be calculated:

$$\begin{aligned} CO &= HR \times SV = 75 \text{ beats/min} \times 70 \text{ mL/beat} \\ &= 5250 \text{ mL/min} = 5.25 \text{ L/min} \end{aligned}$$

The heart rate and hence pulse rate are influenced by various factors acting through neural, chemical and physically induced homeostatic mechanisms (see Figure 11.4 for factors that increase cardiac output).

- Neural changes in heart rate are caused by activation of the sympathetic nervous system which increases heart rate, while parasympathetic activation decreases heart rate (Patton and Thibodeau 2009).
- Chemical regulation of the heart is affected by hormones (adrenaline and thyroxine) and electrolytes (sodium, potassium and calcium) (Patton and Thibodeau 2009). High or low levels of electrolytes, particularly potassium, magnesium and calcium, can cause an alteration in the heart's rhythm and rate.
- Other factors that influence heart rate are age, sex, exercise and body temperature (Marieb and Hoehn 2010).

Table 11.1 **Normal pulse rates per minute at various ages**

Age	Approximate range
1 week–3 months	100–160
3 months–2 years	80–150
2–10 years	70–110
10 years–adult	55–90

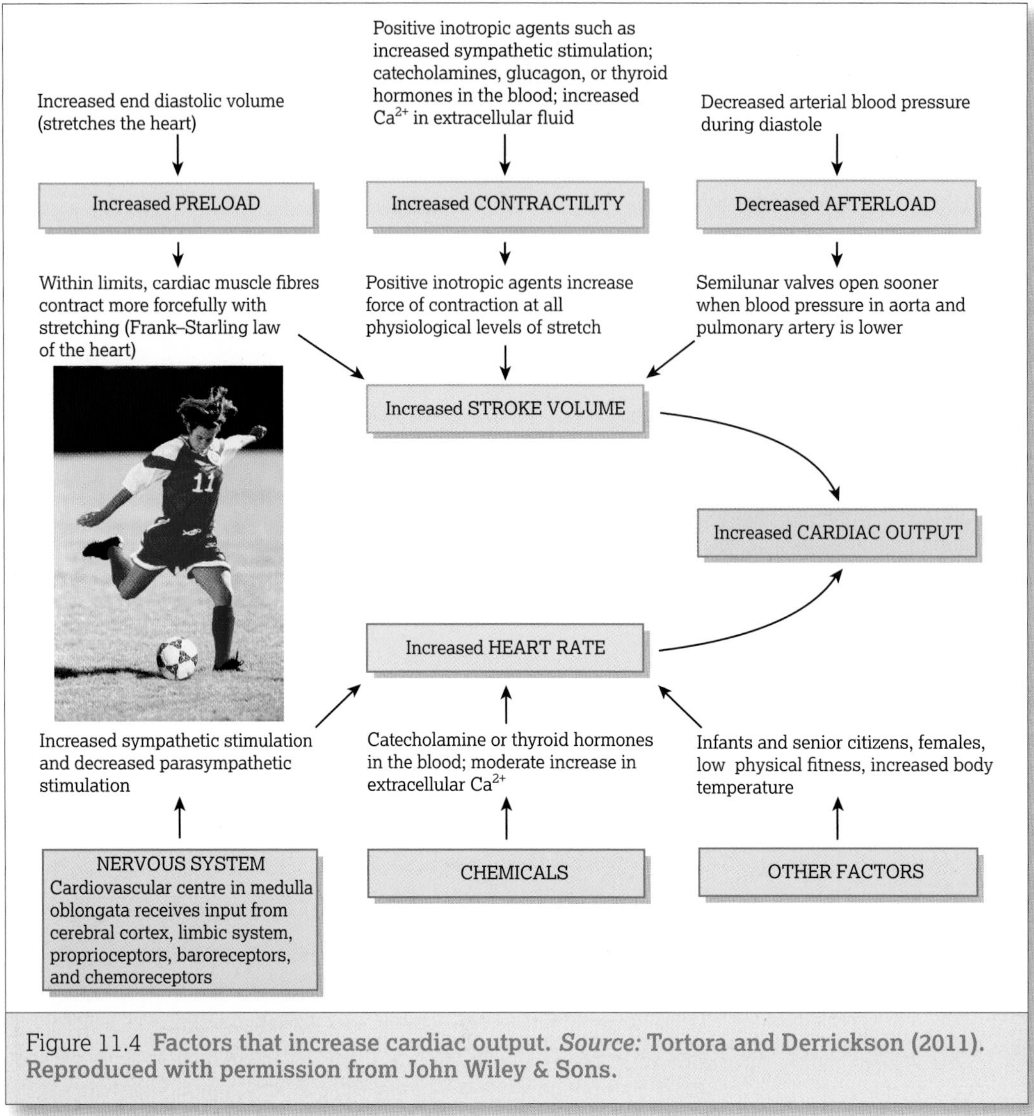

Figure 11.4 **Factors that increase cardiac output.** ***Source:*** **Tortora and Derrickson (2011). Reproduced with permission from John Wiley & Sons.**

Tachycardia

This is an abnormally fast heart rate, over 100 beats per minute in adults. It may result from an elevated body temperature, stress, certain drugs or heart disease (Marieb and Hoehn 2010). Persistent tachycardia is considered pathological because tachycardia occasionally promotes fibrillation (Marieb and Hoehn 2010).

Bradycardia

This is a heart rate slower than 60 beats per minute (Marieb and Hoehn 2010). It may be the result of a low body temperature, certain drugs or parasympathetic nervous system activation. It is also found in fit athletes when physical and cardiovascular conditioning occurs (Marieb and Hoehn 2010). This results in hypertrophy of the heart with an increase in its stroke volume, leading to a lower resting heart rate but with the same cardiac output (Marieb and Hoehn 2010). If persistent bradycardia occurs in an individual as a result of ill health, this may result in inadequate blood circulation to body tissues. Bradycardia is often a warning of brain oedema after head trauma (Marieb and Hoehn 2010) and is one of the indications of raised intracranial pressure.

Rhythm

The pulse rhythm is the sequence of beats. In health, these are regular. The co-ordinated action of the muscles of the heart in producing a regular heart rhythm is due to the ability of cardiac muscle to contract inherently without nervous control (Marieb and Hoehn 2010). The co-ordinated action of the muscles in the heart results from two physiological factors.

- Gap junctions in the cardiac muscles which form interconnections between adjacent cardiac muscles and allow transmission of nervous impulses from cell to cell (Marieb and Hoehn 2010).
- Specialized nerve-like cardiac cells that form the nodal system. These initiate and distribute impulses throughout the heart, so that the heart beats as one unit (Marieb and Hoehn 2010). The nodal system is composed of the sinoatrial node, atrioventricular node, atrioventricular bundle and the Purkinje fibres.

The sinoatrial node is the pacemaker, initiating each wave of contraction. This sets the rhythm for the heart as a whole (Figure 11.5). Its characteristic rhythm is called *sinus rhythm*.

In patients younger than 40 years, irregularity may be linked to breathing, when the heart rate increases on inspiration and decreases on expiration. Although this is rarely noticeable in adults (Higgins 2008a), it is normal and is known as sinus arrhythmia (Woods et al. 2005). Defects in the conduction system of the heart can cause irregular heart rhythms, or arrhythmias, resulting in unco-ordinated contraction of the heart.

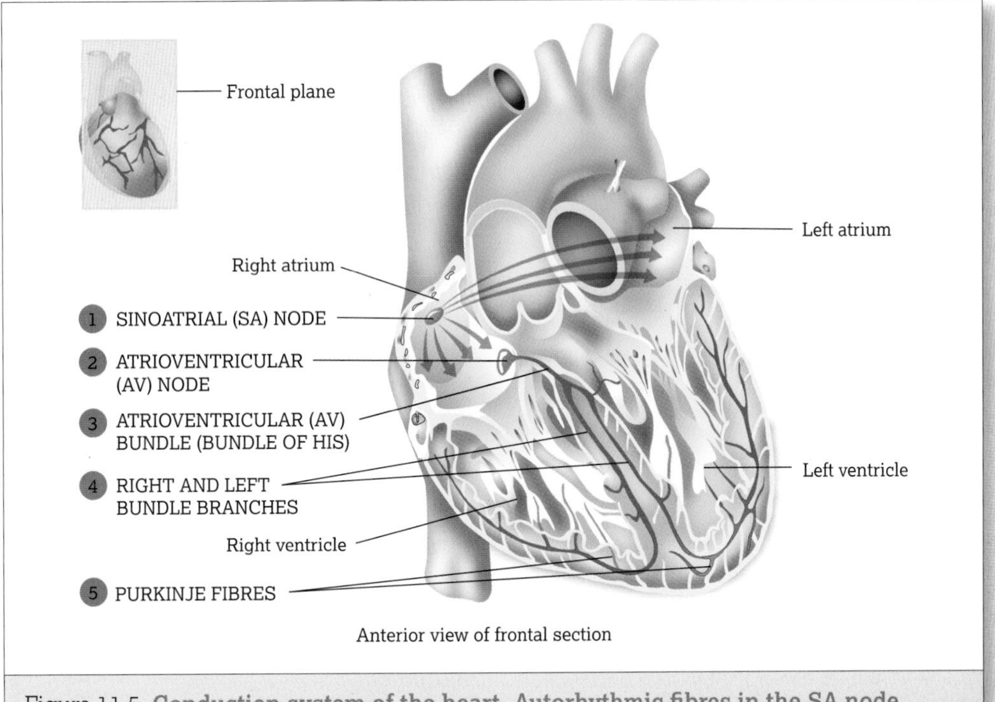

Figure 11.5 **Conduction system of the heart. Autorhythmic fibres in the SA node, located in the right atrial wall, act as the heart's pacemaker, initiating cardiac action potentials that cause contraction of the heart's chambers. The conduction system ensures that the chambers of the heart contract in a co-ordinated manner. *Source:* Tortora and Derrickson (2011). Reproduced with permission from John Wiley & Sons.**

Fibrillation

Fibrillation is a condition of rapid and irregular contractions. A fibrillating heart is ineffective as a pump (Marieb and Hoehn 2010).

Atrial fibrillation is a disruption of rhythm in the atrial areas of the heart occurring at extremely rapid and unco-ordinated intervals. The rapid impulses result in the ventricles not being able to respond to every atrial beat and, therefore, the ventricles contract irregularly (Adam and Osborne 2005). The incidence of atrial fibrillation in the general population is approximately 1%, rising to 10% in people aged over 70 years (Goodacre and Irons 2002).

There are many causes of this condition, but the following are the most common:

- ischaemic heart disease
- acute illness
- electrolyte abnormality
- thyrotoxicosis.

Atrial fibrillation can complicate or cause many other medical conditions, including stroke and heart failure (Navas 2003). If poorly managed, patients are at increased risk of arterial thromboembolism and ischaemic stroke (Jevon 2007a). If the patient has a fast ventricular rate, some contractions may not be strong enough to transmit a pulse wave that is detectable at the radial artery. In this instance, checking the radial pulse is an unreliable method of assessing ventricular rate. Simultaneous monitoring of the apex beat and radial pulse is advisable in patients with atrial fibrillation, because it will determine the ventricular rate more reliably and identify whether there is an apex beat–radial pulse deficit (Jevon 2007a).

This procedure requires two nurses and is described in 'Assessing gross pulse irregularity'.

Ventricular fibrillation is an irregular heart rhythm characterized by chaotic contraction of the ventricles at very rapid rates (Adam and Osborne 2005). Ventricular fibrillation results in cardiac arrest and death if not reversed with defibrillation and the injection of adrenaline. The cause of this condition is often myocardial infarction (MI), electric shock, acidosis, electrolyte disturbances and hypovolaemia (RCUK 2010).

Body fluids are good conductors of electricity so it is possible through electrocardiography to observe how the currents generated are transmitted through the heart. The electrocardiograph provides a graphic representation and record (electrocardiogram [ECG]) of electrical activity as the heart beats – see 'Twelve-lead electrocardiogram (ECG)'. The ECG makes it possible to identify abnormalities in electrical conduction within the heart. Changes in the pattern or timing of the deflection in the ECG may indicate problems with the heart's conduction system, such as those caused by MI (Marieb and Hoehn 2010). For examples of normal and abnormal ECGs, see 'Twelve-lead electrocardiogram (ECG)'.

Amplitude

Amplitude is a reflection of pulse strength and the elasticity of the arterial wall. This varies because of the alternating strong and weak ventricular contractions (Bickley and Szilagyi 2009). The flexibility of the artery of the young adult feels different from the hard artery of the patient suffering from arteriosclerosis. It takes some clinical experience to appreciate the differences in amplitude. However, it is important to be able to recognize major changes such as the faint flickering pulse of the severely hypovolaemic patient or the irregular pulse in cardiac arrhythmias.

Assessing gross pulse irregularity

Paradoxical pulse is a pulse that markedly decreases in amplitude during inspiration. On inspiration, more blood is pooled in the lungs and so decreases the return to the left side of the heart; this affects the consequent stroke volume. A paradoxical pulse is usually regarded as normal, although in conjunction with such features as hypotension and dyspnoea, it may indicate cardiac tamponade (Bickley and Szilagyi 2009), hypovolaemia, and severe airway obstruction or tension pneumothorax (Wong 2007).

When there is a gross pulse irregularity, a stethoscope may be used to assess the apical heartbeat. This is done by placing the diaphragm of the stethoscope over the apex of the heart and counting the beats for 60 seconds. A second nurse should record the radial pulse at the same time. The deficit between the two should be noted using, for example, different colours on the patient's chart to indicate the apex and radial rates (Docherty 2002).

EVIDENCE-BASED APPROACHES

Rationale

The pulse is taken for the following reasons.

- To gather information on the heart rate, pattern of beats (rhythm) and amplitude (strength) of pulse.
- To determine the individual's pulse on admission as a base for comparing future measurements.
- To monitor changes in pulse (Marieb and Hoehn 2010).

Indications

Conditions in which a patient's pulse may need careful monitoring are described below.

- Post-operative and critically ill patients require monitoring of the pulse to assess for cardiovascular stability. The patient's pulse should be recorded pre-operatively in order to establish a baseline and to make comparisons. Hypovolaemic shock post surgery from the loss of plasma or whole blood results in a decrease in circulatory blood volume. The resulting acceleration in heart rate causes a tachycardia that can be felt in the pulse. The greater the loss in volume, the threadier the pulse is likely to feel.
- Blood transfusions require careful monitoring of the pulse as an incompatible blood transfusion may lead to a rise in pulse rate early in the transfusion (British Society for Haematology 2009) (see Chapter 7: Nutrition, fluid balance and blood transfusion) as an incompatible blood transfusion may lead to a rise in pulse rate.
- Patients with local or systemic infections or inflammatory reactions require monitoring of their pulse to detect sepsis/severe sepsis. This is characterized by a decrease in the mean arterial pressure (MAP) and a rise in pulse rate (Marieb and Hoehn 2010).
- Patients with cardiovascular conditions require regular assessment of the pulse to monitor their condition and the efficacy of medications.

Methods of pulse measurement

Manual

The pulse is measured by lightly compressing the artery against firm tissue and counting the number of beats in a minute and/or by auscultation of the apex of the heart with a stethoscope.

Electronic

Automated electronic equipment such as a pulse oximeter, blood pressure recording devices, 12-lead ECG or continuous cardiac monitoring may be used to determine the pulse. However, even where the patient has continuous ECG monitoring, it is still essential to manually feel for a pulse to determine amplitude and volume and whether the pulse is irregular. In pulseless electrical activity (PEA), normal sinus rhythm is shown on the monitor but a pulse is not palpable (Levine et al. 2008).

PRE-PROCEDURAL CONSIDERATIONS

Equipment

Pulse can be measured by:

- *stethoscope* (apical pulse)
- *electronic pulse measurement device* (pulse oximeter): a small electronic device, consisting of a probe which is placed onto the end of a finger to record pulse rate.

Specific patient preparation

Ideally a patient should be at rest for 20 minutes before trying to obtain an accurate pulse. Strenuous activity will result in falsely elevated readings (Rawlings-Anderson and Hunter 2008).

Procedure guideline 11.1 **Pulse measurement**

Essential equipment

- A watch that has a second hand
- Alcohol handrub
- Observations chart
- Black pen
- A stethoscope (if counting the apical beat)
- Electronic pulse measurement device, for example pulse oximeter, blood pressure measuring device or cardiac monitor

Pre-procedure

Action	Rationale
1 Wash hands and dry hands.	To prevent cross-infection (Fraise and Bradley 2009, **E**).
2 Explain and discuss the procedure with the patient.	To ensure that the patient understands the procedure and gives their valid consent (NMC 2013, **C**).

Procedure

Action	Rationale
3 Where possible, measure the pulse under the same conditions each time.	To ensure continuity and consistency in recording (Alexis 2010, **E**).
4 Ensure that the patient is comfortable and relaxed. Ideally the patient should refrain from physical activity for 20 minutes before pulse is measured.	To ensure that the patient is comfortable. **E** Strenous activity will result in falsely elevated readings (Rawlings-Anderson and Hunter 2008, **E**).
5 Place the first and second or in addition the third finger along the appropriate artery and apply light pressure until the pulse is felt (**Action figure 5**).	The fingertips are sensitive to touch. Practitioners should be aware that the thumb and forefinger have pulses of their own and therefore these may be mistaken for the patient's pulse (Docherty and Coote 2006, **E**).
6 Press gently against the peripheral artery being used to record the pulse.	The radial artery is usually used as it is often the most readily accessible (Bickley and Szilagyi 2009, **E**).

7 If the apical heart rate requires recording, place a stethoscope on the left midclavical, 4th–5th intercostal space on left midclavicular line (typically under the breast area) and listen to the heart beat (Alexis 2010).	The apical heart rate is usually used if someone's heart rate is irregular to give a more accurate count of the pulse, in children, and prior to the initiation of some cardiac medications (Alexis 2010, **E**).
8 The pulse should be counted for 60 seconds.	Sufficient time is required to detect irregularities in rhythm or volume. If the pulse is regular and of good volume subsequent readings may be taken for 30 seconds and then doubled to give beats per minute. If the rhythm or volume changes on subsequent readings then pulse must be taken for 60 seconds (Rawlings-Anderson and Hunter 2008, **E**).
9 Record the pulse rate on appropriate documentation. Additional factors such as the rhythm, volume and skin condition (dry, sweaty or clammy) may be described in the patient's nursing notes.	To monitor differences and detect trends; any irregularities should be brought to the attention of the appropriate senior nursing and medical teams (NMC 2010, **C**). Additional qualitative characteristics of the pulse may aid diagnosis of the patient's condition (Rawlings-Anderson and Hunter 2008, **E**).

Post-procedure

10 Discuss result and any further action with the patient.	To involve the patient in their care and provide assurance of a normal result or explain the actions to be undertaken in the event of an abnormal result. **E**, **P**
11 Wash and dry or decontaminate with alcohol handrub hands and/or stethescope.	To prevent cross-infection (Fraise and Bradley 2009, **E**).

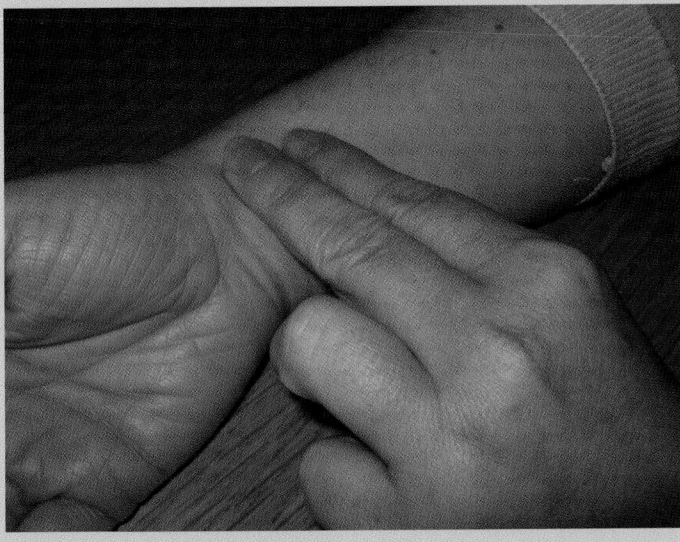

Action Figure 5 Taking a pulse.

Problem-solving table 11.1 **Prevention and resolution (Procedure guideline 11.1)**

Problem	Cause	Prevention	Action
No pulse palpable.	Incorrect positioning of fingers.	Refer to Figure 11.3 for palpation sites.	Place 2 or 3 fingers over the appropriate artery and lightly depress against the tissue or bone. Try alternative sites such as brachial or carotid artery.
Absent or faint pulse.	Poor perfusion.	Assess patient's existing co-morbidities for further information. Identify any causes of hypovolaemia.	Inform medical team if the patient is cardiovascularly compromised.
	Obstruction, for example clot.	Perform a venous thromboembolism (VTE) risk assessment for your patient on admission (NICE 2007b) and ensure appropriate preventive measures in place, for example antiembolism stockings, mechanical devices applying intermittent pneumatic pressure, for example Flowtron, or injections of low molecular weight heparin preparations (Lees and McAuliffe 2010).	Perform a neurovascular assessment, assessing all pulse sites to determine compromised area. Also feel for warmth and sensation and capillary refill to provide further information on the degree of vascular sufficiency.

(continued)

Problem-solving table 11.1 **Prevention and resolution (Procedure guideline 11.1)** ***(continued)***

Problem	Cause	Prevention	Action
Pulse too fast and irregular to palpate manually.	Patient may be in an abnormal rhythm.	Haemodynamic assessment, monitoring and maintenance of electrolyte balance.	Use electronic recording device. New-onset tachycardia and irregular rhythms should prompt a full set of observations: BP, respiratory rate, oxygen saturation and temperature. It is essential to perform a 12-lead ECG and have this reviewed by a doctor.

POST-PROCEDURAL CONSIDERATIONS

Documentation

The pulse should be recorded in the patient's notes on the institution's approved observation chart. The recording should be dated and timed so that the pulse trend may be viewed easily as part of ongoing patient monitoring.

Learning Activity 11.1

Scenario: Pulse measurement

You have been asked to check the pulse rate of a patient who has atrial fibrillation.

How would you go about doing this in order to ensure an accurate measurement?

See the end of the chapter for the answers.

Twelve-lead electrocardiogram (ECG)

DEFINITION

Electrical activity in the heart can be monitored and amplified with an instrument called an electrocardiogram (Marieb and Hoehn 2010). The ECG provides a graphical representation of the heart's electrical conduction and myocardial excitation (Marieb and Hoehn 2010).

The 12-lead ECG is a routine clinical examination which can be performed by a range of healthcare professionals (Crawford and Doherty 2008). When used correctly and in the context of the patient's clinical history, it is a valuable diagnostic tool used to ascertain information about the electrophysiology of the heart (Crawford and Doherty 2008, Marieb and Hoehn 2010). Electrical changes take place as the cardiac muscle contracts and relaxes; the 12-lead ECG records the electrical activity of the heart from 12 viewpoints or 'leads' through 10 cables attached to electrodes on the patient's chest and limbs – note that in this setting 'leads' refers to viewpoints rather than the cables or wires that connect the patient to the machine (Jevon 2009). The 12 different views of cardiac electrical activity show the three-dimensional electrical activity occurring in the heart (Woodrow 2009b).

ANATOMY AND PHYSIOLOGY

All myocardial cells are able to spontaneously generate impulses and initiate the cardiac electrical cycle without the need for external stimulation; this is known as automaticity (Docherty 2005). Cardiac conduction normally begins in the sinoatrial (SA) node, located in the wall of the right atrium. This is the heart's natural pacemaker as it normally initiates impulses at a faster rate than other myocardial cells, generating impulses at a rate of 60–100 beats per minute (Woodrow 2009a). The impulse generated by the SA node spreads through the atrial muscle fibres (depolarization), causing atrial contraction, to the atrioventricular (AV) node. The AV node acts as a gateway into the ventricular conduction system, delaying impulses for approximately 0.1–0.2 seconds and creating a short period of electrical standstill before the depolarization spreads through the AV node into the ventricles, allowing the atria to finish contracting before ventricular contraction commences (Woodrow 2009a).

From the AV node, the impulse travels rapidly through specialized conduction tissue in the ventricles, firstly through the bundle of His, along the left and right bundle branches and then more slowly through the mass of ventricular muscle along the Purkinje fibres, resulting in the powerful ventricular contraction (Tortora and Derrickson 2011). The conduction pathway of the heart is shown in Figure 11.5. The normal ECG waveform depicts five deflections or waves known as P, Q, R, S and T waves (Figure 11.6). The small P wave reflects atrial depolarization, the large QRS reflects the rapid spread of depolarization from the AV node to the Purkinje fibres through the ventricles, and the T wave reflects ventricular repolarization – the return of the ventricular muscle to its resting state. Atrial repolarization is not graphically represented on the ECG as it is hidden in the QRS complex (Sharman 2007).

EVIDENCE-BASED APPROACHES

The 12 leads

The 12-lead ECG shows 12 views of cardiac electrical activity, recording the impulses generated by the heart by recording the electrical energy from electrodes placed on specific areas of the

Figure 11.6 **Normal electrocardiogram or ECG (lead II). P wave = arterial depolarization; QRS complex = onset of ventricular depolarization; T wave = ventricular repolarization.** ***Source:*** **Tortora and Derrickson (2011). Reproduced with permission from John Wiley & Sons.**

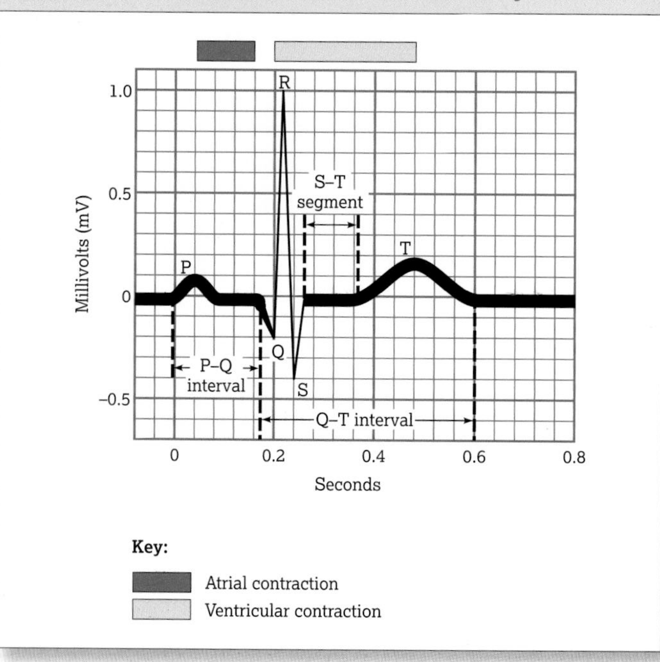

Table 11.2 **Precordial electrode anatomical positions**

Electrode	Position
V1 (C1)	Fourth intercostal space at the right sternal edge
V2 (C2)	Fourth intercostal space at the left sternal edge
V3 (C3)	Midway between V2 and V4
V4 (C4)	Fifth intercostal space in the midclavicular line
V5 (C5)	Left anterior axillary line at same horizontal level as V4
V6 (C6)	Left midaxillary line at same horizontal level as V4 and V5

Source: Reproduced with permission from SCST (2014).

Table 11.3 **Limb electrode positions**

Electrode	Position
Right arm limb lead (RA, red)	Right forearm, proximal to wrist
Left arm limb lead (LA, yellow)	Left forearm, proximal to wrist
Left leg limb lead (LL, green)	Left lower leg, proximal to ankle
Right leg limb lead (RL, black)	Right lower leg, proximal to ankle

Source: Reproduced with permission from SCST (2014).

body (Khan 2004). Six of these views are recorded from the four limb electrodes that use a combination of three electrodes placed on three limbs (right arm, left arm and left leg) along with one neutral electrode placed on the right leg to reduce interference or noise. These three electrodes together create a triangle around the heart, sometimes called Einthoven's triangle (Woodrow 2009b).

The other six views are recorded from the six chest electrodes that are placed in a horizontal plane along the chest wall – these are also known as precordial leads (Khan 2004).

- Limb leads (I, II, III, aVR, aVL, aVF)
- Chest (precordial) leads (V1–V6)

Electrode placement

Table 11.2 describes the anatomical location of each chest electrode and Figure 11.7 shows the standard position of the six chest electrodes (SCST 2014). The limb electrodes should be placed just proximally to the wrist and ankle bones unless there is a clinical reason, such as amputation, burns or surgical wounds, which prevents this; ECGs recorded using any other limb position must be clearly labelled as such to account for any changes that might affect interpretation (SCST 2014). It does not matter if the electrode is positioned on the inside or outside of the limb – position the patient comfortably and use the most accessible aspect for electrode placement (Crawford and Doherty 2010). Table 11.3 describes the anatomical location of each limb electrode.

The 12 different leads (or viewpoints) look at the heart from different directions. Each lead will record a positive or negative wave depending on which direction the impulse is travelling in relation to the observing lead; a positive wave will be recorded if the impulse is travelling towards the observing lead, a negative wave will be recorded if the impulse is travelling away from the observing lead (Docherty 2003). Correct electrode placement

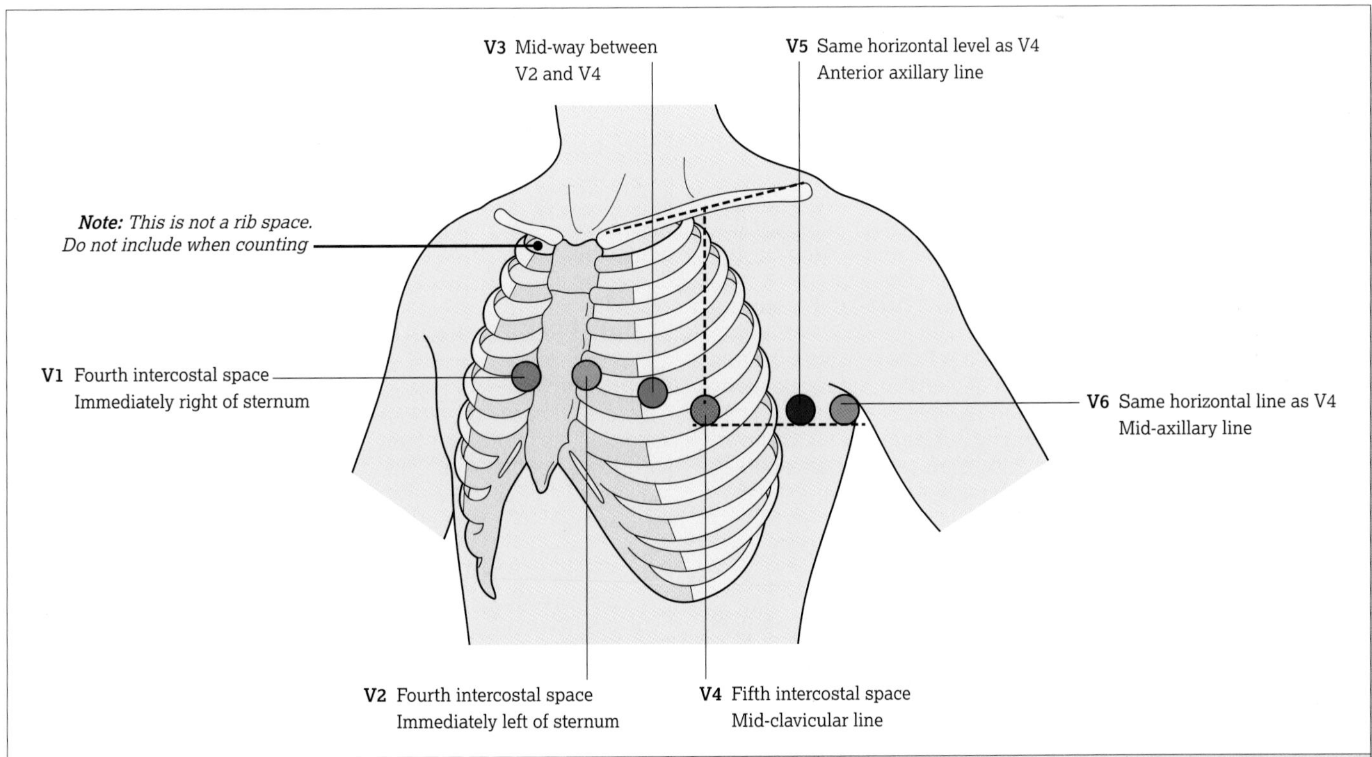

Figure 11.7 **Position of chest electrodes for 12-lead ECG.** ***Source:*** **SCST (2014). Reproduced with permission from The Society for Cardiological Science and and Technology (www.scst.org.uk/)**

Figure 11.8 **Mason–Likar 12-lead ECG system.**

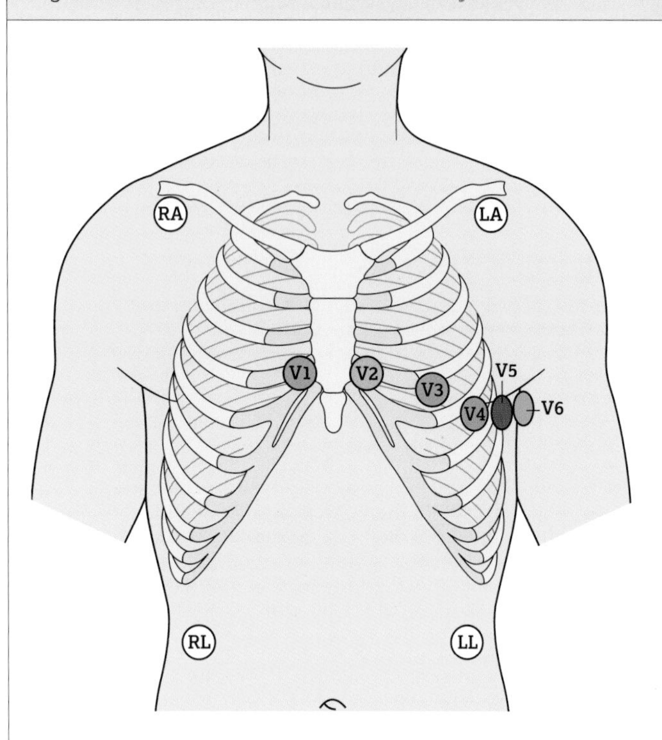

Figure 11.9 **Three-lead ECG electrode placement.**

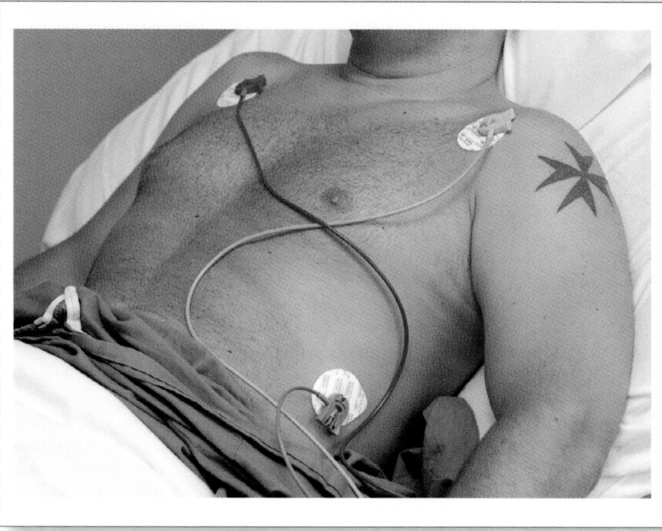

is essential to ensure an accurate ECG recording is obtained. Incorrect electrode placement can lead to morphology changes or alter the amplitude of waves, meaning that ECG changes may be due to artefact rather than physiological abnormalities which may lead to misdiagnosis of apparent abnormalities (Crawford and Doherty 2010).

An alternative positioning of the limb electrodes on the torso, known as the Mason–Likar 12-lead ECG system (Figure 11.8), can however be used in areas where continuous 12-lead ECG monitoring is required, as the waveforms are easily viewed without interference from limb movement (Pelter 2008). However, it should be noted that the QRS complexes are slightly different in amplitude and axis when repositioned on the torso (Drew et al. 2004) and so any deviation from the standard 12-lead electrode placement should be clearly documented on the ECG trace.

In acute clinical areas where continuous cardiac monitoring is required, the three limb electrodes can be placed according to Figure 11.9. The monitor should be set to display lead II as this runs from the right arm to the left foot and so is normally positive, showing the greatest deflection of all the limb leads in a normal heart (Docherty 2002, Khan 2004). The 12-lead ECG is, however, the gold standard for diagnostic purposes and is described in Procedure guideline 11.2: Electrocardiogram.

Rationale

Indications

A 12-lead ECG may be performed electively or to aid diagnosis following any acute deterioration or after any cardiac event such as:

- a baseline prior to surgery or course of medical treatment
- sudden onset of chest pain, shortness of breath
- haemodynamic disturbance
- cardiac rhythm or rate changes
- suspected acute coronary syndrome
- suspected or confirmed myocardial infarction
- cardiac surgery
- percutaneous coronary intervention
- after successful cardiopulmonary resuscitation (Jevon 2010, Woodrow 2009b).

Serial 12-lead ECGs may be required in patients known to have cardiac toxicity, developing myocardial ischaemia or infarction.

Ambulatory ECG monitoring, also known as a 24-hour tape, may be used to record and analyse the patient's heart rhythm during normal daily activities. This is a specialist test and is useful to capture abnormalities that might be missed with a standard 12-lead ECG. Typically the ECG is recorded continuously over a 24–48-hour period (ACC/AHA 2001).

Contraindications

There are no absolute contraindications to performing a 12-lead ECG, but this should not be undertaken in any patient in whom the delay to obtain the ECG would compromise or delay immediate care such as an arrhythmia requiring immediate shock or cardiac arrest (RCUK 2011).

LEGAL, PROFESSIONAL AND RISK ISSUES

Competencies

Any healthcare professional who has been trained and assessed as competent can perform a 12-lead ECG in line with local hospital policy. However, its analysis and diagnosis are usually undertaken by medical staff or specialist nurses (Sharman 2007).

PRE-PROCEDURAL CONSIDERATIONS

Equipment

- *12-lead ECG machine*: consisting of 10 cables which are connected to electrodes fixed to the body. The machine detects and amplifies the electrical impulses that occur at each heart beat and records the waveforms on to graphed paper, by a stylus, or on to a computer. All ECG machines should be tested to ensure accurate data are recorded. Calibration is

Figure 11.10 **ECG calibration verification signal.** ***Source:*** **Crawford and Doherty (2010). Reproduced with permission from Mark Allen Publishing Ltd.**

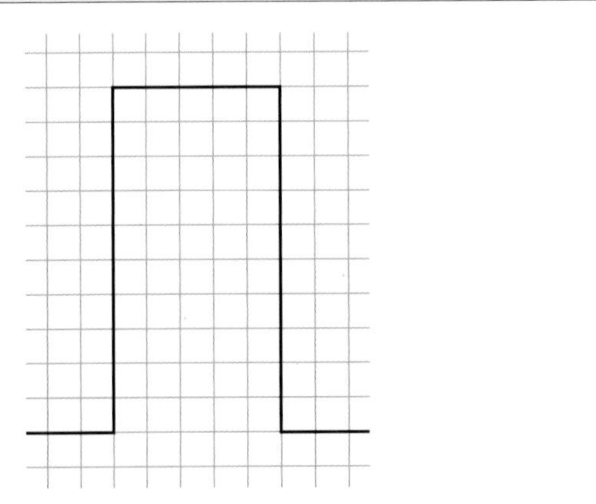

usually undertaken by qualified engineers; however, this should be verified in the clinical setting to confirm that when a voltage of known magnitude (1 mV over 0.2 seconds) is put through the machine, the machine produces an expected deflection (10 mm) and the paper moves at the correct speed (25 mm per second). This calibration verification should be printed at the beginning or end of each line of the ECG as a box shape (Crawford and Doherty 2010, Woodrow 2009b); see Figure 11.10.

- *Electrodes:* the 10 electrodes are attached to the patient's body in the positions described above and in Procedure guideline 11.2: Electrocardiogram. The leads (cables from the ECG machine) clip onto these electrodes and record 12 views of the heart using different combinations of electrodes to measure various signals from the heart.
- *ECG paper:* ECG graph paper is divided into small squares of 1 mm each and five small squares make up a large square. The horizontal axis of the ECG paper represents time and the vertical axis represents amplitude. Standard ECG paper speed is 25 mm per second (mm/s) – each small square equals 0.04 seconds, one large square equals 0.2 seconds and therefore five large squares equal 1 second. ECG machines are calibrated so that the deflection amplitude of cardiac conduction is measured in mm/mV – 10 small squares or two large squares show a deflection of 1 mV (10 mm/mV); see Figure 11.10 (Crawford and Doherty 2010, Khan 2004, Levine et al. 2008).
- *Filter:* filters are electronic devices that remove artefacts from the ECG, improving the tracing obtained. ECG machines have internal pre-programmed filters set by the manufacturer or clinical engineers, which cannot be altered by clinical staff, and control panel filters which can be deployed by clinical staff. Theoretically, if all low-frequency and high-frequency signals were removed, a good-quality ECG would be obtained but the ECG would be of no diagnostic value because the filter distorts the ECG waveforms (Crawford and Doherty 2010). Control panel filters are therefore not recommended for routine use as they distort the waveforms, but they may be required if all other actions to reduce artefact have been unsuccessful (SCST 2014). If the filter is used this must be clearly documented on the ECG.
- *Ambulatory ECG recorder:* a continuous recording of an ECG over a 24–72-hour period, which enables a patient to continue with their daily activities.

All ECG machines should be used and maintained in accordance with the manufacturer's instructions. ECG machines form part of a department's emergency equipment and should always be available in good working order. After use, the ECG machine should be cleaned, returned to its storage location and plugged into a mains electrical supply to charge the internal battery ready for use in an emergency (Metcalfe 2000). Any malfunctioning machine should be taken out of clinical use until repair or service can be undertaken by the relevant department, in accordance with local policy. All clinical incidents relating to ECG machines should be reported through the organization's incident reporting system.

Specific patient preparation

Female patients

The conventional placement of the lateral chest leads (V4, V5 and V6) is beneath the left breast, and whilst there is emerging evidence to support the positioning of these electrodes over the breast, it is currently insufficient to suggest a change of procedure (SCST 2014). It is also worth noting that the fifth intercostal space can only be found by lifting the breast and therefore it is logical to position the electrodes here (Crawford and Doherty 2010).

Dextrocardia

Dextrocardia is any situation where the heart is located within the right side of the chest rather than the left. It may be associated with the condition situs inversus where all of the patient's organs are in a mirror image position.

The SCST (2014) suggests the following approach to ECG recording for patients with suspected or known dextrocardia.

- Dextrocardia should be suspected if the ECG shows an inverted P wave in lead I (P-axis >90°) together with poor R wave progression across the chest leads. In this case a second ECG should be recorded with the chest electrodes positioned on the right side of the chest using the same intercostal spacing and anatomical landmarks to provide a 'true' ECG representation. The limb lead complexes will continue to appear inverted, demonstrating the abnormal location of the heart, but the repositioned chest leads will now show the appropriate R wave progression. The revised electrode positions should be clearly documented on the ECG and both ECGs should be retained for inclusion in the patient's notes.
- Patients who are known to have dextrocardia should have the ECG recorded with the limb electrodes in the usual position and the chest electrodes placed across the right side of the chest as above. Note that swapping of the right and left limb electrodes will 'normalize' the appearance of the limb leads and when repositioning electrodes, it is imperative that the ECG is clearly annotated to describe the new positions of the electrodes (for example, V3R, V4R, etc.) to prevent the possibility of dextrocardia being overlooked.

Education

The patient must give their consent for the ECG to be performed (NMC 2013) and be adequately prepared for the procedure (Jevon 2010). The procedure should be explained and the patient's privacy and dignity ensured; the rationale for the ECG should be given, explaining that it will be useful to aid diagnosis. Reassurance should be provided, explaining that an ECG is not a painful procedure. The patient should be positioned comfortably either lying or sitting, preferably in a semi-recumbent position (at an angle of 45°) with their head supported (Jevon 2010, SCST 2014). It is important that the patient is relaxed and keeps still during the procedure to reduce interference and artefact and facilitate recording of a clear and stable ECG trace (Jevon 2010, SCST 2014).

Procedure guideline 11.2 Electrocardiogram

Essential equipment

- ECG machine with chest and limb leads labelled respectively, for example LA to left arm, V1 to first chest lead
- Disposable electrodes (check that these are in date and not dry prior to use)
- Alcohol handrub

Pre-procedure

Action	Rationale
1 Wash hands using bactericidal soap and water or bactericidal alcohol handrub, and dry.	To minimize the risk of infection (Fraise and Bradley 2009, **E**).
2 Explain the procedure to the patient and gain their consent.	To ensure that the patient understands the procedure and is able to give their valid consent (NMC 2013, **C**; Roberts 2002, **E**).
3 Ensure that the patient is comfortably positioned in semi-recumbent position. Any variations to standard recording techniques must be highlighted on the ECG recording (for example 'ECG recorded whilst patient in wheelchair').	To ensure optimal recording and comfort of the patient (Roberts 2002, **E**). The ECG may vary depending on the patient's position so it is important to note this on the ECG (SCST 2014, **C**).
4 Clean limb and chest electrode sites. If necessary, prepare skin by cleaning with soap and water or clipping hairs.	To ensure good grip and therefore good contact between skin and electrode – this results in less electrical artefact (Roberts 2002, **E**; SCST 2014, **C**). Shaving should be avoided due to the risk of infection if the skin is grazed (Sharman 2007, **E**) or bleeding if the patient is on anticoagulation therapy (Pelter 2008, **E**).

Procedure

Action	Rationale
5 Apply the limb and chest electrodes as described in Tables 11.2 and 11.3 and Figure 11.7. For advice on placement in females and known cardiac abnormalities see 'Specific patient preparation'.	To obtain a three-dimensional view of the electrical activity of the heart (Woodrow 2009b, **E**). Following a standard arrangement ensures consistency between recordings and prevents invalid recordings and misdiagnosis (SCST 2014, **C**).
6 Attach the cables from the ECG machine to the electrodes, checking that the cables are connected correctly and to the relevant electrode.	To obtain the ECG recording (Roberts 2002, **E**). To ensure the correct polarity in the ECG recording (Roberts 2002, **E**).
7 Ensure that the cables are not pulling on the electrodes or lying over each other. Offer the patient a gown or sheet to place over their exposed chest.	To reduce electrical artefact and to obtain a clear ECG recording (Roberts 2002, **E**). To ensure patient dignity and reduce shivering (SCST 2014, **C**).
8 Ask patient to relax and refrain from movement.	To obtain the optimal recording by the reduction of artefact from muscular movement (Jevon 2010, **E**; SCST 2014, **C**).
9 Encourage the patient to breathe normally and not to speak while the recording is being taken.	Speaking can alter the recording (Roberts 2002, **E**).
10 Switch the machine on and enter the patient's details into the machine.	To ensure that it is clear which patient the ECG was taken from (NMC 2010, **C**).
11 Check that the machine is functioning correctly and that calibration is 10 mm/mV.	To ensure standard recording to aid interpretation (Crawford and Doherty 2010, **E**; SCST 2014, **C**).
12 Commence the recording.	To obtain ECG. **E**
13 In the case of artefact or poor recording, check electrodes and connections.	To ensure optimal recording (Jevon 2010, **E**).
14 During the procedure give reassurance to the patient.	To ensure the patient is informed and reassured (Roberts 2002, **E**).
15 Detach the ECG print-out and ensure the recording is labelled with the patient's name, hospital number, date and time. Also include any diagnostic information (i.e. if the patient has chest pain during the recording) and deviations to the standard electrode placement.	To ensure that the ECG forms part of the correct patient's medical record (NMC 2010, **C**). To help with diagnosis and interpretation (Jevon 2010, **E**; SCST 2014, **C**).
16 If the ECG is irregular or abnormal, record a 10-second rhythm strip, usually from lead II.	To assist with interpretation if there have been any acute rhythm disturbances (SCST 2014, **C**).

Post-procedure	
17 Inform patient that the procedure is completed and help to remove the electrodes.	To ensure that the patient can relax and that the electrodes are removed to prevent them drying out and causing any skin irritation. **E**
18 Wash hands using bactericidal soap and water or bactericidal alcohol handrub, and dry.	To minimize the risk of infection (Fraise and Bradley 2009, **E**).
19 Inform relevant nursing and medical staff that the ECG has been completed – show the recording to the person who will analyse the recording.	To enable relevant nursing and medical staff to use the ECG data in their care planning and treatment (NMC 2010, **C**).
20 File the ECG recording in the appropriate documentation.	To ensure appropriate record keeping and aid continuity of care (NMC 2010, **C**).
21 Clean the ECG machine in accordance with manufacturer's recommendations. Return it to its storage place and plug it in to mains electricity to keep the battery fully charged.	The ECG machine forms part of a department's emergency equipment and should always be available and in good working order with a charged battery for use in an emergency (Metcalfe 2000, **E**).

Problem-solving table 11.2 **Prevention and resolution (Procedure guideline 11.2)**

Problem	Cause	Prevention	Action
Unable to turn on the ECG machine.	Low battery.	Ensure the ECG is left on continuous charge when not in use.	Connect to mains electricity – the ECG will function once it is connected to a power supply.
ECG machine is working but the rhythm display is blank.	Loose connection.	Carefully store the cables after use to prevent damage.	Check that each lead is connected to the electrode clip and that the base of the cable is connected to the ECG machine.
	Electrode stickers peel off from the patient's skin.	The patient may have used body lotion or the skin may be clammy, making adhesion difficult.	Cleanse the electrode sites with soap and water to remove the lotion or reduce skin moisture and allow to dry. Reapply new electrode stickers.
		The patient may have a lot of chest hair which makes adhesion difficult.	If the patient has a lot of chest hair, try to push the hair out of the way when applying stickers to make a better contact; reinforcement with tape may be required. If this is unsuccessful, ask the patient for permission to clip the hair at the electrode sites, cleanse to remove loose hair, allow to dry and apply new electrode stickers.
	The electrode stickers may be intact but there is still no rhythm – the patient's skin may be excessively dry and flaky.	Identify underlying causes and severity of dry skin and address them with the multidisciplinary team as appropriate.	With the patient's consent, perform vigorous but gentle rubbing with soap and water to remove the superficial dead skin cells. The skin should be allowed to dry and new electrode stickers applied.
ECG is printing but some of the views are missing.	A loose connection.	Good skin preparation and maintenance of the ECG machine.	Check that the electrode sticker is intact and follow above suggestions for skin preparation. Check that the cables are all securely connected.
ECG is printing but there is interference, making it difficult to interpret safely.	Patient movement.	Ask the patient to remain still and not to speak, but to breathe normally.	Ensure the patient is not moving or talking and repeat the ECG once the displayed rhythm has stabilized.
		The patient may be cold and therefore involuntarily shivering.	Once the electrodes are connected, place a gown, sheet or blanket over the patient to warm them.
	Peripheral interference.	As above – ask the patient to remain still and ensure they are warm.	Place the limb electrodes more centrally as shown in the Mason–Likar placement (see Figure 11.8) to reduce interference from limb movement.

(continued)

Problem-solving table 11.2 **Prevention and resolution (Procedure guideline 11.2)** ***(continued)***

Problem	Cause	Prevention	Action
	General interference/ wandering baseline.	Poor skin contact with the electrodes, poor electrode placement or thoracic movement (Metcalfe 2000).	Ensure good skin preparation. Ask the patient to lie still and breathe normally. Check that the electrodes are properly placed. If necessary, record an additional ECG with the 'filter' function on to limit interference. Write on the ECG that the 'filter' function was used.
		Electrical interference from nearby devices (such as infusion pumps, other monitoring devices or haemodialysis machines).	It may be necessary to temporarily remove or suspend electrical devices if safe and appropriate to do so – repeat the ECG once the displayed rhythm has stabilized. If necessary, record an additional ECG with the 'filter' function on to limit interference. Write on the ECG that the 'filter' function was used.
ECG is working and displays a rhythm but the print-out is blank.	Different manufacturer's ECG paper has been loaded.	Only use the manufacturer's recommended paper for the ECG machine.	Reload using the correct paper and repeat the recording.
	Internal fault.	Ensure manufacturer's recommendations on maintenance and servicing are followed.	Contact in-house engineer, medical device technician or manufacturer for advice in accordance with local policy.

POST-PROCEDURAL CONSIDERATIONS

Immediate care

Any changes on the ECG that might require urgent medical attention should be identified and advice sought from a senior member of nursing or medical staff. If the patient had any cardiac symptoms at the time of recording, such as chest pain or palpitations, this should be noted on the tracing and brought to the immediate attention of a senior member of nursing or medical staff (SCST 2014). Examples of a normal 12-lead ECG and some important abnormal ECG tracings are shown in Figure 11.11 and Figure 11.12.

Documentation

It is good practice for the reviewer, who may be a doctor or senior nurse, to document their interpretation of the ECG directly on to the ECG and to sign and date it. Once reviewed, the ECG should be filed in the patient's medical notes. Nurses should document in the nursing notes when the ECG was recorded, who was asked to review it and the actual time the ECG was reviewed and indicate whether it was normal or, if abnormal, what further action was taken.

Blood pressure

DEFINITION

Blood pressure may be defined as the force of blood inside the blood vessels against the vessel walls (Marieb and Hoehn 2010). Systolic pressure is the peak pressure of the left ventricle contracting and blood entering the aorta, causing it to stretch and therefore in part reflects the function of the left ventricle (Marieb and Hoehn 2010). Diastolic pressure is when the aortic valve closes, blood flows from the aorta into the smaller vessels and the

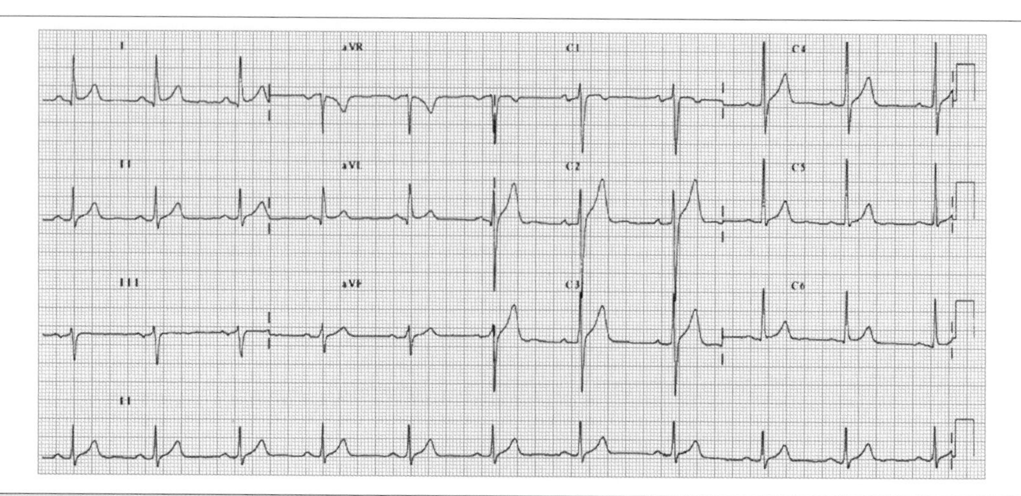

Figure 11.11 **Normal 12-lead ECG.** ***Source:*** **Davey (2008). Reproduced with permission from John Wiley & Sons.**

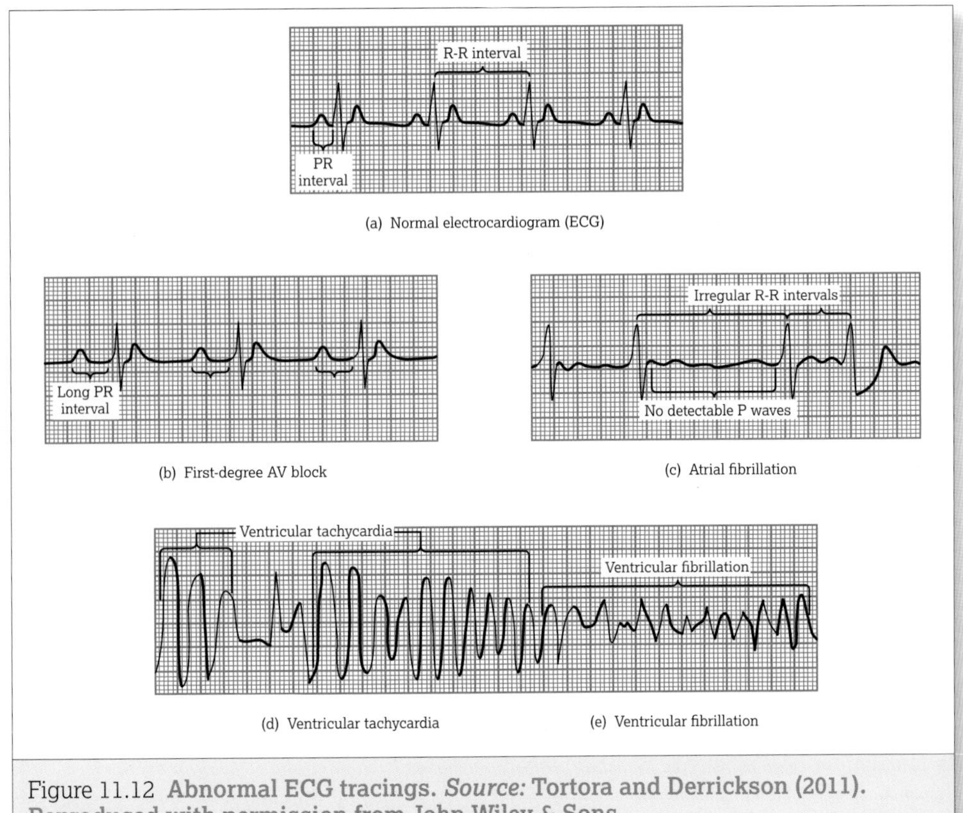

Figure 11.12 **Abnormal ECG tracings.** ***Source:*** **Tortora and Derrickson (2011). Reproduced with permission from John Wiley & Sons.**

aorta recoils back. This is when the aortic pressure is at its lowest and tends to reflect the resistance of the blood vessels (Marieb and Hoehn 2010).

RELATED THEORY

Blood pressure is determined by cardiac output and vascular resistance and can be described as (Woodrow 2004):

$$\underset{\text{(Blood pressure)}}{\text{BP}} = \underset{\text{(Cardiac output)}}{\text{CO}} \times \underset{\text{(Systemic vascular resistance)}}{\text{SVR}}$$

Cardiac output is the volume of blood which flows out of the heart over a specified length of time (Marieb and Hoehn 2010). It is governed by the stroke volume of the heart (the amount of blood pumped out of the ventricles per beat) and the heart rate. The relationship is (Patton and Thibodeau 2009):

$$\underset{\text{(Cardiac output)}}{\text{CO}} = \underset{\text{(Stroke volume)}}{\text{SV}} \times \underset{\text{(Heart rate)}}{\text{HR}}$$

Therefore, if the two equations are combined, blood pressure could be seen as being (Woodrow 2004):

$$\text{BP} = \text{SV} \times \text{HR} \times \text{SVR}$$

In theory, anything which alters one of the above components (stroke volume, heart rate or resistance) will therefore produce a change in blood pressure. However, this is not always the case as a drop in one may be compensated for by an increase in the other (Patton and Thibodeau 2009).

Normal blood pressure

Normal blood pressure ranges between 110–140 mmHg systolic and 70–80 mmHg diastolic at rest (Marieb and Hoehn 2010). However, it varies depending on age (increasing with age), activity and sleep, emotion and positioning, physical condition and fitness (Levick 2010, Tortora and Derrickson 2011). It also varies depending on the time of day, being at its lowest while we sleep (Levick 2010). Blood pressure therefore reflects individual variations but an abnormal blood pressure should not be assumed to be the individual's norm; rather, it will need to be assessed in relation to their previous results, general condition and other observations.

Hypotension

Hypotension is generally defined in adults as a systolic blood pressure below 100 mmHg (Marieb and Hoehn 2010). A low blood pressure may indicate orthostatic hypotension, that is, sudden drop in blood pressure when the patient rises from a supine or sitting position. This is usually compensated for by the baroreceptor reflex and the sympathetic nervous system but especially in older people, this may not work as efficiently (Marieb and Hoehn 2010). Hypotension can also be a symptom of many other conditions including shock, haemorrhage and malnutrition (Marieb and Hoehn 2010). Hypotension results in reduced tissue perfusion leading to hypoxia and an accumulation of waste products (Foxall 2009).

Hypertension

Hypertension is defined as blood pressure of 140/90 mmHg or greater. It can also be defined as a subsequent ambulatory blood pressure monitoring (ABPM) daytime average or home blood pressure monitoring (HBPM) average blood pressure of 135/85 mmHg or higher (NICE 2011b, Patton and Thibodeau 2009). It can be either *primary* hypertension, with no single known cause, or *secondary* hypertension related to another factor such as kidney disease (Patton and Thibodeau 2009). Factors leading to hypertension include gender, genetic factors and age, alongside risk factors such as obesity, lack of exercise, smoking and high caffeine and alcohol intake (Patton and Thibodeau 2009). If hypertension is sustained, the heart will have an increased

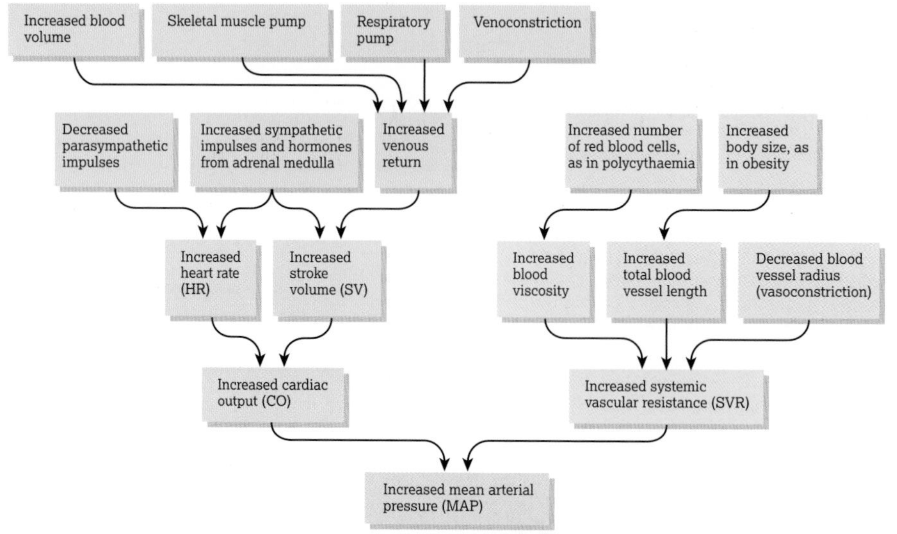

Increased blood volume
Skeletal muscle pump
Respiratory pump
Venoconstriction
Decreased parasympathetic impulses
Increased sympathetic impulses and hormones from adrenal medulla
Increased venous return
Increased number of red blood cells, as in polycythaemia
Increased body size, as in obesity
Increased heart rate (HR)
Increased stroke volume (SV)
Increased blood viscosity
Increased total blood vessel length
Decreased blood vessel radius (vasoconstriction)
Increased cardiac output (CO)
Increased systemic vascular resistance (SVR)
Increased mean arterial pressure (MAP)

Figure 11.13 **Factors that lead to an increase in blood pressure. Changes noted within green boxes increase cardiac output; changes noted within blue boxes increase systemic vascular resistance.** ***Source:*** **Tortora and Derrickson (2011). Reproduced with permission from John Wiley & Sons.**

workload to maintain circulation; greater stress will be placed on the blood vessel walls and cardiac ischaemia can occur (Foxall 2009, NICE 2011a). There are many illnesses and factors which can lead to changes in blood pressure (Figure 11.13) and hypertension is one of the most important preventable causes of premature morbidity and mortality in the UK (NICE 2011a).

Mean arterial pressure

The MAP indicates the average pressure of blood throughout the pulse cycle and thus is a reliable indication of perfusion (Woodrow 2004). Mathematically, the MAP is derived from the diastolic pressure and the pulse pressure (which is the difference between systolic and diastolic blood pressure). The equation is (Marieb and Hoehn 2010):

$$\text{MAP} = \text{diastolic pressure} + (\text{pulse pressure}/3)$$

Therefore, a patient with a blood pressure of 123/90 mmHg has a MAP of 101 mmHg. An adequate MAP is usually deemed to be between 65 mmHg (Hinds and Watson 2009) and 70 mmHg (Woodrow 2004).

Resistance

Resistance is effectively opposition to blood flow (Marieb and Hoehn 2010) and is created by friction between the walls of blood vessels and the blood itself (Patton and Thibodeau 2009). It is termed peripheral or systemic resistance because most of the resistance occurs in the vessels away from the heart (Marieb and Hoehn 2010). Peripheral resistance varies depending on the degree of vasoconstriction or vasodilation and the viscosity of blood and the length of the vessels, although the latter two factors generally remain relatively static (Marieb and Hoehn 2010). Arterioles can dilate or contract; when contracted, peripheral resistance increases and blood flow to the tissues decreases, increasing the arterial blood pressure (Patton and Thibodeau 2009). This can occur systemically, when there is total peripheral resistance, or locally (Patton and Thibodeau 2009). Blood pressure in the vessels of the cardiovascular system can be seen in Figure 11.14.

Blood pressure control

There are many inter-related physiological mechanisms which control blood pressure.

Figure 11.14 **Blood pressure in various parts of the cardiovascular system. The dashed line is the mean (average) blood pressure in the aorta, arteries and arterioles.** ***Source:*** **Peate et al. (2014). Reproduced with permission from John Wiley & Sons.**

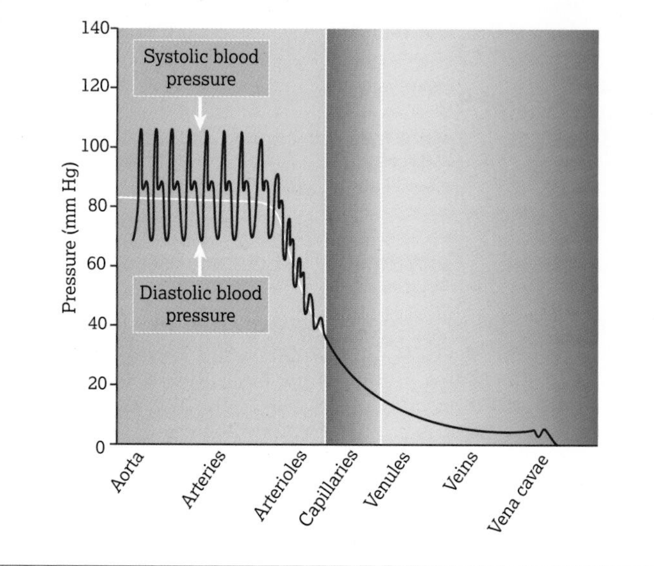

Hormonal control

Many hormones help to regulate blood pressure, including adrenaline and noradrenaline which are released from the adrenal medullae in response to a drop in blood pressure; these hormones increase cardiac contractility and thus cardiac output (Foxall 2009). Atrial natriuretic peptide (ANP) is a hormone which is produced from the atria of the heart in response to hypertension. It works by inhibiting the renin-angiotensin system, raising the glomerular filtration rate by causing specific vasodilation, inhibiting sodium reabsorption and causing fluid transfer into the interstitial space (Levick 2010).

Neural control

When blood pressure increases, the baroreceptors, or stretch receptors, are stimulated and in turn stimulate the cardiac inhibitory centre, reducing sympathetic nerve impulses and increasing parasympathetic nerve impulses (Foxall 2009). This causes a vasodilation and a decrease in cardiac output, thereby reducing the blood pressure (Foxall 2009). When blood pressure is low the opposite occurs. This response is termed a reflex arc, continually maintaining homeostasis (Marieb and Hoehn 2010). Baroreceptors are located in the aortic arch, carotid sinuses and in the walls of most of the large arteries in the thorax and neck (Marieb and Hoehn 2010). Close to these are chemoreceptors which are stimulated when the pH of the blood drops or when the carbon dioxide rises, and when oxygen levels drop significantly, these cause an increase in cardiac output and vasoconstriction, leading to an increase in blood pressure (Marieb and Hoehn 2010).

Renal control

When there is a decrease in blood pressure, adrenaline, increased sympathetic activity and a reduction in the stimulation of stretch receptors stimulate the juxtaglomerular cells within the kidneys to release renin (Levick 2010). This causes angiotensin I to be produced, leading to the production of angiotensin-converting enzyme which converts angiotensin I to angiotensin II (Patton and Thibodeau 2009). Angiotensin II has a potent effect on blood pressure, causing cardiac output and vasoconstriction to increase, stimulating the production of aldosterone and antidiuretic hormone which leads to the reabsorption of water and sodium and stimulates the thirst receptors (Foxall 2009). This increases the circulatory volume of fluid and thereby blood pressure (Foxall 2009). Similarly, the reverse happens when fluid volume in the circulatory system is high.

Other mechanisms which influence blood pressure

Skeletal muscle contractions and respiration promote venous return of blood to the heart and therefore increase cardiac output. The skeletal muscles contract on movement, compressing the veins and pushing the blood towards the heart, and respiration causes a change in thoracic and abdominal pressure which acts to pump venous blood (Patton and Thibodeau 2009). A factor which affects stroke volume is Starling's Law of the heart which states that the force of the contraction of the heart is related to how much blood volume is in the heart (Patton and Thibodeau 2009). The more stretched the muscle fibres are prior to contraction, the stronger the contraction and the greater volume it will pump (Foxall 2009).

Patient positioning can also influence a patient's blood pressure measurement (Cicolini et al. 2010, Eser et al. 2007, Mourad et al. 2003, Netea et al. 2003). It is recommended to measure the blood pressure where possible in the supine or seated position with uncrossed legs, with the back and arms supported, in order to ensure that the middle of the cuff on the upper arm is at the level of the right atrium (the midpoint of the sternum) (Adiyaman et al. 2006).

It is also suggested that a patient's knowledge of their own 'goal blood pressure' is independently associated with improved blood pressure control and any interventions to improve knowledge of specific blood pressure targets may have an important role in optimizing blood pressure management (Wright-Nunes et al. 2012).

EVIDENCE-BASED APPROACHES

Rationale

Indications

Blood pressure measurements should be taken as follows.

- On admission to a ward, in A&E departments when a decision to admit has been made (NICE 2007a).
- When a patient is transferred to a ward setting from intensive or high-dependency care (NICE 2007a).
- At least once every 12 hours while in hospital (NICE 2007a).
- For patients at risk of, or with known, infections (Chalmers et al. 2008).
- To assess response to interventions to correct the patient's blood pressure (Curran 2009, NICE 2011a).
- On patients pre-operatively, to establish a baseline, and post-operatively to assess cardiovascular stability.
- Critically or acutely ill patients, or those who are at risk of rapid deterioration, will require close and potentially continuous monitoring.
- Patients who are being transfused blood or blood products, to establish a baseline, during and after the transfusion (McClelland 2007).
- Any patient showing any signs of shock should have frequent monitoring.
- Any patient who is receiving medications which could alter their blood pressure, such as epidurals or anaesthetics.

Contraindications

There are times when certain methods of blood pressure measurement should be used with caution.

- Oscillometric blood pressure devices may not be accurate in those with weak or thready pulse or patients with pre-eclampsia (MHRA 2005).
- The brachial artery should not be used to measure blood pressure in those with arteriovenous fistulas (Turner et al. 2008).
- Patients with atrial fibrillation should have auscultatory blood pressure measurements taken, rather than oscillometric, and may require multiple readings (Williams et al. 2004).
- Korotkoff sounds are not dependably audible in children under the age of 1 year, and many children under 5 years (Curran 2009). Therefore, ultrasound, Doppler or oscillometric devices are recommended (O'Brien et al. 2003).
- Patients who have had trauma to the upper arm, previous mastectomy or a forearm amputation should not have blood pressure measured on the affected side at the brachial artery (Turner et al. 2008).
- Oscillometric devices should be used with caution in those with atherosclerosis and/or high or low blood pressures, as they may not measure accurately (Bern et al. 2007).
- The manufacturer's guidance should be sought for contraindications specific to the device used.
- Blood pressure should not be measured on an arm that has had brachial artery surgery or is at risk of lymphoedema (Bickley and Szilagyi 2009).

Methods of measuring blood pressure

There are two main methods of measuring blood pressure – direct and indirect.

Direct

The direct method enables continuous monitoring of the blood pressure and so is commonly used for critically ill patients, for example in intensive care units and theatres (Woodrow 2004). To do this, a cannula is inserted into an artery, most commonly the radial artery, as it is easy to access and monitor (Foxall 2009). The cannula has a transducer attached to it and is attached at the external end to a cardiac monitor where the blood pressure is shown as a waveform; it is also attached to a pressurized flush of solution to prevent blood backflow (Foxall 2009). This method has potential risks of severe haemorrhage, thrombosis and air embolism (Foxall 2009); therefore, it must only be used where patients can be continuously observed (Woodrow 2004).

Indirect

For indirect blood pressure measurement, either manual auscultatory sphygmomanometers or automated oscillometric devices are used (Bern et al. 2007). Oscillometric devices electronically measure blood pressure by measuring the oscillation of air pressure in the cuff, so when the artery begins to pulse it causes a corresponding oscillation of cuff pressure (Levick 2010). Manual auscultatory blood pressure involves occluding the artery by use of a pressurized cuff and then gradually releasing the pressure; when the systolic blood pressure exceeds cuff pressure, blood re-enters the arteries briefly, during systole, enabling a pulse to be palpated and producing vibrations in the artery (Levick 2010). As the cuff pressure descends, the sounds cease as the artery remains open throughout the pulse wave (Kacmerek et al. 2005).

Systolic blood pressure is usually defined as being at stage 1 of the Korotkoff sounds and diastolic at stage 5 (Curran 2009, Marieb and Hoehn 2010, NICE 2011b, Patton and Thibodeau 2009). See Box 11.1 for the Korotkoff sounds and the five phases. However, in some patients the Korotkoff sounds may continue until the cuff is completely deflated; in such cases stage 4 will represent the diastolic blood pressure (Williams et al. 2004). The auscultatory gap represents silence between the Korotkoff sounds and may sometimes be present; it is often associated with arterial stiffness, and it is vital not to mistake this for the actual blood pressure (Bickley and Szilagyi 2009). See Figure 11.15 for the Korotkoff sounds.

Alternative sites/methods

BLOOD PRESSURE MEASUREMENT AT THE THIGH

In some patients brachial artery blood pressure measurement is inappropriate; therefore, alternative sites have to be considered. To measure the blood pressure in the thigh, the patient should be prone with the BP bladder centred over the posterior popliteal artery and the stethoscope placed over the artery below the cuff (Bickley and Szilagyi 2009). When the appropriate sized cuffs are used, they should give an equal pressure to that in the arm (Bickley and Szilagyi 2009).

MEASUREMENT OF ORTHOSTATIC BLOOD PRESSURE

Orthostatic blood pressure measurement may be indicated if the patient has a history of dizziness or syncope on changing position (Lahrmann et al. 2006). The patient needs to rest on a bed in the supine position for 10 minutes prior to the initial blood pressure measurement being taken, and then they should stand upright and have their blood pressure taken again within 3 minutes (Bickley and Szilagyi 2009). While in the standing position, the practitioner should support the patient's arm at the elbow, to maintain it at the correct level and ensure accuracy (O'Brien et al. 2003). Orthostatic (postural) hypotension is defined by a drop in arterial BP of at least 20 mmHg for systolic BP and 10 mmHg for diastolic BP after standing (Tyberghein et al. 2013).

Box 11.1 Korotkoff sounds

The sounds heard are called the Korotkoff sounds and have five phases.

1 The first phase is the clear tapping, repetitive sounds which increase in intensity and indicate the systolic pressure.
2 The second phase is murmuring or swishing sounds heard between systolic and diastolic pressures.

Some people may have an auscultatory gap – a disappearance of sounds between the second and third phases.

3 The third phase is sharper and crisper sounds.
4 The fourth phase is the distinct muffling of sounds which may sound soft and blowing.
5 The fifth phase is silence as the cuff pressure drops below the diastolic blood pressure. This disappearance is considered to be the diastolic blood pressure.

Source: NICE (2011a), O'Brien et al. (2003).

Figure 11.15 **Korotkoff sounds.**

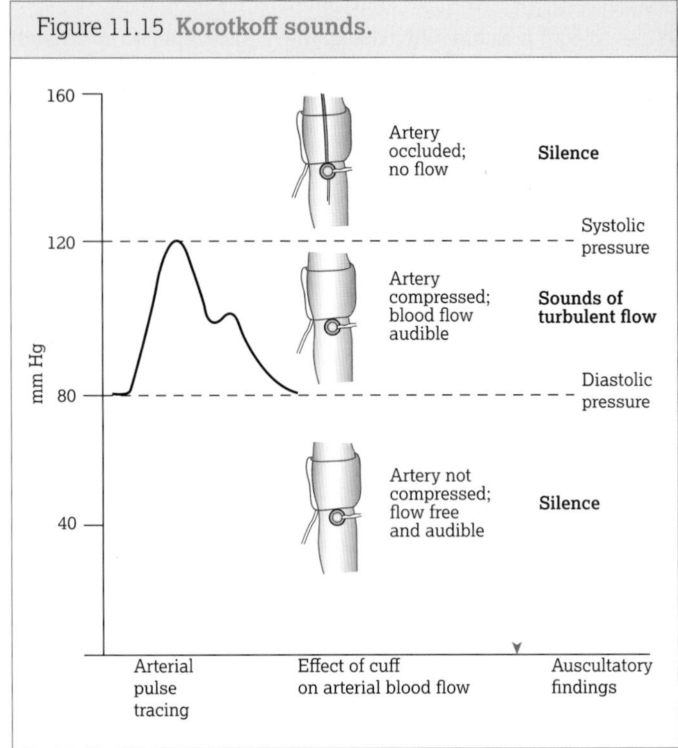

PRE-PROCEDURAL CONSIDERATIONS

Equipment

Sphygmomanometers

The device used to measure blood pressure is called a sphygmomanometer. It consists of a rubber cuff connected to a rubber bulb that is used to inflate the cuff and a meter that registers the pressure in the cuff (Tortora and Derrickson 2011). Sphygmomanometers which are uncalibrated or not working accurately are a cause of potential blood pressure measurement error (Curran 2009). If using a manual sphygmomanometer, check that the dial is set at zero or the mercury level is at zero prior to commencing (O'Brien et al. 2003). In addition, follow the manufacturer's recommendations and local policies regarding servicing and care of the device.

Manual mercury sphygmomanometers have gradually been phased out of mainstream clinical practice and replaced with a dial or electronic manometer (MHRA 2012). This is primarily due to potential mercury leaks which are hazardous to both the environment and humans and secondly because from April 2009 they were no longer available to either members of the public or healthcare professionals (MHRA 2012).

MANUAL ANEROID SPHYGMOMANOMETERS

Aneroid sphygmomanometers measure blood pressure through a lever and bellows system which is more complex than the mercury sphygmomanometer. However, if it is damaged it may become inaccurate (O'Brien et al. 2003). If aneroid sphygmomanometers have a dial gauge then there is a risk of damage with significant errors occurring with the calibration and setting of zero (MHRA 2005). As a result, O'Brien et al. (2003) recommend that these devices are serviced every 6 months to ensure accuracy.

AUTOMATED OSCILLOMETRIC SPHYGMOMANOMETERS

These devices show blood pressure on an electronic display (MHRA 2005). Some studies have found that the results differ between automated and manual blood pressure devices (Bern et al. 2007). Indeed, there are concerns that there is a greater need for validation of the devices so it is recommended that only devices that have passed recognized validation criteria should be used (BHS 2006, MHRA 2005, Stergiou et al. 2010, Williams et al. 2004). If levels of accuracy and reliability can be achieved then they do have certain advantages:

- many devices combine blood pressure with other observations (O'Brien et al. 2003)
- a print-out can be obtained, reducing the risk of bias (O'Brien et al. 2003)
- the preference of terminal digits (0 or 5) should be eradicated (O'Brien et al. 2003)
- data can be stored on the device (O'Brien et al. 2003)
- they enable the setting of alarms (MHRA 2005).

Practitioners must refer to the manufacturer's instructions and be aware of the limitations of the device. If there is any doubt about a measurement then it should be verified by an accurate manual blood pressure reading. Patients who have arrhythmias, hypotension or hypertension or are acutely unwell should have a manual blood pressure taken rather than an automated one (NICE 2011b).

The cuff

The cuff is made of an inelastic material, which encloses an inflatable bladder and encircles the arm. It is important that the correct cuff size is selected for the individual patient (Veiga et al. 2009). Cuffs that are too small yield a reading that is falsely high and large cuffs give a falsely low reading (Williams et al. 2004). With the correct size cuff the bladder should encircle 80% of the patient's arm (Williams et al. 2004). Please see Table 11.4 for guidance on blood pressure cuff sizes.

Alternative adult cuffs (width × length, 12 × 35 cm) have been recommended for all adult patients, but can result in problems with over- and undercuffing. The British Hypertension Society recommends that cuff size be selected based on arm circumference (Williams et al. 2004).

The inflatable bladder, valve, pump and tubing

In a manual sphygmomanometer, the system used to inflate and deflate the bladder consists of a bulb attached to the bladder with rubber tubing. When the bulb is compressed, air is forced into the bladder; to deflate the bladder there is a release valve (O'Brien et al. 2003). The rubber tubes have conventionally been placed so they are inferior to the cuff; however, it is now recommended that they are placed superiorly to prevent them impeding auscultation (O'Brien et al. 2003).

The stethoscope

It is recommended that the stethoscope be of high quality with well-fitting earpieces (O'Brien et al. 2003). It should be placed over the brachial artery at the antecubital fossa (O'Brien et al. 2003). The bell part of the stethoscope may capture the low pitch of the Korotkoff sounds better than the diaphragm but the diaphragm has a larger surface area and is easier to manipulate with one hand (O'Brien et al. 2003).

Table 11.4 **Blood pressure cuff sizes for mercury sphygmomanometer, semi-automatic and ambulatory monitors**

Indication	Bladder width × length (cm)	Arm circumference (cm)
Small adult/child	12 × 18	<23
Standard adult	12 × 26	<33
Large adult	12 × 40	<50
Adult thigh cuff	20 × 42	<53

Source: Reproduced with permission from Williams et al. (2004).

Specific patient preparation

It is important to maintain a standardized environment in which to take the patient's blood pressure (NICE 2011a). The patient should be seated (unless thigh or orthostatic blood pressure measurements are required) in a relaxed, quiet, temperate setting (NICE 2011a). Their arm should be outstretched and supported, as in unsupported arms diastolic blood pressure may be increased by 10% (O'Brien et al. 2003). The brachial artery at the antecubital fossa should be positioned equal to heart level, approximately equal to where the fourth intercostals space meets the sternum (Bickley and Szilagyi 2009).

The patient's back should be supported (Turner et al. 2008) and their feet should be on the floor as systolic blood pressure can increase by an average of 6.6 mmHg in people with their legs crossed (van Groningen et al. 2008). Blood pressure should be taken after a short period of rest, as slight hypertension on standing and moving is initiated by the baroreceptor reflex (Turner et al. 2008). Correct patient positioning can be seen in Figure 11.16.

Blood pressure should initially be measured in both arms as often people have a significant difference in blood pressure measurement between their arms (NICE 2011a). Those patients who have a large and persistent disparity may have underlying conditions such as occlusive artery disease (Eguchi et al. 2007, O'Brien et al. 2003). Differences up to 10 mmHg can be due to random variation (Eguchi et al. 2007). The arm with the highest reading should be the one used for subsequent measurements (NICE 2011a).

Figure 11.16 **Correct blood pressure reading techniques.**

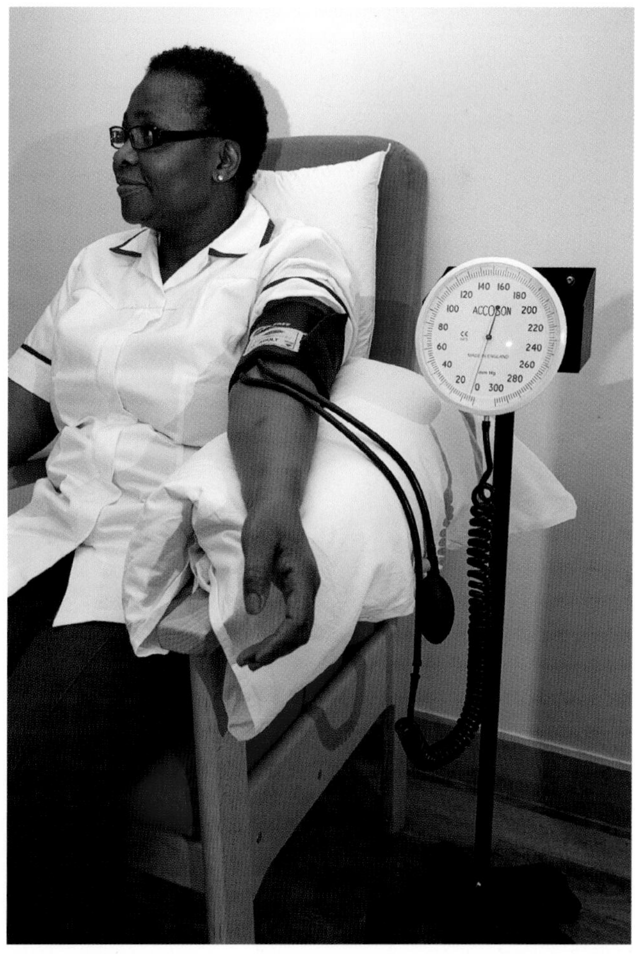

Procedure guideline 11.3 Blood pressure measurement (manual)

Essential equipment

- A range of cuffs
- Sphygmomanometer, working and calibrated
- Stethoscope
- Documentation
- Alcohol handrub
- Detergent wipes

Optional equipment

- Pillow if required to provide extra arm support
- If necessary a bed or examination bench, so the patient can have their blood pressure measured lying down

Pre-procedure

Action	Rationale
1 Explain to the patient that you need to measure their blood pressure, discuss the procedure, and obtain valid consent.	To ensure that the patient understands the procedure and gives their valid consent (NMC 2013, **C**).
2 Wash hands using bactericidal soap and water or bactericidal alcohol handrub, and dry.	To minimize the risk of infection (Fraise and Bradley 2009, **E**).
3 Ask/observe the patient if they have any of the following. • Lymphoedema or are at risk • An arteriovenous fistula • Trauma or surgery to their arm/axilla • Brachial artery surgery. • Intravenous (IV) infusion in progress If there is a contraindication, use other arm or, if bilateral, the lower extremity.	To ensure there are no contraindications to using a particular arm (Bickley and Szilagyi 2009, **E**; Curran 2009, **E**; Turner et al. 2008, **E**). Taking blood pressure is not recommended on a limb with an IV infusion in progress because the pressure could damage the vein, placing the patient at risk of extravasation or infiltration. If there is no other choice, a blood pressure can be taken on a limb with IV catheter *in situ* although the infusion must be temporarily stopped in consultation with registered nursing staff (RCN 2011, **C**).
4 Provide a standardized environment, which should be relaxed and temperate. The patient needs to be seated comfortably, in a chair with back support, for at least 5 min prior to measuring blood pressure.	To enable comparisons to be drawn with prior blood pressure results (NICE 2011a, **C**). Variations in temperature and emotions can alter blood pressure readings (O'Brien et al. 2003, **E**). Resting for 5 minutes will ensure an optimum reading (Bickley and Szilagyi 2009, **E**; O'Brien et al. 2003, **E**; Turner et al. 2008, **E**).
5 Ensure the cuff is the correct size for the arm. The cuff bladder length should be 80% of the arm circumference and its width 40% (BHS 2006).	To prevent falsely high readings that may occur if small cuffs are used or falsely low readings if large cuffs used (Williams et al. 2004, **E**).
6 Check the patient's arm is free from clothing, supported, e.g. with a pillow (whether sitting or standing) and placed at heart level (midsternal level) (Bickley and Szilagyi 2009, NICE 2011a, O'Brien et al. 2003). The patient's bladder should have been recently emptied, their legs uncrossed with their feet flat on the floor if positioned in a chair and ankles uncrossed if in a bed (Turner et al. 2008). See Figure 11.16.	If the arm is lower than heart level it can lead to falsely high readings, and vice versa (O'Brien et al. 2003, **E**). Diastolic pressure can increase by up to 10% if the arm is unsupported (O'Brien et al. 2003, **E**) and alter the systolic pressure by 10 mmHg (Reeves 1995, **E**). Obtaining a measurement before bladder emptying can also increase the systolic blood pressure by up to 10 mmHg (Reeves 1995, **E**). Blood pressure results can be falsely high if the patient has their legs crossed (Handler 2009, **E**; van Groningen et al. 2008, **R3b**). Taking measurements over clothing or with tight clothing pushed up on the arm can cause a tourniquet effect, and also produce significant artefacts (Reeves 1995, **E**).

Procedure

Action	Rationale
7 Wrap the cuff of the sphygmomanometer around the bare arm, with the bladder centred over the brachial artery and superior to the elbow (Marieb and Hoehn 2010, Patton and Thibodeau 2009). The lower edge of the cuff should be 2–3 cm above the brachial artery pulsation (O'Brien et al. 2003).	To obtain an accurate reading (BHS 2006, **C**), and so that the artery can easily be palpated (NICE 2011a, **C**).
8 Ask the patient to stop talking, and eating, during the procedure.	Activity can cause a falsely high blood pressure (BHS 2006, **C**).
9 Palpate the brachial artery while pumping air into the cuff using the bulb. Once the pulse can no longer be felt, rapidly inflate the cuff a further 20–30 mmHg (Bickley and Szilagyi 2009, NICE 2011a).	Palpation of the artery prior to obtaining a blood pressure is recommended as it locates the correct position for stethoscope placement (Valler-Jones and Wedgbury 2005, **E**).

Action	Rationale
	Although the radial artery is also available for palpating, the brachial artery is selected due to its proximity to the most common cuff positioning (superior to the elbow). Inflating the cuff to only 20–30 mmHg above the predicted systolic level prevents undue discomfort (Bickley and Szilagyi 2009, **E**). Therefore the brachial pulse is advocated rather than the radial pulse (NICE 2011a, **C**).
10 Slowly deflate the cuff and note the point at which the pulse becomes detectable again. This approximates the systolic blood pressure.	This provides an indication of systolic pressure and can ensure accurate results in those who have an auscultatory gap (BHS 2006, **C**; Curran 2009, **E**; NICE 2011a, **C**; O'Brien et al. 2003, **E**; Tortora and Derrickson 2011, **E**).
11 Deflate the cuff completely and wait 15–30 seconds (Bickley and Szilagyi 2009).	To allow venous congestion to resolve (O'Brien et al. 2003, **E**).
12 The diaphragm of the stethoscope should be firmly, but without too much pressure, placed on bare skin over the brachial artery where the pulse was palpable.	The bell of the stethoscope may hear the tone of the Korotkoff sounds better (Bickley and Szilagyi 2009, **E**). However, the diaphragm has a larger surface area and is easier to hold in place (O'Brien et al. 2003, **E**). If the stethoscope is in contact with material it may distort the Korotkoff sounds (O'Brien et al. 2003, **E**). Applying pressure with the stethoscope may partially occlude the artery (O'Brien et al. 2003, **E**).
13 Inflate the cuff again to 20–30 mmHg above the predicted systolic blood pressure (Bickley and Szilagyi 2009).	To ensure an accurate measurement (NICE 2011a, **C**).
14 Release the air in the cuff slowly (at an approximate rate of 2–3 mmHg per pulsation) until the first tapping sounds are heard (first Korotkoff sound). This is the systolic blood pressure (Patton and Thibodeau 2009).	The cuff should not be deflated too quickly as this may result in inaccurate readings being taken (O'Brien et al. 2003, **E**).
15 Continue to deflate the cuff slowly, listening to the Korotkoff sounds; the point at which the sound completely disappears is the best representation of the diastolic blood pressure (fifth Korofkoff sound).	To ensure an accurate diastolic blood pressure and that you note any irregularities such as if the sounds never disappear, or disappear significantly below the fourth Korotkoff sound (Bickley and Szilagyi 2009, **E**).
16 Once sounds can no longer be heard, rapidly deflate the cuff.	To prevent venous congestion to the arm (O'Brien et al. 2003, **E**).
17 If you need to recheck the blood pressure, wait 1–2 min before proceeding (BHS 2006).	Venous congestion may make the Korotkoff sounds less audible (Bickley and Szilagyi 2009, **E**).
Post-procedure	
18 Inform patient that the procedure is now finished.	To reassure the patient (Major and Holmes 2008, **R4**).
19 Wash hands using bactericidal soap and water or bactericidal alcohol handrub, and dry. Clean bell and diaphragm of stethoscope and cuff with detergent wipe (no alcohol).	To minimize the risk of infection (Fraise and Bradley 2009, **E**).
20 Document as soon as the measurement has been taken and compare with previous results (O'Brien et al. 2003). Take action as appropriate and document.	Any interruption in the process may result in the measurement being incorrectly remembered (O'Brien et al. 2003, **E**). Records should identify any risks or problems that have arisen and show the action taken to deal with them (NMC 2010, **C**).

Problem-solving table 11.3 **Prevention and resolution (Procedure guideline 11.3)**

Problem	Cause	Prevention	Action
The result is unexpectedly low or high.	This may be due to poor technique or faulty equipment. It may also be due to the patient being incorrectly positioned or post exercise.	Check the sphygmomanometer prior to use to see when it was last serviced. Check all the components for signs of damage. Ensure the patient is correctly positioned, and has rested prior to the procedure.	Wait 1–2 min before repeating the blood pressure measurement (BHS 2006). If the measurement is still unexpected, consider changing devices or asking a colleague to repeat the procedure. If it remains abnormal, notify the medical team of the result.

(continued)

Problem-solving table 11.3 Prevention and resolution (Procedure guideline 11.3) *(continued)*

Problem	Cause	Prevention	Action
On auscultation the Korotkoff sounds disappear after the initial sound, then reappear and then disappear again (Curran 2009).	This is called the auscultatory gap – it may mislead the practitioner into obtaining an incorrect result (Curran 2009).	Palpate the pulse as the cuff is being deflated to gain an approximation of the systolic blood pressure (O'Brien et al. 2003).	Document that the patient has an auscultatory gap and ensure other practitioners are aware to prevent future errors (O'Brien et al. 2003). Recheck using the correct procedure.
On auscultation the Korotkoff sounds are inaudible or very weak.	May be due to poor placement of the stethoscope, a noisy environment, venous congestion or the patient may be in shock (Bickley and Szilagyi 2009, Verrij et al. 2009).	Find a quiet environment in which to measure the patient's blood pressure, listen with the bell of the stethoscope rather than the diaphragm, wait for venous congestion to resolve (Bickley and Szilagyi 2009).	If still inaudible, ask the patient to elevate their arm overhead for 30 seconds, then bring it back to the correct height to inflate the cuff and measure their blood pressure; this increases the loudness of the sounds (Bickley and Szilagyi 2009, Verrij et al. 2009).

POST-PROCEDURAL CONSIDERATIONS

Immediate care

Notify medical staff of an abnormal blood pressure result. As the treatment will depend on what is causing the abnormality, and its severity, it is important that practitioners try to ascertain the possible cause for the physiological change in blood pressure (Kisiel and Perkins 2006). Hypovolaemia will require fluid replacement and, if persistent, then inotropes and other cardiovascular drugs may be necessary (Hinds and Watson 2009). If the hypertension is transient, for example related to anxiety or pain, then it is important to address that issue and monitor the blood pressure until it resolves. However, if the patient is diagnosed as having hypertension, they will require drug therapy to control their condition (NICE 2011a). To determine the cause of the altered blood pressure more information will be required, including:

- gaining a comprehensive medical history from the patient (Steele and Hardin 2007)
- gaining a full set of observations
- an ECG (Steele and Hardin 2007)
- urinalysis including protein, leucocytes, blood and the osmolality of the urine (Steele and Hardin 2007)
- blood tests for full blood count, urea, creatinine and electrolytes (Steele and Hardin 2007) and fasting blood tests for glucose and lipids (Camm and Bunce 2009)
- a chest X-ray or further radiological investigations may be required (Camm and Bunce 2009)
- a septic screen including blood cultures, sputum specimen, swabs of any wounds or potential sites of infection (Hinds and Watson 2009)
- their current fluid balance (Kisiel and Perkins 2006).

Ongoing care

If the patient is hypertensive and in primary care, they will require at least monthly blood pressure measurement and more frequently if it is accelerated hypertension or there are any further concerns (NICE 2011a). Additionally, it will be necessary to give lifestyle advice on, for example, eating healthily and smoking cessation (NICE 2011a). If the hypotension is orthostatic then advise the patient to change position slowly so the baroreceptors and sympathetic nervous system have time to adapt the blood pressure to each stage (Marieb and Hoehn 2010).

Documentation

As well as the accurate recording of the blood pressure measurement, it is also important to record:

- the position the patient was in
- the arm used, and if both arms were used initially, the pressure of each
- arm circumference and the cuff size used
- if there is an auscultatory gap or any difficulties in obtaining a reading, such as the absence of stage 5
- the state of the patient, for example were they in pain, frightened, and so on
- any medication they are on and when they last took it (O'Brien et al. 2003).

When documenting the medication the patient is on, it is important to include not only cardiovascular medication but also other medication which might affect their blood pressure, including tricyclic antidepressants, neuroleptic agents (O'Brien et al. 2003), contraceptives, decongestants, non-steroidal anti-inflammatory drugs (NSAIDs) and cocaine (Steele and Hardin 2007).

Respiration and pulse oximetry

DEFINITION

The major function of the respiratory system is to supply the cells of the human body with oxygen and to remove carbon dioxide, in order that they can continue to function effectively (Tortora and Derrickson 2011). Respiration is composed of four processes:

- *pulmonary ventilation*: the movement of air into and out of the lungs to continually refresh the gases there, commonly called 'breathing'
- *external respiration*: movement of oxygen from the lungs into the blood, and carbon dioxide from the lungs into the blood, commonly called 'gaseous exchange'
- *transport of respiratory gases*: transport of oxygen from the lungs to the cells, and of carbon dioxide from the cells to the lungs, accomplished by the cardiovascular system
- *internal respiration*: movement of oxygen from blood to the cells, and of carbon dioxide from the cells to the blood (Marieb and Hoehn 2010) (see Chapter 9: Respiratory care).

ANATOMY AND PHYSIOLOGY

The organs and structures of the respiratory system can be split into two zones: the conducting zone and the respiratory zone (Marieb and Hoehn 2010). The conducting zone consists of a series of interconnecting passageways, both outside and within the lungs, through which air passes to get to the area of gaseous exchange, such as the nasal cavity, trachea and bronchi. The function of this area is to provide conduits through which air can pass and can also filter, cleanse, warm and humidify the air whilst conducting it to the lungs (Tortora and Derrickson 2011). The respiratory zone consists of the bronchioles, alveolar ducts and alveoli, the main sites where gaseous exchange occurs between air and blood (Marieb and Hoehn 2010).

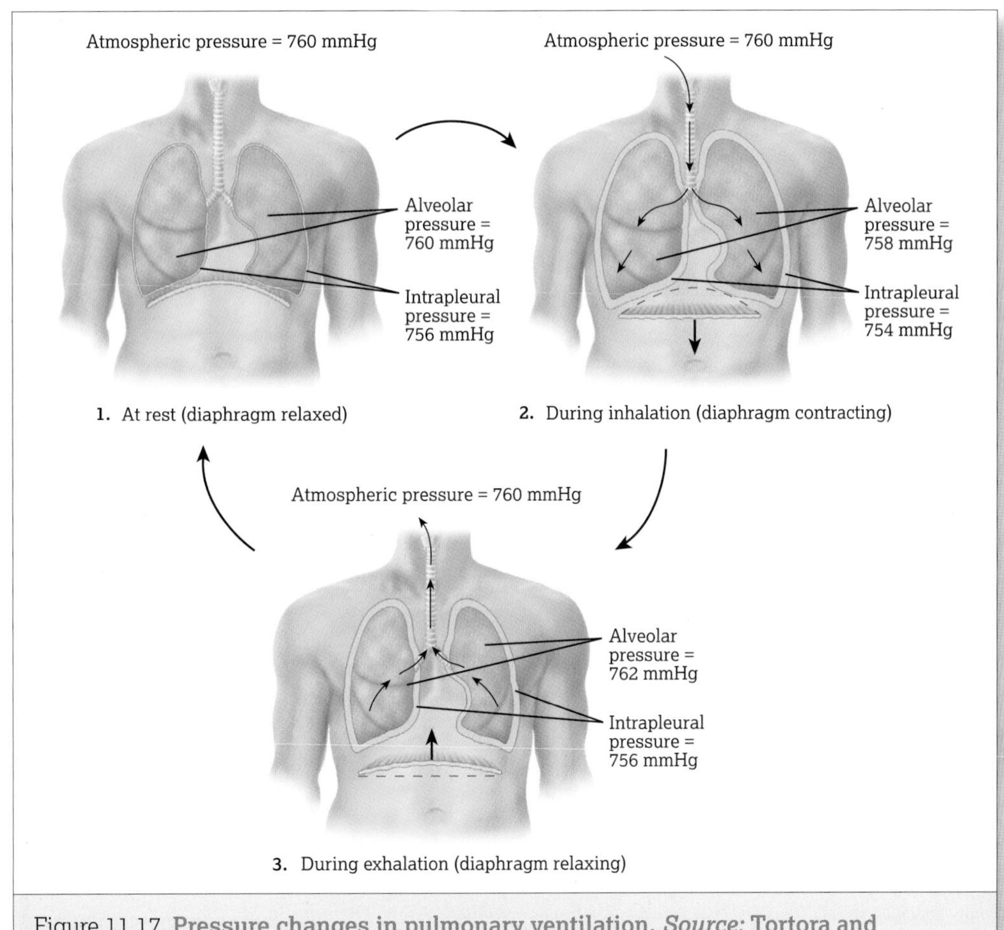

Figure 11.17 **Pressure changes in pulmonary ventilation.** ***Source:*** **Tortora and Derrickson (2011). Reproduced with permission from John Wiley & Sons.**

A variety of efficient inter-relationships exist between the different body systems in order for effective respiration to occur; these include the cardiovascular system, nervous system and musculoskeletal system (Patton and Thibodeau 2010). The respiratory muscles (the diaphragm and intercostal muscles) promote ventilation by causing volume and pressure changes within the respiratory system (Marieb and Hoehn 2010).

The mechanism of breathing

The key mechanism of pulmonary ventilation is that changes of volume within the respiratory system lead to changes in pressure and that these in turn lead to a flow of gases to equalize the pressure (Marieb and Hoehn 2010). The relationship between the pressure and volume of a gas is called Boyle's Law, whereby at a constant temperature the pressure of a gas varies inversely with its volume; in a larger container the pressure of a gas is less than in a smaller one (Marieb and Hoehn 2010). As air will flow from an area of high pressure to an area of lower pressure, air moves into the lungs when the air pressure inside the lungs is lower than the air pressure in the atmosphere, and out of the lungs when the air pressure outside the lungs is greater than the air pressure in the atmosphere (Tortora and Derrickson 2011).

Inspiration

For inspiration to occur, the pressure in the alveoli must be lower than the air pressure in the atmosphere; this is achieved by increasing the size (volume) of the lungs through the contraction of the muscles of inhalation – the diaphragm and the intercostal muscles. The diaphragm flattens and descends and the intercostal muscles lift the ribcage and sternum, causing the ribs to broaden outwards and increasing the diameter of the thoracic cavity, both from side to side and front to back (Patton and Thibodeau 2009).

During normal inspirations, the pressure between the two pleural layers in the pleural cavity (intrapleural pressure) is always just lower than atmospheric pressure (756 mmHg at an atmospheric pressure of 760 mmHg). As the volume of the lungs and pleural cavity increases, the intrapleural pressure drops to 754 mmHg. At the same time, the pressure within the lungs (alveolar or intrapulmonary pressure) drops from 760 mmHg to 758 mmHg, and so a pressure difference between the atmosphere and the alveoli is established and air flows into the lungs (Tortora and Derrickson 2011). The relationship of these pressures can be seen in Figure 11.17.

Expiration

Expiration also occurs due to a pressure gradient but in the opposite direction, whereby the pressure within the lungs is greater than the pressure of the atmosphere. In normal gentle breathing, the process of expiration is largely passive, not involving any muscular contractions but resulting from elastic recoil of the chest wall and lungs (Tortora and Derrickson 2011).

Expiration begins when the inspiratory muscles relax, causing the diaphragm to move superiorly and the ribs to depress, decreasing the diameter of the thoracic cavity and returning it to its normal size. This results in a decrease in lung volume and compression of the alveoli, causing an increase in alveolar (intrapulmonary) pressure to 762 mmHg. This forces gases to flow out from the area of higher pressure in the lungs to the area of lower pressure in the atmosphere (Tortora and Derrickson 2011). A summary of events during inspiration and expiration can be seen in Figure 11.18.

The accessory muscles

The accessory muscles of inspiration further increase the volume of the thoracic cavity and therefore increase the volume of breathing; these include the sternocleidomastoid muscles which elevate the sternum and the scalene muscles and the pectoralis

During normal quiet inhalation, diaphragm and external intercostals contract. During laboured inhalation, sternocleidomastoid, scalenes and pectoralis minor also contract
Alveolar pressure increases to 762 mmHg
Atmospheric pressure is about 760 mmHg at sea level
Thoracic cavity increases in size and volume of lungs expands
Thoracic cavity decreases in size and volume and lungs recoil
Alveolar pressure decreases to 758 mmHg
During normal quiet exhalation, diaphragm and external intercostals relax. During forceful exhalation, abdominal and internal intercostal muscles contract
(a) Inhalation
(b) Exhalation

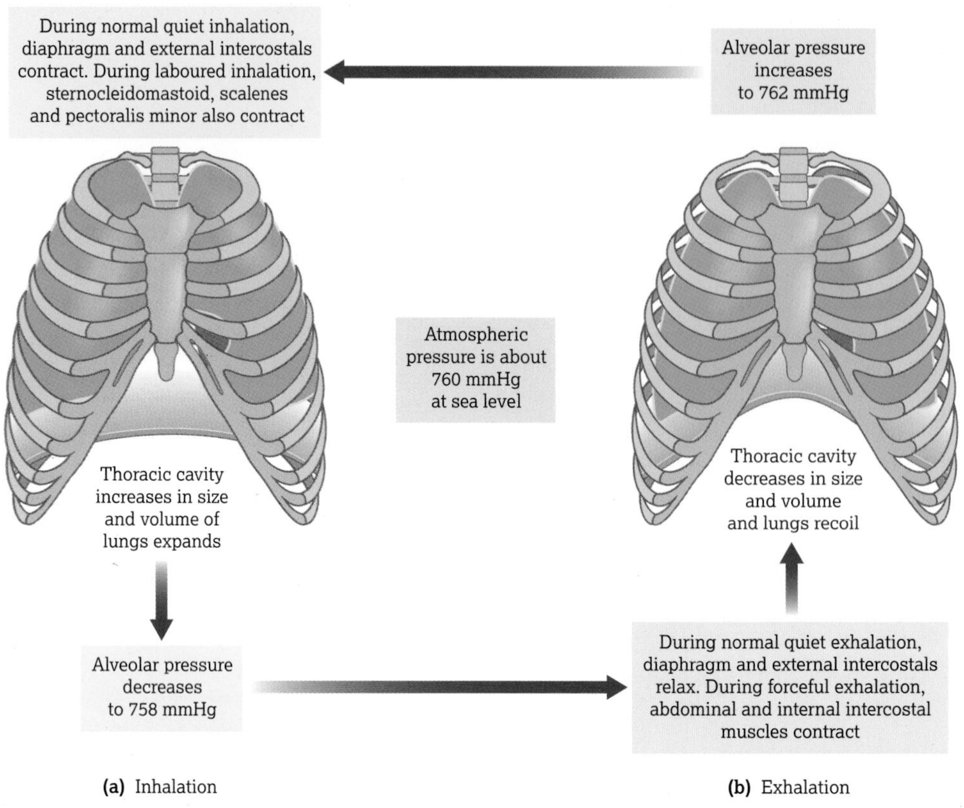

Figure 11.18 **Summary of events of inhalation and exhalation.** ***Source:*** **Peate et al. (2014). Reproduced with permission from John Wiley & Sons.**

minor muscles which elevate the first to the fifth ribs (Tortora and Derrickson 2011). These muscles may be used during exercise or if the individual is in respiratory distress (Marieb and Hoehn 2010).

The accessory muscles of expiration are used only during forceful breathing, such as when playing a wind instrument or during exercise. Contraction of the abdomoinal wall muscles, primarily the oblique and transversus muscles, increases intra-abdominal pressure, forcing the abdominal organs upwards against the diaphragm, and also depresses the ribcage. The internal intercostal muscles also depress the ribcage and decrease thoracic volume, forcing air out of the lungs (Marieb and Hoehn 2010).

Control of respiration

Oxygen consumption increases exponentially during periods of strenuous exercise; several mechanisms help to match respiratory effort to the metabolic demand of the cells (Tortora and Derrickson 2011). Higher brain centres, chemoreceptors and other reflexes modify the basic respiratory rhythms generated in the brainstem. Control of respiration primarily involves neurones in the medulla and pons (Marieb and Hoehn 2010).

The respiratory centres

Within the medulla are two clusters of neurones which are critically important in the co-ordination of the respiratory system: the *dorsal respiratory group* and the *ventral respiratory group* (Marieb and Hoehn 2010).

The ventral respiratory group contains neurones that fire during inspiration, stimulating the diaphragm and the external intercostal muscles to contract, via the phrenic and intercostal nerves, and other neurones which fire during expiration causing the stimulation to stop and the muscles relax. These neurones deliver our normal respiratory rate of 12–15 breaths per minute (Marieb and Hoehn 2010).

The dorsal respiratory group co-ordinates input from the peripheral baroreceptors (or stretch receptors) and chemoreceptors and relays this to the ventral respiratory group to alter respiratory rate as required (Marieb and Hoehn 2010). Baroreceptors monitor the stretch of the bronchi and bronchioles during overinflation of the lungs (Tortora and Derrickson 2011). Chemoreceptors monitor the arterial blood for changes in the partial pressure of carbon dioxide (PCO_2) and pH, but also, to a lesser extent, the partial pressure of oxygen (PO_2) (Patton and Thibodeau 2009). For more information on the chemical factors which affect respiration, see Chapter 9: Respiratory care.

Pontine respiratory centres also relay impulses to the ventral respiratory group to modify breathing rhythms so that there is a smooth transition from inspiration to expiration and so that breathing can be modified to allow for speech, exercise and sleep (Marieb and Hoehn 2010).

Carbon dioxide

Although oxygen is essential for every cell in the body, the body's need to rid itself of carbon dioxide is the most vital stimulus to respiration in a healthy person (Marieb and Hoehn 2010). Arterial PCO_2 is very closely monitored and acceptable levels maintained by a sensitive homeostatic mechanism mediated mainly by the effect that increased CO_2 levels have on the central chemoreceptors of the brainstem. Carbon dioxide passes easily from the blood into the cerebrospinal fluid where it forms carbonic acid, releasing hydrogen ions (H^+). This increase of H^+ causes the pH to drop, stimulating the central chemoreceptors in the brainstem to increase the rate and depth of breathing and so increase the amount of carbon dioxide exhaled (Marieb and Hoehn 2010). Similarly, metabolic causes for low pH levels, such as a build-up of lactic acid, will also provoke alterations in respiration (Marieb and Hoehn 2010). See Figure 11.19 for negative feedback mechanisms by which changes in PCO_2 and

Figure 11.19 **Negative feedback mechanisms by which changes in PCO_2 and blood pH regulate ventilation.** *Source:* **Peate et al. (2014). Reproduced with permission from John Wiley & Sons.**

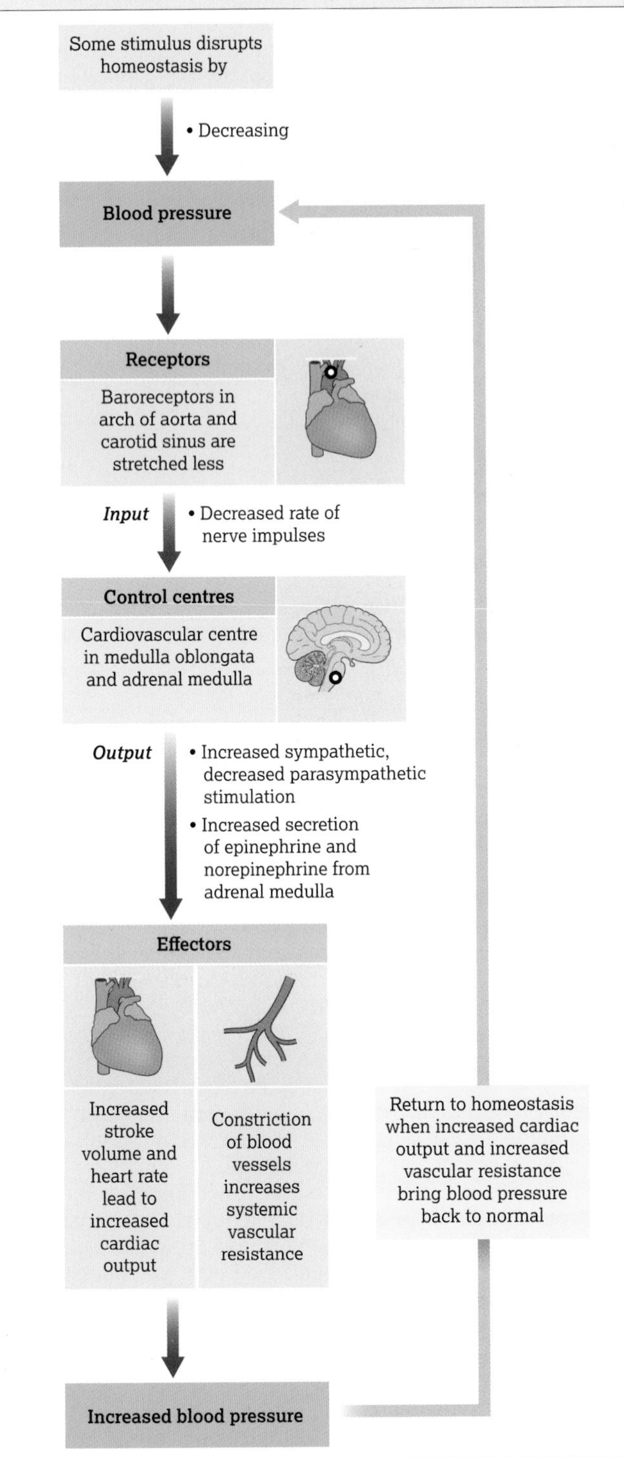

blood pH regulate ventilation. Abnormally low PCO_2 levels cause inhibition of respiration, with breathing becoming slow and shallow, and periods of apnoea may occur, until arterial PCO_2 rises again and stimulates respiration (Marieb and Hoehn 2010).

Oxygen

The peripheral chemoreceptors, found in the aortic arch and carotid arteries, are responsible for sensing the arterial PO_2 (Marieb and Hoehn 2010). Normally, decreasing levels of oxygen only affect respiratory rate by causing the peripheral chemoreceptors to have an increased sensitivity to carbon dioxide (Marieb and Hoehn 2010). Arterial PO_2 must drop substantially, from the normal level of 100 mmHg to at least 60 mmHg, before it stimulates respiratory function; at this point the central receptors become suppressed and at the same time the peripheral receptors stimulate the respiratory centres to increase ventilation even if PCO_2 is normal (Marieb and Hoehn 2010).

Other ways in which respiration is controlled

There are a number of receptors in the lungs which respond to a variety of irritants. Accumulated mucus or inhaled debris stimulates receptors in the bronchioles that cause reflex constriction of those air passages. When stimulated in the bronchi or trachea, a cough is initiated, and a sneeze is triggered when in the nasal cavity (Marieb and Hoehn 2010). These irritant receptors have a protective mechanism to prevent obstruction or aspiration of food or liquids (Patton and Thibodeau 2009). There are also stretch receptors present in the conducting passages and the visceral pleura which are stimulated when the lungs inflate; these then signal the respiratory centres to end inspiration. These receptors are thought to act more as a protective response to prevent excessive stretching of the lungs rather than a normal regulatory mechanism (Marieb and Hoehn 2010).

Respiration can also be altered in the higher cortical centres in response to factors such as strong emotions, pain and alteration of temperature (Patton and Thibodeau 2009, Tortora and Derrickson 2011). The cerebral motor cortex yields a degree of voluntary control over breathing; however, this can be over-ridden by the other mechanisms (Patton and Thibodeau 2009).

Some of the mechanisms through which breathing is controlled are summarized in Figure 11.20.

Figure 11.20 **Factors influencing rate and depth of breathing**

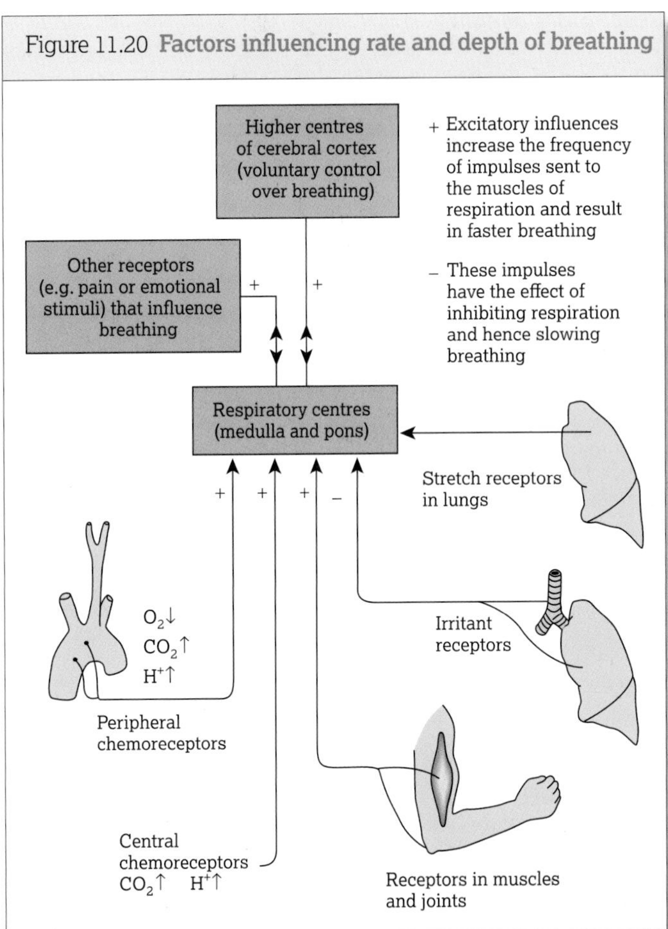

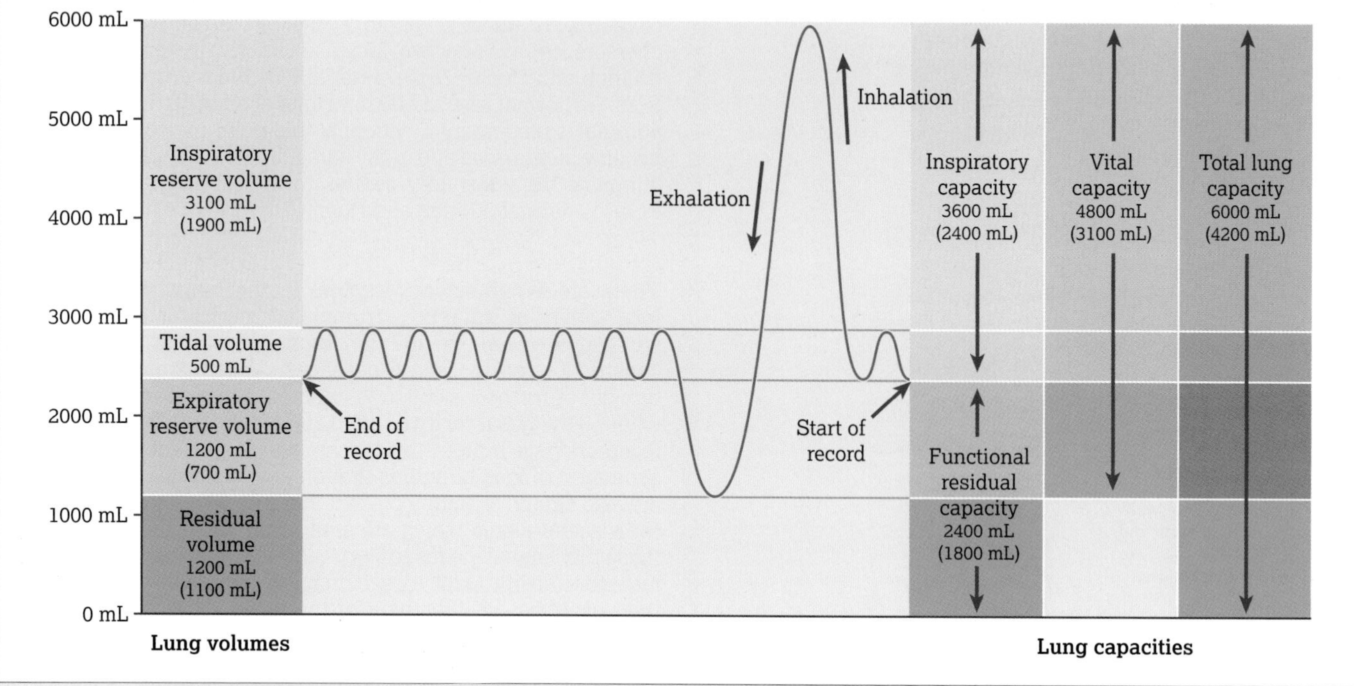

Figure 11.21 **Spirogram of lung volumes and capacities. The average values for a healthy average male and female are indicated, with the values for a female in parenthesis. Note that the spirogram is read from right (start of record) to left (end of record).** ***Source:*** **Peate et al. (2014). Reproduced with permission from John Wiley & Sons.**

RELATED THEORY

Respiratory volumes

The quantity of air that is breathed in and out of the lungs varies depending on the conditions of inspiration and expiration (Marieb and Hoehn 2010). As such, several respiratory volumes can be described, combinations of which (termed respiratory capacities) are measured to gain information about a person's respiratory status (Marieb and Hoehn 2010). A summary of these volumes can be seen in Figure 11.21. See Table 11.5 for a summary of respiratory volumes and capacities for males and females.

Gaseous exchange

Gaseous exchange occurs during *external respiration* where oxygen diffuses from the air in the alveoli of the lungs into blood in the pulmonary capillaries, and carbon dioxide diffuses from the blood into the alveolar air. This occurs as there is a flow of gases from areas of higher pressure to areas of lower pressure; oxygen diffuses from alveolar air where its partial pressure is higher than in the capillary blood, and carbon dioxide diffuses from the blood where its partial pressure is higher than in the alveolar air (Tortora and Derrickson 2011). *Internal respiration,* or systemic gas exchange, takes place where the same gases move into or out of the cells of the body by diffusion, so oxygen moves into the tissues and carbon dioxide moves out of them. See Figure 11.22 for the changes in partial pressures of oxygen and carbon dioxide during internal and external respiration (Tortora and Derrickson 2011). Please see Chapter 9: Respiratory care for further information.

Transport through the blood

Oxygen does not dissolve easily in water and therefore only 1.5% of the oxygen is transported in the blood by being dissolved in the plasma; the other 98.5% is bound to haemoglobin in the red blood cells, forming oxyhaemoglobin ($Hb\text{-}O_2$) (Tortora and Derrickson 2011). The majority of carbon dioxide is transported in the blood as bicarbonate ions (HCO_3^-) within the plasma (70%), approximately 20–23% is bound to haemoglobin forming carbaminohaemoglobin ($Hb\text{-}CO_2$), and the remaining 7–10% is dissolved in the plasma (Marieb and Hoehn 2010). This process is summarized in Figure 11.23; see Chapter 9: Respiratory care.

Hypoxia and hypercapnia

Hypoxia is defined as inadequate oxygen delivery to the tissues. Hypoxia can have various causes and, based on this, can be classified into four types (Marieb and Hoehn 2010, Tortora and Derrickson 2011).

- *Hypoxaemic hypoxia*: caused by a low PO_2 in arterial blood as a result of breathing air with inadequate oxygen (such as at high altitude) or abnormal ventilation/perfusion matching in the lungs (due to airway obstruction or fluid in the lungs). Carbon monoxide poisoning can also cause this.
- *Anaemic hypoxia*: caused by too little functioning haemoglobin being present in the blood which reduces the transport of oxygen to the cells (such as haemorrhage or anaemia).
- *Ischaemic hypoxia*: caused when blood flow to a specific area is inadequate to supply enough oxygen, even though PO_2 and $Hb\text{-}O_2$ levels are normal (due to embolism or thrombosis).
- *Histotoxic hypoxia*: caused by the cells being unable to use the oxygen that has been delivered; this can occur as a result of poisons such as cyanide.

Signs of hypoxia include tachypnoea, dyspnoea, tachycardia, restlessness and confusion, headache, mild hypertension and pallor; in its severe stages the symptoms will worsen, leading to slow, irregular breathing, cyanosis, hypotension, altered level of consciousness, blurred vision and eventual respiratory arrest (Beachey 2012).

Hypercapnia is an elevated level of carbon dioxide level in the blood. Signs include tachypnoea (eventually becoming bradypnoea as it worsens), dyspnoea, tachycardia, hypertension, headaches, vasodilation, drowsiness, sweating and a red colouration (Beachey 2012). Patients with hypercapnia will require

Table 11.5 **Respiratory volumes and capacities**

Respiratory volumes and capacities	Adult male average value	Adult female average value	Description
Tidal volume (V_T)	500mL	500mL	The volume of air inhaled or exhaled in one breath
Minute volume (MV)			The total volume of air inhaled or exhaled each minute = 12 breaths per minute × 500mL/breath = 6 litres/minute
Inspiratory reserve volume (IRV)	3100mL	1900mL	The volume of air that can be forcibly inhaled after a normal tidal volume inhalation
Expiratory reserve volume (ERV)	1200mL	700mL	The volume of air that can be forcibly exhaled after a normal tidal volume exhalation
Residual volume (RV)	1200mL	1100mL	The volume of air left in the lungs after a forced exhalation
Inspiratory capacity (IC)	3600mL	2400mL	The sum of the tidal volume and inspiratory reserve volume = 500 + 3100 = 3600mL (male) =500 + 2400 = 2900mL (female)
Functional residual capacity (FRC)	2400mL	1800mL	The sum of the residual volume and expiratory reserve volume = 1200 + 1200 = 2400mL (male) =1100 + 700 = 1800mL (female)
Vital capacity (VC)	4800mL	3100mL	The sum of inspiratory reserve volume, tidal volume and expiratory reserve volume =3100 + 500 + 1200 = 4800mL (male) = 1900 + 500 + 700 = 3100mL (female)
Total lung capacity (TLC)	6000mL	4200mL	The sum of vital capacity and residual volume = 4800 + 1200 = 6000mL (male) = 3100 + 1100 = 4200mL (female)

Source: Adapted from Tortora & Derrickson (2011).

urgent medical attention and close monitoring as hypercapnia will cause respiratory acidosis (Beachey 2012). Patients with chronic hypercapnia, such as those who have chronic obstructive pulmonary disease (COPD), will have at least partially adapted to the chronically high levels of carbon dioxide; oxygen therapy needs to be administered with caution in these patients as they are at risk of hypercapnic respiratory failure (O'Driscoll et al. 2008).

EVIDENCE-BASED APPROACHES

Rationale

The purpose of respiratory assessment is to determine the respiratory status of the patient (Hunter and Rawlings-Anderson 2008). A thorough respiratory assessment is vital to:

- identify patients who are at risk of deterioration
- commence treatment that may stabilize and improve the patient's condition and outcomes
- help prevent unnecessary admission to critical care units (Higginson and Jones 2009).

Alteration in respiratory observations may indicate a severe derangement in a range of body systems, not simply the respiratory system, so it is a vital indicator of morbidity (Cretikos et al. 2008). Respiratory dysfunction is also a known precursor to adverse events with an associated increase in mortality (NICE 2007a). Breathing, and more specifically respiratory rate, is one of the most sensitive indicators of critical illness and is usually the first vital sign to alter in the deteriorating patient; therefore timely, accurate observations, with early, effective and appropriate interventions may vastly improve patient outcomes (Hunter and Rawlings-Anderson 2008, Moore 2007). Despite this, research shows that respiratory rate is often not recorded or it is just guessed (Jonsson et al. 2011, Leuvan and Mitchell 2008).

Indications

As mentioned previously in this chapter, all patients who are in hospital should have observations taken and recorded regularly (NICE 2007a). In addition, respiratory observations should also be taken and recorded:

- following surgery, investigative procedures, trauma, infections or emergency situations in order to compare and identify any changes to baseline observations (Booker 2009, Hunter and Rawlings-Anderson 2008)
- to monitor before and during blood or blood product transfusions or intravenous fluids (Hunter and Rawlings-Anderson 2008)
- to monitor response to medications, including opiates and bronchodilators (Hunter and Rawling-Anderson 2008).

If the patient is acutely ill or at risk of respiratory deterioration, they will require continuous pulse oximetry and frequent respiratory assessment (Booker 2009, Levine 2007). Similarly, if the patient is receiving oxygen therapy then they will need to be closely monitored to ensure its efficacy (Higginson and Jones 2009). Any patient who has, or is at risk of, chronic hypercapnia should have close monitoring of their respiratory function, with observations performed at least hourly (O'Driscoll et al. 2008).

Any healthcare professional who has been trained and assessed as competent can perform a respiratory assessment and pulse oximetry in accordance with local hospital policy.

Methods of assessing respiration

Airway assessment

It is important to assess whether there is any obstruction to the patient's airway. Such obstruction may be from vomit, foreign bodies or the patient's tongue (Higginson and Jones 2009). In the conscious patient, a quick way to check airway patency is to

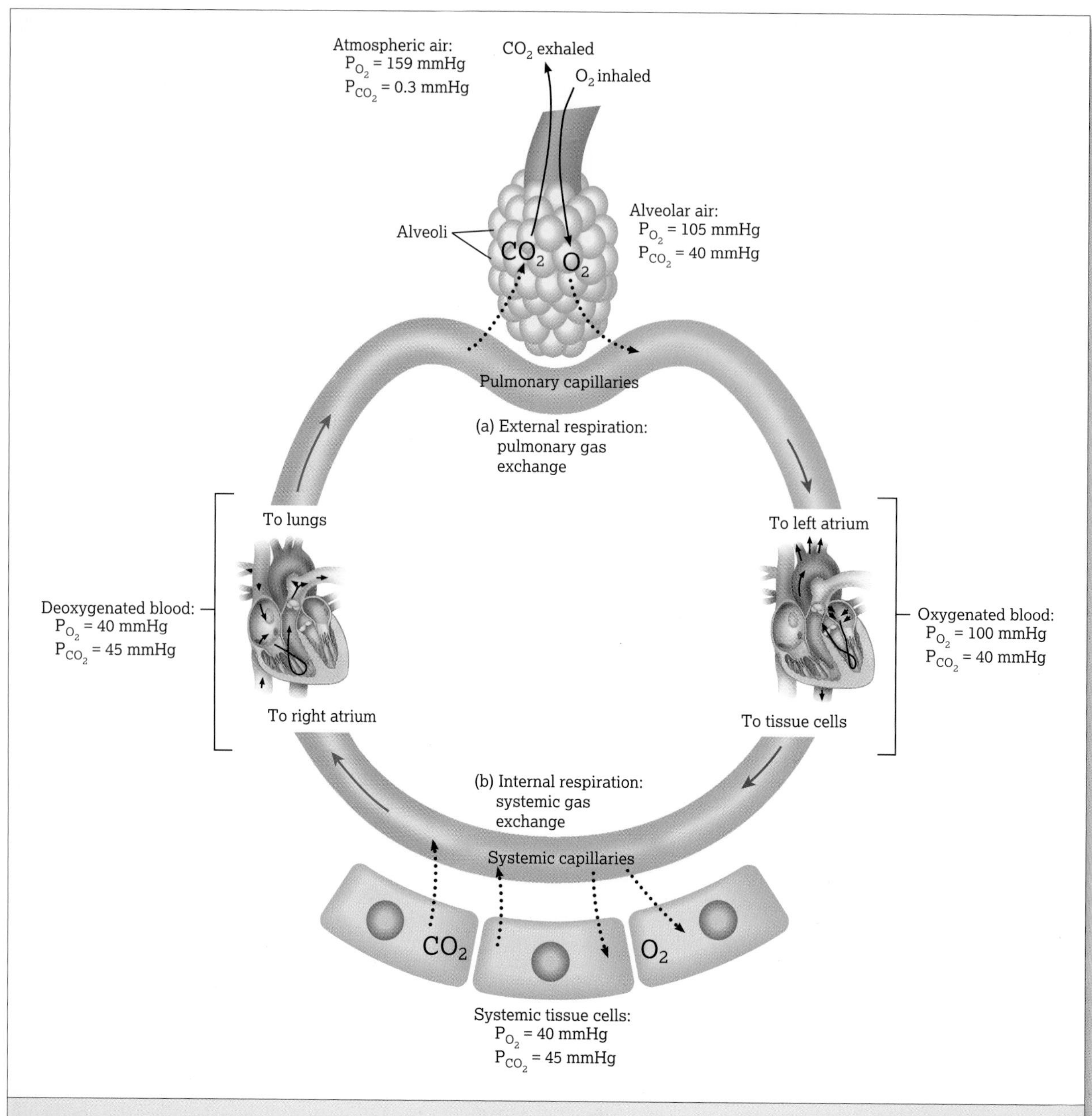

Figure 11.22 **Changes to partial pressures of oxygen and carbon dioxide (in mmHg) during internal and external respiration.** ***Source:*** **Tortora and Derrickson (2011). Reproduced with permission from John Wiley & Sons.**

ask them a question; a normal verbal response confirms that the patient's airway is clear, they are breathing and perfusing their brain (Higginson and Jones 2009) (see Chapter 9: Respiratory care).

Breathing assessment

This is required to assess the patient's ability to adequately ventilate. The initial stage of the breathing assessment is to observe the patient and watch how they breathe, termed inspection. It is important that the following aspects are observed:

- colour of the patient's skin and mucous membranes
- use of accessory muscles or other respiratory signs
- rhythm, rate and depth of respiration
- shape and expansion of the chest (Higginson and Jones 2009).

Skin colour

Cyanosis is a blue tone to the skin and mucous membranes which may occur when high levels of unsaturated haemoglobin are present in the blood; it may be detectable when oxygen saturation of arterial blood drops below 85% (Moore 2007). Cyanosis is, however, often considered a late sign of respiratory deterioration and may be difficult to appreciate, particularly in artificial lighting. There are two types of cyanosis: central, affecting the lips and oral mucosa, usually indicating cardiorespiratory insufficiency, and peripheral, observed in the skin and nail beds, usually indicating poor peripheral circulation if seen in isolation (Moore 2007). Patients who are anaemic may not be cyanotic as there is insufficient haemoglobin to generate the blue tone (Moore 2007); similarly, a pale skin tone may indicate that the patient is anaemic or in shock (Bickley and Szilagyi 2009).

Use of accessory muscles

The use of accessory muscles to increase inspiration such as the sternocleidomastoid, scalene, trapezius and abdominals may suggest that the patient has difficulty breathing and is in

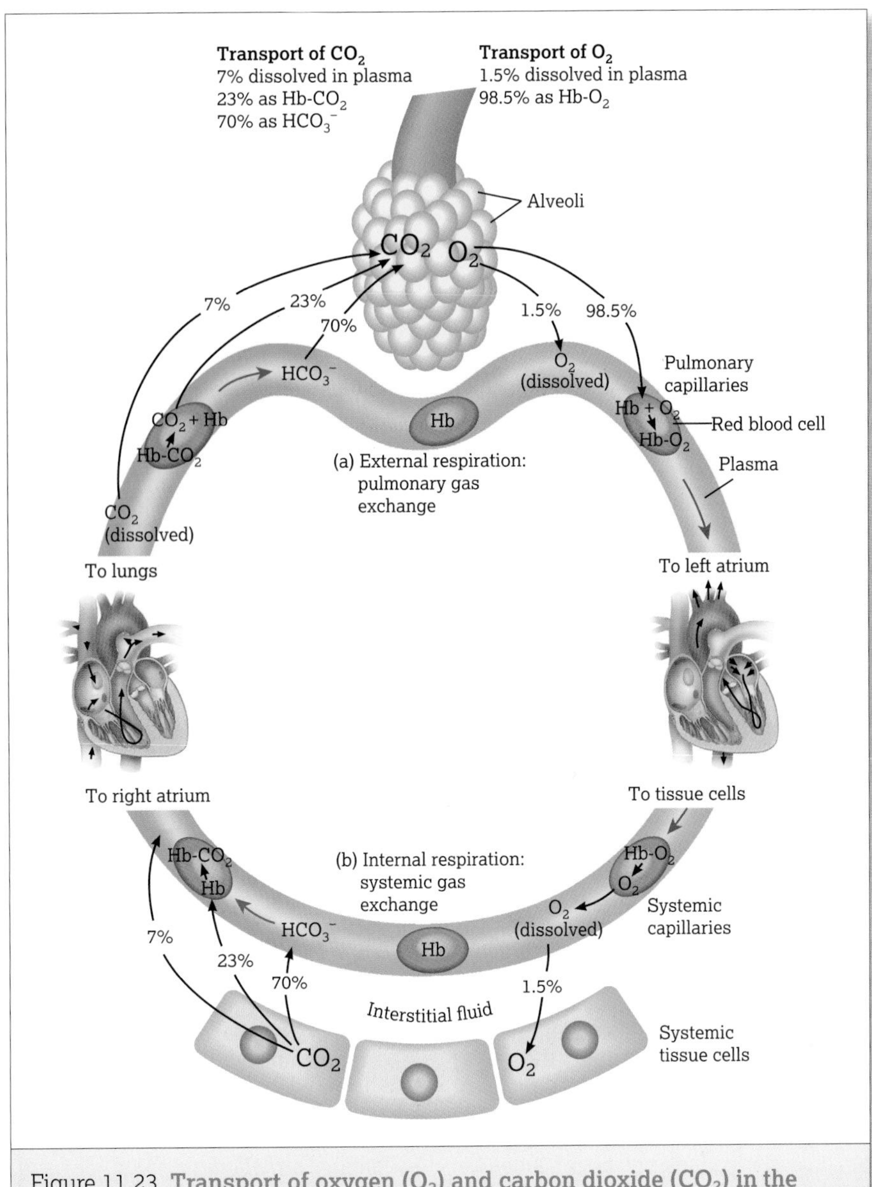

Figure 11.23 **Transport of oxygen (O_2) and carbon dioxide (CO_2) in the blood.** ***Source:*** **Tortora and Derrickson (2011). Reproduced with permission from John Wiley & Sons.**

respiratory distress (Higginson and Jones 2009, Moore 2007). Observe the patient's neck during inspiration to see if there is any contraction of the sternomastoid or other accessory muscles (Bickley and Szilagyi 2009). In addition, some patients may breathe through pursed lips on expiration as they try to force air out of overdistended alveoli, or have nasal flaring as they attempt to force more air into the lungs (Moore 2007).

Rhythm, rate and depth of respiration

The normal respiratory rate in adults is 12–18 breaths per minute with expiration lasting approximately twice as long as inspiration (Higginson and Jones 2009). The rate should be counted for one full minute to fully assess both the rate and the rhythm (Morton and Rempher 2009). An increase from the patient's normal respiratory rate by as little as 3–5 breaths per minutes is an early and important sign of respiratory distress (Field 2006). Patients with a respiratory rate greater than 24 breaths per minute should have frequent observations and be closely monitored; if they also have other physiological alterations, they should receive prompt medical attention, as should all patients with a respiratory rate greater than 27 breaths per minute (Cretikos et al. 2008). Respiratory rates of eight or less also require urgent medical care (Docherty 2002).

Respiratory rate can be classified into one of the following.

- *Eupnoea*: unconscious, gentle respiration, the normal respiratory rate and rhythm, usually between 12–17 breaths per minute (Patton and Thibodeau 2009).
- *Bradypnoea*: a respiratory rate which is slower than the normal range – less than 10 breaths per minute; this may signify depression of the respiratory centre, opioid overdose, increased intracranial pressure or a diabetic coma; regardless of the cause, this indicates a severe deterioration in the patient's condition (Bickley and Szilagyi 2009, Moore 2007).
- *Tachypnoea*: a respiratory rate which is faster than the normal range and shallow – greater than 18–24 breaths per minute; this may indicate a number of conditions including anxiety, pain, restrictive lung disease, cardiac or circulatory problems, or pyrexia and is the first indication of respiratory distress (Bickley and Szilagyi 2009, Moore 2007, Simpson 2006).

- *Dyspnoea*: breathing where the individual is conscious of the effort to breathe and finds it more difficult; when dyspnoea occurs when the patient lies flat, it is termed orthopnoea (Patton and Thibodeau 2009).
- *Apnoea*: is a temporary cessation of breathing (Patton and Thibodeau 2009).
- *Biot's breathing*: irregular respiratory rate and depth – alternating periods of deep gasping with periods of apnoea, seen in patients with increased intracranial pressure, head trauma, brain abscess, spinal meningitis and encephalitis (Patton and Thibodeau 2009, Simpson 2006).
- *Cheyne–Stokes breathing*: regular pattern of alternating periods of deep breathing with periods of apnoea; this may have many causes including heart failure, renal failure, brain damage, drug overdose or increased intracranial pressure, and may also be present at the end-stage of life (Bickley and Szilagyi 2009, Simpson 2006).
- *Kussmaul breathing:* rapid deep breathing resulting from stimulation of the respiratory centre caused by metabolic acidosis and occurs in diabetic ketoacidosis (Moore 2007).
- *Hyperventilation*: increase in respiratory rate and depth and can be caused by anxiety, exercise, metabolic acidosis, diabetic ketoacidosis or alteration in blood gas concentrations (Bickley and Szilagyi 2009, Simpson 2006).
- *Hypoventilation*: is shallow and irregular breathing and can be caused by an overdose of certain anaesthetic agents or opiate drugs; it may also occur with prolonged bedrest or conscious splinting of the chest to avoid respiratory pain (Simpson 2006).

Shape and expansion of the chest

The respiratory assessment should also consider the shape and expansion of the chest. The anteroposterior (AP) diameter of the chest wall may give an indication of underlying respiratory conditions or other problems (Higginson and Jones 2009); it may change with ageing or increase in chronic pulmonary disease (Bickley and Szilagyi 2009). It is also important to view the way the chest expands with each breath; when normal, it should be equal and bilateral (Higginson and Jones 2009). Any paradoxical movements such as only one side of the chest moving, greater movement on one side or one side moving up and the other moving down should be noted as they can indicate a particular problem with one side of the chest (Higginson and Jones 2009). Asymmetrical chest expansion is abnormal and may indicate pleural disease, pulmonary fibrosis, collapse of upper lobes or bronchial obstruction; spinal deformities such as kyphosis also influence lung expansion (Moore 2007).

General condition or distress of the patient

Respiratory assessment also involves assessing the entire patient for other signs or symptoms of respiratory insufficiency; high temperature may be suggestive of pneumonia, increased pulse may indicate cardiovascular disease and low blood pressure may indicate sepsis. The patient's level of consciousness should also be assessed, along with how alert and orientated they are and if they appear distressed (Moore 2007). If the patient can only speak in very short sentences or only a few words without needing to stop to breathe then they are in respiratory distress (Higginson and Jones 2009).

Pulse oximetry

Pulse oximetry provides continuous and non-invasive monitoring of the oxygen saturation from haemoglobin in arterial blood (Moore 2007). Pulse oximetry is an effective method of monitoring for hypoxaemia and will immediately alert the practitioner to a fall in arterial oxygen saturation, often even before any obvious symptoms are displayed (Higginson and Jones 2009, Moore 2007). It also provides useful information about heart rate (Jevon and Ewens 2000). Normal oxygen saturation ranges between 95% and 100%; however, patients with chronic respiratory conditions may have adjusted to lower oxygen saturation levels (Higginson and Jones 2009) and therefore the aim should be to keep oxygen saturations as near to the patient's normal range as possible (Levine 2007, O'Driscoll et al. 2008). In general terms, a level below 90% is of concern, but the trend of oxygen saturations may be of more importance than individual readings as this gives an indication of whether the patient is responding to therapy or deteriorating (Higginson and Jones 2009, Jevon and Ewens 2007). The British Thoracic Society states that oxygen saturation should be kept at 94–98% for acutely ill adults and 88–92% for those at risk of hypercapnic respiratory failure (O'Driscoll et al. 2008). It also states that in patients who are not hypoxic, a sudden drop of greater than 3% in oxygen saturation within the target saturation range should prompt the nurse to check that the device is working correctly and to undertake further assessment of the patient's condition (O'Driscoll et al. 2008).

Arterial blood gas analysis has been the gold standard for monitoring arterial oxygen saturation, but it is invasive, time consuming, costly and involves repeated arterial blood sampling and only provides intermittent information (Jevon and Ewens 2007). The use of pulse oximetry may therefore reduce the need for arterial samples to be taken (Simpson 2006).

Although pulse oximetry is a useful tool in the assessment of respiratory status, its limitations should be recognized. One of the main limitations is its inability to reliably detect hypoventilation (particularly in patients receiving supplemental oxygen) and carbon dioxide retention (Higginson and Jones 2009, Jevon and Ewens 2007); this is usually confirmed by measurement of $PaCO_2$ by arterial blood gas analysis. Likewise, pulse oximetry does not give an indication of haemoglobin so if the patient is profoundly anaemic then their oxygen saturation may be normal but they may still be hypoxic (Levine 2007). Other factors which may impact on the pulse oximetry readings include the following.

- *Nail polish:* particularly dark colours such as black, blue and green will affect the accuracy of readings (Moore 2007).
- *Intravenous dyes:* pulse oximetry may be inaccurate in patients who have received dye treatment such as methylene blue, indiocyanine green and indiocarmine (Levine 2007).
- *Poor peripheral perfusion:* to work effectively, an adequate peripheral blood flow is required. This may be impaired by factors such as hypovolaemia, hypotension, hypothermia, vasoconstriction or heart failure (Elliott and Coventry 2012) and may result in falsely low readings.
- *Cardiac arrhythmias:* such as atrial fibrillation can cause inadequate or irregular perfusion resulting in falsely low readings (Jevon and Ewens 2007).
- *Recording blood pressure:* inflation of the blood pressure cuff will cause the readings to be inaccurate; the probe should be positioned on a finger of the opposite arm to where blood pressure is being taken (Moore 2007).
- *Carbon monoxide poisoning:* pulse oximetry should not be used on patients with suspected or confirmed carbon monoxide poisoning as the sensor cannot differentiate between oxyhaemoglobin and carboxyhaemoglobin and will therefore provide falsely elevated oxygen saturation readings; arterial blood gas analysis should be undertaken instead (Levine 2007, Moore 2007).
- *Methaemoglobinaemia:* changes in the structure of haemoglobin, caused by lignocaine, nitrates, metoclopramide and local anaesthetics, can inhibit oxygen release from the haemoglobin, resulting in tissue hypoxia and unreliable oxygen saturation measurements (Jevon and Ewens 2007).
- *Bright external light:* fluorescent lighting or light interference from surgical lamps, infra-red warming lamps or direct sunlight can give falsely high readings (Adam and Osborne 2005, Jevon and Ewens 2007).
- *Movement:* sudden movement, due to shivering or seizures, or restlessness may dislodge the sensor or cause motion artefact affecting the ability of light to travel from the light-emitting diode to the detector in the probe (Moore 2007).

PRE-PROCEDURAL CONSIDERATIONS

Equipment

Pulse oximeter

A pulse oximeter is a device that measures the amount of haemoglobin saturation in the tissue capillaries. The probe consists of two light-emitting diodes (one red and one infra-red) on one side of the probe and a photodetector on the other side. The device projects light through the tissue to the detector measuring absorption in pulsatile blood by saturated haemoglobin (visible red) and desaturated haemoglobin (infra-red wavelength). This is translated by the receiver into a percentage of oxygen saturation of the blood, symbolized as SpO_2 (McMorrow and Mythen 2006, Moore 2007).

In order to achieve a successful reading, the sensor of the pulse oximeter should be placed on an appropriate site with an adequate pulsating vascular bed (the probe must be designed for use on the chosen site). Therefore the sensor may be attached to the patient's fingers, ears, toes or nose (Goodell 2012, Higginson and Jones 2009, Jevon and Ewens 2007, Johnson et al. 2012, Yönt et al. 2011).

Pulse oximeters should be serviced and calibration checked according to the manufacturer's recommendations to ensure accurate and reliable data are recorded (Booker 2008). They should be used and maintained in accordance with the manufacturer's instructions. Any malfunctioning probes or machines should be taken out of clinical use until repair or service can be undertaken by the relevant department, in accordance with local policy.

Pulse oximeters are essential in all areas where emergency oxygen is given (O'Driscoll et al. 2008). Pulse oximeters form part of a department's emergency equipment and so should always be available in good working order. After use, the probe and machine should be cleaned, returned to its storage location and plugged into a mains electrical supply to charge the internal battery ready for use in an emergency.

Specific patient preparation

Appropriate positioning of the patient can help to ease any respiratory distress and facilitate the assessment and observation of their breathing (Moore 2009b). The patient should have rested and not have engaged in any strenuous physical activity prior to the assessment (Hunter and Rawlings-Anderson 2008). If this is not contraindicated, the patient should be positioned upright or lying in bed with the head section elevated to an angle of 45–60° to allow good lung expansion; pillows can help to support the patient in this position (Hunter and Rawlings-Anderson 2008). With the patient's consent, it may be useful to remove clothing from their thorax to aid with observation of breathing (Moore 2007, 2009b). Positioning can also help to relax the patient and therefore potentially reduce the distress resulting from breathlessness (Gosselink et al. 2008). The patient should give their consent to the assessment and be asked to keep still while pulse oximetry is being performed so that an accurate result can be obtained (Hunter and Rawlings-Anderson 2008). Similarly, blood pressure measurement should not be performed whilst pulse oximetry recording is under way and nail polish should be removed from the probe site (Moore 2007).

Procedure guideline 11.4 **Respiratory assessment and pulse oximetry**

Essential equipment

- Pulse oximeter
- Power source
- Cleaning materials (according to manufacturer's recommendations and local policy)
- Sensor (probe) applicable to the chosen site
- A watch with a second hand
- Appropriate method of documentation and a pen

Optional equipment

- Variety of sensors (probes) available for different sites

Pre-procedure

Action	Rationale
1 Wash hands thoroughly with soap and water and dry.	To reduce the risk of cross-contamination (Fraise and Bradley 2009, **E**; Hunter and Rawlings-Anderson 2008, **E**).
2 Explain the procedure to the patient, answering any questions they may have, and gain their consent.	Consent must be gained prior to commencing any procedure (NMC 2013, **C**).
3 Ask the patient to remain as still as possible during the procedure and ensure that a constant temperature is maintained in the patient's environment.	Artefacts from movement such as shivering may adversely affect the accuracy of measurement (Barnett et al. 2012, **E**).
4 While talking to the patient, assess their respiratory status, including their ability to talk in full sentences, the colour of their skin, whether they appear to be in distress or not, and whether they are alert and orientated.	This initial assessment can give important information about the patient's respiratory function and any potential problems (Higginson and Jones 2009, **E**; Kallet 2012, **E**).
5 Determine the site to be used to perform pulse oximetry. The site should have a good blood supply, determined by checking it is warm, with a proximal pulse and brisk capillary refill.	To ensure the sensor will get strong enough signals to produce a result by being located in a well-perfused area (Adam and Osborne 2005, **E**; Jevon and Ewens 2000, **E**; Levine 2007, **E**).
6 Ensure that the area to be used is clean and free from dirt, and that the sensor is also clean (Moore 2009a). If using the patient's fingers, ensure that all nail polish and any artificial nails have been removed.	Dirt or nail polish may interfere with the transmission of the light signals, causing inaccurate results (Booker 2008, **E**; Moore 2009a, **E**).

(continued)

Procedure guideline 11.4 **Respiratory assessment and pulse oximetry *(continued)***

Action	Rationale
7 Select the correct pulse oximeter sensor for the site which is most appropriate for your patient, dependent on circulation and the manufacturer's instructions.	The correct sensor should be used for each site to ensure good contact, that excessive pressure is not applied (Levine 2007, **E**) and that an accurate reading from the chosen site is obtained (Johnson et al. 2012, **E**).
Procedure	
8 Position the sensor securely but do not secure it with tape, unless specifically recommended by the manufacturer (MHRA 2010) (**Action figure 8**). If the pulse oximetry is to be continuous then the site should be changed at least every 4 hours.	If the probe is too tight it may impede the blood flow, leading to inaccurate results and the potential for pressure ulcer formation to the site, particularly in patients whose conditions can compromise skin integrity (Goodell 2012, **E**; Moore 2009a, **E**).
9 Turn the pulse oximeter on and, if using continuously, set the alarms on the device dependent on the patient's condition and within locally agreed limits.	To ensure that it is ready to use (Adam and Osborne 2005, **E**).
10 Ask the patient not to talk while you palpate their pulse. Check that the pulse reading on the device corresponds with the patient's actual pulse.	Any large deviations in pulse may show that the device is not measuring accurately or is being affected by movement (Levine 2007, **E**; Moore 2007, **E**).
11 Assess respiration by keeping your fingers on the patient's wrist once the pulse rate has been obtained. Count their respiratory rate for a full minute – one breath is equal to one inspiration and expiration and is done by watching the abdomen or chest wall move in and out (Hunter and Rawlings-Anderson 2008). Assess the regularity and depth of breathing, the shape and expansion of the chest, and look for any use of accessory muscles.	The patient should ideally not be aware that their respiratory rate is being counted as this may produce inaccurate results (Kallet 2012, **E**; Moore 2007, **E**).
Post-procedure	
12 Document results clearly, including the time and date of the reading.	Records must be kept of all assessments made and care provided (NMC 2010, **C**).
13 Clean the pulse oximeter according to manufacturer's recommendations and local policy.	It may become colonized and be a source of infection to another patient (Goodall and Allan 2009, **E**).
14 Wash hands thoroughly with soap and water and dry.	To reduce the risk of cross-contamination (Fraise and Bradley 2009, **E**).

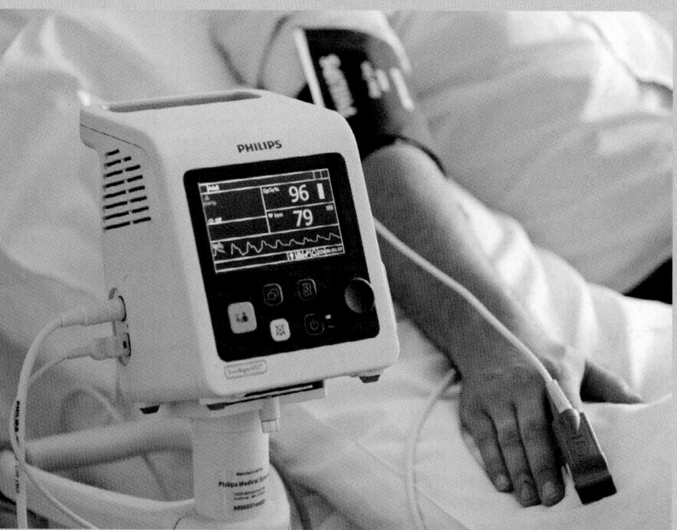

Action Figure 8 Position of an oxygen saturation probe.

Problem-solving table 11.4 **Prevention and resolution (Procedure guideline 11.4)**

Problem	Cause	Prevention	Action
Unable to turn on the pulse oximeter.	Low battery.	Ensure the pulse oximeter is left on continuous charge when not in use.	Connect to mains electricity – the pulse oximeter will function once it is connected to a power supply.
Pulse oximeter is working but the heart rate and saturations display is blank.	Loose connection.	Carefully store the cables after use to prevent damage.	Check that the probe is securely connected to the machine.
Poor trace or inconsistent reading.	Movement from shivering, seizures or tremors can affect the accuracy of the reading (Levine 2007, Moore 2007).	Encourage the patient to keep as still as possible. If still unable to obtain an accurate reading, try to use a site which is less affected by movement, for example an ear lobe (Levine 2007, Moore 2007).	If the finger has been used, compare the pulse rate as given by the oximeter with the palpated radial pulse – if there is a difference then the oxygen saturation reading will not be accurate and arterial blood gases may be required to monitor the patient's oxygen saturation, if accurate pulse oximetry cannot be obtained from an alternative site (Levine 2007).
Unexpectedly low result which does not correlate with the patient's clinical condition.	The site chosen may not have an adequate blood supply (Adam and Osborne 2005).	Check for perfusion by palpating for a pulse and checking the area is warm with good capillary refill.	Reposition sensor to new site. If it remains low, arterial blood gases may need to be considered (Adam and Osborne 2005).
Pulse oximetry heart rate does not correlate with palpated pulse.	Not all pulsations are being detected.	Check for perfusion by palpating for a pulse and checking the area is warm with good capillary refill.	Obtain a replacement probe and/ or monitor (Moore 2007).

POST-PROCEDURAL CONSIDERATIONS

Immediate care

Any abnormalities of respiration discovered during the respiratory assessment should prompt rapid action (Higginson and Jones 2009) as early intervention is essential to improve patient outcomes (Moore 2007). If there is risk of a compromised airway or respiratory insufficiency/failure then senior nursing and medical assistance, including an anaesthetist, should be requested urgently (RCUK 2011). Further information will be needed, including obtaining:

- a full set of observations including temperature, blood pressure and heart rate (Higginson and Jones 2009)
- a history of the patient's current condition and any past medical history, including a list of the medications they are taking (Bickley and Szilagyi 2009).

Other tests may also be required depending on the condition of the patient. These may include the following.

- Arterial blood gases to check for level of carbon dioxide, oxygen level, pH, acid/base balance (Higginson and Jones 2009).
- Sputum collection to assess for infection and/or specific diseases such as tuberculosis (Moore 2007, Simpson 2006).
- Chest X-ray or CT scan (Simpson 2006).
- Blood tests including a full blood count, urea and electrolytes, clotting screen and cross-match (Docherty 2002).
- Fluid balance to monitor for signs of fluid overload or dehydration (Docherty 2002).

Airway management and administration of oxygen

If a patient's condition necessitates the administration of oxygen, this should be provided as quickly and efficiently as possible. Although oxygen should be prescribed, in an emergency situation the absence of a prescription should not delay its adminstration (Higginson and Jones 2009). For further information see Chapter 9: Respiratory care.

Ongoing care

As well as involving senior nurses, the medical team and potentially anaesthestists in the care of the patient, it may also be useful to refer the patient to the physiotherapy team for further support and appropriate interventions (Docherty 2002).

Documentation

It is vital that all documentation on oxygen saturations should state whether the patient was breathing air or oxygen, and the flow of oxygen and method of administration (O'Driscoll et al. 2008). If the oxygen is being given in an emergency situation without a prescription then subsequent documentation must state the rationale for the administration of oxygen and the flow rate (O'Driscoll et al. 2008).

Education of patient and relevant others

One of the key focuses of education of patients with respiratory conditions should be to ascertain if they smoke and, if they do, to encourage them to stop as smoking cessation may help to improve their prognosis (Tonnesen et al. 2007). For more information on this topic see Chapter 9: Respiratory care.

COMPLICATIONS

It is recommended that to prevent any tissue damage, the pulse oximeter sensor is not taped in place (unless recommended by the manufacturer) and that the sensor should be resited routinely every 4 hours or more frequently if necessary, depending on the patient's condition and the manufacturer's recommendation. Assess tissues integrity before siting the probe and avoid placement on damaged tissue (Goodell 2012).

Peak flow

DEFINITION

Peak expiratory flow (PEF) is the highest flow achieved on forced expiration from a position of maximum lung inflation expressed in litres per minute (L/min) (Miller et al. 2005). PEF is a simple test of lung function, commonly used to help detect and monitor moderate and severe respiratory disease, and is particularly useful in the diagnosis and monitoring of patients with asthma to assess the degree of airway obstruction, the severity of an asthma attack and response to treatment (Booker 2007, British Thoracic Society/Scottish Intercollegiate Guidelines Network 2012, NICE 2013).

ANATOMY AND PHYSIOLOGY

In healthy individuals without any pathological conditions of the airways, factors which determine PEF include:

- the quality of the large airways
- the volume of the lungs (a function of thoracic dimensions and the individual's stature)
- the elastic properties of the lungs (the degree of stretch the lungs have been subjected to previously and the recoil ability of the lungs)
- the power and co-ordination of the expiratory muscles, primarily abdominal muscles (related to lung inflation and the speed with which maximum alveolar pressure is reached)
- the resistance of the instrument used to measure peak expiratory flow (Quanjer et al. 1997).

Any condition which alters any of the above factors could affect PEF. However, a reduction in one of these factors may be compensated for by an increase in one of the others, meaning that PEF may not alter, resulting in staff potentially underestimating the severity of the condition (Quanjer et al. 1997).

RELATED THEORY

530 Peak expiratory flow reflects a range of physiological characteristics of the lungs, airways and neuromusculature; the most common disorders which affect PEF are those which increase the resistance to air flow in the large conducting intrathoracic airways, such as asthma (Booker 2009, Quanjer et al. 1997). However, PEF may also be impaired by:

- disorders which limit chest movement and respiratory musculoskeletal problems
- obstruction of the extrathoracic airways
- impairment of nerves supplying the respiratory system (Quanjer et al. 1997).

Peak expiratory flow readings are subject to individual variation depending on the patient's age, gender, ethnic origin and stature (Quanjer et al. 1997). Therefore, the patient's results should be compared against normal reference values for people of the same age, gender and height (Figure 11.24) and, more importantly, against previous results for that individual (Higgins 2005, Jevon 2007b).

Figure 11.24 **Normal peak expiratory flow rate measurements.** ***Source:*** **Reproduced with permission from Clement Clarke International, Ltd (www.peakflow.com).**

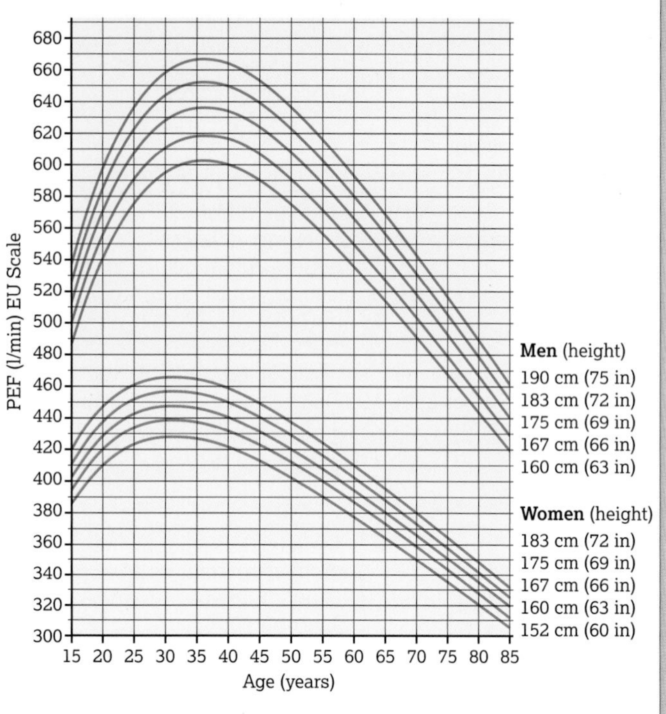

Peak expiratory flow is similar to forced expired volume in 1 second (FEV_1) measurements but the two are not interchangeable and both measure different aspects of lung function (Ruffin 2004). FEV_1 measures the volume of air exhaled during the first second of forced vital capacity (FVC), which occurs when an individual exhales forcefully to their maximum capacity following a deep inspiration (Marieb and Hoehn 2010). FEV_1 is usually 80% of FVC in healthy participants (Marieb and Hoehn 2010). FEV_1 is felt to be more sensitive in detecting mild airway obstruction as peak expiratory flow is effort dependent and so can have a greater degree of intrasubject variability (Hansen et al. 2001). However, both FEV_1 and PEF were found to have similar predictive ability in relation to mortality in patients with COPD, although FEV_1 was found to be a better predictor in patients with asthma (Booker 2009, Hansen et al. 2001).

EVIDENCE-BASED APPROACHES

Rationale

Peak expiratory flow is a simple, objective procedure which can be used to measure the degree of air flow limitation and, although it may not give a full representation of lung function, it can monitor efficacy of treatment and progression of the condition (Frew and Doffman 2012).

Indications

Peak expiratory flow can be used to:

- confirm a diagnosis of asthma and identify asthma control (Booker 2009, Ruffin 2004)
- determine the severity of an asthma exacerbation (Booker 2009)
- monitor the severity of the condition in patients with chronic severe asthma (Reddel 2006)
- identify exacerbating factors (Reddel 2006)

- monitor progression of respiratory disease (Frew and Doffman 2012)
- evaluate effectiveness of treatment (Frew and Doffman 2012).

Contraindications

There are no absolute contraindications for peak expiratory flow measurement but PEF should be used and interpreted with caution in the following situations.

- Patients who are acutely breathless, as the procedure requires physical effort (Higgins 2005)
- Patients with severe air flow obstruction, as included in the measurement may be air coming from the collapsing airway, yielding an erroneously high result (Quanjer et al. 1997).
- Patients unable to take a full inspiration, for example if they have a persistent cough, as the results will be inaccurate (Quanjer et al. 1997).
- Consecutive results producing a reduction in scoring – the procedure itself may cause an exacerbation of the air flow limitation (Quanjer et al. 1997).
- Young children may not understand or be able to comply with the procedure correctly (Gorelick et al. 2004).

Methods for measuring peak flow

Treatment is often based on PEF measurements and so it is vital that these are as accurate as possible. Patients should be advised to perform PEF measurements in accordance with their monitoring regimen even if symptom free (Buist et al. 2006) as trends can be more important than isolated results (unless the isolated results reflect an exacerbation) (Booker 2009). The patient should repeat the procedure three times with the best result of the three being documented (Miller et al. 2005). Unless the procedure induces an exacerbation, there should be consistency between the three results. If the top two results have a greater disparity than 40 L/min then, as long as the patient is not fatigued, a further two attempts can be made to reach a greater level of consistency (Miller et al. 2005).

Timing of peak flow readings

Whilst an isolated PEF measurement can indicate a restriction in air flow, in general sequential measurements are of more value, displaying trends essential to understanding the severity and progression of the disease (Booker 2009, Quanjer et al. 1997). However, there may be significant diurnal variations, with higher values obtained in the evenings and the lowest measurements occurring during the night and first thing in the morning (Jevon 2007b, Quanjer et al. 1997). Therefore, it is recommended that measurements should be taken and documented on waking, in the afternoon and prior to going to bed (Frew and Doffman 2012). If it is suspected that the patient may have restricted air flow due to occupational causes, the patient should take measurements for a minimum of 2 weeks while at work and 2 weeks while not at work to enable a comparison (Frew and Doffman 2012).

LEGAL AND PROFESSIONAL ISSUES

Competencies

All healthcare professionals who measure PEF must have received appropriate approved training and undertaken supervised practice; this role should be undertaken in accordance with local hospital policy (Higgins 2005, Jevon 2007b).

PRE-PROCEDURAL CONSIDERATIONS

Equipment

Wright and mini-Wright peak flow meter

Peak flow is measured by the patient exhaling as quickly and forcefully as possible following maximal inspiration; the maximum expiratory flow is measured by the PEF meter and usually occurs early in expiration (Bongers and O'Driscoll 2006).The Wright peak flow meter was developed in 1959 as a portable, simple device for monitoring PEF in the home. It has since been redesigned as the mini-Wright peak flow meter which is commonly used today (Ruffin 2004). In September 2004 the scales of measurement used on peak flow meters were changed from the non-linear Wright scale, which was found to overestimate PEF by up to 30%, to a new EU scale (Bongers and O'Driscoll 2006). The EU scale specifies one measurement range from 60 L/min to 800 L/min and increases the accuracy of the assessment, enhancing the ability to compare measurements with conventional spirometry (Higgins 2005). All new prescriptions and sales of peak flow meters in the European Union after this time have been for this new model which is labelled as 'EN 13826' or 'EU scale'.

Patients with their own meter should be encouraged to bring it with them to appointments. If the patient does not have their own meter then most hospitals and clinics have multiple patient use PEF meters which are valved and have disposable single patient use mouthpieces to prevent infection (Booker 2009). Most hand-held PEF meters do not need day-to-day calibration (Miller et al. 2005) but all PEF meters should be replaced annually as with regular use the spring becomes slack and so the meter becomes inaccurate (Booker 2007).

All PEF meters should be used and maintained in accordance with the manufacturer's instructions. In settings where meters are used between patients, a log should be kept of cleaning and disinfection procedures and disposable one-way mouthpieces that prevent patients inhaling through the meter should be used (Booker 2007).

Spirometers

Spirometers can produce a reading for PEF alongside other lung function measurements such as FVC. However, these results may not be comparable to those obtained using a mini-Wright meter due to both the equipment and technique used. Therefore, the patient should use the same equipment and technique each time to enable comparisons with previous results (Bongers and O'Driscoll 2006).

Assessment and recording tools

Recording peak flow measurements on individualized action plans/booklets gives patients a greater degree of control and awareness about when they need to access medical care. The use of these recording tools is strongly advocated (British Thoracic Society/Scottish Intercollegiate Guidelines Network 2012, Gibson et al. 2003).

Specific patient preparation

The procedure should be performed when the patient is at rest (unless otherwise specified) and may be performed with them sitting upright or standing as long as their neck is not flexed (Quanjer et al. 1997). To increase reliability and enable comparisons to be drawn, it is advisable that the patient uses the same posture each time (Booker 2009).

Education

The practitioner must ensure that the patient is fully informed about how to perform the procedure and performs it accurately, as even small alterations in technique may produce inaccurate results. If the patient has not performed the procedure previously then they will need a full explanation of what PEF is, what it measures and how they should interpret and act on the results (Higgins 2005). Patients should have the opportunity to have the procedure demonstrated for them and have their own practice attempts (Quanjer et al. 1997).

Procedure guideline 11.5 **Peak flow reading using a manual peak flow meter**

Essential equipment

- Peak flow meter
- Disposable mouthpiece
- Peak flow chart to document results and a pen
- Other respiratory function tests including pulse oximetry
- Oxygen mask and oxygen source
- Equipment to give a nebulizer
- Emergency resuscitation equipment

Pre-procedure

Action	Rationale
1 Explain the procedure to the patient and obtain their consent.	To ensure the patient understands the procedure and gives valid consent (NMC 2013, **C**).
2 Ask the patient what their best peak flow measurements have been and what their current peak flow readings are.	This will enable a comparison to be drawn between their current and previous results (British Thoracic Society/Scottish Intercollegiate Guidelines Network 2012, **C**).
3 Wash and dry hands or use alcohol handrub.	To minimize the spread of cross-infection (Fraise and Bradley 2009, **E**).
4 Assemble equipment; ask the patient to use their own meter, if it is in good working order and less than 1 year old. If using a multiple patient use device, ensure that it is valved and has a disposable single patient use mouthpiece.	As different equipment might have slight variations in results (Bongers and O'Driscoll 2006, **E**). Regular use causes the spring to become slack and so the meter may become inaccurate (Booker 2007, **E**). To prevent cross-infection (Booker 2009, **E**).
5 Ask the patient to adopt the position in which they normally undertake the procedure; this can be either standing or sitting. They should be advised not to flex their neck.	In order that their maximal lung volume can be reached and so that there is no positional obstruction which could affect the results, and to enable comparisons between results (Booker 2009, **E**; Quanjer et al. 1997, **E**).
6 Push needle on the gauge down to zero.	To ensure the results are accurate (Booker 2009, **E**).
Procedure	
7 Ask the patient to hold the peak flow meter horizontally, ensuring their fingers do not impede the gauge.	So that the movement of the needle is not obstructed and can move easily (Booker 2009, **E**; Frew and Doffman 2012, **E**).
8 Ask the patient to take a deep breath in through their mouth to full inspiration.	To ensure they achieve the greatest measurement (Frew and Doffman 2012, **E**; Quanjer et al. 1997, **E**).
9 Ask the patient to immediately place their lips tightly around the mouthpiece. The inspiration should be held for no longer than 2 seconds at total lung capacity.	To ensure a good seal around the mouthpiece and to prevent their tongue and teeth from obstructing it (Booker 2009, **E**; Quanjer et al. 1997, **E**).
10 Ask the patient to blow out through the meter in a short sharp 'huff' as forcefully as they can. See **Action figure 10**.	This can be very quick and need only take about 1 second, to enable accuracy of results (Booker 2009, **E**; Quanjer et al. 1997, **E**).
11 Take a note of the reading and return the needle on the gauge to zero. Ask the patient to take a moment to rest and then repeat the procedure twice, noting the reading each time. Ideally there should be less than 20 L/min difference between the three readings. If there is more than 40 L/min difference in the recordings, two additional blows can be performed. Document the highest of the three acceptable readings, stating the specific time or previous medication.	To ensure that the best possible result is achieved (Frew and Doffman 2012, **E**; Miller et al. 2005, **E**; Quanjer et al. 1997, **E**).
Post-procedure	
12 Document the readings on the patient's record chart, comparing measured values against predicted values or patient trends and report any abnormality to medical or senior nursing staff.	Records must be kept of all assessments made, treatment or care provided and the outcome of this (NMC 2010, **C**).
13 Dispose of the mouthpiece and clean the meter in line with local policies and the manufacturer's recommendation.	To prevent the risk of cross-infection (Fraise and Bradley 2009, **E**).
14 Wash and dry hands or use alcohol handrub.	To minimize the spread of cross-infection (Fraise and Bradley 2009, **E**).

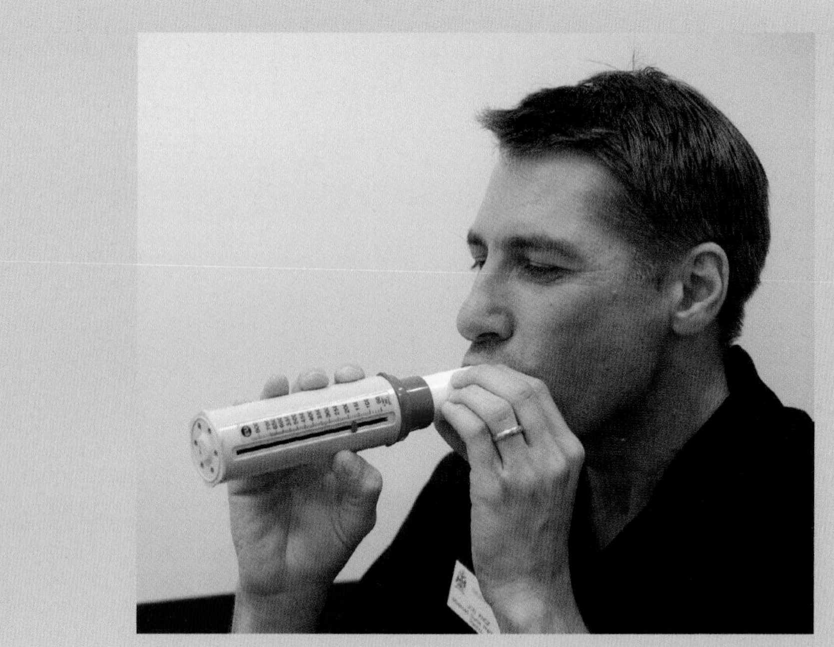

Action Figure 10 Manual peak flow meter technique.

Problem-solving table 11.5 **Prevention and resolution (Procedure guideline 11.5)**

Problem	Cause	Prevention	Action
A higher than expected result is obtained.	May be caused by the needle not being pushed back to zero prior to commencement, or by poor technique leading to 'explosive decompression' whereby there is sudden opening of the glottis, or release of the tongue occluding the mouthpiece, or caused by coughing or spitting into the mouthpiece (Quanjer et al. 1997).	Allow practice runs prior to the procedure and ensure that the patient is educated on technique.	Reset the needle back to zero, educate the patient on the correct technique, and if they appear fatigued, allow them to rest prior to repeating the procedure.
A lower than expected result is obtained.	Failing to take a maximal inhalation. Holding breath at maximal inhalation and delaying blowing into the meter. Failure to make maximum effort. Mouthpiece leaks due to blowing out cheeks, loose-fitting dentures or facial palsy (Booker 2007).	Allow practice runs prior to the procedure and ensure that the patient is educated on the correct technique.	Reset the needle back to zero, educate the patient on the correct technique, and if they appear fatigued, allow them to rest prior to repeating the procedure.

POST-PROCEDURAL CONSIDERATIONS

Immediate care

A reduction in peak flow may indicate a life-threatening situation and so should receive urgent medical attention. For example, a PEF<50% of the reference value incidates acute severe asthma and <33% indicates acute life-threatening asthma (British Thoracic Society/Scottish Intercollegiate Guidelines Network 2012). The treatment provided will be aimed at increasing air flow and oxygenation. Oxygen therapy is usually applied with the aim of keeping oxygen saturations at 94–98% (British Thoracic Society/Scottish Intercollegiate Guidelines Network 2012). In patients who are known, or suspected, to have hypercapnia, oxygen should be initially administered at 28% via a Venturi mask out of hospital, and in hospital at 24% via a Venturi mask, unless their condition is of such severity to require a greater flow (O'Driscoll et al. 2008). However, if the patient's oxygen saturation exceeds 92% then the flow of oxygen should be reduced (O'Driscoll et al. 2008).

All these patients will require arterial blood gas samples to be taken at the earliest opportunity to enable their condition to be more thoroughly assessed (O'Driscoll et al. 2008). Medication will be used to try and reverse the air flow reduction and will usually include a combination of inhaled bronchodilators and steroids (British Thoracic Society/Scottish Intercollegiate Guidelines Network 2012).

Ongoing care

It should be noted if the patient has experienced or been in contact with any of the following prior to the exacerbation.

- Cold air.
- Heightened levels of emotion.
- Exposure to allergens.
- Viral infection.
- Inhaled irritants such as pollution or dust.
- Medication or drugs, including anti-inflammatories and beta-adrenoreceptor blocking agents.
- Occupational sensitizers (Frew and Doffman 2012).

The patient will probably require other medical tests to assess their condition; these may include chest X-ray, blood and sputum tests (Frew and Doffman 2012).

Education of patient and relevant others

Patient education is vital so that patients can manage their own condition (Buist et al. 2006). This will include information on exacerbating factors, smoking cessation and when to access medical help. Written personalized action plans as part of self-management education have been shown to improve health outcomes for people with asthma, with particularly good evidence for those with moderate-to-severe disease. It is also useful for those who have had recent exacerbations where successful interventions have reduced hospitalizations and emergency department attendances in people with severe asthma; patients also report improvement in outcomes such as self-efficacy, knowledge and confidence (British Thoracic Society/Scottish Intercollegiate Guidelines Network 2012).

Learning Activity 11.2 Case study: Breathing assessment

Mr Lyle is a 74-year-old man who has been admitted with exacerbation of his chronic obstructive pulmonary disease (COPD). He is finding it hard to catch his breath, particularly after walking short distances around the ward. He usually finds that sitting in certain positions makes it more comfortable to breathe. He is having regular nebulizers and is finding these are helping to ease his breathing.

1 You wish to assess Mr Lyle's breathing, how might you prepare him?
2 In carrying out an assessment of his breathing, what observations should you be making?
3 What additional parameters will help you to determine his respiratory status?

See the end of the chapter for the answers.

Temperature

DEFINITION

Body temperature represents the balance between heat production and heat loss (Marieb and Hoehn 2010). If the rate of heat generated equates to the rate of heat lost, the core body temperature will be stable (Tortora and Derrickson 2011). All body tissues produce heat depending on how metabolically active they are. When the body is resting, most heat is generated by the heart, liver, brain and endocrine organs (Marieb and Hoehn 2010).

ANATOMY AND PHYSIOLOGY

Core body temperature measurements are taken to assess for deviation from the normal range of 36–37.5°C, to maintain cell metabolic activity. The core body temperature is set and closely regulated by the thermoregulatory centre of the hypothalamus in the brain (Tortora and Derrickson 2011).

Body temperature is a regulated function of the hypothalamus, and is the balance between heat gain (metabolism) and heat loss (respiration). All tissues produce heat as a result of cell metabolism, and this is increased by exercise and activity (Marieb and Hoehn 2010). Humans have the ability through homeostasis to maintain a constant core temperature in spite of environmental changes. The body core generally has the highest temperature while the skin is the coolest (Figure 11.25). Core temperature reflects the heat of arterial blood and represents the balance between the heat generated by body tissues in metabolic activity and that lost through various mechanisms (Marieb and Hoehn 2010).

Figure 11.25 **Body core and skin temperature.**

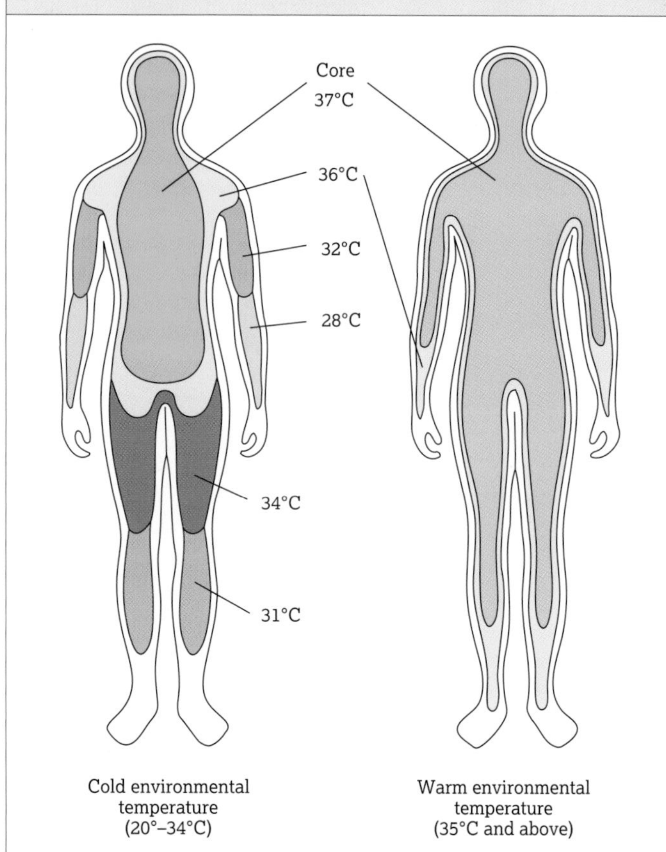

The hypothalamus comprises a group of neurones in the anterior and posterior portions, referred to as the preoptic area (Tortora and Derrickson 2011), which works as a thermostat (Figure 11.26). A relatively constant temperature is maintained by homeostasis, which is a constant process of heat gain and heat loss. The body requires stability of its temperature to produce an optimum environment for biochemical and enzymic reactions to maintain cellular function. Body temperature above or below this normal range affects total body function (Marieb and Hoehn 2010). A temperature above 41°C can cause convulsions and a temperature of 43°C renders life unsustainable.

Heat is a by-product of the metabolic reactions of all cells in the body, especially of the muscles and liver (Jenkins and Tortora 2013). Heat loss is achieved through the skin by the processes of radiation, convection, conduction and evaporation (Marieb and Hoehn 2010). Various factors cause fluctuations of temperature.

- The body's circadian rhythms cause daily fluctuations. The body temperature is higher in the evening than in the morning (Marieb and Hoehn 2010). Minor and Waterhouse (1981) recorded a difference of 0.5–1.5°C between morning and evening measurements.
- Ovulation can elevate the body's temperature as it influences the basal metabolic rate (Tortora and Derrickson 2011).
- Exercise and eating cause an elevation in temperature (Marieb and Hoehn 2010).
- Extremes of age affect a person's response to environmental change. While young people will shiver at a temperature of 36°, most people over the age of 80 will not shiver until the body temperature falls to 35.1° (Kenney and Munce 2003). Thermoregulation is inadequate in the newborn and especially in low-birthweight babies. In older people, there is an increased sensitivity to cold and the body temperature is generally lower (Nakamura et al. 1997).

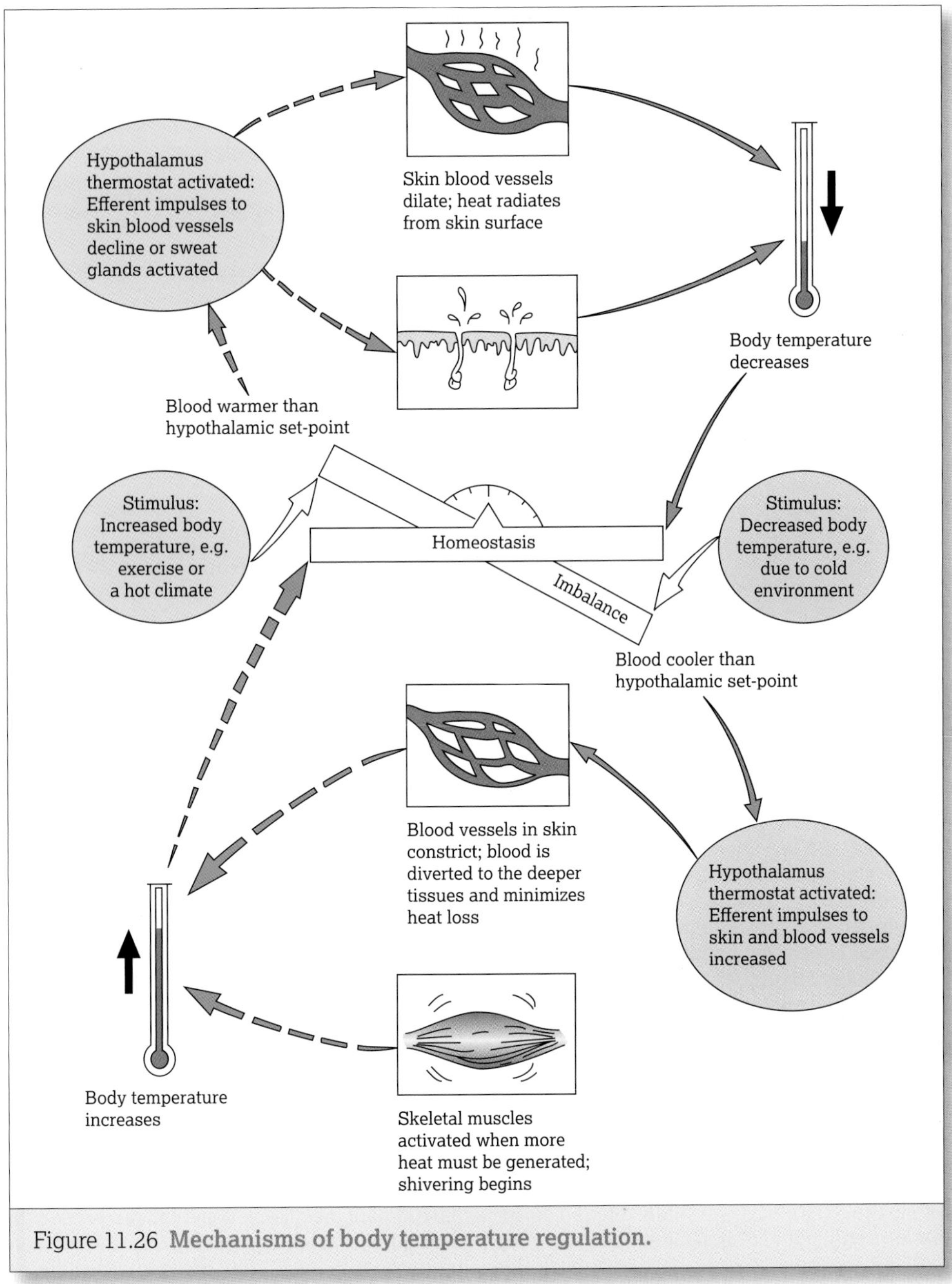

Figure 11.26 **Mechanisms of body temperature regulation.**

RELATED THEORY

Hypothermia

Hypothermia (lowered body temperature) is defined as a core temperature of 35°C (Frink et al. 2012) that causes the metabolic rate to decrease (Trim 2005). Hypothermia may be classified as mild (32–35°C), moderate (28–32°C) and severe (less than 28°C) (Cuddy 2004). Hypothermia occurs when the body loses more heat and is subsequently unable to maintain homeostasis (Neno 2005). In contrast to a raised temperature, during hypothermia cellular metabolism slows, and the need for oxygen is reduced as more oxygen remains bound to haemoglobin (Jenkins and Tortora 2013). This can lead to a reduction in respiratory rate.

If the temperature does fall below 35°C, the patient will start to shiver severely (Edwards 1997). However, hypothermia frequently escapes detection due to symptoms being non-specific and an oral thermometer's failure to record in the appropriate range (Marini and Wheeler 2012). It can occur in all ages, although the elderly are at particular risk, and is often multifactorial in origin with other risk factors including a Body Mass Index lower than 30 or an ambient temperature lower than 20°C (68°F) (Winslow et al. 2012).

Hypothermia can arise as a result of:

- environmental exposure
- medications that can alter the perception of cold, increase heat loss through vasodilation or inhibit heat generation, for example alcohol or paracetamol
- metabolic conditions, for example hypoglycaemia and adrenal insufficiency
- the exposure of the body and internal organs during surgery and the use of drugs which dampen the vasoconstrictor response (Marini and Wheeler 2012).

There are three known entities of hypothermia: induced, endogenous and accidental (Frink et al. 2012). Induced hypothermia is commonly used in elective cardiac surgery and in the management of patients with brain injuries (Yokobori et al.

2011). This is due to the theorized protective effects on apoptosis and the post-traumatic immune response (Frink et al. 2012).

Endogenous hypothermia results from a metabolic dysfunction with decreased heat production (e.g. hypothyroidism, hypoglycaemia, hypoadrenalism) or disturbed thermoregulation (e.g. intracranial tumour or degenerative neurological disorders). Finally, accidental hypothermia is characterized by an unintentional decrease of the core temperature, due to exposure to a cold environment without a thermoregulative dysfunction (Frink et al. 2012).

Surgical patients having procedures longer than 1 hour have increased disruption to normal homeostatic mechanisms, resulting in a drop in temperature. Complications can include cardiovascular ischaemia, delayed wound healing and increased risk of wound infections and increase in postoperative recovery time (Wagner 2006). To prevent unplanned perioperative hypothermia, aggressive use of convective and conductive warming measures and an increased ambient temperature is recommended, especially for the following patients:

- those undergoing major surgery
- those with compromised thermoregulatory systems (such as older adults)
- those undergoing surgery considered to be exceptionally painful (such as total knee arthroscopy) (Benson et al. 2012, Winslow et al. 2012).

Hyperthermia

Sudden temperature elevations usually indicate infection, making it prudent to perform a directed physical examination and, if indicated, obtain appropriate cultures and institute antibiotics. However, although infection is the most common explanation, several life-threatening non-infectious causes of fever are frequently overlooked (Marini and Wheeler 2012) (Table 11.6).

Fever caused by pyrexia (elevated body temperature) is the result of the internal thermostat resetting to higher levels. This is the result of the action of pyrogens, which are chemical substances now known to be cytokines. Cytokines are chemical mediators, which are involved in cellular immunity (Marieb and Hoehn 2010). They enhance the immune response and are released from white blood cells, injured tissues and macrophages. This causes the hypothalamus to release prostaglandins, which in turn reset the hypothalamic thermostat (Scrase and Tranter 2011). The body then promotes heat-producing mechanisms such as vasoconstriction. As a result of vasoconstriction, heat loss from the body surface declines, the skin cools and shivering begins to generate heat. These 'chills' are a sign that body temperature is rising (Marieb and Hoehn 2010) and are often referred to as 'rigors'. Shivering marks a rigor and the patient complains of feeling cold. The temperature quickly rises as a result of the normal physiological response to cold; see the grades of pyrexia in Table 11.7. This results in the following physiological changes.

- Thermoreceptors in the skin are stimulated, resulting in vasoconstriction. This decreases heat loss through conduction and convection.
- Sweat gland activity is reduced to minimize evaporation.
- Shivering occurs; muscles contract and relax out of sequence with each other, thus generating heat.

Table 11.6 Non-infectious causes of hyperthermia

Agonist drugs	Malignancy
Alcohol withdrawal	Malignant hyperthermia
Anticholinergic drugs	Neuroleptic malignant syndrome
Allergic drug or transfusion reaction	Phaeochromocytoma
Autonomic insufficiency	Salicylate intoxication
Crystalline arthritis (gout)	Status epilepticus
Drug allergy	Stroke or central nervous system damage
Heat stroke	Vasculitis hyperthyroidism

- The body increases catecholamine and thyroxine levels, elevating the metabolic rate in an attempt to increase temperature (Marieb and Hoehn 2010).

All these changes contribute to a rise in metabolism and a faster rate of diffusion, with an increase in carbon dioxide excretion and the need for oxygen (Jenkins and Tortora 2013). This leads to an increased respiratory rate. When the body temperature reaches its new 'setpoint', the patient no longer complains of feeling cold, shivering ceases and sweating commences.

There are several grades of pyrexia, and these are described in Table 11.7. However, the intensity of a pyrexia is not an indicator of the severity of infection (NICE 2007a), which varies from person to person.

EVIDENCE-BASED APPROACHES

Rationale

Core body temperature measurements are taken to assess for deviation from the normal range that may indicate disease, deterioration in condition, infection or reaction to treatment.

Body temperature measurement is part of routine care in clinical practice and can influence important decisions regarding tests, diagnosis and treatment (Lefrant et al. 2003). Temperature needs to be measured accurately and monitored effectively to enable changes to be detected quickly and any necessary intervention commenced (NICE 2007a, van Vliet et al. 2010). Temperature assessment accuracy depends on several factors: measurement technique, device type, body site and a healthcare professional's training (McCallum and Higgins 2012). Temperature recording is a core assessment (and reassessment) in nursing practice, but can create clinical issues if not performed appropriately (Docherty 2000).

Indications

Conditions in which a patient's temperature requires careful monitoring include the following.

- Patients with conditions that affect basal metabolic rate, such as disorders of the thyroid gland, require monitoring of body

Table 11.7 Grades of pyrexia

Level of pyrexia	Temperature	Remarks
Low-grade pyrexia	Normal to 38°C	Indicative of an inflammatory response due to a mild infection, allergy, disturbance of body tissue by trauma, surgery, malignancy or thrombosis
Moderate to high-grade pyrexia	38–40°C	May be caused by wound, respiratory or urinary tract infections
Hyperpyrexia	40°C and above	May arise because of bacteraemia, damage to the hypothalamus or high environmental temperatures

temperature. Hypothyroidism is a condition where inadequate secretion of hormones from the thyroid gland results in slowing of physical and metabolic activity; thus the individual has a decrease in body temperature. Hyperthyroidism is excessive activity of the thyroid gland; a hypermetabolic condition results, with an increase in all metabolic processes. The patient complains of a low heat tolerance. Thyrotoxic crisis is a sudden increase in thyroid hormones and can cause a hyperpyrexia (Walsh and Crumbie 2007).

- Post-operative and critically ill patients require monitoring of temperature. The patient's temperature should be observed pre-operatively in order to make any significant comparisons. In the post-operative period the nurse should observe the patient for hyperthermia or hypothermia as a reaction to the surgical procedures (Wagner 2006).
- Patients with a susceptibility to infection, for example those with a low white blood cell count (less than 1000 cells/mm^3) or those undergoing radiotherapy, chemotherapy or steroid treatment will require more frequent observation of temperature. The fluctuation in temperature is influenced by the body's response to pyrogens. Immunocompromised patients are less able to respond to infection. Bacteraemia means a bacterial invasion of the bloodstream. Septic shock is a circulatory collapse as a result of severe infection. Pyrexia may be absent in those who are immunosuppressed or in the elderly (Neno 2005).
- Patients with a systemic or local infection require monitoring of temperature to assess development or regression of infection.
- Pyrexia can occur when patients are receiving a blood transfusion but severe transfusion reactions usually occur within the first 15 minutes of starting (British Society for Haematology 2009).

Methods of recording temperature

All metabolizing body cells manufacture heat in varying amounts. Therefore, temperature is not evenly distributed across the body (Childs 2011). The measurement of core body temperature may seem simple, but several issues affect the accuracy of the reading (McCallum and Higgins 2012); these include the measurement site, the reliability of the instrument and user technique (Pusnik and Miklavec 2009). True core temperature readings can only be measured by invasive means, such as placing a temperature probe into the oesophagus, pulmonary artery or urinary bladder (Childs 2011), and are therefore used most in the critical care setting. This must be undertaken by specialists or nurses who have received additional training that incorporates anatomical imaging technology (Makic et al. 2012).

Traditionally, the mouth, axilla, rectum and external auditory canal have been the preferred sites for obtaining temperature readings, due to their accessibility. As temperature between these sites can vary greatly, ideally the same site should be used continuously throughout patient assessments to allow for comparison, and the location of the site must be recorded on the observation chart (Davie and Amoore 2010). Unfortunately, an accurate, non-invasive method to measure core temperature has yet to be established, as current instruments produce a wide range of temperatures (Hooper and Andrews 2006).

Oral

To most accurately measure the temperature orally, the thermometer is placed in the posterior sublingual pocket of tissue at the base of the tongue (Torrance and Semple 1998). It is important that the thermometer is placed in this region and not in the area under the front of the tongue, as there may be a temperature difference of up to 1.7°C between these areas. This temperature difference is due to the sublingual pockets being protected from the air currents, which cool the frontal areas (Neff et al. 1989). This area is in close proximity to the thermoreceptors which respond rapidly to changes in the core temperature, hence changes in core temperatures are reflected quickly here (Carroll 2000, Stevenson 2004).

Oral temperatures are thought to be affected by ingested foods and fluids, smoking, the muscular activity of chewing, exercise and the environment such as draughts (Mazerolle et al. 2011). A respiratory rate that exceeds 18 breaths per minute, together with a patient who smokes, will also reduce the core temperature values (Knies 2003).

Rectal

The rectal temperature is often higher than the oral temperature because this site is more sheltered from the external environment. Rectal thermometry has been demonstrated in clinical trials to be more accurate than oral or axillary thermometry; however, it is not advocated due to its invasive nature (Trim 2005).

Aspects relating to privacy, dignity and patient choice should be considered when assessing temperature via this route. While other more precise methods can still detect fever, the rectal method offers greater precision in terms of obtaining the core temperature. However, the presence of soft stool may separate the thermometer from the bowel wall and give a false reading, especially if the central temperature is changing rapidly. In infants and the immunosuppressed, this method is not recommended as it carries a risk of rectal ulceration or perforation (Price and Gwin 2008).

A rectal thermometer should be inserted at least 4 cm into the rectum in an adult to obtain the most accurate reading.

Axillary

The axilla is considered less desirable than the other sites because of the difficulty in achieving accurate and reliable readings (Evans and Kenkre 2006) as it is not close to major vessels, and skin surface temperatures vary more with changes in temperature of the environment (Woollons 1996). It is usually only used for patients who are unsuitable for, or who cannot tolerate, oral thermometers, for example after general anaesthetic or patients with mouth injuries (Edwards 1997).

To take an axillary temperature reading, the thermometer should be placed in the centre of the armpit, with the patient's arm firmly against the side of the chest. It is important that the same arm is used for each measurement, as there is often a variation in temperature between left and right (Heindenreich and Giuffe 1990).

Whichever route is used for temperature measurement, it is important that this is then used consistently, as switching between sites can produce a record that is misleading or difficult to interpret.

Consideration is required when interpreting variations in 4–6 hourly observations, and when taking once-only daily temperatures as the average person experiences circadian rhythms, with the highest body temperature occurring in the late afternoon or early evening, that is between 4 pm and 8 pm. The most sensitive time for detecting pyrexias appears to be between 7 pm and 8 pm (Angerami 1980). Samples et al. (1985) found the highest temperature between 5 pm and 7 pm. These studies suggest that the most useful time to measure and detect an abnormal temperature would be approximately 6 pm.

Tympanic

The tympanic membrane is an increasingly popular method, as it is less invasive and provides rapid results (<1 minute) (McCallum and Higgins 2012). It has been suggested by some that tympanic membrane thermometers give an accurate representation of actual body temperature. This is because the tympanic membrane lies close to the temperature regulation centre in the hypothalamus, shares the same artery and is therefore considered to directly reflect core temperature in adults (Chue et al. 2012).

In 2003, the MHRA published a medical device alert following reports of tympanic thermometers providing low temperature readings and these were attributed to a dirty probe and probe covers and user error (MHRA 2003). A soiled probe or probe cover would record a low temperature because the infra-red emissions from the tympanic membrane will be affected.

Anticipated patient outcomes

To determine the patient's temperature on admission as a baseline for comparison with future measurements and to monitor fluctuations in temperature.

PRE-PROCEDURAL CONSIDERATIONS

Temperature can be measured at a number of different sites, using different tools for measurement. When assessing the body temperature it is important to consider the methods and tools used for measurement (Docherty and Foudy 2006).

The critical issue to consider when using any thermometer is whether you are controlling the factors that affect the accuracy and precision of the measurement. These factors must be addressed when educating staff on the use of different temperature measurement methods. It is therefore important to recall that therapeutic decisions should not be made on the basis of a single vital sign (Bridges and Thomas 2009).

Equipment

There are a number of devices on the market, including electronic contact thermometers, chemical thermometers and infra-red-sensing thermometers, each obtaining temperatures in differing time frames and working in different ways. If the device can be used on multiple sites the programming will need to be altered to reflect the chosen site per manufacturer's guidelines. Clinical thermometry is governed by the International Standard BS EN ISO 80601-2-56 (British Standards Institution 2012) which stipulates the need for regular calibration and maintenance.

In terms of health and safety, the MHRA advised that equipment with mercury should be replaced, primarily due to the potential for mercury leaks (MHRA 2012). Coupled with the fact that mercury thermometers respond slowly to temperature changes, this has meant that use of an electronic device is preferable when recording temperature extremes and rapid fluctuations (Marini and Wheeler 2012). In clinical practice other types of thermometer should be used instead.

- Single-use plastic-coated strips with heat-sensitive recorders (dots) which change colour to indicate the temperature (record from 35.5 to 40.4°C).
- Digital analogue probe thermometers with plastic disposable sheets (record from 32 to 42°C).
- Invasive thermometers attached to a pulmonary artery catheter (record from 0 to 50°C) (Braun et al. 1998, O'Toole 1997).

Tympanic membrane thermometer

Tympanic thermometers are small hand-held devices that have a disposable probe cover that is inserted into the patient's ear canal. The sensor at the end of the probe records the infra-red radiation (IRR) that is emitted by the tympanic membrane, as a result of its warmth, and converts this into a temperature reading presented on a digital screen (Davie and Amoore 2010). The probe is protected by a disposable cover, which is changed between patients to prevent cross-infection (Gallimore 2004). Advantages of tympanic membrane thermometry are speed (temperature reading available within seconds), safety and ease of use (Gasim et al. 2013).

Figure 11.27 **Tympanic membrane thermometer.**

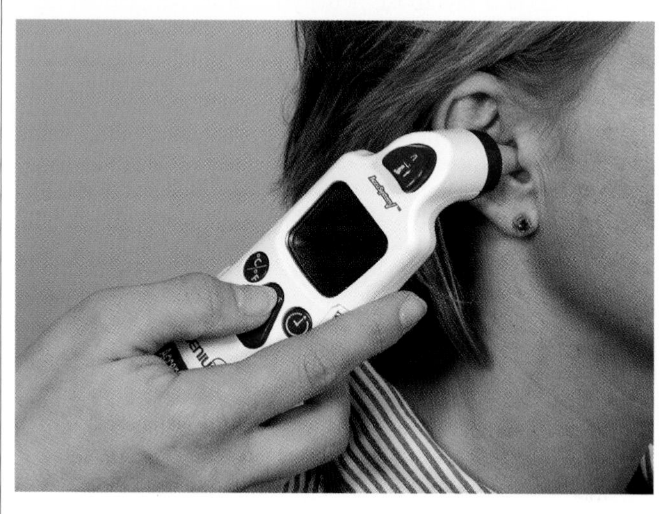

A common problem with using tympanic thermometers is poor technique leading to inaccurate temperature measurements (Farnell et al. 2005, Gilbert et al. 2002). The placement of the probe to fit snugly within the ear canal (Figure 11.27) is crucial as differences between the opening of the ear canal and the tympanic membrane can be as much as 2.8°C (Munro 2009). Jevon and Jevon (2001) highlight other causes of false readings, which include dirty or cracked probe lens, incorrect installation of the probe cover and short time intervals between measurements (less than 2–3 minutes). Ear infections and wax are reported to influence the true temperature of the tympanum (Callejo et al. 2004, Farnell et al. 2005), therefore the ear should be inspected prior to obtaining a reading and if wax or evidence of an infection is present, an alternative route for obtaining the temperature should be sought. For infection prevention and control purposes, the appropriate disposable probe cover should be used and the nurse should inspect the cover to ensure that it has been fitted correctly and that there are no wrinkles over the tip end. This will ensure an accurate reading is achieved (Davie and Amoore 2010).

Specific patient preparation

Ask the patient when they last ate, smoked and had a drink as these may influence their temperature.

Procedure guideline 11.6 **Temperature measurement**

Essential equipment

- Tympanic membrane thermometer
- Disposable probe covers
- Alcohol handrub

Pre-procedure

Action	Rationale
1 Explain and discuss procedure with the patient. If patient is wearing a hearing aid, remove the device from the ear and wait 10 minutes before taking a reading.	To ensure that the patient understands the procedure and gives their valid consent (NMC 2013, **C**).
2 Wash and dry hands.	To minimize the risks of cross-infection and contamination (Fraise and Bradley 2009, **E**).

Procedure	
3 Inspect the ear canal for the presence of ear drainage, blood, cerebrospinal fluid, vernix, cerumen (compacted ear wax) or foreign bodies.	The presence of these substances can affect the accuracy of the reading (Covidien 2011, **C**). Ear wax does not affect accuracy but cerumen plugs or impactions containing debris can lower the temperature measurement by several tenths of a degree (Covidien 2011, **C**).
4 Remove thermometer from the base unit and ensure the lens is clean, not cracked and that the probe lens is free of smudge/debris. Use a dry lint-free swab to wipe clean if required and calibrate according to the manufacturer's guidelines.	Alcohol-based wipes should not be used as this can lead to a false low temperature measurement (Jevon and Jevon 2001, **E**).
5 Verify the mode setting on LCD display to show the route by which the temperature is due to be measured, e.g. ear, oral, core, rectal or axillary.	To ensure accuracy when interpreting the result (Covidien 2011, **C**).
6 Place disposable probe cover on the probe tip, ensuring the manufacturer's instructions are followed, e.g. ensuring the cover is flush with the thermometer end and not touching the plastic film on the distal tip of the probe cover.	The probe cover protects the tip of the probe and is necessary for the functioning of the instrument (Jevon and Jevon 2001, **E**).
7 Obtain a reading from both ears and take the greater of the readings. A new probe cover must be used for each reading to ensure the highest degree of accuracy and to prevent cross-contamination between ears.	Recent evidence suggests there are no anatomical differences between the two ears with the newer generation of infra-red tympanic thermometers (Haugan et al. 2013, **R3d**). However, previous evidence has suggested a difference of up to 1°C (Heusch and McCarthy 2005, **R1b**; Jevon and Jevon 2001, **E**).
8 Ensure the patient has not been lying on either ear in the 20-minute interval immediately preceding temperature measurement (Bridges and Thomas 2009). If a patient is lying on their side, always take the temperature in the exposed ear.	There are significant differences in tympanic temperature caused when the patient has been lying on their ear (Arslan et al. 2011, **R.3b**).
9 Align the probe tip with the ear canal and gently advance into the ear canal until the probe lightly seals the opening, ensuring a snug fit. See Figure 11.27.	To prevent air at the opening of the ear from entering it, causing a false low temperature measurement (Covidien 2011, **C**; Jevon and Jevon 2001, **E**).
10 Press and release SCAN button.	To commence the scanning (Covidien 2011, **C**).
11 Remove probe tip from the ear as soon as the thermometer display reads DONE or displays the temperature reading, usually indicated by beeps.	To ensure procedure is carried out for allocated time. Measurement is usually complete within seconds (Gasim et al. 2013, **E**).
12 Read the temperature display and document in the patient's records and compare with previous results along with the ear used. Take action as appropriate.	Any interruption in the process may result in the measurement being incorrectly remembered (O'Brien et al. 2003, **E**). Deviations from normal temperature ranges may result in urgent medical/clinical attention (Jevon and Jevon 2001, **E**; NMC 2010, **C**).
Post-procedure	
13 Press RELEASE/EJECT button to discard probe cover into a waste bin per local infection control guidelines.	Probe covers are for single use only (Covidien 2011, **C**; Jevon and Jevon 2001, **E**).
14 Wipe thermometer clean as per manufacturer's guidelines and return to the base unit for storage.	To reduce the risk of cross-infection (Fraise and Bradley 2009, **E**).

Problem-solving table 11.6 **Prevention and resolution (Procedure guideline 11.6)**

Problem	Cause	Prevention	Action
Thermometer is not working properly, for example 'error' is showing.	The battery may be low.	At the first level, the low battery sign is lit and approximately 100 more temperatures may be taken.	Replace the battery.
If the 'wait' indicator is on.	'Wait' indicator will appear if you attempt to take successive temperatures in too short a period of time.	Wait briefly until the 'wait' indicator disappears before taking another temperature.	Retry and if still instructing to 'wait', send for repair.
'Use new cover' showing even though probe cover has been installed.	Probe cover replaced too quickly.	Check that probe cover has been fitted correctly.	Press RELEASE/EJECT button and reinstall probe cover.

POST-PROCEDURAL CONSIDERATIONS

Immediate care

Hyperthermia

A rise in temperature can be regarded as a cure, in that it is part of the autonomic response to remove infection and create a favourable environment for antibiotics (Gardner 2012). A post-operative fever is often a normal inflammatory response to surgery; however, it can also be a manifestation of a serious underlying infectious or non-infectious aetiology (Burke 2010). If a temperature rises above 40°C (hyperthermia), it is dangerous and may indicate that the patient's regulatory systems have failed.

It remains common practice to try to reduce fever with medication such as antipyretics and physical cooling methods. Antipyretics, including paracetamol or ibuprofen, can mask the function of the hypothalamus by reducing the temperature while hiding the underlying signs of disease (Cuddy 2004). It is thought that these drugs inhibit the inflammatory action of prostaglandins, affecting the hypothalamus by temporarily resetting the thermostat to normal levels. Currently the evidence on how to reduce fever in practice is weak and does not support the routine administration of antipyretic therapies (Carey 2010, Outzen 2009). Therefore nurses should assess patients individually, using antipyretic therapies selectively and with caution. Physical cooling methods alone should never be used (Carey 2010).

Consideration of a patient's comfort is also important (although caution and individualized assessment are also needed when considering physical cooling methods). Fanning is of benefit for moderate-to-high pyrexia but fanning and tepid sponging are not recommended while the patient's temperature is still rising as this will only make the patient feel colder, and could cause distress (Sharber 1997). Fanning during this time can actually increase a person's body temperature as it can stimulate a compensatory response by the hypothalamus, initiating heat-gaining activities such as shivering and peripheral vasoconstriction that could compromise unstable patients by depleting their metabolic reserve (Brooker and Nicol 2003, Carey 2010).

Nurses should be aware of the side-effects associated with cooling techniques, such as:

- arrhythmias, bradycardia
- coagulation pathway impairment
- electrolyte disorders from intracellular shifts and renal excretion (calcium, magnesium, phosphate and potassium levels can be affected)
- insulin resistance with hyperglycaemia
- patient discomfort from shivering and skin breakdown (Polderman and Herold 2009).

Comfort measures in addition to reassurance may include:

- providing dry clothing and bedlinen
- offering oral hygiene to keep the mouth moist
- limit patient exertion to minimize heat production, particularly during the flush stage

> **Learning Activity 11.3**
>
> **Scenario: Temperature measurement and hyperthermia**
>
> You have just checked your patient's temperature using a tympanic thermometer and note that it is 39.2°C.
>
> 1 Who should you report this to?
> 2 What measures can you take to help to reduce the temperature?
> 3 What else should you do?
>
> See the end of the chapter for the answers.

- offering sufficient nutrition and fluids (2.5–3 L daily) to meet the patient's higher metabolic demands to avoid dehydration
- providing extra blankets when the patient feels cold, but remove surplus blankets when the patient complains of too much warmth (Kozier et al. 2008).

Hypothermia

The immediate management of a low temperature needs to address potential emergency conditions, such as cardiac arrhythmias and hypotension, as well as fluid and electrolyte shifts (Davis 2012). Nursing management should therefore focus on preventing further heat loss and rewarming the body core temperature because there is an increased risk of mortality and morbidity below 34°C (Frink et al. 2012).

Davis (2012) suggests there are three basic types of hypothermia treatment: passive external, active external and active internal rewarming. Passive treatments include removing wet clothing and providing a greater insulation. Passive external rewarming is used for patients with mild hypothermia (34–35°C), who are neither neurologically nor cardiovascularly compromised and are still able to generate heat. Active external methods are advised for moderate (30–33.9°C) accidental hypothermia and poor cardiac performance and include forced-air/warm blankets and water circulating suits (Davis 2012). Active internal methods are reserved for patients who have severe hypothermia (<30°C) and are haemodynamically unstable. Active internal methods include the use of warmed intravenous fluids such as saline or blood, because a 2 litre crystalloid bag administered at a temperature of 18°C will decrease a patient's core temperatures about 0.6°C (Hohlrieder et al. 2007). Other active internal techniques include warmed oxygen administration, and bladder, peritoneal or thoracic lavage (Davis 2012).

During any rewarming process attention must be paid to the speed because patients who are warmed slowly have a higher mortality rate (Vassal et al. 2001) and rewarming that results in hyperthermia has been reported to cause ischaemia and hypoxia (Kjaergaard and Bach 2006). For both active external and internal treatment types, specific training and knowledge of the associated devices and products are necessary.

Documentation

Recordings of body temperature are an index of biological function and a valuable indicator of a patient's health.

Urinalysis

DEFINITION

Urinalysis is the analysis of the volume and physical, chemical and microscopic properties of urine (Tortora and Derrickson 2011) and can provide valuable information about a patient's condition, allowing detection of systemic disease and infection (Bishop 2008).

ANATOMY AND PHYSIOLOGY

Urine is formed in the kidneys, which process approximately 180 litres of blood-derived fluid a day. Approximately 1% of this total actually leaves the body as urine, the rest returns to the circulation (Marieb and Hoehn 2010). Urine formation, and the simultaneous adjustment of blood composition, involves three processes (Figure 11.28):

- glomerular filtration
- tubular reabsorption
- tubular secretion (Marieb and Hoehn 2010).

Glomerular filtration

This occurs in the glomeruli of the kidney, which act as non-selective filters. Filtration occurs as a result of increased

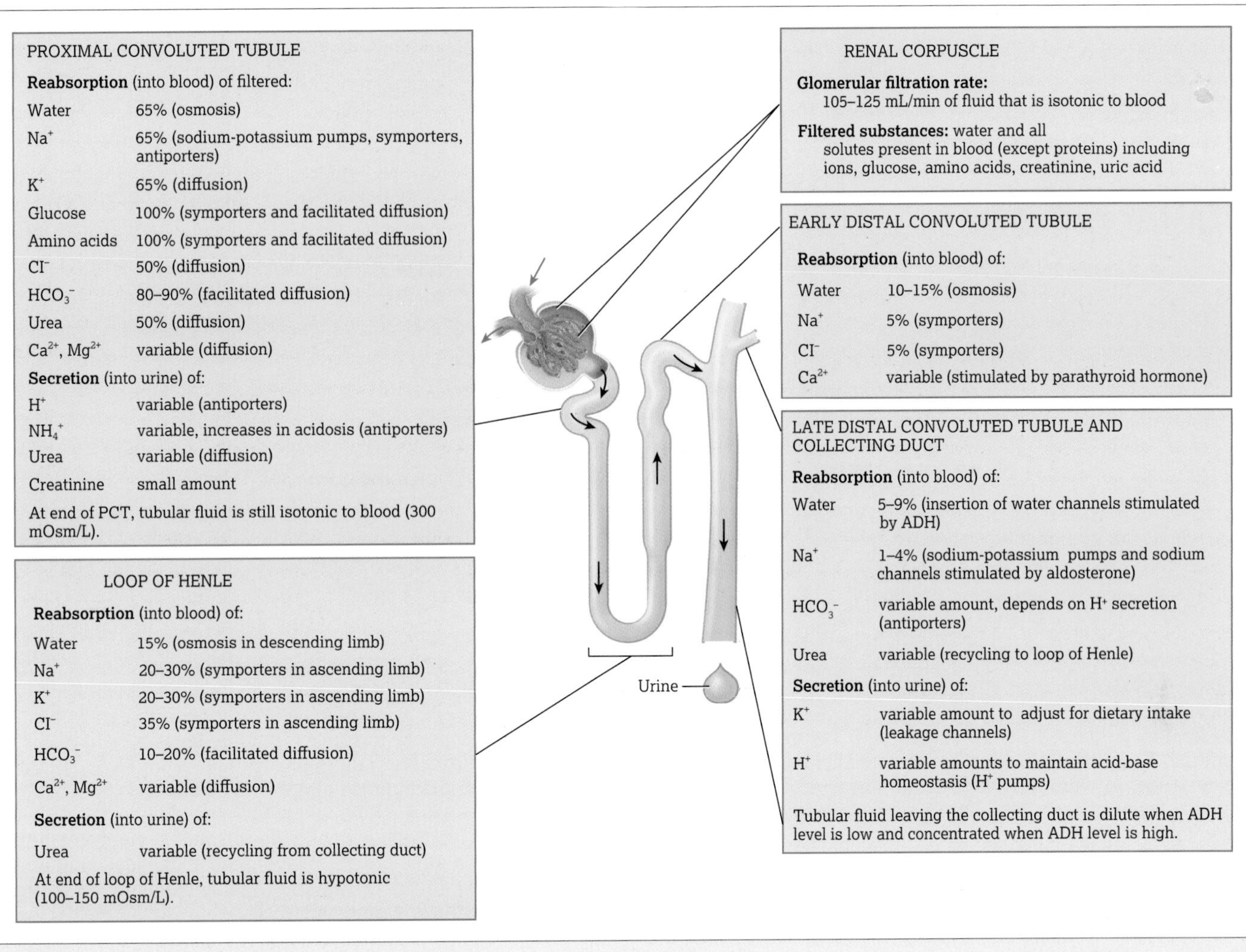

PROXIMAL CONVOLUTED TUBULE
Reabsorption (into blood) of filtered:
Water 65% (osmosis)
Na+ 65% (sodium-potassium pumps, symporters, antiporters)
K+ 65% (diffusion)
Glucose 100% (symporters and facilitated diffusion)
Amino acids 100% (symporters and facilitated diffusion)
Cl− 50% (diffusion)
HCO3− 80–90% (facilitated diffusion)
Urea 50% (diffusion)
Ca2+, Mg2+ variable (diffusion)
Secretion (into urine) of:
H+ variable (antiporters)
NH4+ variable, increases in acidosis (antiporters)
Urea variable (diffusion)
Creatinine small amount
At end of PCT, tubular fluid is still isotonic to blood (300 mOsm/L).
LOOP OF HENLE
Reabsorption (into blood) of:
Water 15% (osmosis in descending limb)
Na+ 20–30% (symporters in ascending limb)
K+ 20–30% (symporters in ascending limb)
Cl− 35% (symporters in ascending limb)
HCO3− 10–20% (facilitated diffusion)
Ca2+, Mg2+ variable (diffusion)
Secretion (into urine) of:
Urea variable (recycling from collecting duct)
At end of loop of Henle, tubular fluid is hypotonic (100–150 mOsm/L).
RENAL CORPUSCLE
Glomerular filtration rate:
105–125 mL/min of fluid that is isotonic to blood
Filtered substances: water and all solutes present in blood (except proteins) including ions, glucose, amino acids, creatinine, uric acid
EARLY DISTAL CONVOLUTED TUBULE
Reabsorption (into blood) of:
Water 10–15% (osmosis)
Na+ 5% (symporters)
Cl− 5% (symporters)
Ca2+ variable (stimulated by parathyroid hormone)
LATE DISTAL CONVOLUTED TUBULE AND COLLECTING DUCT
Reabsorption (into blood) of:
Water 5–9% (insertion of water channels stimulated by ADH)
Na+ 1–4% (sodium-potassium pumps and sodium channels stimulated by aldosterone)
HCO3− variable amount, depends on H+ secretion (antiporters)
Urea variable (recycling to loop of Henle)
Secretion (into urine) of:
K+ variable amount to adjust for dietary intake (leakage channels)
H+ variable amounts to maintain acid-base homeostasis (H+ pumps)
Tubular fluid leaving the collecting duct is dilute when ADH level is low and concentrated when ADH level is high.
Urine

Figure 11.28 **Summary of filtration, reabsorption and secretion in the nephron and collecting duct.** ***Source:*** **Tortora and Derrickson (2011). Reproduced with permission from John Wiley & Sons.**

glomerular blood pressure caused by the difference in diameter between afferent and efferent arterioles. The effect is a simple mechanical filter that permits substances smaller than plasma proteins to pass from the glomeruli to the glomerular capsule (Marieb and Hoehn 2010).

Tubular reabsorption

Tubular reabsorption then occurs, removing necessary substances from the filtrate and returning them to the peritubular capillaries. Tubular reabsorption is an active process that requires protein carriers and energy. Substances reabsorbed include nutrients and most ions. It is also a passive process, however, driven by electrochemical gradients. Substances reabsorbed in this way include sodium ions and water. Creatinine and the metabolites of drugs are not reabsorbed because of their size, insolubility or a lack of carriers. Most of the nutrients, 65% of the water and sodium ions, and the majority of actively transported ions are reabsorbed in the proximal convoluted tubules (Marieb and Hoehn 2010).

Reabsorption of additional sodium ions and water occurs in the distal tubules and collecting ducts and is hormonally controlled. Aldosterone increases the reabsorption of sodium, and antidiuretic hormone (ADH) enhances water reabsorption by the collecting ducts (Marieb and Hoehn 2010).

Tubular secretion

Tubular secretion is an active process that is important in eliminating drugs, certain wastes and excess ions and in maintaining the acid/base balance of blood (Marieb and Hoehn 2010).

Regulation of urine concentration and volume occurs in the loop of Henle, where the osmolarity of the filtrate is controlled. As the filtrate flows through the tubules, the permeability of the walls controls how dilute or concentrated the resulting urine will be. In the absence of ADH, dilute urine is formed because the filtrate is not reabsorbed as it passes through the kidneys. As levels of ADH increase, the collecting tubules become more permeable to water, and water moves out of the filtrate back into the blood. Consequently, more concentrated urine is produced, and in smaller amounts (Marieb and Hoehn 2010).

Urine is a clear, straw-coloured fluid. The normal composition of urine includes water, urea, creatinine, sodium, potassium, organic acids, protein, small traces of glucose and cellular components. The colour of urine is due to a pigment called urochrome which is derived from the body's destruction of haemoglobin. The more concentrated urine is, the deeper yellow it becomes. An abnormal colour such as pink or brown may result from eating certain foods (beetroot or rhubarb), or may be due to the presence of bile products or blood (Marieb and Hoehn 2010). Often fresh urine appears turbid (cloudy), indicating that there may be an infection of the urinary tract. The urinary tract is the most common site of bacterial infection. Risk factors for urinary tract infections (UTI) include presence of a urinary catheter, female gender, diabetes and advanced age (Marini and Wheeler 2012). See Figure 11.29 for other UTI predisposing factors.

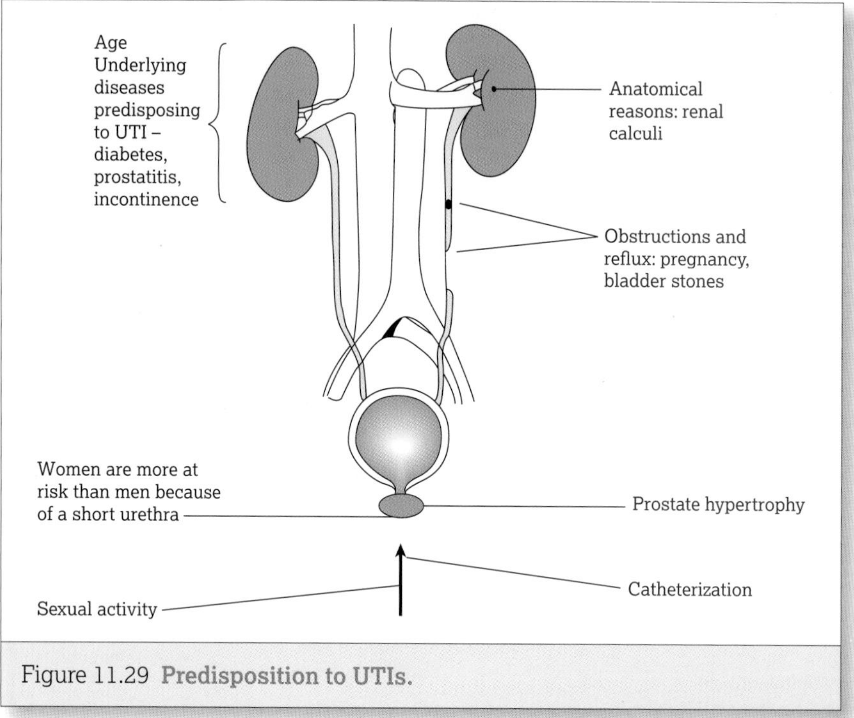

Figure 11.29 **Predisposition to UTIs.**

Bacteriuria is defined as the presence of bacteria in the urine (Rigby and Gray 2005). Urine specimens are rarely sterile, as a result of contamination with periurethral flora during collection. Infection is distinguished by counting the number of bacteria. Significant bacteriuria is defined as the presence of more than 10^5 organisms per mL of urine in the presence of clinical symptoms (Marini and Wheeler 2012). See Figure 11.30 for illustration of significant bacteriuria.

Fresh urine is slightly aromatic. This can change as a result of disease processes such as diabetes mellitus, when acetone is present in the urine, giving it a fruity smell (Marieb and Hoehn 2010). The composition of urine can change dramatically as a result of disease, and abnormal substances may be present. Urinalysis can identify many of these substances, and should be part of every physical assessment (Cook 1996, Torrance and Elley 1998).

EVIDENCE-BASED APPROACHES

Rationale

Urinalysis (urine testing) is commonly undertaken in general practice as a non-invasive means of:

Figure 11.30 **Significant bacteriuria. Specimens of urine are rarely sterile. A cut-off point is identified to distinguish true infection (significant bacteriuria) from effects of contamination from surrounding tissues.**

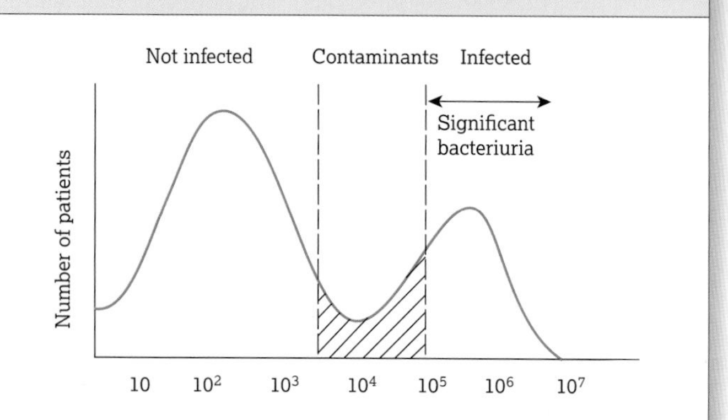

- measuring response to certain treatments
- assessing particular symptoms
- assisting in the diagnosis of medical conditions

and as a part of routine health assessments. Interpretation of urinalysis is generally based on reviewing all the test components and correlating them with the physical examination and the patient's clinical signs and symptoms.

Urinalyses are performed for several reasons.

- To detect renal and metabolic diseases.
- To diagnose diseases or disorders of the kidneys or urinary tract.
- To monitor patients with diabetes mellitus.
- To assess for pregnancy.
- To detect the presence of drug metabolites or alcohol.
- To contribute to the assessment of hydration.

A sensible approach to urine collection is advised dependent on the clinical situation (Schmiemann et al. 2010). The collection of urine for sampling may be obtained via natural voiding, a pad, a catheter specimen of urine (CSU) or a suprapubic aspirate (SPA) collected via the rubber specimen side port (Struthers et al. 2012). An initial urine investigation with a dipstick, from a fresh spontaneous urine sample, will be sufficient in most clinical situations. In other circumstances, a clean-catch midstream urinalysis (MSU) will be required as contamination is frequent in 'spontaneous' urine collected without any special hygiene precautions (Roche Diagnostics 2010). This is especially the case in women, where urine contains leucocytes in the presence of discharge and erythrocytes in the presence of menstruation. For this reason, no urine testing should be attempted in women for 2–3 days after menstruation finishes (Roche Diagnostics 2010).

When collecting an MSU it is necessary to clean the genitals to ensure the culture specimen is processed with as little contamination as possible. This is to minimize the presence of contaminating elements, such as bacteria, analytes and formed particles (Lifshitz and Kramer 2000, Manoni et al. 2011).

Consideration should be given to whether a urine sample should be obtained at the first or second morning void (before noon). This will be guided by referring to local guidelines and liaising with the requesting party. First morning voids have proven worthwhile for most test purposes (Roche Diagnostics 2010), although clinical circumstances where the first morning void may be necessary include testing for microalbuminuria (Genova Diagnostics 2012, Witte et al. 2009) or spot urine testing for evaluating daily salt intake (Kawamura et al. 2006). This is because the urine has been in the bladder for a reasonably long period, and its composition is independent of daily variations in food and fluid intake and physical activity (Roche Diagnostics 2010).

Indications

The composition of urine can change dramatically as a result of disease processes. Urine may contain red blood cells, glucose, proteins, white blood cells or bile (Marieb and Hoehn 2010). It can reveal diseases that have gone unnoticed because they do not produce striking symptoms, and may also be used in ongoing management of conditions (Higgins 2008b).

- *Screening and prevention*: for systemic disease, for example, diabetes mellitus, renal conditions such as kidney or urogenital diseases, liver disease and haemolytic disorders.
- *Diagnosis*: to confirm or exclude suspected conditions, for example urinary tract infection.
- *Management and planning*: to ascertain as a baseline, monitor progress of an existing condition and/or plan programme of care and medication (Roche Diagnostics 2010).

Methods of urinalysis

There are three main methods by which urinalysis is performed.

- Using urine reagent test strips (dipstick).
- Light microscopy.
- Timed collection.

Reagent test strips

Before using a reagent strip to analyse a sample of urine, the following observations should be made to support the overall assessment.

- Colour
- Clarity/debris
- Odour

These properties should be considered with reference to the clinical condition, urine output and fluid balance records over the past 24 hours.

The main advantages of urine dipstick are that it is convenient, quick and non-invasive with results usually determined in a few minutes. The main disadvantages are in terms of accuracy, both with colour changes being affected by the factors listed below and a certain degree of subjectivity during interpretation.

The following are a few examples of factors that can affect the analysis of results and could lead to false positives or negatives.

- Bilirubin and urobilinogen are relatively unstable when subjected to light and at room temperature, so it is important to use fresh urine to obtain the most accurate result (Roche Diagnostics 2010).
- Exposure of unpreserved urine at room temperature for a considerable period of time (>4 hours) may result in an increase in micro-organisms in the urine and change in pH (Veljkovic et al. 2012).
- Bacterial growth of contaminated organisms in urine may produce a positive blood reaction (Roche Diagnostics 2010).
- Urine that is highly alkaline may show false-positive results for the presence of protein (Roche Diagnostics 2010).
- Glucose in urine may reduce its pH as a result of metabolism of glucose by organisms present in the urine (Roche Diagnostics 2010).
- The presence of urea-splitting organisms that convert urea to ammonia may cause urine to become more alkaline (Roche Diagnostics 2010).
- *Drug and chemical intereferences*: such as false-positive influence with the leucocyte reading from cefoxitin, levodopa or tetracycline, or false negatives with nitrates from high concentrations of trimethoprim or mesna (Roche Diagnostics 2010).

Light microscopy

Having undertaken a urine dipstick and discovered adverse results, further testing may be necessary under laboratory conditions. This may include culture and sensitivity testing to identify organisms responsible for infection and to determine the most effective treatment (Wilson 2005) (Table 11.8). Optical or light microscopy involves passing visible light transmitted through or reflected from the sample through single or multiple

Table 11.8 **Routine observations of urine: possible indications and plan of action**

Observation	Possible indications	Plan of action
Colour		
Green	*Pseudomonas* infection, presence of bilirubin	Culture and microscopy
	Excretion of cytotoxic agents, for example mitomycin, or substances, for example methylene blue	Discard with care
Pink/red	Blood	Culture and microscopy. If currently receiving chemotherapy, for example ifosfamide, further mesna may need to be given
	Excretion of cytotoxic agents, for example doxorubicin	Discard with care
Orange	Excess urobiliogen, rifampicin	Discard
Yellow	Bilirubin	Discard
Brown	Bilirubin	Discard
Odour		
Fishy	Infection	Culture and microscopy
Sweet smelling	Ketones	Culture and microscopy
Debris		
Cloudy	Infection, stale urine	Culture and microscopy
Sediment	Infection, contamination	Culture and microscopy

Source: Rigby and Gray (2005). Reproduced with permission from EMAP Publishing, Ltd.

lenses to allow for a magnified view of the sample. The image generated can then be read and interpreted by the eye, imaged on a photographic plate, or captured digitally. The light microscopy will examine the number and types of cells and/or material in the urine and can yield a great detail of information and suggest a more specific diagnosis. For light microscopy, an MSU should be used as opposed to a fresh spontaneous sample so that any contaminating bacteria in the urethra are flushed out first, and the sample represents the bladder contents. This reduces the chance of contamination of the specimen with epithelial cells, especially vaginal flora (Struthers et al. 2012).

In the microbiology laboratory, urine samples constitute about 40% of the total workload; of these, 70–80% of samples are not infected (Manickam et al. 2013). This means that much time, energy and finances are wasted on unnecessary sample processing and investigation (Manickam et al. 2013), which is why it is so vital to only send samples where urine dipstick has indicated cause for concern.

Timed urinalysis

Timed urine collection is typically undertaken over an 8-, 12- or 24-hour period. It simply requires a person to collect their urine in a special container over the set period, although it is important to follow local guidelines in terms of the time of day to commence collection, storage and processing requirements. During collection, the sample is usually stored in a cool/refrigerated environment or on ice. This test typically focuses on renal creatinine clearance, sodium and protein. Renal clearance refers to the volume of plasma that is cleared of a particular substance in a given time, usually 1 minute. Renal clearance tests are done to determine the glomerular filtration rate (GFR), which allows us to detect glomerular damage and follow the progress of renal disease (Marieb and Hoehn 2010). Timed urinalysis may also examine hormone levels, urea nitrogen or copper as well as measuring substances such as steroids, white cells and electrolytes or determining urine osmolarity (Tortora and Derrickson 2011).

PRE-PROCEDURAL CONSIDERATIONS

Equipment

Dipstick (reagent) tests

Dipstick reagents have been primarily used as screening tools for components in the urine such as protein, glucose or ketones. More sophisticated reagents are now available which test for nitrites and leucocyte esterase as indicators of bacterial infection. Leucocyte esterase is an enzyme from neutrophils not normally found in urine and can be a marker of infection (Reynard et al. 2013). Nitrites are produced by the bacterial breakdown of dietary nitrate, which is a waste product of protein metabolism (Rigby and Gray 2005). Other reagent dipsticks also test for presence of blood, urobilinogen and bilirubin, test the specific gravity and determine the urine pH.

The urine dipstick is usually a narrow plastic strip, which has several squares on it impregnated with chemicals and represented by different colours. Each small square represents one of the components described above. When dipped in urine, the chemicals react with abnormal substances and change colour. Once the strip is quickly dipped into the urine sample and the necessary time has lapsed for the colour changes to take place, the strip is then compared either visually (manually) or electronically (automated) to a standardized colour chart, which will display results in terms of parameters. It is essential to use the strips according to the manufacturer's instructions and be aware of factors that may affect the results, including specific drugs (Table 11.9), the quality of the urine specimen itself and the possibility of false-negative results. There are many different urinalysis test strips available, each testing a different combination of components.

Table 11.9 **How drugs may influence the results of reagent sticks**

Drug	Reagent test	Effect on the results
Ascorbic acid	Glucose, blood, nitrite	High concentrations may diminish colour
L-dopa	Glucose	High concentrations may give a false-negative reaction
	Ketones	Atypical colour
Nalidixic acid	Urobilinogen	Atypical colour – probenacid
Phenazopyridine (pyridium)	Protein	May give atypical colour
	Ketones	Coloured metabolites may mask a small reaction
	Urobilinogen, bilirubin	May mimic a positive reaction
	Nitrite	Causes false positive result
Rifampicin	Bilirubin	Coloured metabolites may mask a small reaction
Salicylates (aspirin)	Glucose	High doses may give a false-negative reaction

Specific patient preparation

Education

Most patients need advice on hygiene and technique before the procedure to prevent contamination from hands or the genital area (Higgins 2008b) and to ensure that the midstream sample is collected correctly. Midstream urine specimens are indicated in adults and children who are continent and can empty their bladder on request (Gilbert 2006).

Procedure guideline 11.7 **Urinalysis: reagent strip procedure**

Essential equipment

- Non-sterile disposable gloves
- Apron
- Urine dipsticks, that are in date and have been stored according to the manufacturer's recommendations
- Appropriate urine specimen pot

Pre-procedure

Action	Rationale
1 Explain and discuss the procedure with the patient.	To ensure that the patient understands the procedure and gives their valid consent (NMC 2013, **C**).

2 Wash and dry hands and put on gloves and apron.	To maintain infection control and prevent cross-infection (Fraise and Bradley 2009, **E**).
Procedure	
3 If taking the specimen from a urinary catheter, it should be collected using an aseptic technique via the catheter side port. For women, the labia should be separated with cotton wool or a sponge moistened with water, and the vulva should be wiped from the front to the back although disinfectant must never be used. Men should clean the glans penis with soap and water.	To reduce sample contamination (Fraise and Bradley 2009, **E**; Roche Diagnostics 2010, **C**).
4 Obtain a clean specimen of fresh urine from the patient, which is to be analysed within 2 hours from collection. Women should separate the labia.The patient should commence micturition, and when a few millilitres of urine have been passed into the toilet, a container or sterile receptacle should be introduced into the urine stream, and then the remaining urine can pass into the toilet.	Urine that has been stored deteriorates rapidly and can lead to false results (Roche Diagnostics 2010, **C**).
5 Check reagent sticks have been stored in accordance with manufacturer's instructions. This is usually a dark dry place in an airtight container.	To ensure reliable results. Tests may depend on enzymic reaction so expired, contaminated or improperly stored strips can give false-positive results such as leucocyte and blood readings (Roche Diagnostics 2010, **C**). Prolonged exposure to the air (nitrous gases) can also affect result accuracy (Roche Diagnostics 2010, **C**).
6 Dip the reagent strip into the urine for no longer than 1 second. The strip should be completely immersed in the urine and then removed immediately. Run edge of strip along the container.	To remove any excess urine and prevent mixing of chemicals from adjacent reagent areas (Roche Diagnostics 2010, **C**).
7 Hold the stick at an angle.	Urine reagent strips should not be held upright when reading them because urine may run from square to square, mixing various reagents (Roche Diagnostics 2010, **C**).
8 Wait the required time before reading the strip against the colour chart, usually 60 seconds (see **Action figure 8**).	The strips must be read at exactly the time interval specified or the reagents will not have time to react, or may be inaccurate (Roche Diagnostics 2010, **C**).
Post-procedure	
9 Dispose of urine sample appropriately in either sluice or toilet. Dispose of urinalysis stick and gloves in correct wastage bin. Ensure cap to urine reagent strips is replaced immediately and closed tightly.	To ensure strips are in airtight container according to storage guidelines (Roche Diagnostics 2010, **C**).
10 Wash and dry hands.	To maintain infection control and prevent cross-infection (Fraise and Bradley 2009, **E**).
11 Document urinalysis readings and inform medical staff of any abnormal readings.	To allow prompt action if change to treatment plan required (NMC 2010, **C**).

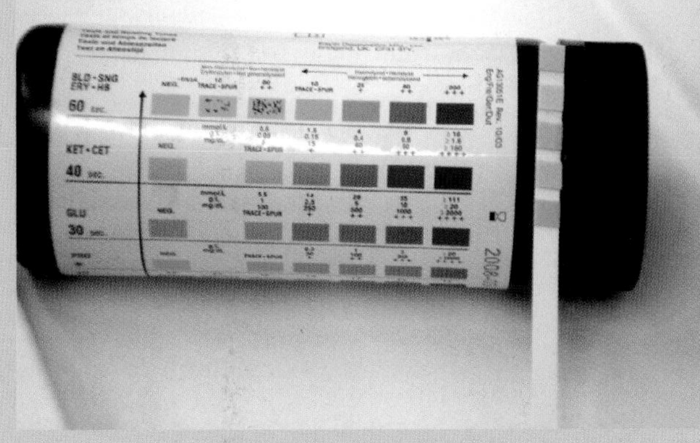

Action Figure 8 Compare urinalysis results and document results on appropriate forms.

POST-PROCEDURAL CONSIDERATIONS

When sending a urine specimen to the laboratory, check that the laboratory form is completed and that all relevant information is included. Take care not to contaminate the outside of the container or the request forms (Bishop 2008).

Reagent strips are a quick and easy method of testing urine and can provide valuable information about a patient's condition. However, patients should be made aware that further tests and investigations may be required if the urine sample indicates any abnormality (Steggall 2007).

Blood glucose

DEFINITION

Blood glucose is the amount of glucose in the blood (Brooker 2010). See Table 11.10 for normal target ranges, which are expressed as millimoles per litre (mmol/L) (NICE 2004).

Normally blood glucose levels stay within narrow limits throughout the day: 4–8 mmol/L. But they are higher after meals and usually lowest in the morning.

ANATOMY AND PHYSIOLOGY

Blood glucose is regulated by insulin and glucagon. Insulin is synthesized and secreted from the beta cells within the islets of Langerhans found in the pancreas (Wallymahmed 2007). It is produced in response to high blood glucose levels (i.e. after meals), promoting the uptake and storage of sugar by fat and muscle tissue as glycogen (Crosser and McDowell 2007). Glucagon is secreted by the alpha cells in response to low blood glucose levels and results in the release of stored sugar back into the blood (Wallymahmed 2007). These processes maintain blood glucose stability within the body (homeostasis) (Crosser and McDowell 2007).

Diabetes mellitus (DM) is a heterogeneous disorder characterized by chronic hyperglycaemia due to lack of insulin or complete insulin deficiency or the body's resistance to it (Blake and Nathan 2004, WHO/IDF 2006). There are two main types of DM: type 1 and type 2. Type 1 is believed to be triggered by an autoimmune process causing destruction of the beta cells in the pancreas, which produce insulin, resulting in complete loss of insulin production. Type 2 diabetes is characterized by a resistance to insulin (Thornton 2009).

People with type 1 or type 2 diabetes will have total or partial disruption to this normal metabolic regulatory system. Type 1 diabetes normally occurs in the younger population (Gillibrand et al. 2009) and means that they will need replacement-injected insulin to compensate (Crosser and McDowell 2007). Type 2 diabetes is strongly linked to obesity, age and family history (Gillibrand et al. 2009) but can also be a result of steroid use and pancreatic cancer (Schwab and Porter 2007). Both these can result in hyperglycaemia (high blood glucose) which may cause degenerative changes affecting the kidneys, nerves and eyes (Wallymahmed 2007), resulting in blindness, renal failure and neuropathies. Further complications including coronary artery and peripheral vascular disease, stroke, renal disease, central and peripheral nerve damage, amputations and blindness are also serious consequences of uncontrolled blood glucose (Gillibrand et al. 2009, WHO/IDF 2006).

Table 11.10 Normal target blood glucose ranges

Children and young people <18 years of age	Adults ≥18 years of age
Pre-prandial blood glucose levels 4–8 mmol/L	Pre-prandial blood glucose levels 4–7 mmol/L
Post-prandial blood glucose levels of less than 10 mmol/L	Post-prandial blood glucose levels of less than 9 mmol/L

Source: NICE (2004; updated 2014) Reproduced with permission from NICE (www.nice.org.uk/CG15).

A diagnosis of diabetes can primarily be based on a fasting blood glucose of more than or equal to 7 mmol/L or a random plasma glucose of more than or equal to 11.1 mmol/L accompanied by symptoms associated with diabetes such as polydipsia, polyuria and weight loss (Blake and Nathan 2004, WHO/IDF 2006). These features of diabetes do not appear until 80% of beta cells are lost and so it is possible to reverse type 2 diabetes if it is picked up early enough (Schwab and Porter 2007).

Furthermore, during infection, major surgery or critical illness such as sepsis, pancreatitis or respiratory distress, counter-regulatory or stress hormones (adrenaline, noradrenaline, cortisol, growth hormone and glucagon) are released causing significant metabolic alterations. These hormones increase insulin resistance that decreases peripheral intake of glucose and also promotes glucogenesis by stimulating glycogen and fat breakdown, causing hyperglycaemia (Crosser and McDowell 2007). For this reason, patients with diabetes may need treatment of insulin or antidiabetic medication during acute illness, in order to replicate this homeostasis or improve the body's ability to produce insulin or use it.

Hyperglycaemia

Hyperglycaemia is distinctly associated with poor clinical outcomes, increased mortality and extended time of discharge from hospital (Lipska and Kosiborod 2011, Pichardo-Lowden and Gabbay 2012). It is defined as a random blood glucose of more than 11.1 mmol/L (WHO/IDF 2006). When insulin is deficient or absent as in type 1 or 2 diabetes, blood glucose levels will remain high after a meal, in times of illness or stress because glucose is unable to enter most cells (Wallymahmed 2007). Therefore cells are starved of glucose and the body reacts inappropriately by producing stress hormones that cause glycogenolysis (the breakdown of glycogen to release glucose), lipolysis (the breakdown of stored fat into glycerol and fatty acids) and gluconeogenesis (the conversion of glycerol and amino acids into glucose) (D'Hondt 2008, Marieb and Hoehn 2010) (Figure 11.31).

This causes the blood glucose to rise further which results in a number of signs and symptoms. Water reabsorption in the kidneys becomes inhibited, resulting in frequent, large volumes of urine (polyuria). This will cause the person to feel excessive thirst (polydipsia) and may also result in extreme hunger (polyphagia). Polyuria and polydipsia will cause dehydration, a fall in blood pressure and electrolyte imbalance (Marini and Wheeler 2012). Moreover, the subsequent loss of sodium (hyponatraemia) and potassium (hypokalaemia) leads to muscle cramps, nausea, vomiting and diarrhoea, confusion, blurred vision, lethargy, cardiac events, coma and death.

Despite the excessive glucose in the body, the body cannot utilize it, so the body starts to break down its fat and protein stores for energy, which leads to high levels of fatty acids in the blood (lipidaemia) (Marieb and Hoehn 2010). This can also cause sudden and dramatic weight loss. These fatty acids are converted to ketones. They accumulate in the blood more quickly than they can be excreted or used and cause the blood pH to fall, resulting in ketoacidosis. Ketones will also be present in the urine. If ketoacidosis is allowed to continue it can become life threatening, disrupting all physiological processes, including oxygen transportation and heart activity and depression of the nervous system, leading to coma and death (Marieb and Hoehn 2010).

Reasons for hyperglycaemia include:

- inadequate doses of insulin
- stress
- infection/sepsis
- surgery
- medications, for example steroids

Organs/tissue involved	Organ/tissue responses to insulin deficiency	Resulting conditions		Signs and symptoms
		In blood	In urine	
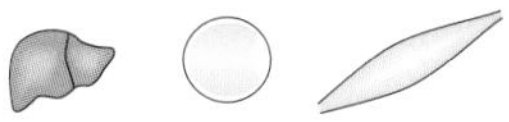	Decreased glucose uptake and utilization	Hyperglycaemia	Glycosuria	
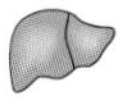	Glycogenolysis		Osmotic diuresis	Polydipsia (and fatigue, weight loss)
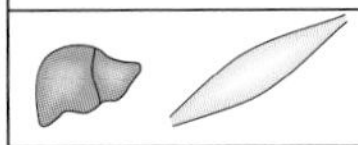	Protein catabolism and gluconeogenesis			Polyphagia
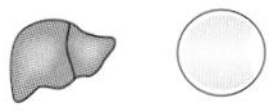	Lipolysis and ketogenesis	Lipidaemia and ketoacidosis	Ketonuria Loss of Na^+, K^+; electrolyte and acid–base imbalances	Acetone breath Hyperpnoea Nausea/vomiting/ abdominal pain Cardiac irregularities Central nervous system depression; coma

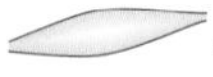

= Muscle = Adipose tissue 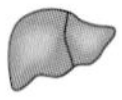 = Liver

Figure 11.31 **Consequences of insulin deficiency.**

- variability in oral or nutritional intake
- nutritional support, for example parenteral nutrition (PN) or enteral nutrition
- critical illness (Marieb and Hoehn 2010).

It has been found that enteral and parenteral feeding contributes to hyperglycaemia both in patients with a diagnosis of diabetes and those without (McKnight and Carter 2008). This is particularly true of patients receiving PN which bypasses the gut and therefore the incretin hormones that also help to maintain glucose homeostasis (McKnight and Carter 2008, Pichardo-Lowden and Gabbay 2012). Hyperglycaemia in response to steroids, for example dexamethasone, is another consideration and some researchers believe that their hypermetabolic action decreases glucose uptake, increases hepatic glucose production and may directly inhibit insulin release (Delaunay et al. 1997, Ogawa et al. 1992, Wallymahmed 2007). For this reason these patients will need blood glucose monitoring and potential changes to their insulin needs or to temporarily commence insulin.

Hypoglycaemia

Hypoglycaemia is described as a blood glucose level that is unable to meet the metabolic needs of the body (Marini and Wheeler 2012), normally lower than 4 mmol/L (Wallymahmed 2007). Hypoglycaemia is an acute complication of diabetes that increases morbidity, mortality and economic costs of diabetes and can decrease quality of life (Fidler et al. 2011, Liu et al. 2012). Often young, healthy individuals can be asymptomatic during this inadequate level of glucose in the blood but early symptoms can be sweating, tremor, weakness, nervousness, tachycardia and hypertension (Wallymahmed 2007), although these depend on not only the absolute blood glucose but also its rate of decline (Tortora and Derrickson 2011). Severe hypoglycaemia can lead to mental disorientation, convulsions, unconsciousness and death and blood glucose less than 3 mmol can start to affect the brain.

The most common causes of hypoglycaemia are missed or delayed meals, not eating enough, exercise without carbohydrate compensation, too much glucose-lowering medication (e.g. insulin) and excessive alcohol (Wallymahmed 2007). Other causes could be infection, muscle and fat depletion (e.g. anorexia), diarrhoea and vomiting, hepatic failure due to tumour or cirrhosis, salicylate poisoning, insulin-secreting tumours, ventilation, congestive heart failure, cerebral vascular accident, concurrent medications (beta-blockers, adrenaline) and surgery (D'Hondt 2008, Lui et al. 2012, Marini and Wheeler 2012).

There are several ways to reduce hypoglycaemia risk which include frequent monitoring of blood sugars with home blood glucose tests and occasionally continuous glucose monitoring (McCall 2012).Treatment should ideally be the administration of glucose. The route will depend on the consciousness level of the patient, their treatment and their ability to take oral substances (Marini and Wheeler 2012). If they can tolerate an oral or enteral intake, they should be given a fast-acting carbohydrate such as 3–6 glucose tablets, 150 mL sugary fizzy drink or 50–100 mL Lucozade followed by a longer acting carbohydrate such as a sandwich or biscuits. If unconscious or unable to take food and drink then they can receive intramuscular glucagon or intravenous dextrose (Wallymahmed 2007). Blood glucose needs to be checked 5–10 minutes after treatment and then as necessary. Diabetic treatment should not be omitted because of a single episode of hypoglycaemia but, if it remains a consistent problem, treatment should be reviewed (Wallymahmed 2007).There is a three-fold increased risk of severe hypoglycaemia which occurs in both type 1 and type 2 diabetes with tight glucose control and there is therefore a need to individualize therapy and glycaemia goals to minimize this risk (McCall 2012).

EVIDENCE-BASED APPROACHES

Rationale

Blood glucose monitoring provides an accurate indication of how the body is controlling glucose metabolism and provides feedback to guide clinicians and patients about their treatment adjustments in order to achieve optimal glucose control. In the short term, it can prevent hypo- and hyperglycaemia and in the long term it can significantly reduce the risk of prolonged, life-threatening microvascular complications (Dailey 2011, Lipska and Kosiborod 2011, Rizvi and Saunders 2006, Snell-Bergeon and Wadwa 2012).

Capillary blood glucose monitoring is preferred due to the immediacy of results and its ability to inform us whether blood sugar is high or low, whereas urine testing only indicates instances of high blood sugar (Wallymahmed 2007). Capillary blood glucose monitoring is also referred to as point-of-care testing (POCT).

Indications

Conditions in which blood glucose monitoring will need to take place include the following.

- To make a diagnosis of diabetes indicated by signs and symptoms of polyuria, polydipsia, weight loss for type 1 or weight gain, family history for type 2 (WHO/IDF 2006).
- To monitor and manage the day-to-day treatment of known type 1 and type 2 diabetes (Wallymahmed 2007).
- In acute management of unstable diabetes, that is, evidence of hyperglycaemia, hypoglycaemia, diabetic ketoacidosis, hyperosmolar non-ketotic coma (once severe dehydration is corrected) (Wallymahmed 2007).
- Hospitalized patients with diabetes according to morbidity and treatment, that is, sliding scales, nutritional intake/support (McKnight and Carter 2008, Wallymahmed 2007).
- Initial parenteral and enteral nutritional support of all patients (McKnight and Carter 2008).
- Patients taking steroids and other drugs that cause raised blood glucose (Schwab and Porter 2007).

Contraindications

The following conditions can affect the accuracy of blood glucose monitoring and it may be necessary to obtain a venous sample for more accurate results (MHRA 2011), especially where treatment, e.g. insulin, is due to be initiated on the acquired result.

- Peripheral circulatory failure and severe dehydration, for example diabetic ketoacidosis, hyperosmolar non-ketotic coma, shock, hypotension. These conditions cause peripheral shutdown, which can cause artificially low capillary readings.
- Haematocrit values above 55% may lead to inaccurate levels if the blood glucose level is more than 11 mmol/L.
- Intravenous infusion of ascorbic acid.
- Pre-eclampsia.
- Some renal dialysis treatments.
- *Hyperlipidaemia*: cholesterol levels above 13 mmol/L may lead to artificially raised capillary blood glucose readings.

Principles of care

Although capillary blood glucose monitoring is an essential part of diabetic management, it can have severe consequences if not done correctly (Wallymahmed 2007). The Department of Health issued a hazard warning in 1987 and a safety notice in 1996 highlighting the need for formal training and strict quality control (MHRA 1996), which has been emphasized since by the MHRA (2011).

Blood glucose monitoring needs to be performed regularly enough for patterns to be established on which treatment changes can be based (Walker 2004). 'Regularly' will vary in different circumstances and any unusual situation, for example illness, change of daily routine, hospitalization, will affect diabetes control and therefore require more frequent testing (Walker 2004). Generally people with type 1 diabetes will need to test blood glucose several times a day or more depending on treatment while those with type 2 will require less testing due to a lower risk of such great fluctuations in blood glucose levels (Goldie 2008). Blood glucose monitoring should be individualized dependent on the type of treatment (diet versus oral medication versus insulin), level of haemoglobin A1c and treatment goals.

There is variation in the literature surrounding the frequency of blood glucose monitoring for type 2 diabetes (IDF 2012), although for well-educated patients with type 1 diabetes it is suggested that monitoring four or more times daily is necessary (Minder et al. 2013). With both types of diabetes, more regular testing will be required in certain circumstances, for example illness, steroid treatment, changes in diet, exercise and routine where there is impaired hypoglycaemia awareness, and in the terminal care setting (Minder et al. 2013).

Within the hospital setting. self-monitoring of blood glucose (SMBG) may be appropriate for the competent adult patient who is medically stable and successfully self-managing their diabetes at home (IDF 2012). However, SMBG in the hospital setting would need to be supported by local policy and supportive assessment documentation.

For all patients (irrespective of previous diabetic diagnosis) receiving nutritional support, that is enteral or parenteral feeding, blood glucose levels should be checked once or twice daily (or more if needed) until stable and then weekly (NICE 2008).

Methods of blood glucose testing

Blood glucose testing involves obtaining a drop of capillary blood and putting it on a testing strip that is read by a blood glucose meter (Farmer et al. 2012). Most meters offer the option of using blood from the fingertips, palm of the hand, upper arm, forearm, calf or thigh (Dale 2006). The most commonly used site is the finger tip as the blood from this area responds rapidly to changes in blood glucose level, as does the blood from the palm of the hand, and therefore delivers the most accurate results (Dale 2006, Goldie 2008). However, the fingertips contain nerve endings, which can become sore and less sensitive with frequent testing. The outer parts of the finger are less painful to prick and the thumb and forefinger should be used sparingly due to their continual use in apposition (Goldie 2008). It is important to rotate areas used for blood glucose testing to avoid infection from multiple stabbings, areas becoming toughened and to reduce pain (Roche Diagnostics 2013).

Anticipated patient outcomes

There have been several trials investigating the benefits of tight glycaemic control to near normal levels. D'Hondt (2008) refers to three randomized controlled trials in which intensive insulin treatment was used in hospitalized patients. The trials showed that intensive insulin treatment to achieve tight glycaemic control did result in reductions in length of stay, sepsis, dialysis and hospital mortality and morbidity (Furnary et al. 2000, Krinsley 2004, van den Berghe et al. 2001). Blood glucose testing is integral to achieving this tight control but there is currently no absolute conclusion for the standardization of this treatment (D'Hondt 2008). It does, however, indicate that keeping blood sugar levels as near normal as possible should be the ultimate aim of blood glucose testing.

Accurate blood glucose monitoring and management are vital and poor control and management are known to lead to increased hospital admissions and longer length of stays (NHS Diabetes 2011).

LEGAL AND PROFESSIONAL ISSUES

The DH report (MHRA 1996) and a subsequent MHRA alert (2011) highlight that there must be standardization in training, reliability and quality control for blood glucose testing and staff should be updated at appropriate intervals. In order to achieve this, the following aspects must be considered when selecting monitoring devices.

- Equipment is designed for use by non-laboratory staff and is suitable for use in the clinical environment.
- All equipment is compatible and will give reliable results.
- The biochemistry laboratory is involved in the purchase and maintenance of the equipment. This may involve the purchase of one type of device from one company for the whole hospital, to reduce costs and provide standardization.
- The equipment should be easy to use and staff should be involved in the choice of device (Hall 2005).
- The ongoing cost and maintenance of the device need to be considered, including buying strips, control solutions and replacement devices (Hall 2005).
- Written standard operating procedures should be available and kept with the device.

- Training is given to the operators of the equipment and records are kept of this. After training, the following learning outcomes should be demonstrated by the operator:
  - basic principles of measurement
  - expected results in normal and pathological states
  - demonstration of the proper use of the equipment in accordance with the manufacturer's specification
  - demonstration of the consequences of improper use
  - knowledge of operator-dependent steps
  - instruction in the collection of appropriate blood samples
  - health and safety aspects
  - instruction in the importance of complete documentation of all data produced
  - appropriate calibration and quality control techniques
  - practical experience of the procedures, including a series of analyses to satisfy the instructor that the trainee is competent
  - information regarding contraindications
  - information on basic troubleshooting, error messages and potential sources of error (MHRA 2011).

It is a hospital and government directive to keep records of training and quality testing results and the frequency of these quality control tests may vary according to manufacturer or hospital policy (Walker 2004). Independent quality control should be carried out with the collaboration of the biochemistry laboratory and external auditing of quality control should be undertaken, which may be provided by the company providing the equipment.

PRE-PROCEDURAL CONSIDERATIONS

Equipment

Errors can occur in any phase of the testing process: pre-analytic, analytic or post-analytic. Common sources of meter error include patient or methodology interferences, operator mistakes, environmental exposure and device malfunction (Nichols 2011).

All equipment should be checked for expiry dates (according to individual hospital trust policy) and successful calibration, and stored according to manufacturer's guidelines.

- *Blood glucose monitor*: a medical device which measures the concentration of glucose in a human blood sample using a blood glucose test strip.
- *Testing strip*: strip with a small window used to collect a sample of the patient's blood to be inserted into the blood glucose monitor. The strips must be calibrated with the monitor prior to use.
- *Lancet*: a device used to draw out a small amount of blood from the patient for testing of glucose level. Single-use lancets are used to minimize the risk of cross-infection and accidental needlestick injury and set to the correct depth according to the skin turgor (Roche Diagnostics 2013). Disposable lancets are advisable following an outbreak of hepatitis B in French and US hospitals (European Agency for Safety and Health at Work 2010, MHRA 1996, Roche Diagnostics 2013).

The accuracy of glucose meters is a factor for consideration when purchasing or renting glucose meters. This is especially true in the post-operative setting where, in recent years, clinicians have been looking for tight control of glucose to assist in improving recovery and outcomes (Rice et al. 2010). Home glucose meters that have been adopted for use in some hospitals without additional testing may not give the high level of accuracy that anaesthetists require and that is available when using a central laboratory device or an automated blood gas analyser (Rice et al. 2010).

Specific patient preparation

Patients should be advised to wash their hands prior to testing or the test area should be cleaned with soap and water and then dried. Use of alcohol gel should be avoided to ensure non-contamination of the result. The patient should be encouraged to warm their hands before sampling to encourage blood flow and to obtain an adequate amount of blood to cover the test strip (Dale 2006, Wallymahmed 2007).

Procedure guideline 11..8 **Blood glucose monitoring**

Essential equipment

- Blood glucose monitor
- Test strips
- Control solution
- Single-use safety lancets
- Non-sterile gloves
- Cotton wool/low-linting gauze
- Sharps box

Pre-procedure

Action	Rationale
1 Turn the machine on and ensure the correct date and time are presented on screen, and that there is adequate battery life. Where applicable, enter or scan operator number, e.g. number or bar code on name badge, as per manufacturer's guidelines.	To ensure accuracy in the result record and patient safety (Roche Diagnostics 2013, **C**).
2 Check the unit of measure and ensure that it is reading in mmol/L prior to each use.	Units of measure may change from mmol/L to mg/dL, which could result in the meter user thinking that the blood glucose level is higher than it actually is (MHRA 2011, **C**).
3 Before taking the device to the patient, the monitor and testing strips need to be checked for the following (where applicable to the device. Newer automated systems will self-calibrate when turned on). • Testing strips are in date and have not been left exposed to air. • The monitor and test strips have been calibrated together. • If a new pack of strips is required, the monitor is recalibrated.	As any device can fail under the right conditions (Nichols 2011, **E**).

(continued)

Procedure guideline 11.8 Blood glucose monitoring *(continued)*

Action	Rationale
• Internal quality control carried out with both high and low or level 1 and 2 solutions, in accordance with trust and manufacturer's guidelines. Ensure the LOT number is recorded, either manually or via bar code scanning system. • Result (pass or fail) of internal quality control is to be recorded in equipment log book and signed. Where an automated device is used, ensure the device is docked in its base unit for the centrally held electronic records to be maintained. • The meter has previously been decontaminated per local guidelines and is fit for use. • The meter service record is in date according to local policy. • That the screen/display is intact and the 'screen safety check' has been completed in accordance with manufacturer's guidelines.	
4 Identify the patient, i.e. verbally and against their hospital identity band, and explain the procedure.	The patient should give consent to the procedure. Explanation may allay any fear or anxieties (NMC 2013, **C**).
5 Select a site that is warm, pink and free of any calluses, burns, cuts, scars, bruises or rashes. Avoid skin areas that have evidence of previous punctures. The usual site for lancing is the palmar surface of the distal segment of the third or fourth finger, ideally of the non-dominant hand as they are usually less calloused.	It is important to avoid previous punctures by rotating the site lanced to avoid fingertip soreness and reduce callous formation (WHO 2010, **C**). Fingers on the non-dominant hand and the index finger are generally less calloused. The index finger is also potentially more sensitive to pain due to additional nerve endings. The thumb also may be calloused and has a pulse, indicating arterial presence, and the distance between the skin surface and the bone in the fifth finger also makes it unsuitable for puncture (WHO 2010, **C**). Tips and pads of fingers should be avoided as they are denser with nerve supply and can be more painful (WHO 2010, **C**).
Procedure	
6 Ask patient to sit or lie down.	To ensure the patient's safety and minimize the risks if they feel faint when blood is taken (Roche Diagnostics 2013, **C**).
7 Ask the patient to wash their hands with soap and water and dry thoroughly with low-linting gauze.	To avoid sample contamination (CDC 2013, **C**). Not washing hands can lead to a difference in the glucose concentration, especially with fingers exposed to fruit or a sugar-containing product (Hortensius et al. 2011, **R1b**).
8 Wash your hands and put on gloves.	To minimize the risk of cross-infection and contamination (Fraise and Bradley 2009, **E**).
9 Take a single-use lancet and, if it has depth settings, ensure the correct setting is used (most commonly middle one).	To minimize the risk of cross-infection and accidental needlestick injury (FDA 2010, **C**; Fraise and Bradley 2009, **E**). The correct depth setting will ensure patient comfort (Roche Diagnostics 2013, **C**).
10 Activate the single-use, auto-disabling fingerstick device/lancet or reusable device, as per manufacturer's guidelines, at the chosen site, e.g. the side of the finger. Ensure the site of piercing is rotated (see **Action figure 10**), avoiding frequent use of index finger and thumb. Other areas may be used if finger or palm of hand are unusable. The fingertip may need 'milking' from palm of hand towards finger to gain a large enough droplet of blood but avoid milking the finger alone.	In settings where assisted monitoring of blood glucose is performed, single-use, auto-disabling fingerstick devices should be used. Although reusable devices may be used in the patient's own environment, they should never be used for more than one person due to the risk of bloodborne viruses (CDC 2013, **C**). The side of the finger is less painful and easier to obtain a hanging droplet of blood. Sites are rotated to avoid infection from multiple stabbings, area becoming toughened and to reduce pain (Roche Diagnostics 2013, **C**). Milking the finger can cause tissue fluid contamination and a false low reading (Hortensius et al. 2011, **R1b**), cause haemolysis and impede blood flow (WHO 2010, **C**).
11 Activate safety-engineered medical device (where applicable and if not automated), dispose of lancet and testing strip in a sharps container.	A cost-effective way to reduce the risk of needlestick injury (European Agency for Safety and Health at Work 2010, **C**; Roche Diagnostics 2013, **C**; Tan et al. 2001, **R1a**).
12 Insert testing strip into blood glucose monitor and apply the first drop of blood to the testing strip. Some strips are hydrophilic and are dosed/filled from the side instead of dropping blood directly onto the strip. Ensure that the window on the test strip is entirely covered with blood (see **Action figure 12**).	To ensure accurate results, the window on the test strip needs to be adequately filled as per manufacturer's guidelines (Roche Diagnostics 2013, **C**).

13 Place gauze over puncture site, apply firm pressure and monitor for excess bleeding.	To ensure patient safety (Wallymahmed 2007, **E**) and to stop the bleeding (WHO 2010, **C**).
14 Remove gloves, place in clinical waste and perform hand hygiene again.	To prevent healthcare-associated infections and spread of antimicrobial resistance (WHO 2013, **C**).
Post-procedure	
15 Once result is obtained (see **Action figure 15**), document and sign.	To ensure centralized records are maintained (Roche Diagnostics 2013, **C**).
16 Where applicable, dock machine.	To ensure accuracy in record keeping (NMC 2010, **C**; Roche Diagnostics 2013, **C**).
17 Report any unexpected results.	To ensure appropriate treatment and obtain optimal blood glucose range (Wallymahmed 2007, **E**).

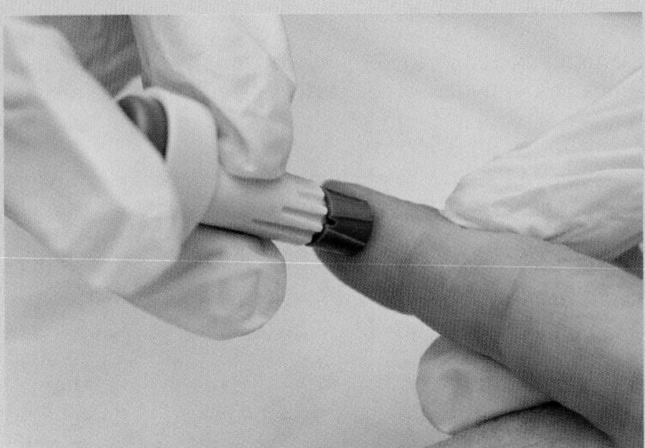

Action Figure 10 Blood glucose taking: Step 1. Take a blood sample from the side of the finger using a lancet, ensuring that the site of piercing is rotated.

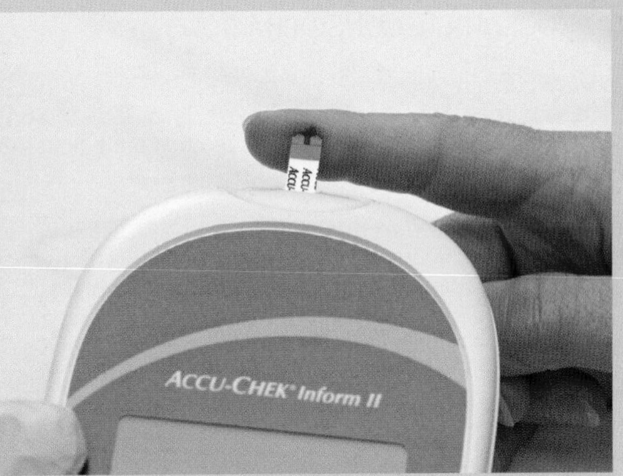

Action Figure 12 Blood glucose taking: Step 2. Insert the test strip into the blood glucose monitor and apply the blood to the test strip. Ensure that the window on the test strip is entirely covered with blood.

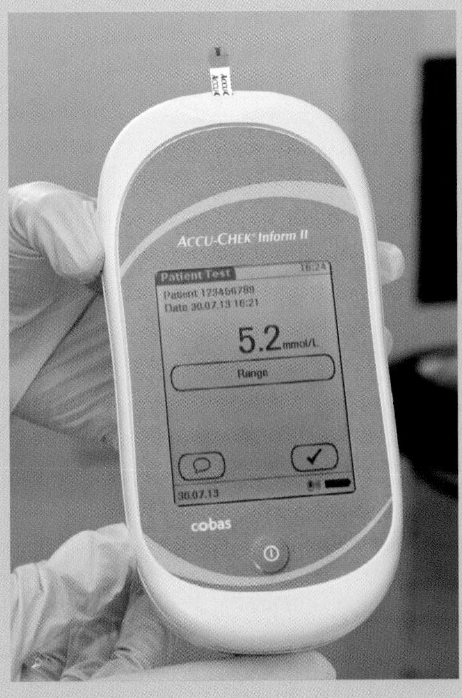

Action Figure 15 Blood glucose taking: Step 3. Read the result.

Problem-solving table 11.7 **Prevention and resolution (Procedure guideline 11.8)**

Problem	Cause	Prevention	Action
Inaccurate results.	User error including: • inadequate meter calibration • failure to code correctly • poor meter maintenance • incorrect user technique. 50% of errors are due to an inadequate amount of blood on the test strip, which can lead to a falsely low reading (Blake and Nathan 2004). Out-of-date or incorrectly stored test strips are other common errors leading to lower glucose levels.	Staff training and education about diabetes are essential in prevention of these errors (Heinemann 2010, Janssen and Delanghe 2010).	Contact colleague to repeat test and, if error persists, report glucose meter to technician and use another machine.

POST-PROCEDURAL CONSIDERATIONS

Immediate care

If a true abnormal blood glucose result is detected then the appropriate action should be taken according to medical advice and hospital policy.

Education of patient and relevant others

Diabetes mellitus is a long-term, often lifelong condition affecting all aspects of a person's life. Ninety-five percent of diabetes care is self-care and all people with type 1 and type 2 diabetes should have access to self-monitoring. Research has found that diabetes self-management education improves quality of life (Thorpe et al. 2013). The nurse has a role in educating and promoting self-management of diabetes and advising patients on the type and frequency of monitoring based on individual clinical need so that patients can monitor and adjust their own treatment (Diabetes UK 2008). NICE and the Department of Health also recommend that people are given annual updates to ensure they are still able to perform tests accurately and learn about any new developments (DH 2008, NICE 2004, NICE 2008). Healthcare professionals should advocate a healthy lifestyle for patients with diabetes, including regulating blood pressure, low-sugar diet and exercise (NICE 2008).

Neurological observations

DEFINITION

Neurological observation is the collection of information about the patient's central nervous system (Mooney and Comerford 2003). Despite advances in neuromonitoring, clinical observation of the patient remains the most sensitive measure of neurological function (Adam and Osbourne 2005).

ANATOMY AND PHYSIOLOGY

The nervous system is the most complex of the body systems, responsible for the co-ordination of all body functions, adapting to changes in internal and external environments. The activites of the nervous system can be grouped into three basic functions (Tortora and Derrickson 2011).

- *Sensory (input):* detection of internal or external stimuli; this information is carried to the brain and spinal cord through cranial and spinal nerves.
- *Integrative (process):* analysis of sensory information and deciding on appropriate responses.
- *Motor (output):* eliciting an appropriate motor response by activating effectors (muscles and glands) through cranial and spinal nerves.

The intricate network of neurones and neuroglia which comprise the nervous system are divided into two main subdivisions: the central nervous system and the peripheral nervous system.

The central nervous system

The central nervous system consists of the brain and spinal cord (Tortora and Derrickson 2011).

The brain

Located within the skull, the brain is the control centre for registering sensations, correlating them with one another and stored information, making decisions and taking actions; it is also the centre for intellect, emotions, behaviour and memories (Tortora and Derrickson 2011). The adult brain consists of four regions: the brainstem, the cerebellum, the diencephalon and the cerebrum (Figure 11.32).

The cerebrum is the largest part of the brain and provides us with the ability to read, write and speak, to make calculations, and to remember the past, plan for the future and imagine things.

The cerebral hemispheres contain the greatest mass of brain tissue. Each hemisphere is subdivided into several lobes named after the bones that cover them: frontal, parietal, temporal and occipital lobes (Figure 11.33). Each of these lobes has a particular function.

- The *frontal lobe* is located at the front of the brain and is associated with cognitive function (orientation, memory, insight, judgement, calculation and abstraction), expressive language (verbal and written) and voluntary motor function (through skeletal muscle).
- The *parietal lobe* is located in the middle section of the brain and is associated with sensory function, including integration of sensory information, awareness of body parts, interpretation of touch, pressure and pain, and recognition of object size, shape and texture.
- The *occipital lobe* is located at the back of the brain and is associated with interpreting visual stimuli and receives impulses from the optic nerve.
- The *temporal lobe* is located in the bottom section of the brain and is primarily associated with hearing, speech, behaviour and memory (Adam and Osbourne 2005, Baumann 2009).

The spinal cord

The spinal cord is a cylindrical mass of nerve tissue encased within the vertical canal of the vertebral column extending from the medulla oblongata of the brainstem to the superior border of the second lumbar vertebra (Tortora and Derrickson 2011). It contains important motor and sensory nerve pathways that exit and enter the cord through anterior and posterior nerve roots and spinal and peripheral nerves, and also mediates reflex activity of the deep tendon reflexes from the spinal nerves (Bickley and Szilagyi 2009).

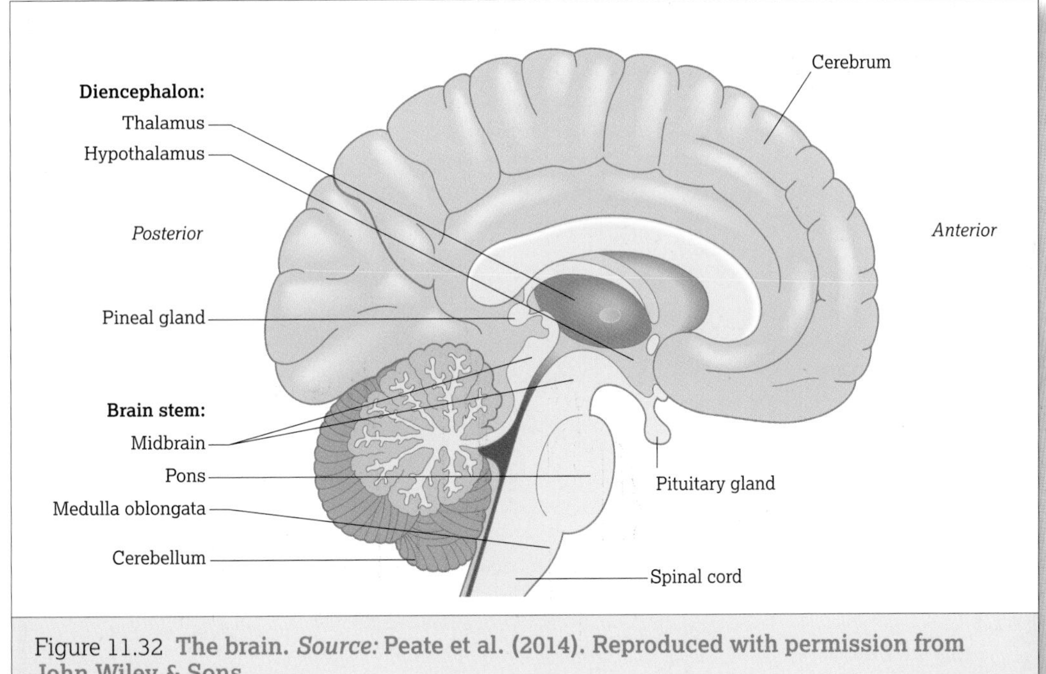

Figure 11.32 **The brain.** ***Source:*** **Peate et al. (2014). Reproduced with permission from John Wiley & Sons.**

The spinal cord is divided into five segments: cervical, from C1 to C8; thoracic, from T1 to T12; lumbar, from L1 to L5; sacral, from S1 to S5; and coccygeal (Bickley and Szilagyi 2009) (Figure 11.34).

The peripheral nervous system

The peripheral nervous system consists of the 12 pairs of cranial nerves and the 31 pairs of spinal and peripheral nerves (Tortora and Derrickson 2011).

The cranial nerves

Twelve pairs of special nerves called cranial nerves emerge from the brain. They are named according to their distribution and are numbered I to XII in order of their attachment to the brain (Tortora and Derrickson 2011). Cranial nerves II–XII arise from the diencephalon and the brainstem (Table 11.11). Cranial nerves I and II are actually fibre tracts emerging from the brain. Some cranial nerves are limited to general motor or sensory functions whereas others are specialized, producing smell, vision or hearing (I, II, VIII) (Bickley and Szilagyi 2009).

The peripheral nerves

In addition to the cranial nerves, the peripheral nervous system also includes spinal and peripheral nerves that carry impulses to and from the spinal cord. The 31 pairs of spinal nerves are named and numbered in accordance with the region and level of the spinal cord from which they emerge: eight cervical, 12 thoracic, five lumbar, five sacral and one coccygeal. Spinal nerves are typically connected to the spinal cord by a posterior root (containing sensory fibres) and an anterior root (containing motor fibres) (Tortora and Derrickson 2011).

RELATED THEORY

Changes in neurological status can be rapid and dramatic or subtle, developing over minutes, hours, days, weeks or even longer (Aucken and Crawford 1998). The frequency of neurological observations will depend upon the patient's condition and the rapidity with which changes are occurring or expected to occur. Neurological assessment must include (Adam and Osbourne 2005):

- assessment of level of consciousness
- pupil size and reaction to light
- limb assessments (including both motor and sensory function)
- vital signs.

Level of consciousness

Level of consciousness is the most sensitive indicator of neurological deterioration and is therefore the most important aspect of any neurological assessment (Waterhouse 2005). Consciousness is a state of awareness of self and the environment and is dependent upon two components: arousal and awareness (Baumann 2009). These correspond to two brain structures, the reticular activating system (RAS) and the cerebral cortex. Consciousness depends on the interaction between the neurones in the RAS in the brainstem and the neurones in the cerebral cortex (Adam and Osbourne 2005).

Arousal

This is a primitive state managed by the RAS (Figure 11.35). The core of nuclei which make up the RAS extends from the brainstem with projections upwards to the cortex and downwards to the spinal cord. The RAS receives auditory, visual and sensory impulses (such as pain, touch, movement of limbs, bright light or noise), and because of its connections is ideal for governing arousal of the brain as a whole (Adam and Osbourne 2005). Unless inhibited by other areas of the brain, the reticular neurones send a continuous stream of impulses to the cerebral cortex, maintaining the cortex in an alert, conscious state; the RAS is selective, however, forwarding only essential information to the cortex and filtering out unnecessary information. Certain drugs have a direct effect on the RAS – alcohol, sleep-inducing drugs and tranquillizers depress the RAS and drugs such as LSD remove the RAS filter system, leading to heightened sensory arousal (Adam and Osbourne 2005).

Awareness

This is the more sophisticated part of consciousness and requires an intact cerebral cortex to interpret sensory input and respond accordingly (Adam and Osbourne 2005).

Assessing consciousness

Consciousness cannot be measured directly but is assessed by observing behaviour in response to different stimuli; the

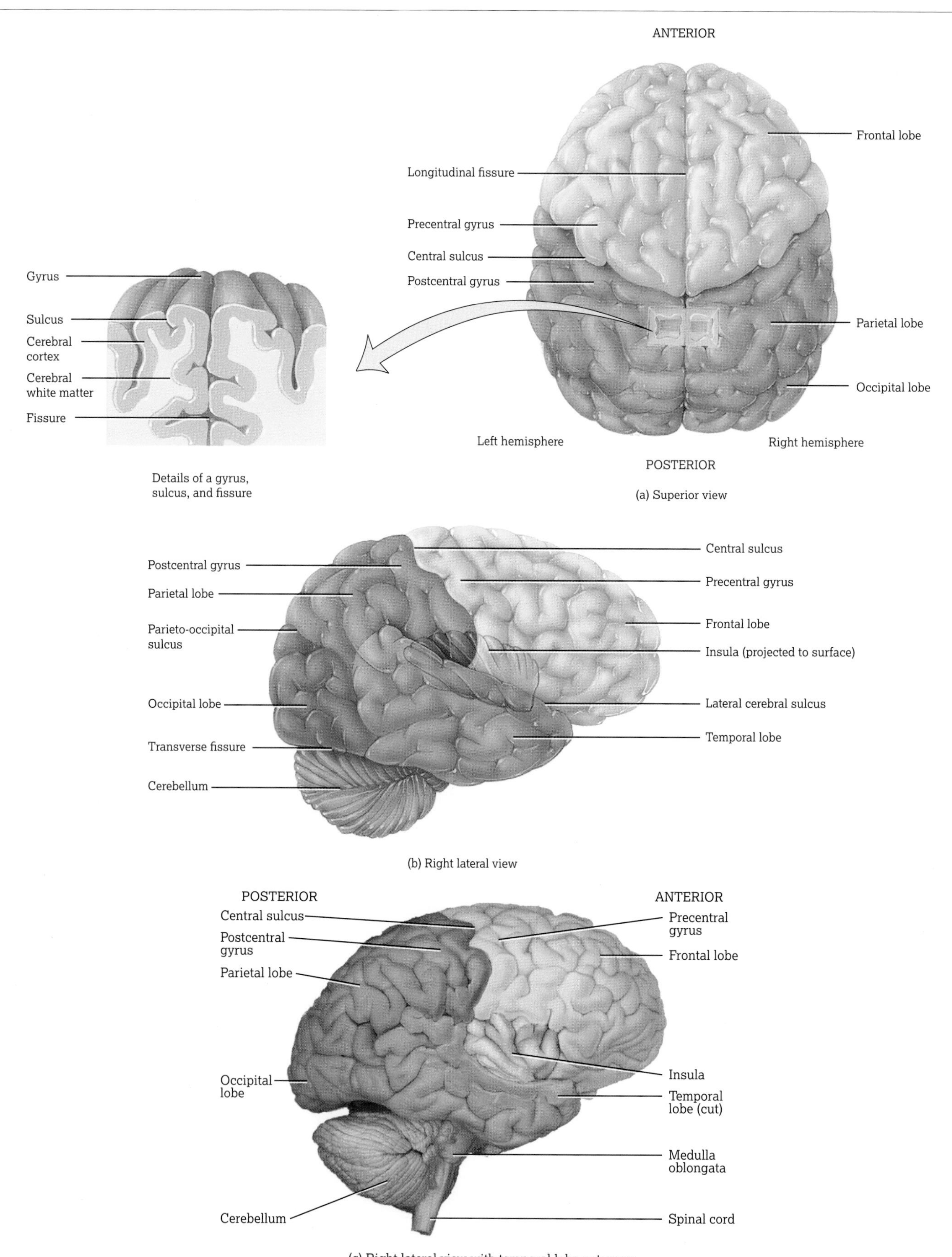

Figure 11.33 **The cerebrum.** ***Source:*** **Tortora and Derrickson (2011). Reproduced with permission from John Wiley & Sons.**

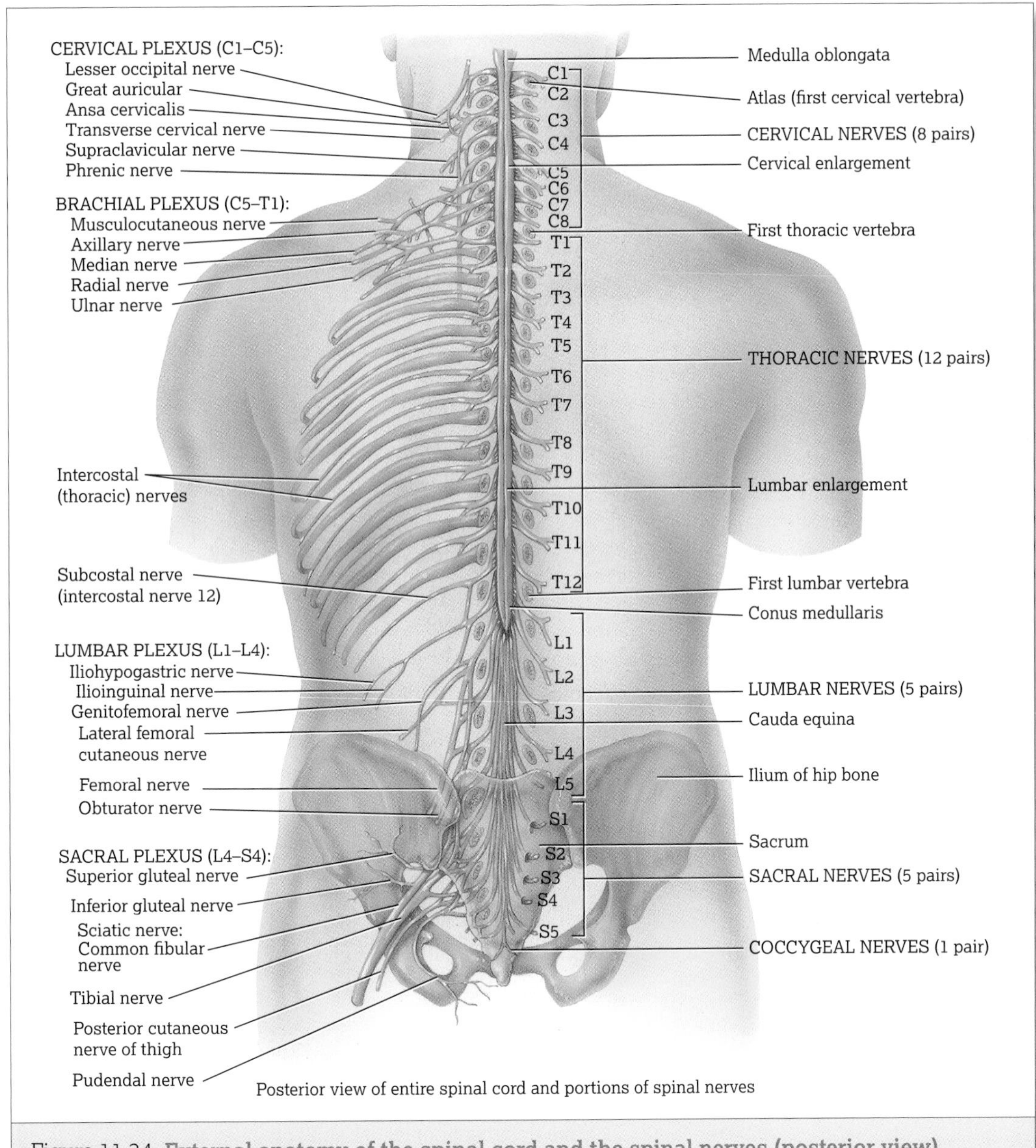

Figure 11.34 **External anatomy of the spinal cord and the spinal nerves (posterior view).** ***Source:*** **Tortora and Derrickson (2011). Reproduced with permission from John Wiley & Sons.**

response indicates the level at which the sensory information has been translated within the central nervous system (Adam and Osbourne 2005).

Assessment of arousal focuses on the patient's ability to respond appropriately to verbal or non-verbal stimuli and begins with verbal stimulus in a normal tone and if there is no response the stimulus is progressively increased, firstly by raising the voice, followed by gently shaking the patient and finally by applying noxious (painful) stimuli (Baumann 2009).

Assessment of awareness is concerned with the patient's orientation to person, place and time; changes in responses that indicate increasing degrees of confusion and disorientation may be the first sign of neurological deterioration (Baumann 2009).

Previous and/or co-existing problems should be considered when assessing levels of consciousness, for example deafness, hemiparesis/hemiplegia. A manifestation of altered consciousness implies an underlying brain dysfunction. Its onset may be sudden, for example following an acute head injury, or it may occur more gradually, such as in hypoglycaemia (Jevon 2008). Similarly, alterations in level of consciousness can vary from slight to severe changes, indicating the degree of brain dysfunction (Aucken and Crawford 1998).

Consciousness ranges on a continuum from alert wakefulness to deep coma with no apparent responsiveness. Therefore, nurses must ensure that families and friends are involved at the initial history taking and throughout care so as to accurately note any change in neurological symptoms. Terms such as 'fully conscious', 'semi-conscious' or 'stuporous', previously used to describe levels of consciousness, are subjective and open to misinterpretation and therefore level of consciousness should be measured using the Glasgow Coma Scale (GCS) or, during a rapid assessment of an acutely unwell patient, the AVPU scale (see Assessment and recording tools') (Adam and Osbourne 2005, Jevon 2008).

Application of painful stimuli

Painful stimuli should be employed only if the patient does not respond to firm and clear commands (Jevon and Ewens 2007).

Table 11.11 **Summary of cranial nerves***

Cranial nerve	Components	Principal functions
Olfactory (I)	**Special sensory**	Olfaction (smell)
Optic (II)	**Special sensory**	Vision (sight)
Oculomotor (III)	**Motor**	
	Somatic	Movement of eyeballs and upper eyelid
	Motor (autonomic)	Adjusts lens for near vision (accommodation) Constriction of pupil
Trochlear (IV)	**Motor**	
	Somatic	Movement of eyeballs
Trigeminal (V)	**Mixed**	
	Sensory	Touch, pain, and thermal sensations from scalp, face, and oral cavity (including teeth and anterior two-thirds of tongue)
	Motor (branchial)	Chewing and controls middle ear muscle
Abducens (VI)	**Motor**	
	Somatic	Movement of eyeballs
Facial (VII)	**Mixed**	
	Sensory	Taste from anterior two-thirds of tongue Touch, pain, and thermal sensations from skin in external ear canal
	Motor (branchial)	Control of muscles of facial expression and middle ear muscle
	Motor (autonomic)	Secretion of tears and saliva
Vestibulocochlear (VIII)	Special sensory	Hearing and equilibrium
Glossopharyngeal (IX)	**Mixed**	
	Sensory	Taste from posterior one-third of tongue Proprioception in some swallowing muscles Monitors blood pressure and oxygen and carbon dioxide levels in blood Touch, pain, and thermal sensations from skin of external ear and upper pharynx
	Motor (branchial)	Assists in swallowing
	Motor (autonomic)	Secretion of saliva
Vagus (X)	**Mixed**	
	Sensory	Taste from epiglottis Proprioception from throat and voice box muscles Monitors blood pressure and oxygen and carbon dioxide levels in blood Touch, pain, and thermal sensations from skin of external ear Sensations from thoracic and abdominal organs
	Motor (branchial)	Swallowing, vocalization, and coughing
	Motor (autonomic)	Motility and secretion of gastrointestinal organs Constriction of respiratory passageways Decreases heart rate
Accessory (XI)	**Motor**	
	Branchial	Movement of head and pectoral girdle
Hypoglossal (XII)	**Motor**	
	Somatic	Speech, manipulation of food, and swallowing

Source: Tortora and Derrickson (2011). Reproduced with permission from John Wiley & Sons.

*Mnemonic for Cranial Nerves:

oh	**o**h	**o**h	**T**o	**T**ouch	**A**nd	**F**eel	**V**ery	**G**reen	**V**egetables	**AH!**	
Olfactory	**O**ptic	**O**culomotor	**T**rochlear	**T**rigeminal	**A**bducens	**F**acial	**V**estibulocochlear	**G**lossopharyngeal	**V**agus	**A**ccessory	**H**ypoglossal

Figure 11.35 **The reticular activating system.** ***Source:*** **Tortora and Derrickson (2011). Reproduced with permission from John Wiley & Sons.**

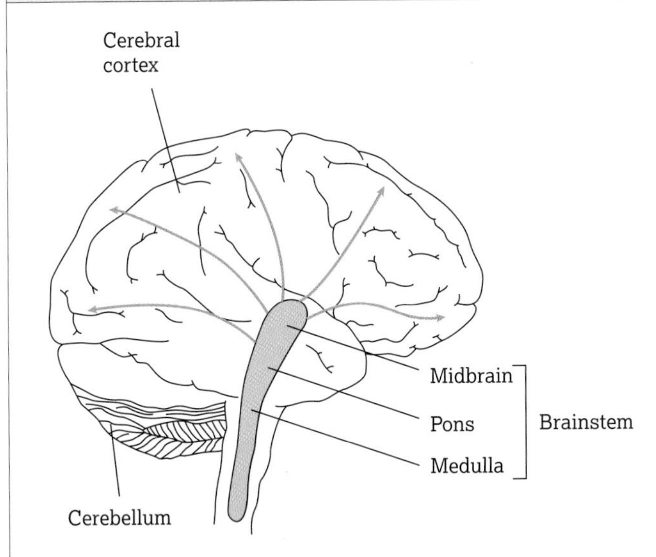

The stimulus should be applied in a standard way, increasing from light pressure and being maintained until a response is elicited, for a maximum of 10 seconds to avoid soft tissue injury or causing the patient pain (Adam and Osbourne 2005, Jevon and Ewens 2007). As such, it should only be undertaken by appropriately qualified and experienced professionals.

As the ability to localize pain is lost, various responses may be observed when painful stimuli are applied (Baumann 2009). It is important to note, when applying a painful stimulus, that peripherally it may only elicit a spinal reflex which does not involve cerebral function and, therefore, evaluation of cerebral function requires the application of central stimuli (Jevon and Ewens 2007).

Central stimuli can be applied in the following ways (Baumann 2009, Jevon and Ewens 2007).

- *Trapezium squeeze*: using the thumb and two fingers, hold 5 cm of the trapezius muscle where the neck meets the shoulder and twist the muscle.
- *Supraorbital pressure*: by running a finger along the supraorbital margin (the bony ridge along the top of the eye) a notch is felt. Applying pressure to the notch stimulates the supraorbital nerve and causes an ipsilateral (on that side) sinus headache-type pain. This method should not be used if the facial or cranial bones are unstable, facial fractures are suspected or after facial surgery. Using supraorbital pressure as a painful stimulus may also make the patient grimace and lead to closing the eye rather than eye opening (Fairley et al. 2005).
- *Sternal rub*: using the knuckles of a clenched fist to grind on the centre of the sternum. When applied adequately, marks are left on the skin as sternal tissue is tender and bruises easily. Please note that because of the risk of bruising, this should not be used for repeated assessment but may be indicated to guide medical decisions about the patient's management.

If there is no response to central stimuli then a peripheral stimulus should be applied to assess limbs that have not moved (Adam and Osbourne 2005). The patient's finger should be placed between the assessor's thumb and a pencil or pen. Pressure is gradually increased over a few seconds until the slightest response is seen. Due to the risk of bruising, pressure should not be applied to the nailbed.

Table 11.12 **Examination of pupils**

Observation	Pupil size	Pupil reactiveness	Possible indication
Pupils equal	Pinpoint	–	Opiates or pontine lesion
	Small	Reactive	Metabolic encephalopathy
	Mid-sized	Fixed	Midbrain lesion
		Reactive	Metabolic lesion
Pupils unequal	Dilated	Unreactive	3rd nerve palsy
	Small	Reactive	Horner's syndrome

Source: Fuller (2008). Reproduced with permission from Churchill Livingstone.

Pupillary activity

Careful examination of the reactions of the pupils to light is an important part of neurological assessment (Table 11.12). The size, shape, equality, reaction to light (in both the eye directly exposed to light [direct] and the eye not directly exposed to it [consensual]) and position of the eyes should be noted as well as whether the eyes are deviated upwards or downwards, and whether the eyes are conjugate (moving together) or dysconjugate (not moving together). Pupillary response to light is dependent upon intact afferent (optic nerve) and efferent (oculomotor nerve) function transmitting the light impulse from the retina to the midbrain and the pupillary musculature (Adam and Osbourne 2005). Pupillary pathways are relatively resistant to metabolic insults and therefore response to light is the single most important sign in distinguishing structural from metabolic coma. Impaired pupillary response to light signifies that the midbrain itself may be suffering from pressure exerted by an expanding mass in the brain and is therefore important as a localizing sign; pupillary constriction and dilation are controlled by cranial nerve III (oculomotor) and any changes may indicate pressure on this nerve or brainstem damage (Adam and Osbourne 2005, Fuller 2008).

Limb assessment

MOTOR FUNCTION

Damage to any part of the motor nervous system can affect the ability to move. After assessing motor function on one side of the body, the contralateral muscle group should also be evaluated to detect asymmetry. Motor function assessment involves an evaluation of the following.

- Muscle strength
- Muscle tone
- Muscle co-ordination
- Reflexes
- Abnormal movements (Aucken and Crawford 1998, Fuller 2008)

MUSCLE STRENGTH

This involves testing the patient's muscle strength against the pull of gravity and then against one's own resistance. Changes in motor strength, especially between right and left sides, may indicate imminent neurological failure (Baumann 2009).

MUSCLE TONE

This involves flexing and extending the patient's limbs on both sides and noting how well such movements are resisted; increased resistance would denote increased muscle tone and decreased resistance decreased tone (Baumann 2009).

MUSCLE CO-ORDINATION

Any disease or injury that involves the cerebellum or basal ganglia will affect co-ordination. Assessment of hand and leg co-ordination can be achieved by testing the rapidity and rhythm of alternating movements and point-to-point movements (Baumann 2009).

Reflexes

Amongst the most important reflexes are blink, gag and swallow, oculocephalic and plantar.

- *Blink (corneal)*: this is a protective reflex and can be affected by damage to the Vth cranial nerve (trigeminal) and the VIIth cranial nerve (facial). Facial weakness (VIIth cranial nerve) will affect eye closure and absence of the corneal reflex may result in corneal damage (Fuller 2008).
- *Gag and swallow*: damage to the IXth cranial nerve (glossopharyngeal) and Xth cranial nerve (vagus) may impair protective reflexes. These two cranial nerves are always assessed together as their functions overlap. Muscle innervation of the palate is from the vagus, while sensation is supplied by the glossopharyngeal nerves (Aucken and Crawford 1998, Fuller 2008).
- *Oculocephalic*: this reflex is an eye movement that occurs only in patients with a severely decreased level of consciousness (in conscious patients this reflex is not present). When the reflex is present, the patient's eyes will move in the opposite direction from the side to which the head is turned. However, in patients with absent brainstem reflexes, the eyes will appear to remain stationary in the centre. This reflex should not be assessed if there is suspected instability of the cervical spine as the necessary head movement could exacerbate any spinal injury (Baumann 2009).
- *Plantar*: abnormalities of plantar reflex will help to locate the anatomical site of the lesion. Upgoing plantar (extension) reflex is termed 'positive Babinski' (dorsiflexion of the big toe and fanning of the other toes) and indicates an upper motor neurone lesion. Note that upgoing plantar is normal in babies under 1 year of age (Baumann 2009).

Abnormal movements

When carrying out neurological observations, any abnormal movements such as seizures, tics and tremors must be noted.

Sensory functions

Constant sensory input enables an individual to alter responses and behaviour to suit the environment. When disease or injury damages the sensory pathways, the sensory responses are always affected. Any assessment of sensory function should include an evaluation of the following.

- Central and peripheral vision
- Hearing and ability to understand verbal communication
- Superficial sensations (light touch, pain) and deep sensations (muscle and joint pain, muscle and joint position) (Baumann 2009, Fuller 2008)

Visual acuity

The clarity or clearness of vision may be tested with a Snellen chart, which uses decreasing letter size, or newspaper prints, with glasses if worn.

Visual fields

Lesions at different points in the visual pathways affect vision. It should be noted that loss of vision is always described with reference to the visual fields rather than the retinal fields (Weldon 1998).

Vital signs

It is recommended that assessments of vital signs should be made in the following order.

1. Respirations
2. Temperature
3. Blood pressure
4. Pulse

Please see relevant sections in this chapter.

RESPIRATIONS

Of these four vital signs, respiratory patterns give the clearest indication of how the brain is functioning because the complex process of respiration is controlled by more than one area of the brain – the cerebral hemispheres, the cerebellum and the brainstem (Adam and Osbourne 2005, Jevon and Ewens 2007). Any disease or injury that affects these areas may produce respiratory changes. The rate, character and pattern of a patient's respiration must be noted. Abnormal respiratory patterns are listed in Table 11.13.

Constant re-evaluation of the patient's ability to maintain and protect their airway is essential when there is evidence of reduced consciousness or coma (GCS score is less than 8). At this stage, muscles often become flaccid and use of the recovery position may need to be considered. Patients whose neurological function has deteriorated may require adjuncts to protect the airway and possibly artificial ventilation (RCUK 2011). Close liaison with physiotherapists and speech and language therapists is important to minimize the danger of chest infections due to the inability to clear secretions or aspiration.

TEMPERATURE

Damage to the hypothalamus, the temperature-regulating centre, may result in grossly fluctuating temperatures (Adam and Osbourne 2005).

Table 11.13 **Abnormal respiratory patterns**

Type	Pattern	Significance
Cheyne–Stokes	Rhythmic waxing and waning of both rate and depth of respirations, alternating regularly with briefer periods of apnoea. Greater than normal respiration, that is 16–24 breaths per minute	May indicate deep cerebral or cerebellar lesions, usually bilateral; may occur with upper brainstem involvement
Central neurogenic hyperventilation	Sustained, regular, rapid respirations, with forced inspiration and expiration	May indicate a lesion of the low midbrain or upper pons areas of the brainstem
Apneustic	Prolonged inspiration with a pause at full inspiration; there may also be expiratory pauses	May indicate a lesion of the lower pons or upper medulla, hypoglycaemia or drug-induced respiratory depression
Cluster breathing	Clusters of irregular respirations alternating with longer periods of apnoea	May indicate a lesion of lower pons or upper medulla
Ataxic breathing	A completely irregular pattern with random deep and shallow respirations; irregular pauses may also appear	May indicate a lesion of the medulla

BLOOD PRESSURE AND PULSE

Hypertension with a widening pulse pressure, bradycardia and a fall in respiratory rate may be indicative of rising intracranial pressure (ICP) and is part of the Cushing's reflex (Adam and Osbourne 2005, Jevon and Ewens 2007). Abnormalities of blood pressure and pulse usually occur late (and may not appear at all in some patients); usually the patient's level of consciousness will have begun to deteriorate before there is any alteration in their vital signs (Adam and Osbourne 2005).

EVIDENCE-BASED APPROACHES

Rationale

Indications

An accurate neurological assessment is essential in planning appropriate patient care. The information gained from a neurological assessment can be used in the following ways.

- To aid diagnosis (Pentland et al. 2009).
- As a baseline for observations (Meurier et al. 2005, Mooney and Comerford 2003).
- To determine both subtle and rapid changes in an individual's condition (Meurier et al. 2005).
- To monitor neurological status following a neurological procedure or trauma (Mooney and Comerford 2003).
- To observe for deterioration and establish the extent of a traumatic head injury (Walsh 2006).
- To detect life-threatening situations (Alcock et al. 2002).

Frequency of observations

There is no published consensus on how frequently neurological observations should be recorded (Mooney and Comerford 2003, Price 2002). It is therefore impossible to be prescriptive, as the frequency will depend on the patient's presenting condition, medical diagnosis, underlying pathology and possible consequences. Clinicians' professional knowledge and judgement will dictate the necessary timing interval for the assessment. If the patient's condition is deteriorating, observations may need to be carried out as frequently as every 10–15 minutes for the first few hours and then 1–2-hourly observations for a further 48 hours.

The nurse must be competent to take appropriate action if changes in the patient's neurological status occur, as well as reporting any subtle signs that may indicate deterioration; for example, patients will often become increasingly restless or a previously restless patient may become atypically quiet. It should never be assumed that difficulty to rouse a patient is due to night-time sleep as even a deeply asleep patient with no focal deficit should respond to pain. If the patient requires an increased amount of stimulus to achieve the same response, this may be an indication of subtle deterioration (Table 11.14) (Aucken and Crawford 1998, Waterhouse 2005).

PRE-PROCEDURAL CONSIDERATIONS

Equipment

The following equipment may be used as part of the neurological assessment.

- *Pen torch*: used to assess the reaction of the pupils to light and consensual light reflex (Fairley and Pearce 2006a).
- *Tongue depressor*: a device used to depress the tongue to allow for examination of mouth and throat (Fuller 2008).
- *Patella hammer*: a tendon hammer used to strike the patella tendon below the knee to assess the deep knee jerk/reflex (Fuller 2008).
- *Neuro tips*: a sharp instrument used to apply pressure and test for superficial sensations to pain. Can be replaced by a safety pin or other suitable sharp object (Fuller 2008).
- *Snellen chart*: a letter chart used to measure visual acuity.

Assessment and recording tools

The initial assessment of a patient should include a history (taken from relatives or friends if appropriate), noting changes in mood, intellect, memory and personality, since these may be indicators of a long-standing problem (Baumann 2009).

Assessment of level of consciousness can be carried out using the GCS or the AVPU scale.

Glasgow Coma Scale

The GCS, first developed by Teasdale and Jennett (1974), is a widely used tool to assess level of consciousness and should be used to assess all patients with head injuries (NICE 2007c). It forms a quick, objective and easily interpreted mode of neurological assessment. The GCS measures arousal and awareness, by assessing three different areas of the patient's behaviour: eye opening, verbal response and motor response (Dawes and Durham 2007). Each area is allocated a score, enabling objectivity, ease of recording and comparison between recordings. The total sum provides a score out of 15, whereby a score of 15 indicates a fully alert and responsive patient and a score of 3 (the lowest possible score) indicates unconsciousness (Dawes and Durham 2007). When used consistently, the GCS provides a graphical representation that shows any improvement or deterioration of the patient's conscious level at a glance (Figure 11.36 and Table 11.15).

Assessment using the GCS involves three phases (Teasdale and Jennett 1974).

1 Eye opening.
2 Evaluation of verbal response.
3 Evaluation of motor response.

EVALUATION OF EYE OPENING

Eye opening indicates that the arousal mechanism in the brain is active (Waterhouse 2005). Eye opening may be spontaneous; to speech; to painful stimulus; or not at all. Arousal (eye opening) is always the first measurement undertaken when performing the GCS, as without arousal, cognition cannot occur (Aucken and Crawford 1998).

- *Spontaneous:* the patient is observed to be awake with their eyes open without any speech or touch (allocated a score of 4).
- *To speech:* the patient opens their eyes to loud, clear commands (allocated a score of 3).

Table 11.14 **Frequency of observations**

Category	Frequency	Rationale
All patients diagnosed as suffering from neurological or neurosurgical conditions	At least 4-hourly, affected by the patient's condition	To monitor the condition of the patient so that any necessary action can be instigated
Unconscious patients (including ventilated and anaesthetized)	Frequency indicated by patient's condition	To monitor the condition closely and to detect trends so that appropriate action may be taken

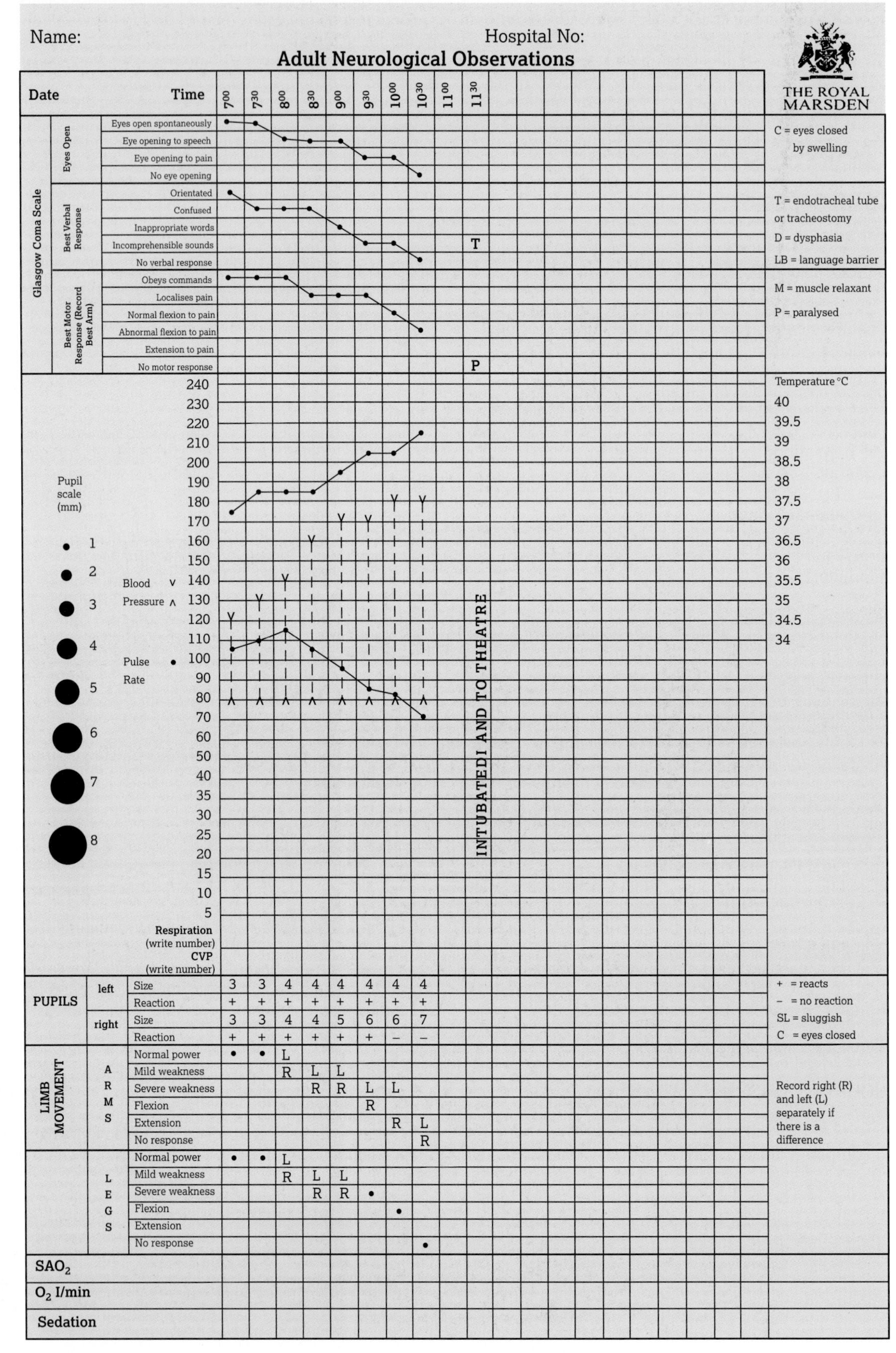

Figure 11.36 The Glasgow Coma Scale.

Table 11.15 **Scoring activities of the Glasgow Coma Scale. Scores are added, with the highest score 15 indicating full consciousness**

Category	Score	Response
Eye opening		
Spontaneous	4	Eyes open spontaneously without stimulation
To speech	3	Eyes open to verbal stimulation (normal, raised or repeated)
To pain	2	Eyes open with painful/noxious stimuli
None	1	No eye opening regardless of level of stimulation
Verbal response		
Orientated	5	Able to give accurate information regarding time, person and place
Confused	4	Able to answer in sentences using correct language but cannot answer orientation questions appropriately
Inappropriate words	3	Uses incomprehensible words in a random or disorganized fashion
Incomprehensible sounds	2	Makes unintelligible sounds, for example moans and groans
None	1	No verbal response despite verbal or other stimuli
Best motor response		
Obeys commands	6	Obeys and can repeat simple commands, for example arm raise
Localizes to pain	5	Purposeful movement to remove painful stimuli
Normal flexion	4	Withdraws extremity from source of pain, for example flexes arm at elbow without wrist rotation in response to painful stimuli
Abnormal flexion	3	Decorticate posturing (flexion of arms, hyperextension of legs) spontaneously or in response to noxious stimuli
Extension	2	Decerebrate posturing (limbs extended and internally rotated) spontaneously or in response to noxious stimuli
None	1	No response to noxious stimuli. Flaccid limbs

Source: Adapted from Aucken and Crawford (1998), Baumann (2009).

- *To pain:* the patient opens their eyes to a painful stimulus (allocated a score of 2).
- *None:* the patient does not open their eyes to painful stimuli (allocated a score of 1) (Fairley et al. 2005, Fairley and Pearce 2006b, Mooney and Comerford 2003, Waterhouse 2005).

A patient with flaccid ocular muscles may lie with their eyes open all the time; this is not a true arousal response and should be recorded as 'none' (Fairley and Pearce 2006b). If a patient's eyes are closed as a result of swelling or facial fractures, eye opening cannot be used to determine a falling conscious level (Fairley et al. 2005). This should be recorded as a 'C' on the chart.

EVALUATION OF VERBAL RESPONSE

- *Orientated*: the patient can correctly identify who they are (person), where they are (place) and the current year (time) (allocated a score of 5).
- *Confused*: the patient's responses to the above questions are incorrect and they are unaware of person, place or time (allocated a score of 4).
- *Inappropriate words:* the patient responds using intelligible words which are unsuitable as conversational responses; swearing is common, as are single word responses (allocated a score of 3).
- *Incomprehensible*: the patient may mumble, moan or groan without recognizable words (allocated a score of 2).
- *Absent*: the patient does not speak or make sounds at all (allocated a score of 1) (Fairley et al. 2005, Fairley and Pearce 2006b, Waterhouse 2005).

The absence of speech may not always indicate a falling level of consciousness; for example, the patient may not speak English (though they can still speak). A patient with an endotracheal tube should be recorded as 'T' on the chart under no response and allocated a score of 1 (Fairley and Pearce 2006b). Likewise, if the patient is dysphasic the best verbal response cannot be determined accurately. The patient may have a motor (expressive) dysphasia, and therefore be able to understand but be unable to find the right word, or a sensory (receptive) dysphasia, being unable to comprehend what is being told to them (Aucken and Crawford 1998, Shah 1999). At times patients with expressive dysphasia may also have receptive problems; therefore it is important to make an early referral to a speech and language therapist. This should be recorded as a 'D' on the chart under no response and allocated a score of 1 (Fairley and Pearce 2006b).

If a patient cannot follow the instruction due to a language barrier or unconsciousness, observe spontaneous movements and note how strong they appear. Then, if necessary, apply painful stimuli.

The nurse should also consider that some patients may need a lot of stimulation to maintain their concentration to answer questions, even though they can answer them correctly. It is, therefore, important to note the amount of stimulation that the patient required as part of the baseline assessment (Aucken and Crawford 1998, Waterhouse 2005).

EVALUATION OF MOTOR RESPONSE

Motor response is the most important prognostic aspect of the GCS after traumatic brain injury (Adam and Osbourne 2005). To obtain an accurate picture of brain function, motor response is tested by using the upper limbs because responses in the lower limbs reflect spinal function (Aucken and Crawford 1998, Adam and Osbourne 2005). The patient should be asked to obey a couple of simple commands; for example, they should be asked to squeeze the examiner's hands (both sides) – the nurse should note power in the hands and the patient's ability to release the grip in order to discount a reflex action (Fairley et al. 2005). In addition, the patient should be asked to raise their eyebrows or stick out their tongue with the best motor response recorded (Fairley et al. 2005, Waterhouse 2005). If movement is spontaneous, the nurse should note which limbs move and whether the movement is purposeful. If the patient is able to obey commands they should be allocated a score of 6.

If the patient is unresponsive to simple commands, their response to painful stimuli should be assessed. This may be:

- *localized*: the patient moves their hand to the site of the stimulus – either up beyond the chin or across the midline of the body (allocated a score of 5)
- *normal flexion:* no localization is seen, instead the patient bends their arms at the elbow in response to painful stimuli – this is a rapid response associated with abduction of the shoulder (allocated a score of 4)
- *abnormal flexion:* internal rotation, adduction of the shoulder and flexion of the elbow in response to painful stimuli – this is much slower than normal flexion and may be accompanied by spastic flexion of the wrist (allocated a score of 3)
- *extension*: no abnormal flexion is seen, the patient has straightening of the elbow joint, adduction and internal rotation of the shoulder, and inward rotation and spastic flexion of the wrist limb in response to painful stimuli (allocated a score of 2)
- *flaccid/none*: no motor response is seen at all in response to painful stimuli (allocated a score of 1) (Fairley et al. 2005, Fairley and Pearce 2006b, Waterhouse 2005).

The AVPU scale

The AVPU scale is a simple, rapid and effective method to assess consciousness, and now forms part of the National Early Warning Score (NEWS) (Royal College of Physicians 2012). It is particularly useful during the rapid assessment of an acutely unwell patient (RCUK 2011).

AVPU is a mnemonic for a simple neurological scoring system which quantifies the response to stimulation and assesses the level of consciousness (Jevon and Ewens 2007); it stands for Alert, response to Voice, response to Pain, Unresponsive. Assessment using the AVPU method is done in sequence and only one outcome is recorded; for example, if the patient responds to voice, it is not necessary to assess the response to pain.

- *Alert*: a fully awake (although not necessarily orientated) patient. Such patients will have spontaneous opening of the eyes, will respond to voice (although may be confused) and will have motor function.
- *Voice:* the patient makes some kind of response when you talk to them, which could be in any of the three component measures of eyes, voice or motor, for example, the patient's eyes open on being asked, 'Are you OK?'. The response could be as little as a grunt, moan, or slight movement of a limb when prompted by voice.
- *Pain:* the patient makes a response to a pain stimulus. A patient who is not alert and who has not responded to voice is likely to exhibit only withdrawal from pain, or even involuntary flexion or extension of the limbs from the pain stimulus.
- *Unresponsive:* this is also commonly referred to as 'unconscious'. This outcome is recorded if the patient does not give any eye, voice or motor response to voice or pain (Royal College of Physicians 2012).

Procedure guideline 11.9 **Neurological observations and assessment**

Essential equipment

- Pen torch
- Thermometer
- Sphygmomanometer
- Tongue depressor
- Patella hammer
- Neuro tips
- Alcohol handrub

Optional equipment

- Low-linting swabs
- Two test tubes
- Snellen chart
- Ophthalmoscope

Pre-procedure

Action	Rationale
1 Inform the patient of the procedure, whether conscious or not, and explain and discuss the observations.	Sense of hearing is frequently unimpaired even in unconscious patients. It is important, as far as is possible, that the patient understands the procedure and gives their valid consent (NMC 2013, **C**).

Procedure

Action	Rationale
2 Wash and dry hands.	To minimize the risk of cross-contamination (Fraise and Bradley 2009, **E**).
3 Observe the patient without speech or touch.	To assess eye opening as part of the GCS and level of consciousness as part of the AVPU (Fairley et al. 2005, **E**; Royal College of Physicians 2012, **C**).
4 Talk to the patient. Note whether they are alert and giving their full attention or restless or lethargic and drowsy. Ask the patient who they are, where they are and what day, month and year it is. Also ask them to give details about their family.	To establish whether the patient's level of consciousness is deteriorating. If the patient is becoming disorientated, changes will occur in this order: **(a)** disorientation as to time **(b)** disorientation as to place **(c)** disorientation as to person (Aucken and Crawford 1998, **E**).

5 Ask the patient to squeeze and release your fingers (both sides should be assessed) and then to stick out their tongue or raise their eyebrows.	To evaluate motor responses and to ensure that the responses are equal and are not reflexive (Baumann 2009, **E**; Fairley et al. 2005, **E**; Waterhouse 2005, **E**).
6 If the patient does not respond, apply painful stimuli. Suggested methods have been discussed earlier.	Responses grow less purposeful as the patient's level of consciousness deteriorates. As the condition worsens, the patient may no longer localize pain and respond to it in a purposeful way (Baumann 2009, **E**).
7 Record the findings precisely, recording the patient's best response. Write exactly what stimulus was used, where it was applied, how much pressure was needed to elicit the response, and how the patient responded.	Vague terms can be easily misinterpreted. Accurate recording will enable continuity of assessment and comply with NMC guidelines (NMC 2010, **C**; Waterhouse 2005, **E**).
8 Extend both hands and ask the patient to squeeze your fingers as hard as possible. Compare grip and strength.	To test grip and ascertain strength. Record best arm in GCS chart to reflect best outcome (Baumann 2009, **E**).
9 Reduce any external bright light by darkening the room, if necessary, or shield the patient's eyes with your hands.	To allow accurate monitoring of pupil reaction and enable a better view of the eye (Fairley and Pearce 2006a, **E**).
10 Ask the patient to open their eyes. If the patient cannot do so, hold the eyelids open and note the size, shape and equality of both pupils simultaneously.	To assess the size, shape and equality of the pupils as an indication of brain damage (Waterhouse 2005, **E**). Normal pupils are round and equal in size with a diameter ranging from 2 to 5 mm (Fairley et al. 2005, **E**; Fairley and Pearce 2006a, **E**).
11 Hold each eyelid open in turn. Shine a bright light into each eye as above, moving from the outer corner of each eye towards the pupil. This should cause the pupil to constrict immediately and cause an immediate and brisk dilation of the pupil once the light is withdrawn.	To assess the direct light reflex of the pupils (Fairley et al. 2005, **E**; Fairley and Pearce 2006a, **E**).
12 Hold both eyelids open but shine the light into one eye only. Both pupils should constrict immediately and immediately and briskly dilate once the light is withdrawn.	To assess consensual light reflex (Fairley et al. 2005, **E**; Fairley and Pearce 2006a, **E**).
13 Record pupillary size (in mm) and reactions on observation chart. Brisk reaction is documented as '+', no reaction as '-', sluggish response of one pupil compared to the other as 'S'.	Accurate recording will enable continuity of assessment and comply with NMC guidelines (Fairley et al. 2005, **E**; Fairley and Pearce 2006a, **E**; NMC 2010, **C**).
14 Record unusual eye movements such as nystagmus or deviation to the side.	To assess cranial nerve damage (Waterhouse 2005, **E**).
15 Note the rate, character and pattern of the patient's respirations.	Respirations are controlled by different areas of the brain. When disease or injury affects these areas, respiratory changes may occur (Adam and Osbourne 2005, **E**; Baumann 2009, **E**; Jevon and Ewens 2007, **E**).
16 Take and record the patient's temperature at specified intervals.	Damage to the hypothalamus, the temperature-regulating centre in the brain, will be reflected in grossly abnormal temperatures (Adam and Osbourne 2005, **E**).
17 Take and record the patient's blood pressure and pulse at specified intervals.	To monitor signs of increased intracranial pressure. Hypertension and bradycardia usually occur late, after the patient's level of consciousness has begun to deteriorate. Call for medical assistance as soon as it is evident that there is a deterioration in the patient's level of consciousness (Adam and Osbourne 2005, **E**; Jevon and Ewens 2007, **E**; Tortora and Derrickson 2011, **E**).
18 Ask the patient to close the eyes and hold the arms straight out in front, with palms upwards, for 20–30 seconds. Observe for any sign of weakness or drift.	To show weakness and difference in limbs (Baumann 2009, **E**; Waterhouse 2005, **E**).
19 Stand in front of the patient and extend your hands. Ask the patient to push and pull against your hands. Ask the patient to lie on their back in bed. Place the patient's leg with knee flexed and foot resting on the bed. Instruct the patient to keep the foot down as you attempt to extend the leg. Then instruct the patient to straighten the leg while you offer resistance.	To test arm strength. If one arm drifts downwards or turns inwards, it may indicate hemiparesis. To test flexion and extension strength in the patient's extremities by having the patient push and pull against your resistance (Baumann 2009, **E**; Waterhouse 2005, **E**).
20 Flex and extend all the patient's limbs in turn. Note how well the movements are resisted.	To test muscle tone (Baumann 2009, **E**).

(continued)

Procedure guideline 11.9 **Neurological observations and assessment *(continued)***	
21 Ask the patient to pat their thigh as fast as possible. Note whether the movements seem slow or clumsy. Ask the patient to turn the hand over and back several times in succession. Evaluate co-ordination. Ask the patient to touch the back of the fingers with the thumb in sequence rapidly.	To assess hand and arm co-ordination. The dominant hand should perform better (Baumann 2009, **E**; Bickley and Szilagyi 2009, **E**).
22 Extend one of your hands towards the patient. Ask the patient to touch your index finger, then their nose, several times in succession. Repeat the test with the patient's eyes closed.	To assess hand and arm co-ordination/cerebellar function (Baumann 2009, **E**).
23 Ask the patient to place a heel on the opposite knee and slide it down the shin to the foot. Check each leg separately.	To assess leg co-ordination (Fuller 2008, **E**).
24 Ask the patient to look up or hold the eyelid open. With your hand, approach the eye unexpectedly or touch the eyelashes.	To test the corneal (blink) reflex (Fuller 2008, **E**).
25 Ask the patient to open the mouth, and hold down the tongue with a tongue depressor. Touch the back of the pharynx, on each side, with a low-linting swab.	To test the gag reflex (Fuller 2008, **E**).
26 Ask the patient to lie on their back in bed. Place your hand under the knee, raise and flex it. Tap the patellar tendon. Note whether the leg responds.	To assess the deep tendon knee-jerk reflex (Bickley and Szilagyi 2009, **E**; Fuller 2008, **E**).
27 Stroke the lateral aspect of the sole of the patient's foot. If the response is abnormal (Babinski's response), the big toe will dorsiflex and the remaining toes will fan out.	To assess for upper motor neurone lesion (Baumann 2009, **E**; Bickley and Szilagyi 2009, **E**; Fuller 2008, **E**).
28 Ask the patient to read something aloud. Check each eye separately. If vision is so poor that the patient is unable to read, ask the patient to count your upraised fingers or distinguish light from dark.	To test for visual acuity (Fuller 2008, **E**).
29 Occlude one ear with a low-linting swab. Stand a short way from the patient. Whisper numbers into the open ear. Ask for feedback. Repeat for the other ear.	To test hearing and comprehension (Fuller 2008, **E**).
30 Ask the patient to close the eyes. Using the point of a Neuro tip (sharp instrument for applying pressure), stroke the skin. Use the blunt end occasionally. Ask patient to tell you what is felt. See if the patient can distinguish between sharp and dull sensations.	To test superficial sensations to pain (Fuller 2008, **E**).
31 Ask the patient to close their eyes. Fill two test tubes with water – one warm, one cold. Touch the patient's skin with each test tube and ask patient to distinguish between them.	To test superficial sensations to temperature (Fuller 2008, **E**).
32 Stroke a low-linting swab lightly over the patient's skin. Ask the patient to say what they feel.	To test superficial sensations to touch (Fuller 2008, **E**).
33 Ask the patient to close the eyes. Hold the tip of one of the patient's fingers between your thumb and index finger. Move it up and down and ask the patient to say in which direction it is moving. Repeat with the other hand. For the legs, hold the big toe.	To test proprioception (Bickley and Szilagyi 2009, **E**). *Proprioception* is the receipt of information from muscles and tendons in the labyrinth that enables the brain to determine movements and position of the body (Tortora and Derrickson 2011, **E**).
Post-procedure	
34 Document the observation recordings on the patient's observation chart; record only what you see. Do not be influenced by previous observations.	To ensure adequate records and enable continued care of the patient (NMC 2010, **C**).
35 Report any abnormal findings to medical staff.	To prevent further deterioration and allow timely intervention. **E**
36 Wash and dry hands or use alcohol handrub.	To minimize the spread of cross-infection (Fraise and Bradley 2009, **E**).
37 Clean the equipment after use.	To prevent cross-infection (Fraise and Bradley 2009, **E**).

Problem-solving table 11.8 **Prevention and resolution (Procedure guideline 11.9)**			
Problem	**Cause**	**Prevention**	**Action**
Language difficulties or dysphasia.	Difficulty making accurate assessment of consciousness.	Knowledge of language difficulties.	Use of interpreter for language barrier. Consideration when taking into account overall assessment process.
Patient unable to open eye(s).	Result of swelling.	Unable to prevent.	Does not necessarily indicate a low or falling conscious level.

POST-PROCEDURAL CONSIDERATIONS

Documentation

A validated observation chart is the most common method of monitoring and recording neurological observations. Although the layout may differ from chart to chart, in essence all neurological observation charts measure and record the same clinical information, including the level of consciousness, pupil size and response, motor and sensory response and vital signs (Dawes and Durham 2007).

Observation charts ensure a systematic approach to collecting and analysing essential information regarding a patient's condition. Such charts also act as a means of communication between nurses and other healthcare professionals (Dawes and Durham 2007).

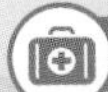
Learning Activity 11.4

Learning in practice: Neurological observations

In your clinical area, review a copy of the neurological observations chart that is used. Practise undertaking a neurological assessment on a colleague, following Procedure guideline 11.9: Neurological observations and assessment.

- Is this procedure any different to that you may have observed in practice?
- Particularly practise checking pupil size and reactions, assessment of conscious level using the Glasgow Coma Scale and assessment of motor function.
- Reflect on aspects of the assessment that you found most challenging; what do you need to practise/clarify prior to undertaking this assessment on one of your patients?

Learning for practice

After studying this chapter, list three key points you have learnt about observations that you will be able to apply to your clinical practice.

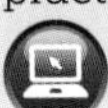
For further learning exercises visit **www.royalmarsdenmanual.com/student**.

Now Test Yourself

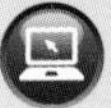
This section provides a range of exercises/activities to further test your learning. For additional exercises visit **www.royalmarsdenmanual.com/student**.

What have you learnt?

1 How often does NICE (2007) recommend that observations should be taken for patients in hospital?
A At least 4 hourly
B At least 8 hourly
C At least 12 hourly
D At least daily

2 Which tool has been found to help with structuring and standardizing communication when reporting a concern about a patient?
A SBAR
B NEWS
C MET
D PART

3 Which of the following describes the amount of blood pumped out by each ventricle in 1 minute?
A Stroke volume
B Heart rate
C Pulse rate
D Cardiac output

4 In a normal ECG waveform the five waves are known as P, Q, R, S and T; which wave reflects ventricular repolarization?
A P
B Q
C R
D S
E T

5 Hypertension is defined as a blood pressure that is equal or greater than:
A 140/90
B 140/100
C 150/90
D 150/100

6 What are the four key components of a breathing assessment?

7 List five factors which may impact on the accuracy of pulse oximetry readings.

8 In patients with a pyrexia, fanning and tepid sponging are not recommended while their temperature is still rising.
A True
B False

9 If urine has a 'sweet' smell about it what might this indicate?
A Infection
B Blood
C Ketones
D Bilirubin

10 As one of the most sensitive indicators of critical illness, which vital sign is usually the first to alter in the deteriorating patient?
A Pulse
B Respiratory rate
C Blood pressure
D Temperature

See the end of the chapter for the answers.

Key points

- The taking of patient observations forms a fundamental part of the assessment process.
- Observations are generally undertaken to act as a baseline to help determine the patient's usual range and to help identify if a patient's condition is deteriorating or improving.
- Professional accountability demands more than nurses just undertaking observations. It is about nurses being able to interpret them and then to take appropriate action (Kisiel and Perkins 2006).

REFERENCES

ACC/AHA (2001) ACC/AHA Clinical Competence Statement on Electrocardiography and Ambulatory Electrocardiography: a report of the ACC/AHA/ACP-ASIM task force on Clinical Competence. *Circulation*, 104, 3169–3178.

Adam, S.K. & Osborne, S. (2005) *Critical Care Nursing: Science and Practice*, 2nd edn. Oxford: Oxford University Press.

Adiyaman, A., Verhoeff, R., Lenders, J.W., Deinum, J. & Thien, T. (2006) The position of the arm during blood pressure measurement in sitting position. *Blood Pressure Monitoring*, 11(6), 309–313.

Alcock, K., Clancy, M. & Crouch, R. (2002) Physiological observations of patients admitted from A&E. *Nursing Standard*, 16(34), 33–37.

Alexis, O. (2010) Providing best practice in manual pulse measurement. *British Journal of Nursing*, 19(4), 228–234.

Angerami, E.L. (1980) Epidemiological study of a body temperature in patients in a teaching hospital. *International Journal of Nursing Studies*, 17(2), 91–99.

Arslan, G.G., Eser, I. & Khorshid, L. (2011) Analysis of the effect of lying on the ear on body temperature measurement using a tympanic thermometer. *Journal of Pakistan Medical Association*, 61(11), 1065–1068.

Aucken, S. & Crawford, B. (1998) Neurological assessment. In: Guerrero, D. (ed.) *Neuro-oncology for Nurses*. London: Whurr, pp.29–65.

Barnett, E., Duck, A. & Barraclough, R. (2012) Effect of recording site on pulse oximetry readings. *Nursing Times*, 108(1–2), 22–23.

Baumann, J.J. (2009) Neurologic clinical assessment and diagnostic procedures. In: Urden, L., Stacy, K. & Lough, M. (eds) *Critical Care Nursing: Diagnosis and Management*, 6th edn. St Louis, MO: Mosby, pp.700–723.

Beachey, W. (2012) Acid base balance. In: Kacmarek, R.M., Stoller, J.K. & Heuer, A.H. (eds) *Egan's Fundamentals of Respiratory Care*, 10th edn. St Louis, MO: Mosby.

Benson, E.E., McMillan, D.E. & Ong, B. (2012) The effects of active warming on patient temperature and pain after total knee arthroplasty. *American Journal of Nursing*, 112(5), 26–33.

Bern, L., Brandt, M., Mbelu, N., et al. (2007) Differences in blood pressure values obtained with automated and manual methods in medical inpatients. *Medsurg Nursing*, 16(6), 356–361.

BHS (2006) Blood Pressure Measurement. Ware: British Hypertension Society. Available at: www.bhsoc.org/files/5213/3363/9181/Factfile_2006_1_blood_pressure_measurement.pdf

Bickley, L.S. & Szilagyi, P.G. (2009) *Bates' Guide to Physical Examination and History Taking*, 10th edn. Philadelphia: Lippincott Williams & Wilkins.

Bishop, T. (2008) Urine testing. *Practice Nurse*, 35(12), 18–20.

Blake, D.R. & Nathan, D.M. (2004) Point-of-care testing for diabetes. *Critical Care Nursing Quarterly*, 27(2), 150–161.

Bongers, T. & O'Driscoll, B.R. (2006) Effects of equipment and technique on peak flow measurements. *BMC Pulmonary Medicine*, 6, 14.

Booker, R. (2007) Peak expiratory flow measurement. *Nursing Standard*, 21(39), 42–43.

Booker, R. (2008) Pulse oximetry. *Nursing Standard*, 22(30), 39–41.

Booker, R. (2009) Interpretation and evaluation of pulmonary function tests. *Nursing Standard*, 23(39), 46–56; quiz 58.

Braun, S.K., Preston, P. & Smith, R.N. (1998) Getting a better read on thermometry. *RN*, 61(3), 57–60.

Bridges, E. & Thomas, K. (2009) Noninvasive measurement of body temperature in critically ill patients. *Critical Care Nurse*, 29, 94–97.

British Society for Haematology (2009) *Guideline on the Administration of Blood Components*. London: British Society for Haematology. Available at: www.bcshguidelines.com/documents/Admin_blood_components_bcsh_05012010.pdf

British Thoracic Society & Scottish Intercollegiate Guidelines Network (2012) *British Guideline on the Management of Asthma: A National Clinical Guideline*. London: British Thoracic Society. available at: www.brit-thoracic.org.uk/guidelines-and-quality-standards/asthma-guideline/

Brooker, C. (2010) *Mosby's Dictionary of Medicine, Nursing and Health Professions*. London: Mosby Elsevier.

Brooker, C. & Nicol, M. (2003) *Nursing Adults: The Practice of Caring*. Edinburgh: Mosby.

BSI (2012) *Medical Electrical Equipment. Particular Requirements for Basic Safety and Essential Performance of Clinical Thermometers for Body Temperature Measurement*. London: British Standards Institution.

Buist, A.S., Vollmer, W.M., Wilson, S.R., Frazier, E.A. & Hayward, A.D. (2006) A randomized clinical trial of peak flow versus symptom monitoring in older adults with asthma. *American Journal of Respiratory and Critical Care Medicine*, 174(10), 1077–1087.

Burke, L.J. (2010) Postoperative fever: a normal inflammatory response or cause for concern? *Journal of American Academy of Nurse Practitioners*, 22(4), 192–197.

Callejo, G.F.J., Zamarreño, P.A., Gil, S.E., Sanz, M.M., Lacruz, A.R.J. & Beneyto, M M.P. (2004) Otologic determining factors on infra-red tympanic thermometry in children. *Acta Otorrinolaringologia Espanola*, 55(3), 107–113.

Camm, A.J. & Bunce, N. (2009) Cardiovascular disease. In: Kumar, P. & Clarke, M. (eds) *Clinical Medicine*. 7th edn. London: Elsevier.

Carey, J.V. (2010) Literature review: should antipyretic therapies be routinely administered to patients with fever? *Journal of Clinical Nursing*, 19(17–18), 2377–2393.

Carroll, M. (2000) An evaluation of temperature measurement. *Nursing Standard*, 14(44), 39–43.

CDC (2013) *Infection Prevention during Blood Glucose Monitoring and Insulin Administration*. Atlanta, GA: Centers for Disease Control and Prevention.

Chalmers, J.D., Singanayagam, A. & Hill, A.T. (2008) Systolic blood pressure is superior to other haemodynamic predictors of outcome in community acquired pneumonia. *Thorax*, 63(8), 698–702.

Childs, C. (2011) Maintaining body temperature. In: Brooker, C. & Nicol, M. (eds) *Alexander's Nursing Practice*, 4th edn. Oxford: Elsevier.

Chue, A.L., Moore, R.L., Cavey, A., et al. (2012) Comparability of tympanic and oral mercury thermometers at high ambient temperatures. *BMC Research Notes*, 16(5), 356.

Cicolini, G., Gagliardi, G. & Ballone, E. (2010) Effect of Fowler's body position on blood pressure measurement. *Journal of Clinical Nursing*, 19(23–24), 3581–3583.

Cook, R. (1996) Urinalysis: ensuring accurate urine testing (continuing education credit). *Nursing Standard*, 10(46), 49–52; quiz 54–55.

Covidien (2011) *Genius 2 Tympanic Thermometer and Base Operating Manual*. Mansfield, MA: Covidien. Available at: http://www.patientcare-edu.com/imageServer.aspx?contentID=14135&contenttype=application/pdf

Crawford, J. & Doherty, L. (2008) Recording a standard 12-lead ECG: filling in gaps in knowledge. *British Journal of Cardiac Nursing*, 3(12), 572–577.

Crawford, J. & Doherty, L. (2010) Ten steps to recording a 12-lead ECG. *Practice Nursing*, 21(12), 622–630.

Cretikos, M.A., Bellomo, R., Hillman, K., Chen, J., Finfer, S. & Flabouris, A. (2008) Respiratory rate: the neglected vital sign. *Medical Journal of Australia*, 188(11), 657–659.

Critical Care Stakeholders Forum and National Outreach Forum (2007) *Clinical Indicators for Critical Care Outreach Services*. Available at: www.dh.gov.uk.

Crosser, A. & McDowell, J.R. (2007) Nurses' rationale for blood glucose monitoring in critical care. *British Journal of Nursing*, 16(10), 576–580.

Crouch, A. & Meurier, C. (2005) *Vital Notes for Nurses: Health Assessment*. Oxford: Blackwell Publishing.

Cuddy, M.L. (2004) The effects of drugs on thermoregulation. *AACN Clinical Issues*, 15(2), 238–253.

Curran, R. (2009) The vital signs, part 1: blood pressure. *EMS Magazine*, 38(3), 62–66.

Dailey, G. (2011) Overall mortality in diabetes mellitus: where do we stand today? *Diabetes Technology & Therapeutics*, S1, 65–74.

Dale, L. (2006) Make a point about alternate site blood glucose sampling. *Nursing*, 36(2), 52–53.

Davey, P. (2008) *ECG at a Glance*. Oxford: John Wiley & Sons.

Davie, A. & Amoore, J. (2010) Best practice in the measurement of body temperature. *Nursing Standard*, 24(42), 42–49.

Davis, R.A. (2012) The big chill: accidental hypothermia. *American Journal of Nursing*, 112(1), 38–46.

Dawes, E. & Durham, L. (2007) Monitoring and recording patients' neurological observations. *Nursing Standard*, 22(10), 40–45.

Delaunay, F., Khan, A., Cintra, A., et al. (1997) Pancreatic beta cells are important targets for the diabetogenic effects of glucocorticoids. *Journal of Clinical Investigation*, 100(8), 2094–2098.

DH (2000) *Comprehensive Critical Care: A Review of Adult Critical Care Services*. London: Department of Health.

DH (2001) *The Nursing Contribution to the Provision of a Comprehensive Critical Care for Adults*. London: Department of Health.

DH (2008) *Five Years On: Delivering the Diabetes National Service Framework*. London: Department of Health.

D'Hondt, J.N. (2008) Continuous intravenous insulin ready for prime time. *Diabetes Spectrum*, 21(4), 255–261.

Diabetes UK (2008) *Position Statement: Self Monitoring of Blood Glucose*. Available at: www.diabetes.org.uk/Documents/Position%20statements/Diabetes-UK-position-statement-SMBG-Type2-0413.pdf

Docherty, B. (2000) Temperature recording. *Professional Nurse*, 16(3), 943.

Docherty, B. (2002) Cardiorespiratory physical assessment for the acutely ill: 1. *British Journal of Nursing*, 11(11), 750–758.

Docherty, B. (2003) 12-lead ECG interpretation and chest pain management. *British Journal of Nursing*, 12, 1248–1255.

Docherty, B. (2005) The arteriovenous system: part one, the anatomy. *Nursing Times*, 101(34), 28–29.

Docherty, B. & Coote, S. (2006) Monitoring the pulse as part of the track and trigger. *Nursing Times*, 102(43), 28–29.

Docherty, B. & Foudy, C. (2006) Homeostasis part 3: temperature regulation. *Nursing Times*, 102(16), 20–21.

Drew, B., Califf, R. M., Funk, M., et al. (2004) Practice Standards for Electrocardiographic Monitoring in Hospital Settings: An American Heart Association Scientific Statement from the Councils on Cardiovascular Nursing, Clinical Cardiology, and Cardiovascular Disease in the Young. *Circulation*, 110, 2721–2746.

Edwards, S.L. (1997) Measuring temperature. *Professional Nurse*, 13(2 Suppl), S5–7.

Eguchi, K., Yacoub, M., Jhalani, J., Gerin, W., Schwartz, J.E. & Pickering, T.G. (2007) Consistency of blood pressure differences between the left and right arms. *Archives of Internal Medicine*, 167(4), 388–393.

Elliott, M. & Coventry, A. (2012) Critical care: the eight vital signs of patient monitoring. *British Journal of Nursing*, 21(10), 621–625.

Eser, I., Khorshid, L., Gunes, U.Y. & Demir, Y. (2007) The effect of different body positions on blood pressure. *Journal of Clinical Nursing*, 16(1), 137–140.

European Agency for Safety and Health at Work (2010) *Directive 2010/32/EU Prevention from Sharp Injuries in the Hospital and Healthcare Sector*. Brussels: European Agency for Safety and Health at Work.

Evans, J. & Kenkre, J. (2006) Current practice and knowledge of nurses regarding patient temperature measurement. *Journal of Medical Engineering and Technology*, 30(4), 218–223.

Fairley, D. & Pearce, A. (2006a) Assessment of consciousness. Part one. *Nursing Times*, 102(4), 26–27.

Fairley, D. & Pearce, A. (2006b) Assessment of consciousness. Part two. *Nursing Times*, 102(5), 26–27.

Fairley, D., Timothy, J., Donaldson-Hugh, M., Stone, M., Warren, D. & Cosgrove, J. (2005) Using a coma scale to assess patient consciousness levels. *Nursing Times*, 101(25), 38–41.

Farmer, A.J., Perera, R., Ward, A., et al. (2012) Meta-analysis of individual patient data in randomised trials of self monitoring of blood glucose in people with non-insulin treated type 2 diabetes. *BMJ*, 344, e486.

Farnell, S., Maxwell., L., Tan, S., Rhodes, A. & Philips, B. (2005) Temperature measurement: comparison of non-invasive methods in critical care *Journal of Clinical Nursing*, 14(5), 632–639.

FDA (2010) *Public Health Notification: Use of Fingerstick Devices on More than One Person Poses Risk for Transmitting Bloodborne Pathogens: Initial Communication*. US Food and Drug Administration. Available at: www.fda.gov/medicaldevices/safety/alertsandnotices/ucm224025.htm

Fidler, C., Elmelund, C.T. & Gillard, S. (2011) Hypoglycemia: an overview of fear of hypoglycemia, quality-of-life, and impact on costs. *Journal of Medicine Economics*, 14(5), 646–655.

Field, D. (2006) Respiratory care. In: Sheppard, M. & Wright, M. (eds) *Principles and Practice of High Dependency Nursing*, 2nd edn. Edinburgh: Baillière Tindall.

Field, L. (2008) *Nursing Care: An Essential Guide*. Harlow, Essex: Pearson Prentice Hall.

Foxall, F. (2009) *Haemodynamic Monitoring and Manipulation: An Easy Learning Guide*. Keswick, Cumbria: M & K Publishing.

Fraise, A.P. & Bradley, T. (eds) (2009) *Ayliffe's Control of Healthcare-associated Infection: A Practical Handbook*, 5th edn. London: Hodder Arnold.

Frew, A.J. & Doffman, S. (2012) Respiratory disease. In: Kumar, P. & Clarke, M. (eds) *Clinical Medicine*, 8th edn. London: Elsevier.

Frink, M., Flohé, S., Griensven, M., Mommsen, P. & Hildebrand, F. (2012) Facts and fiction: the impact of hypothermia on molecular mechanisms following major challenge. *Mediators of Inflammation*, 2012, 1–13.

Fuller, G. (2008) *Neurological Examination Made Easy*, 4th edn. Edinburgh: Churchill Livingstone.

Furnary, A.P., Chaugle, H., Kerr, K.J. & Grunkmeier, G.L. (2000) Postoperative hypoglycaemia prolongs length of stay in diabetic CABG patients. *Circulation*, 102(11), 556.

Gallimore, D. (2004) Reviewing the effectiveness of tympanic thermometers. *Nursing Times*, 100(32), 32–34.

Gardner, J. (2012) Is fever after infection part of the illness or the cure? *Emergency Nurse*, 19(10), 20–25.

Gasim, G.I., Musa, I.R., Abdien, M.T. & Adam, I. (2013) Accuracy of tympanic temperature measurement using an infrared tympanic membrane thermometer. *BMC Research Notes*, 6, 194.

Genova Diagnostics (2012) *First Morning Void vs. 24-Hour Collection Options for Urine Hormone Collection*. Available at: www.gdx.net/core/support-guides/24Hr-vs-FMV-Support-Guide.pdf

Gibson, P.G., Powell, H., Coughlan, J., et al. (2003) Self-management education and regular practitioner review for adults with asthma. *Cochrane Database of Systematic Reviews*, 1, CD001117.

Gilbert, M., Barton, A.J. & Counsell, C.M. (2002) Comparison of oral and tympanic temperatures in adult surgical patients. *Applied Nursing Research*, 15(1), 42–47.

Gilbert, R. (2006) Taking a midstream specimen of urine. *Nursing Times*, 102(18), 22–23.

Gillibrand, W., Holdich, P. & Covill, C. (2009) Managing type 2 diabetes: new policy and interventions. *British Journal of Community Nursing*, 14(7), 285, 288–291.

Goldie, L. (2008) Insulin injection and blood glucose monitoring. *Practice Nurse*, 36(2), 11–14.

Goodacre, S. & Irons, R. (2002) ABC of clinical electrocardiography: atrial arrhythmias. *BMJ (Clinical research ed.)*, 324(7337), 594–597.

Goodall, J.R. & Allan, W.B.D. (2009) Pulse-oximetry in intensive care: hazard warning or potential hazard? *Intensive Care Medicine*, 35(S269). Available at: http://poster-consultation.esicm.org/ModuleConsultationPoster/posterDetail.aspx?intIdPoster=412

Goodell, T.T. (2012) An in vitro quantification of pressures exerted by earlobe pulse oximeter probes following reports of device-related pressure ulcers in ICU patients. *Ostomy Wound Management*, 58(11), 30–34.

Gorelick, M.H., Stevens, M.W., Schultz, T. & Scribano, P.V. (2004) Difficulty in obtaining peak expiratory flow measurements in children with acute asthma. *Pediatric Emergency Care*, 20(1), 22–26.

Gosselink, R., Bott, J., Johnson, M., et al. (2008) Physiotherapy for adult patients with critical illness: recommendations of the European Respiratory Society and European Society of Intensive Care Medicine Task Force on Physiotherapy for Critically Ill Patients. *Intensive Care Medicine*, 34(7), 1188–1199.

Hall, G. (2005) Choosing and teaching the use of blood glucose monitors. *Practice Nurse*, 30(7), 46–50.

Handler, J. (2009) The importance of accurate blood pressure measurement. *Permanente Journal*, 13(3), 51–54.

Hansen, E.F., Vestbo, J., Phanareth, K., Kok-Jensen, A. & Dirksen, A. (2001) Peak flow as predictor of overall mortality in asthma and chronic obstructive pulmonary disease. *American Journal of Respiratory and Critical Care Medicine*, 163(3 Pt 1), 690–693.

Haugan, B., Langerud, A.K., Kalvøy, H., Frøslie, K.F., Riise, E. & Kapstad, H. (2013) Can we trust the new generation of infrared tympanic thermometers in clinical practice? *Journal of Clinical Nursing*, 22(5–6), 698–709.

Heindenreich, T. & Giuffe, M. (1990) Postoperative temperature measurement. *Nursing Research*, 39(3), 153–155.

Heinemann, L. (2010) Quality of glucose measurement with blood glucose meters at the point-of-care: relevance of interfering factors. *Diabetes Technology and Therapeutics*, 12(11), 847–857.

Heusch, A.I. & McCarthy, P.W. (2005) The patient: a novel source of error in clinical temperature measurement using infrared aural thermometry. *Journal of Alternative Complement Medicine*, 11(3), 473–476.

Higgins, D. (2005) Measuring PEFR. *Nursing Times*, 101(10), 32–33.

Higgins, D. (2008a) Patient assessment part 5 – measuring pulse. *Nursing Times*, 104(11), 24–25.

Higgins, D. (2008b) Specimen collection: obtaining a midstream specimen of urine. *Nursing Times*, 104(17), 26–27.

Higginson, R. & Jones, B. (2009) Respiratory assessment in critically ill patients: airway and breathing. *British Journal of Nursing*, 18(8), 456, 458–461.

Hinds, C.J. & Watson, D. (2009) Intensive care medicine. In: Kumar, P. & Clarke, M. (eds) *Clinical Medicine*, 7th edn. London: Elsevier.

Hodgetts, T., Kenward, G., Vlackonikolis, I.G., Payne, S. & Castle, N. (2002) The identification of risk factors for cardiac arrest and formulation of activation criteria to alert a medical emergency team. *Resuscitation*, 54, 125–131.

Hohlrieder, M., Kaufmann, M., Moritz, M. & Wenzel, V. (2007) Management of accidental hypothermia. *Anaesthesist*, 56(8), 805–811.

Hooper, V.D. & Andrews, J.O. (2006) Accuracy of noninvasive core temperature measurement in acutely ill adults: the state of the science. *Biological Research for Nursing*, 8(10), 24–34.

Hortensius, J., Slingerland, R.J., Kleefstra, N., et al. (2011) Self-monitoring of blood glucose: the use of the first or the second drop of blood. *Diabetes Care*, 34(3), 556–560.

Hunter, J. & Rawlings-Anderson, K. (2008) Respiratory assessment. *Nursing Standard*, 22(41), 41–43.

IDF (2012) *Clinical Guidelines Task Force Global Guideline for Type 2 Diabetes*. Brussels: International Diabetes Federation.

Institute for Innovation and Improvement (2008) *SBAR – Situation – Background – Assessment*. Available from: www.institute.nhs.uk/quality_and_service_improvement_tools/quality_and_service_improvement_tools/sbar_-_situation_-_background_-_assessment_-_recommendation.html

Janssen, K. & Delanghe, J. (2010) Importance of the pre-analytical phase in blood glucose analysis. *Acta Clinica Belgica*, 65(5), 311–318.

Jenkins, G. & Tortora, G.J. (2013) *Anatomy and Physiology: From Science to Life*, 3rd edn. London: Wiley.

Jevon, P. (2007a) Cardiac monitoring. Part 4 – Monitoring the apex beat. *Nursing Times*, 103(4), 28–29.

Jevon, P. (2007b) Respiratory procedures. Part 2 – Measuring peak expiratory flow. *Nursing Times*, 103(33), 26–27.

Jevon, P. (2008) Neurological assessment. Part 1—-assessing level of consciousness. *Nursing Times*, 104(27), 26–7.

Jevon, P. (2009) *ECGs for Nurses*, 2nd edn. Oxford: John Wiley & Sons.

Jevon, P. (2010) Procedure for recording a standard 12-lead electrocardiogram. *British Journal of Nursing*, 9(10), 64.

Jevon, P. & Ewens, B. (2000) Pulse oximetry – 1. *Nursing Times*, 96(26), 43–44.

Jevon, P. & Ewens, B. (2007) *Monitoring the Critically Ill Patient*. Oxford: Blackwell Science Limited.

Jevon, P. & Jevon, M. (2001) Using a tympanic thermometer. *Nursing Times*, 97(9), 43–44.

Johnson, C L., Anderson, M.A. & Hill, P.D. (2012) Comparison of pulse oximetry measures in a healthy population. *Medsurg Nursing*, 21(2), 70–75; quiz 76.

Jonsson, T., Jonsdottir, H., Moller, A.D. & Baldursdottir, L. (2011) Nursing documentation prior to emergency admissions to the intensive care unit. *Nursing in Critical Care*, 16(4), 164–169.

Kacmerek, R.M., Dimas, S. & Mack, C.W. (2005) *The Essentials of Respiratory Care*, 4th edn. St Louis, MO: Elsevier Mosby.

Kallet, R.H. (2012) Bedside assessment of the patient. In: Kacmarek, R.M., Stoller, J.K. & Heuer, A.H. (eds) *Egan's Fundamentals of Respiratory Care*, 10th edn. St Louis, MO: Mosby.

Kawamura, M., Kusano, Y., Takahashi, T., Owada, M. & Sugawara, T. (2006) Effectiveness of a spot urine method in evaluating daily salt intake in hypertensive patients taking oral antihypertensive drugs. *Hypertension Research*, 29(6), 397–402. Available at: www.ncbi.nlm.nih.gov/pubmed/16940701

Kenney, W.L. & Munce, T.A. (2003) Invited review: aging and human temperature regulation. *Journal of Applied Physiology*, 95(6), 2598–2603.

Khan, E. (2004) Clinical skills: the physiological basis and interpretation of the ECG. *British Journal of Nursing*, 13(8), 440–446.

Kisiel, M. & Perkins, C. (2006) Nursing observations: knowledge to help prevent critical illness. *British Journal of Nursing*, 15(19), 1052–1056.

Kjaergaard, B. & Bach, P. (2006) Warming of patients with accidental hypothermia using warm water pleural lavage. *Resuscitation*, 68(2), 203–207.

Knies, R. (2003) *Research Applied to Clinical Practice: Temperature Measurement in Acute Care: The Who, What, Where, When, Why and How*. Available at: http://enw.org/Research--Thermometry.htm

Kozier, B., Erb, G., Berman, A. & Snyder, S. (2008) *Fundamentals of Nursing: Concepts, Process and Practice*, 8th edn. Harlow, Essex: Pearson.

Krinsley, J.S. (2004) Effect of an intensive glucose management protocol on the mortality of critically ill adult patients. *Mayo Clinic Proceedings*, 79(8), 992–1000.

Kyriacos, U., Jelsma, J. & Jordan, S. (2011) Monitoring vital signs using early warning scoring systems: a review of the literature. *Journal of Nursing Management*, 19(3), 311–330.

Lahrmann, H., Cortelli, P., Hilz, M., Mathias, C.J., Struhal, W. & Tassinari, M. (2006) EFNS guidelines on the diagnosis and management of orthostatic hypotension. *European Journal of Neurology*, 13(9), 930–936.

Lees, L. & McAuliffe, M. (2010) Venous thromboembolism risk assessments in acute care. *Nursing Standard*, 24(22), 35–41.

Lefrant, J.Y., Muller, L., de la Coussaye, J.E., et al. (2003) Temperature measurement in intensive care patients: comparison of urinary bladder, oesophageal, rectal, axillary, and inguinal methods versus pulmonary artery core method. *Intensive Care Medicine*, 29(3), 414–418.

Leuvan, C.H. & Mitchell, I. (2008) Missed opportunities? An observational study of vital sign measurements. *Critical Care and Resuscitation*, 10(2), 111–115.

Levick, J.R. (2010) *An Introduction to Cardiovascular Physiology*, 5th edn. London: Hodder Arnold.

Levine, D. (2007) Respiratory monitoring. In: Kaplow, R. & Hardin, S.R. (eds) *Critical Care Nursing: Synergy for Optimal Outcomes*. Sudbury, MA: Jones and Bartlett, p.iv

Levine, J., Munden, J. & Thompson, G. (2008) *ECG Interpretation Made Incredibly Easy*. London: Lippincott Williams & Wilkins.

Lifshitz, E. & Kramer, L. (2000) Outpatient urine culture: does collection technique matter? *Archives of Internal Medicine*, 160(16), 2537–2540.

Lipska, K.J. & Kosiborod, M. (2011) Hypoglycemia and adverse outcomes: marker or mediator? *Reviews in Cardiovascular Medicine*, 12(3), 132–135.

Liu, S., Zhao, Y., Hempe, J.M., Fonseca, V. & Shi, L. (2012) Economic burden of hypoglycemia in patients with Type 2 diabetes. *Expert Review of Pharmacoeconomics and Outcomes Research*, 12(1), 47–51.

Major, G. & Holmes, J. (2008) How do nurses describe health care procedures? Analysing nurse–patient interaction in a hospital ward. *Australian Journal of Advanced Nursing*, 25(4), 58–70.

Makic, M.B., Lovett, K. & Azam, M.F. (2012) Placement of an oesophageal temperature probe by nurses. *Advanced Critical Care*, 23(1), 24–31.

Manickam, K., Karlowsky, J.A., Adam, H., et al. (2013) CHROMagar orientation medium reduces urine culture workload. *Journal of Clinical Microbiology*, 51(4), 1179–1183.

Manoni, F., Gessoni, G., Alessio, M.G., et al. (2011) Mid-stream vs. first-voided urine collection by using automated analyzers for particle examination in healthy subjects: an Italian multicenter study. *Clinical Chemistry and Laboratory Medicine*, 50(4), 679–684.

Marieb, E.N. & Hoehn, K. (2010) *Human Anatomy & Physiology*, 10th edn. San Francisco: Pearson Benjamin Cummings.

Marini, J.J. & Wheeler, A.P. (2012) *Critical Care Medicine: The Essentials*, 4th edn. Philadelphia: Lippincott Williams & Wilkins.

Mazerolle, S.M., Ganio, M.S., Casa, D.J., Vingren, J. & Klau, J. (2011) Is oral temperature an accurate measurement of deep body temperature? A systematic review. *Journal of Athletic Training*, 46(5), 566–573.

McCall, A.L. (2012) Insulin therapy and hypoglycemia. *Endocrinology and Metabolism Clinics of North America*, 41(1), 57–87.

McCallum, L. & Higgins, D. (2012) Measuring body temperature. *Nursing Times*, 108(45), 20–22.

McClelland, D.B.L. (2007) *Handbook of Transfusion Medicine*, 4th edn. Norwich: Stationery Office.

McKnight, K.M. & Carter, L. (2008) From trays to tube feedings: overcoming the challenges of hospital nutrition and glycemic control. *Diabetes Spectrum*, 21(4), 233–240.

McMorrow, R.C. & Mythen, M.G. (2006) Pulse oximetry. *Current Opinion in Critical Care*, 12(3), 269–271.

Metcalfe, H. (2000) Recording a 12-lead electrocardiogram – 1. *Nursing Times*, 96(19), 43–44.

Meurier, C., Brown, J. & Crouch, A. (2005) Physical assessment of the nervous system. In: Crouch, A. & Meurier, C. (eds) *Vital Notes for Nurses: Health Assessment*. Oxford: Blackwell Publishing, pp.178–186

MHRA (1996) *Extra-Laboratory Use of Blood Glucose Meters and Test Strips: Contraindications, Training and Advice to Users*. London: Medicines and Healthcare Products Regulatory Agency.

MHRA (2003) *Infra-red Ear Thermometer – Home Use*. London: Medicines and Healthcare Products Regulatory Agency.

MHRA (2005) *Report of the Independent Advisory Group on* Blood Pressure *Monitoring in Clinical Practice*. London: Medicines and Healthcare Products Regulatory Agency.

MHRA (2006) *Device Bulletin: Managing Medical Devices Guidance for Healthcare and Social Services Organisations*. London: Medicines and Healthcare Products Regulatory Agency. Available at: www.mhra.gov.uk/home/groups/dts--bs/documents/publication/con2025143.pdf

MHRA (2010) *Top Tips for Pulse Oximetry*. London: Medicines and Healthcare Products Regulatory Agency.

MHRA (2011) *Point of Care Testing – Blood Glucose Meters*. London: Medicines and Healthcare Products Regulatory Agency.

MHRA (2012) *Mercury in Medical Devices*. London: Medicines and Healthcare Products Regulatory Agency. Available at: www.mhra.gov.uk/Safetyinformation/Generalsafetyinformationandadvice/Product--specificinformationandadvice/Product--specificinformationandadvice%E2%80%93M%E2%80%93T/Mercuryinmedicaldevices/index.htm

Miller, M.R., Hankinson, J., Brusasco, V., et al. (2005) Standardisation of spirometry. *European Respiratory Journal*, 26(2), 319–338.

Minder, A.E., Albrecht, D., Schäfer, J. & Zulewski, H. (2013) Frequency of blood glucose testing in well educated patients with diabetes mellitus type 1: how often is enough? *Diabetes Research and Clinical Practice*, 101(1), 57–61.

Minor, D.G. & Waterhouse, J.M. (1981) *Circadian Rhythms and the Human*. Bristol: Butterworth-Heinemann.

Mooney, G.P. & Comerford, D.M. (2003) Neurological observations. *Nursing Times*, 99(17), 24–25.

Moore, T. (2007) Respiratory assessment in adults. *Nursing Standard*, 21(49), 48–56; quiz 58.

Moore, T. (2009a) Pulse oximetry. In: Moore, T. & Woodrow, P. (eds) *High Dependency Nursing Care: Observation, Intervention and Support for Level 2 Patients*. Oxford: Routledge.

Moore, T. (2009b) Respiratory assessment. In: Moore, T. & Woodrow, P. (eds) *High Dependency Nursing Care: Observation, Intervention and Support for Level 2 Patients*. Oxford: Routledge.

Morton, P. & Rempher, K. (2009) Patient assessment: respiratory system. In: Morton, P. & Fontaine, D. (eds) *Critical Care Nursing: A Holistic Approach*, 9th edn. Philadelphia: Lippincott.

Mourad, A., Carney, S., Gillies, A., Jones, B., Nanra, R. & Trevillian, P. (2003) Arm position and blood pressure: a risk factor for hypertension? *Journal of Human Hypertension*, 17(6), 389–395.

Mulligan, A. (2010) Validation of a physiological track and trigger score to identify developing critical illness in haematology patients. *Intensive and Critical Care Nursing*, 26(4), 196–206.

Munro, N. (2009) Cardiac surgery. In: Morton, P. & Fontaine, D. (eds) *Critical Care Nursing: A Holistic Approach*, 9th edn. Philadelphia: Lippincott.

Nakamura, K., Tanaka, M., Motohashi, Y. & Maeda, A. (1997) Oral temperatures of the elderly in nursing homes in summer and winter in relation to activities of daily living. *International Journal of Biometeorology*, 40(2), 103–106.

Navas, S. (2003) Atrial fibrillation: part 2. *Nursing Standard*, 17(38), 47–54; quiz 55–56.

Neff, J., Ayoub, J., Longman, A. & Noyes, A. (1989) Effect of respiratory rate, respiratory depth, and open versus closed mouth breathing on sublingual temperature. *Research in Nursing and Health*, 12(3), 195–202.

Neno, R. (2005) Hypothermia: assessment, treatment and prevention. *Nursing Standard*, 19(20), 47–52; quiz 54, 56.

Netea, R.T., Lenders, J.W., Smits, P. & Thien, T. (2003) Both body and arm position significantly influence blood pressure measurement. *Journal of Human Hypertension*, 17(7), 459–462.

NHS Diabetes (2011) *Inpatient Care for People with Diabetes: the Economic Case for Change. Insight Health Economics*. Available at: http://www.diabetes.org.uk/upload/News/Inpatient%20Care%20for%20People%20with%20Diabetes%20%20The%20Economic%20Case%20for%20Change%20Nov%202011.pdf

NICE (2004) *Guidelines for the Diagnosis and Management of Type 1 Diabetes in Children, Young People and Adults, CG15*. London: National Institute for Health and Clinical Excellence.

NICE (2007a) *Acutely Ill Patients in Hospital: Recognition of and Response to Acute Illness in Adults in Hospital, CG50*. London: National Institute for Health and Clinical Excellence.

NICE (2007b) *Venous Thromboembolism: Reducing the Risk of Venous Thromboembolism (Deep Vein Thrombosis and Pulmonary Embolism) in Inpatients Undergoing Surgery, CG92*. London: National Institute for Health and Clinical Excellence.

NICE (2007c) *Head Injury: Triage, Assessment, Investigation and Early Management of Head Injury in Infants, Children and Adults*. London: National Institute for Health and Clinical Excellence.

NICE (2008) *Type 2 Diabetes: The Management of Type 2 Diabetes, CG66*. London: National Institute for Health and Clinical Excellence.

NICE (2011a) *Hypertension: Clinical Management of Primary Hypertension in Adults, CG127*. London: National Institute for Health and Clinical Excellence. Available at: http://publications.nice.org.uk/hypertension--cg127

NICE (2011b) *Quick Reference Guide: Hypertension: Clinical Management of Primary Hypertension in Adults, CG127*. London: National Institute for Health and Clinical Excellence.

NICE (2013) *Quality Standard for Asthma, QS25*. London: National Institute for Health and Clinical Excellence.

Nichols, J.H. (2011) Blood glucose testing in the hospital: error sources and risk management. *Journal of Diabetes Science and Technology*, 5(1), 173–177.

NMC (2010) *Record Keeping: Guidance for Nurses and Midwives*. London: Nursing and Midwifery Council.

NMC (2013) *Consent*. London: Nursing and Midwifery Council.

NMC (2015) *The Code: Standards of Conduct, Performance and Ethics for Nurses and Midwives*. London: Nursing and Midwifery Council.

O'Brien, E., Asmar, R., Beilin, L., et al. (2003) European Society of Hypertension recommendations for conventional, ambulatory and home blood pressure measurement. *Journal of Hypertension*, 21(5), 821–848.

O'Driscoll, B.R., Howard, L.S., Davison, A.G. & British Thoracic Society (2008) BTS guideline for emergency oxygen use in adult patients. *Thorax*, 63(Suppl 6), vi1–68.

Ogawa, A., Johnson, J.H., Ohneda, M., et al. (1992) Roles of insulin resistance and beta-cell dysfunction in dexamethasone-induced diabetes. *Journal of Clinical Investigation*, 90(2), 497–504.

O'Toole, S. (1997) Alternatives to mercury thermometers. *Professional Nurse*, 12(11), 783–786.

Outzen, M.J. (2009) Management of fever in older adults. *Gerontology Nursing*, 35(5), 17–23.

Patton, K.T. & Thibodeau, G.A. (2009) *Anatomy and Physiology*, 7th edn. St Louis, MO: Mosby Elsevier.

Peate, I., Nair, M. & Wild, K. (2014) *Nursing Practice: Knowledge and Care.* Oxford: John Wiley & Sons.

Pelter, M.M. (2008) Electrocardiographic monitoring in the medical–surgical setting: clinical implications, basis, lead configurations, and nursing implications. *Medsurg Nursing*, 17(6), 421–428.

Pentland, B., Davenport, R. & Cowie, R. (2009) The nervous system. In: Douglas, G., Nicol, F. & Robertson, C. (eds) *MacLeod's Clinical Examination*, 12th edn. London: Churchill Livingstone, pp.267–306.

Pichardo-Lowden, A. & Gabbay, R.A. (2012) Management of hyperglycemia during the perioperative period. *Current Diabetes Reports*, 12(1), 108–118.

Polderman, K.H. & Herold, I. (2009) Therapeutic hypothermia and controlled normothermia in the intensive care unit: practical considerations, side effects, and cooling methods. *Critical Care Medicine*, 37(3), 1101–1120.

Price, D.L. & Gwin, J.F. (2008) *Paediatric Nursing: An Introductory Text*, 10th edn. Philadelphia: Saunders.

Price, T. (2002) Painful stimuli and the Glasgow Coma Scale. *Nursing in Critical Care*, 7(1), 17–23.

Prytherch, D.R., Smith, G.B., Schmidt, P., et al. (2006) Calculating early warning scores – a classroom comparison of pen and paper and hand-held computer methods. *Resuscitation*, 70(2), 173–178.

Pusnik, I. & Miklavec, A. (2009) Dilemmas in measurement of human body temperature. *Instrument Science Technology*, 37(5), 516–530.

Quanjer, P.H., Lebowitz, M.D., Gregg, I., Miller, M.R. & Pedersen, O.F. (1997) Peak expiratory flow: conclusions and recommendations of a Working Party of the European Respiratory Society. *European Respiratory Journal*, 24(Suppl), 2S–8S.

Rawlings-Anderson, K. & Hunter, J. (2008) Monitoring pulse rate. *Nursing Standard*, 22(31), 41–43.

RCN (2011) *Accountability and Delegation: What You Need to Know. The Principles of Accountability and Delegation for Nurses, Students, Health Care Assistants and Assistant Practitioners.* London: Royal College of Nursing. Available at: www.rcn.org.uk/__data/assets/pdf_file/0003/381720/003942.pdf

RCUK (2010) *Resuscitation Guidelines.* London: Resuscitation Council UK Publications.

RCUK (2011) *Advanced Life Support*, 6th edn. London: Resuscitation Council UK.

Reddel, H.K. (2006) Peak flow monitoring in clinical practice and clinical asthma trials. *Current Opinion in Pulmonary Medicine*, 12(1), 75–81.

Reeves, R.A. (1995) The rational clinical examination. Does this patient have hypertension? How to measure blood pressure. *JAMA*, 273(15), 1211–1218.

Reynard, J., Brewster, S. & Biers, S. (2013) *Oxford Handbook of Urology*, 3rd edn. Oxford: Oxford University Press.

Rice, M.J., Pitkin, A.D. & Coursin, D.B. (2010) Glucose measurement in the operating room: more complicated than it seems. *Anesthesia and Analgesia*, 110(4), 1056–1065.

Rigby, D. & Gray, K. (2005) Understanding urine testing. *Nursing Times*, 101(12), 60–62.

Rizvi, A.A. & Sanders, M.B. (2006) Assessment and monitoring of glycemic control in primary diabetes care: monitoring techniques, record keeping, meter downloads, tests of average glycemia, and point-of-care evaluation. *Journal of the American Academy of Nurse Practitioners*, 18(1), 11–21.

Roberts, A. (2002) The role of anatomy and physiology in interpreting ECGs. *Nursing Times*, 98(20), 34–36.

Roche Diagnostics (2010) *Compendium of Urinalysis. Urine Test Strips and Microscopy.* Geneva: Roche Diagnostics.

Roche Diagnostics (2013) *ACCU-CHEK® Safe-T-Pro Plus lancet.* Geneva: Roche Diagnostics.

Royal College of Physicians (2012) *National Early Warning Score (NEWS). Standardising the Assessment of Acute Illness Severity in the NHS.* London: Royal College of Physicians. Available at: www.rcplondon.ac.uk/sites/default/files/documents/national--early--warning--score--standardising--assessment--acute--illness--severity--nhs.pdf

Ruffin, R. (2004) Peak expiratory flow (PEF) monitoring. *Thorax*, 59(11), 913–914.

Samples, J.F., van Cott, M.L., Long, C., King, I.M. & Kersenbrock, A. (1985) Circadian rhythms: basis for screening for fever. *Nursing Research*, 34(6), 377–379.

Schmiemann, G., Kniehl, E., Gebhardt, K., Matejczyk, M.M. & Hummers-Pradier, E. (2010) The diagnosis of urinary tract infection: a systematic review. *Deutsches Arzteblatt International*, 107(21), 361–367.

Schwab, N. & Porter, M. (2007) Inpatient diabetes mellitus in the oncology setting. *Clinical Journal of Oncology Nursing*, 11(4), 489–492.

Scrase, W. & Tranter, S. (2011) Improving evidence-based care for patients with pyrexia. *Nursing Standard*, 25(29), 37–41.

SCST (2014) *Clinical Guidelines by Consensus: Recording a Standard 12-lead Electrocardiogram: An Approved Methodology by The Society for Cardiology Science and Technology.* London: Society for Cardiology Science and Technology.

Shah, S. (1999) Neurological assessment. *Nursing Standard*, 13(22), 49–54; quiz 55–56.

Sharber, J. (1997) The efficacy of tepid sponge bathing to reduce fever in young children. *American Journal of Emergency Medicine*, 15(2), 188–192.

Sharman, J. (2007) Clinical skills: cardiac rhythm recognition and monitoring. *British Journal of Nursing*, 16(5), 306–311.

Simpson, H. (2006) Respiratory assessment. *British Journal of Nursing*, 15(9), 484–488.

Snell-Bergeon, J.K. & Wadwa, R.P. (2012) Hypoglycemia, diabetes, and cardiovascular disease. *Diabetes Technology Therapeutics*, 14(1), S51–58.

Steele, J.R. & Hardin, S.R. (2007) Hypertension. In: Kaplow, R. & Hardin, S.R. (eds) *Critical Care Nursing: Synergy for Optimal Outcomes.* Sudbury, MA: Jones and Bartlett.

Steggall, M.J. (2007) Urine samples and urinalysis. *Nursing Standard*, 22(14–16), 42–45.

Stergiou, G.S., Karpettas, N., Atkins, N. & O'Brien, E. (2010) European Society of Hypertension International Protocol for the validation of blood pressure monitors: a critical review of its application and rationale for revision. *Blood Pressure Monitoring*, 15(1), 39–48.

Stevenson, T. (2004) Achieving best practice in routine observation of hospital patients. *Nursing Times*, 100(30), 34–35.

Struthers, J.K., Weinbren, M.J., Taggart, C. & Wiberg, K.J. (2012) *Medical Microbiology Testing in Primary Care.* London: Mason Publishing.

Tan, L., Hawk, J.C. & Sterling, M.L. (2001) Report of the Council on Scientific Affairs: Preventing Needlestick Injuries in Health Care Settings. *JAMA Archive of Internal Medicine*, 161(7), 929–936.

Teasdale, G.M. (2012) National early warning score (NEWS) is not suitable for all patients. *BMJ*, 345, e5875.

Teasdale, G. & Jennett, B. (1974) Assessment of coma and impaired consciousness. A practical scale. *Lancet*, 2(7872), 81–84.

Thornton, H. (2009) Type 1 diabetes, part 1: an introduction. *British Journal of Nursing*, 4(5), 223.

Thorpe, C.T., Fahey, L.E., Johnson, H., Deshpande, M., Thorpe, J.M. & Fisher, E.B. (2013) Facilitating healthy coping in patients with diabetes: a systematic review. *Diabetes Education*, 39(1), 33–52.

Tonnesen, P., Carrozzi, L., Fagerstrom, K.O., et al. (2007) Smoking cessation in patients with respiratory diseases: a high priority, integral component of therapy. *European Respiratory Journal*, 29(2), 390–417.

Torrance, C. & Elley, K. (1998) Urine testing – 2. urinalysis. *Nursing Times*, 94(5), suppl 1–2.

Torrance, C. & Semple, M. (1998) Recording temperature – 1. *Nursing Times*, 94(2), suppl 1–2.

Tortora, G.J. & Derrickson, B.H. (2011) *Principles of Anatomy & Physiology*, 13th edn. Hoboken, NJ: John Wiley & Sons.

Trim, J. (2005) Monitoring temperature. *Nursing Times*, 101(20), 30–31.

Turner, M., Burns, S.M., Chaney, C., et al. (2008) Measuring blood pressure accurately in an ambulatory cardiology clinic setting: do patient position and timing really matter? *Medsurg Nursing*, 17(2), 93–98.

Tyberghein, M., Philips, J.C., Krzesinski, J.M. & Scheen, A.J. (2013) Orthostatic hypotension: definition, symptoms, assessment and pathophysiology. *Revue Medicale de Liege*, 68(2), 65–73.

Valler-Jones, T. & Wedgbury, K. (2005) Measuring blood pressure using the mercury sphygmomanometer. *British Journal of Nursing*, 14(3), 145–150.

van den Berghe, G., Wouters, P., Weekers, F., et al. (2001) Intensive insulin therapy in critically ill patients. *New England Journal of Medicine*, 345(19), 1359–1367.

van Groningen, L.F., Adiyaman, A., Elving, L., Thien, T., Lenders, J.W. & Deinum, J. (2008) Which physiological mechanism is responsible for the increase in blood pressure during leg crossing? *Journal of Hypertension*, 26(3), 433–437.

van Vliet, M., Donnelly, J.P., Potting, C.M. & Blijlevens, N.M. (2010) Continuous non-invasive monitoring of the skin temperature of HSCT recipients. *Support and Care in Cancer*, 18(1), 37–42.

Vassal, T., Benoit-Gonin, B., Carrat, F., Guidet, B., Maury, E. & Offenstadt, G. (2001) Severe accidental hypothermia treated in an ICU: prognosis and outcome. *Chest*, 120(6), 1998–2003.

Veiga, E.V., Arcuri, E.A., Cloutier, L. & Santos, J. L. (2009) Blood pressure measurement: arm circumference and cuff size availability. *Revista Latino-Americana de Enfermagem*, 17(4), 455–461.

Veljkovic, K., Rodríguez-Capote, K., Bhayana, V., et al. (2012) Assessment of a four hour delay for urine samples stored without preservatives at

room temperature for urinalysis. *Clinical Biochemistry*, 45(10–11), 856–858.
Verrij, E.A., Nieuwenhuizen, L. & Bos, W.J.W. (2009) Raising the arm before cuff inflation increases the loudness of Korotkoff sounds. *Blood Pressure Monitoring*, 14(6), 268–273.
Wager, K.A., Schaffner, M.J., Foulois, B., Swanson Kazley, A., Parker, C. & Walo, H. (2010) Comparison of the quality and timeliness of vital signs data using three different data-entry devices. *Computers, Informatics, Nursing*, 28(4), 205–212.
Wagner, D.V. (2006) Unplanned perioperative hypothermia. *AORN Journal*, 83(2), 470, 473–476.
Walker, R. (2004) Capillary blood glucose monitoring and its role in diabetes management. *British Journal of Community Nursing*, 9(10), 438–440.
Wallymahmed, M. (2007) Capillary blood glucose monitoring. *Nursing Standard*, 21(38), 35–38.
Walsh, M. (2006) *Nurse Practitioners: Clinical Skills and Professional Issues*, 2nd edn. Edinburgh: Butterworth–Heinemann.
Walsh, M. & Crumbie, A. (2007) *Watson's Clinical Nursing and Related Sciences*, 7th edn. London: Baillière Tindall.
Waterhouse, C. (2005) The Glasgow Coma Scale and other neurological observations. *Nursing Standard*, 19(33), 55–64; quiz 66–67.
Weldon, K. (1998) Neurological observations. In: Guerrero, D. (ed.) *Neuro-oncology for Nurses*. London: Whurr.
Wheatley, I. (2006) The nursing practice of taking level 1 patient observations. *Intensive and Critical Care Nursing*, 22, 115–121.
WHO (2010) *WHO Guidelines on Drawing Blood: Best Practices in Phlebotomy*. Geneva: World Health Organization.
WHO (2013) *The Evidence for Clean Hands*. Geneva: World Health Organization.
WHO/IDF (2006) *Definition and Diagnosis of Diabetes Mellitus and Intermediate Hyperglycaemia*. Geneva: World Health Organization/ International Diabetes Federation.
Williams, B., Poulter, N., Brown, M., et al. (2004) Guidelines for management of hypertension: report of the fourth working party of the British Hypertension Society 2004 – BHS IV. *Journal of Human Hypertension*, 18(3), 139–185.
Wilson, L.A. (2005) Urinalysis. *Nursing Standard*, 19(35), 51–54.
Winslow, E.H., Cooper, S.K., Haws, D.M., et al. (2012) Unplanned perioperative hypothermia and agreement between oral, temporal artery, and bladder temperatures in adult major surgery patients. *Journal of PeriAnesthesia Nursing*, 27(3), 165–180.
Witte, E.C., Lambers Heerspink, H J., de Zeeuw, D., Bakker, S.J.L., de Jong, P.E. & Gansevoort, R. (2009) First morning voids are more reliable than spot urine samples to assess microalbuminuria. *Journal of the American Society of Nephrology*, 20(2), 436–443.
Wong, F.W. (2007) Pulsus paradoxus in ventilated and non-ventilated patients. *Dynamics*, 18(3), 16–18.
Woodhall, L. (2008) Implementation of the SBAR communication technique in a tertiary centre. *Journal of Emergency Nursing*, 34(4), 314–317.
Woodrow, P. (2004) Arterial blood pressure monitoring. In: Moore, T. & Woodrow, P. (eds) *High Dependency Nursing Care: Observation, Intervention and Support*. London: Routledge.
Woodrow, P. (2009a) An introduction to electrocardiogram interpretation: part 1. *Nursing Standard*, 24(12), 50–57.
Woodrow, P. (2009b) An introduction to electrocardiogram interpretation: part 2. *Nursing Standard*, 24(13), 48–56.
Woods, S.L., Froelicher, E.S., Motzer, S.A. & Bridges, E.J. (2005) *Cardiac Nursing*, 5th edn. Philadelphia: Lippincott Williams & Wilkins.
Woollons, S. (1996) Temperature measurement devices. *Professional Nurse*, 11(8), 541–542, 544, 547.
Wright-Nunes, J.A., Luther, J.M., Ikizler, T.A. & Cavanaugh, K.L. (2012) Patient knowledge of blood pressure target is associated with improved blood pressure control in chronic kidney disease. *Patient Education and Counselling*, 88(2), 184–188.
Yokobori, S., Frantzen, J., Bullock, R., et al. (2011) The use of hypothermia therapy in traumatic ischemic/reperfusional brain injury: review of the literature. *Therapeutic Hypothermia and Temperature Management*, 1(4), 185–192.
Yont, G.H., Korhan, E.A. & Khorshid, L. (2011) Comparison of oxygen saturation values and measurement times by pulse oximetry in various parts of the body. *Applied Nursing Research*, 24(4), e39–43.
Zietz, K. & McCutcheon, H. (2006) Observations and vital signs: ritual or vital for the monitoring of postoperative patients? *Applied Nursing Research*, 19, 204–211.

Answers

Learning Activity 11.1 Scenario: Pulse measurement

You have been asked to check the pulse rate of a patient who has atrial fibrillation.

How would you go about doing this in order to ensure an accurate measurement?

- Simultaneous monitoring of the apex beat and radial pulse is advisable in patients with atrial fibrillation.
- Use a stethoscope to assess the apical heartbeat. The diaphragm of the stethoscope should be placed over the apex of the heart and beats counted for 60 seconds.
- Ask a second nurse to record the radial pulse at the same time. The deficit between the two should be noted using, for example, different colours on the patient's chart to indicate the apex and radial rates (Docherty 2002).

Learning Activity 11.2 Case study: Breathing assessment

Mr Lyle is a 74-year-old man who has been admitted with exacerbation of his chronic obstructive pulmonary disease (COPD). He is finding it hard to catch his breath, particularly after walking short distances around the ward. He usually finds that sitting in certain positions makes it more comfortable to breathe. He is having regular nebulizers and is finding these are helping to ease his breathing.

1 You wish to assess Mr Lyle's breathing, how might you prepare him?
- Provide information to Mr Lyle and obtain verbal consent for the assessment.
- With permission, remove his shirt as this will help you to observe his chest movements more accurately.
- Encourage an upright position. Leaning slightly forwards, using a pillow to rest his arms on, may assist further in achieving a comfortable position and maximize chest expansion.

2 In carrying out an assessment of his breathing, what observations should you be making?
- The colour of his skin and mucous membranes.
- The degree to which he is using his accessory muscles, whether he has nasal flaring on inspiration or pursed lips on expiration.
- The rate, rhythm and depth of his respirations, with the rate being counted for a full minute.
- Shape and expansion of his chest, noting any asymmetry.

3 What additional parameters will help you to determine his respiratory status?
- Pulse oximetry, peak expiratory flow reading.
- Medical and smoking history; co-morbidities.
- Refer to Procedure guidelines 11.4: Respiratory assessment and pulse oximetry and 11.5: Peak flow reading using an manual peak flow meter.

Learning Activity 11.3 Scenario: Temperature measurement and hyperthermia

You have just checked your patient's temperature using a tympanic thermometer and note that it is 39.2°C.

1 Who should you report this to?
- Report to your supervising nurse in the first instance and explain your observations with the patient.

2 What measures can you take to help to reduce the temperature?
- Reduce amount of bedding/clothing.
- Consider antipyretic therapy.
- Consider cooling methods, although use with caution if temperature still rising.

3 What else should you do?
- Ask the patient if there is anything that would make them feel more comfortable.

Now Test Yourself What have you learnt?

1 How often does NICE (2007) recommend that observations should be taken for patients in hospital?
A At least 4 hourly
B At least 8 hourly
C At least 12 hourly
D At least daily

2 Which tool has been found to help with structuring and standardizing communication when reporting a concern about a patient?
A SBAR
B NEWS
C MET
D PART

3 Which of the following describes the amount of blood pumped out by each ventricle in 1 minute?
A Stroke volume
B Heart rate
C Pulse rate
D Cardiac output

4 In a normal ECG waveform the five waves are known as P, Q, R, S and T; which wave reflects ventricular repolarization?
A P
B Q
C R
D S
E T

5 Hypertension is defined as a blood pressure that is equal or greater than:
A 140/90
B 140/100
C 150/90
D 150/100

6 What are the four key components of a breathing assessment?
- The colour of the patient's skin and mucous membranes
- The use of accessory muscles or other respiratory signs
- The rhythm, rate and depth of respiration
- The shape and expansion of the chest

7 List five factors which may impact on the accuracy of pulse oximetry readings.
- For example: nail polish, intravenous dyes, poor peripheral perfusion, cardiac arrhythmias, recording blood pressure, carbon monoxide poisoning, bright external light, movement

8 In patients with a pyrexia, fanning and tepid sponging are not recommended while their temperature is still rising.
A True – fanning during this time can increase a person's body temperature by initiating compensatory responses such as shivering and peripheral vasoconstriction.
B False

9 If urine has a 'sweet' smell about it what might this indicate?
A Infection
B Blood
C Ketones
D Bilirubin

10 As one of the most sensitive indicators of critical illness, which vital sign is usually the first to alter in the deteriorating patient?
A Pulse
B Respiratory rate
C Blood pressure
D Temperature

Part Four
Supporting the patient through treatment

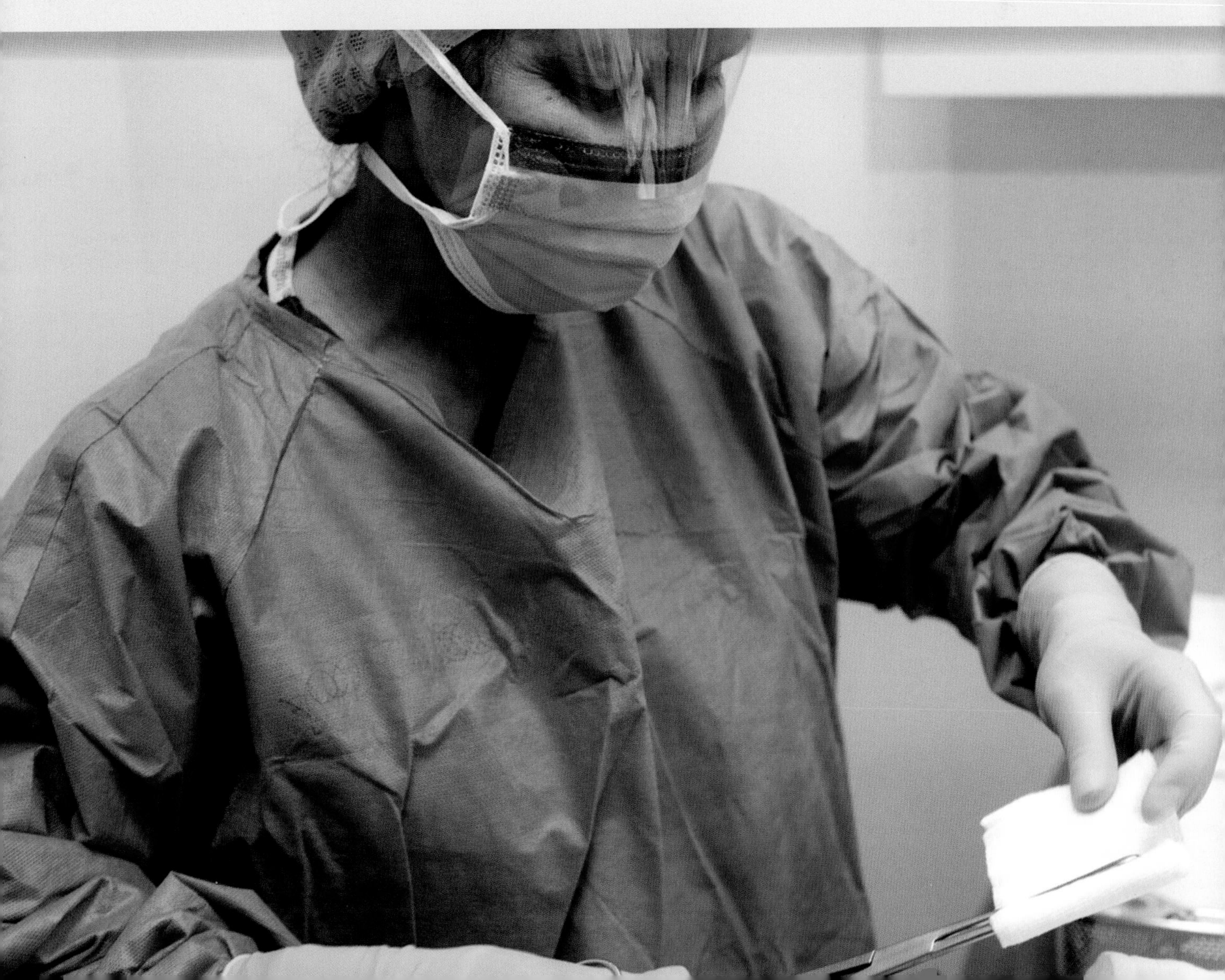

Medicines management

12

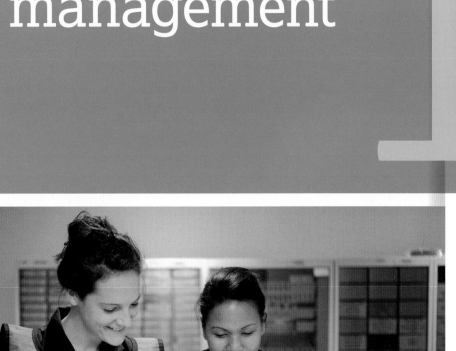

By reading this chapter and undertaking the learning activities within it, you should be able to:

1. Demonstrate an understanding of the safe, effective and appropriate use of medicines in partnership with the patient.
2. Identify the importance of safe prescribing, supply and storage of medicines.
3. Analyse the principles of safe administration of medicines via different routes and how their effectiveness can be monitored.
4. Demonstrate knowledge of how to effectively support patients to manage their own medications both within the hospital setting and following their discharge.

Procedure guidelines

The Royal Marsden Manual of Clinical Nursing Procedures: Student Edition, Ninth Edition. Edited by Lisa Dougherty, Sara Lister and Alexandra West-Oram

Overview

In this chapter the safe, effective and appropriate use of medicines in partnership with the patient will be discussed. This will include prescribing, supply, administration and supporting patients in their own environment to manage their medicines effectively. The terms medicine and drugs will be used interchangeably throughout the chapter and mean the same.

DEFINITIONS

Medicines management

> 'Medicines management in hospitals encompasses the entire way that medicines are selected, procured, delivered, prescribed, administered and reviewed to optimise the contribution that medicines make to producing informed and desired outcomes of patient care' (Audit Commission 2001, p.5).

The Medicines and Healthcare Products Regulatory Agency (MHRA 2004) defines medicines management as 'the clinical, cost-effective and safe use of medicines to ensure patients get the maximum benefit from the medicines they need, while at the same time minimising potential harm'. All Registered Nurses have a professional responsibility with regard to procurement, prescription, supply and disposal of medicines as defined in the NMC *Standards for Medicines Management* (NMC 2010a). They must ensure the patient understands what medicines they are taking, the indication for the medication and any likely side-effects.

Medicinal products and medical devices

The definition of a medicine is:

- any substance or combination of substances presented as having properties for treating or preventing disease in human beings; or
- any substance or combination of substances which may be used in or administered to human beings either with a view to restoring, correcting or modifying physiological functions by exerting a pharmacological, immunological or metabolic action, or to making a medical diagnosis.

The definition of a medical device is any instrument, apparatus, appliance, material or other article, whether used alone or in combination, including the software necessary for its proper application intended by the manufacturer to be used for human beings for the purpose of:

- diagnosis, prevention, monitoring, treatment or alleviation of disease
- diagnosis, monitoring, treatment, alleviation of or compensation for an injury or handicap
- investigation, replacement or modification of the anatomy or of a physiological process
- control of conception

and which does not achieve its principal intended action in or on the human body by pharmacological, immunological or metabolic means, but which may be assisted in its function by such means.

There are three main types of medical device which incorporate or are used to administer a medicinal product.

- Devices which are used to administer medicinal product, e.g. medicine spoon, dropper.
- Devices for administering medicinal products where the device and the medicinal product form a single integral product designed to be used exclusively in the given combination and which are not reusable or refillable, e.g. pre-filled syringe.
- Devices incorporating, as an integral part, a substance which, if used separately, may be considered to be a medicinal product and which is such that the substance is liable to act upon the body with action ancillary to that of the device, e.g. wound dressings with antimicrobial agents.

Pharmacology

- *Pharmacology* can be defined as the study of the effects of drugs on the function of living systems. Its purpose is to understand what drugs do to living organisims and, more practically, how their effects can be applied to the treatment of diseases (Rang and Dale 2012).
- *Pharmacokinetics* looks at the absorption, distribution, metabolism and excretion of drugs within the body, i.e. what the body does to the drug. When these four factors are considered, with the dose of a drug given, the concentration of drug in the body over a period of time can be determined. Pharmacokinetics is most useful when considered with *pharmacodynamics* which is the study of the mechanisms of action of drugs and other biochemical and physiological effects, i.e. what the drug does to the body (Rang and Dale 2012).
- The *indication* for a drug refers to the use of that drug for treating a particular disease. Drugs often have more than one indication, which means that there is more than one disease for which it could be used. Indications may be diagnostic, prophylactic or for therapeutic purposes.
- A *contraindication* to a medicine is a specific situation in which a medicine should not be used, because it may be harmful to the patient. This could be due to the patient's allergy status, co-morbidities, current disease state or other medicines they are taking.
- A *drug interaction* is when a substance (e.g. another medicine, food) affects the activity of a drug when both are administered together. This action can be synergistic (when the drug's effect is increased) or antagonistic (when the drug's effect is decreased) or a new effect can be produced that neither drug produces on its own. Interactions between drugs are termed drug–drug interactions and interactions between drugs and foods are known as drug–food interactions (Stockley's Drug Interactions: www.medicinescomplete.com). It is important not to forget over-the-counter, herbal and complementary medicines when considering potential interactions.
- *Side-effects* of a medicine are defined as 'any effect that is in addition to its intended primary effect that can be harmful, unpleasant or in some cases beneficial to the patient'. The harmful or unpleasant side-effects are more commonly described as adverse drug reactions (ADRs) (Aronson 2006).

EVIDENCE BASE FOR MEDICINES MANAGEMENT IN PRACTICE

Good medicines management is essential to assure high standards in the clinical care of patients. When delivered effectively, it can reduce the risk of medication errors and serious adverse drug reactions and prevent unneccesary delays for the patient at the point of discharge. It also enables the spending on medicines to be more effectively managed (Audit Commission 2001).

All aspects of a medicine's use must be managed with a multidisciplinary approach to ensure it is supported by a strong evidence base and that the safety and well-being of the patient remain paramount (NMC 2015, Shepherd 2002a).

Key principles of medicines management

Legislation

Legislative frameworks, government guidelines and professional regulations govern medicines management in the UK. The primary pieces of legislation are the Medicines Act 1968 and the European Directives and the Misuse of Drugs Act 1971 (HMSO 1971). European Community Council Directives and Regulations and the Medicines Act 1968 (HMSO 1968) regulate the manufacture, distribution and importation of medicines for human use.

THE MEDICINES ACT 1968

The Medicines and Health Care Products Regulatory Agency (MHRA) in the UK and the European Medicines Agency (EMEA) are responsible for the licensing procedures for medicinal products. The availability of products is restricted by defining which of the following legal categories they are in:

- prescription-only medicines (POM)
- pharmacy-only medicines (P)
- general sales list medicines (GSL).

Different requirements apply to the sale, supply and labelling of medicines in each category. In hospitals, medicines can be supplied in line with patient-specific directions, from an appropriate practitioner in relation to the medicine, which in most cases will be an instruction on the patient ward drug chart. The legislation also allows the supply of prescription-only medicines to be made under a Patient Group Direction (PGD). A PGD needs to be signed by a doctor and a pharmacist. The regulations permit certain registered professionals to supply or administer under a PGD.

In addition to the above, there are also a range of exemptions from the regulations which allow certain groups of health professionals to sell, supply and administer particular medicines direct to patients. For example, in an emergency and under certain conditions, a pharmacist working in a registered pharmacy can supply a prescription-only medicine to a patient without a prescription if requested by a prescriber or patient (Appelbe and Wingfield 2005, RPSGB 2012).

Legal methods for prescribing medicines

The Medicines Act 1968 states that only authorized healthcare practitioners can legally prescribe medicines in the UK. It provides all prescribers with a framework for which medicines require a prescription and which medicines can be available to the public without a prescription and under what circumstances. All medicines administered in hospital must be considered prescription only. This is because administration, whether by a nurse or by a patient to themselves, may only take place in accordance with one or more of the following processes:

- patient-specific direction
- patient medicines administration chart (also called a medicines administration record [MAR])
- Patient Group Direction (PGD)
- Medicines Act exemplar
- standing orders
- homely remedy protocol
- prescription form (NMC 2010a, pp.13–19).

Prescriptions can be handwritten on a chart, a prescription pad or provided electronically. E-prescribing has been defined as the 'utilisation of electronic systems to facilitate and enhance the communication of a prescription or medicine order, aiding the choice, administration and supply of a medicine through knowledge and decision support and providing a robust audit trail for the entire medicines use process' (NHS Connecting for Health 2009, p.9). There are many benefits of e-prescribing systems, summarized in Box 12.1.

A growing number of UK hospitals have introduced e-prescribing systems. One major motivation for this is to improve the safety of medicines used and reduce the current and unacceptable levels of adverse drug events. In a systematic review, nine of the 13 studies demonstrated a significant reduction in prescribing errors for all or some drug types when e-prescribing was used (Reckmann et al. 2009).

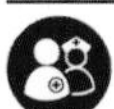

Box 12.1 **Benefits of e-prescribing systems**

The Connecting for Health programme has outlined the benefits of e-prescribing systems as:

- computerized entry and management of prescriptions
- knowledge support, with immediate access to medicines information, for example *British National Formulary*
- decision support, aiding the choice of medicines and other therapies, with alerts such as drug interactions
- computerized links between hospital wards/departments and pharmacies
- ultimately, links to other elements of patients' individual care records
- improvements in existing work processes
- a robust audit trail for the entire medicines use process
- a reduction in the risk of medication errors as a result of several factors, including:
  - more legible prescriptions
  - alerts for contraindications, allergic reactions and drug interactions
  - guidance for inexperienced prescribers
  - improved communication between different departments and care settings
  - reduction in paperwork-related problems, for example fewer lost or illegible prescriptions
  - clearer, and more complete, audit trails of medication administration
  - improved formulary guidance and management and appropriate reminders within care pathways.

Source:

Nurse prescribing and Patient Group Directions

As nurses have undertaken increasingly specialized roles, the need for them to have powers to prescribe has become more apparent. The report of the Advisory Committee on Nurse Prescribing (DH 1989) initially recommended a limited nurses' formulary for community nurses and health visitors. The Medicinal Products: Prescription by Nurse, etc. Act 1992 granted the statutory authority for this to occur. The Crown Report (DH 1989) also recommended that doctors and nurses collaborate in drawing up local protocols for the administration of medicines in situations that would benefit specific groups of patients, for example those requiring vaccinations.

The practice of prescribing under group protocols became widespread across the NHS, and they were used to support initiatives such as nurse-led clinics (Laverty et al. 1997, Mallett et al. 1997). The legality of this practice was then questioned. Section 58 of the Medicines Act 1968 states that 'no one should administer any medication (other than to himself) unless he is the appropriate practitioner or a person who is acting according to directions from an appropriate practitioner'. The terms *direction* and *administration* were open to interpretation and how they were used varied across the country (McHale 2002).

Nurse prescribing was therefore reviewed and two further reports were published.

- *Review of Prescribing, Supply and Administration of Medicines. A Report on the Supply and Administration of Medicines under Group Protocols* (DH 1998).
- *Review of Prescribing, Supply and Administration of Medicines. Final Report* (DH 1999).

The first specifically offered guidance about group protocols, including changing the name to Patient Group Directions (PGD) (Box 12.2 and Figure 12.1).

Box 12.2 Patient Group Directions

The legal definition of a Patient Group Direction is 'a written instruction for the supply and/or administration of a licensed medicine (or medicines) in an identified clinical situation signed by a doctor or dentist and a pharmacist' (NPC 2009). It is drawn up locally by doctors, pharmacists and other appropriate professionals and must be approved by the employer, advised by the relevant professional advisory committee. It applies to groups of patients or other service users who may not be individually identified before presentation for treatment (DH 2004). The Health and Safety Commission (HSC) advised that the majority of medication 'should be prescribed and administered on an individual patient specific basis', but that it is appropriate to use PGDs for the supply and administration of medicines in situations where this offers an advantage for patient care (DH 2000b). Shepherd suggests that this means 'where medical staff are either inaccessible or unavailable' (Shepherd 2002b, p.44). The flowchart in Figure 12.1 aims to assist practitioners in deciding the appropriate system for the prescription, supply or administration of medicines. Using a PGD is not a form of prescribing (NICE 2014a).

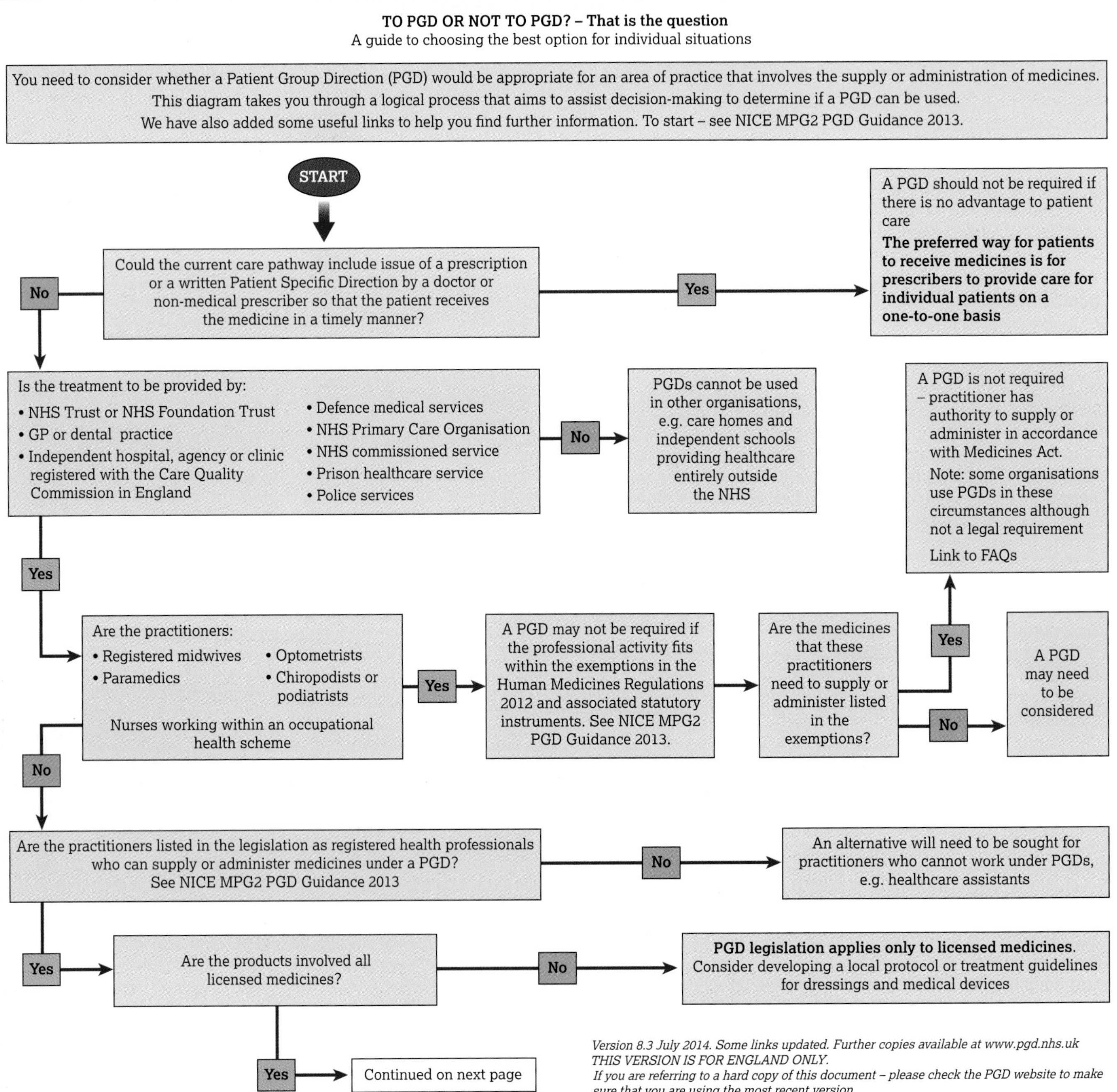
TO PGD OR NOT TO PGD? – That is the question
A guide to choosing the best option for individual situations
You need to consider whether a Patient Group Direction (PGD) would be appropriate for an area of practice that involves the supply or administration of medicines. This diagram takes you through a logical process that aims to assist decision-making to determine if a PGD can be used. We have also added some useful links to help you find further information. To start – see NICE MPG2 PGD Guidance 2013.
START
Could the current care pathway include issue of a prescription or a written Patient Specific Direction by a doctor or non-medical prescriber so that the patient receives the medicine in a timely manner?
Yes
A PGD should not be required if there is no advantage to patient care
The preferred way for patients to receive medicines is for prescribers to provide care for individual patients on a one-to-one basis
No
Is the treatment to be provided by:
• NHS Trust or NHS Foundation Trust
• GP or dental practice
• Independent hospital, agency or clinic registered with the Care Quality Commission in England
• Defence medical services
• NHS Primary Care Organisation
• NHS commissioned service
• Prison healthcare service
• Police services
No
PGDs cannot be used in other organisations, e.g. care homes and independent schools providing healthcare entirely outside the NHS
A PGD is not required – practitioner has authority to supply or administer in accordance with Medicines Act.
Note: some organisations use PGDs in these circumstances although not a legal requirement
Link to FAQs
Yes
Are the practitioners:
• Registered midwives
• Paramedics
• Optometrists
• Chiropodists or podiatrists
Nurses working within an occupational health scheme
Yes
A PGD may not be required if the professional activity fits within the exemptions in the Human Medicines Regulations 2012 and associated statutory instruments. See NICE MPG2 PGD Guidance 2013.
Are the medicines that these practitioners need to supply or administer listed in the exemptions?
Yes
No
A PGD may need to be considered
No
Are the practitioners listed in the legislation as registered health professionals who can supply or administer medicines under a PGD? See NICE MPG2 PGD Guidance 2013
No
An alternative will need to be sought for practitioners who cannot work under PGDs, e.g. healthcare assistants
Yes
Are the products involved all licensed medicines?
No
PGD legislation applies only to licensed medicines.
Consider developing a local protocol or treatment guidelines for dressings and medical devices
Yes
Continued on next page
Version 8.3 July 2014. Some links updated. Further copies available at www.pgd.nhs.uk
THIS VERSION IS FOR ENGLAND ONLY.
If you are referring to a hard copy of this document – please check the PGD website to make sure that you are using the most recent version

Figure 12.1 Patient Group Directions (PGDs) flowchart. The diagram takes the practitioner through a logical process that aims to assist in determining if a PGD can be used. *Source:* Patient Group Directions (England) (www.pgd.nhs.uk). Please check the PGD website for the most recent version of this tool and for further resources and guidance relating to PGDs. www.medicinesresources.nhs.uk/en/Communities/NHS/PGDs/PGD-Legislation-Guidance/PGD-Website-Tools/To-PGD-or-not-to-PGD-that-is-the-question/

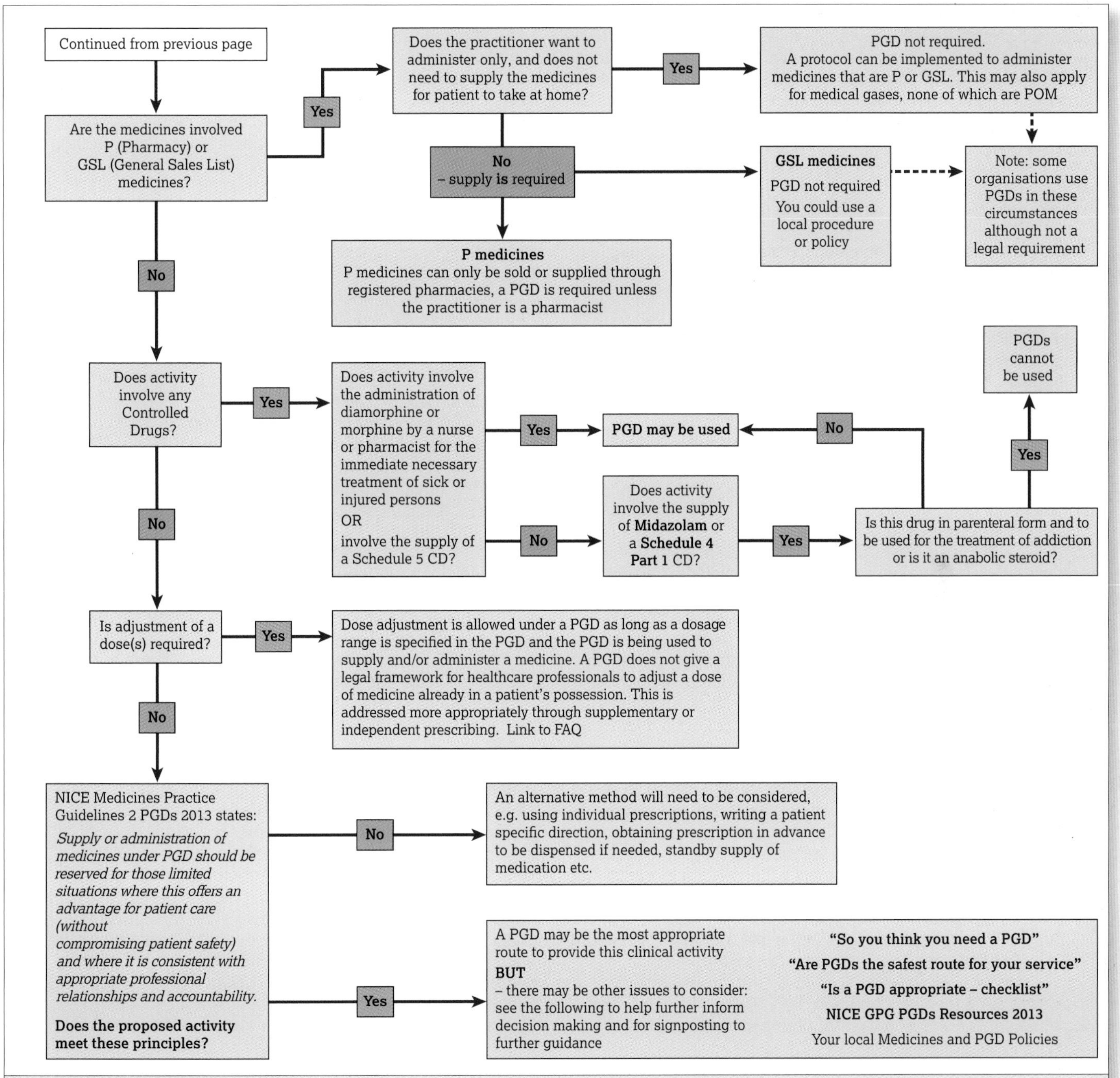

Continued from previous page

Are the medicines involved P (Pharmacy) or GSL (General Sales List) medicines?

Yes → Does the practitioner want to administer only, and does not need to supply the medicines for patient to take at home?

Yes → PGD not required. A protocol can be implemented to administer medicines that are P or GSL. This may also apply for medical gases, none of which are POM

No – supply is required → GSL medicines: PGD not required. You could use a local procedure or policy → Note: some organisations use PGDs in these circumstances although not a legal requirement

No – supply is required → **P medicines**: P medicines can only be sold or supplied through registered pharmacies, a PGD is required unless the practitioner is a pharmacist

No → Does activity involve any Controlled Drugs?

Yes → Does activity involve the administration of diamorphine or morphine by a nurse or pharmacist for the immediate necessary treatment of sick or injured persons OR involve the supply of a Schedule 5 CD?

Yes → **PGD may be used**

No → Does activity involve the supply of **Midazolam** or a **Schedule 4 Part 1** CD?

Yes → Is this drug in parenteral form and to be used for the treatment of addiction or is it an anabolic steroid?

Yes → PGDs cannot be used

No → **PGD may be used**

No → Is adjustment of a dose(s) required?

Yes → Dose adjustment is allowed under a PGD as long as a dosage range is specified in the PGD and the PGD is being used to supply and/or administer a medicine. A PGD does not give a legal framework for healthcare professionals to adjust a dose of medicine already in a patient's possession. This is addressed more appropriately through supplementary or independent prescribing. Link to FAQ

No → NICE Medicines Practice Guidelines 2 PGDs 2013 states: *Supply or administration of medicines under PGD should be reserved for those limited situations where this offers an advantage for patient care (without compromising patient safety) and where it is consistent with appropriate professional relationships and accountability.* **Does the proposed activity meet these principles?**

No → An alternative method will need to be considered, e.g. using individual prescriptions, writing a patient specific direction, obtaining prescription in advance to be dispensed if needed, standby supply of medication etc.

Yes → A PGD may be the most appropriate route to provide this clinical activity **BUT** – there may be other issues to consider: see the following to help further inform decision making and for signposting to further guidance

"So you think you need a PGD"
"Are PGDs the safest route for your service"
"Is a PGD appropriate – checklist"
NICE GPG PGDs Resources 2013
Your local Medicines and PGD Policies

Figure 12.1 *Continued*

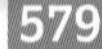

The second report looked at the existing arrangements for prescribing, supply and administration of medicines and suggested the introduction of a new form of prescribing to be undertaken by non-medical health professionals (DH 2003a). Independent nurse prescribing was initially allowed from an extremely limited formulary (Shuttleworth 2005). It was then extended a number of times until finally, appropriately qualified nurses were allowed to prescribe from the whole *British National Formulary* (BNF).

- *Independent prescribing:* this allows nurses who are registered as independent prescribers to prescribe any licensed medicine (and now unlicensed; DH 2009) for any medical condition (this also includes some controlled drugs; see section on 'Controlled drugs') but only within their own level of experience and competence, and acting in accordance with the NMC *Code* (Public Health England 2006, NMC 2015). Only those who have undergone appropriate training and are registered with the NMC as an independent prescriber can prescribe (NMC 2006). It must also be considered to be part of that nurse's role.
- *Supplementary prescribing* has been defined as: 'A voluntary prescribing partnership between an independent prescriber and a supplementary prescriber to implement an agreed patient specific clinical management plan with the patient's agreement' (DH 2003a). Amendments to the Prescription Only Medicines Order and the NHS regulations allowed supplementary prescribing by suitably trained nurses from April 2003. Supplementary prescribers prescribe in partnership

with a doctor or dentist (the independent prescriber) and are able to prescribe any medicine, including controlled drugs and unlicensed medicines that are listed in an agreed clinical management plan. The plan is drawn up with the patient's agreement, following diagnosis of the patient by an independent prescriber and following consultation and agreement between the independent and supplementary prescribers (DH 2003a, pp.6 and 7).

The key principles that underpin supplementary prescribing are:

- the importance of communication between prescribing partners
- the need for access to shared patient records
- the patient is treated as a partner in their care and is involved at all stages in decision making, including whether part of their care is delivered via supplementary prescribing (NPC 2003a).

Preparation for both independent nurse prescribing and supplementary prescribing is at least 26 days in length and must follow the standards set out in the NMC *Circular 25/2002* (NMC 2001b). Any preparation must enable independent and supplementary non-medical prescribers to reach the competencies outlined in *Maintaining Competency in Prescribing: An Outline Framework to Help Nurse Prescribers* (NPC 2001), *Maintaining Competency in Prescribing: An Outline Framework to Help Nurse Supplementary Prescribers* (NPC 2003b) and the competences in shared decision making within the Medicines Partnership document (Medicines Partnership Programme 2007).

The addition of prescriptive authority to the nurse role has not only been a positive way of making a service more responsive for service users, but also has helped to meet increasing demands on health services (Bridge et al. 2005). Patients are satisfied with nurse prescribing (Latter et al. 2005) and it is also generally viewed positively by other healthcare professionals (Latter et al. 2010). In 2005 it was estimated that there were 28,000 nurses who were able to prescribe from the limited formulary and 4000 extended prescribers (MHRA 2005). Latter et al. (2010) found that 2–3% of both the nursing and pharmacist workforce are qualified to prescribe medicines independently, in both primary and secondary care settings. A national survey of 246 nurse prescribers concluded that nurse prescribing is largely successful in both practice and policy terms (Latter et al. 2005): this is discussed in more detail in Box 12.3.

A range of competencies and skills are required to ensure quality and safe prescribing; the nurse prescriber:

- identifies main medical condition
- explores patient's presenting symptoms and their management
- explores past medical history, current medication, including over-the-counter (OTC), allergies and family history
- is able to initiate a physical examination
- is able to request and interpret diagnostic tests.

The evidence is that nurses need to be more consistent in the frequency with which they apply these skills (Latter 2008).

Box 12.3 **An evaluation of nurse prescribing**

- Most nurse prescribers were confident in their prescribing practice.
- Most felt extended prescribing had a positive impact on patient care and enabled them to make better use of their skills.
- Most felt that the limited nurse formulary imposed unhelpful limitations on their practice.
- Nurses were satisfied with the support received from their medical practitioner.
- Patients were positive about their experience of nurse prescribing.
- Doctors were positive about the development of nurse prescribers in their teams.

Source: Latter et al. (2005).

Unlicensed and 'off-label' medicines

Under European medicines legislation, a medicinal product placed on the market is required to have a marketing authorization (product licence) granted following demonstration of safety, quality and efficacy. However, member states can put in place arrangements to allow an authorized healthcare professional to gain access to an unlicensed medicine, that is, a medicine that does not have a marketing authorization, to meet the special needs of individual patients. In the UK, this occurs via the arrangements for 'specials' manufactured in the UK and the notification scheme for products imported into the UK.

'Specials' can be supplied if there is an order for them, a registered doctor has requested the product and the product will be used for a patient under the care of that doctor and under that doctor's supervision. A 'special' cannot be supplied if an equivalent licensed product is available which will meet the patient's needs. If a 'special' is manufactured in the UK, the manufacturer must hold a manufacturer's (special) licence issued by the MHRA. An unlicensed medicine may also be imported if the importer holds the appropriate wholesaler dealer licence or wholesaler dealer import licence issued by the MHRA. The importer will need to inform the MHRA on each occasion that they intend to import the product. 'Off label' refers to the use of a medicine outside the terms of its licence.

For herbal medicines, there are three possible regulatory routes by which they can reach the market in the UK: as an unlicensed herbal remedy; as a registered traditional herbal medicine (identified as the product container or packaging will include a nine-digit registration number starting with the letters THR) (MHRA 2009); and as a licensed herbal medicine.

Unlicensed medicines can be prescribed by doctors, dentists and nurse independent prescribers (DH 2009). 'Off-label' medicines can be prescribed by doctors, dentists, independent nurse prescribers, independent pharmacist prescribers and independent optometrist prescribers. The MHRA has published advice for prescribers on the use of unlicensed and off-label medicines because the responsibility for prescribing such medicines is potentially greater than for licensed products (Box 12.4).

Nurse independent prescribers can also mix medicines prior to administration and direct others to mix, for example for use within syringe pumps (DH 2009).

As discussed later in this chapter, the MHRA advises that healthcare professionals have a responsibility to help monitor the safety of medicines in clinical use through submission of suspected adverse drug reactions to the MHRA and the Commission on Human Medicines (CHM) via the Yellow Card Scheme (www.yellowcard.mhra.gov.uk). Such reporting is equally important for unlicensed medicines or those used off label as for those that are licensed.

Verbal orders

The NMC (2010a) clearly states that a verbal order is not acceptable on its own. 'In exceptional circumstances, where the medication (NOT including controlled drugs) has been previously prescribed and the prescriber is unable to issue a new prescription, but where changes to the dose are considered necessary, the use of information technology (such as fax or e-mail) may be used but the prescriber must confirm any changes to the original prescription' (NMC 2010a, p.28). This should be followed up by a new prescription, signed by the prescriber confirming the changes, within a maximum

Box 12.4 **MHRA advice for prescribers on the use of unlicensed and off-label medicines**

- Before prescribing an unlicensed medicine, be satisfied that an alternative, licensed medicine would not meet the patient's needs.
- Before prescribing a medicine off label, be satisfied that such use would better serve the patient's needs than an appropriately licensed alternative.
- Before prescribing an unlicensed medicine or using a medicine off-label:
  - be satisfied that there is a sufficient evidence base and/ or experience of using the medicine to show its safety and efficacy
  - take responsibility for prescribing the medicine and for overseeing the patient's care, including monitoring and follow-up
  - record the medicine prescribed and, where common practice is not being followed, the reasons for prescribing this medicine; you may wish to record that you have discussed the issue with the patient.

The MHRA also advises that best practice suggests that:

- you give patients, or those authorizing treatment on their behalf, sufficient information about the proposed treatment, including known serious or common adverse reactions, to enable them to make an informed decision
- where current practice supports the use of a medicine outside the terms of its licence, it may not be necessary to draw attention to the licence when seeking consent. However, it is good practice to give as much information as patients or carers require or which they may see as relevant
- you explain the reasons for prescribing a medicine off label or an unlicensed medicine where there is little evidence to support its use, or where such use of a medicine is innovative.

of 24 hours. The changes must be authorized before the new dosage is administered (NMC 2010a).

Learning Activity 12.1

Scenario: Verbal orders

You have been asked to ring the doctor on-call, as one of your patients, who has just been admitted to the ward, is complaining of pain and there is currently no analgesia prescribed on their medication chart. The doctor asks you if you can give the patient some paracetamol and he will come down shortly to prescribe it.

What would you do? Discuss this scenario with your mentor/ supervising nurse.

See the end of the chapter for the answers.

Supply of medicines

Medicines reconciliation

Medicines reconciliation forms part of the medicines management process. It impoves patient safety and contributes to the Quality, Innovation, Productivity and Prevention (QIPP) programme by reducing length of stay and the risk of readmission to hospital. It has been defined by the Institute for Healthcare Improvement as 'the process of creating the most accurate list possible of all medications the patient is taking – including drug name, dosage, frequency and route – and comparing that list against the physician's admission, transfer, and/or discharge orders, with the goal of providing correct medications to the patient at all transition points within the hospital' (www.ihi.org).

The National Prescribing Centre (NPC) guidance recommends specific competencies required for undertaking medicines reconciliation. These include effective communication skills, technical knowledge of relevant medicines management processes and therapeutic knowledge (NPC 2007b). Medicines reconciliation requires clinical judgement and should only be undertaken by competent healthcare staff. In most hospital settings medicines reconciliation is performed by a member of the pharmacy team who has completed the necessary local accreditation processes deemed essential to perform this role safely and accurately.

Dispensing

Dispensing is defined as 'to label from stock and supply a clinically appropriate medicine to a patient/client/carer usually against a written prescription, for self-administration or administration by another professional and to advise on safe and effective use' (NMC 2010a, p.20). The majority of these activities in hospitals are undertaken by the pharmacy department. They can supply medicines as stock to a ward or for specific patients who are inpatients, daycase patients or outpatients. Pharmacists are professionally accountable for all decisions to supply a medicine and offer advice. As part of this accountability, they must ensure that if any tasks are to be delegated, they are delegated to persons competent to perform them. Nurses may only dispense in exceptional circumstances (NMC 2010a).

A pharmaceutical assessment of a prescription, which is the point at which pharmacists apply their knowledge to establish the safety, quality, efficacy and perhaps cost-effective use of drug treatments specified by a prescriber, must be performed by a pharmacist and must be carried out on every prescription (RPSGB 2007a). Following this assessment, the assembly of the prescription can be delegated to a pharmacy technician or a pharmacy assistant. Once the prescription is assembled, it will be presented for accuracy checking by a pharmacist or a suitably qualified pharmacy technician.

Many pharmacies have also now adopted practices of one-stop dispensing and robotic dispensing. One-stop dispensing involves medicines for inpatients being supplied in a form ready for discharge. Robotic and automated systems can be used to pick and label medicines in order to reduce errors in these areas (RPSGB 2007a).

Use of patient's own drugs

Patients are encouraged to bring their medication into hospital with them to facilitate a comprehensive medicines reconciliation process. This can also be useful if the organization has a policy of using the patient's own drugs.

These medicines remain the property of the patient and should not be destroyed without prior consent from the patient or their representative. If the patient does agree to the destruction of the medicines, they must be sent to the pharmacy for destruction. If the patient does not want the medicines to be stored in the hospital or sent to pharmacy for destruction, they must be sent home with the patient's representative. Patients' medicines should only be used if they can be positively identified, are of a suitable quality and are labelled according to labelling requirements. They should be stored to the same security standards as other medicine stock on the ward. They should be used for the sole use of the patient whose property they remain (RPSGB 2005).

Learning Activity 12.2

Learning in practice: Patients' own medicines

In your clinical area:

- Find out what the local procedure is for safe storage of a patient's own drugs whilst they remain in hospital.
- What is the recommended practice for administration of such medications while the patient is in hospital?
- Discuss this with the pharmacist linked to your clinical area, or your mentor/supervising nurse.

Safe storage of medicines

The report *The Safe and Secure Handling of Medicines: A Team Approach* (RPSGB 2005) details that the responsibility for establishing and maintaining a system for the security of medicines should be that of the senior pharmacist in the hospital. They should do this in consultation with senior nursing staff and appropriate medical staff. The appointed nurse in charge of the area will have the responsibility of ensuring that this system is followed and that the security of medicines is maintained. The nurse in charge may delegate some of these duties but always remains responsible for this task. The safe and secure handling of medicines on the ward is governed by the following principles.

SECURITY

All drugs should be stored in locked cupboards with separate storage for internal medicines, external medicines, controlled drugs and medicines needing refrigeration or storage in a freezer.

Diagnostic reagents, intravenous and topical agents should also be kept separately in individual storage.

STABILITY

No medicinal preparation should be stored where it may be subject to substantial variations in temperature, for example not in direct sunlight.

The normal temperature ranges for storage are as follows.

- *Cold storage*: products to be stored between 2°C and 8°C. Refrigerators should be placed in an area where the ambient temperature does not affect the temperature control within it. Most refrigerators will function effectively in an environment of 10–32°C. Refrigerators should have a minimum and maximum thermometer fitted which should be read and reset daily (MHRA 2001).
- *Cool storage*: products that need to be stored in a cool place or between 8°C and 15°C. If these temperatures cannot be achieved, these products should be stored in a fridge provided that temperatures below 8°C do not affect the stability of the product. If lower temperatures do affect the stability, it is recommended that they are stored in an area where the temperature will not exceed 18°C (MHRA 2001).
- *Room temperature*: for products that need to be stored at room temperature or not above 25°C (MHRA 2001).

CONTAINERS

The type of container used may have been chosen for specific reasons. Therefore all medicines should be stored in the containers in which they were supplied by pharmacy. Medicinal preparations should never be transferred (in bulk) from one container to another except in the pharmacy.

STOCK CONTROL

A system of stock rotation must be operated (e.g. first in, first out) to ensure that there is no accumulation of old stocks. Only one pack/container of a named medicine should be in use at any one time. A list of stock medicines to be kept on the ward should be regularly reviewed according to usage figures. The medicines to be held on the ward should be discussed between the nurse in charge and a pharmacist with relevant medical staff.

STORAGE REQUIREMENTS OF SPECIFIC PREPARATIONS

- *Aerosol containers* should not be stored in direct sunlight or over radiators: there is a risk of explosion if they are heated.
- *Creams* may deteriorate rapidly if subjected to extremes of temperature.
- *Eye drops and ointments* may become contaminated with microorganisms during use and thus pose a danger to the recipient. Therefore, in hospitals, eye preparations should be discarded 7 days after they are first opened. For use at home, this limit is extended to 28 days.
- *Mixtures* may have a relatively short shelf-life. Most antibiotic mixtures require refrigerated storage and even then have a shelf-life of only 7–14 days. Always check the label for details.
- *Tablets and capsules* are relatively stable but are susceptible to moisture unless correctly packed. They should be stored only in the containers in which they were supplied by the pharmacy.
- *Vaccines* and similar preparations usually require refrigerated storage and may deteriorate rapidly if exposed to heat.

SAFE AND SECURE HANDLING OF MEDICINES

Handling of medicines is a frequent everyday nursing activity that carries great responsibility.

The effective and safe prescribing, dispensing and administration of medicines to patients demands a partnership between the various health professionals concerned, that is doctors, pharmacists and nurses. The revised Duthie Report, *The Safe and Secure Handling of Medicines: A Team Approach* (RPSGB 2005), defined a medicine as 'a substance administered by mouth, applied to the body or introduced into the body for the purpose of treating or preventing disease, diagnosing disease or ascertaining the existence, degree or extent of a physiological condition, contraception, inducing anaesthesia, or otherwise preventing or interfering with the normal operation of a physiological function' (p.103). It follows from this definition that infusions or injections of sodium chloride 0.9% and water for injection are included, as are all medicinal products covered by the European Directive on Medicines. This report details how the key principles of compliance with legislation, adherence to guidance and safety of patients and staff should be applied to the management and handling of medicines. In order to achieve this, organizations should have in place Standard Operating Procedures (SOPs) for each activity in the medicines trail, also indicating clear responsibilities, training, competencies and performance standards for each member of staff. Processes for validation, audit and risk assessment of the activities also need to be included.

The activities defined in the medicines trail are detailed in Box 12.5.

Box 12.5 **Activities defined in the medicines trail**

- Prescribing/initiation of treatment
- Procurement/acquisition of medicines
- Manufacture/manipulation of medicines
- Receipt of medicines
- Issue to point of use/dispensing or supply
- Preparation/manipulation of medicines for administration
- Use of medicines/administration
- Removal/disposal of surplus/waste medicines from wards and departments
- Removal/disposal of surplus/waste medicines or related materials from the hospital

Safe administration of medicines

All nurses who administer medicines must be familiar with and adhere to the *Standards for Medicines Management* (NMC 2010a). The nurse is accountable for the safe administration of medicines which is arguably one of the most common clinical procedures that a nurse will undertake. This can be regarded as the greatest area of risk in nursing practice. To achieve safe administration, the nurse must have a sound knowledge of the therapeutic use, usual dose, side-effects, precautions and contraindications of the drug being administered. If the nurse lacks knowledge of a particular medicine, s/he must not administer the medicine and must seek advice from a senior colleague

Institutional policies and procedures will assist the nurse to administer drugs safely and a sound working knowledge of these is essential. Medicines administration requires thought and the exercise of professional judgement (NMC 2010a, p.3). There are a number of 'rights' – five rights (Federico 2011, MacDonald 2010), six rights (Potter 2011), eight rights (Bonsell 2011) and nine rights (Elliott & Liu 2010) (see Table 12.1).

NEVER EVENTS

Never events are 'serious, largely preventable patient safety incidents that should not occur if the available preventative measures have been implemented by health care providers' (DH 2012). To be a Never Event, an incident must have clear potential for or has previously caused severe harm, is a known source of risk, there is existing national guidance on how to prevent it and it is largely preventable if the guidance is implemented. Finally it must be easily defined, identified and measured (DH 2012). Occurrence of a Never Event indicates that an organization may not have put the right systems and processes in place to prevent incidents from happening (DH 2012).

For examples of Never Events related to medications, see Box 12.6.

DEFINITION AND CAUSES OF MEDICATION ERRORS

Medication administration errors occur frequently and are more likely to result in serious harm and death than other types of medication errors (Westbrook et al. 2011). Direct observational

Table 12.1 **The rights**

5	6	8	9
Patient • Check name on prescription and the patient • Use 2 identifiers • Ask patient to identify themselves • Use technology when available (bar codes)	Patient	Patient	Patient
Medicine • Check the prescription • Check medication label	Medicine	Medicine	Medicine
Route • Check the prescription and appropriateness • Confirm the patient can take or receive the medication by the prescribed route	Route	Route	Route
Time • Check the frequency on prescription • Check you are giving at the right time • Confirm when the last dose was given	Time	Time	Time
Dose • Check name on prescription • Check appropriateness • Calculate dose if necessary	Dose	Dose	Dose
	Documentation • Document AFTER giving the prescribed medication • Chart the time and route, your signature and any other specific information as necessary	Documentation	Documentation
		Reason • Confirm the rationale for the prescribed medication • Review the long-term medications	Action
		Response • Has the drug had the desired effect? • Document monitoring	Form
			Requirement

Source: Adapted from Bonsell (2011), Elliott & Liu (2010), Federico (2011), MacDonald (2010), Potter (2011).

Box 12.6 **List of Never Events related to medications 2012–13**

- Wrongly prepared high-risk injectable medications
- Maladministration of a potassium-containing solution
- Wrong route of chemotherapy
- Intravenous administration of epidural medication
- Overdose of midazolam for conscious sedation
- Air embolism
- Misidentification of patients
- Maladministration of insulin
- Opioid overdose in an opioid-naïve patient
- Inappropriate administration of daily oral methotrexate

Source: DH (2012).

studies in hospitals estimate error rates in 19–27% of drugs administered to patients (Westbrook et al. 2011). Studies have demonstrated that interruptions are common and that these and other distractions can increase error and accident rates related to drug adminstration (Relihan et al. 2010, Westbrook et al. 2010) (Box 12.7).

Key principles for administration of medicines

Patient identification

When administering a medicine, the nurse must be certain of the identity of the patient to whom the medicine is to be administered (NMC 2010a), i.e. check name, hospital number and date of birth. To avoid misidentification of patients, staff should check the patient's identity using an identification wristband, following the NPSA (2007b) guidance on the use of a wristband for patient identification.

Patient misidentification can occur at any stage of a patient's journey and, as it is under-reported, its 'true' incidence unknown (Rosenthal 2003). Not identifying the patient correctly can result in the administration of a wrong drug or dose and can sometimes be fatal (Schulmeister 2008). The patient's prescription chart should be taken to the bedside to ensure verification against two patient identifiers, e.g. patient name, date of birth and/or hospital number (Grissinger 2008, Gunningberg et al. 2014).

Allergy status

Accurate and up-to-date allergy information is important in reducing medicine-related harm to patients. The patient's allergy status must be up to date at all times. It is the responsibility of all healthcare professionals involved in the patient's care to update and document any identified allergies, hypersensitivities, anaphylaxis or drug intolerances (Jevon 2008, Shelton and Shivnan 2011).

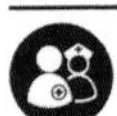

Box 12.7 **Key areas of risk for medication error**

- Wrong drug/diluent
- Calculation errors
- Level of knowledge
- Administration to wrong patient
- Administration via wrong route
- Unsafe handling/poor aseptic technique

Source: NPSA (2007a). For updates see www.england.nhs.uk/.

Table 12.2 **Types of allergic reactions**

Type of reaction	Result of reaction	Example of reaction
Type I IgE-mediated reactions	Urticaria, angio-oedema, anaphylaxis and bronchospasm	Anaphylaxis from beta-lactam antibiotic
Type II IgG/M-mediated cytotoxic reaction	Anaemia, cytopenia and thrombocytopenia	Haemolytic anaemia from penicillin
Type III IgG/M-mediated immune complexes	Vasculitis, lymphadenopathy, fever, arthropathy and rashes	
	Can also be known as serum sickness	Serum sickness from antithymocyte globulin
Type IV Delayed hypersensitivity reactions	Dermatitis, bullous exanthema, maculopapular and pustular xanthemata	Contact dermatitis from topical antihistamine

Source: Adapted from Beijnen and Schellens (2004), Riedl and Casillas (2003).

Allergic reactions are immune mediated and can be classified as in Table 12.2. There are many risk factors that increase the likelihood of an allergic reaction. These can be split into those that are specific to the patient and those that are specific to the drug. The patient-related factors and drug-related factors are listed in Box 12.8 and Box 12.9 respectively.

Although the incidence of true allergic drug reactions is low, the potential morbidity and mortality related to these reactions can be high, so it is important that drug allergies are accurately diagnosed and treated. The first step towards an accurate diagnosis is a detailed history (Mirakian et al. 2009). Guidance on what information should be collated and accurately recorded is detailed in the British Society for Allergy and Clinical Immunology (BSACI)

Box 12.8 **Allergic reactions: patient-related risk factors**

- *Immune status:* previous reaction to the same or related compound.
- *Age:* younger adults are more likely to have an allergic reaction than infants or the elderly.
- *Gender:* women are more likely than men to suffer skin reactions.
- *Genetic:* atopic predisposition is more likely to result in a severe reaction and genetic polymorphisms may predispose to drug hypersensitivity, e.g. G6PD deficiency, slow acetylators.
- *Concomitant disease:* viral infections such as HIV and herpes are associated with an increased risk of allergic reactions; cystic fibrosis is associated with an increased risk of allergic reactions to antibiotics, which is thought to be due to the prolonged use in this group of patients.

Source: Mirakian et al. (2009).

 Box 12.9 **Allergic reactions: drug-related risk factors**

- *Drug chemistry:* some drugs are more likely to cause drug reactions than others. These are high molecular weight compounds, for example insulin. Also, drugs that bind to proteins called haptens, forming complexes that can cause an immune response, for example beta-lactam antibiotics.
- *Route of administration:* the topical route is most likely to cause an allergic reaction, with the oral route being least likely. The intramuscular route is more likely than the intravenous route.
- *Dose:* a large single dose is less likely to cause a reaction than prolonged or frequent doses.

Source: Mirakian et al. (2009). Reproduced with permission from John Wiley & Sons.

drug allergy guidelines which can be found at www.bsaci.com and NICE guidance (NICE 2014b) and include the following.

- Detailed description of reaction:
  - symptom sequence and duration
  - treatment provided
  - outcome.
- Timing of symptoms in relation to drug administration.
- Has the patient had the suspected drug before this course of treatment?
  - How long had the drug(s) been taken before onset of reaction?
  - When was/were the drug(s) stopped?
  - What was the effect?
- Witness description (patient, relative, doctor).
- Is there a photograph of the reaction?
- Illness for which suspected drug was being taken, that is, underlying illness (this may be the cause of the symptoms, rather than the drug).
- List of all drugs taken at the time of the reaction (including regular medication, OTC and 'alternative' remedies).
- Previous history:
  - other drug reactions
  - other allergies
  - other illnesses (Mirakian et al. 2009, NICE 2014b).

This guideline also gives details on further investigations which may be required in order to accurately diagnose an allergic

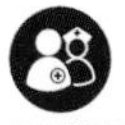 Box 12.10 **Treatment of acute drug reaction**

An acute drug reaction must be treated promptly and appropriately.

1 Stop the suspected drug.
2 Treat the reaction.
3 Identify and avoid potential cross-reacting drugs.
4 Record precise details of the reaction and its treatment.
5 Identify a safe alternative. In some cases this may not be possible so where the case is less severe, it may be decided to continue with the medication with suppression of the symptoms with, for example, a corticosteroid and an antihistamine.

Source: Mirakian et al. (2009). Reproduced with permission from John Wiley & Sons.

reaction (Box 12.10). In some cases, desensitization may be considered but this is rarely indicated.

Following an allergic reaction, it is extremely important that the patient is given information regarding what substances they should avoid. This information should be recorded clearly in the patient's medical records, including paper and electronic records. All inpatients should have their allergy indicated by wearing a red-coloured identity band (NPSA 2007b). The allergic drug reaction should also be reported using the Yellow Card Scheme (Mirakian et al. 2009) (see 'Adverse drug reactions', below).

Prior to administering any medication, the nurse must confirm the patient's allergy status and where necessary document any changes.

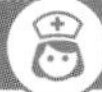 Learning Activity 12.3

Scenario: Allergy status

You have been looking after a female patient who has had an allergic reaction to her antibiotics, in the form of a raised, itchy, skin rash.

1 What actions should be taken to ensure that such a reaction is avoided in the future?
2 Consider which actions are the responsibility of the nurse, doctor, pharmacist and also the patient themselves.

See the end of the chapter for the answers.

Medication

The nurse must know the therapeutic uses of the medicine to be administered, its normal dosage, side-effects, precautions and contraindications. If the nurse has concerns regarding the prescription or the prescription is not clear, the prescriber or pharmacist must be contacted. If weight and/or height are required for calculation of the dose, ensure a recent height or weight has been used.

Calculating the required dose is vital as any miscalculation of medication dosage represents a potential threat to both patient safety and clinical effectiveness (Weeks et al. 2000). Acquisition and maintenance of mathematical competency for nurses in practice is an important issue in prevention of medication errors (Brady et al. 2009) although, when Wright (2010) reviewed studies, she found insufficient evidence to suggest that medication errors are caused by nurses' poor calculation skills. There are a number of computer-based programmes on infection control and IV therapy, infusion pumps (NHSCLU 2009) and medication dosage calculation problem-solving skills (Weeks et al. 2001) which provide information for nurses, facilitate assessment of their competency and can be used as part of induction or mandatory training.

To ensure the patient receives the correct intended treatment, the following checks must be performed:

- correct medicine and formulation selected
- correct dose prepared
- medicine within expiry date
- correct route, administration time and rate if applicable.

If a delivery device is required, ensure that the correct device is used, i.e. vascular access device for intravenous therapy or an epidural catheter for epidural drug administration.

Additional factors to consider

DRUG INTERACTIONS

Consideration should also be given to potential interactions between concomitant drugs and/or food. These interactions can result in an increased effect, causing toxicity, or a decreased

Table 12.3 Types of pharmacokinetic interactions

Type of interaction	Interaction caused by	Example of when to consider in clinical practice
Drug absorption interactions	Changes in the gastrointestinal (GI) pH Adsorption or chelation in the GI tract Changes in GI motility Induction or inhibition of transporter proteins or malabsorption	Allopurinol and mercaptopurine – allopurinol inhibits xanthane oxidase, an enzyme which metabolizes mercaptopurine to an inactive metabolite, thereby resulting in increased mercaptopurine toxicity such as bone marrow suppression. If used together, the mercaptopurine dose should be decreased to a third of the original dose (Baxter 2008)
Drug distribution interactions	Protein binding or inhibition or induction of drug transporter proteins	Therapeutic drug monitoring as drugs that can be displaced in this way can appear subtherapeutic when monitored but doses would not need to be increased (Baxter 2008)
Drug metabolism interactions	Changes in first-pass metabolism, enzyme induction, enzyme inhibition and genetic factors The hepatic cytochrome P450 enzyme system is the major site of drug metabolism and most drug–drug interactions occur at this site	Grapefruit juice can inhibit the cytochrome P450 isoenzyme CYP3A4, thus reducing the metabolism of calcium channel blockers (Baxter 2008)
Drug excretion interactions	Changes in urinary pH, active renal tubular excretion, renal blood flow and biliary excretion or the enterohepatic shunt	Probenecid and penicillin compete for the same active transport systems in the renal tubules. As a result, probenecid reduces the excretion of penicillin which can lead to penicillin toxicity (Baxter 2008)

effect, resulting in decreased efficacy of the drug. Drug interactions can be divided into pharmacokinetic (Table 12.3) and pharmacodynamic interactions (Table 12.4).

Herbal and complementary medicines have been increasingly used in the UK over recent years and as a result there has been an increase in the reporting of interactions between these agents and conventional drugs. Some of the most common herbal interactions are those involving St John's wort, a popular herbal product used as an antidepressant. Concomitant use should be avoided with, for example, antiepileptics, antivirals, warfarin.

Interactions can also occur between drugs and food. Food can have an effect on drugs by changing gastrointestinal motility or by binding to drugs whilst in transit in the gastrointestinal tract. An example of interactions between food and a drug can be seen with monoamine oxidase inhibitors and tyramine-containing foods such as mature cheese, pickled herring or broad bean pods. Tyramine is a chemical present in certain foods that are rich in protein and can interact with monoamine oxidase inhibitors (MAOIs). As procarbazine has mild MAOI properties, it is possible that taking both together could result in a hypertensive reaction which can cause symptoms of raised blood pressure, headache, pounding heart, neck stiffness, sweating, flushing and vomiting. Patients should therefore be advised to avoid tyramine-rich foods such as mature and aged cheeses, yeast or meat extracts, pickled fish, salami and heavy red wines (Baxter 2008).

Table 12.4 Types of pharmacodynamic interactions

Type of interaction	Interaction caused by	Example of when to consider in clinical practice
Additive or synergistic interactions	Two drugs have the same pharmacological effect and therefore the results can be additive	Opioids with benzodiazepines causing increased drowsiness (Baxter 2008)
Antagonistic or opposing interactions	Two drugs have opposing activities	Vitamin K and warfarin resulting in the effects of the anticoagulant being opposed (Baxter 2008)

Source: Beijnen and Schellens (2004). Reproduced with permission from Elsevier.

ADVERSE DRUG REACTIONS

Although we use drugs to diagnose, prevent or treat disease, no drug is administered without risk. It is important when choosing a drug treatment that consideration is given to the balance between clinical effect and undesired effects. The World Health Organization definition of ADRs is 'harmful, unintended reactions to medicines that occur at doses normally used for treatment' (WHO 2008). ADRs can be classified as type A or type B reactions. Type A ('augmented') reactions are considered to be an exaggeration of the medicine's normal effect when given at the usual dose. This category includes unwanted reactions that are predictable from the drug's pharmacology and are usually dose dependent (e.g. respiratory depression with opioids and bleeding with warfarin) (Rawlins and Thompson 1977). In many instances this type of unwanted effect is reversible and the problem can often be dealt with by reducing the dose (Rang and Dale 2012). Type B ('bizarre') reactions are effects that are not pharmacologically predictable and can include hypersensitivity reactions (e.g. anaphylaxis with beta-lactam antibiotics). These cannot be related to the pharmacological action of the drug, are not dose related and therefore cannot be controlled by dose reduction. Type A reactions are more common than type B but type B reactions tend to cause a higher rate of serious illness and mortality (Rawlins and Thompson 1977).

The WHO states that 'ADRs are among the leading causes of death in many countries. At least 60% of ADRs are preventable and in some countries ADR-related costs, such as hospitalisation, surgery and lost productivity, exceed the cost of the medications' (WHO 2008).

Although the effect of a drug cannot always be predicted, it is important that when a drug is given to a patient, the risk of harm is minimized by ensuring that prescribed medicines are of good quality, safe, effective and used by the right patient in the right dose at the right time. Consideration should always be given to predisposing factors that drugs or a patient may have which could increase the risk of ADRs, including:

- polypharmacy
- age of the patient
- gender
- co-morbidities, e.g. renal disease
- race
- genetic factors
- allergies
- drug–drug interactions (Koda-Kimble et al. 2005, Walker and Edwards 2003).

Preventing and detecting adverse effects from medicines is termed pharmacovigilance. It is an important aspect for all healthcare professionals to consider in order to identify potential new hazards related to medicines and prevent harm to patients (MHRA 2010a).

Although medicines are widely tested within clinical trials before they become commercially available, trials do not provide information about how different patient populations may respond to the medicines. The only way for this information to be collected is through careful patient monitoring and further collection of data through post-marketing surveillance. In the UK this information is collected through the Yellow Card Scheme which is run by the MHRA and the Commission on Human Medicines (CHM). The scheme is used to collect information from both health professionals and patients about suspected ADRs with prescribed medicines, OTC medicines and herbal medicines. Yellow Cards can be completed by using the MHRA website (www.yellowcard.mhra.gov.uk) or by completing the paper card found in the BNF.

Record of administration

The nurse must document a clear, accurate and immediate record of all medicines administered, intentionally withheld or refused by the patient, ensuring all written entries and signatures are clear and legible (NMC 2010b). If any medication is withheld or refused by a patient, the reasons must be documented.

Single or double checking of medicines

Medicines can be prepared and administered by a single qualified nurse or by two nurses checking (known as double checking). There are certain times when double or second checking is required. It is recommended that for the administration of controlled drugs, a secondary signature is required (NMC 2010a). The NMC *Standards for Medicines Management* also states that 'wherever possible two registrants should check medication to be administered intravenously, one of whom should also be the registrant who then administers the intravenous medication' (NMC 2010a, p.34). Where the administration of a medicine requires complex calculations, it is deemed good practice for a second practitioner (a registered professional) to check the calculation independently in order to minimize the risk of error (NMC 2010a).

In the Jarman et al. (2002) review of 129 nurses, using questionnaires and reviewing incidents, both during double checking and then once single checking had been introduced, demonstrated no increase in drug errors following the change. Single checking provided satisfaction for nurses and more effective use of time and the nurses felt that single checking allowed them more autonomy and that it was more beneficial to patients and enabled them to be more responsive to their needs. Armitage (2008) suggested that double checking is a common but inconsistent process. Athough often seen to be integral to safe practice, it is often sacrificed when there is a shortage of time or staff (Armitage 2008). He listed the issues with double checking as:

- deference to authority
- reduction of responsibility
- auto-processing (familiarity)
- lack of time (to check properly)
- solutions (how to do it).

Another study viewed independent double checking as an alternative. This is when two nurses check a drug independently of each other. In this study nurses were observed during the setting up of ambulatory chemotherapy pumps. When compared with the old system of double checking, the new system showed no significantly statistical difference in reducing errors in dose, rate or documentation but did show a reduction in errors related to patient identification (Savage and Tripp 2008).

Those nurses who wish or need to have their administration supervised will retain the right to do so until such time as all parties agree that the requested level of proficiency has been achieved. The nurse checking the medicine must be able to justify any action taken and be accountable for the action taken. This is in keeping with the principles of *The Code* (NMC 2015).

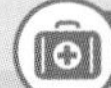 Learning Activity 12.4

Learning in practice: Double checking of medicines

There are certain times where double or second checking is required in order to ensure safe administration of medicines. Within your own clinical area:

- Identify on what occasions double/second checking of medications is used.
- Discuss why this is the case with your mentor/supervising nurse.
- Identify those situations in which you as a student nurse are able/not able to double/second check.

Delegation of medicines administration

If a Registered Nurse delegates any aspect of the administration of a medicinal product, they are also accountable for ensuring that the patient or carer/care assistant is competent to carry out the task (NMC 2010a). In delegating to unregistered practitioners, it is the Registered Nurse who must apply the principles of administration and they may then delegate the unregistered practitioner to assist the patient in the ingestion or application of the medicinal product (NMC 2010a, p.33). Student nurses must never administer/supply medicinal products without direct supervision and both the student and Registered Nurse must sign the medication chart or document the administration in the notes (NMC 2010a).

LEGAL AND PROFESSIONAL ISSUES

Medicines governance and risk management

A medication incident involves an error in the process of prescribing, dispensing, preparing, administering, monitoring or providing medicine advice, regardless of whether any harm occurred or was possible. This is a broad definition and the majority of errors reported to the National Reporting and Learning Service (NRLS) result in no or low harm (NPSA/NRLS Safety in Doses 2009). Incidents involving medicines were the third largest of all incidents reported to the NRLS. Nearly half of the reports describe incidents involved with the administration or supply of a medicine in a clinical area. The effective and safe prescribing, dispensing and administration of medicines to patients demands partnership between the various health professionals concerned, that is doctors, pharmacists and nurses.

The most frequently reported types of medication incidents accounting for approximately 70% of fatal and serious harms were:

- unclear/wrong dose or frequency
- wrong medicine
- omitted/delayed medicines.

Box 12.11 details seven key actions to improve medication safety.

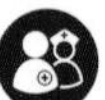

Box 12.11 **Seven key actions to improve medication safety**

- Increase reporting and learning from medication incidents.
- Implement NPSA safer medication practice recommendations.
- Improve staff skills and competencies.
- Minimize dosing errors.
- Ensure medicines are not omitted.
- Ensure the correct medicines are given to the correct patients.
- Document patients' medicine allergy status.

Source: NPSA (2007a). © Crown copyright. Reproduced under the Open Government Licence v2.0. For updates see www.england.nhs.uk/.

The Department of Health document *An Organization with a Memory* (DH 2000a) highlighted the importance of reporting and acting on reports of adverse healthcare events and potential adverse events. The document recognizes that the majority of incidents could be avoided if only the lessons of experience were properly learned.

Procedures for reporting and investigating near misses and patient safety incidents should aim to support active learning and ensure that the positive lessons learnt from these events are embedded into the organization's culture and practices. Learning from incidents is an essential part of integrated governance and risk management.

All employees have a duty to report incidents. It is recognized that fear of reprisal, blame and/or disciplinary action may deter staff from reporting an incident (or potential incident). Creating a learning environment to allow an open 'fair blame' culture for incident reporting is therefore essential.

The NMC believes that all errors and incidents require a thorough and careful investigation at a local level, taking full account of the context, circumstances and position of the practitioner involved. Such incidents require sensitive management and a comprehensive assessment of all the circumstances before a professional and managerial decision is reached on the appropriate way to proceed (NMC 2010a).

The Department of Health NHS Commissioning Board Special Health Authority (the Board Authority) requires the mandatory reporting of specific accidents, incidents and patient safety incidents by all healthcare organizations. All incidents classified as Serious Incidents Requiring Investigation must also be reported to the Commissioners, the Strategic Health Authority and Monitor.

Self-administration of medicines

EVIDENCE-BASED APPROACHES

Rationale

The Audit Commission report *A Spoonful of Sugar – Medicines Management in NHS Hospitals* (2001) recommended self-administration of medicines by patients. This report detailed how studies have shown that only one-half of patients take their medicines properly when they get home. The National Institute for Health and Clinical Excellence (NICE) published Clinical Guideline 76 on medicines adherence (NICE 2009) which states that between a third and a half of medicines that are prescribed for long-term conditions are not used. This non-adherence has quality and cost implications for the NHS due to wasted medicines and readmissions for patients.

The Audit Commission states that self-administration is beneficial to patients because it empowers the patient and allows them to take medication at the right time, for example analgesics when they are in pain and medicines to be taken before and after food. Self-administration allows patients to take an active role in managing their own care, improves patient compliance and has the potential to reduce admission to hospital due to problems with medicines (Audit Commission 2001). It allows patients to practise taking their medicines in hospital under supervision so that any problems can be dealt with. It has also been found that patients who had administered their own medications in hospital were more likely to report that their overall care was excellent and that they were satisfied with the discharge process than patients who had not (Deeks and Byatt 2000).

The Healthcare Commission report *The Best Medicine – The Management of Medicines in Acute and Specialist Trusts* (2007) states that, where patients are self-administering, it is important that medicines are stored securely in suitable storage near to the bedside, and that procedures and training need to be in place which should cover the assessment process and the patient's suitability for self-administration. Although, by definition, self-administration of medicines shifts the balance of responsibility for this part of care towards the patient, it in no way diminishes the fundamental professional duty of care. It is therefore essential that local policies, procedures and records are adequate to ensure that this duty is, and can be shown to be, discharged. The revised Duthie Report (RPSGB 2005) states that any transfer of responsibility should occur on the basis of an assessment of the patient's ability to manage the tasks involved and with the patient's consent. The patient's consent should be recorded with the date and time.

The NMC sets out the responsibilities of the nurse regarding the self-administration of medicines. These include viewing the medicines, checking the suitability for reuse, that they have been prescribed, assessment of the patient, what should be documented and how they should be stored (NMC 2010a).

Assessment of patients for self-administration normally results in the allocation of a level of supervision. Examples of levels of supervision can be seen in Table 12.5. All patients should be

Table 12.5 **Examples of levels of supervision for self-administration of medicines**

Level of supervision	Role of patient	Role of nurse
Level 1	None	Nurse administers medicine from cabinet Key locked in cabinet and nurse uses master Nurse signs drug administration chart
Level 2	Patient administers medicine with nurse supervision	Cabinet is opened by nurse Nurse supervises patient administration Nurse signs drug administration chart
Level 3	Key kept by patient Patient administers their own medicines	Nurse must check that the appropriate medication was taken and endorse the chart with an identifier to indicate that the patient is self-administering and their initials

Source: NPC (2007a). Reproduced with permission from NICE (www.nice.org.uk).

assessed on a regular basis, using local policies to ensure that the individual patient is able to self-administer. The nurse is responsible for recognizing and acting upon changes in the patient's clinical condition which may affect their ability to self-administer. This information should be documented in their records (NMC 2010b).

PRE-PROCEDURAL CONSIDERATIONS

A medicines reconciliation needs to be carried out with the patient and they will be assessed for their ability to self-administer. Any constraint such as physical or visual handicap must be addressed. Changes in performance status may result from the underlying condition or its treatment, and must be allowed for (NMC 2010a, Shepherd 2002a).

If a compliance aid such as a 'dosette' box is to be used, responsibility for filling and labelling the aid, especially whilst used on the ward, must be agreed and approved by the organization and documented in the patient's notes (NMC 2010a, Shepherd 2002a).

Procedure guideline 12.1 **Medication: self-administration**

Essential equipment

- Drugs to be administered
- Recording sheet or book as required by law or hospital policy
  - Consent form
  - Patient information leaflet explaining the self-administration scheme
- Patient's prescription chart, to check dose, route and so on
- Any protective clothing required by hospital policy for specified drugs, such as antibiotics or cytotoxic drugs

Pre-procedure

Action	Rationale
1 Carry out a medicines reconciliation with the patient on admission by reviewing proposed (inpatient) prescription in liaison with the pharmacist and compare with details given by the patient and medicines in their possession. Any differences should be investigated and highlighted with the medical team.	To ensure an accurate record of all medicines being taken (prescribed or otherwise); dietary supplements, for example multivitamins, herbal remedies, complementary therapies; allergies or hypersensitivities; understanding of current medicines; possible problems with self-administration (Jordan et al. 2003, **E**; NMC 2010a, **C**; NMC 2010b, **C**; NICE/NPSA 2007, **C**; Shepherd 2002b, **E**).
2 Carry out an assessment of the patient's ability to self-administer medication using an assessment form with the criteria in Table 12.6.	Technical patient safety solutions for medicines reconciliation on admission of adults to hospital (NICE/NPSA 2007, **C**).
3 Consider whether there are any constraints on self-administration and, if so, how they might be overcome. Discuss this with appropriate members of the multidisciplinary team.	To promote successful and safe self-administration and ensure that medicines are dispensed and labelled appropriately for the patient's needs (DH 2003b, **C**; NMC 2010a, **C**; Shepherd 2002a, **E**).
4 Following the assessment, a level of supervision will be recommended and entered on the assessment form. The assessment form and the consent will be filed in the patient records. For examples of levels see Table 12.5.	To ensure that the correct level of supervsion is selected and communicated to other staff. **E**

Procedure

Action	Rationale
5 Discuss with the patient their medication and any problems they may be having with the regimen. Document discussions in the care plan. Teach any special skills required, for example correct use of aerosol inhalers. Reassess whether they need any changes to their levels of supervision, either up or down.	To promote the informed commitment and involvement of patients in their own care, where appropriate. To ensure that treatment is received as intended (NMC 2010a, **C**).

Post-procedure

Action	Rationale
6 Check every day that drugs are taken as intended, and that the necessary records are kept.	To ensure that the patient is taking the medication as the nurse continues to take overall responsibility for patient care and well-being. To maintain a record of responsibilities undertaken (NMC 2010a, **C**; NMC 2010b, **C**; NMC 2015, **C**).
7 Monitor changes in the patient's prescription.	To ensure that changes are put into effect promptly; drugs are properly relabelled or redispensed; any discontinued drugs are retrieved from the patient (DH 2003b, **C**; NMC 2010a, **C**; Shepherd 2002b, **E**).
8 Check when drug supplies are expected to run out and make arrangements for resupply. Order drugs to take out (TTO) as far in advance as possible.	To ensure that drugs are represcribed and dispensed in time to allow uninterrupted treatment and to facilitate planned discharge (DH 2003b, **C**; NMC 2010a, **C**; Shepherd 2002b, **E**).
9 Evaluate the effectiveness of the self-administration teaching programme and record any difficulties encountered and interventions made.	To identify further learning and teaching needs and modify care plan accordingly (NMC 2010a, **C**; NMC 2010b, **C**; NMC 2015, **C** Shepherd 2002b, **E**).

Table 12.6 **Assessment form**

Assessment criteria	Rationale
• Is the patient willing to participate in self-administration after being given information explaining the scheme with associated time to read and understand it?	Patient's agreement should be recorded with a date and time (RPSGB 2005)
• Has the patient signed a consent form agreeing to self-administration?	Patient's agreement should be recorded with a date and time (RPSGB 2005)
• Is the patient sufficiently well to take part in the scheme?	Patients who are not well enough or who are undergoing surgery will not be able to self-administer until they have recovered and have been reassessed. If frequent changes of drug or dose are expected, immediate self-administration may be undesirable and/or impractical
• Is the patient confused, forgetful or disorientated?	Patients who are confused, forgetful or disorientated will need to have their medicines administered by a nurse in the usual way. This may be assessed by asking relatives or carers or by asking specific questions for assessing state of mind
• Does the patient have a history of drug/alcohol abuse/self-harm?	Patients with this history can self-administer under the supervision of a nurse
• Does the patient self-administer medicines at home?	Patients who are not responsible for self-administering their medicines in the community will need to have their medicines administered by a nurse in the usual way
• Can the patient read the labels on the medicines?	These patients can either self-administer with supervision or have their medicines administered by a nurse. Referral can be made to pharmacy around assessment of labels. Can they be given extra large or Braille labels if necessary?
• Can the patient open the medicine bottles and foil strips?	These patients can either self-administer with supervision or have their medicines administered by a nurse. Referral can be made to pharmacy for assessment and provision of appropriate containers
• Can the patient open the locker where the medicines are stored while they are in hospital?	Patients who cannot open the locker can self-administer with nurse supervision
• Does the patient know what their medicines are for, their dosage, instructions and potential side-effects (Shepherd 2002b)?	Patients who don't know this can be allowed to self-administer with nurse supervision. Re-education can take place in order to achieve full self-administration

POST-PROCEDURAL CONSIDERATIONS

Ongoing care

The nurse must monitor for any changes in the patient's prescription and condition. They must check when drugs supplied are expected to run out and ensure that drugs are ordered along with any TTOs. The effectiveness of the self-administration teaching programme must be evaluated (Shepherd 2002b).

Documentation

Particular care with record keeping is needed in the period of gradual transition from nurse administration to self-administration. Any problems encountered must be addressed (NMC 2010a, NMC 2010b, NMC 2015).

The detail and format of the record may vary according to the patient's needs and performance status, the complexity of treatment, and local circumstances and policy (NMC 2010a, NMC 2010b, NMC 2015).

Controlled drugs

DEFINITION

Controlled drugs are those drugs that are listed in Schedule 2 of the Misuse of Drugs Act 1971 and are subject to the controls stipulated in the Act, for example diamorphine, morphine, amphetamines, benzodiazepines. The use of controlled drugs in medicine is permitted by the Misuse of Drugs Regulations and related regulations, as detailed in the next section, Legal and professional issues.

LEGAL AND PROFESSIONAL ISSUES

Legislation

Medicines Act 1968

The Act and the regulations made under the Act set out the requirements for the legal sale, supply and administration of medicines. It also allows certain exemptions for the general restrictions on the sale, supply and administration of medicines which, for example, enable midwives to supply and/or administer diamorphine, morphine, pethidine or pentazocine.

A number of healthcare professionals are permitted to supply and/or administer medicines generally in accordance with a PGD. Some of these professional groups, but not all, are permitted to possess, supply or administer controlled drugs in accordance with a PGD under the Misuse of Drugs legislation.

Misuse of Drugs Act 1971

For reasons of public safety, the Misuse of Drugs Act controls the export, import, supply and possession of dangerous or otherwise harmful drugs to prevent abuse as most are potentially addictive or habit forming as well as harmful. The Act dictates what constitutes an unlawful activity. Drugs controlled under the Misuse of Drugs Act 1971 are divided into three classes, A, B and C, for the purposes of establishing the maximum penalties which can be imposed. The Misuse of Drugs Act 1971 also controls the manufacture of controlled drugs. Other regulations of the Act govern safe storage, destruction and supply to known addicts.

Misuse of Drugs (Safe Custody) Regulations 1973

These regulations control the storage of controlled drugs. The level of control of storage depends on the premises in which they are being stored and the schedule of the drug.

Misuse of Drugs Regulations 2001

Under these regulations, controlled drugs are classified into five schedules, each representing a different level of control (Table 12.7). The Schedule in which a CD is placed depends upon its medicinal or therapeutic benefit balanced against its harm when misused. Schedule 1 CDs are subject to the highest level of control, whereas Schedule 5 CDs are subject to a much lower level of control. A comprehensive list of drugs included within the Schedules is given in the Misuse of Drugs Regulations 2001 and can be accessed at www.opsi.gov.uk.

The requirements of the Act as they apply to nurses working in a hospital with a pharmacy department are described in Table 12.8.

Controlled Drugs (Supervision of Management and Use) Regulations 2006

These regulations set out the requirements for certain NHS bodies and independent hospitals to appoint an accountable officer. The duties and responsibilities of the accountable officer are to improve the management and use of controlled drugs. These regulations also allow the periodic inspection of premises.

Misuse of Drugs and Misuse of Drugs (Safe Custody) (Amendment) Regulations 2007

These regulations give accountable officers authority to nominate persons to witness the destruction of controlled drugs within their organization. They also allow operating department practitioners to order, possess and supply controlled drugs.

In addition, they set out changes to the record keeping for controlled drugs, with requirements for recording in the controlled drugs register the person (the patient, patient's representative or a healthcare professional) collecting the Schedule 2 controlled drug. If it is a healthcare professional, there is a requirement for the name and address of that person. Records need to be kept regarding whether proof of identity was requested of the patient or the patient's representative and whether this proof of identity was provided. These requirements also changed midazolam from Schedule 4 to Schedule 3.

Implications of the regulations for nursing practice

Accountability and responsibility

The nurse in charge of an area is responsible for the safe and appropriate management of controlled drugs in that area. Certain tasks such as holding of the keys can be delegated to a Registered Nurse but the overall responsibility remains with the nurse in charge.

Table 12.7 **Legal requirements for the schedules of controlled drugs (CDs)**

	Schedule 2	Schedule 3	Schedule 4 Part I	Schedule 4 Part II	Schedule 5
	Includes opioids and major stimulants, for example amphetamines	Includes minor stimulants, temazepam, barbiturates, tramadol	Includes benzodiazepines, zopiclone	Includes anabolic steroids, growth hormones	Includes low-dose opioids
Designation	CD	CDs With no register entry	CDs Benzodiazepines	CDs-Anabolic steroids	CDs-Needing invoice retention
Safe custody	Yes, except quinalbarbitone	Yes, except certain exemptions listed in the Medicines, Ethics and Practices including phenobarbitone	No	No	No
Prescription requirements	Yes	Yes, except temazepam	No	No	No
Requisitions necessary	Yes	Yes	No	No	No
Records to be kept in CD register	Yes	No	No	No	No
Pharmacist must ascertain the identity of the person collecting the CD	Yes	No	No	No	No
Emergency supplies allowed	No	No, except phenobarbitone for epilepsy	Yes	Yes	Yes
Validity of prescription	28 days	28 days	28 days	28 days	6 months
Maximum duration that can be prescribed	30 days as good practice	30 days as good practice	30 days as good practice	30 days as good practice	

Source: DH (2007). © Crown copyright. Reproduced under the Open Government Licence v2.0.
Further details can be found in The Misuse of Drugs and Misuse of Drugs (Safe Custody) (Amendment) (England, Wales and Scotland) Regulations (2014).

Table 12.8 **Summary of legal requirements for handling of controlled drugs (CDs) as they apply to nurses in hospitals with a pharmacy**

	Schedule 1: CDs Home Office licence	Schedule 2: CDs subject to full controls	Schedule 3: CDs with no register entry	Schedule 4: CDs anabolic steroids/ benzodiazepines	Schedule 5: CDs needing invoice retention
Drugs in the schedule	Cannabis + derivatives but excluding nabilone, LSD (lysergic acid diethylamide)	Most opioids in common use including: alfentanyl; amphetamines; cocaine; diamorphine; methadone; morphine papaveretum; fentanyl; phenoperidine; pethidine; codeine; dihydrocodeine injections; pentazocine	Minor stimulants; barbiturates (but excluding hexobarbitone, thiopentone); diethylpropion; buprenorphine; midazolam; temazepam*, tramadol	Part 1: anabolic steroids, zopiclone Part 2: benzodiazepines	Some preparations containing very low strengths of cocaine; codeine; morphine; pholcodine and some other opioids
Ordering	Possession and supply permitted only by special licence from the Secretary of State issued (to a doctor only) for scientific or research purposes	A requisition must be signed in duplicate by the nurse in charge. The requisition must be endorsed to indicate that the drugs have been supplied. Copies should be kept for 2 years	As Schedule 2	No requirement†	No requirement†
Storage	Must be kept in a suitable locked cupboard to which access is restricted	As Schedule 1	Buprenorphine and diethylpropion: as Schedule 1 drugs. All other drugs, no requirement	No requirement†	No requirement†
Record keeping	Controlled drugs register must be used	As Schedule 1	No requirement†	No requirement†	No requirement†
Prescription	Prescription must include: • the name and address of patient • the drug, the dose, the form of preparation • the total quantity of drug or the total number of dosage units to be supplied. This quantity must be stated in words and figures The prescription must be written indelibly and signed and dated by the prescriber	As Schedule 1	As Schedule 1 except for phenobarbitone (this includes all preparations of phenobarbitone and phenobarbitone sodium). Because of its use as an antiepileptic, it does not need to comply with prescription requirements	No requirement†	No requirement†
Administration to patients	Under special licence only A doctor or dentist or anyone acting on their instructions may administer these drugs to anyone for whom they have been prescribed	A doctor or dentist or anyone acting on their instructions may administer these drugs to anyone for whom they have been prescribed	A doctor or dentist or anyone acting on their instructions may administer these drugs to anyone for whom they have been prescribed	No requirement†	No requirement†

*Temazepam preparations are exempt from record-keeping and prescription requirements, but are subject to storage requirements.
†'No requirement' indicates that the Misuse of Drugs Act 1971 imposes no legal requirements additional to those imposed by the Medicines Act 1968 (HMSO 1968).
Source: The Misuse of Drugs and Misuse of Drugs (Safe Custody) (Amendment) (England, Wales and Scotland) Regulations (2014).

Figure 12.2 **Controlled drugs record book.**

68 NAME, FORM OF PREPARATION AND STRENGTH Morphine Sulphate Injection 10mg / 1 mL

AMOUNT(S) OBTAINED			AMOUNT(S) ADMINISTERED						
Amount	Date Received	Serial No. of Requisition	Date	Time	Patient's Name	Amount given	Given by (Signature)	Witnessed by (Signature)	STOCK BALANCE
10 amps	26/5/2010	12	26/5/2010	14:00	Received from Pharmacy		[signature]	[signature]	10
			27/5/10	14:15	Mr. John Smith	10 mg	[signature]	[signature]	9
			27/5/10	18:00	Mrs. Daisy Rose	5mg given/5mg wasted	[signature]	[signature]	8

Requisition

The nurse in charge of an area is responsible for the requisition of controlled drugs for that area. This task can be delegated to a Registered Nurse but the overall responsibility remains with the nurse in charge. Orders should be written on suitable stationery and must be signed by an authorized signatory. All those who are authorized to order should have a copy of their signatures kept in pharmacy for validation. All stationery which is used to order, return or distribute controlled drugs (CD stationery) must be stored securely, and access to it should be restricted.

Receipt

When controlled drugs are delivered to the ward they must be handed to an appropriate individual and not left unattended. A Registered Nurse in charge should check the order against the requisition, including the number ordered and received, and if all is correct they should sign the 'received by' section of the order book.

The controlled drug should be entered in the controlled drugs register, recording the following information: date, number of requisition, quantity, name, formulation and strength of drug, name and signature of person making the entry, name and signature of witness and the balance of stock. The updated balance should be checked against the controlled drugs physically present and that these are the same. The number of units received should be written in words not figures. The controlled drugs will then be placed in the controlled drugs cupboard.

Storage/equipment

Controlled drugs should be stored in controlled drugs cupboards that conform to British Standard BS2881. If the amount of controlled drugs that are stored is large or in areas where there is not a 24-hour staff presence, a security cabinet that has been evaluated against the SOLD SECURE standard SS304 should be used.

Cupboards should be locked when not in use. The lock must not be common to any other lock in the hospital. Keys must only be available to authorized members of staff and at any time the key holder should be readily identifiable. The cupboard must be dedicated to the storage of controlled drugs. Controlled drugs must be locked away when not in use. There must be arrangements for keeping keys secure, especially in areas that are not operational at all times.

Key holding and access

The nurse in charge is responsible for the controlled drugs keys. Key holding may be delegated but the legal responsibility lies with the nurse in charge. The controlled drug keys should be returned to the nurse in charge immediately after use.

For the purpose of stock checking, the key may be handed to an authorized member of pharmacy staff. If keys are lost, the senior nurse, the pharmacy manager and accountable officer must be contacted. Spare keys can be issued to ensure that patient care is not impeded.

Record keeping

Each ward that holds controlled drugs should keep a record of received and administered controlled drugs in a controlled drugs record book (Figure 12.2). The nurse in charge is responsible for keeping the controlled drugs record book up to date and in good order.

The controlled drugs record book should have sequentially numbered pages, have a separate page for each drug and strength, entries should be in chronological order and in ink. The entries in the controlled drugs record book should be signed by a Registered Nurse and then witnessed by a second Registered Nurse. If a second nurse is unavailable, the transaction can be witnessed by another registered practitioner such as a doctor, pharmacist or pharmacy technician.

When the end of a page is reached, the balance should be transferred to another page. The new number should be written on the bottom of the finished page and, as a matter of good practice, the transfer should be witnessed. If a mistake is made in the record book, the mistake should be bracketed so that the original entry is still clear and then signed, dated and witnessed by another nurse or registered professional who will also do the same for the correction.

Stock checks and discrepancies

The stock balance entered in the controlled drugs record book should be checked against the amounts in the cupboard. In addition, regular stock checks should be carried out by pharmacy. The nurse in charge is responsible for ensuring that the stock checks are carried out. The stock checks should be carried out by two Registered Nurses. When checking the balance, the record book should be checked against the contents of the cupboard, not the reverse. Packs with unopened tamper-evident seals do not need to be opened during the check. Stock balances of liquid medicines may be checked by visual inspection but the balance must be confirmed to be correct on completion of a bottle. Any discrepancy should be reported to the nurse in charge who should inform the pharmacist. A record should be made in the record book that the stock has been checked with words such as 'check of stock level' and a signature of the Registered Nurse and the witness.

If a discrepancy is found, it should be checked that all requisitions have been entered, that all drugs administered have been entered, that items have not been recorded in the wrong place in the record book, that the drugs have not been placed in the wrong cupboard and that the balances have been added correctly. If an error is found, the nurse in charge should make an entry to correct the balance which should be witnessed. If the error cannot be found, the chief pharmacist and the accountable officer should be contacted immediately.

Archiving

Controlled drugs record books should be stored for a minimum of 2 years from the date the last entry was made/date of use.

Administration

Any registered practitioner can administer any drug specified as Schedule 2, 3 and 4 provided they are acting in accordance with the directions of an appropriately qualified prescriber. Two practitioners must be involved in the administration of controlled drugs, and both practitioners should be present during the whole administration procedure (NMC 2010a). The two practitioners should have clearly defined roles. One should be the checker and the other should take responsibility for taking the drug out of the cupboard, preparing and administering the drug. These roles should not be interchangeable during the procedure as this can result in errors. They should both witness the preparation, the controlled drug being administered and the destruction of any surplus drug. An entry should be made in the controlled drugs record book recording the following information (see Figure 12.2):

- the date and time the dose was administered
- the name of the patient
- quantity administered
- the name of the controlled drug
- the formulation
- the dose being administered (and any amount being destroyed if only a part vial is required)
- the name and signature of the person administering
- the name and signature of the witness
- the balance in stock (see Procedure guideline 12.2 Medication: controlled drug administration.

Return and disposal including part vials

Unused controlled drug stock should be returned to pharmacy. Controlled drugs that are expired should also be returned to pharmacy for safe destruction. An entry should be made in the relevant page of the record book recording the following information:

- date
- reason for return
- name and signature of Registered Nurse
- name and signature of witness
- quantity removed
- name, form and strength
- the balance remaining.

Disposal of controlled drugs can take place on the ward if a part vial is administered to the patient or if individual doses of controlled drugs were prepared and not administered. If destroying a part vial, the Registered Nurse should record the amount given and the amount wasted under the administration entry in the record book; for example, if the patient is prescribed diamorphine 2.5 mg and only a 5 mg preparation is available, the record should show '2.5 mg given and 2.5 mg wasted'. The entry and destruction should be witnessed by a Registered Nurse or other registered professional. If destroying an unused prepared controlled drug, this should also be recorded in the record book and the entry and destruction witnessed by another registered professional.

Stationery

Controlled drugs stationery should be stored in a locked cupboard or drawer. Controlled drugs stationery will be issued from pharmacy against a written requisition signed by an appropriate member of staff. Only one requisition book should be in use by a ward. If a new record book is started, the stock balance transfer should be witnessed by a Registered Nurse.

Transport

Controlled drugs should be transferred in a secure, locked or sealed, tamper-evident container. A person collecting controlled drugs should be aware of safe storage and security and the importance of handing over to an authorized person to obtain a signature. They must also have a valid ID badge.

Supply under PGD

When acting in their capacity as such under a PGD, nurses are authorized to supply, or offer to supply, diamorphine and morphine where administration of such drugs is required for the immediate, necessary treatment of sick or injured persons (excluding the treatment of addiction) in any setting.

They can also supply or administer any Schedule 3 or 4 controlled drug in accordance with a PGD (except anabolic steroids in Schedule 4 Part 2 and injectable formulations for the purpose of treating a person who is addicted to a drug).

Prescribing

A supplementary prescriber, when acting in accordance with a clinical management plan, can prescribe a controlled drug provided the drug is included in the clinical management plan. Nurse independent prescribers may prescribe any controlled drug listed in Schedules 2–5 for any medical condition, except diamorphine, cocaine and dipipanone for the treatment of addiction (other controlled drugs are prescribable by nurse independent prescribers for the treatment of addiction). The authority to prescribe any controlled drug is given on the basis that nurses must only prescribe within their competence.

In response to seven case reports, published between 2000 and 2005, regarding deaths due to the administration of high-dose (30 mg or greater) morphine or diamorphine to patients who had not previously received doses of opiates, the NPSA released a safer practice notice in 2006, *Ensuring Safer Practice with High Dose Ampoules of Morphine and Diamorphine* (NPSA 2006). In line with this safer practice notice, the following guidance should be adhered to (Box 12.12).

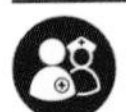

Box 12.12 **High-dose opiate guidance**

- High-strength preparations of morphine or diamorphine (30 mg or above) should be stored in a location separate from lower-strength preparations (10 mg) within the controlled drugs cupboard.
- Awareness should be raised of the similarities of drug packaging, and consider use of alert stickers being attached to high-strength preparations by pharmacy.
- A review of stock levels should be undertaken in all clinical areas where morphine and diamorphine are stored to assess whether high-strength preparations need to be kept on a permanent basis or whether they could be ordered according to specific patient requirements.
- Clear guidance should be provided to ensure that the correct doses of diamorphine and morphine are prepared in the appropriate clinical situation. For example, diamorphine 5 mg and 10 mg ampoules could be used for both bolus administration and patients newly commenced on diamorphine infusions; diamorphine 30 mg ampoules could be reserved for patients already receiving diamorphine infusions and who require higher daily doses.
- Patients should be observed for the first hour after receiving their first dose of diamorphine or morphine injection.
- Naloxone injections should be available in all clinical areas where morphine and diamorphine are stored.

Source: NPSA (2006). For updates see www.england.nhs.uk/.

Box 12.13 **Opioid dose/strength guidance**

- Confirm any recent opioid dose, formulation, frequency of administration and any other analgesic medicines prescribed for the patient. This may be done, for example, through discussion with the patient or their representative (although not in the case of treatment for addiction), the prescriber or through medication records.
- Where a dose increase is intended, ensure that the calculated dose is safe for the patient (e.g. for oral morphine or oxycodone in adult patients, not normally more than 50% higher than the previous dose).
- Ensure they are familiar with the following characteristics of that medicine and formulation: usual starting dose, frequency of administration, standard dosing increments, symptoms of overdose, common side-effects.

Source: NPSA (2008a). For updates see www.england.nhs.uk/.

Between 2005 and 2008, 4223 incidents were reported to the NRLS involving opioid medicines and the 'wrong/unclear dose or strength' or 'wrong frequency' of medication. As a result, the NPSA released a Rapid Response Report in July 2008. The guidance shown in Box 12.13 has been given.

The NPSA was notified of 498 midazolam patient safety incidents between November 2004 and November 2008 where the dose prescribed or administered to the patient was inappropriate. Three midazolam-related incidents have resulted in death. As a result, the NPSA released a Rapid Response Report in December 2008. The guidance in Box 12.14 has been given.

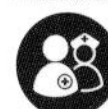

Box 12.14 **Midazolam guidance**

- Ensure that the storage and use of high-strength midazolam (5 mg/mL in 2 mL and 10 mL ampoules, or 2 mg/mL in 5 mL ampoules) are restricted to general anaesthesia, intensive care, palliative medicine and clinical areas/situations where its use has been formally risk assessed, for example, where syringe drivers are used.
- Ensure that in other clinical areas, storage and use of high-strength midazolam are replaced with low-strength midazolam (1 mg/mL in 2 mL or 5 mL ampoules).
- Review therapeutic protocols to ensure that guidance on use of midazolam is clear and that the risks, particularly for the elderly or frail, are fully assessed.
- Ensure that all healthcare practitioners involved directly or participating in sedation techniques have the necessary knowledge, skills and competences.
- Ensure that stocks of flumazenil are available where midazolam is used and that the use of flumazenil is regularly audited as a marker of excessive dosing of midazolam.
- Ensure that sedation is covered by organizational policy and that overall responsibility is assigned to a senior clinician who, in most cases, will be an anaesthetist.

Source: NPSA (2008b). For updates see www.england.nhs.uk/.

Procedure guideline 12.2 **Medication: controlled drug administration**

Essential equipment

- Prescription chart
- Controlled drugs record book
- Appropriate medication container, for example medicine pot or syringe
- Red 'Do Not Disturb' medication tabard

Pre-procedure

Action	Rationale
1 Apply red tabard.	To prevent nurse being disturbed during the process. **E**
2 Look at the patient's prescription chart: check the name, date of birth, hospital number, allergy status and then read the following.	To ensure that the correct patient is given the correct drug, in the correct formulation, in the prescribed dose using the appropriate diluent and by the correct route (DH 2003b, **C**; NMC 2010a, **C**).
(a) Drug name (generic)	
(b) Dose	
(c) Date and time of administration	
(d) Frequency	
(e) Route and method of administration	
(f) Formulation of oral preparation, e.g. modified release, immediate release	To ensure the correct formulation is given as many different formulations are available for the same drug. **E**
(g) Diluent as appropriate	
(h) Validity of prescription	To ensure prescription is legal (DH 2003b, **C**).
(i) Legible signature and contact details of prescriber.	To ensure prescription is legal and complies with hospital policy (DH 2003b, **C**).
(j) Check when the drug was last administered	To ensure that the patient requires the drug at this time. **E**

(continued)

Procedure guideline 12.2 Medication: controlled drug administration *(continued)*

Action	Rationale
If any of these pieces of information are missing, are unclear or illegible then the nurse should not proceed with administration and should consult with the prescriber.	To prevent any errors occurring. **E**
Procedure	
3 With the second Registered Nurse, take the keys and open the controlled drugs cupboard. Take the ward controlled drug record book that contains the prescribed controlled drugs, check the contents page to ascertain and turn to the relevant page headed with the name and strength of the controlled drug.	To check the stock and to enter the details into the controlled drugs record book (DH 2003b, **C**).
4 With the second Registered Nurse, take the correct drug out of the controlled drugs cupboard.	To comply with hospital policy and to ensure the patient receives the correct medicine (DH 2003b, **C**; NMC 2010a, **C**; NPSA 2006, **C**).
5 With the second Registered Nurse, check the stock level against the last entry in the controlled drugs record book.	To comply with hospital policy (DH 2003b, **C**; NMC 2010a, **C**; NPSA 2006, **C**).
6 With the second Registered Nurse, check the appropriate dose and concentration/strength (e.g. 10 mg in 1 mL or 5 mg in 5 mL) and formulation against the prescription chart and remove the dose from the box/bottle and place into an appropriate container, e.g. medicine pot or syringe.	To comply with hospital policy and to ensure the patient receives the correct dose and strength of medicine (DH 2003b, **C**; NMC 2010a, **C**; NPSA 2006, **C**).
7 Return the remaining stock to the cupboard and lock the cupboard.	To comply with hospital policy (DH 2003b, **C**; NMC 2010a, **C**; NPSA 2006, **C**).
8 Enter the date, dose, new stock level and the patient's name in the controlled drugs record book, ensuring that both you and the second Registered Nurse sign the entry (**Action figure 8**). NB: May require entry into different sections if the dose is to be made up of different doses, e.g. 70 mg = 1 × 50 mg and 2 × 10 mg). If any is wasted then ensure it is documented correctly, e.g. 5 mg given and 5 mg wasted.	To comply with hospital policy (DH 2003b, **C**; NMC 2010a, **C**; NPSA 2006, **C**).
9 (a) With the second Registered Nurse, take the prepared dose to the patient and check the patient's identity by asking them to verbally identify themselves (where possible) and check the information the patient gives against the identification wristband the patient is wearing. (b) Ask the patient if they have any allergies, checking their response against the prescription chart.	To prevent error and confirm patient's identity (NPSA 2005, **C**; NPSA 2007b, **C**).
(c) Check when the patient last had the medication against the prescription chart.	To ensure that the patient has not already received the medication. **E**
10 Administer the drug. If given orally, wait until the patient has swallowed the medication.	To ensure the patient receives the medicines (DH 2003b, **C**).
Post-procedure	
11 Once the drug has been administered, the prescription chart is signed by the nurse responsible for administering the medication and the Registered Nurse who witnessed the administration.	To comply with hospital policy (DH 2003b, **C**; NMC 2010a, **C**; NPSA 2006, **C**). To maintain accurate records, provide a point of reference in the event of any queries and prevent any duplication of treatment (NMC 2010a, **C**; NMC 2010b, **C**; NMC 2015, **C**).
12 Check the patient after administration for effectiveness and/or toxicity.	To ensure that the drug has been effective and to administer a breakthrough dose if necessary. To check that the patient has not experienced any toxicity that may require interventions. **E**
13 If the drug is given via a syringe pump, return to check the infusion (for rate) and site (for signs of any local complications) and document in the appropriate records.	To ensure that the infusion is infusing at the correct rate and the site is suitable. **E**

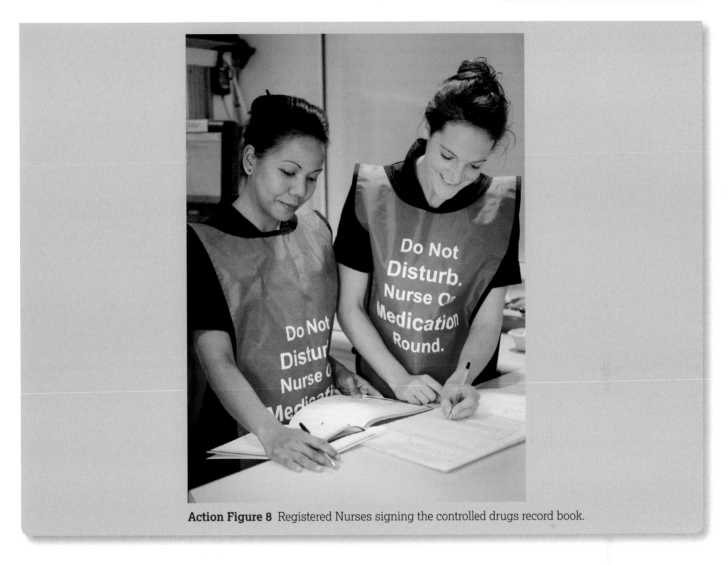

Action Figure 8 Registered Nurses signing the controlled drugs record book.

POST-PROCEDURAL CONSIDERATIONS

Ongoing care

Patients should be monitored for signs of adverse effects from opioids and for signs of toxicity. The most common side-effects are constipation, nausea and vomiting and drowsiness. All patients who are prescribed an opioid regularly should be prescribed laxatives concurrently to prevent constipation. Nausea and vomiting should subside after a few days but patients should be prescribed antiemetics and given reassurance. Drowsiness due to opioids should also subside after a few days so if patients experience these symptoms, they should be given reassurance that they will pass in time (Regnard and Hockley 2004).

The warning signs of toxicity due to opioids are:

- pin-point pupils
- confusion
- myoclonus
- hallucinations and nightmares
- respiratory depression.

If patients are showing signs of toxicity, the opioid dose should be reduced or stopped and as-required opioid pain relief given (Regnard and Hockley 2004). Changing to an alternative opioid can also be considered (Regnard and Hockley 2004).

Naloxone, a specific opioid antagonist, has a high affinity for opioid receptors and reverses the effect of opioid analgesics. It is rarely needed but may be required in the case of opioid-induced respiratory depression (with respiration rate of 8 or below).

Care must be taken not to give naloxone to patients who have opioid-induced drowsiness, confusion or hallucinations that are not life threatening as this may risk reversing the opioid analgesic effect (Twycross et al. 2007).

Naloxone should be given in stat doses of 400 micrograms every 2 minutes until respiratory function is satisfactory and doses should be titrated against respiratory function and not the level of consciousness of the patient in order to avoid total reversal of the analgesic effect (Twycross et al. 2007). Registered Nurses administering opioids should be aware of local policy procedures and protocols. Flumazenil is used for reversal of the effects of benzodiazepine toxicity.

Routes of administration

The three basic routes of administration are enteral, parenteral and topical (Table 12.9, Table 12.10). The enteral route uses the gastrointestinal (GI) tract for absorption of drugs. The parenteral route bypasses the GI tract and is associated with all forms of injections. The topical route also bypasses the GI tract and is associated with drugs that are administered to the skin and mucous membranes.

Table 12.9 **Advantages and disadvantages of the routes of administration**

Route	Advantages	Disadvantages
Oral	Convenient	Compliance
	Easy to administer	Some drugs not suitable for oral route
	Least expensive	May not be able to swallow or take oral medications
Topical	Easy to apply	Can stain clothing
	Local effects	Local irritation
Injections	Absorbed quickly	Invasive
	Avoids gastrointestinal tract	Pain
		Complications such as infection
		May be difficult to self-administer
Site specific, for example eye, ear, nasal, vaginal, rectal, pulmonary	Often for local effects	Discomfort and embarrassment May be difficult to self-administer

Oral administration

DEFINITION

Medication taken by mouth, that is swallowed by the patient, e.g. liquid, tablets or capsules (Merck Manual 2014), or administered via a feeding tube, for example nasogastric, percutaneous endoscopic gastrostomy (PEG) (Potter 2011). See Figure 12.3.

Oral administration is the most convenient route for drug administration and may result in better compliance (Kelly and Wright 2009). It is usually the safest and least expensive. Due to the widespread use of oral drugs, they are prepared in a variety of dosage forms.

RELATED THEORY

Tablets

These come in a great variety of shapes, sizes, colours and types. The formulation may be very simple, presenting as a plain, white, uncoated tablet, or complex, designed with specific therapeutic aims, for example sustained-release preparations. Sugar coatings are used to improve appearance and palatability. In cases where the drug is a gastric irritant or is broken down by gastric acid, an enteric coating may be used; this is designed to allow the tablet to remain intact in the stomach and to pass unchanged into the small bowel where the coating dissolves and the drug is released and absorbed.

Tablets may be formulated specifically to control the rate of release of drug from the tablet as it passes through the GI tract. Terms such as 'sustained release', 'controlled release' and

Table 12.10 **Considerations for specific types of administration**

Consideration	Rationale
Administer irritant drugs with meals or snacks	To minimize their effect on the gastric mucosa (Jordan et al. 2003, Shepherd 2002a)
Administer drugs that interact with food, or that are destroyed in significant proportions by digestive enzymes, between meals or on an empty stomach	To prevent interference with the absorption of the drug (Jordan et al. 2003, Shepherd 2002a)
Do not break a tablet unless it is scored and appropriate to do so. Break scored tablets with a file or a tablet cutter. Wash after use	Breaking may cause incorrect dosage, gastrointestinal irritation or destruction of a drug in an incompatible pH. To reduce risk of contamination between tablets (DH 2007, Jordan et al. 2003, NMC 2010a, Shepherd 2002a)
Do not interfere with time-release capsules and enteric-coated tablets. Ask patients to swallow these whole and not to chew them	The absorption rate of the drug will be altered (Jordan et al. 2003, Perry 2007)
Sublingual tablets must be placed under the tongue and buccal tablets between gum and cheek	To allow for correct absorption (Perry 2007)
When administering liquids to babies and young children, or when an accurately measured dose in multiples of 1 mL is needed for an adult, an oral syringe should be used in preference to a medicine spoon or measure	An oral syringe is much more accurate than a measure or a 5 mL spoon Use of a syringe makes administration of the correct dose much easier in an unco-operative child Oral syringes are available and are designed to be washable and reused for the same patient. However, in the immunocompromised patient single use only is recommended. Oral syringes must be clearly labelled for oral or enteral use only (DH 2007, NPSA 2007d)
In babies and children especially, correct use of the syringe is very important. The tip should be gently pushed into and towards the side of the mouth. The contents are then *slowly* discharged towards the inside of the cheek, pausing if necessary to allow the liquid to be swallowed. If children are unco-operative it may help to place the end of the barrel between the teeth	To prevent injury to the mouth and eliminate the danger of choking the patient (Watt 2003) To get the dose in and to prevent the patient spitting it out (Watt 2003)
When administering gargling medication, throat irrigations should not be warmer than body temperature	Liquid warmer than body temperature may cause discomfort or damage tissue

Figure 12.3 **Examples of oral medication.**

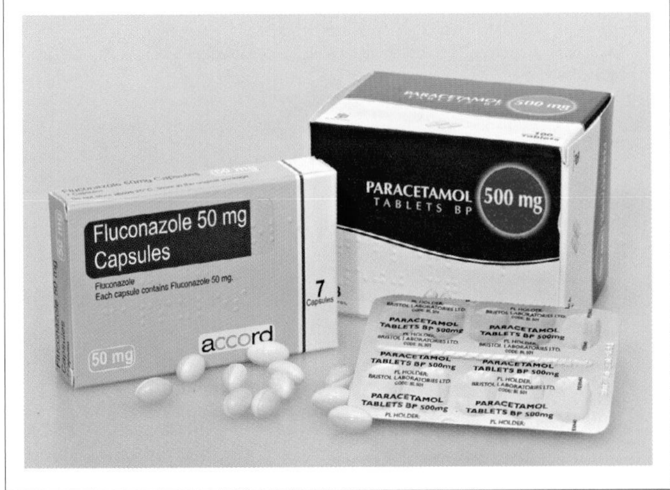

'modified release' are used by manufacturers to describe these preparations. Tablets may also be formulated specifically to dissolve readily ('soluble' or 'effervescent'), to be chewed or to be held under the tongue ('sublingual') or placed between the gum and inside of the mouth ('buccal'). Unscored or coated tablets should not be crushed or broken, nor should most 'modified-release' tablets, since this can affect the pharmacokinetic profile of the drug and may result in excessive peak plasma concentrations and side-effects (Smyth 2006).

Capsules

These offer a useful method of formulating drugs which are difficult to make into a tablet or are particularly unpalatable.

The capsule shells are usually made of gelatine and the contents of the capsules may be solid, liquid or of a paste-like consistency. The contents do not cause deterioration of the shell. The shell, however, is attacked by the digestive fluids and the contents are then released. Delayed-release capsule formulations also exist. Gastro-resistant capsules are delayed-release capsules that are intended to resist the gastric fluid and to release their active substance or substances in the intestinal fluid (British Pharmacopoeia 2007). If for any reason the capsule is unpalatable or the patient is unable to take it, the contents should not routinely be removed from the shell without first seeking advice from a pharmacist. Removing contents from the capsule could destroy their properties and cause gastric irritation or premature release of the drug into an incompatible pH (Downie et al. 2003).

Lozenges and pastilles

Lozenges and pastilles are solid, single-dose preparations intended to be sucked to obtain a local or systemic effect to the mouth and/or throat (British Pharmacopoeia 2007).

Linctuses, elixirs and mixtures

Linctuses

These are viscous oral liquids that may contain one or more active ingredients; the solution usually contains a high proportion of sucrose. Linctuses are intended for use in the treatment or relief of cough.

Elixirs

These are clear, flavoured oral liquids containing one or more active ingredients dissolved in a vehicle that usually contains a high proportion of sucrose. A vehicle is a substance usually without therapeutic action used to give bulk for the administration of medicines. If the active drug is sensitive to moisture, it may be formulated as a flavoured powder or granulation and then dissolved in water just before use.

Mixtures

Mixtures are usually aqueous preparations, containing one or more drug, which can be in the form of either a solution or a suspension. Mixtures are normally made up when required as they have a shelf-life of 2 weeks from preparation. Suspended drugs may slowly separate on standing but are easily redispersed by shaking so this should be done before every use.

Drugs suspended, mixed or dispersed in liquids are often referred to as syrups. However, syrups do not contain active ingredients but are used as a vehicle for medications in order to decrease crystallization, increase solubility and provide aromatic and flavouring properties (British Pharmacopoeia 2007).

EVIDENCE-BASED APPROACHES

Observational studies suggest that medication administration errors for oral medicine range from 3% to 8% (Ho et al. 1997, Taxis et al. 1999) but the rate has been found to be twice as high in mental health patients who have swallowing difficulties (Haw et al. 2007). A proportion of these difficulties are due to an aversion to swallowing tablets, the most common cause being dysphagia (Kelly and Wright 2009). Guidance on medicines management related to dysphagia can be found within the NMC *Standards for Medicines Management* (NMC 2010a). When giving medicines to patients with dysphagia, both the patient and the medicine should be reviewed on a regular basis. If patients cannot swallow tablets then liquid or dispersible medications should be the first consideration (Kelly and Wright 2009). If the oral route is not patent then alternative routes should be used.

Covert drug administration

The NMC recognizes that 'this is a complex issue', as covert drug administration involves the fundamental principles of patient and client autonomy and consent to treatment, which are set out in common law and statute and underpinned by the Human Rights Act 1998 (NMC 2010a). The covert administration of medicines should not be confused with the administration of medicines against someone's will, which in itself may not be deceptive but may be unlawful (NMC 2010a).

Some vulnerable groups of patients, such as those who are confused, may refuse to take medication. Traditionally, in some places, medication has therefore been hidden or disguised in food. The NMC (2001a, 2001b, 2010a) offered the following position statement.

> 'As a general principle, by disguising medication in food or drink, the patient or client is being led to believe that they are not receiving medication when in fact they are. The registered nurse, midwife or health visitor will need to be sure that what they are doing is in the best interests of the patient or client and be accountable for this decision.'

Disguising medication in food and drink is acceptable under exceptional circumstances in which covert administration may be considered to prevent a patient, who is incapable of informed consent, from missing out on essential treatment (NMC 2001a, NMC 2010a). The following principles should be followed when making such a decision.

- The medication must be considered essential for the patient's health and well-being.
- The decision to administer medication covertly should be considered only as a contingency in an emergency, not as regular practice.

- The registered practitioner must make the decision only after discussion and with the support of the multiprofessional team and, if appropriate, the patient's relatives, carers or advocates.
- The pharmacist must be involved in these decisions as adding medication to food or drink can alter its pharmacological properties and thereby affect its performance.
- The decision and action taken must be fully documented in the patient's care plan and regularly reviewed.
- Regular attempts should continue to be made to encourage the patient to take the medication voluntarily (NMC 2001a, NMC 2010a, Treloar et al. 2000).

PRE-PROCEDURAL CONSIDERATIONS

Equipment

Medicine pots

Medicine pots (Figure 12.4) allow a dosage form to be taken from its original container for immediate administration to a patient. The person who removes medication from its original container and places it into a medicine pot must oversee the administration of this medication. This responsibility cannot be transferred to someone else.

Tablet splitters

Commercially available tablet splitters (Figure 12.5) may increase the accuracy of tablet splitting when this activity is necessary. Tablets that are unscored, unusually thick or oddly shaped, sugar coated, enteric coated and modified-release tablets are not suitable for splitting. Areas for consideration when using a tablet splitter include the following.

- Can the tablets be split? This must always be discussed with the pharmacy department.
- Do patients have the manual dexterity to use a tablet splitter when at home?
- Will splitting the tablets affect patient adherence when they are at home? Will patients skip or double dose rather than split tablets?

Figure 12.4 **Medicine pot.**

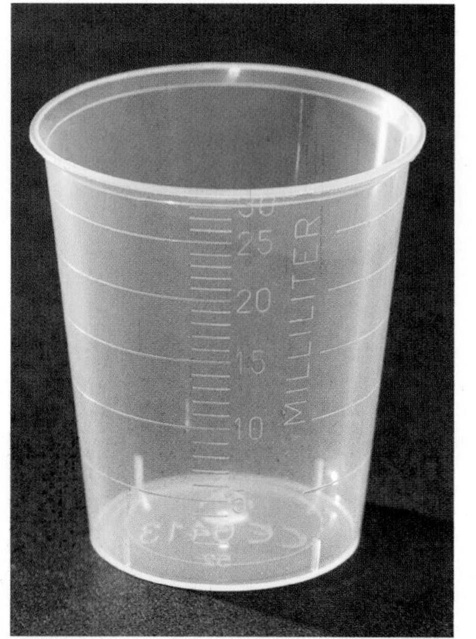

Figure 12.5 **Tablet splitter.**

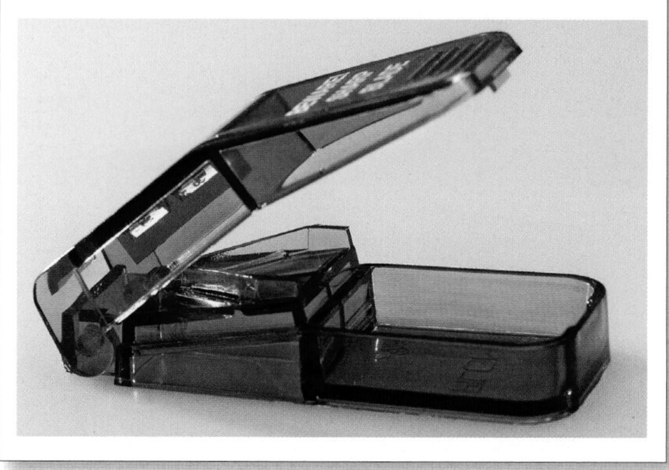

- How will the storage of split tablets affect the stability of the tablets? What about the effect of light and air (Marriott and Nation 2002)?

Tablet crushers

Tablet crushers (Figure 12.6) can be used when a patient has swallowing difficulties and no alternative dosage form exists. Crushing tablets is usually outside the product licence. The Medicines Act 1968 states that unlicensed medicines can only be authorized by a medical or dental practitioner, so if tablets are going to be crushed, there should be discussion and agreement between the prescriber and the person who will administer the medicine. Discussion should also take place with the pharmacist to check that the tablet is suitable for crushing and that the efficacy of the medication is not changed as a result. Tablets that are enteric coated, sustained release or chewable cannot be crushed. Areas for consideration when crushing a tablet include the following.

- Can the tablet be crushed? This must always be discussed with the pharmacy department.
- Will crushing make the tablet unpalatable?
- Will crushing the tablet cause any adverse effects for the patient, for example burning of the oral mucosa?

Figure 12.6 **Tablet crusher.**

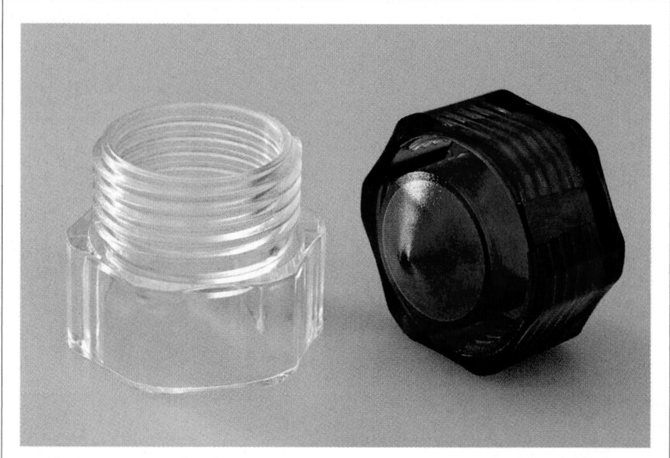

Figure 12.7 **Dosette box.**

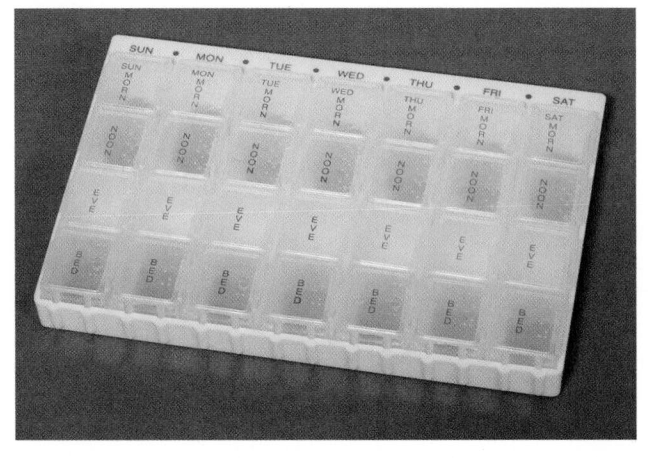

Figure 12.8 **Oral syringe (compliant with NPSA guidance).**

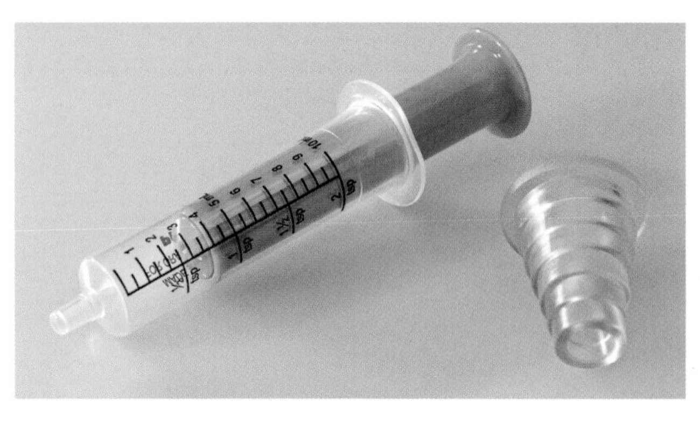

- Will crushing the tablet result in inaccurate dosing (Kelly and Wright 2009)?

When a tablet crusher is used, water should be added to the crushed tablet and the resulting solution drawn up using an oral syringe. The crusher should then be rinsed and the process repeated. Tablet crushers should be rinsed before and after use to prevent cross-contamination with other medicines (Fair and Proctor 2007, Smyth 2006).

When a tablet crusher has been used, it should be opened and washed under running water, dried with a tissue and left to air dry on a tissue or paper towel.

Monitored dosage systems and compliance aids

Monitored dosage systems and compliance aids, for example dosette boxes (Figure 12.7), are designed to help patients remember when to take their medication. They can also let carers know whether patients have taken their medication. The following should be considered when using these systems.

- They can only be used for tablets and capsules.
- Medicines that are susceptible to moisture should not be put in these systems.
- Light-sensitive medicines should not be put in these systems.
- Medicines that are harmful when handled should not be put in these systems.
- If the patient is on medications that cannot be stored in these systems, precautions should be put in place to ensure that they can cope with two systems.
- If the patient's drug regimen is not stable, consideration should be given to how easy it will be to make changes to the system.
- As-required medication cannot be placed in these systems.
- These systems comply with labelling and leaflet legislation so they must always be dispensed by a pharmacy department (RPSGB 2007b).

Oral syringes

If a syringe is needed to measure and administer an oral dose, an oral syringe (Figure 12.8) that cannot be attached to intravenous catheters or ports should be used. These syringes are purple in colour. All oral syringes containing oral liquid medicines must be labelled by the person who prepared the syringe with the name and strength of the medicine, the patient name and the time it was prepared. Labelling is unnecessary if the preparation and administration is one uninterrupted process and the labelled syringe does not leave the hands of the person who prepared it. Only one unlabelled syringe should be handled at any one time (NPSA 2007d).

Specific patient preparation

Before administering oral medication, the nurse should assess for:

- the patient's ability to understand the purpose of the medication being administered
- any medication allergies and hypersensitivities
- nil by mouth status
- the patient's ability to swallow the form of medication
- the patient's cough and gag reflexes
- any contraindications to oral medications including nausea and vomiting, absence of bowel sounds/reduced peristalsis, nasogastric suctioning or any circumstance affecting bowel motility or absorption of medication, for example general anaesthesia, GI surgery, inflammatory bowel disease
- any possibility of drug–drug or drug–food interactions
- any pre-administration assessment for specific medications, for example pulse or blood pressure (Chernecky et al. 2002, Potter 2011).

Procedure guideline 12.3 **Medication: oral drug administration**

Essential equipment

- Drugs to be administered
- Recording sheet or book as required by law or hospital policy
- Patient's prescription chart, to check dose, route and so on
- Glass of water
- Any protective clothing required by hospital policy for specified drugs, such as antibiotics or cytotoxic drugs, for example gloves
- Medicine container (disposable if possible)

(continued)

Procedure guideline 12.3 **Medication: oral drug administration *(continued)***

Action	Rationale
Pre-procedure	
1 Wash hands with bactericidal soap and water or bactericidal alcohol handrub.	To minimize the risk of cross-infection (DH 2007, **C**; Fraise and Bradley 2009, **E**).
2 Before administering any prescribed drug, check that it is due and has not already been given. Make any required assessments such as pulse, BP or respiration. Check that the information contained in the prescription chart is complete, correct and legible.	To protect the patient from harm (DH 2003b, **C**; NMC 2010a, **C**). These are required to ensure the patient is fit enough to receive medication, for example BP before antihypertensives (Chernecky et al. 2002, **E**).
3 Before administering any prescribed drug, look at the patient's prescription chart and check the following. (a) The correct patient (b) Drug (c) Dose (d) Date and time of administration (e) Route and method of administration (f) Diluent as appropriate (g) Validity of prescription (h) Signature of prescriber (i) The prescription is legible	To ensure that the correct patient is given the correct drug in the prescribed dose using the appropriate diluent and by the correct route (DH 2003b, **C**; NMC 2010a, **C**). To protect the patient from harm (DH 2003b, **C**; NMC 2010a, **C**).
If any of these pieces of information are missing, are unclear or illegible then the nurse should not proceed with administration and should consult with the prescriber.	To prevent any errors occurring. **E**
Procedure	
4 Select the required medication and check the expiry date.	Treatment with medication that is outside the expiry date is dangerous. Drugs deteriorate with storage. The expiry date indicates when a particular drug is no longer pharmacologically efficacious (DH 2003b, **C**; NMC 2010a, **C**).
5 Empty the required dose into a medicine container. Avoid touching the preparation.	To minimize the risk of cross-infection. To minimize the risk of harm to the nurse (DH 2007, **C**; Fraise and Bradley 2009, **E**).
6 Take the medication and the prescription chart to the patient. Check the patient's identity by asking the patient to state their full name and date of birth. If the patient is unable to confirm details then check patient identity band against prescription chart. Check the patient's allergy status by asking them or by checking the nameband.	To ensure that the medication is administered to the correct patient and prevent any errors related to drug allergies (NPSA 2005, **C**).
7 Evaluate the patient's knowledge of the medication being offered by asking them to tell you what the medication is for and what side-effects to expect. If this knowledge appears to be faulty or incorrect, offer an explanation of the use, action, dose and potential side-effects of the drug or drugs involved.	A patient has a right to information about treatment (NMC 2010a, **C**; NMC 2015, **C**). To ensure that the patient understands the procedure and gives their valid consent (Griffith and Jordan 2003, **E**; NMC 2013, **C**; NMC 2015, **C**).
8 Assist the patient to a sitting position where possible. A side-lying position may also be used if the patient is unable to sit.	To ease swallowing and prevent aspiration (Chernecky et al. 2002, **E**).
9 Administer the drug as prescribed.	To meet legal requirements and hospital policy (DH 2003b, **C**; NMC 2010a, **C**; NMC 2010b, **C**; NMC 2015, **C**).
10 Offer a glass of water, if allowed, assisting the patient where necessary.	To facilitate swallowing of the medication (Chernecky et al. 2002, **E**; Jordan et al. 2003, **E**).
11 Stay with the patient until they have swallowed all the medication.	To ensure that medication has been taken on time (Chernecky et al. 2002, **E**).
Post-procedure	
12 Record the dose given and sign the prescription chart and in any other place made necessary by legal requirement or hospital policy.	To meet legal requirements and hospital policy (DH 2003b, **C**; NMC 2010a, **C**; NMC 2010b, **C**; NMC 2015, **C**).

Problem-solving table 12.1 **Prevention and resolution (Procedure guideline 12.3)**

Problem	Cause	Prevention	Action
Patient vomits when taking or after taking tablets.	Patient suffering from nausea.	Administer antiemetics prior to administration of tablets. These may need to be given via rectal, IM or IV route.	If patient vomits immediately after tablet swallowed then it may be given again (maybe after antiemetics). If patient vomits some time after tablet taken, it may depend on type and frequency of medication as to whether it can be retaken. Patients are advised to retake their medication if they can see a whole tablet in vomit.
Patient unable to swallow tablets.	Patient suffering from dysphagia or has issues swallowing tablets.	Discuss with pharmacy regarding availability of medication in liquid form.	Discuss with prescriber as to administering the medicine in another form or route.

Learning Activity 12.5

Scenario: Drug administration

You have been asked to give some oral medication to a patient you are looking after.

What should you check before administering the medication?

See the end of the chapter for the answers.

Topical administration

DEFINITION

Medication applied onto the skin and mucous membranes primarily for its local effects, for example creams, ointments and patches (Potter 2011).

RELATED THEORY

Creams

Creams are emulsions of oil and water and are generally well absorbed into the skin. They are usually more cosmetically acceptable than ointments because they are less greasy and easier to apply (BNF 2014). They may be used as a 'base' in which a variety of drugs may be applied for local therapy (BNF 2014).

Ointments

Ointments are greasy preparations, which are normally anhydrous and insoluble in water, and are more occlusive than creams (BNF 2014). They are absorbed more slowly into the skin and leave a greasy residue. They have similar uses to creams and are particularly suitable for dry, scaly lesions (BNF 2014).

Lotions

Lotions have a cooling effect and may be preferred to ointments or creams for application over a hairy area (BNF 2014).

Pastes

These are stiff preparations containing a high proportion of finely powdered solids such as zinc oxide suspended in ointment. They are less occlusive than ointments and can be used to protect inflamed or excoriated skin (BNF 2014, Potter 2011).

Wound products

See Chapter 14: Wound management.

EVIDENCE-BASED APPROACHES

The risk of serious effects is generally low but systemic effects can occur if the skin is thin, if drug concentration is high or contact is prolonged (Potter 2011).

PRE-PROCEDURAL CONSIDERATIONS

Specific patient preparation

The condition of the affected site should be assessed for altered skin integrity as applying medicines to broken skin could cause them to be absorbed too rapidly, resulting in systemic effects (Chernecky et al. 2002, Potter 2011). The affected area must be washed and dried before applying the topical medicines where appropriate, unless the prescription directs otherwise.

Procedure guideline 12.4 **Medication: topical applications**

Essential equipment

- Disposable plastic apron
- Clean non-sterile gloves
- Sterile topical swabs
- Applicators

Pre-procedure

Action	Rationale
1 Wash hands with bactericidal soap and water or bactericidal alcohol handrub.	To minimize the risk of cross-infection (DH 2007, **C**; Fraise and Bradley 2009, **E**).
2 Before administering any prescribed drug, look at the patient's prescription chart and check the following. (a) The correct patient (b) Drug	To ensure that the correct patient is given the correct drug in the prescribed dose using the appropriate diluent and by the correct route (DH 2003b, **C**; NMC 2010a, **C**). To protect the patient from harm (DH 2003b, **C**; NMC 2010a, **C**).

(continued)

Procedure guideline 12.4 Medication: topical applications *(continued)*

Action	Rationale
(c) Dose (d) Date and time of administration (e) Route and method of administration (f) Diluent as appropriate (g) Validity of prescription (h) Signature of prescriber (i) The prescription is legible	
If any of these pieces of information are missing, are unclear or illegible then the nurse should not proceed with administration and should consult with the prescriber.	To prevent any errors occurring. **E**
3 Explain and discuss the procedure with the patient.	To ensure that the patient understands the procedure and gives their valid consent (Griffith and Jordan 2003, **E**; NMC 2013, **C**; NMC 2015, **C**).
Procedure	
4 Put on a plastic apron and assist the patient into the required position.	To protect the patient from infection and the nurse from the topical agent as well as allowing access to the affected area of skin. **E**
5 Close room door or curtains if appropriate.	To ensure patient privacy and dignity. **E**
6 Expose the area that requires the lotion and where necessary cover the patient with a towel or sheet.	To gain access to affected area and to ensure patient dignity. **E**
7 Apply gloves and assess the condition of the skin using aseptic technique if the skin is broken.	To prevent local or systemic infection (DH 2007, **C**; Fraise and Bradley 2009, **E**).
8 If the medication is to be rubbed into the skin, the preparation should be placed on a sterile topical swab.	To minimize the risk of cross-infection. To protect the nurse (DH 2007, **C**; Fraise and Bradley 2009, **E**).
9 If the preparation causes staining, advise the patient of this.	To ensure that adequate precautions are taken beforehand such as removal of clothing and to prevent stains (NMC 2015, **C**).
10 Apply the ointment.	To ensure the medication is applied. **E**
11 Apply a sterile dressing if required.	To ensure the ointment remains in place (Chernecky et al. 2002, **E**).
Post-procedure	
12 Remove gloves and apron and dispose of waste appropriately.	To ensure safe disposal and prevent reuse of equipment (DH 2005, **C**; MHRA 2004, **C**).
13 Record the administration on appropriate charts.	To maintain accurate records, provide a point of reference in the event of any queries and prevent any duplication of treatment (NMC 2010a, **C**; NMC 2010b, **C**).

POST-PROCEDURAL CONSIDERATIONS

Educate the patient to inform the nurse if there is any itching, skin colour change or signs of a rash following application.

COMPLICATIONS

Local skin reaction

The skin site may appear inflamed and oedema with blistering indicates that subacute inflammation or eczema has developed from worsening of skin lesions. Patients may also complain of pruritus and tenderness which could indicate slow or impaired healing and should be referred to the prescriber; alternative therapies may be required (Potter 2011).

Transdermal administration

DEFINITION

Medication applied to the outermost layer of the skin, the stratum corneum, usually as an adhesive medicated disc that allows the medication to be absorbed at a slow and constant rate in order to produce a systemic effect (Chernecky et al. 2002).

RELATED THEORY

Conventional transdermal systems

These consist of a gel or ointment which is measured and placed directly onto the skin. Drugs that are used in this way include

Figure 12.9 **Transdermal patches.**

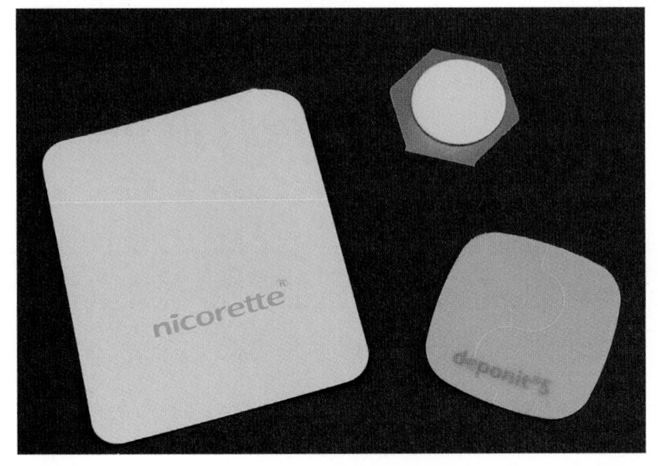

glyceryl trinitrate and oestradiol. Delivering drugs in this way can be messy for patients and can also result in variations of the dose delivered due to the amount applied, the amount of rubbing in of the product, the amount of product transferred onto clothing and so on.

Transdermal patches

A transdermal patch (Figure 12.9) contains a certain amount of drug and delivers it in a quantity which is sufficient to cause the desired pharmacological effect when it crosses the skin and into the systemic system. Drugs which can be delivered in a transdermal system include fentanyl, hyoscine, nicotine and oestradiol (Hillery et al. 2001).

Three types of transdermal patch are available.

Adhesive

These are simply designed patches which consist of a drug-containing adhesive and a backing material. These patches do not provide much control over the rate of delivery and in most cases the stratum corneum controls the rate (Hillery et al. 2001).

Layered or matrix patches

Layered patches consist of a drug-containing matrix, an adhesive layer and a backing material. The drug-containing matrix controls the release of drug from the system (Hillery et al. 2001).

Reservoir

Reservoir patches consist of an enclosed reservoir of drug, a membrane layer, an adhesive layer and a backing material. The membrane layer controls the rate of drug delivery from the reservoir of drug.

EVIDENCE-BASED APPROACHES

The advantages of transdermal systems are the avoidance of the presystemic metabolism, the drug effects can be maintained within the therapeutic window for longer which reduces side-effects and maintains constant dosing, there can be improved patient compliance and drug effects can be stopped with the withdrawal of the patch and avoidance of first-pass metabolism (Hillery et al. 2001). First-pass metabolism occurs when a drug passes through the digestive system and enters the hepatic portal system and the liver before it reaches the rest of the body. The liver metabolizes many drugs, thus reducing their bioavailability before reaching the rest of the circulatory system (Hardman et al. 1996).

A disadvantage of transdermal systems is the limited number of drugs for which the system is suitable; for example, drugs have to have a suitable potency to allow them to absorb across the skin and cause an effect. Tolerance-inducing drugs would need a period during which they were not administered, which is not always possible with transdermal systems. In addition, drugs to be used in transdermal systems cannot be irritating to the skin otherwise they would not be tolerated by patients (Hillery et al. 2001).

PRE-PROCEDURAL CONSIDERATIONS

Specific patient preparation

The condition of the affected site should be assessed for altered skin integrity as applying medicines to broken skin could cause too rapid absorption, resulting in systemic effects (Chernecky et al. 2002, Potter 2011). The affected area must be washed and dried before applying the patch, which should be attached to hairless areas of skin. The upper chest, upper arms and upper back are recommended sites and the distal areas of extremities should be avoided (Chernecky et al. 2002). Patches should not be trimmed or cut.

Procedure guideline 12.5 **Medication: transdermal applications**

Essential equipment

- Clean non-sterile gloves
- Disposable plastic apron
- Transdermal patch

Pre-procedure

Action	Rationale
1 Wash hands with bactericidal soap and water or bactericidal alcohol handrub.	To minimize the risk of cross-infection (DH 2007, **C**; Fraise and Bradley 2009, **E**).
2 Before administering any prescribed drug, look at the patient's prescription chart and check the following. (a) The correct patient (b) Drug (c) Dose (d) Date and time of administration (e) Route and method of administration (f) Diluent as appropriate (g) Validity of prescription (h) Signature of prescriber (i) The prescription is legible	To ensure that the correct patient is given the correct drug in the prescribed dose using the appropriate diluent and by the correct route (DH 2003b, **C**; NMC 2010a, **C**). To protect the patient from harm (DH 2003b, **C**; NMC 2010a, **C**).

(continued)

Procedure guideline 12.5 Medication: transdermal applications *(continued)*

Action	Rationale
If any of these pieces of information are missing, are unclear or illegible then the nurse should not proceed with administration and should consult with the prescriber.	To prevent any errors occurring. **E**
3 Explain and discuss the procedure with the patient.	To ensure that the patient understands the procedure and gives their valid consent (Griffith and Jordan 2003, **E**; NMC 2013, **C**; NMC 2015, **C**).
Procedure	
4 Put on a plastic apron and assist the patient into the required position.	To allow access to the affected area of skin. **E**
5 Close room door or curtains if appropriate.	To ensure patient privacy and dignity. **E**
6 Expose the area where the patch will be applied and where necessary cover the patient with a towel or sheet.	To gain access to affected area and to ensure patient privacy and dignity. **E**
7 Apply gloves and assess the condition of the skin and do not apply to skin that is oily, burnt, cut or irritated in any way.	To prevent local or systemic infection (DH 2007, **C**; Fraise and Bradley 2009, **E**). To prevent local or systemic effects and to ensure the patch will remain in place (DH 2007, **C**; Potter 2011, **E**).
8 Where necessary, remove the used patch and fold it in half, adhesive side inwards, place in the original sachet and dispose into clinical waste.	To ensure that the release membrane is not exposed. **E**
9 Remove any drug residue from the former site before placing the next patch.	To avoid any skin irritation (Chernecky et al. 2002, **E**).
10 Carefully remove the patch from its protective cover and hold it by the edge without touching the adhesive edges.	To ensure the patch will adhere and the medication dose will not be affected (Potter 2011, **E**).
11 Apply the patch immediately, pressing firmly with the palm of the hand for up to 10 seconds, making sure the patch sticks well around the edges.	To ensure adequate adhesion and prevent loss of patch which would result in reduced dose and effectiveness (Potter 2011, **E**).
12 Date and initial the patch.	To ensure all staff know when it must be changed (Potter 2011, **E**).
Post-procedure	
13 Remove and dispose of waste in appropriate waste bags.	To ensure safe disposal and prevent reuse of equipment.
14 Record the administration on appropriate charts.	To maintain accurate records, provide a point of reference in the event of any queries and prevent any duplication of treatment (NMC 2010a, **C**; NMC 2010b, **C**).

POST-PROCEDURAL CONSIDERATIONS

Ongoing care

A different skin site should be used each time to avoid skin irritation (Chernecky et al. 2002). After use, the patch still contains substantial quantities of active ingredients which may have harmful effects if they reach the aquatic environment. Hence, after removal, the used patch should be folded in half, adhesive side inwards so that the release membrane is not exposed, placed in the original sachet and then discarded safely out of reach of children. Any used or unused patches should be discarded according to local policy or returned to the pharmacy. Used patches should not be flushed down the toilet or placed in liquid waste disposal systems (www.medicines.org.uk).

COMPLICATIONS

See 'Topical applications'.

Rectal administration

DEFINITION

These preparations are administered via the rectum which may exert a local effect on the GI mucosa, e.g. anti-inflammatory in ulcerative colitis or systemic effects, e.g. analgesics or to relieve vomiting (Potter 2011).

RELATED THEORY

Suppositories

Suppositories are solid preparations which may contain one or more drug. The drugs are normally ground or sieved and then dissolved or dispersed into a glyceride-type fatty acid or water-soluble base. These suppositories will either melt after insertion into the body or dissolve and mix with the available volume of rectal fluid (Aulton 1988).

Enemas

Enemas are solutions or dispersions of a drug in a small volume of water or oil. These preparations are presented in a small plastic container made of a bulb which contains the drug and an application tube. The bulb can be compressed when the tube has been inserted in the rectum to deliver the drug. Enemas can be difficult for patients to use by themselves compared to suppositories and therefore their use is not as widespread (Aulton 1988).

EVIDENCE-BASED APPROACHES

The advantages of rectal administration include the following.

- The drug can be administered when the patient cannot use the oral route, for example if the patient is vomiting or is post-operative and therefore either unconscious or unable to ingest via the oral route.
- In some categories of patient, it may be easier to use the rectal route than the oral one as it does not require swallowing, for example children, the elderly.
- The drug may be less suited to the oral route; for example, the oral route can cause severe local GI side-effects. The drug may not be stable after GI administration or it may have an unacceptable taste which makes it unpalatable via the oral route.
- Rarely cause local irritation or side-effects (Chernecky et al. 2002, Potter 2011).

The disadvantages of the rectal route include the following.

- Strong feelings against the rectal route by some patients in some countries and also feelings of discomfort and embarrassment.
- There can be slow and incomplete absorption via the rectal route.
- The development of proctitis has been reported with rectal drug administration.
- Contraindicated in patients who have had rectal surgery or have active rectal bleeding (Chernecky et al. 2002, Downie et al. 2003, Potter 2011).

After a suppository is inserted into the rectum, body temperature melts the suppository so the medication can be distributed. Proper placement is important to promote retention of the medication until it dissolves and is absorbed into the mucosa (Potter 2011).

For further information about the administration of rectal medication, see Chapter 5, Procedure guideline 5.15: Suppository administration.

Vaginal administration

DEFINITION

Medications are inserted into the vaginal canal usually for local effects such as treatment of infections (e.g. *Trichomonas* and *Candida* infections) and contraceptive purposes. They are used less commonly for systemic effects (such as oestrogens and progesterones) (Chernecky et al. 2002, Potter 2011).

RELATED THEORY

Vaginal preparations can be delivered in a wide variety of dosage forms including pessaries, creams, aerosol foams, gels and tablets (Chernecky et al. 2002, Potter 2011).

EVIDENCE-BASED APPROACHES

The advantages of the vaginal route include the following.

- The vagina offers a large surface area for drug absorption.
- A rich blood supply ensures a rapid absorption of drug.
- This route can act as an alternative for drugs that cannot be delivered via the oral route (as for suppositories).
- This route can be used when patients cannot take drugs via the oral route (as for suppositories).
- The vaginal route can deliver drug over a controlled period of time, thus avoiding peaks and troughs which result in less toxicity and risk of ineffectiveness.

The disadvantages include the following.

- The route is limited to drugs that are potent molecules and are therefore easily absorbed.
- The vagina can be easily irritated by the use of devices or locally irritating drugs.
- Care must be taken with the use of vaginal devices to ensure they are sterilized and not acting as a growth medium for bacteria.
- The vaginal bioavailability can be affected by hormone levels and can therefore change during menstrual cycles, with age and during pregnancy.
- Leakage can occur with vaginal preparations. This can be alleviated by using the preparation at night.
- This route may not be acceptable to some patients (Hillery et al. 2001).

PRE-PROCEDURAL CONSIDERATIONS

Specific patient preparation

Check patient for any allergies and also whether they have recently given birth or undergone vaginal surgery as this may alter tissue integrity and the level of discomfort. The nurse should also review the patient's willingness and ability to self-administer the medication (Chernecky et al. 2002, Potter 2011).

Procedure guideline 12.6 **Medication: vaginal administration**

Essential equipment

- Disposable gloves
- Topical swabs
- Disposable sanitary pad
- Lubricating jelly
- Prescription chart
- Warm water
- Pen torch
- Disposable plastic apron

Medicinal products

- Pessary

Pre-procedure

Action	Rationale
1 Wash hands with bactericidal soap and water or bactericidal alcohol handrub.	To minimize the risk of cross-infection (DH 2007, **C**; Fraise and Bradley 2009, **E**).
2 Explain and discuss the procedure with the patient.	To ensure that the patient understands the procedure and gives her valid consent (Griffith and Jordan 2003, **E**; NMC 2013, **C**; NMC 2015, **C**).

(continued)

Procedure guideline 12.6 Medication: vaginal administration *(continued)*

Action	Rationale
3 Before administering any prescribed drug, look at the patient's prescription chart and check the following. (a) The correct patient (b) Drug (c) Dose (d) Date and time of administration (e) Route and method of administration (f) Diluent as appropriate (g) Validity of prescription (h) Signature of prescriber (i) The prescription is legible	To ensure that the correct patient is given the correct drug in the prescribed dose using the appropriate diluent and by the correct route (DH 2003b, **C**; NMC 2010a, **C**). To protect the patient from harm (DH 2003b, **C**; NMC 2010a, **C**).
If any of these pieces of information are missing, are unclear or illegible then the nurse should not proceed with administration and should consult with the prescriber.	To prevent any errors occurring. **E**
4 Select the appropriate pessary and check it with the prescription chart.	To ensure that the correct medication is given to the correct patient at the appropriate time (NMC 2010a, **C**).
Procedure	
5 Close room door or curtains, keeping the patient covered as much as possible.	To ensure patient privacy and dignity. **E**
6 Apply an apron and assist the patient into the appropriate position, either left lateral with buttocks to the edge of the bed or supine with the knees drawn up and legs parted. May require a light source, e.g. lamp or torch.	To facilitate easy access to the vaginal canal, visualize the external genitalia and vaginal canal and facilitate correct insertion of the pessary (manufacturer's instruction, **C**; Chernecky et al. 2002, **E**; Potter 2011, **E**).
7 Wash hands with bactericidal soap and water or bactericidal alcohol handrub, and put on gloves.	To minimize the risk of cross-infection (DH 2007, **C**; Fraise and Bradley 2009, **E**).
8 Clean the area with warm water if necessary.	To remove any previously applied creams (Downie et al. 2003, **E**).
9 Remove the pessary from the wrapper and apply lubricating jelly to a topical swab and from the swab on to the pessary. Lubricate gloved index finger of dominant hand.	To facilitate insertion of the pessary and ensure the patient's comfort (manufacturer's instruction, **C**).
10 With non-dominant gloved hand, gently retract labial folds to expose vaginal orifice.	To enable insertion of pessary into correct orifice (Potter 2011, **E**).
11 Insert the rounded end of the pessary along the posterior vaginal wall and into the top of the vagina (entire length of finger).	To ensure the pessary is inserted into the correct position to ensure equal distribution of medication (Potter 2011, **E**). To ensure that the pessary is retained and that the medication can reach its maximum efficiency (manufacturer's instruction, **C**; Chernecky et al. 2002, **E**).
12 Wipe away any excess lubricating jelly from the patient's vulval and/or perineal area with a topical swab.	To promote patient comfort (Potter 2011, **E**).
13 Make the patient comfortable and explain to her that there may be a small amount of discharge and apply a clean sanitary pad.	To absorb any excess discharge (Potter 2011, **E**).
Post-procedure	
14 Remove and dispose of gloves and apron safely and in accordance with locally approved procedures.	To ensure safe disposal (DH 2005, **C**; MHRA 2004, **C**).
15 Record the administration on appropriate charts.	To maintain accurate records, provide a point of reference in the event of any queries and prevent any duplication of treatment (NMC 2010a, **C**; NMC 2010b, **C**).

POST-PROCEDURAL CONSIDERATIONS

The patient needs to retain the medication so it is recommended that the medication is administered prior to going to bed or the patient should remain supine for 5–10 minutes after instilling the pessary (Chernecky et al. 2002, Potter 2011). It should be explained to the patient that she may also notice a discharge following administration and that it is nothing to be concerned about.

Pulmonary administration

DEFINITION

'Dosage forms introduced into the body via the lungs in an aerosol form to achieve local effects such as to improve bronchodilation or to improve clearance of pulmonary secretions' (Chernecky et al. 2002, Potter 2011). Systemic effects can also be achieved through the pulmonary route, for example volatile anaesthetics (Hillery et al. 2001). Some are inhaled via the mouth, some via the nose and some via nose and mouth (Downie et al. 2003).

RELATED THEORY

In order for drugs to reach the lungs, they must be delivered in an aerosol form. The aerosol penetrates the lung airways and the deeper passages of the respiratory tract provide a large surface area for drug absorption and the alveolar-capillary network absorbs medication rapidly (Potter 2011).

There are three ways in which this aerosol can be produced: by nebulizer, by pressurized metered dose inhalers and by drug powder inhalers.

- *Nebulization* involves the passage of air or oxygen driven through a solution of a drug. The resulting fine mist is then inhaled via a facemask (Trounce and Gould 2000). Some antibiotics and bronchodilators may be given in this way (Figure 12.10).
- *Metered dose inhalers* (MDI) involve a drug being suspended in a propellant in a small hand-held aerosol can in the form of a spray, mist or fine powder. Metered doses can then be delivered from the aerosol by the use of a metering valve within the device which is designed to release a fixed volume, for example Ventolin. Steroid medications are often administered by MDI to treat long-term reactive airway disease (Chernecky et al. 2002, Potter 2011) (Figure 12.11).

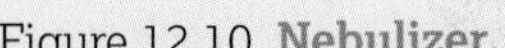

Figure 12.10 **Nebulizer.**

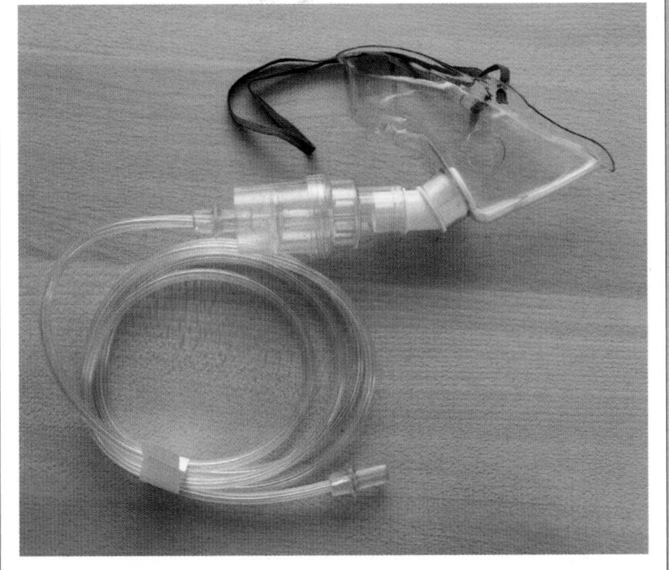

Figure 12.11 **Metered dose inhaler (MDI).**

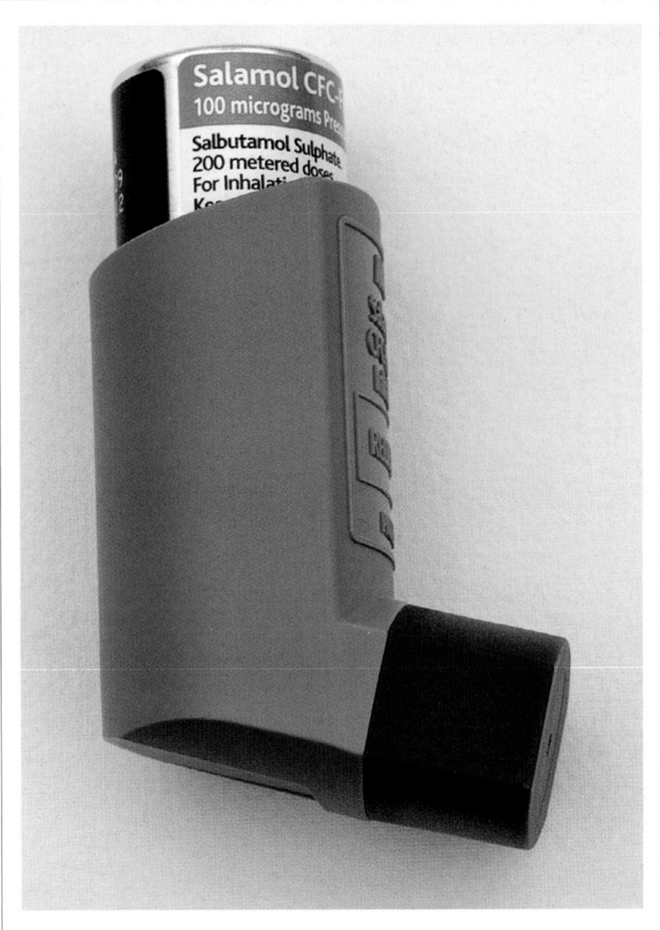

- *Dry powder inhalers* (DPI) involve a powder being delivered to the lung via a breath-actuated device. Examples of inhalers in this group are the Accuhaler (Figure 12.12) and the Turbohaler (Figure 12.13).

PRE-PROCEDURAL CONSIDERATIONS

Equipment

Nebulizer

The advantage of nebulizers is that they can deliver more drug to the lungs than standard inhalers because of the smaller particles that are generated. They also do not require any co-ordination in order to deliver the drug to the lungs. The disadvantages are that they are expensive, they are not easily portable and the delivery of drug can be difficult to control, for example due to loss in the tubing and mouthpiece.

Metered dose inhaler (MDI)

The advantages of MDIs are that they are convenient, can deliver a fixed dose and are inexpensive. The disadvantage can be the co-ordination needed to use one. In order to be effective, the patient needs to trigger the MDI during a deep slow inhalation and then hold their breath for around 10 seconds. This need for co-ordination between actuation of the dose and inhalation can be removed by using a spacer device (Figure 12.14). The spacer device reduces the speed with which the dose is delivered and the resultant 'cold freon' effect that can occur, which can prevent a patient from continuing to inhale after actuation of the

Figure 12.12 **Accuhaler.**

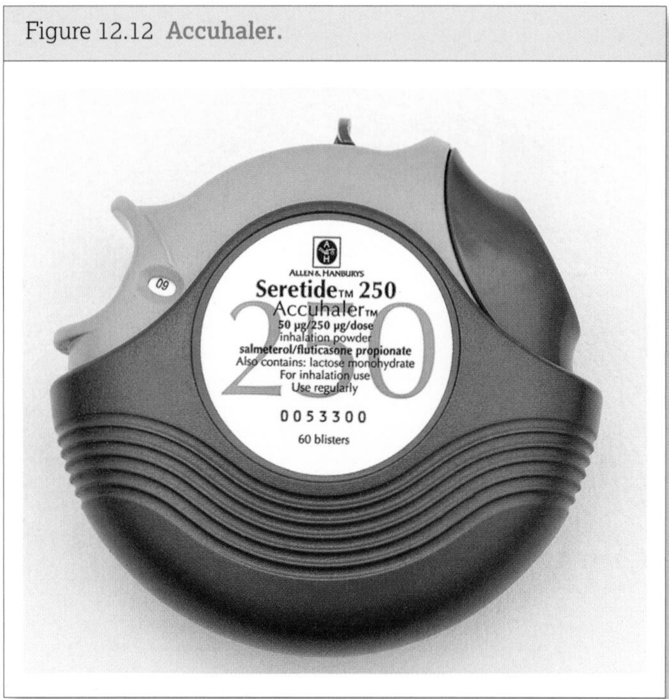

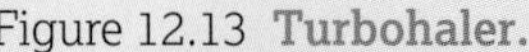

Figure 12.13 **Turbohaler.**

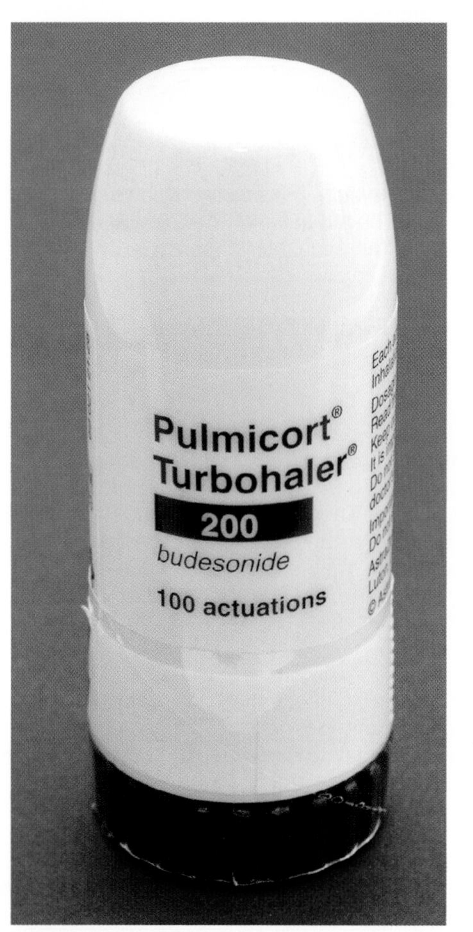

Figure 12.14 **Spacer device.**

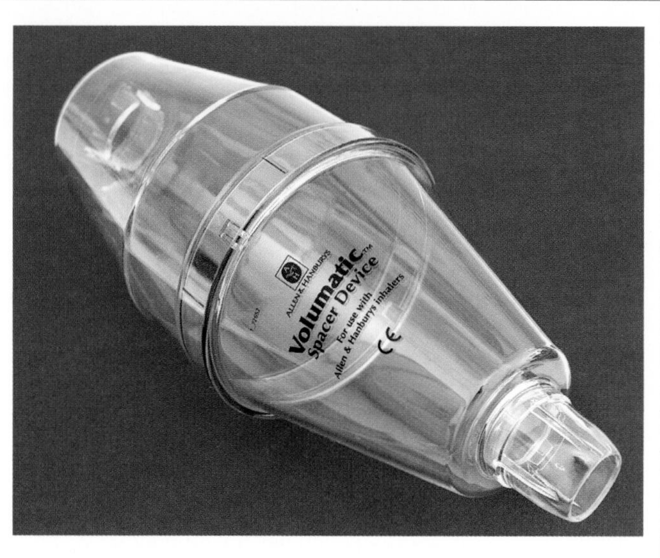

MDI. Spacers are also useful for patients on high-dose inhaled steroids in order to prevent oral candidiasis, for children and patients requiring higher doses, and can improve dose delivery to 15% (Downie et al. 2003). Spacer devices are designed to be compatible with specific inhalers and therefore care should be taken to ensure the correct spacer device is used.

Medication in MDIs is under pressure and so they should not be punctured or stored near heat or in hot conditions (e.g. patients must be informed not to leave their MDI in a hot car) (Chernecky et al. 2002).

Dry powder inhalers (DPI)

Dry powder inhalers are also useful when there are problems with co-ordination. However, they can initiate a cough reflex and patients need to have sufficient breath inhalation to activate the device.

It is also important to remember that because these medications are absorbed rapidly through the pulmonary circulation, most create systemic side-effects (Chernecky et al. 2002, Potter 2011).

Specific patient preparation

Patients who suffer from chronic respiratory disease and require airway management frequently receive inhalational medications. Maximum benefit is obtained only when the correct technique of inhalation is used so it is vital that patients are taught how to use these devices correctly and safely. Periodic checks should be carried out to ensure that efficiency is being maintained. Use of an MDI requires co-ordination during the breathing cycle and impairment of grasp or presence of tremors of the hands interferes with patient ability to depress the canister within the inhaler (Chernecky et al. 2002, Potter 2011). Studies have shown that both adults and children have difficulties with aerosol inhalers and problems include co-ordinating activation and inhalation, too rapid inhalation and too short breaths after inspiration (Hilton 1990). Baseline observations of pulse, respirations and breath sounds should be performed before beginning treatment to use as a comparison during and after treatment (Potter 2011). Patients who are to receive nebulized medicines should be in a sitting position either in bed or a chair (Downie et al. 2003).

Education

Compliance is more likely to be achieved if the patient is well informed. It is the responsibilty of the nurse, doctor and pharmacists to ensure that patients have adequate teaching and demonstration and are monitored at intervals. The patient should know the following.

- About the disease, the purpose of the therapy, how to recognize and report deterioration in the condition.
- How to use and care for the inhaler.
- The dose to be taken.
- The time interval.
- The maximum number of inhalations which should be taken in 24 hours (Downie et al. (2003).

Procedure guideline 12.7 Medication: administration by inhalation using a metered dose inhaler

Essential equipment

- MDI device
- Spacer device

Pre-procedure

Action	Rationale
1 Wash hands with bactericidal soap and water or bactericidal alcohol handrub.	To minimize the risk of cross-infection (DH 2007, **C**; Fraise and Bradley 2009, **E**).
2 Explain and discuss the procedure with the patient.	To ensure that the patient understands the procedure and gives their valid consent (Griffith and Jordan 2003, **E**; NMC 2013, **C**; NMC 2015, **C**).
3 Correct use of inhalers is essential (see manufacturer's information leaflet) and will be achieved only if this is carefully explained and demonstrated to the patient. If further advice is required, contact the hospital pharmacist.	Incorrect use may result in most of the dose remaining in the mouth and/or being expelled almost immediately. This renders treatment ineffective (Watt 2003, **E**; manufacturer's instructions, **C**).
Procedure	
4 Sit the patient in an upright position if possible in the bed or a chair.	To permit full expansion of the diaphragm. **E**
5 Before administering any prescribed drug, look at the patient's prescription chart and check the following. (a) The correct patient (b) Drug (c) Dose (d) Date and time of administration (e) Route and method of administration (f) Diluent as appropriate (g) Validity of prescription (h) Signature of prescriber (i) The prescription is legible	To ensure that the correct patient is given the correct drug in the prescribed dose using the appropriate diluent and by the correct route (DH 2003b, **C**; NMC 2010a, **C**). To protect the patient from harm (DH 2003b, **C**; NMC 2010a, **C**).
If any of these pieces of information are missing, are unclear or illegible then the nurse should not proceed with administration and should consult with the prescriber.	To prevent any errors occurring. **E**
6 Remove mouthpiece cover from inhaler.	To expose the area for use. **E**
7 Shake inhaler well for 2–5 seconds.	To ensure mixing of medication in canister (Potter 2011, **E**).
8 *Without a spacer device:* Ask patient to take a deep breath and exhale completely, open lips and place inhaler mouthpiece in mouth with opening toward back of throat, closing lips tightly around it.	Prepares airway to receive medication and directs aerosol towards airway (Potter 2011, **E**).
With a spacer device: Insert MDI into end of the spacer device. Ask the patient to exhale and then grasp spacer mouthpiece with teeth and lips while holding inhaler.	To enable the medication to reach the airways instead of hitting the back of the throat. The spacer improves delivery of correct dose of inhaled medication. **E**
9 Ask the patient to tip head back slightly, inhale slowly and deeply through the mouth whilst depressing canister fully.	To allow medication to be distrubted to airways during inhalation. **E**
10 Instruct the patient to breathe in slowly for 2–3 seconds and hold their breath for approximately 10 seconds, then remove MDI from mouth (if not using spacer) before exhaling slowly through pursed lips.	To enable aerosol spray to reach deeper branches of airways (Chernecky et al. 2002, **E**).

(continued)

Procedure guideline 12.7 Medication: administration by inhalation using a metered dose inhaler *(continued)*

Action	Rationale
11 Instruct the patient to wait 20–30 seconds between inhalations (if same medication) or 2–5 minutes between inhalations (if different medication). Always administer bronchodilators before steroids.	To ensure that the medication has optimum effect and minimal side-effects. **E**
12 If steroid medication is administered, ask the patient to rinse their mouth with water approximately 2 minutes after inhaling the dose.	To remove any medication residue from oral cavity area. Steroids may alter the normal flora of the oral mucosa and lead to development of fungal infection (Lilley et al. 2007, **E**).
Post-procedure	
13 Clean any equipment used and discard all disposable equipment in appropriate containers.	To minimize the risk of infection (Fraise and Bradley 2009, **E**).
14 Record the administration on appropriate charts.	To maintain accurate records, provide a point of reference in the event of any queries and prevent any duplication of treatment (NMC 2010a, **C**; NMC 2010b, **C**; NPSA 2007c, **C**).

Procedure guideline 12.8 Medication: administration by inhalation using a nebulizer

Essential equipment
- Facemask or mouthpiece
- Nebulizer and tubing

Medicinal products
- Medication required

Pre-procedure

Action	Rationale
1 Wash hands with bactericidal soap and water or bactericidal alcohol handrub.	To minimize the risk of cross-infection (DH 2007, **C**; Fraise and Bradley 2009, **E**).
2 Explain and discuss the procedure with the patient.	To ensure that the patient understands the procedure and gives their valid consent (Griffith and Jordan 2003, **E**; NMC 2013, **C**; NMC 2015, **C**).
3 Sit the patient in an upright position if possible in the bed or a chair.	To permit full expansion of the diaphragm and facilitate effective inhalation (Jevon et al. 2010, **E**).
4 Before administering any prescribed drug, look at the patient's prescription chart and check the following. (a) The correct patient (b) Drug (c) Dose (d) Date and time of administration (e) Route and method of administration (f) Diluent as appropriate (g) Validity of prescription (h) Signature of prescriber (i) The prescription is legible	To ensure that the correct patient is given the correct drug in the prescribed dose using the appropriate diluent and by the correct route (DH 2003b, **C**; NMC 2010a, **C**). To protect the patient from harm (DH 2003b, **C**; NMC 2010a, **C**).
If any of these pieces of information are missing, are unclear or illegible then the nurse should not proceed with administration and should consult with the prescriber.	To prevent any errors occurring. **E**
Procedure	
5 Administer only one drug at a time unless specifically instructed to the contrary.	Several drugs used together may cause undesirable reactions or may inactivate each other (Jordan et al. 2003, **E**).
6 Assemble the nebulizer equipment as per manufacturer's instructions.	To ensure correct administration (manufacturer's instructions, **C**).
7 Measure any liquid medication with a syringe. Add the prescribed medication and diluent (if needed) to the nebulizer.	To ensure the correct dose (DH 2007, **C**).

Action	Rationale
8 Attach the mouthpiece or facemask via the tubing to medical piped air or oxygen as prescribed. (a) If a patient has a clinical need for supplementary oxygen therapy, oxygen therapy must *not* be discontinued whilst the nebulizer is in progress. In this situation the drug should be nebulized with oxygen therapy. The patient should receive continuous pulse oximetry for at least the duration of the nebulizer treatment. (b) If a patient is hypercapnic or acidotic (e.g. COPD) the nebulizer should be driven by medical air, not oxygen.	To ensure it is ready to use when switched on. **E** To ensure patient maintains their target saturation (Jevon et al. 2010, **E**). To avoid worsening hypercapnia (NICE 2010, **C**).
9 Ask the patient to hold the mouthpiece between the lips or apply the facemask and take a slow deep breath.	To promote greater deposition of medication in the airways (Potter 2011, **E**).
10 After inspiration, the patient should pause briefly and then exhale.	Improves effectiveness of medication. **E**
11 Turn on the piped air/O_2 and ensure sufficient mist is formed. A minimum flow rate of 6–8 litres per minute is required.	To ensure effective nebulization of the medication (Downie et al. 2003, **E**; Jevon et al. 2010, **E**).
12 The patient should continue to breathe as above until all the nebulized medication is completed (0.5 mL will remain in chamber).	To ensure all medication has been received. **E**
13 Optimal nebulization of 4 mL takes approximately 10 minutes.	To ensure it is effective. **E**.
Post-procedure	
14 If appropriate and prescribed, recommence oxygen therapy at the appropriate dose.	To continue with patient's required therapy (Jevon et al. 2010, **E**).
15 Clean any equipment used and/or discard all single-use disposable equipment in appropriate containers.	To minimize the risk of infection (DH 2007, **C**; Fraise and Bradley 2009, **E**; Jevon et al. 2010, **E**).
16 Record the administration on appropriate charts.	To maintain accurate records, provide a point of reference in the event of any queries and prevent any duplication of treatment (NMC 2010a, **C**; NMC 2010b, **C**).

POST-PROCEDURAL CONSIDERATIONS

If the nebulizer is marked as single use then it must be discarded after each use. However, nebulizers should not be used for single patient use unless clearly indicated by the manufacturer. If it can be reused, then the nebulizer chamber and mask should be washed in hot soapy water, rinsed thoroughly and dried with paper towels to reduce bacterial contamination and also to prevent any build-up of crystallized medication in the nebulizer (Downie et al. 2003). Spacer devices should be washed, rinsed and allowed to dry naturally on a weekly basis and replaced after 6–12 months (Downie et al. 2003).

COMPLICATIONS

There is a risk of patients developing oral candidiasis when using an MDI. This can be reduced by using a spacer device. Overuse of some inhalers can result in cardiac dysrhythmias and patients may suffer from tachycardia, palpitations, headache, restlessness and insomnia. The doctor should be informed and observations commenced (Potter 2011).

Ophthalmic administration

DEFINITION

Dosage forms introduced into the eye for local effects, for example, to treat infections, to dilate or constrict the pupil, or to treat eye conditions such as glaucoma (Potter 2011).

RELATED THEORY

The topical route is the most popular way to introduce drugs into the eye in the form of eye drops or eye ointment. Most types of drops are instilled into the inferior fornix, the pocket formed by gently pulling on the lower eyelid, as the conjunctiva in this area is less sensitive than that overlying the cornea and will aid the retention of the medication (Jevon et al. 2010).

There are many factors that affect how much of this drug will have an effect on the eye. The eye has a highly selective corneal barrier which can prevent absorption of drug. It also has a tear film which provides an effective clearance mechanism. When an excess volume of fluid is present in the eye, this fluid will either be spilled onto the cheeks and eyelashes or will enter the nasolacrimal drainage system with a potential for systemic absorption of drug. Drugs also need to be introduced to the eye at a neutral pH, as acidic or alkaline preparations will result in reflex lacrimation which will remove the drug from the eye.

EVIDENCE-BASED APPROACHES

In order to optimize the effects of topical eye preparations, attempts should be made to ensure that there is proper placement of eye drops and ointments and that the volume applied is kept to a minimum. The number of drops instilled depends on the type of solution used and its purpose. Usually one drop only is ordered and will be sufficient if it is instilled in the correct manner. The exceptions to the 'one drop' rule are as follows.

- *Oil-based solutions*: these are used for lubricating the eyeball. Usually one drop is instilled and repeated as required.
- *Anaesthetic drops*: used to anaesthetize the eye; one drop should be instilled at a time. This is repeated until the drop cannot be felt on the eye.

Figure 12.15 **How to instil eye drops.**

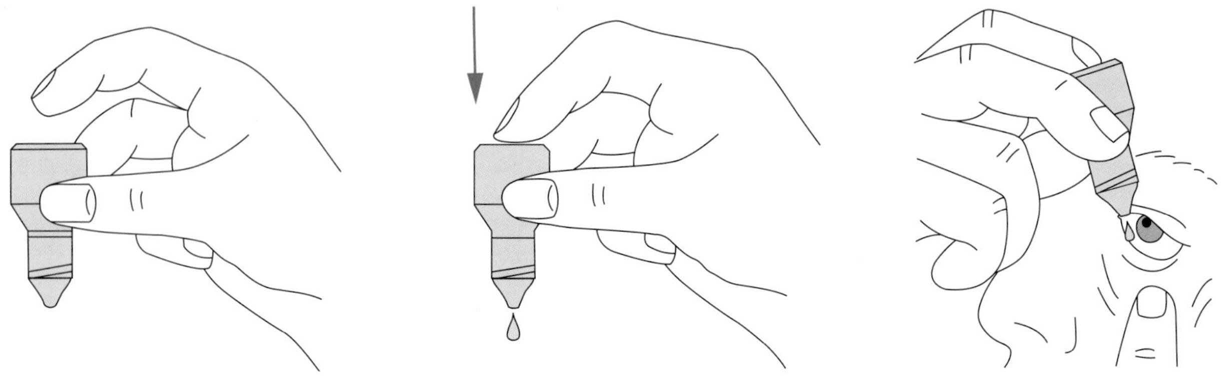

The dropper should be held as close to the eye as possible without touching the lids or the cornea. This will avoid corneal damage and reduce the risk of cross-infection. If the drop falls from too great a height, it is difficult to control and will be uncomfortable for the patient. The eye should be closed for as long as possible after application, preferably for 1–2 minutes.

Useful properties of eye ointment include:

- longer duration of action than eye drops
- a soothing emollient action
- easy to apply
- long shelf-life (Downie et al. 2003).

Ointments are applied to the upper rim of the inferior fornix using a similar technique to eye drops (Figure 12.15, Figure 12.16). A 2 cm line of ointment should be applied from the nasal canthus outwards. Similarly to the instillation of eye drops, the nozzle should be held approximately 2.5 cm above the eye to avoid contact with the cornea and eyelids (Aldridge 2010, Alexander et al. 2007).

PRE-PROCEDURAL CONSIDERATIONS

Equipment

A variety of droppers and bottles are available for the instillation of eye preparations. These include pipettes, bottles incorporating pipettes, plastic bottles with a dropper attachment and single-dose packs. Pipettes are easy to use but need to be dried and sterilized between doses. Plastic bottles can be squeezed and so avoid the need for a pipette and they are also cheaper than glass bottles with a dropper. Each patient should have their own individual eye drop container for each eye and single-dose containers should be used for all patients in eye clinics or in accident and emergency departments (BNF 2014).

It is important that eye preparations are sterile before use and attempts are made to reduce microbial contamination. Eye preparations being used at home should be discarded after 4 weeks whereas eye preparations being used in hospital should be discarded after 1 week. If concerns exist around cross-contamination from one eye to another, separate bottles should be issued.

A number of patients experience problems instilling eye medication. This may be due to difficulty aiming eye drops or squeezing the bottle. Aids are available to assist patients with both these problems. Patients will need guidance in how to use any aids (Downie et al. 2003).

If patients are going to use more than one eye drop preparation, they may experience overflow and dilution when one immediately follows the other so they should be advised to leave an interval of at least 5 minutes between the two (BNF 2014). If both drops and ointments are prescribed, the drops should be applied before the ointment as ointment will leave a film on the eye and hamper the absorption of the medication in drop form (Aldridge 2010).

Figure 12.16 **How to instil eye ointment.**

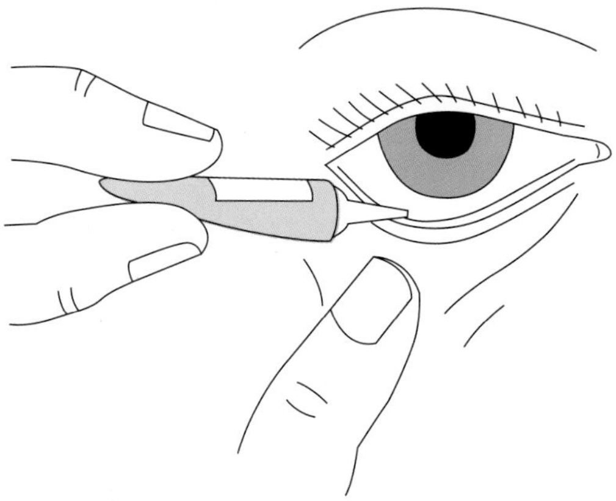

Pharmacological support

Drugs may be given either systemically or topically to exert an effect on the eye (BNF 2014). However, if given systemically, the prescribing doctor needs to take account of the blood–aqueous barrier which exists within the eye. This barrier is selective in allowing drugs to pass into the intraocular fluids. The permeability of this barrier may increase during inflammatory conditions or following paracentesis – the removal of excess fluid with a needle or cannula (Andrew 2006).

Medications applied topically meet some resistance at the barrier presented by the lacrimal system (tear film barrier). A further barrier is the cornea which is selectively permeable and only allows the passage of water and not drugs. However, corneal resistance may alter if there is damage to the corneal epithelium (Kirkwood 2006). Many drugs will produce a similar effect on both the healthy and diseased eye.

Drugs for use in the eye are usually classified according to their action.

Figure 12.17 **Effects of mydriatics.**

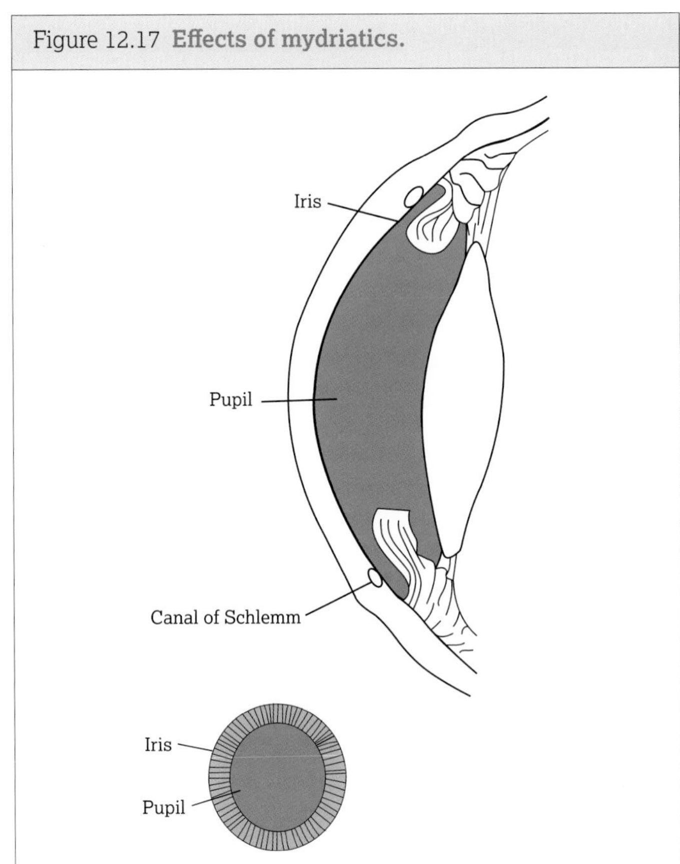

Mydriatics and cycloplegics

These drugs cause pupil dilation and produce their effects by paralysing the ciliary muscle, stimulating the dilator muscle of the pupil (Figure 12.17) or by a combination of both. They are used mainly for diagnostic purposes and most have an anticholinergic action. The most commonly used preparations are cyclopentolate hydrochloride, tropicamide and atropine (BNF 2014).

Miotics

These drugs produce their effects by contracting the ciliary muscle and constricting the pupil (Figure 12.18). They open the inefficient drainage channels in the trabecular meshwork (BNF 2014). Miotics help in the drainage of aqueous humour and are used mainly in the treatment of primary angle-closure glaucoma. An example is pilocarpine (BNF 2014).

Local anaesthetics

These render the eye and the inner surfaces of the lids insensitive. They are used before minor surgery, removal of foreign bodies and tonometry (measurement of intraocular pressure). The most widely used eye anaesthetics are oxybuprocaine and tetracaine (BNF 2014).

Anti-inflammatories

Anti-inflammatory drugs include steroids, antihistamines, lodoxamide and sodium cromoglycate. The most commonly used steroid preparations are dexamethasone, prednisolone and betamethasone (BNF 2014).

Corticosteroid eye drops should be used with caution as they can cause cataract formation or a gradual rise in intraocular pressure in a small percentage of people, particularly if they have a history of glaucoma (Forrester et al. 2002).

Antibacterials/antivirals/antifungals

Antibacterials and antivirals can be used for the active treatment of eye infections or as prophylactic treatment for eye surgery, after removal of a foreign body or following an eye injury. Antibiotic preparations in common use are chloramphenicol, fusidic acid and gentamicin. Aciclovir is the most commonly used antiviral eye preparation and is licensed for local treatment of herpes simplex infections (BNF 2014).

Artificial tears

Artificial tears are used when there is a deficiency in natural tear production. This can be due to a disease process, post radiotherapy treatment, as a side-effect of certain drugs or when the eye-blink reflex is absent. These artificial lubricants commonly contain hypromellose or hydroxyethylcellulose (BNF 2014). Additionally, pilocarpine can be given orally. The severity of the problem and the patient's choice will determine the treatment.

Specific patient preparation

The eye to be treated must be ascertained and the unaffected eye should not be dosed. Ascertain if the patient is wearing contact lenses as contact of the medication with the lens can lead to increased drug absorption, visual distortion and discolouration of the lens (Chernecky et al. 2002). It may be necessary for the patient to remove the lenses and replace them with glasses for the duration of their treatment.

Figure 12.18 **Effect of miotics.**

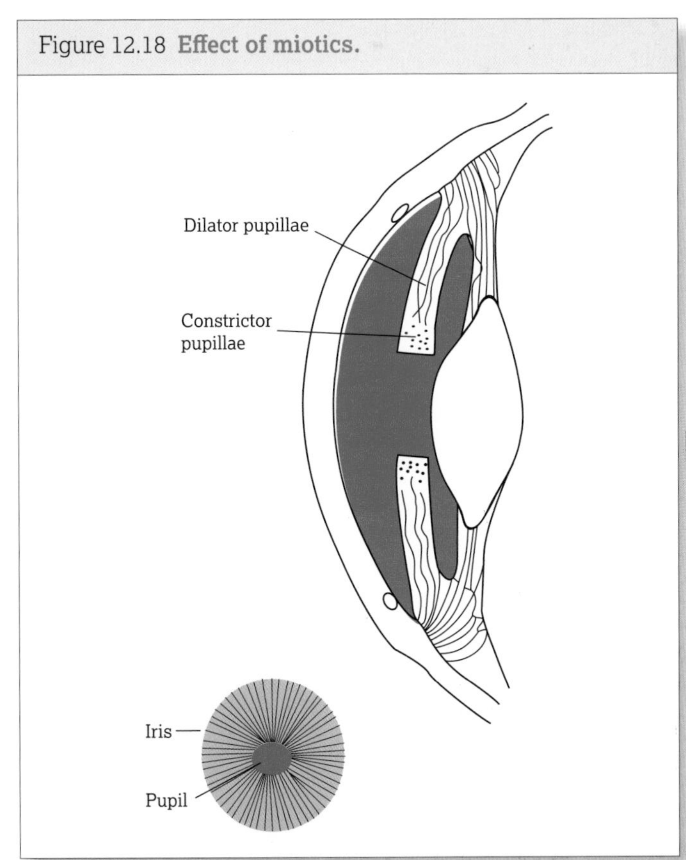

Procedure guideline 12.9 Medication: eye administration

Essential equipment

- Non-sterile powder-free gloves
- Low-linting swabs
- Sterile 0.9% sodium chloride or warm water
- Eye drops at room temperature or eye ointment

Optional equipment

- Eye swab

Pre-procedure

Action	Rationale
1 Explain and discuss the procedure with the patient. Ask the patient to explain how their eyes feel, if they are able to.	To ensure that the patient understands the procedure and gives their valid consent (Griffith and Jordan 2003, **E**; NMC 2013, **C**; NMC 2015, **C**). To gain a baseline understanding of current problems or changes the patient is experiencing. **E**
2 Before administering any prescribed drug, look at the patient's prescription chart and check the following. (a) The correct patient (b) Drug (c) Dose (d) Date and time of administration (e) Route and method of administration (f) Diluent as appropriate (g) Validity of prescription (h) Signature of prescriber (i) The prescription is legible	To ensure that the correct patient is given the correct drug in the prescribed dose using the appropriate diluent and by the correct route (DH 2003b, **C**; NMC 2010a, **C**). To protect the patient from harm (DH 2003b, **C**; NMC 2010a, **C**).
If any of these pieces of information are missing, are unclear or illegible then the nurse should not proceed with administration and should consult with the prescriber.	To prevent any errors occurring. **E**
3 Wash hands and apply well-fitting gloves.	To reduce the risk of cross-infection (DH 2007, **C**; Fraise and Bradley 2009, **E**).

Procedure

Action	Rationale
4 Ask the patient to sit back with neck slightly hyperextended or lie down.	To ensure a position that allows easy access for medication instillation and to avoid excess running down the patient's cheek (Stollery et al. 2005, **E**). Correct positioning minimizes drainage of eye medication into the tear duct (Potter 2011, **E**).
5 If there is any discharge, proceed as for eye swabbing (see Chapter 10: Interpreting diagnostic tests). If any crusting or drainage is present around the eye, gently wash away with warm water or 0.9% sodium chloride and a swab. Always wipe clean from inner to outer canthus.	To prevent the introduction of micro-organisms into the lacrimal ducts (Potter 2011, **E**).
6 Ask the patient to look at the ceiling and carefully pull the skin below the affected eye using a wet swab to expose the conjunctival sac.	To move the sensitive cornea up and away from the conjunctival sac and reduce stimulation of blink reflex (Potter 2011, **E**).
7 If administering both drops and ointment, administer drops first.	Ointment will leave a film in the eye which may hamper the absorption of medication in drop form (Jevon et al. 2010, **E**).
8 *Either:*	
Administer the prescribed number of drops, holding the eye dropper 1–2 cm above the eye. If the patient blinks or closes their eye, repeat the procedure.	To provide even distribution of medication across the eye. Therapeutic effect of drug is obtained only when drops enter conjunctival sac (Potter 2011, **E**).
Or:	
Apply a thin stream of ointment evenly along the inner edge of lower eyelid on conjunctiva from the nasal corner outwards. If there is excess medication on the eyelid, gently wipe it from inner to outer canthus.	To provide even distribution of medication across the eye and lid margin and reduce the risk of cross-infection, contamination of the tube and trauma to the eye (Fraise and Bradley 2009, **E**; Potter 2011, **E**; Stollery et al. 2005, **E**). To avoid excess ointment irritating the suroounding skin (Stollery et al. 2005, **E**).

9 Ask the patient to close their eyes and keep them closed for 1–2 minutes.	To help distribute medication (Aldridge 2010, **E**; Potter 2011, **E**).
10 Explain to the patient that they may have blurred vision for a few minutes after application.	To ensure the patient understands why they have blurred vision and to refrain from driving or operating machinery until their vision returns to normal (Aldridge 2010, **E**).
Post-procedure	
11 Clean any equipment used and discard all disposable equipment in appropriate containers.	To minimize the risk of infection (DH 2007, **C**; Fraise and Bradley 2009, **E**).
12 Record the administration on appropriate charts.	To maintain accurate records, provide a point of reference in the event of any queries and prevent any duplication of treatment (NMC 2010a, **C**; NMC 2010b, **C**).

POST-PROCEDURAL CONSIDERATIONS

Immediate care

After using any eye medications, any excess medication should be wiped off from inner to outer canthus. If an eye patch is to be worn, it should be secured without putting any pressure on the eye. Patients should be warned not to drive for 1–2 hours, until their vision is clear, after instillation of mydriatics (which dilate the pupil and paralyse the ciliary muscle) (BNF 2014). Patients should be taught how to instil eye medication. If it is difficult for them to do so then it may be necessary for a community nurse to attend and administer the eye medications (Chernecky et al. 2002).

Nasal administration

DEFINITION

Medication introduced to the cavity of the nose for local or systemic effects (Aldridge 2010).

RELATED THEORY

The nasal passages are lined with highly vascular mucous membranes covered with ciliated epithelium which warms and moistens air and traps dust. Medication can be delivered directly to the nasal cavity to relieve local symptoms such as allergic rhinitis in the form of nasal drops or nasal sprays (Aldridge 2010).

The nasal cavity can also be used to allow the delivery of drugs systemically. Examples include sumatriptan for migraine, desmopressin for the treatment of diabetes insipidus and nocturia and fentanyl for the treatment of breakthrough pain.

EVIDENCE-BASED APPROACHES

The advantages of the delivery of drugs using the nasal route include the large vascular surface of the nasal cavity which allows rapid absorption, the avoidance of first-pass metabolism, the accessibility of the nose, the ease of administration and the fact that this route can be used when patients are unable to swallow. There are some disadvantages to the nasal route, including the presence of mucus which acts as a barrier to absorption and the mucociliary clearance which reduces the time that drugs are held in the nasal cavity. Colds can affect absorption from the nasal cavity, and some drugs may irritate the nasal cavity.

PRE-PROCEDURAL CONSIDERATIONS

Specific patient preparation

The patient should be encouraged to clear their nostrils by blowing or manually cleaning with a tissue or damp cotton bud to ensure that the drug has access to the nasal mucosa (Aldridge 2010).

Procedure guideline 12.10 **Medication: nasal drop administration**

Essential equipment

- Tissues
- Clean non-sterile gloves

Medicinal product

- Nasal spray or drops

Optional equipment

- Cotton bud

Pre-procedure

Action	Rationale
1 Wash hands with bactericidal soap and water or bactericidal alcohol handrub.	To minimize the risk of cross-infection (DH 2007, **C**; Fraise and Bradley 2009, **E**).
2 Explain and discuss the procedure with the patient.	To ensure that the patient understands the procedure and gives their valid consent (Griffith and Jordan 2003, **E**; NMC 2013, **C**; NMC 2015, **C**).

(continued)

Procedure guideline 12.10 Medication: nasal drop administration *(continued)*

Action	Rationale
3 Before administering any prescribed drug, look at the patient's prescription chart and check the following. (a) The correct patient (b) Drug (c) Dose (d) Date and time of administration (e) Route and method of administration (f) Diluent as appropriate (g) Validity of prescription (h) Signature of prescriber (i) The prescription is legible	To ensure that the correct patient is given the correct drug in the prescribed dose using the appropriate diluent and by the correct route (DH 2003b, **C**; NMC 2010a, **C**). To protect the patient from harm (DH 2003b, **C**; NMC 2010a, **C**).
If any of these pieces of information are missing, are unclear or illegible then the nurse should not proceed with administration and should consult with the prescriber.	To prevent any errors occurring. **E**
4 Have paper tissues available.	To wipe away secretions and/or medication. **E**
Procedure	
5 Ask the patient to blow their nose to clear the nasal passages, if appropriate.	To ensure maximum penetration for the medication (Chernecky et al. 2002, **E**).
6 Place the patient in a supine position and hyperextend the neck (unless clinically contraindicated, for example cervical spondylosis).	To obtain a safe optimum position for insertion of the medication. **E**
7 Wash hands and put on gloves.	To reduce the risk of cross-infection (DH 2007, **C**; Fraise and Bradley 2009, **E**).
8 With the non-dominant hand, gently push upward on the end of the patient's nose.	To aid in opening the nostrils. **E**
9 Avoid touching the external nares with the dropper and instil the drops just inside the nostril of affected side.	To prevent the patient from sneezing. **E**
10 Ask the patient to sniff back any liquid into the back of the nose or to maintain their position for 2 or 3 minutes.	To ensure full absorption of the medication. **E**
11 Discard any remaining medication in the dropper into the sink before returning it to the container.	To minimize the risk of cross-infection (Chernecky et al. 2002, **E**; DH 2007, **C**; Fraise and Bradley 2009, **E**).
12 Instruct patient not to blow their nose.	To maintain the medication in contact with nasal passages. **E**
13 Each patient should have their own medication and dropper.	To minimize the risk of cross-infection (DH 2007, **C**; Fraise and Bradley 2009, **E**).
Post-procedure	
14 Record the administration on appropriate charts.	To maintain accurate records, provide a point of reference in the event of any queries and prevent any duplication of treatment (NMC 2010a, **C**; NMC 2010b, **C**).

POST-PROCEDURAL CONSIDERATIONS

The patient should be discouraged from sniffing too vigorously post administration as this can cause 'run-off' of the medication down the nasopharynx. This can cause an unpleasant taste in the throat and affect absorption of the medication (Aldridge 2010).

Otic administration

DEFINITION

Medication introduced into the ear for local effects such as treatment of ear infections and softening of ear wax (cerumen) prior to ear syringing (Aldridge 2010, Chernecky et al. 2002, Nichols and O'Brien 2012).

RELATED THEORY

Drugs administered via this route are intended to have a localized effect and act within the anatomy of the ear and auditory canal (Aldridge 2010). Ear preparations can be presented in the form of drops, sprays, ointments and solutions. Certain factors can affect the absorption or action of drugs in the ear, including ear wax and the acidic environment around the ear skin surface.

EVIDENCE-BASED APPROACHES

Internal ear structures are very sensitive to temperature extremes and so solutions should be administered at room temperature. When drops are instilled cold, patients may experience vertigo, ataxia or nausea (Chernecky et al. 2002, Potter 2011). Solutions should never be forced into the ear canal as medication administered under pressure can injure the eardrum. The ear drop solution should be labelled for the ear it is intended to treat. The dropper should be held as close to the ear as possible without touching to reduce the risk of cross-infection.

PRE-PROCEDURAL CONSIDERATIONS

Specific patient preparation

The nurse should examine the ear, taking note of any discharge, redness, swelling and the amount and texture of any ear wax present as these will give an indication of the general health of the ear (Harkin 2008). The nurse should also discuss with the patient their current level of hearing. It should be explained to the patient that they must lie still as sudden movements could cause injury from the ear dropper.

Procedure guideline 12.11 **Medication: ear drop administration**

Essential equipment

- Clean non-sterile gloves
- Tissues

Medicinal products

- Ear drops
- Disposable plastic apron

Pre-procedure

Action	Rationale
1 Wash hands with bactericidal soap and water or bactericidal alcohol handrub.	To minimize the risk of cross-infection (DH 2007, **C**; Fraise and Bradley 2009, **E**).
2 Explain and discuss the procedure with the patient.	To ensure that the patient understands the procedure and gives their valid consent (Griffith and Jordan 2003, **E**; NMC 2013, **C**; NMC 2015, **C**).
3 Before administering any prescribed drug, look at the patient's prescription chart and check the following. (a) The correct patient (b) Drug (c) Dose (d) Date and time of administration (e) Route and method of administration (f) Diluent as appropriate (g) Validity of prescription (h) Signature of prescriber (i) The prescription is legible	To ensure that the correct patient is given the correct drug in the prescribed dose using the appropriate diluent and by the correct route (DH 2003b, **C**; NMC 2010a, **C**). To protect the patient from harm (DH 2003b, **C**; NMC 2010a, **C**).
If any of these pieces of information are missing, are unclear or illegible then the nurse should not proceed with administration and should consult with the prescriber.	To prevent any errors occurring. **E**
Procedure	
4 Ask the patient to lie on their side with the ear to be treated uppermost.	To ensure the best position for insertion of the drops. **E**
5 Warm the drops to near body temperature by holding the container in the palm of the hand for a few minutes.	To prevent trauma to the patient (ASHP 1982, **C**; Harkin 2008, **E**; Potter 2011, **E**).
6 Wash hands and apply gloves.	To reduce the risk of cross-infection (DH 2007, **C**; Fraise and Bradley 2009, **E**).
7 Pull the cartilaginous part of the pinna backwards and upwards (**Action figure 7**).	To prepare the auditory meatus for instillation of the drops (Harkin 2008, **E**).
8 If cerumen (ear wax) or drainage occludes outermost portion of the ear canal, wipe out gently with cotton-tipped applicator.	To enable the medication to enter the ear. **E**
9 Allow the drop(s) to fall in direction of the external canal. The dropper should not touch the ear.	To ensure that the medication reaches the area requiring therapy. **E**
10 Gently massage over tragus to help work in the drops.	To aid the passage of medication into the ear and prevent escape of medication. **E**
11 It may be necessary to temporarily place a gauze swab over the ear canal.	To prevent escape of the medication (Chernecky et al. 2002, **E**).

(continued)

Procedure guideline 12.11 Medication: ear drop administration *(continued)*

Action	Rationale
12 Request the patient to remain in this position for 2–3 minutes.	To allow the medication to reach the eardrum and be absorbed. To prevent escape of the medication (Aldridge, 2010, **E**; Potter 2011, **E**).
Post-procedure	
13 Record the administration on appropriate charts.	To maintain accurate records, provide a point of reference in the event of any queries and prevent any duplication of treatment (NMC 2010a, **C**; NMC 2010b, **C**).

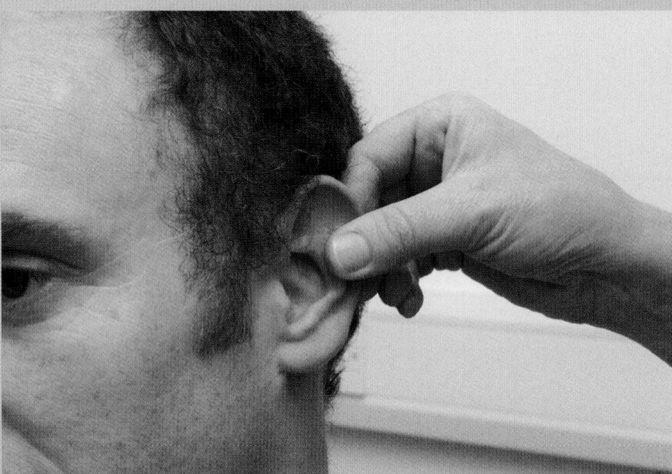

Action Figure 7 Holding ear for ear drops.

POST-PROCEDURAL CONSIDERATIONS

The nurse should ask the patient if there are any changes in order to monitor effectiveness of the intervention. Consideration should also be given to the patient's hearing aids and assistance given to help clean these.

Injections and infusions

DEFINITIONS

Injections are sterile solutions, emulsions or suspensions. They are prepared by dissolving, emulsifying or suspending the active ingredient and any added substances in either water for injections or a suitable non-aqueous liquid or in a mixture of these vehicles (British Pharmacopoeia 2007). Box 12.15 lists the types of injections and infusions.

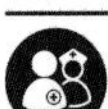

Box 12.15 **Types of injections and infusions**

- Intradermal injection
- Subcutaneous injection and infusion
- Intramuscular injection
- Intra-arterial injection
- Intraosseous injection
- Intra-articular injection
- Intrathecal injection and infusion
- Intravenous:
  - bolus injection
  - intermittent and continuous infusion

Injections can be described as the act of giving medication by use of a syringe and needle. An infusion is defined as an amount of fluid in excess of 100 mL designated for parenteral infusion because the volume must be administered over a long period of time. However, medications may be given in small volumes (50–100 mL) or over a shorter period (30–60 minutes) (Weinstein and Plumer 2007).

ANATOMY AND PHYSIOLOGY

The skin is made up of two layers: the dermis and epidermis. Within the dermis there is the papillary layer (upper dermal region) which contains capillaries, pain and touch receptors. The reticular layer contains blood vessels, sweat and oil glands. Both collagen and elastic fibres are found throughout the dermis. Collagen fibres are responsible for the toughness of the dermis. The skin also has a rich nerve supply (Marieb and Hoehn 2007).

There are three types of muscles – skeletal, cardiac and smooth. Skeletal muscles are attached to the body's skeleton and are also known as striated muscle because the fibres appear to be striped (Marieb and Hoehn 2007). For specific muscles used for injections, see 'Intramuscular injection site and volume of injection'.

EVIDENCE-BASED APPROACHES

Medicines should only be administered by injection when no other route is suitable or available. As injections avoid the GI tract, this is described as parenteral administration. Injections would be administered when the medications might be destroyed by the stomach; rapid first-pass metabolism may be extensive; the drug is not absorbed when given orally; precise control over dosage is required; unable to be given by mouth; need to achieve high drug plasma levels (Downie et al. 2003, Ostendorf 2012). There are disadvantages as injections are invasive, cause pain

Figure 12.19 **Ampoules.**

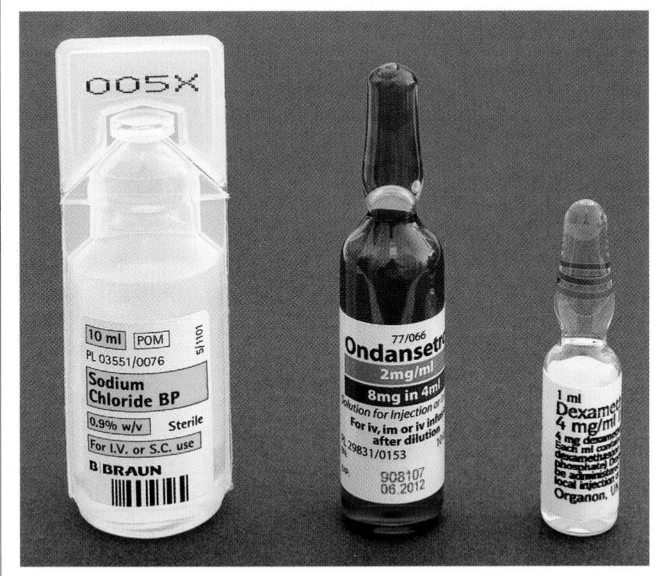

Figure 12.20 **Vials.**

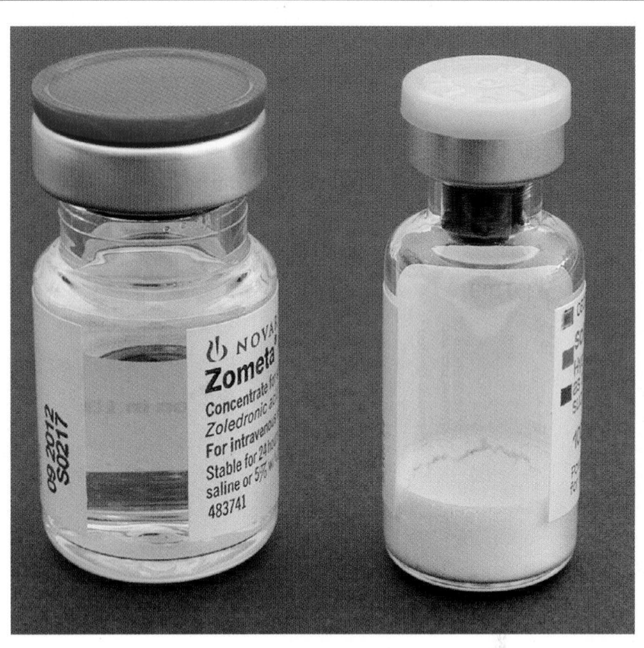

and discomfort, and can put the patient at risk of infection and, in the case of intravenous injections, infiltration and extravasation.

PRE-PROCEDURAL CONSIDERATIONS

Equipment

Ampoule

Ampoules (Figure 12.19) are single-dose glass containers although plastic ampoules are now used for certain products (Downie et al. 2003). They have a wide-ranging capacity and are sealed by heat fusion to exclude any contamination. They have a thin wall which allows rupture of the glass to expose the contents of liquid or powder. There is a narrow constriction leading to the neck which is often marked with a white ring which indicates the place where the neck can be snapped off (Downie et al. 2003). Ampoule opening devices of various designs are available. Ampoules are available in several sizes from 1 to 20 mL (Ostendorf 2012).

Vials

Vials (Figure 12.20) are glass containers which have a rubber closure which can be penetrated to allow the addition of a diluent to dissolve powder contents and withdrawal of a dose via the needle. The exposed rubber surface is usually covered by a protective pull-off metal or plastic cap which prevents tampering or damage but does not provide sterility (Downie et al. 2003, Ostendorf 2012). The vials may be packaged with a specific transfer needle, and the nurse should follow the manufacturer's instructions in these instances.

Syringes

Syringes are commonly plastic and disposable, although occasionally a medicine must be administered via a glass syringe, e.g. adenosine. They consist of a graduated barrel and a plunger and a tip. It is the tip that classifies the type of syringe as Luer-Lok or Luer-Slip (Figure 12.21). Syringes come in various sizes from 1 to 60 mL. The choice of syringe is made according to the volume of medication to be administered so it is important to choose the smallest syringe possible to ensure accuracy (Downie et al. 2003, Ostendorf 2012). For Luer-Lok, syringes, the needle must be twisted onto the tip and 'locked' into position. This provides security and these syringes are recommended for use with intravenous medicines, especially cytotoxic medications and any medicines administered via a syringe pump. Luer-Slip syringes tend to be used for intramuscular and subcutaneous injections. Insulin syringes are low-dose syringes often calibrated in units and are only used for insulin administration (Downie et al. 2003, Ostendorf 2012, NPSA 2010). They should be stored and distinguished from IV syringes (MHRA 2008, Reid 2012). Injection pens are pre-filled syringes that contain a disposable cartridge. They provide a convenient delivery method and allow patients to self-administer their medications subcutaneously, e.g. insulin, adrenaline (Ostendorf 2012).

Following intrathecal incidents, the NPSA (2009) issued a safety alert that all spinal (intrathecal) bolus doses and lumbar puncture samples (part A) and all epidural, spinal (intrathecal) and regional anaesthesia infusions and bolus doses (part B) should

Figure 12.21 **Syringes: Luer-Lok and Luer-Slip.**

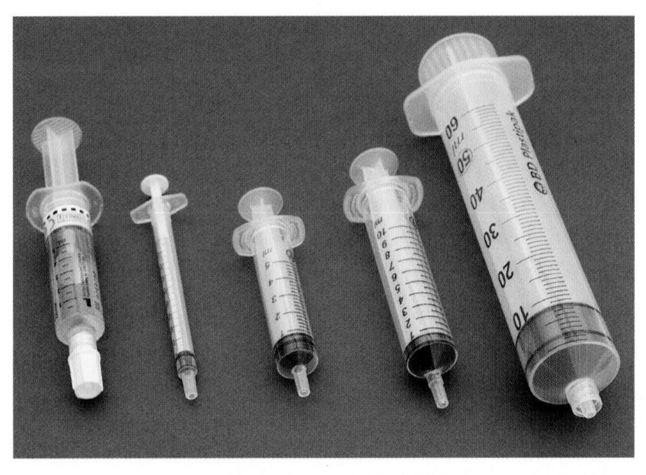

Figure 12.22 **Needles.**

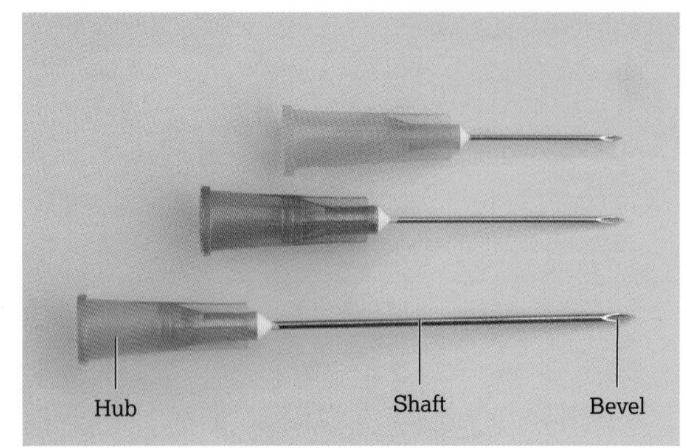

Figure 12.23 **Safety needles.**

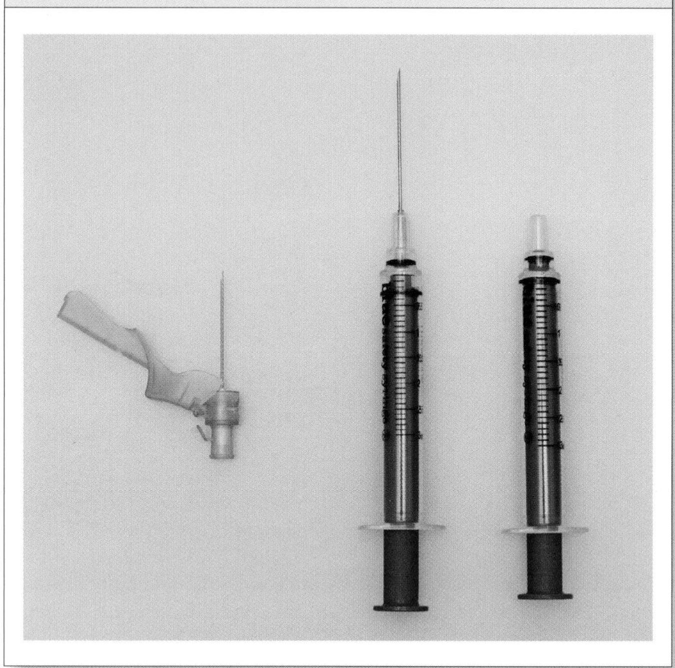

be performed using syringes, needles and other devices with connectors that *will not* also connect with intravenous equipment.

There are now a number of pre-prepared syringes that contain 0.9% sodium chloride specifically for flushing or ready-to-administer medicines often used in emergency situations.

Needles

A hypodermic needle is composed of three parts (see Figure 12.22):

- the hub which fits onto the tip of a syringe
- the shaft which connects the hub
- the bevel or slanted tip or eye of the needle (different bevels are required depending on use of needle).

Needle sizes are known as gauges, for example 19 G, 21 G (used for intramuscular [IM] injections), 23 G (subcutaneous [SC] injections) and 25 G (intradermal injections). This indicates their diameter. The higher the gauge, the finer the needle and selection is made depending on the viscosity of the liquid to be injected (Downie et al. 2003, Ostendorf 2012). Needles vary in length from 10 to 16 mm and selection of length will depend on the size and weight of the patient, and the type of tissue into which the drug is to be injected, for example longer for IM and shorter for SC. Each needle is enclosed in a removable plastic guard and then sealed in a sterile pack. Filter needles may be used to prevent drawing up glass and rubber particles into the syringe (Downie et al. 2003, Ostendorf 2012).

There are now a variety of safety needles available to prevent needlestick injury where a plastic guard or sheath slips over the needle after an injection (EU Directive 2010) (Figure 12.23).

Three categories of needle bevel are available.

- *Regular*: for all intramuscular and subcutaneous injections.
- *Intradermal*: for diagnostic injections and other injections into the epidermis.
- *Short*: rarely used.

Medication preparation

Medicines presented as liquids can be drawn up directly from the vial or ampoule. If the medicine has been presented in a powder form it will need to be reconstituted. This is usually done using water for injections but some medications will require special diluents which are often supplied with the medication. When adding diluent to a powder, for example 2 mL to a 100 mg vial, the final volume will exceed 2 mL although this is usually not of any consequence if the total dose is to be administered (Downie et al. 2003). In order to ensure that the correct volume is withdrawn, it will be necessary to perform a calculation.

Medication calculations

The drug volume required from stock strength:

$$\frac{\text{Strength required}}{\text{Stock strength}} \times \text{volume of stock solution} = \text{volume required}$$

What you want/what you have got × volume of stock solution

Displacement values

Displacement values are when you take a drug and dissolve it in a solution, e.g. water. The resulting solution will have a greater volume than before. Displacement value volumes can vary from drug to drug and may be so small that the increased volume is not considered in calculating doses (Lapham and Agar 2003). However, the total volume may be increased significantly and, if this is not taken into account when calculating a dose, errors in dosage may occur, particularly when small doses are involved, e.g. for neonates (Lapham and Agar 2003). Displacement volumes may be stated in the relevant drug information sheets.

To calculate dose using displacement volumes:

Volume to be added = diluent volume – displacement volume

It is important to note that the 'use of calculators to determine the volume or quantity of medication should not act as a substitute for arithmetical knowledge and skill' (NMC 2010a).

Single-dose preparations

The volume of the injection in a single-dose container is sufficient to permit the withdrawal and administration of the nominal dose using a normal technique.

Multidose preparations

Multidose aqueous injections contain a suitable antimicrobial preservative at an appropriate concentration except when the preparation itself has adequate antimicrobial properties. When it is necessary to present a preparation for parenteral use in a multidose container, the precautions to be taken for its administration and more particularly for its storage between successive withdrawals are given.

Parenteral infusions

Parenteral infusions are sterile, aqueous solutions or emulsions with water; they are free from pyrogens and are usually made isotonic with blood. They are principally intended for administration in large volume. Parenteral infusions do not contain any added antimicrobial preservative (British Pharmacopoeia 2007, Hillery et al. 2001).

Specific patient preparation

Reducing pain of injections

Patients are often afraid of receiving injections because they perceive the injection will be painful (Downie et al. 2003). Torrance (1989) listed a number of factors that cause pain.

- The needle.
- The chemical composition of the drug/solution.
- The technique.
- The speed of the injection.
- The volume of drug.

Applying manual pressure to an injection site before performing an injection can be an effective means of reducing pain intensity (Chung et al. 2002). A small study carried out by Chan (2001) showed that administering subcutaneous heparin slowly (over 30 seconds rather than 10) can reduce site pain intensity as well as bruising. Pain may also be reduced when using retractable needles (Lamblet et al. 2011).

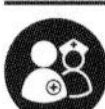

Box 12.16 **Reducing the pain of injections**

- Correct length and gauge of needle (use smallest possible).
- Correct site.
- Correct angle (90° for IM).
- Correct volume (no more than 3 mL at a site for IM).
- Rotate sites to prevent formation of indurations or abscesses.
- Consider using ice, freezing spray or topical local anaesthetic to numb the skin.
- Listen to views of the experienced patient.
- Explain the benefits of the injection.
- Positioning of the patient so that the muscles are relaxed.
- Use distraction.
- If appropriate, ask the patient to turn their foot inwards (IM).
- Insert and remove the needle smoothly and quickly.
  - Hold the syringe steady once the needle is in the tissue to prevent tissue damage.
- Inject medication slowly but smoothly.

Source: Adapted from Dickerson (1992), Downie et al. (2003), Potter (2011).

Other ways of reducing pain during injections are covered in Box 12.16.

Procedure guideline 12.12 **Medication: single-dose ampoule: solution preparation**

Essential equipment

- Medication ampoule
- Needle
- Syringe
- Sterile topical swab
- Sharps container
- Ampoule opening aid

Action	Rationale
Pre-procedure	
1 Wash hands with bactericidal soap and water or bactericidal alcohol handrub.	To prevent contamination of medication and equipment (DH 2007, **C**).
2 Inspect the solution for cloudiness or particulate matter. If this is present, discard and follow hospital guidelines on action to take; for example, return drug to pharmacy.	To prevent the patient from receiving an unstable or contaminated drug (NPSA 2007d, **C**).
Procedure	
3 Tap the neck of the ampoule gently.	To ensure that all the solution is in the bottom of the ampoule (NPSA 2007d, **C**).
4 Cover the neck of the ampoule with a sterile topical swab and snap it open. If there is any difficulty, a file or ampoule opening aid may be required.	To minimize the risk of contamination. To prevent aerosol formation or contact with the drug which could lead to a sensitivity reaction. To reduce the risk of injury to the nurse (NPSA 2007d, **C**).
5 Inspect the solution for glass fragments; if present, discard.	To minimize the risk of injection of foreign matter into the patient (NPSA 2007d, **C**).
6 Open packaging and attach the needle onto the syringe.	To assemble equipment. **E**
7 Withdraw the required amount of solution, tilting the ampoule if necessary.	To avoid drawing in any air (NPSA 2007d, **C**).
8 Replace the sheath on the needle using one-handed scooping method (Figure 12.24) and tap the syringe to dislodge any air bubbles. Expel air (replacing the sheath should not be confused with resheathing used needles).	To prevent needlestick injury and aerosol formation (NPSA 2007d, **C**). To ensure that the correct amount of drug is in the syringe (NPSA 2007d, **C**).

(continued)

Procedure guideline 12.12 Medication: single-dose ampoule: solution preparation *(continued)*

Action	Rationale
Or: An alternative to expelling the air with the needle sheath in place would be to use the ampoule or vial to receive any air and/or drug.	
9 Attach a new needle if required (and discard used needle into appropriate sharps container) or attach a plastic end cap or insert syringe into the syringe packet.	To reduce the risk of contamination of the syringe tip. To avoid tracking medications through superficial tissues and to ensure that the correct size of needle is used for intramuscular or subcutaneous injection. To reduce the risk of injury to the nurse (NPSA 2007d, **C**).
10 Attach a label to the syringe.	To ensure practitioner can identify medication in syringe (NPSA 2007d, **C**).
11 Keep all ampoules/vials and diluents in the tray with the syringe	To enable checking at the bedside. **E**

Figure 12.24 **Scooping.**

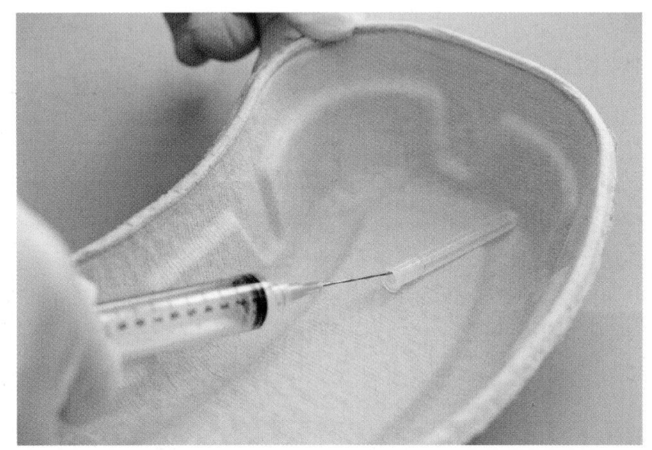

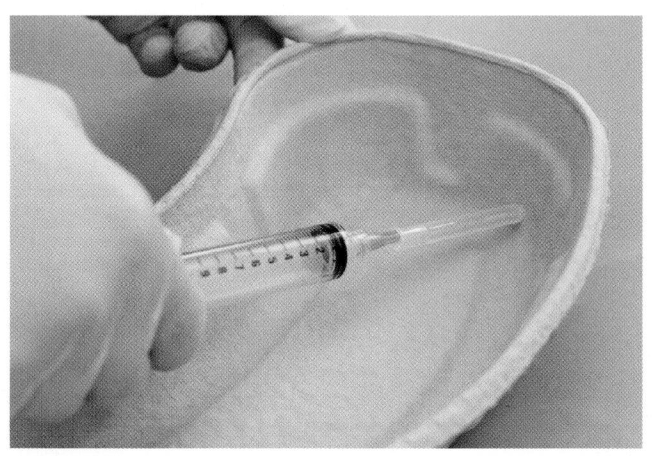

Procedure guideline 12.13 Medication: single-dose ampoule: powder preparation

Essential equipment

- Medication ampoule
- Diluent
- Needle
- Syringe
- Sharps container
- Swab

Pre-procedure

Action	Rationale
1 Wash hands with bactericidal soap and water or bactericidal alcohol handrub.	To prevent contamination of medication and equipment (DH 2007, **C**).
2 Open packaging and attach needle to the syringe.	To assemble the equipment. **E**

Procedure

Action	Rationale
3 Open the diluent and draw up required volume.	To ensure the correct volume of diluent. **E**
4 Tap the neck of the ampoule gently.	To ensure that any powder lodged here falls to the bottom of the ampoule (NPSA 2007d, **C**).
5 Cover the neck of the ampoule with a sterile topical swab and snap it open. If there is any difficulty, an ampoule opening device may be required.	To minimize the risk of contamination. To prevent contact with the drug which could cause a sensitivity reaction. To prevent injury to the nurse (NPSA 2007d, **C**).

Action	Rationale
6 Inject the correct diluent slowly into the powder within the ampoule.	To ensure that the powder is thoroughly wet before agitation and is not released into the atmosphere (NPSA 2007d, **C**).
7 Agitate the ampoule.	To dissolve the drug (NPSA 2007d, **C**).
8 Inspect the contents.	To detect any glass fragments or any other particulate matter. If present, continue agitation or discard as appropriate (NPSA 2007d, **C**).
9 When the solution is clear, withdraw the prescribed amount, tilting the ampoule if necessary.	To ensure the powder is dissolved and has formed a solution with the diluent. To avoid drawing in air (NPSA 2007d, **C**).
10 Replace the sheath on the needle using a one-handed scooping method (see Figure 12.24) and tap the syringe to dislodge any air bubbles. Expel air.	To prevent aerosol formation. To ensure that the correct amount of drug is in the syringe (NPSA 2007d, **C**).
11 Attach a new needle if required (and discard used needle into appropriate sharps container) or attach a plastic end cap or insert syringe into the syringe packet.	To reduce the risk of contamination of the syringe tip. To avoid possible trauma to the patient if the needle has barbed (become bent/hooked), to avoid tracking medications through superficial tissues and to ensure that the correct size of needle is used for intramuscular or subcutaneous injection. To reduce the risk of injury to the nurse (NPSA 2007d, **C**).
12 Attach a label to the syringe.	To ensure practitioner can identify medication in syringe (NPSA 2007d, **C**).
13 Keep all ampoules/vials and diluents in the tray with the syringe.	To enable checking at the bedside. **E**

Procedure guideline 12.14 Medication: multidose-vial: powder preparation using a venting needle

Essential equipment

- Medication ampoule
- Diluent
- Needles × 2
- Syringe
- Alcohol swab

Pre-procedure

Action	Rationale
1 Wash hands with bactericidal soap and water or bactericidal alcohol handrub.	To prevent contamination of medication and equipment (DH 2007, **C**).
2 Open packaging and attach needle to the syringe.	To assemble the equipment. **E**
Procedure	
3 Open the diluent and draw up required volume.	To ensure the correct volume of diluent. **E**
4 Remove the tamper-evident seal on the vial and clean the rubber septum with alcohol swab and let it air dry for at least 30 seconds.	To prevent bacterial contamination of the drug, as the plastic lid prevents damage but does not ensure sterility (NPSA 2007d, **C**).
5 Insert a 21 G needle into the cap to vent the bottle (**Action figure 5a**).	To prevent pressure differentials, which can cause separation of needle and syringe (NPSA 2007d, **C**).
6 Insert the needle bevel up, at an angle of 45–60°. Before completing the insertion of the needle tip, lift the needle to 90° and proceed (**Action figure 6**).	To minimize the risk of coring when inserting the needle into the cap. **E**
7 Inject the correct diluent slowly into the powder within the ampoule.	To ensure that the powder is thoroughly wet before it is mixed and is not released into the atmosphere (NPSA 2007d, **C**).
8 Remove the needle and the syringe.	To enable adequate mixing of the solution. **E**
9 Place a sterile topical swab over the venting needle (see **Action figure 5b**) and gently swirl to dissolve the powder.	To prevent contamination of the drug or the atmosphere. To mix the diluent with the powder and dissolve the drug (NPSA 2007d, **C**).
10 Inspect the solution for cloudiness or particulate matter. If this is present, discard. Follow hospital guidelines on what action to take, for example return drug to pharmacy.	To prevent patient from receiving an unstable or contaminated drug (NPSA 2007d, **C**).
11 Withdraw the prescribed amount of solution, and inspect for pieces of rubber which may have 'cored out' of the cap (see **Action figure 5c**).	To ensure that the correct amount of drug is in the syringe (NPSA 2007d, **C**). To prevent the injection of foreign matter into the patient (NPSA 2007d, **C**).

(continued)

Procedure guideline 12.14 Medication: multidose-vial: powder preparation using a venting needle *(continued)*

Action	Rationale
12 Remove air from syringe without spraying into the atmosphere by injecting air back into the vial (see **Action figure 5d**) or replace the sheath on the needle using a one-handed scooping method (see Figure 12.24) and tap the syringe to dislodge any air bubbles. Expel air.	To reduce risk of contamination of practitioner. To prevent aerosol formation (NPSA 2007d, **C**).
13 Attach a new needle if required (and discard used needle into appropriate sharps container) or attach a plastic end cap or insert syringe into the syringe packet.	To reduce the risk of contamination of the syringe tip. To avoid possible trauma to the patient if the needle has barbed (become bent/hooked), to avoid tracking medications through superficial tissues and to ensure that the correct size of needle is used for intramuscular or subcutaneous injection. To reduce the risk of injury to the nurse (NPSA 2007d, **C**).
14 Attach a label to the syringe.	To ensure practitioner can identify medication in syringe (NPSA 2007d, **C**).
15 Keep all ampoules/vials and diluents in the tray with the syringe.	To enable checking at the bedside. **E**

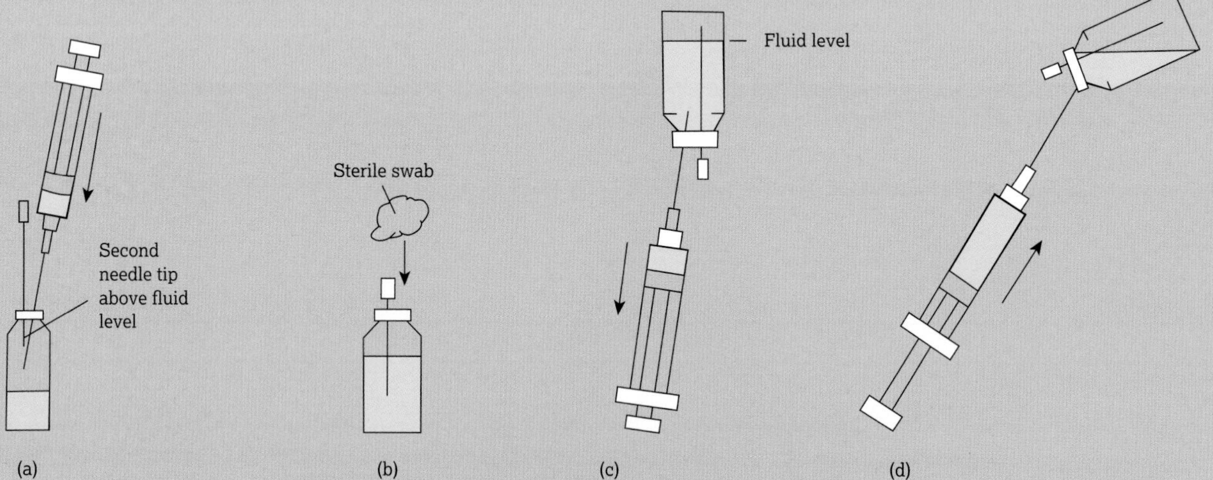

Action Figure 5 Suggested method of vial reconstitution to avoid environmental exposure. (a) When reconstituting vial, insert a second needle to allow air to escape when adding diluent for injection. (b) When gently swirling the vial to dissolve the powder, push in second needle up to Luer connection and cover with a sterile swab. (c) To remove reconstituted solution, insert syringe needle and then invert vial. Ensuring that tip of second needle is above fluid, withdraw the solution. (d) Remove air from syringe without spraying into the atmosphere by injecting air back into vial.

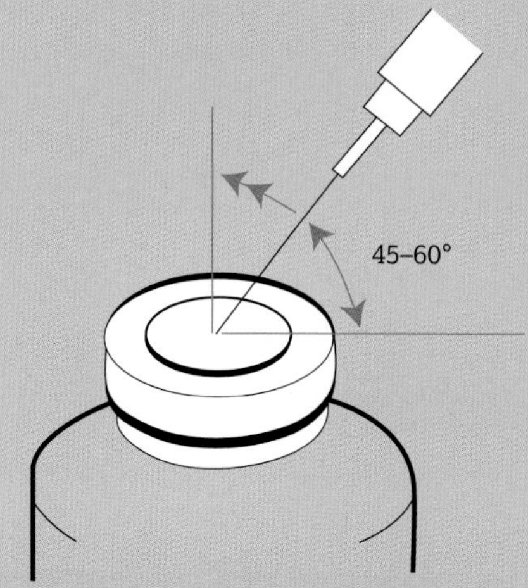

Action Figure 6 Method to minimize coring.

Procedure guideline 12.15 Medication: multidose vial: powder preparation using equilibrium method

Essential equipment

- Medication vial
- Diluent
- Needle
- Syringe
- Alcohol swab

Pre-procedure

Action	Rationale
1 Wash hands with bactericidal soap and water or bactericidal alcohol handrub.	To prevent contamination of medication and equipment (DH 2007, **C**).
2 Open packaging and attach needle to the syringe.	To assemble the equipment. **E**

Procedure

Action	Rationale
3 Open the diluent and draw up required volume.	To ensure the correct volume of diluent. **E**
4 Remove the tamper-evident seal on the vial and clean the rubber septum with an alcohol swab and let it air dry for at least 30 seconds.	To prevent bacterial contamination of the drug, as the plastic lid prevents damage but does not ensure sterility (NPSA 2007d, **C**).
5 Inject the diluent into the vial. Keeping the tip of the needle above the level of the solution in the vial, release the plunger. The syringe will fill with air which has been displaced by the solution.	To prevent bacterial contamination of the drug (NPSA 2007d, **C**).
6 With the syringe and needle still in place, gently swirl the vial to dissolve all the powder.	To mix the diluent with the powder and dissolve the drug (NPSA 2007d, **C**).
7 Inspect the solution for cloudiness or particulate matter. If this is present, discard. Follow hospital guidelines on what action to take; for example, return drug to pharmacy.	To prevent patient from receiving an unstable or contaminated drug (NPSA 2007d, **C**).
8 Invert the vial. Keep the needle in the solution and slowly depress the plunger to push the air into the vial.	To create an equilibrium in the vial (NPSA 2007d, **C**).
9 Release the plunger so that the solution flows back into the syringe (if a large volume of solution is to be withdrawn, use a push-pull technique).	To create an equilibrium in the vial (NPSA 2007d, **C**).
10 Inject the diluent into the vial. Keeping the tip of the needle above the level of the solution in the vial, release the plunger. The syringe will fill with the air which has been displaced by the solution.	This 'equilibrium method' helps to minimize the build-up of pressure in the vial (NPSA 2007d, **C**).
11 Withdraw the prescribed amount of solution, and inspect for pieces of rubber which may have 'cored out' of the cap (see **Action figure 5c** in Procedure guideline 12.14).	To ensure that the correct amount of drug is in the syringe (NPSA 2007d, **C**). To prevent the injection of foreign matter into the patient (NPSA 2007d, **C**).
12 Remove air from syringe without spraying into the atmosphere by injecting air back into the vial (see **Action figure 5d** in Procedure guideline 12.14) or replace the sheath on the needle using a one-handed scooping method (see Figure 12.24) and tap the syringe to dislodge any air bubbles.	To reduce risk of contamination of practitioner. To prevent aerosol formation (NPSA 2007d, **C**).
13 Attach a new needle if required (and discard used needle into appropriate sharps container) or attach a plastic end cap or insert syringe into the syringe packet.	To reduce the risk of contamination of the syringe tip. To avoid possible trauma to the patient if the needle has barbed (become bent/hooked), to avoid tracking medications through superficial tissues and to ensure that the correct size of needle is used for intramuscular or subcutaneous injection. To reduce the risk of injury to the nurse (NPSA 2007d, **C**).
14 Attach a label to the syringe.	To ensure practitioner can identify medication in syringe (NPSA 2007d, **C**).
15 Keep all ampoules/vials and diluents in the tray with the syringe.	To enable checking at the bedside. **E**

Procedure guideline 12.16 Medication: injection administration

Essential equipment

- Clean tray or receiver in which to place drug and equipment
- 21 G needle(s) to ease reconstitution and drawing up, 23 G if from a glass ampoule
- 21, 23 or 25 G needle, size dependent on route of administration
- Syringe(s) of appropriate size for amount of drug to be given
- Swabs saturated with isopropyl alcohol 70%
- Sterile topical swab, if drug is presented in ampoule form
- Drug(s) to be administered
- Patient's prescription chart, to check dose, route and so on
- Recording sheet or book as required by law or hospital policy
- Any protective clothing required by hospital policy for specified drugs, such as antibiotics or cytotoxic drugs, such as goggles or gloves.

Pre-procedure

Action	Rationale
1 Collect and check all equipment.	To prevent delays and enable full concentration on the procedure. **E**.
2 Check that the packaging of all equipment is intact.	To ensure sterility. If the seal is damaged, discard (NPSA 2007d, **C**).
3 Wash hands with bactericidal soap and water or bactericidal alcohol handrub.	To prevent contamination of medication and equipment (DH 2007, **C**).
Procedure	
4 Prepare needle(s), syringe(s) and so on, on a tray or receiver.	To contain all items in a clean area. **E**
5 Inspect all equipment.	To check that none is damaged; if so, discard or report to MHRA. **C**
6 Explain and discuss the procedure with the patient.	To ensure that the patient understands the procedure and gives their valid consent (Griffith and Jordan 2003, **E**; NMC 2013, **C**; NMC 2015, **C**).
7 Before administering any prescribed drug, look at the patient's prescription chart and check the following. (a) The correct patient (b) Drug (c) Dose (d) Date and time of administration (e) Route and method of administration (f) Diluent as appropriate (g) Validity of prescription (h) Signature of prescriber (i) The prescription is legible	To ensure that the patient is given the correct drug in the prescribed dose using the appropriate diluent and by the correct route (DH 2003b, **C**; NMC 2010a, **C**). To protect the patient from harm (DH 2003b, **C**; NMC 2010a, **C**).
If any of these pieces of information are missing, are unclear or illegible then the nurse should not proceed with administration and should consult with the prescriber.	To prevent any errors occurring. **E**
8 Check all details with another nurse if required by hospital policy.	To minimize any risk of error (NMC 2010a, **C**).
9 Select the drug in the appropriate volume, dilution or dosage and check the expiry date.	To reduce wastage. Treatment with medication that is outside the expiry date is dangerous. Drugs deteriorate with storage. The expiry date indicates when a particular drug is no longer pharmacologically efficacious (NPSA 2007d, **C**).
10 Proceed with the preparation of the drug, using protective clothing if advisable.	To protect practitioner during preparation (NPSA 2007d, **C**).
11 Take the prepared dose to the patient and close the door or curtains as appropriate.	To ensure patient privacy and dignity. **E**
12 Check patient's identity.	To prevent error and confirm patient's identity (NPSA 2005, **C**).

13 Evaluate the patient's knowledge of the medication being offered. If this knowledge appears to be faulty or incorrect, offer an explanation of the use, action, dose and potential side-effects of the drug or drugs involved.	A patient has a right to information about treatment (NMC 2010a, **C**).
14 Administer the drug as prescribed.	To ensure patient receives treatment. **E**
Post-procedure	
15 Dispose of all equipment in the appropriate waste containers/sharps bins.	To ensure safe disposal of all equipment.
16 Record the administration on appropriate charts.	To maintain accurate records, provide a point of reference in the event of any queries and prevent any duplication of treatment (NMC 2010a, **C**; NMC 2010b, **C**; NPSA 2007d, **C**).

METHODS FOR INJECTION OR INFUSION

There are a number of routes for injection or infusion (see Box 12.15). The selection may be pre-determined, for example intra-arterial, intra-articular injections. The choice of other routes will normally depend on the desired therapeutic effect and the patient's safety and comfort.

Intra-arterial

This special technique allows the delivery of a high concentration of drug to the tissues or organ supplied by a particular artery if the medications are rapidly metabolized or systematically toxic (Downie et al. 2003). This route can be used for the administration of chemotherapy and vasodilators and for diagnostic purposes. Injection of drugs into an artery is a rare and hazardous procedure. The introduction of the cannula or catheter must be performed with care as the vessel may go into spasm, causing pain and occlusion. This could result in necrosis of an organ or part of a limb.

Intra-articular

In inflammatory conditions of the joints, corticosteroids are given by intra-articular injection to relieve inflammation and increase joint mobility (Downie et al. 2003).

Intrathecal administration of medication

Intrathecal administration is the administration of drugs into the central nervous system (CNS) via the cerebrospinal fluid. This is usually achieved using a lumbar puncture (Polovich et al. 2014, Stanley 2002, Wilkes and Barton Burke 2011).

Medications can be administered intrathecally if they have poor lipid solubility and therefore do not pass the blood–brain barrier (Downie et al. 2003). Only medication specially prepared for the intrathecal route should be used; doses should be carefully calculated and are usually much smaller than would be given by intramuscular or intravenous injection. Water-soluble antibiotics are administered by the intrathecal route to achieve adequate concentrations in the cerebrospinal fluid (CSF) in the treatment of meningitis. Other medicines administered via this route include antifungal agents, opioids, cytotoxic therapy and radiopaque substances (used in the diagnosis of spinal lesions) (Downie et al. 2003).

Intradermal injection

DEFINITION

An intradermal injection is given into the dermis of the skin just below the epidermis where the blood supply is reduced and drug absorption can occur slowly (Chernecky et al. 2002). The intradermal route provides a local rather than systemic effect and is used primarily for administering small amounts of local anaesthetic and skin testing, for example allergy or tuberculin testing (Potter 2011).

EVIDENCE-BASED APPROACHES

Observation of the skin for an inflammatory reaction is a priority, so the best sites are those that are lowly pigmented, thinly keratinized and hairless. Chosen sites are the inner forearms and the scapulae. The injection site most commonly used for skin testing is the medial forearm area as this allows for easy inspection (Downie et al. 2003). Volumes of 0.5 mL or less should be used (Chernecky et al. 2002).

PRE-PROCEDURAL CONSIDERATIONS

Equipment

The injections are best performed using a 25 or 27 G needle inserted at a 10–15° angle, bevel up, just under the epidermis. Usually a TB (tuberculosis) or 1 mL syringe is used to ensure accuracy of dose.

Procedure guideline 12.17 Medication: intradermal injection

Essential equipment

- Needle 25–27 G
- 1 mL syringe containing medication
- Alcohol swab
- Apron
- Non-sterile gloves

Pre-procedure

Action	Rationale
1 Explain and discuss the procedure with the patient.	To ensure that the patient understands the procedure and gives their valid consent (Griffith and Jordan 2003, **E**; NMC 2013, **C**; NMC 2015, **C**).

(continued)

Procedure guideline 12.17 Medication: intradermal injection *(continued)*

Action	Rationale
2 Before administering any prescribed drug, look at the patient's prescription chart and check the following. (a) The correct patient (b) Drug (c) Dose (d) Date and time of administration (e) Route and method of administration (f) Diluent as appropriate (g) Validity of prescription (h) Signature of prescriber (i) The prescription is legible	To ensure that the patient is given the correct drug in the prescribed dose using the appropriate diluent and by the correct route (DH 2003b, **C**; NMC 2010a, **C**). To protect the patient from harm (DH 2003b, **C**; NMC 2010a, **C**).
If any of these pieces of information are missing, are unclear or illegible then the nurse should not proceed with administration and should consult with the prescriber. Prepare medication as described in Procedure guidelines 12.12, 12.13, 12.14 and 12.15.	To prevent any errors occurring. **E**
Procedure	
3 Apply apron, close the curtains or door and assist the patient into the required position. Wash hands.	To ensure patient privacy and dignity. **E** To allow access to the appropriate injection site (Workman 1999, **E**).
4 Remove appropriate garments to expose the injection site.	To gain access for injection (Workman 1999, **E**).
5 Assess the injection site for signs of inflammation, oedema, infection and skin lesions.	To promote effectiveness of administration (Workman 1999, **E**). To reduce the risk of infection (Fraise and Bradley 2009, **E**; Workman 1999, **E**). To avoid skin lesions and avoid possible trauma to the patient (Workman 1999, **E**).
6 Choose the correct needle size and attach the needle.	To minimize the risk of missing the subcutaneous tissue and any ensuing pain (Workman 1999, **E**).
7 Apply gloves and clean the injection site with a swab saturated with isopropyl alcohol 70% and apply gloves.	To reduce the number of pathogens introduced into the skin by the needle at the time of insertion. (For further information on this action see 'Skin preparation'.)
8 Remove the needle sheath and hold syringe with the dominant hand with the bevel of needle pointing up.	To facilitate needle placement (Ostendorf 2012, **E**).
9 With the non-dominant hand, stretch skin over the site with forefinger and thumb.	To facilitate the needle piercing the skin more easily (Ostendorf 2012, **E**).
10 With the needle almost against the patient's skin, insert the needle into the skin at an angle of 10–15° and advance through the epidermis so the needle tip can be seen through the skin.	To ensure the needle tip is in the dermis (Ostendorf 2012, **E**).
11 Inject medication slowly. It is not necessary to aspirate as the dermis is relatively avascular.	To minimize the discomfort at site (Ostendorf 2012, **E**).
12 While injecting medication, a bleb (resembling a mosquito bite) will form (**Action figure 12**).	To indicate medication is in dermis (Ostendorf 2012, **E**).
13 Withdraw the needle rapidly and apply pressure gently. Do not massage the site.	To prevent dispersing medication into underlying tissue layers and altering test results (Chernecky et al. 2002, **E**; Ostendorf 2012, **E**).
Post-procedure	
14 Where appropriate, activate safety device. Ensure that all sharps and non-sharp waste are disposed of safely and in accordance with locally approved procedures. For example, sharps into sharps bin and syringes into an orange clinical waste bag.	To ensure safe disposal and to avoid laceration or other injury to staff (DH 2005, **C**; EU 2010, **C**; MHRA 2004, **C**).
15 Record the administration on appropriate sheets.	To maintain accurate records, provide a point of reference in the event of any queries and prevent any duplication of treatment (NMC 2010a, **C**; NMC 2010b, **C**; NPSA 2007d, **C**).

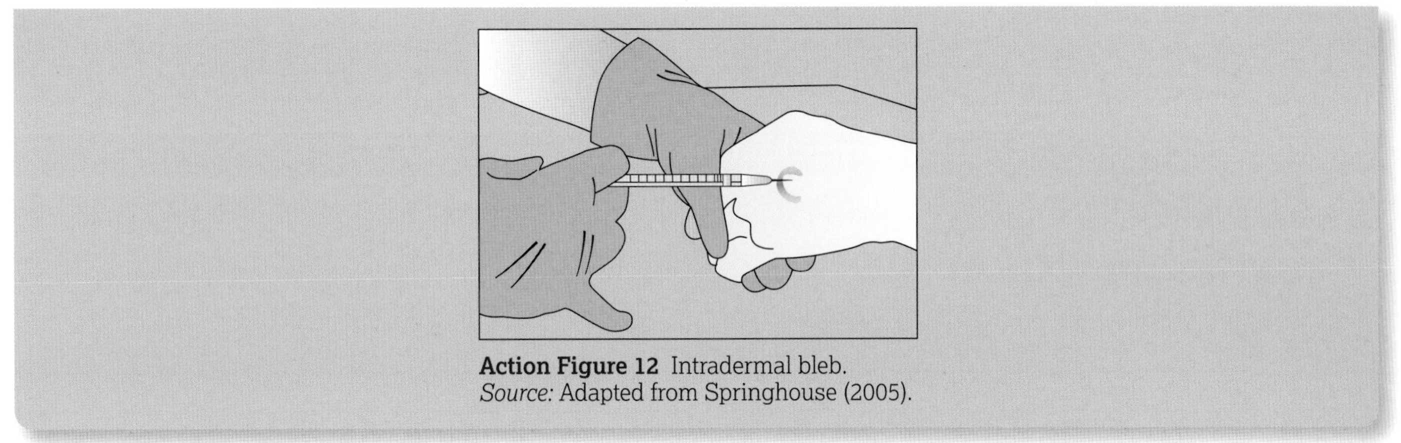

Action Figure 12 Intradermal bleb.
Source: Adapted from Springhouse (2005).

Subcutaneous injection

DEFINITION

These are given beneath the epidermis into the loose fat and connective tissue underlying the dermis and are used for administering small doses of non-irritating water-soluble substances such as insulin or heparin (Downie et al. 2003).

RELATED THEORY

Subcutaneous tissue is not richly supplied with blood vessels and so medication is absorbed more slowly than when given intramuscularly. The rate of absorption is influenced by factors that affect blood flow to tissues such as physical exercise or local application of hot or cold compresses (Ostendorf 2012). Other conditions can prevent or delay absorption due to an impaired blood flow so in these conditions, subcutaeous injections are contraindicated, for example circulatory shock, occlusive vascular disease (Ostendorf 2012).

EVIDENCE-BASED APPROACHES

Injection sites

Sites recommended are the abdomen in the umbilical region, the lateral or posterior aspect of the lower part of the upper arm, the thighs (under the greater trochanter rather than midthigh) and the buttocks (Downie et al. 2003) (Figure 12.25). It has been found that the amount of subcutaneous tissue varies more than was previously thought; this is particularly significant for administration of insulin as inadvertent intramuscular administration can result in rapid absorption and hypoglycaemic episodes (King 2003). Rotation of sites can decrease the likelihood of irritation and ensure improved absorption. If using the abdominal area then try to inject each subsequent injection 2.5 cm from the previous one (Chernecky et al. 2002). Injection sites should be free of infection, skin lesions, scars, birthmarks, bony prominences and large underlying muscles or nerves (Ostendorf 2012).

The skin should be gently pinched into a fold to elevate the subcutaneous tissue which lifts the adipose tissue away from the underlying muscle (FIT 2011). The practice of aspirating to ensure a blood vessel has not been pierced is no longer recommended as it has been shown that this is unlikely to occur (Ostendorf 2012, Peragallo-Dittko 1997). The maximum volume tolerable using this route for injection is 2 mL and drugs should be highly soluble to prevent irritation (Downie et al. 2003).

PRE-PROCEDURAL CONSIDERATIONS

Equipment

Injections are usually given using a 25 G needle. To ensure medication reaches the subcutaneous tissue, the rule is: if you can grasp 2 inches of tissue, insert the needle at a 90° angle; for 1 inch, insert needle at a 45° angle (Chernecky et al. 2002, Ostendorf 2012). With the introduction of shorter needles (4–8 mm), it is recommended that insulin injections be given at an angle of 90° (FIT 2011, King 2003). The length of the needle should be selected by pinching the skin tissue and selecting a needle one-half the width of the skinfold (Chernecky et al. 2002, FIT 2011). Shorter needles should also be used at a 45° angle in children and underweight adults.

Figure 12.25 **Sites recommended for subcutaneous injection.** ***Source:*** **Adapted from Elkin et al. (2007).**

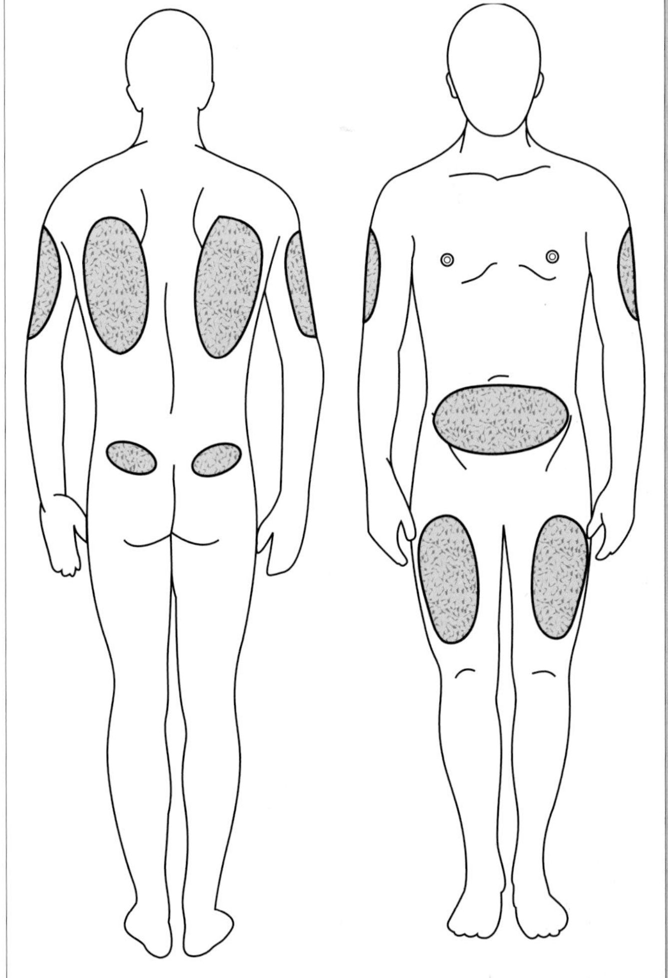

Specific patient preparation

It has been stated that it is not necessary to use an alcohol swab to clean the skin prior to administration of injections providing the skin is socially clean (FIT 2011). If unsure or in immunocompromised patients, the skin should be prepared using an antiseptic swab (Dann 1969, Downie et al. 2003, FIT 2011).

Procedure guideline 12.18 Medication: subcutaneous injection

Essential equipment

- Gloves and apron
- Alcohol swab
- Needle
- Syringe containing prepared medication
- Sterile gauze

Pre-procedure

Action	Rationale
1 Explain and discuss the procedure with the patient.	To ensure that the patient understands the procedure and gives their valid consent (Griffith and Jordan 2003, **E**; NMC 2013, **C**; NMC 2015, **C**).
2 Before administering any prescribed drug, look at the patient's prescription chart and check the following: (a) The correct patient (b Drug (c) Dose (d) Date and time of administration (e) Route and method of administration (f) Diluent as appropriate (g) Validity of prescription (h) Signature of prescriber (i) The prescription is legible	To ensure that the correct patient is given the correct drug in the prescribed dose using the appropriate diluent and by the correct route (DH 2003b, **C**; NMC 2010a, **C**). To protect the patient from harm (DH 2003b, **C**; NMC 2010a, **C**).
If any of these pieces of information are missing, are unclear or illegible then the nurse should not proceed with administration and should consult with the prescriber.	To prevent any errors occurring. **E**
Prepare medication as described in Procedure guidelines 12.12, 12.13, 12.14 and 12.15.	
3 Wash hands and apply an apron.	To prevent contamination of medication and equipment (DH 2007, **C**). To prevent possible cross-contamination (Fraise and Bradley 2009, **E**).

Procedure

Action	Rationale
4 Close the curtains or door and assist the patient into the required position.	To ensure patient's privacy and dignity. **E** To allow access to the appropriate injection site (Ostendorf 2012, **E**).
5 Remove appropriate garments to expose the injection site.	To gain access for injection. **E**
6 Assess the injection site for signs of inflammation, oedema, infection and skin lesions.	To promote effectiveness of administration (Ostendorf 2012, **E**). To reduce the risk of infection (Fraise and Bradley 2009, **E**; Workman 1999, **E**). To avoid skin lesions and possible trauma to the patient (Ostendorf 2012, **E**).
7 Wash and dry hands and apply non-sterile gloves.	To prevent contamination of medication and equipment (DH 2007, **C**). To prevent possible cross-contamination (Fraise and Bradley 2009, **E**).
8 Pinch the skin and select the correct needle size (this is commonly a 23 G needle).	To minimize the risk of missing the subcutaneous tissue and any ensuing pain (FIT 2011, **C**; Ostendorf 2012, **E**).
9 Where appropriate, clean the injection site with a swab saturated with isopropyl alcohol 70%.	To reduce the number of pathogens introduced into the skin by the needle at the time of insertion (FIT 2011, **C**). (For further information on this action see 'Skin preparation'.)
10 Remove the needle sheath.	To prepare the syringe for use. **E**

11 Gently pinch the skin up into a fold.	To elevate the subcutaneous tissue, and lift the adipose tissue away from the underlying muscle (FIT 2011,**C**; Ostendorf 2012, **E**).
12 Hold the syringe between thumb and forefinger of dominant hand as if grasping a dart.	To enable a quick smooth injection (Ostendorf 2012, **E**).
13 Insert the needle into the skin at an angle of 45° and release the grasped skin (unless administering insulin when an angle of 90° should be used). Inject the drug slowly over 10–30 seconds.	Injecting medication into compressed tissue irritates nerve fibres and causes the patient discomfort (Ostendorf 2012, **E**). The introduction of shorter insulin needles makes 90° the more appropriate angle (FIT 2011,**C**; Trounce and Gould 2000, **E**).
14 Withdraw the needle rapidly. Apply gentle pressure with sterile gauze. Do not massage area.	To aid absorption. Massage can injure underlying tissue (Ostendorf 2012, **E**).
Post-procedure	
15 Where appropriate, activate safety device. Ensure that all sharps and non-sharp waste are disposed of safely and in accordance with locally approved procedures.	To ensure safe disposal and to avoid laceration or other injury to staff (DH, 2005b, **C**; MHRA, 2004, **C**).
16 Record the administration on appropriate sheets.	To maintain accurate records, provide a point of reference in the event of any queries and prevent any duplication of treatment (NMC 2010a, **C**; NMC 2010b, **C**; NPSA 2007d, **C**).

POST-PROCEDURAL CONSIDERATIONS

Education of patient and relevant others

Patients often have to administer their own subcutaneous injections, for example insulin for diabetics. The nurse must teach the patient how to prepare and administer self-injection, including aspects such as equipment, storage, hand washing, injection technique, rotation of sites and safe disposal of equipment and sharps (FIT 2011, Ostendorf 2012).

COMPLICATIONS

Medications collecting within the tissues can cause sterile abscesses, which appear as hardened, painful lumps (Ostendorf 2012) or in rare cases lipohypertrophy (wasting of the subcutaneous tissue at injection sites) can develop (FIT 2011). The nurse must monitor and report these and avoid using these areas for further injections (FIT 2011).

Subcutaneous infusion

DEFINITION

Continuous infusion of fluids or medication into the subcutaneous tissues (Ostendorf 2012).

EVIDENCE-BASED APPROACHES

Methods for subcutaneous infusions of fluids (hypodermoclysis)

Hypodermoclysis is a method of infusing fluid into subcutaneous tissue that is easier than administering intravenous fluids (Sasson and Shvartzman 2001). Subcutaneous fluids can be given to maintain adequate hydration in patients with mild or moderate dehydration (Scales 2011, Walsh 2005) and have been shown to be as effective as the intravenous route for replacing fluid and electrolytes (Barton et al. 2004, Barua and Bhowmick 2005, Luk et al. 2008). The use of this route is generally limited to palliative care or elderly patients (Scales 2011, Walsh 2005). It is not recommended for patients needing rapid administration of fluids, and is also contraindicated in patients with clotting disorders or who have problems with fluid overload (such as those with cardiac failure) (Mei and Auerhahn 2009, Walsh 2005).

A volume of 1000–2000 mL can be given over 24 hours; this can be given as a continuous infusion, over a number of hours (such as overnight) or as intermittent boluses (Moriarty and Hudson 2001, Scales 2011, Walsh 2005). More than one site can be used if greater volumes are required. It is recommended that electrolyte-containing fluids such as sodium chloride 0.9% or dextrose saline be used although 5% glucose has also been used (Hypodermoclysis Working Group 1998, Sasson and Shvartzman 2001).

Advantages of this route include the following.

- Side-effects are few and not generally significant.
- It is a relatively easy procedure which can be carried out at home, reducing the need for hospitalization.
- May be set up and administered by nurses in almost any setting.
- Low cost.
- Less likely to cause fluid overload.
- Intravenous access can be problematic in elderly or debilitated patients; avoidance of this can reduce anxiety and distress (Mei and Auerhahn 2009, Scales 2011).

Side-effects of subcutaneous fluid administration include pain, bruising, local oedema, erythema and local inflammation, which can be reduced by changing the site of infusion (Mei and Auerhahn 2009, Scales 2011).

Hyaluronidase is an enzyme which temporarily increases the permeability of subcutaneous connective tissue by degrading hyaluronic acid and has been shown to increase the dispersion and absorption of co-administered molecules (Thomas et al. 2009). It can be given as a subcutaneous injection before commencing fluids or added to infusion bags (Sasson and Shvartzman 2001). A randomized study compared absorption and side-effects of administration of subcutaneous fluids with or without hyaluronidase. No significant differences were found although patients not receiving hyaluronidase showed an increase in the size of the limb in which the fluid had been administered, but no differences in pain or local discomfort were found so no clear benefit to the use of hyaluronidase was demonstrated (Constans et al. 1991). Most agree that it is not necessary to use hyaluronidase if the infusion rate is 1 mL/min or less (Mei and Auerhahn 2009).

Methods for subcutaneous infusions of drugs

This may be the route of choice in patients with problems such as vomiting, diarrhoea or dysphagia and who are unable to tolerate drugs by the oral route; patients with bowel obstruction whose gut absorption may be impaired may also benefit. It is also commonly used for patients who are dying and no longer able to manage medication orally (Dickman et al. 2007, Dychter et al. 2012, Menahem and Shvartzman 2010, Ostendorf 2012). Continuous subcutaneous infusion of insulin is used in a small number of diabetic patients, particularly when adequate control cannot be achieved with multiple daily insulin doses. Such patients need to be under the care of a multidisciplinary team familiar with the use of such infusions (NICE 2003).

Infusions of a single drug, such as an antiemetic or analgesic, do not generally cause problems with stability. The drug should be diluted with a suitable diluent (sodium chloride is recommended for most drugs) and given over 12–24 hours (Dickman et al. 2007). The use of a combination of drugs can be problematic; there is anecdotal evidence regarding combinations of drugs but not many pharmaceutical studies confirming compatibility. Combinations of up to four drugs have been reported but if compatibility is uncertain, it may be best to use a second syringe pump. It is also important to ensure that the diluent used is compatible with all the drugs in the infusion. It is recommended that infusions are not exposed to direct sunlight or to increased temperatures as drug instability may result (Dickman et al. 2007). Hyaluronidase may be used to enhance the pharmacokinetics of drugs such as subcutaneous morphine (Menahem and Shvartzman 2010, Thomas et al. 2009).

PRE-PROCEDURAL CONSIDERATIONS

Equipment

Access devices

Research has shown that the use of peripheral cannulas rather than steel winged infusion devices results in sites remaining viable for longer (Torre 2002). Incidence of needlestick injuries may also be reduced (Dawkins et al. 2000). It is now recommended that subcutaneous infusion be given via a plastic cannula. Administration of infusions of drugs or fluids requires the insertion of a 25 G winged infusion set or a 24 G cannula (RCN 2010, Scales 2011). These should be inserted at an angle of 45° and secured with a transparent dressing to enable inspection of the site. This may also be appropriate for patients not receiving a continuous infusion but requiring frequent subcutaneous injections; this is common practice in palliative care in order to reduce the number of needles inserted into the patient and the subsequent trauma caused.

Syringe driver/pump

A syringe driver/pump is a portable battery-operated infusion device. It is used to deliver drugs at a predetermined rate via the appropriate parenteral route (e.g. subcutaneous) and is suitable for symptom management and palliative care (Dickman et al. 2007, Quinn 2008). It should be used for patients who are unable to tolerate oral medication, for example, in nausea and vomiting, dysphagia, intestinal obstruction, local disease or sometimes in intractable pain which is unrelieved by oral medications and where rapid dose titration is required. Drugs administered by subcutaneous infusion include opioid analgesics, antiemetics, anxiolytic sedatives, corticosteroids, non-steroidal anti-inflammatory drugs and anticholinergic drugs (Dickman et al. 2007, Dychter et al. 2012).

Examples include the Graseby MS16A (calibrated in millimetres per hour) and MS26 (calibrated in millimetres per day) syringe drivers (currently being phased out of use) and the McKinley T34 syringe pump (mL/h). Other types are available and nurses should follow the manufacturer's instruction manual for details of their use.

Most sizes and brands of plastic syringes can be used with these devices; however, it is recommended to use Luer-Lok syringes to avoid leakage or accidental disconnection.

The advantages of the syringe driver are as follows.

- It avoids the necessity of intermittent injections.
- Mixtures of drugs may be administered.
- Infusion timing is accurate, which is particularly advantageous in the community where it is not possible to constantly monitor the rate.
- The device is lightweight and compact, allowing mobility and independence.
- Rate can be increased.
- Simple calculations of dosage are required over a 12- or 24-hour period.
- It allows patients to spend more time at home with their symptoms managed effectively.

The disadvantages are as follows.

- The patient may become psychologically dependent on the device.
- Inflammation or infection may occur at the insertion site of the subcutaneous cannula.
- The rate calculation differs between certain syringe drivers which can be confusing for the nurse.
- The alarm system of some devices operates only if the plunger is obstructed. It does not alert the nurse if the flow is too rapid or too slow (Dickman et al. 2007).

Specific patient preparation

Infusion sites

Choice of site should be based on both thickness of subcutaneous tissue and patient convenience. Sites recommended for subcutaneous infusion of drugs or fluids are the lateral aspects of the upper arms and thighs, the abdomen, the chest and the scapula (Walsh 2005). If the patient is ambulant then the chest or abdomen is the preferred site (Dickman et al. 2007). The following areas should not be used.

- Lymphoedematous areas, as absorption may be impaired and infection may be introduced.
- Sites over bony prominences, as there may be insufficient subcutaneous tissue.
- Previously irradiated skin areas, as absorption may be impaired.
- Sites near a joint, as movement may cause the cannula to become dislodged.
- Any areas of inflamed, infected or broken skin (Mitten 2001, Ostendorf 2012).

Rotation of the site every 3 days should be routine in order to minimize site reactions although in some patients this may not be feasible so the infusion site must be monitored regularly and the device resited as necessary (Dickman et al. 2007).

Procedure guideline 12.19 Medication: subcutaneous infusion of fluids

Essential equipment

- Clinically clean receiver or tray
- Sharps box
- Isopropyl alcohol 70% swab
- Apron
- Non-sterile gloves
- Transparent adhesive dressing
- Winged infusion set or 24 G cannula
- Infusion fluid
- Administration set

Pre-procedure

Action	Rationale
1 Explain and discuss the procedure with the patient.	To ensure that the patient understands the procedure and gives their valid consent (Griffith and Jordan 2003, **E**; NMC 2013, **C**; NMC 2015, **C**).
2 Before administering any prescribed fluid, check that it is due and has not already been given.	To protect the patient from harm (NPSA 2007d, **C**).
3 Before administering any prescribed fluid, look at the patient's prescription chart and check the following. (a) The correct patient (b) Drug/fluid (c) Dose (d) Date and time of administration (e) Route and method of administration (f) Diluent as appropriate (g) Validity of prescription (h) Signature of prescriber (i) The prescription is legible	To ensure that the correct patient is given the correct fluid in the prescribed dose using the appropriate diluent and by the correct route (DH 2003b, **C**; NMC 2010a, **C**). To protect the patient from harm (DH 2003b, **C**; NMC 2010a, **C**).
If any of these pieces of information are missing, are unclear or illegible then the nurse should not proceed with administration and should consult with the prescriber.	To prevent any errors occurring. **E**
4 Wash hands with bactericidal soap and water or bactericidal alcohol handrub, and assemble the necessary equipment.	To minimize the risk of infection (Fraise and Bradley 2009, **E**; Loveday et al. 2014, **C**).

Procedure

Action	Rationale
5 Check the name and volume of infusion fluid against the prescription chart.	To ensure that the correct type and quantity of fluid are administered (NMC 2010a, **C**; NPSA 2007d, **C**).
6 Check the expiry date of the infusion bag.	To prevent an ineffective or toxic compound being administered to the patient (NPSA 2007d, **C**).
7 Check that the packaging is intact and inspect the container and contents in a good light for cracks, punctures or air bubbles.	To check that no contamination of the infusion container has occurred (NPSA 2007d, **C**).
8 Inspect the fluid for discoloration, haziness and crystalline or particulate matter. If this occurs, discard.	To prevent any toxic or foreign matter being infused into the patient (NPSA 2007d, **C**). To detect any incompatibility or degradation (NPSA 2007d, **C**).
9 Establish the correct drip rate setting using the correct calculation.	To monitor rate and ensure fluid is infused safely (Pickstone 1999, **E**).
10 Place the infusion bag and administration set in a clean receptacle. Wash hands and proceed to the patient.	To minimize the risk of contamination (Loveday et al. 2014, **C**).
11 Check the identity of the patient against the prescription chart, and with the patient.	To minimize the risk of error and ensure the correct fluid is administered to the correct patient (NMC 2010a, **C**; NPSA 2007d, **C**).
12 Place the infusion bag on a flat surface, remove the seal and insert the spike of the administration set fully into the infusion bag port.	To prevent puncturing the side of the infusion and to reduce the risk of contamination (DH 2007, **C**).
13 Hang the infusion bag from a drip stand.	To allow gravity flow. **E**
14 Open the roller clamp and allow the fluid through the set to prime it. Close clamp.	To remove air from the set. **E**
15 Apply apron and assist the patient into a comfortable position.	To ensure patient comfort during the proedure. **E**
16 Expose the chosen site for infusion.	To expose the area. **E**
17 Apply gloves and clean the chosen site with a swab saturated with 70% isopropyl alcohol. Wait until the alcohol evaporates.	To reduce the risk of infection and prevent stinging sensation on insertion of needle (Fraise and Bradley 2009, **E**; Loveday et al. 2014, **C**).
18 Grasp the skin firmly.	To elevate the subcutaneous tissue. **E**

(continued)

Procedure guideline 12.19 Medication: subcutaneous infusion of fluids *(continued)*

Action	Rationale
19 Insert the infusion needle into the skin at an angle of 45°, bevel up, and release the grasped skin. (If using a cannula, remove the stylet.)	To gain access to the subcutaneous tissue (Walsh 2005, **E**).
20 Connect the administration set to the device.	To commence the infusion. **E**
21 Apply transparent dressing to secure infusion device.	To prevent movement and reduce the risk of mechanical phlebitis and infection (Fraise and Bradley 2009, **E**; Loveday et al. 2014, **C**; Weinstein and Plumer 2007, **E**).
22 Open the roller clamp and adjust until the flow rate is achieved. The rate is usually 1 mL/min per site by gravity.	To ensure the correct rate is set. **E**
Post-procedure	
23 Complete the patient's prescription chart and other hospital and/or legally required documents.	To comply with local drug administration policies and provide a record in the event of any queries (NMC 2010b, **C**). To prevent any duplication of treatment (NMC 2010a, **C**).
24 Monitor the patient for any infusion- or site-related complications and document these in the patient's notes.	To detect complications promptly (Sasson and Shvartzman 2001, **E**).
25 Ask the patient to report any pain or tenderness at the infusion site.	To ascertain whether there are any problems that may require nursing care and refer to medical staff where appropriate. **E**.
26 Discard waste, making sure that it is placed in the correct containers, for example sharps into a designated receptacle.	To ensure safe disposal and avoid injury to staff. To prevent reuse of equipment (DH 2005, **C**; MHRA 2004, **C**).

Procedure guideline 12.20 Medication: subcutaneous administration using a McKinley T34 syringe pump

Essential equipment

- Clinically clean receiver or tray containing the prepared drug
- Syringe pump
- Battery (PP3 size, 9 volt alkaline)
- Plastic peripheral cannulas (e.g. 24 G) and microbore extension set (100 cm) with needle-free Y connector injection site (or 100 cm winged infusion set)
- Luer-Lok syringe of suitable size (minimum size 20 mL)
- Swab saturated with isopropyl alcohol 70%
- Transparent adhesive dressing
- Drugs and diluent
- Needle (to draw up drug)
- Drug additive label
- Patient's prescription chart
- Recording chart or book as required by law or hospital policy
- Sharps box
- Apron
- Non-sterile gloves

Pre-procedure

Action	Rationale
1 Explain and discuss the procedure with the patient.	To ensure that the patient understands the procedure and gives their valid consent (Griffith and Jordan 2003, **E**; NMC 2013, **C**; NMC 2015, **C**).
2 Before administering any prescribed drug, check that it is due and has not already been given.	To protect the patient from harm (NPSA 2007d, **C**).
3 Before administering any prescribed drug, look at the patient's prescription chart and check the following. (a) The correct patient (b) Drug (c) Dose (d) Date and time of administration	To ensure that the correct patient is given the correct drug in the prescribed dose using the appropriate diluent and by the correct route (DH 2003b, **C**; NMC 2010a, **C**). To protect the patient from harm (DH 2003b, **C**; NMC 2010a, **C**).

Action	Rationale
(e) Route and method of administration (f) Diluent as appropriate (g) Validity of prescription (h) Signature of prescriber (i) The prescription is legible If any of these pieces of information are missing, are unclear or illegible then the nurse should not proceed with administration and should consult with the prescriber.	To prevent any errors occurring. **E**
4 Calculate and check dosage of drugs required over a 24-hour period.	To establish correct dosages of drugs (Pickstone 1999, **E**).
5 Wash hands with bactericidal soap and water or bactericidal alcohol handrub, and assemble the necessary equipment.	To minimize the risk of infection (Fraise and Bradley 2009, **E**; Loveday et al. 2014, **C**).
Procedure	
6 Check the name, strength and volume of subcutaneous drug(s) against the prescription chart.	To ensure that the correct type and quantity of fluid are administered (NMC 2010a, **C**; NPSA 2007d, **C**).
7 Check the expiry date of the drug(s).	To prevent an ineffective or toxic compound being administered to the patient (NPSA 2007d, **C**).
8 Check that the packaging is intact and inspect the container and contents in a good light for cracks, punctures, air bubbles.	To check that no contamination of the infusion container has occurred (NPSA 2007d, **C**).
9 Check the identity and amount of drug to be prepared.	To minimize any risk of error. To ensure safe and effective administration of the drug (NPSA 2007d, **C**).
Consider: (a) compatibility of drugs (b) stability of mixture over the prescription time (c) any special directions for dilution, for example pH, optimum concentration (d) sensitivity to external factors such as light (e) any anticipated allergic reaction. If any doubts exist about the listed points, consult the pharmacist or appropriate reference works.	To enable anticipation of toxicities and the nursing implications of these (NPSA 2007d, **C**).
10 Prepare medication as described in Procedure guidelines 12.12, 12.13, 12.14 and 12.15. Using a Luer-Lok syringe, draw up drugs required with diluent to measure a total volume (this will depend on type of syringe pump used). See Box 12.17 for McKinley T34 recommended volumes and **Action figure 10** for a McKinley T34 syringe pump.	To ensure accuracy and avoid any infusion errors. To ensure the drug is prepared correctly (NPSA 2007d, **C**).
11 Inspect the fluid for discoloration, haziness and crystalline or particulate matter. If this occurs, discard and re-evaluate drug compatability. *Note*: This can occur even if the mixture is theoretically compatible, thus making vigilance essential.	To prevent any toxic or foreign matter being infused into the patient (NPSA 2007d, **C**). To detect any incompatibility or degradation (NPSA 2007d, **C**).
12 Establish the correct rate setting of the pump using the correct calculation.	To monitor rate and ensure drug is infused safely (Dickman et al. 2007, **E**; Pickstone1999, **E**).
13 Complete the drug additive label and fix it onto the syringe without obscuring the markings.	To identify which drug has been added, when and by whom and be able to visually inspect the amount in the syringe (NPSA 2007d, **C**).
14 Wash hands with bactericidal soap and water or bactericidal alcohol handrub.	To minimize the risk of infection (Fraise and Bradley 2009, **E**; Loveday et al. 2014, **C**).
15 Connect prepared syringe to a 100 cm microbore driver set with needle-free Y connector injection site.	This length of tubing allows patient greater freedom of movement. **E**
16 Prime the infusion by gently depressing the plunger of the syringe until the fluid is visible at the end of the infusion set. Priming the infusion set after calculation will reduce the delivery time by approximately half an hour for the first infusion. Do not alter previously calculated rate setting despite volume reduction in barrel of syringe.	This removes extraneous air from the system. **E** Ensures patient receives drugs immediately and accurately. **E**

(continued)

Procedure guideline 12.20 Medication: subcutaneous administration using a McKinley T34 syringe pump *(continued)*

Action	Rationale
17 Place the syringe and infusion set in a clean receptacle. Wash hands and proceed to the patient.	To minimize the risk of contamination (Loveday et al. 2014, **C**).
18 Check the identity of the patient against the prescription chart, syringe drug additive label and with the patient if possible.	To minimize the risk of error and ensure the correct drug is administered to the correct patient (NMC 2010a, **C**; NPSA 2007d, **C**).
19 Apply apron and assist the patient into a comfortable position.	To aid patient comfort. **E**
20 Expose the chosen site for infusion.	To gain access to the site. **E**
21 Apply gloves and clean the chosen site with a swab saturated with 70% isopropyl alcohol. Wait until the alcohol evaporates.	To reduce the risk of infection and prevent stinging sensation on insertion of needle (Fraise and Bradley 2009, **E**; Loveday et al. 2014, **C**).
22 Grasp the skin firmly.	To elevate the subcutaneous tissue. **E**
23 Insert the infusion needle into the skin at an angle of 45° and release the grasped skin. (If using a cannula, remove the stylet and connect the extension set.)	Positioning shallower than 45° may shorten the life of the infusion site. **E**
24 Apply transparent dressing to secure infusion device.	To prevent movement and reduce the risk of mechanical phlebitis and infection (Fraise and Bradley 2009, **E**; Loveday et al. 2014, **C**; Weinstein and Plumer 2007, **E**).
25 Check that the infusion set and syringe are securely connected.	To ensure that there is no disconnection so that the drug(s) are administered correctly. **E**
26 Connect the syringe to the syringe pump.	To ensure the syringe is connected correctly to the syringe pump. **E**
27 Press the >Back key to adjust the actuator to accommodate the syringe. Lift the barrel arm and ensure the syringe is loaded correctly. If not loaded into the barrel, collar and plunger correctly, this will be identified on the LED screen.	To ensure the syringe is in the correct position (manufacturer's instructions, **C**).
28 The pump will detect size and brand of syringe. Check and confirm by pressing YES key.	To enable the pump mechanism to operate correctly (manufacturer's instructions, **C**).
29 Set a new programme for each syringe.	To clear previous programme and reduce risk of error (manufacturer's instructions, **C**).
30 Pump measures deliverable volume in syringe.	To check the volume is as required. **E**
31 Press YES to confirm volume to be infused. Press YES to confirm infusion duration. Pump displays rate calculated on volume and duration set by user. Then press YES to confirm.	To complete set-up of device (manufacturer's instructions, **C**).
32 Secure in the clear Perspex lock box (for syringes 30 mL or larger only).	To ensure extra security and minimize the risk of errors in infusional rates. **E**
33 Discard waste, making sure that it is placed in the correct containers, for example sharps into a designated receptacle.	To ensure safe disposal and avoid injury to staff. To prevent reuse of equipment (DH 2005, **C**; MHRA 2004, **C**).
Post-procedure	
34 Complete the patient's prescription chart and other hospital and/or legally required documents. This should include infusion device serial number and infusion device and site checks.	To comply with local drug administration policies and ensure the safe administration and monitoring of the infused drug and accurate records. To provide a record in the event of any queries (NMC 2010b, **C**). To prevent any duplication of treatment (NMC 2010b, **C**).
35 Monitor the patient for any infusion-related complications.	To detect complications promptly (Dickman et al. 2007, **E**; Dougherty 2002, **E**; MHRA 2010b, **C**; Pickstone 1999, **E**; Quinn 2000, **E**).
36 Ask the patient to report any pain and tenderness at the infusion site and if they experience any change in their symptoms or have new symptoms.	To ascertain whether there are any problems that may require nursing care and refer to medical staff where appropriate. **E**

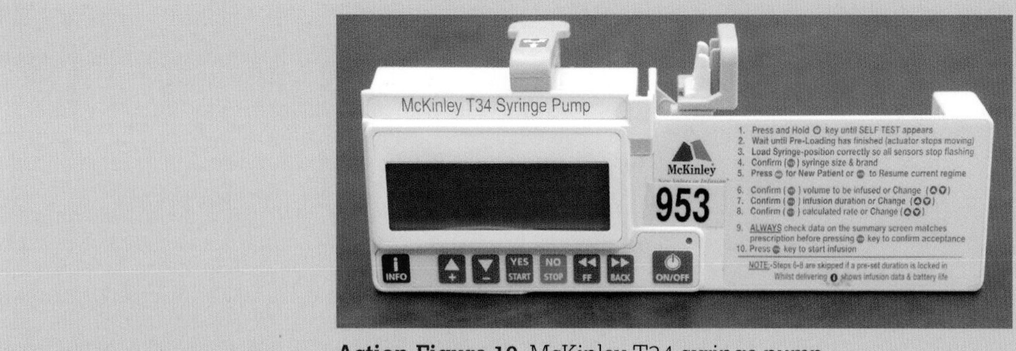

Action Figure 10 McKinley T34 syringe pump.

Problem-solving table 12.2 **Prevention and resolution (Procedure guideline 12.20)**

Problem	Cause	Prevention	Action
Precipitation or cloudiness in the syringe.	Indicates incompatibility.	Check compatibility prior to mixing. Use http://book.pallcare.info for up-to-date advice.	Remove syringe, dispose of contents and prepare a new syringe.

POST-PROCEDURAL CONSIDERATIONS

Ongoing care

Accurate documentation of the site, rate, flow, start time and drugs used is imperative in order to avoid confusion and errors amongst staff (Dickman et al. 2007, Dougherty 2002, MHRA 2010b, NMC 2010a, NMC 2010b, Quinn 2000, Sasson and Shvartzman 2001). Sites and tubing will need to be changed every 1–4 days.

The frequency of checks should be as follows.

- At start of infusion – record date, time, start volume, infusion rate setting, name of person setting up infusion.
- Based upon the type of infusion and patient's condition; however, at a minimum these should be carried out 15 minutes and 1 hour after the initial set-up and thereafter a minimum of every 4 hours.
- Device must be checked at the start of each shift and/or when setting up an infusion.

Infusion device and infusion checks

- Check and record the date, time, rate and volume remaining and that the battery/syringe pump is working.
- Record any reasons for changing of the drug, dose, rate setting of syringe pump or site.
- Check subcutaneous site for:
  - pain/discomfort
  - swelling/induration
  - erythema
  - leakage of fluid
  - bleeding.

Box 12.17 **Volumes for syringe pumps**

- 10 mL syringe must be drawn up to 10 mL (approx. rate = 0.42 mL per 24 hours)
- 20 mL syringe must be drawn up to 17 mL (approx. rate = 0.71 mL per 24 hours)
- 30 mL syringe must be drawn up to 22 mL (approx. rate = 0.92 mL per 24 hours)
- 60 mL syringe must be drawn up to 32 mL (approx. rate = 1.33 mL per 24 hours)

COMPLICATIONS

Skin reactions

Some drugs are particularly likely to cause irritation and may need to be diluted in a greater volume of diluent; cyclizine and levomepromazine are amongst these. This may result in skin sites that break down rapidly or site reactions. The following methods can help to prevent this.

- Check compatibility of drugs and diluents and consider changing the drug combination.
- Dilute the solution as much as possible or change the diluent.
- Rotate the site at least every 72 hours.
- Use of a non-metal cannula.
- Use a different site cleanser.
- Change the dressing used.
- Consider adding dexamethasone 1 mg to the pump; this may be helpful but is not currently recommended for routine use. Care should also be taken as dexamethasone is incompatible with a number of drug combinations (Dickman et al. 2007).

Intramuscular injections

DEFINITION

An intramuscular injection deposits medication into deep muscle tissue under the subcutaneous tissue (Chernecky et al. 2002). The vascularity of muscle aids the rapid absorption of medication (Ostendorf 2012).

EVIDENCE-BASED APPROACHES

Site and volume of injection

Selecting the site requires correct identification of the muscle groups by using landmarks to identify the correct anatomical features (Hunter 2008). Choice will be influenced by the patient's physical condition and age. Intramuscular injections should be given into the densest part of the muscle (Pope 2002). An active patient will probably have a greater muscle mass than older or emaciated patients (Hunter 2008).

The injectable volume will depend on the muscle bed. In children, injectable volumes should be halved because muscle mass is less (Workman 1999). However, it appears that it is the medicine rather than just the volume that affects how a patient tolerates the injection. Malkin (2008) uses Botox injections as an example where a volume of 1–3 mL can be injected into facial muscle groups, supporting the view that tolerance of the drug is more important than the volume.

Current research evidence suggests that there are five sites that can be utilized for the administration of intramuscular injections (Rodger and King 2000, Tortora and Derrickson 2011).

- The *ventrogluteal site* (Figure 12.26a) is relatively free of major nerves and blood vessels and the muscle is large and well defined, making it easy to locate (Greenway 2004). It is located by placing the palm of the hand on the patient's opposite greater trochanter (right hand on left hip). The index finger is then extended to the anterior superior iliac spine to make a V. Injection in the centre of the V will ensure the injection is given into the gluteus medius muscle (Hunter 2008). This is the site of choice for intramuscular injections (Rodger and King 2000) and used for antibiotics, antiemetics, deep intramuscular and Z-track injections in oil, narcotics and sedatives. Up to 2.5 mL can be safely injected into the ventrogluteal site (Rodger and King 2000).
- The *deltoid site* (Figure 12.26b) has the advantage of being easily accessible whether the patient is standing, sitting or lying down. It is found by visualizing a triangle where the horizontal line is located 2.5–5 cm below the acromial process and midpoint of the lateral aspect of the arm, in line with the axilla to form the apex (Hunter 2008). The injection is then given 2.5 cm down from the acromial process, avoiding the radial and brachial nerves. Owing to the small area of this site, the number and volume of injections which can be given into it are limited. Drugs such as narcotics, sedatives and vaccines, which are usually small in volume, tend to be administered into the deltoid site (Workman 1999). Rodger and King (2000) state that the maximum volume that should be administered at this site is 1 mL.
- The *dorsogluteal site* (Figure 12.26c) or upper outer quadrant is the traditional site of choice and is used for deep intramuscular and Z-track injections. It is located by using imaginary lines to divide the buttocks into four quarters. However, this site carries the danger of the needle hitting the sciatic nerve and the superior gluteal arteries (Workman 1999). The gluteus muscle has the lowest drug absorption rate and this can result

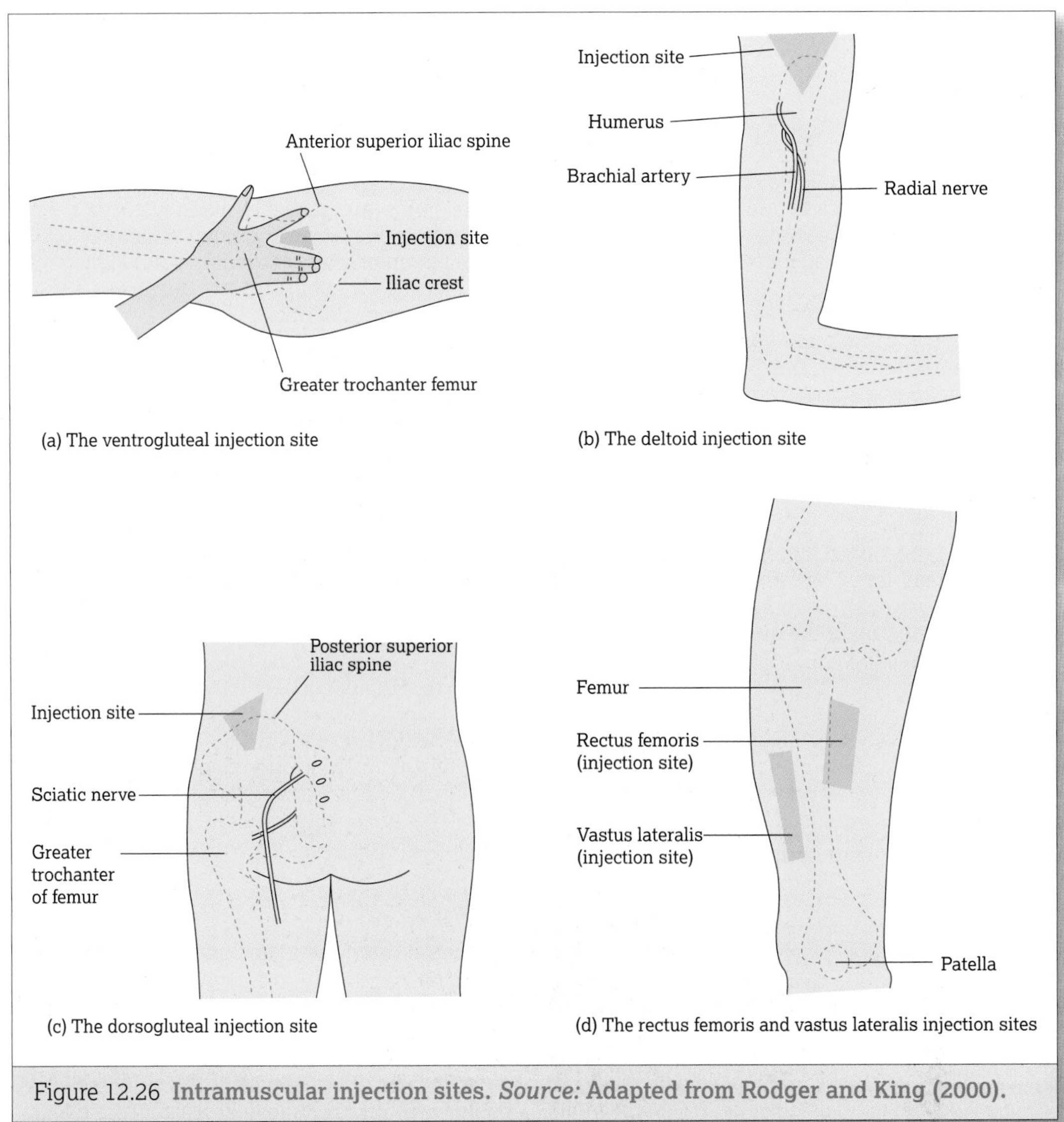

Figure 12.26 Intramuscular injection sites. ***Source:*** **Adapted from Rodger and King (2000).**

in a build-up in the tissues, increasing the risk of overdose (Malkin 2008). The muscle mass is also likely to have atrophied in elderly, non-ambulant and emaciated patients. Finally, it appears that there is a risk that the medication will not reach the muscle due to the amount of subcutaneous tissue in this area (Greenway 2004) and so it is not recommended for routine immunizations due to the poor absorption and risk of nerve injury (Public Health England 2006, WHO 2004). In adults, up to 4 mL can be safely injected into this site (Rodger and King 2000).

- The *rectus femoris site* (Figure 12.26d) is a well-defined muscle found by measuring a hand's breadth from the greater trochanter and the knee joint, which identifies the middle third of the quadriceps muscle (Hunter 2008). It is used for antiemetics, narcotics, sedatives, injections in oil, deep intramuscular and Z-track injections. It is rarely used by nurses, but is easily accessed for self-administration of injections or for infants (Workman 1999). 1–5 mL can be injected (1–3 mL in children).
- The *vastus lateralis site* (Figure 12.26d) is used for deep intramuscular and Z-track injections. One of the advantages of this site is its ease of access and, more importantly, there are no major blood vessels or significant nerve structures associated with this site. It is the better option in the obese patient (Nisbet 2006). Up to 5 mL can be safely injected (Rodger and King 2000).

There is debate over which site to use. The two recommended are the vastus lateralis and the ventrogluteal, but most nurses tend to use the dorsogluteal as it is more familiar (Greenway 2004).

Rate of administration

It is recommended that the plunger is depressed at a rate of 10 seconds per millilitre.

Technique

The syringe should be held like a pen to insert with a dart-like motion. Aspiration is still an accepted part of an IM injection to ensure that the medication does not enter the capillaries or is inadvertently given intravenously (Hunter 2008), but there is no evidence to support this. The Z-track method reduces the leakage of medication through the subcutaneous tissue and decreases skin lesions at the injection site and may hurt less.

It involves pulling the skin downwards or laterally of the injection site and inserting the needle at a 90° angle to the skin, which moves the cutaneous and subcutaneous tissues by approximately 2–3 cm (Antipuesto 2010, Take 5 2006). The injection is given and the needle withdrawn, while releasing the retracted skin at the same time. This manoeuvre seals off the puncture track.

PRE-PROCEDURAL CONSIDERATIONS

Equipment

The most common size of needle is 21 G (23 G may also be used in a thin patient) but it does depend on the viscosity of the medication. The important aspect of the needle is the length. The correct use of needle length will result in fewer adverse events and reduce complications of absecess, pain and bruising (Malkin 2008). Needles should be long enough to penetrate the muscle and still allow a quarter of the needle to remain external to the skin (Workman 1999). Lenz (1983) states that when choosing the correct needle length for intramuscular injections, it is important to assess the muscle mass of the injection site, the amount of subcutaneous fat and the weight of the patient. It may be necessary to calibrate the BMI to calculate body fat (Public Health England 2006). Without such an assessment, most injections intended for gluteal muscle are deposited in the gluteal fat. The following are suggested as ways of determining the most suitable size of needle to use.

Deltoid and vastus lateralis muscles

The muscle to be used should be grasped between the thumb and forefinger to determine the depth of the muscle mass or the amount of subcutaneous fat at the injection site.

Gluteal muscles

The layer of fat and skin above the muscle should be gently lifted with the thumb and forefinger for the same reasons as before.

The patient's weight indicates the length of needle to use.

- Children 16 mm needle
- 31.5–40.0 kg 25 mm needle
- 40.5–90.0 kg 25 mm needle
- 90 kg 38 mm needle

Remember women have more subcutaneous tissue than men so a longer needle will be needed (Pope 2002).

Specific patient preparation

Skin preparation

There are differences in opinion regarding skin cleaning prior to subcutaneous or intramuscular injections. Previous studies have suggested that cleaning with an alcohol swab is not always necessary, as not cleaning the site does not result in infections and may predispose the skin to hardening (Dann 1969, Koivistov and Felig 1978, Workman 1999).

Dann (1969), in a study over a period of 6 years involving more than 5000 injections, found no single case of local and/or systemic infection. Koivistov and Felig (1978) concluded that whilst skin preparations did reduce skin bacterial count, they are not necessary to prevent infections at the injection site. Some hospitals accept that if the patient is physically clean and the nurse maintains a high standard of hand hygiene and asepsis during the procedure, skin disinfection is not necessary (Workman 1999).

In the immunosuppressed patient, the skin should be cleaned as such patients may become infected by inoculation of a relatively small number of pathogens (Downie et al. 2003). The practice at the Royal Marsden Hospital is to clean the skin prior to injection in order to reduce the risk of contamination from the patient's skin flora. The skin is cleaned using an 'alcohol swab' (containing 70% isopropyl alcohol) for 30 seconds and then allowed to dry. If the skin is not dry before proceeding, skin cleaning is ineffective and the antiseptic may cause irritation by being injected into the tissues (Downie et al. 2003).

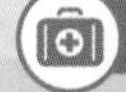
Learning Activity 12.6

Learning in practice: Skin preparation prior to injection

In your clinical area:

- Find out what the local guidance is for skin preparation prior to intramuscular injection.
- How does this compare to the evidence presented within this manual?
- Discuss the evidence with your mentor/supervising nurse.

Procedure guideline 12.21 Medication: intramuscular injection

Essential equipment

- Clinically clean receiver or tray containing prepared drug
- Apron
- Non-sterile gloves
- 70% Alcohol swab
- Needle
- Syringe containing prepared IM medication

Pre-procedure

Action	Rationale
1 Explain and discuss the procedure with the patient.	To ensure that the patient understands the procedure and gives their valid consent (Griffith and Jordan 2003, **E**; NMC 2013, **C**; NMC 2015, **C**).
2 Before administering any prescribed drug, look at the patient's prescription chart and check the following. (a) The correct patient (b) Drug (c) Dose (d) Date and time of administration (e) Route and method of administration (f) Diluent as appropriate (g) Validity of prescription (h) Signature of prescriber (i) The prescription is legible	To ensure that the correct patient is given the correct drug in the prescribed dose using the appropriate diluent and by the correct route (DH 2003b, **C**; NMC 2010a, **C**). To protect the patient from harm (DH 2003b, **C**; NMC 2010a, **C**).
If any of these pieces of information are missing, are unclear or illegible then the nurse should not proceed with administration and should consult with the prescriber.	To prevent any errors occurring. **E**
Prepare medication as described in Procedure guidelines 12.12, 12.13, 12.14 and 12.15.	
Procedure	
3 Apply apron, close the curtains or door and assist the patient into the required position. Wash hands.	To ensure patient privacy and dignity. **E** To allow access to the injection site and to ensure the designated muscle group is flexed and therefore relaxed (Workman 1999, **E**).
4 Remove the appropriate garment to expose the injection site.	To gain access for injection (Workman 1999, **E**).
5 Apply gloves and assess the injection site for signs of inflammation, oedema, infection and skin lesions.	To promote effectiveness of administration (Workman 1999, **E**). To reduce the risk of infection (Fraise and Bradley 2009, **E**; Workman 1999, **E**). To avoid skin lesions and avoid possible trauma to the patient (Ostendorf 2012, **E**; Workman 1999, **E**).
6 Clean the injection site with a swab saturated with isopropyl alcohol 70% for 30 seconds and allow to dry for 30 seconds (Workman 1999).	To reduce the number of pathogens introduced into the skin by the needle at the time of insertion and to prevent stinging sensation if alcohol is taken into the tissues upon needle entry (Antipuesto 2010, **E**; Hunter 2008, **E**). (For further information on this action see 'Skin preparation'.)
7 With the non-dominant hand, stretch the skin slightly around the injection site.	To displace the underlying subcutaneous tissues, facilitate the insertion of the needle and reduce the sensitivity of nerve endings (Antipuesto 2010, **E**; Hunter 2008, **E**).
8 Holding the syringe in the dominant hand like a dart, inform the patient and quickly plunge the needle at an angle of 90° into the skin until about 1 cm of the needle is left showing.	To ensure that the needle penetrates the muscle (Hunter 2008, **E**; Workman 1999, **E**).
9 Pull back the plunger. If no blood is aspirated, depress the plunger at approximately 1 mL every 10 seconds and inject the drug slowly. If blood appears, withdraw the needle completely, replace it and begin again. Explain to the patient what has occurred.	To confirm that the needle is in the correct position and not in a vein (Antipuesto 2010, **E**). This allows time for the muscle fibres to expand and absorb the solution (Hunter 2008, **E**; Workman 1999, **E**). To prevent pain and ensure even distribution of the drug (Ostendorf 2012, **E**).
10 Wait 10 seconds before withdrawing the needle.	To allow the medication to diffuse into the tissue (Ostendorf 2012, **E**; Workman 1999, **E**).
11 Withdraw the needle rapidly. Apply gentle pressure to any bleeding point but do not massage the site.	To ensure that the injected medication is not forced out of the tissues (Antipuesto 2010, **E**).
12 Apply a small plaster over the puncture site.	To prevent tissue injury and haematoma formation (Ostendorf 2012, **E**).

Post-procedure	
13 Where appropriate, activate safety device. Ensure that all sharps and non-sharp waste are disposed of safely and in accordance with locally approved procedures, for example put sharps into sharps bin and syringes into orange clinical waste bag.	To ensure safe disposal and to avoid laceration or other injury to staff (DH 2005, **C**; EU 2010, **C**; MHRA 2004, **C**).
14 Record the administration on appropriate charts.	To maintain accurate records, provide a point of reference in the event of any queries and prevent any duplication of treatment (NMC 2010a, **C**; NMC 2010b, **C**; NPSA 2007d, **C**).

Intravenous injections and infusions

DEFINITION

The introduction of medication or solutions into the circulatory system via a peripheral or central vein (Chernecky et al. 2002).

ANATOMY AND PHYSIOLOGY

Anatomy of veins

Veins consist of three layers.

Tunica intima

The tunica intima is a smooth endothelial lining, which allows the passage of blood cells (Jenkins and Tortora 2013). If it becomes damaged, the lining may become roughened and there is an increased risk of thrombus formation (Hadaway 2010, Scales 2008). Within this layer are thin folds of endothelium called valves (flap-like cusps), which keep blood moving towards the heart by preventing backflow (Jenkins and Tortora 2013). Valves are present in larger vessels and at points of branching and are present as noticeable bulges in the veins (Weinstein and Plumer 2007).

Tunica media

The middle layer of the vein wall is composed of muscular tissue and nerve fibres, both vasoconstrictors and vasodilators, which can stimulate the vein to contract or relax. This layer is not as strong or stiff as in an artery and therefore veins can distend or collapse as the pressure rises or falls (Jenkins and Tortora 2013). Stimulation of this layer by a change in temperature (cold), mechanical or chemical stimulus can produce venous spasm, which can make insertion of a needle more difficult.

Tunica adventitia/externa

The tunica adventitia is the outer layer and consists of connective tissue, which surrounds and supports the vessel (Tortora and Derrickson 2011).

RELATED THEORY

Intravenous therapy is now an integral part of the majority of nurses' professional practice (RCN 2010). The nurse's role has progressed considerably from being able to add drugs to infusion bags (DHSS 1976) to now assessing patients and inserting the appropriate vascular access device (VAD) prior to drug administration (Gabriel et al. 2005).

Any nurse administering intravenous drugs must be competent in all aspects of intravenous therapy and act in accordance with *The Code* (NMC 2015), that is, to maintain knowledge and skills (Hyde 2008, RCN 2010). Training and assessment should comprise both theoretical and practical components and include legal and professional issues, fluid balance, pharmacology, drug administration, local and systemic complications, infection control issues, use of equipment and risk management (Hyde 2008, RCN 2010).

The nurse's responsibilities in relation to intravenous drug administration include the following.

- Knowing the therapeutic use of the drug or solution, its normal dosage, side-effects, precautions and contraindications.
- Preparing the drug aseptically and safely, checking the container and drug for faults, using the correct diluent and only preparing it immediately prior to administration.
- Identifying the patient and checking allergy status.
- Checking the prescription chart.
- Checking and maintaining patency of the VAD.
- Inspecting the site of the VAD and managing/reporting complications where appropriate.
- Controlling the flow rate of infusion and/or speed of injection.
- Monitoring the condition of the patient and reporting changes.
- Making clear and immediate records of all drugs administered (Finlay 2008, NMC 2010b, NMC 2015, RCN 2010).

EVIDENCE-BASED APPROACHES

Methods of administering intravenous drugs

There are three methods of administering intravenous drugs: continuous infusion, intermittent infusion and direct intermittent injection.

Continuous infusion

Continuous infusion may be defined as the intravenous delivery of a medication or fluid at a constant rate over a prescribed time period, ranging from several hours to several days to achieve a controlled therapeutic response (Turner and Hankins 2010). The greater dilution also helps to reduce venous irritation (Weinstein and Plumer 2007, Whittington 2008).

A continuous infusion may be used when:

- the drugs to be administered must be highly diluted
- maintenance of steady blood levels of the drug is required (Turner and Hankins 2010).

Pre-prepared infusion fluids with additives such as those containing potassium chloride should be used whenever possible. This reduces the risk of extrinsic contamination, which can occur during the mixing of drugs (Weinstein and Plumer 2007). Only one addition should be made to each bottle or bag of fluid after the compatibility has been ascertained. More additions can increase the risk of incompatibility occurring, for example precipitation (Weinstein and Plumer 2007, Whittington 2008). The additive and fluid must be mixed well to prevent a layering effect which can occur with some drugs (Whittington 2008). The danger is that a bolus injection of the drug may be delivered. To safeguard against this, any additions should be made to the infusion fluid and the container inverted a number of times to ensure mixing of the drug, before the fluid is hung on the infusion stand (NPSA 2007d). The infusion container should be labelled clearly after the addition has been made. Constant monitoring of the infusion fluid mixture (Weinstein and Plumer 2007, Whittington 2008) for cloudiness or presence of particles should occur, as well as checking the patient's condition and intravenous site for patency, extravasation or infiltration (Downie et al. 2003).

Intermittent infusion

Intermittent infusion is the administration of a small-volume infusion, that is, 25–250 mL, over a period of between 15 minutes and 2 hours (Turner and Hankins 2010). This may be given as a specific dose at one time or at repeated intervals during 24 hours (Pickstone 1999).

An intermittent infusion may be used when:

- a peak plasma level is required therapeutically
- the pharmacology of the drug dictates this specific dilution
- the drug will not remain stable for the time required to administer a more dilute volume
- the patient is on a restricted intake of fluids (Whittington 2008).

Delivery of the drug by intermittent infusion can be piggy-backed (via a needle-free injection port), if the primary infusion is of a compatible fluid; this may utilize a system such as a 'Y' set or a burette set with a chamber capacity of 100 or 150 mL (Turner and Hankins 2010). This is when the drug can be added to the burette and infused while the primary infusion is switched off. A small-volume infusion may also be connected to a cannula specifically to keep the vein open and maintain patency.

All the points considered when preparing for a continuous infusion should be taken into account here, for example pre-prepared fluids, single additions of drugs, adequate mixing, labelling and monitoring.

Direct intermittent injection

Direct intermittent injection (also known as intravenous push or bolus) involves the injection of a drug from a syringe into the injection port of the administration set or directly into a VAD (Chernecky et al. 2002, Turner and Hankins 2010). Most are administered over a time span anywhere from 3 to 10 minutes depending upon the drug (Weinstein and Plumer 2007, Whittington 2008).

A direct injection may be used when:

- a maximum concentration of the drug is required to vital organs. This is a 'bolus' injection which is given rapidly over seconds, as in an emergency, for example adrenaline
- the drug cannot be further diluted for pharmacological or therapeutic reasons or does not require dilution. This is given as a controlled 'push' injection over a few minutes
- a peak blood level is required and cannot be achieved by small-volume infusion (Turner and Hankins 2010).

Rapid administration could result in toxic levels and an anaphylactic-type reaction. Manufacturer's recommendations of rates of administration (i.e. millilitres or milligrams per minute) should be adhered to. In the absence of such recommendations, administration should proceed slowly, over 5–10 minutes (Dougherty 2002).

Delivery of the drug by direct injection may be via the cannula through a resealable needle-less injection cap, extension set or via the injection site of an administration set.

- If a peripheral device is *in situ*, the bandage and dressing must be removed to inspect the insertion of the cannula, unless a transparent dressing is in place (Finlay 2008).
- Patency of the vein must be confirmed prior to administration and the vein's ability to accept an extra flow of fluid or irritant chemical must also be checked (Dougherty 2008).

Administration into the injection site of a fast-running drip may be advised if the infusion in progress is compatible in order to dilute the drug further and reduce local chemical irritation (Dougherty 2002). Alternatively, a stop–start procedure may be employed if there is doubt about venous patency. This allows the nurse to constantly check the patency of the vein and detect early signs of extravasation. If the infusion fluid is incompatible with the drug, the administration set may be switched off and a compatible solution may be used as a flush (NPSA 2007d).

If a number of drugs are being administered, 0.9% sodium chloride must be used to flush in between each drug to prevent interactions. In addition, 0.9% sodium chloride should be used at the end of the administration to ensure that all the drug has been delivered. The device should then be flushed to ensure patency is maintained (Dougherty 2008).

The following principles are to be applied throughout preparation and administration.

Asepsis and reducing the risk of infection

Microbes on the hands of healthcare personnel contribute to healthcare-associated infection (Weinstein and Plumer 2007). Therefore aseptic technique must be adhered to throughout all intravenous procedures. The nurse must employ good hand-washing and drying techniques using a bactericidal soap or bactericidal alcohol handrub. If asepsis is not maintained, local infection, septic phlebitis or septicaemia may result (Hart 2008, Loveday et al. 2014, RCN 2010).

The insertion site should be inspected at least once a day for complications such as infiltration, phlebitis or any indication of infection, for example redness at the insertion site or pyrexia (RCN 2010). These problems may necessitate the removal of the device and/or further investigation (Finlay 2008).

It is desirable that a closed system of infusion is maintained wherever possible, with as few connections as is necessary for its purpose (Finlay 2008, Hart 2008). This reduces the risk of bacterial contamination. Any extra connections within the administration system increase the risk of infection. Three-way taps have been shown to encourage the growth of micro-organisms. They are difficult to clean due to their design, as micro-organisms can become lodged and are then able to multiply in the warm, moist environment (Finlay 2008, Hart 2008). This reservoir of micro-organisms may then be released into the circulation.

The injection sites on administration sets or injection caps should be cleaned using a 2% chlorhexidine alcohol-based antiseptic, allowing time for it to dry (Loveday et al. 2014). Connections should be cleaned before changing administration sets and manipulations kept to a minimum. Administration sets should be changed according to use (intermittent/continuous therapy), type of device and type of solution, and the set must be labelled with the date and time of change (NPSA 2007d, RCN 2010).

To ensure safe delivery of intravenous fluids and medication:

- replace all tubing when the vascular device is replaced (Loveday et al. 2014)
- replace solution administration sets and stopcocks used for continuous infusions every 96 hours unless clinically indicated, for example, if drug stability data indicate otherwise (Loveday et al. 2014, RCN 2010). A Cochrane review of 13 randomized controlled trials found no evidence that changing intravenous administration sets more often than every 96 hours reduces the incidence of bloodstream infection (Loveday et al. 2014)
- replace solution administration sets used for lipid emulsions and parenteral nutrition at the end of the infusion or within 24 hours of initiating the infusion (Loveday et al. 2014, RCN 2010)
- replace blood administration sets at least every 12 hours and after every second unit of blood (Loveday et al. 2014, McClelland 2007, RCN 2010)
- all solution sets used for intermittent infusions, for example antibiotics, should be discarded immediately after use and not allowed to hang for reuse (RCN 2010)

- if administering more than one infusion via a multilumen extension set or multiple ports, be aware of the risk of back-tracking of medication and consider using sets with one-way, non-return or antireflux valves (MHRA 2010a).

Inspection of fluids, drugs, equipment and their packaging must be undertaken to detect any points where contamination may have occurred during manufacture and/or transport. This intrinsic contamination may be detected as cloudiness, discoloration or the presence of particles (BNF 2014, RCN 2010, Weinstein and Plumer 2007). Infusion bags should not be left hanging for longer than 24 hours. In the case of blood and blood products, this is reduced to 5 hours (McClelland 2007, RCN 2010).

Safety

All details of the prescription and all calculations must be checked carefully in accordance with hospital policy in order to ensure safe preparation and administration of the drug(s).

The nurse must also check the compatibility of the drug with the diluent or infusion fluid. The nurse should be aware of the types of incompatibilities and the factors which could influence them. These include pH, concentration, time, temperature, light and the brand of the drug. If insufficient information is available, a reference book (e.g. *British National Formulary*) or the product data sheet must be consulted (NPSA 2007d, Whittington 2008). If the nurse is unsure about any aspect of the preparation and/or administration of a drug, they should not proceed and should consult with a senior member of staff (NMC 2010a). Constant monitoring of both the mixture and the patient is important. The preferred method and rate of intravenous administration must be determined.

Drugs should never be added to the following: blood; blood products, that is plasma or platelet concentrate (see Chapter 7: Nutrition, fluid balance and blood transfusion); mannitol solutions; sodium bicarbonate solution; and so on. Only specially prepared additives should be used with fat emulsions or amino acid preparations (Downie et al. 2003).

Accurate labelling of additives and records of administration are essential (NPSA 2007d, RCN 2010).

Any protective clothing which is advised should be worn, and vinyl gloves should be used to reduce the risk of latex allergy (Hart 2008). Healthcare professionals who use gloves frequently or for long periods face a high risk of allergy from latex products. All healthcare facilities should develop policies and procedures that determine measures to protect staff and patients from latex exposure and outline a treatment plan for latex reactions (RCN 2010).

Preventing needlestick injuries should be key in any health and safety programme and organizations should introduce safety devices and needle-free systems wherever possible (EU Directive 2010). Basic rules of safety include not resheathing needles, disposal of needles immediately after use into a recognized sharps bin and convenient location of sharps bins in all areas where needles and sharps are used (Hart 2008, MHRA 2004, RCN 2010).

Comfort

Both the physical and psychological comfort of the patient must be considered. Comprehensive explanation of the practical aspects of the procedure together with information about the effects of treatment will contribute to reducing anxiety and will need to be tailored to each patient's individual needs.

LEGAL AND PROFESSIONAL ISSUES

At least one patient will experience a potentially serious intravenous (IV) drug error every day in an 'average' hospital. IV drug errors have been estimated to be a third of all drug errors. 'Fifteen million infusions are performed in the NHS every year and 700 unsafe incidents are reported each year with 19% attributed to user error' (NPSA 2004, p.1). Between 2005 and 2010, the MHRA investigated 1085 reports involving infusion pumps (MHRA 2011). In 69% of incidents no cause was established. However, of the remaining incidents, 21% were attributed to user error (e.g. misloading of the administration set or syringe, setting the wrong rate, confusing pump type) and 11% to device-related issues (e.g. poor maintenance, cleaning) (MHRA 2011). Syringe pumps have given rise to the most significant problems in terms of patient mortality and morbidity (Fox 2000, MHRA 2010b, NPSA 2003).

The high frequency of human error has highlighted the need for more formalized, validated, competency-based training and assessment (MHRA 2010b, NPSA 2003, 2004, Pickstone 2000, Quinn 2000). Nurses must be familiar with the device they are using and not attempt to operate any device that they have not been fully trained to use (MHRA 2011, Murray and Glenister 2001, NPSA 2003). As a minimum, the training should cover the device, drugs and solutions, and the practical procedures related to setting up the device and problem solving (MHRA 2010b, MHRA 2011, MHRA 2014). Staff should also be made aware of the mechanisms for reporting faults with devices and procedures for adverse incident reporting within their trust and to the MHRA (MHRA 2006b, MHRA 2011).

A useful checklist (Box 12.18) has been produced by the Medical Devices Agency for staff to follow prior to using a medical device to ensure safe practice (MHRA 2010b, MHRA 2014).

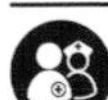

Box 12.18 **Checklist: how safe is your practice?**

- Have I been trained in the use of the infusion device?
- Was the training formalized and recorded or did I just pick it up as I went along?
- How was my competency in relation to the infusion device assessed?
- Have I read the user instructions on how to use the infusion device and am I familiar with any warning labels?
- When was the infusion device last serviced?
- Are there any signs of wear, damage or faults?
- Do I know how to set up and use the infusion device?
- Is the infusion device and any additional equipment in good working order?
- Do I know how the infusion device should perform and the monitoring that needs to be done to check its performance?
- Am I using the correct additional equipment, for example the appropriate disposable administration set for the infusion pump?
- Do I know how to recognize whether the infusion device has failed?
- Do I know what to do if the infusion device fails?
- Do I know how and to whom to report an infusion device-related adverse incident?
- Does checking the infusion device indicate it is functioning correctly and to the manufacturer's specification?
- What action should be taken if the infusion device is not functioning properly?
- Is there up-to-date documentation to record regular checking of the infusion device?
- What are the details (name and serial number) of the infusion device being used?
- What is the cleaning and/or decontamination procedure for the infusion device and what are my responsibilities in this process?
- Do I know how to report an adverse incident?
- Do I have access to MHRA device bulletins of relevance to my area of practice and do I read and take note of hazard and safety notices?

Source: Medical Devices Agency (2000).

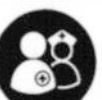

Box 12.19 Groups at risk of complications associated with flow control

- Infants and young children
- The elderly
- Patients with compromised cardiovascular status
- Patients with impairment or failure of organs, for example kidneys
- Patients with major sepsis
- Patients suffering from shock, whatever the cause
- Post-operative or post-trauma patients
- Stressed patients, whose endocrine homeostatic controls may be affected
- Patients receiving multiple medications, whose clinical status may change rapidly

Source: Quinn (2008). Reproduced with permission from John Wiley & Sons.

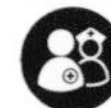

Box 12.21 Criteria for selection of an infusion device

- Rationalization of devices
- Clinical requirement
- Education
- Compatibility with other equipment
- Disposables
- Product support
- Costs
- Service and maintenance
- Regulatory issues, for example compliance with European Community Directives

Source: Adapted from Department of Health, Social Services and Public Safety (2006), Health Care Standards Unit (2007a, 2007b), MHRA (2010b), NHS Litigation Authority (2007), Quinn (2000).

The nurse must have knowledge of the solutions, their effects, rate of administration, factors that affect flow of infusion, as well as the complications which could occur when flow is not controlled (Weinstein and Plumer 2007). The nurse should have an understanding of which groups require accurate flow control in order to prevent complications (Box 12.19) and how to select the most appropriate device for accuracy of delivery to best meet the patient's flow control needs (according to age, condition, setting and prescribed therapy) (Weinstein and Plumer 2007).

The identification of risks is crucial, for example complex calculations, prescription errors (Dougherty 2002, Weinstein and Plumer 2007) and the risks associated with infusions, such as neonatal risk infusions, high-risk infusions, low-risk infusions and ambulatory infusions (MHRA 2010b, Quinn 2000). The early detection of errors and infusion-related complications, for example over- and underinfusion (Box 12.20), is imperative in order to instigate the appropriate interventions in response to an error or to manage any complications, as serious errors or complications can result in patient death (Dougherty 2002, NPSA 2003, Quinn 2008). Overinfusion accounts for about half of the reported errors involving infusion pumps, with 80% due to user error rather than a fault with the device (MHRA 2014). The use of infusion devices, both mechanical and electronic, has increased the level of safety in intravenous therapy. However, it is recommended that a clearly defined structure for management of infusion systems must exist within a hospital (Department of Health, Social Services and Public Safety 2006, MHRA 2010b, MHRA 2011, NHS Litigation Authority 2013, NPSA 2004) (Box 12.21).

Box 12.20 Complications of inadequate flow control

Complications associated with overinfusion

- Fluid overload with accompanying electrolyte imbalance.
- Metabolic disturbances during parenteral nutrition, mainly related to serum glucose levels.
- Toxic concentrations of medications, which may result in a shock-like syndrome ('speed shock').
- Air embolism, due to containers running dry before expected.
- An increase in venous complications, for example chemical phlebitis, caused by reduced dilution of irritant substances (Weinstein and Plumer 2007).

Complications associated with underinfusion

- Dehydration.
- Metabolic disturbances.
- A delayed response to medications or below therapeutic dose.
- Occlusion of a cannula/catheter due to slow flow or cessation of flow.

Source: Quinn (2008). Reproduced with permission from John Wiley & Sons.

Strategies need to be developed for replacement of old, obsolete or inappropriate devices (Department of Health, Social Services and Public Safety 2006, Health Care Standards Unit 2007a, Health Care Standards Unit 2007b, MHRA 2010b, NHS Litigation Authority 2013, Quinn 2000), planned service maintenance programmes and acceptance testing (MHRA 2010b, MHRA 2011).

Healthcare professionals are personally accountable for their use of infusion devices and they must therefore ensure they have appropriate training before using the pump (MHRA 2008, MHRA 2011, Quinn 2008). Records of training must also be maintained.

Improving infusion device safety

A high frequency of human error is reported in the use of infusion device systems, so competence-based training is advocated for users of these systems (MHRA 2010b, NPSA 2004). By rationalizing the range of infusion device types within organizations and the establishment of a centralized equipment library, the number of patient safety incidents will be reduced (MHRA 2010b, NPSA 2004). Smart infusion pumps reduce pump programming errors by the setting of pre-programmed upper and lower dose limits for specific drugs. The pump will alert the nurse when setting the infusion device if the pump has been set outside the pre-set dose limits (Keohane et al. 2005, MHRA 2011,Weinstein and Plumer 2007, Wilson and Sullivan 2004). Whatever infusion device is used, the need to monitor the patient and the device remains paramount for patient safety (Quinn 2008, RCN 2010).

PRE-PROCEDURAL CONSIDERATIONS

Equipment

Peripheral cannulas

A cannula is a flexible tube containing a needle (stylet) which may be inserted into a blood vessel (Dougherty 2008, RCN 2010). Cannulas are usually placed in the peripheral veins in the lower arm but may also be placed in the veins of the foot (an area used particularly in paediatric care) (Weinstein and Plumer 2007). However, veins of the lower extremities should not be routinely used in adults due to the risk of embolism and thrombophlebitis (INS 2011, RCN 2010).

The advantages of using a peripheral cannula are that they are usually easy to insert and have few associated complications; however, they are associated with phlebitis (either mechanical or chemical) and require constant resiting (Dougherty 2008, INS 2011, RCN 2010).

INDICATIONS

- Short-term therapy of less than a week.
- Bolus injections or short infusions in the outpatient/day unit setting (Hadaway 2010, RCN 2010).

CONTRAINDICATIONS

- Long-term intravenous therapy.
- Longer or continous infusions of medications that are vesicant or those that have a pH >9 (Hadaway 2010).

IMMEDIATE CARE

Once sited, the peripheral cannula should be flushed using a pulsatile flush, ending with positive pressure (Dougherty 2008, RCN 2010, Weinstein and Plumer 2007). The cannula should be secured using clean tape or a securing device (Figure 12.27). Non-sterile tape should not cover the insertion site and taping should enable the site to remain visible and the cannula stable (Figure 12.28). Securement devices are now available and reduce the risk of dislodgement and other complications (Bausone-Gazda et al. 2010, Moureau and Iannucci 2003). A dressing should be applied: this can be either a transparent dressing or low-linting gauze (Perucca 2010). Once the gauze is in place, a bandage may be applied. However, transparent dressings, particularly moisture-permeable dressings, should not be bandaged as the visibility and moisture permeability are obscured.

Figure 12.27 **Peripheral cannula secured with Statlock.**

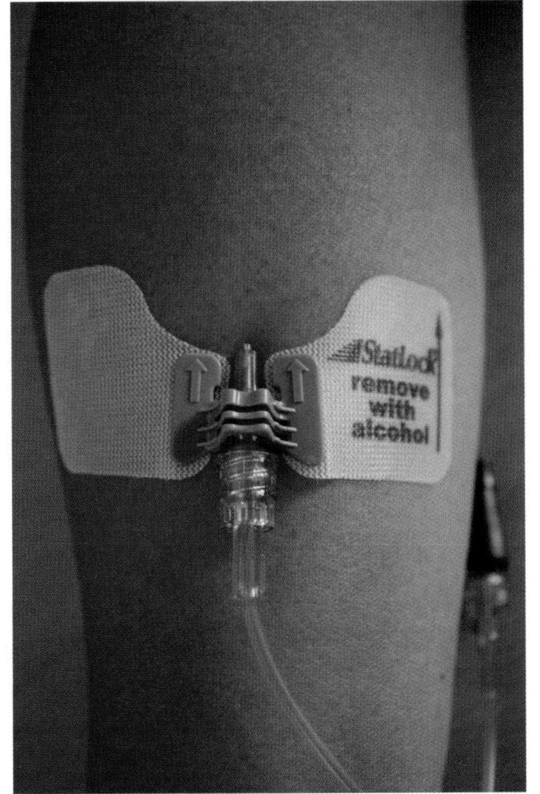

Figure 12.28 **Cannula *in situ*.**

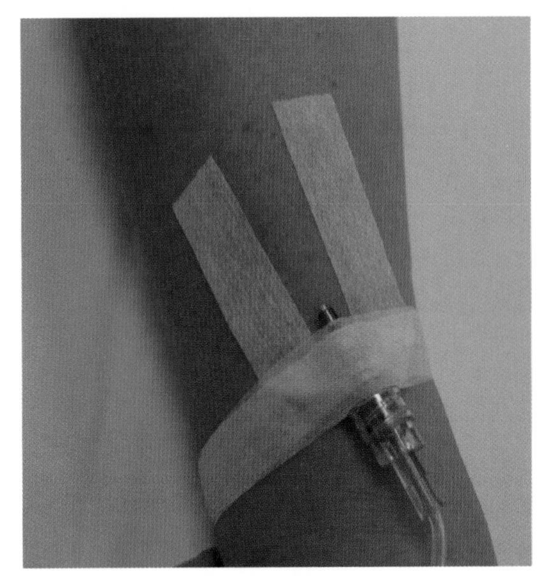

ONGOING CARE

A peripheral cannula should be flushed before and after each use to check for patency prior to administration of a medication, and at least daily if not in use, using 0.9% sodium chloride. The dressing should be changed as required (if transparent) or each time the device is manipulated (gauze). The site should be monitored daily or when the device is used. The site should be inspected for signs of infiltration, extravasation and leakage and using a scale such as the VIP Scale for signs of phlebitis (DH 2010). The Visual Infusion Phlebitis Scale (VIP) (Figure 12.29) was developed by Jackson (1998) and measures the signs and symptoms of phlebitis, matching them to the appropriate management. Each stage has a numbered score and this is recorded by nursing staff at regular intervals and, where necessary, the corresponding action is taken (Groll et al. 2010, Morris 2011). However, there is now debate as to the efficacy of these phlebitis assessment scales (Ray-Barruel et al. 2013).

REMOVAL

It has been recommended that peripheral devices should be resited every 48–72 hours (Barker et al. 2004, DH 2012) but some literature supports dwell times (length of time cannula *in situ*) of up to 96 hours with no significant complications providing that non-irritants are administered (Homer and Holmes 1998, McGoldrick 2010, Palese et al. 2011). Other studies have found that drug irritation is the most significant predictor of phlebitis and infiltration, rather than dwell time, and that extending the dwell time up to 144 hours could be considered under certain circumstances (Bregenzer et al. 1998, Catney et al. 2001).

The Rickard et al. (2012) study of over 5000 peripheral cannulas found no difference in phlebitis, infection or failure rates between replacing cannulas every 3 days compared with leaving *in situ* and replacing when clinically indicated. They concluded that peripheral devices need only be removed as clinically indicated and that this would save millions of unecessary resites, associated discomfort and a reduction in cost of both equipment and staff time. This is supported by van Donk et al. (2009) and Webster et al. (2008) who recommend resiting cannulas based on clinical indication instead of time *in situ*. Lee et al. (2009) also state that this approach does not increase infection rate but they do recommend that insertion is done by highly skilled IV

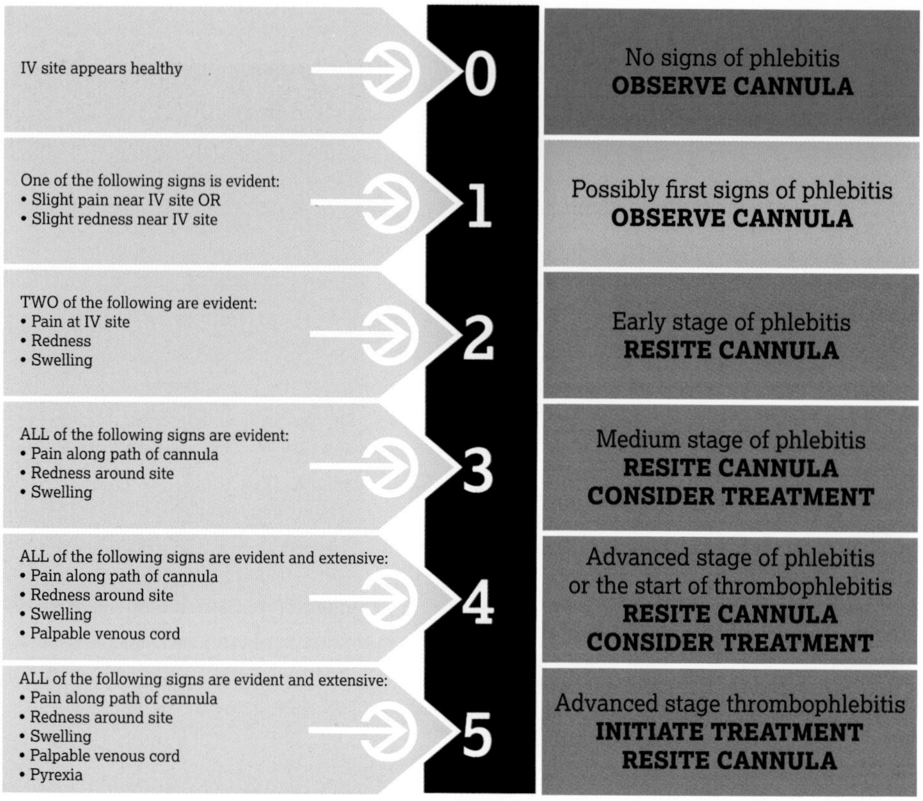

Signs	Score	Assessment / Action
IV site appears healthy	0	No signs of phlebitis **OBSERVE CANNULA**
One of the following signs is evident: • Slight pain near IV site OR • Slight redness near IV site	1	Possibly first signs of phlebitis **OBSERVE CANNULA**
TWO of the following are evident: • Pain at IV site • Redness • Swelling	2	Early stage of phlebitis **RESITE CANNULA**
ALL of the following signs are evident: • Pain along path of cannula • Redness around site • Swelling	3	Medium stage of phlebitis **RESITE CANNULA** **CONSIDER TREATMENT**
ALL of the following signs are evident and extensive: • Pain along path of cannula • Redness around site • Swelling • Palpable venous cord	4	Advanced stage of phlebitis or the start of thrombophlebitis **RESITE CANNULA** **CONSIDER TREATMENT**
ALL of the following signs are evident and extensive: • Pain along path of cannula • Redness around site • Swelling • Palpable venous cord • Pyrexia	5	Advanced stage thrombophlebitis **INITIATE TREATMENT** **RESITE CANNULA**

Figure 12.29 **Vein Infusion Phlebitis (VIP) Scale.** ***Source:*** **Jackson (1998). Reproduced with permission from EMAP Publishing Ltd.**

teams or rates could increase. Finally, Epic3 now recommend that peripheral cannulas should only be resited when clinically indicated and not routinely (Loveday et al. 2014).

Removal of the intravenous device or cannula should be an aseptic procedure. The device should be removed carefully using a slow, steady movement and pressure should be applied until haemostasis is achieved. This pressure should be firm and not involve any rubbing movement. A haematoma will occur if the device is carelessly removed, causing discomfort and a focus for infection (Perucca 2010). The site should be inspected to ensure bleeding has stopped and should then be covered with a sterile dressing (INS 2011). The cannula integrity should be checked to ensure the complete device has been removed (Dougherty 2008, INS 2011, RCN 2010). The date, time and reason for removal of the cannula must be documented in the patient's notes (DH 2011, Dougherty 2008, RCN 2010). This documentation ensures adequate records for the continued care of the device and patient as well as enabling audit and gathering of statistics on rates of phlebitis and infiltration.

Administration sets

An administration set is used to administer fluids, blood or medications via an infusion bag into a VAD. The set comprises a number of components (Figure 12.30, Figure 12.31, Figure 12.32). At the top is a spike which is inserted into the infusion container via an entry port. This is covered by a sterile plastic lid which is removed just prior to insertion into the container (Downie et al. 2003). The plastic tubing continues from the spike to a drip chamber which may contain a filter. This is filled by squeezing it when attached to the fluid and waiting for the chamber to fill halfway, thus allowing the practitioner to observe the drops. Along the tubing is a roller clamp which allows the tubing to be incrementally occluded by pinching the tubing as the clamp is tightened; this is used to adjust the rate of flow (Hadaway 2010). It is usually positioned on the upper third of the administration set but should be repositioned along the set at intervals as the tubing can develop a 'memory' and not regain its shape, making it difficult to regulate (Hadaway 2010). It is opened to allow the fluid along the tubing to remove the air and then closed until attached to the patient's VAD. Finally the Luer-Lok end is covered with a plastic cap to maintain sterility until ready to be attached (Downie et al. 2003).

There is a variety of sets. A solution set is used to administer crystalloid solutions (it can be used as a primary or secondary set and is also available as a Y-set to allow for dual administration of compatible solutions). Parenteral nutrition is also administered

Figure 12.30 **Fluid administration set.**

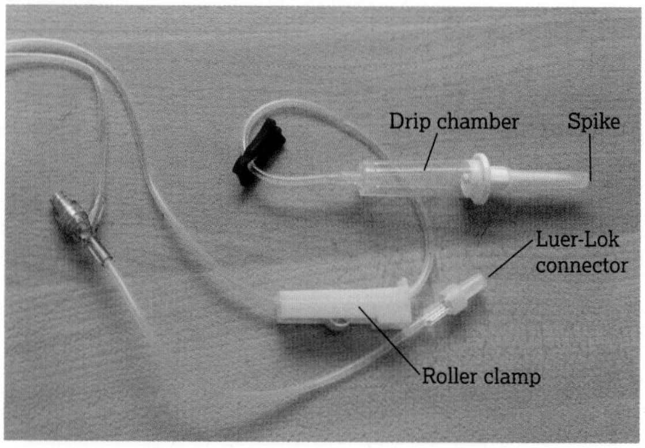

Drip chamber
Spike
Luer-Lok connector
Roller clamp

Figure 12.31 **Roller clamp.**

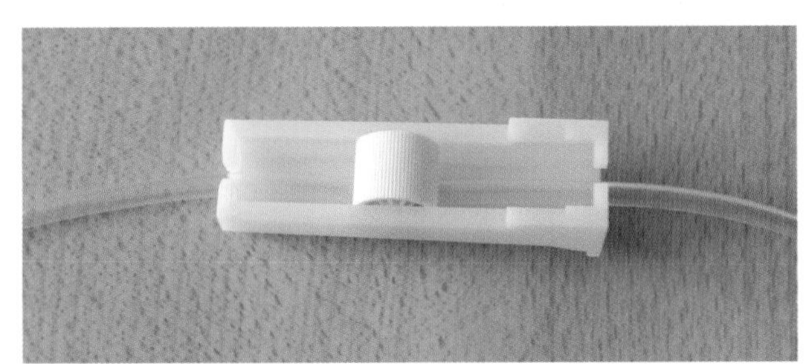

via solution sets. Solution sets may have needle-free injection ports which allow for the administration of bolus injections or connection of secondary infusions. Sets may also have back check valves which allow solutions to flow in one direction only and are used especially when a secondary set is used (Hadaway 2010).

Blood and blood products are administered via a blood administration set (Figure 12.33) which has a special filter. Platelets can be administered via blood sets (check with manufacturer) or specialist platelet administration sets. Some medications such as taxanes must be administered via special taxane administration sets as they have a 0.22 micron filter.

Extension sets

Extension sets are used to add length (Hadaway 2010). The short extension sets tend to have a needle-free connector (Figure 12.34) and are attached directly to the VAD to provide a closed system and other equipment is then attached via the needle-free connector. The long (50–200 cm) extension sets are used to connect from syringe pumps to a VAD and usually have a back-check or antisiphon valve. They can be single, double or triple and may contain a slide or pinch clamp but do not regulate flow (Hadaway 2010).

Needleless connectors/injection caps

These are caps that are attached to the end of a VAD or extension set (see Figure 12.34) to provide a closed system and remove the

Figure 12.32 **Labelled administration set.**

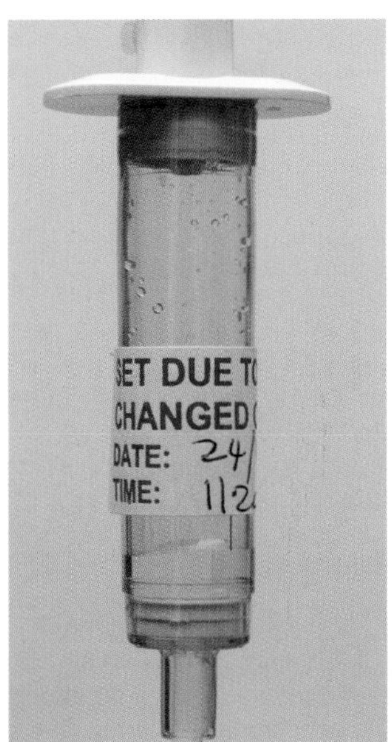

Figure 12.33 **Blood administration set.**

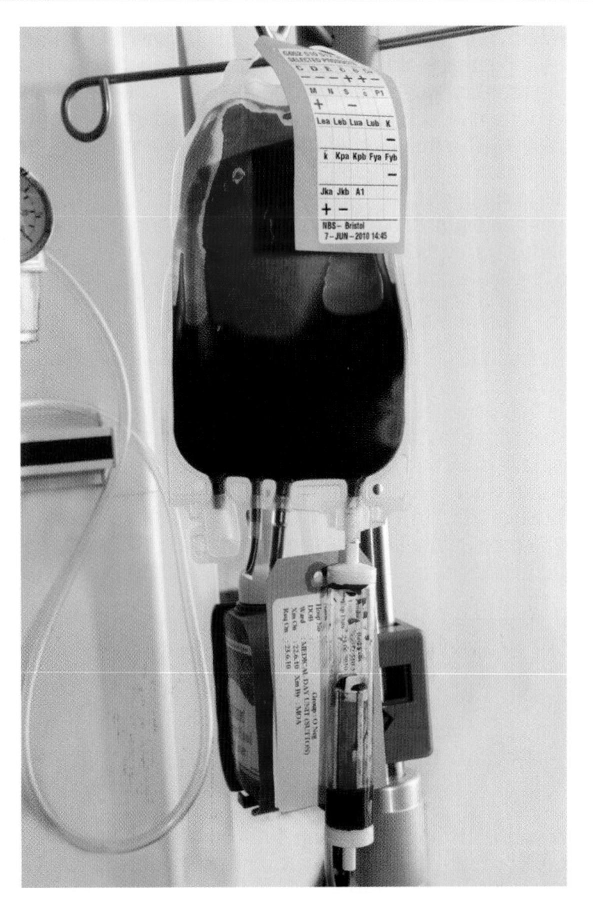

Figure 12.34 **Extension set with needle-free injection cap.**

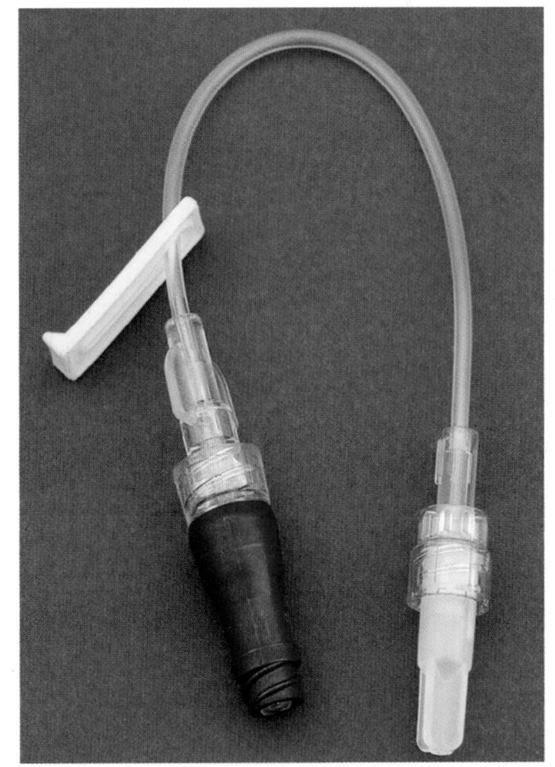

need for needles when administering medications, thus removing the risk of needlestick injury. There are various types available categorized by (a) the internal mechanisms (split septum or mechanical valve) (Hadaway 2010) and (b) how they function – that is, the presence of fluid displacement inside the device. There are three main types: negative (blood will be pulled back into the catheter lumen which occurs, for example, when an empty fluid container is left connected which can lead to occlusion), positive (these valves have a reservoir for holding a small amount of fluid; upon disconnection this fluid is pushed out to the catheter lumen to overcome the reflux of blood that has occurred) or neutral (prevents blood reflux upon connection and disconnection) (Hadaway 2010). Others are coated with antimicrobial or antibactericidal solutions on external or internal parts to reduce the risk of infection (Hadaway 2010). These require regular changing in accordance with the manufacturer's instructions as well as cleaning before and after each use (MHRA 2007, MHRA 2008).

It has been suggested that needle-free systems can increase the risk of bloodstream infections (Danzig et al. 1995). However, most studies have found no difference in microbial contamination when comparing conventional and needle-free systems (Brown et al. 1997, Luebke et al. 1998, Mendelson et al. 1998). It appears that an increased risk is only likely where there is lack of compliance with cleaning protocols or changing of equipment (Loveday et al. 2014).

Other equipment

Other IV equipment includes stopcocks (used to direct flow), usually three- or four-way devices. These tend to be used in critical care but are discouraged in the general setting due to misuse and contamination issues. If used, they should be capped off (Hadaway 2010).

Infusion devices

An infusion device is designed to accurately deliver measured amounts of fluid or drug via a number of routes (intravenous, subcutaneous or epidural) over a period of time. The infusion device is set at an appropriate rate to achieve the desired therapeutic response and prevent complications (Dougherty 2002, MHRA 2010b, MHRA 2011).

Gravity infusion devices

Gravity infusion devices depend entirely on gravity to deliver the infusion. The system consists of an administration set containing a drip chamber and a roller clamp to control the flow, which is usually measured by counting drops (Pickstone 1999). The indications for use are:

- delivery of fluids without additives
- administration of drugs or fluids where adverse effects are not anticipated and which do not need to be infused with absolute precision
- where the patient's condition does not give cause for concern and no complication is predicted (Quinn 2008).

The flow rate is calculated using a formula that requires the following information: the volume to be infused; the number of hours the infusion is running over; and the drop rate of the administration set (which will differ depending on type of set). The number of drops per millilitre is dependent on the type of administration set used and the viscosity of the infusion fluid. Increased viscosity causes the size of the drop to increase. For example, crystalloid fluid administered via a solution set is delivered at the rate of 20 drops/mL; the rate of packed red cells given via a blood set will be calculated at 15 drops/mL (Quinn 2008).

The rate of administration of a continuous or intermittent infusion may be calculated from the following equation (Pickstone 1999):

$$\frac{\text{Volume to be infused}}{\text{Time in hours}} \times \frac{\text{Drop rate}}{\text{60 minutes}} = \text{Drops per minute}$$

In this equation, 60 is a factor for the conversion of the number of hours to the number of minutes.

Factors influencing flow rates are as follows.

TYPE OF FLUID

The composition, viscosity and concentration of the fluid affect flow (Pickstone 1999, Quinn 2000, Springhouse 2005, Weinstein and Plumer 2007). Irritating solutions may result in venospasm and impede the flow rate, which may be resolved by the use of a warm pack over the cannula site and the limb (Springhouse 2005, Weinstein and Plumer 2007).

HEIGHT OF THE INFUSION CONTAINER

Intravenous fluids run by gravity and so any changes in the height of the container will alter the flow rate. The container can be hung up to 1.5 m above the infusion site which will provide a hydrostatic pressure of 110 mmHg (MHRA 2010b, Springhouse 2005). One metre above the infusion site would create 70 mmHg of pressure, which is adequate to overcome venous pressure (normal range in an adult is 25–80 mmHg) (Pickstone 1999). If it is hung too high then it can create too great a pressure within the vein, leading to infiltration of the medication (MHRA 2006a). Therefore any alterations in the patient's position may alter the flow rate and necessitate a change in the speed of the infusion to maintain the appropriate rate of flow (Hadaway 2010, MHRA 2011, Weinstein and Plumer 2007). Positioning of the patient will affect flow and patients should be instructed to keep the arm lower than the infusion, if the infusion is reliant on gravity (Quinn 2008).

ADMINISTRATION SET

The flow rate of the infusion may be affected in several ways.

- Roller clamps (see Figure 12.31) or screw clamps, used to adjust and maintain rates of flow on gravity infusions, vary considerably in their efficiency and accuracy which are often dependent on a number of variables such as patient movement and height of infusion container (Hadaway 2010). The roller clamp should be used as the primary means of occluding the tubing even if there is an anti-free flow device (MHRA 2010b).
- The inner diameter of the lumen and the length of tubing will also affect flow. Microbore sets have a narrow lumen, so flow is restricted to some degree. However, these sets may be used as a safeguard against 'runaway' or bolus infusions by either an integrated antisiphon valve or anti-free flow device (Hadaway 2010, Quinn 2000, Weinstein and Plumer 2007).
- Inclusion of other in-line devices, for example filters, may also affect the flow rate (Hadaway 2010, MHRA 2010b).

VASCULAR ACCESS DEVICE

The flow rate may be affected by any of the following.

- *The condition and size of the vein*: for example, phlebitis can reduce the lumen size and decrease flow (Quinn 2008, Weinstein and Plumer 2007).
- *The gauge of the cannula/catheter* (MHRA 2010b, Springhouse 2005, Weinstein and Plumer 2007).
- *The position of the device within the vein*: that is, whether it is up against the vein wall (Quinn 2008).
- *The site of the vascular access device*: for example, the flow may be affected by the change in position of a limb, such as a decrease in flow when a patient bends their arm if a cannula is sited over the elbow joint (Springhouse 2005).
- *Kinking, pinching or compression* of the cannula/catheter or tubing of the administration set may cause variation in the set rate (MHRA 2010b, Springhouse 2005).
- *Restricted venous circulation*: for example, a blood pressure cuff or the patient lying on the limb increases the risk of occlusion and may result in clot formation (Quinn 2008).

THE PATIENT

Patients occasionally adjust the control clamp or other parts of the delivery system, for example, change the height of the container, thereby making flow unreliable. Some pumps have tamper-proof features to minimize the risk of accidental manipulation of the infusion device (Hadaway 2010) or unauthorized changing of infusion device controls (Amoore and Adamson 2003).

ADVANTAGES AND DISADVANTAGES OF GRAVITY INFUSION DEVICES

A gravity flow system is simple to set up. It is low cost and the infusion of air is less likely than with electronic devices (Pickstone 1999). However, the system does require frequent observation and adjustment due to:

- the tubing changing shape over time
- creep or distortion of tubing made of polyvinyl chloride (PVC)
- fluctuations of venous pressure which can affect the flow of the solution
- the roller clamp can be unreliable, leading to inconsistent flow rates.

There can also be variability of drop size and, if the roller clamp is inadvertently left open, free flow will occur. Infusion rates with viscous fluids can be reduced (particularly if administered via small cannulas) and there is a limitation on the type of infusion as it is not suitable for arterial infusions: this is because viscosity and arterial flow offer a high resistance to flow which cannot be overcome by gravity (Pickstone 1999, Quinn 2008). If more than one infusion is infusing and one is slower than the other or there is no flow in the second set then there is a risk of back-tracking which leads to underinfusion or bolus delivery of medicines. The MHRA recommends that in these systems, the sets should include antireflux valves (MHRA 2007).

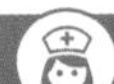 Learning Activity 12.7

Scenario: Calculating flow rate

One of the patients you are looking after has an intravenous infusion of fluids (sodium chloride 0.9%), which is being administered using a gravity solution set. Your supervising nurse has just put up a new 1 L bag of fluids which needs to infuse over 8 hours and you have been asked to calculate the flow rate based on the principle that crystalloid fluids administered via a solution set is delivered at the rate of 20 drops/mL.

1 What should the flow rate be?
2 What else should you consider to help ensure the accuracy of the flow rate?

See the end of the chapter for the answers.

Gravity drip rate controllers

A controller is a mechanical device that operates by gravity. These devices use standard solution sets and, although they look much like a pump, they have no pumping mechanism. The desired flow rate is set in drops per minute and controlled by battery- or mains-powered occlusion valves (MHRA 2010b).

ADVANTAGES AND DISADVANTAGES OF GRAVITY DRIP RATE CONTROLLERS

Although they can maintain a drip rate within 1%, volumetric accuracy is not guaranteed and many of the disadvantages associated with gravity flow still remain. The main advantages are that they are relatively inexpensive and can usually use standard gravity sets. They also incorporate some audible and visual alarm systems (MHRA 2010b).

Infusion pumps

These devices use pressure to overcome resistance from many causes along the fluid pathway, for example length and bore of tubing or particulate matter in the tubing (Hadaway 2010). There are a number of general features required in infusion pumps.

ACCURACY OF DELIVERY

In order to meet requirements for high-risk and neonatal infusions, pumps must be accurate to within ±5% of the set rate when measured over a 60-minute period although some may be as accurate as ±2% (Hadaway 2010, MHRA 2010b). They also have to satisfy short-term, minute-to-minute accuracy requirements, which demand smoothness and consistency of output (MHRA 2010b).

OCCLUSION RESPONSE AND PRESSURE

Flow will occur if the pressure at the tip of an intravascular device is just fractionally above the pressure in the vein; the pressure does not need to be excessive. In an adult peripheral vein, pressure is approximately 25 mmHg while in a neonate it is 5 mmHg (Quinn 2000). Most pumps have a variable pressure setting which allows the user to use their own judgement about the pressure needed to deliver therapy safely. The normal pumping pressure is only slightly lower than the occlusion pressure (Hadaway 2010). Flow is dependent upon pressure divided by resistance. If long extension sets of small internal bore are used, the resistance to flow will increase (Pickstone 1999, Quinn 2000).

If an administration set occludes, the resistance increases and the infusion will not flow into the vein. The longer the occlusion occurs, the greater the pressure and the pump will continue to pump until an occlusion alarm is activated. There are two types of occlusions: upstream, between the pump and the container, and downstream, between the pump and the patient. An upstream occlusion alarms when a vacuum is created in the upstream tubing or full reservoir, due to a collapsed or empty plastic fluid container or clamped/kinking tubing. A downstream occlusion is when the pressure required by the pump exceeds a certain pounds per square inch (psi) limit to overcome the pressure created by the occlusion. Downstream occlusion pressures range from 1.5 to 15 psi (Hadaway 2010).

Pumps alarm at 'occlusion alarm pressure' and many pumps allow the user to set the pressure within a range (MHRA 2010b). Therefore, the time it takes to alarm depends on the rate of flow: high rates alarm more quickly. When the alarm is activated, a certain amount of stored medication will be present and it is important that what could be a potentially large bolus is not released into the vein. The release of the stored bolus could lead to rupture of the vein or constitute overinfusion, which may be detrimental to the patient, particularly if it is a critical medication (Amoore and Adamson 2003, MHRA 2010b). With a syringe pump, to prevent a bolus being delivered to the patient, the clamp should not be opened as this will release the bolus: the first action is to remove the pressure by opening the syringe plunger clamp and then deal with the occlusion.

A pump's downstream occlusion alarm must not be relied upon to detect infiltration or extravasation (Huber and Augustine 2009, Marders 2012, MHRA 2011) and routine assessment of IV sites is still vital to prevent these complications. Single-unit variable pressure pump settings which allow an earlier alarm alert are used in neonatal and paediatric units (Quinn 2008).

AIR IN LINE

Air-in-line detectors are designed to detect only visible or microscopic 'champagne' bubbles. They should not create anxiety over small particles of air but alert the nurse to the integrity of the system (MHRA 2011). Most air bubbles detected are too small to have a harmful effect but the nurse should clarify the cause of any alarms (MHRA 2010b).

ANTISIPHONAGE

Uncontrolled flow from a syringe is called siphonage; this is a result of gravity or leakage of air into the syringe and administration set. Siphonage can occur whether or not the syringe is fixed into an infusion device (Quinn 2008). It has been reported that 'in practice, a 50 mL syringe attached to a length of administration set with an internal diameter of 3 mm has been shown to empty by siphonage in less than 1 minute' (Pickstone 1999, p.57).

To minimize the risk of siphonage, the following safe practice should be undertaken.

- The syringe (plunger and barrel) should be correctly located and secured (MHRA 2011).
- Intravenous administration extension sets should always be micro/narrow bore in diameter to increase the resistance to flow; wide-bore extension sets should be avoided.
- The syringe pump should always be positioned at the same level as the infusion site (MHRA 2011).
- Extension sets with an integral antisiphonage/antireflux valve should be used (MHRA 2007, MHRA 2010b, Quinn 2008).

SAFETY SOFTWARE

Smart pump technology incorporates safeguards such as a list of high alert medications, soft and hard dosage limits and a drug library that can be tailored to specific patient care areas (Agius 2012, Harding 2012, Hertzel and Sousa 2009). A number of studies have evaluated the effectiveness of using smart pumps to prevent medication errors, showing the success of these systems (Dennison 2007, Fields and Peterson 2005, Larson et al. 2005, Rothschild et al. 2005). It is now recommended that nurses use this technology when administering intravenous fluids and medications (Harding 2011) but careful selection and training are vital for compliance and to ensure safety outcomes (Longshore et al. 2010).

Volumetric pumps

Volumetric pumps (Figure 12.35) pump fluid from an infusion bag or bottle via an administration set and work by calculating the volume delivered (Quinn 2008). This is achieved when the pump measures the volume displaced in a 'reservoir'. The reservoir is an integral component of the administration set (Hadaway 2010). The mechanism of action may be piston or peristaltic (Hadaway 2010). The indications for use are all large-volume infusions, both venous and arterial.

All are mains and battery powered, with the rate selected in millilitres per hour. The accuracy of flow is usually within 5% when measured over a period of time, which is more than adequate for most clinical applications (MHRA 2010b, Pickstone 1999).

ADVANTAGES AND DISADVANTAGES OF VOLUMETRIC PUMPS

These pumps are able to overcome resistance to flow by increased delivery pressure and do not rely on gravity. This generally makes the performance of pumps predictable and capable of accurate delivery over a wider range of flow rates (MHRA 2010b).

The pumps also incorporate a wide range of features, including air-in-line detectors, variable pressure settings and comprehensive alarms such as end of infusion, keep vein open (KVO, where the pump switches to a low flow rate, for example 5 mL/h, in order to continue flow to prevent occlusion of the device) and low battery. Many have a secondary infusion facility, which allows for intermittent therapy, for example antibiotics. The pump is programmed to switch to a secondary set and, when completed, it reverts back to the primary infusion at the previously set rate. The changing hospital environment has led to an increased demand on volumetric pumps, which in turn has resulted in the development of multichannel and dual-channel infusion pumps. These may consist of two devices with an attached housing or of several infusion channels within a single device (Hadaway 2010).

The disadvantages are that these are usually relatively expensive and often dedicated administration sets are required. The use of the wrong set could result in error even if the pump appears to work. Some are complicated to set up, which can also lead to errors (MHRA 2010b).

Figure 12.35 **Volumetric pump.**

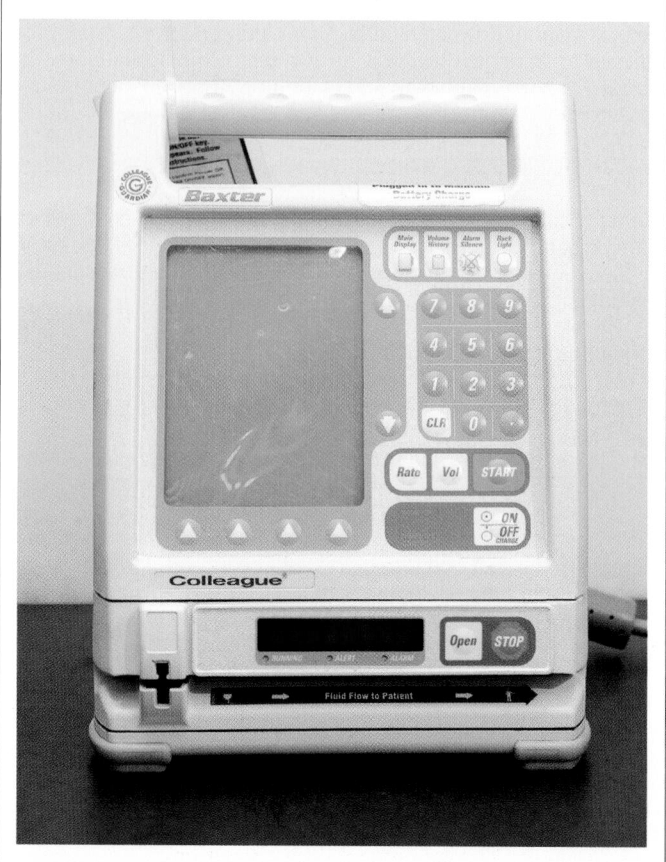

Syringe pumps

Syringe pumps (Figure 12.36) are low-volume, high-accuracy devices designed to infuse at low flow rates. The plunger of a syringe containing the substance to be infused is driven forward by the syringe pump at a controlled rate to deliver it to the patient (MHRA 2010b).

Syringe pumps are useful where small volumes of highly concentrated drugs need to be infused at low flow rates (Quinn 2008). The volume for infusion is limited to the size of the syringe used in the device, which is usually 60 mL, but most pumps will accept different sizes and brands of syringe.

These devices are calibrated for delivery in millilitres per hour (Weinstein and Plumer 2007).

ADVANTAGES AND DISADVANTAGES OF SYRINGE PUMPS

Syringe pumps are mains and/or battery powered, are usually easy to operate, and tend to cost less than volumetric pumps. The alarm systems are becoming more comprehensive and include low battery, end of infusion and syringe clamp open alarms. Most of the problems associated with the older models, for example free flow, mechanical backlash (slackness which delays the start-up time of the infusion) and incorrect fitting of the syringe, have been eliminated in the newer models (MHRA 2010b, Quinn 2008). The risk of free flow is minimized by the use of an antisiphonage valve which may be integral to the administration set (Pickstone 1999). Despite the use of an antisiphonage valve, the clamp of the administration set must still be used (MHRA 2010b). Where mechanical backlash is an issue and there is a prime or purge option, this should be used at the start of the infusion to take up the mechanical slack (Amoore et al. 2001).

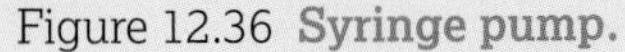
Figure 12.36 **Syringe pump.**

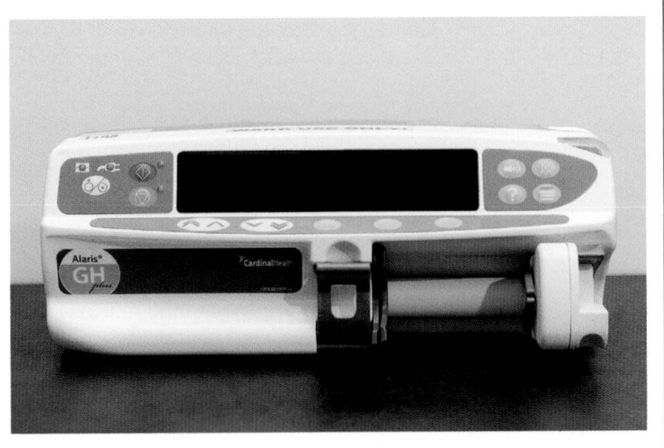

Specialist pumps

PATIENT-CONTROLLED ANALGESIA PUMPS

Patient-controlled analgesia (PCA) devices are typically syringe pumps (although some are based on volumetric designs) (MHRA 2010b) (Figure 12.37). The syringe pump forces down on the syringe piston, collapsing the syringe at a pre-set rate, but the distinguishing feature is the ability of the pump to deliver doses on demand, which occurs when the patient pushes a button (Hadaway 2010). Whether or not the dose is delivered is determined by pre-set parameters in the pump. That is, if the maximum amount of drug over a given period of time has already been delivered, a further dose cannot be delivered.

Patient-controlled analgesia pumps are useful for patients who require pain control. They are used more in the acute setting but are also useful in ambulatory situations (Chumbley and Mountford 2010).

Infusion options of a PCA pump are usually categorized into three types.

- *Basal*: a 'baseline' rate can be accompanied by intermittent doses requested by patients. This aims to achieve pain relief with minimal medication, but not necessarily to achieve a pain-free state (Hadaway 2010).

Figure 12.37 **PCA pump used generally in acute hospital settings.**

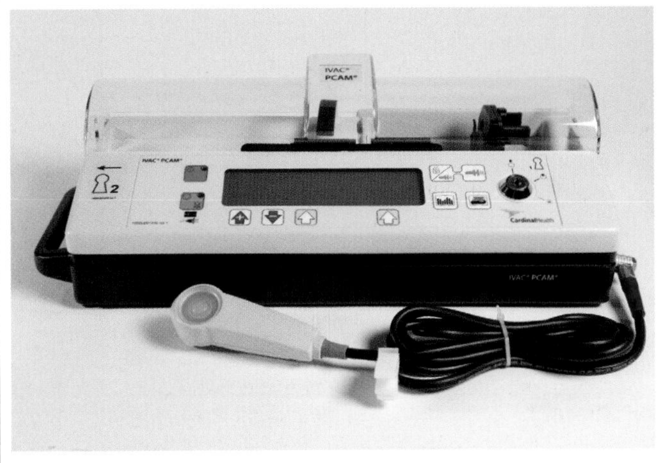

- *Continuous*: designed for the patient who needs maximum pain relief without the option of demand dosing, for example epidural.
- *Demand*: drug delivered by intermittent infusion when a button is pushed and can be used alone or supplemented by the basal rate. Doses can be limited by a designated maximum amount (Hadaway 2010).

The PCA pump can dispense a bolus dose, with an initial bolus being called a loading dose. This may benefit patients as the one-time dose is significantly higher than a demand dose in order to achieve immediate pain relief (see Chapter 8: Patient comfort and end-of-life care).

ADVANTAGES AND DISADVANTAGES OF PCA PUMPS

These devices offer a 'lock-out' feature (when a key or a combination of numbers is necessary to gain access to pump controls), which is designed for patient safety. They have an extensive memory capability which can be accessed through the display via a printer or computer (MHRA 2010b). This facility is critical for the pump's effective use in pain management (Hadaway 2010), as it enables the clinician to determine when and how often demand is made by a patient and what total volume has been infused (Hadaway 2010). It has also been shown that they increase patient satisfaction, patients require less sedation, their anxiety is reduced and so are their nursing needs and time in hospital (Ripamonti and Bruera 1997).

Anaesthesia pumps

These are syringe pumps designed for delivery of anaesthesia or sedation and must only ever be used for that purpose. They should be restricted to operating theatres or critical care units and should be clearly labelled. They are designed to allow rapid changes in flow rate and bolus to be made while the pump is infusing (Quinn 2008). Total intravenous anaesthesia (TIVA) and target-controlled infusion (TCI) pumps are now available, designed to control the induction, maintenance and reversal phases of anaesthesia (Absalom and Struys 2006).

Syringe drivers

See 'Subcutaneous infusion equipment'.

Specific patient preparation

Selecting the appropriate infusion device for the patient

The nurse has a responsibility to determine when and how to use an infusion device to deliver hydration, drugs, transfusions and nutritional support, and how to select the appropriate device in order to manage the needs of the patient. The following factors should be considered when selecting an appropriate infusion delivery system (Quinn 2008).

- Risk to the patient of:
  - overinfusion
  - underinfusion
  - uneven flow
  - inadvertent bolus
  - high-pressure delivery
  - extravascular infusion.
- Delivery parameters:
  - infusion rate and volume required
  - accuracy required (over a long or short period of time)
  - alarms required
  - ability to infuse into site chosen (venous, arterial, subcutaneous)
  - suitability of device for infusing drug (e.g. ability to infuse viscous drugs).
- Environmental features:
  - ease of operation
  - frequency of observation and adjustment
  - type of patient (neonate, child, critically ill)
  - mobility of patient.

Table 12.11 **Therapy categories and performance parameters**

Therapy category	Therapy description	Patient group	Critical performance parameters
A	Drugs with narrow therapeutic margin	Any	Good long-term accuracy Good short-term accuracy
	Drugs with short half-life	Any	Rapid alarm after occlusion Small occlusion bolus
	Any infusion given to neonates	Neonates	Able to detect very small air embolus (volumetric pumps only)
			Small flow rate increments
			Good bolus accuracy
			Rapid start-up time (syringe pumps only)
B	Drugs other than those with a short half-life	Any except neonates	Good long-term accuracy Alarm after occlusion
	Parenteral nutrition	Volume sensitive except neonates	Small occlusion bolus
	Fluid maintenance Transfusions		Able to detect small air embolus (volumetric pumps only)
			Small flow rate increments
C	Diamorphine	Any except neonates	Bolus accuracy
	Parenteral nutrition Fluid maintenance	Any except volume sensitive or neonates	Long-term accuracy Alarm after occlusion Small occlusion bolus
	Transfusions		Able to detect air embolus (volumetric pumps only) Incremental flow rates

Source: MHRA (2010b). © Crown copyright. Reproduced under the Open Government Licence v2.0.

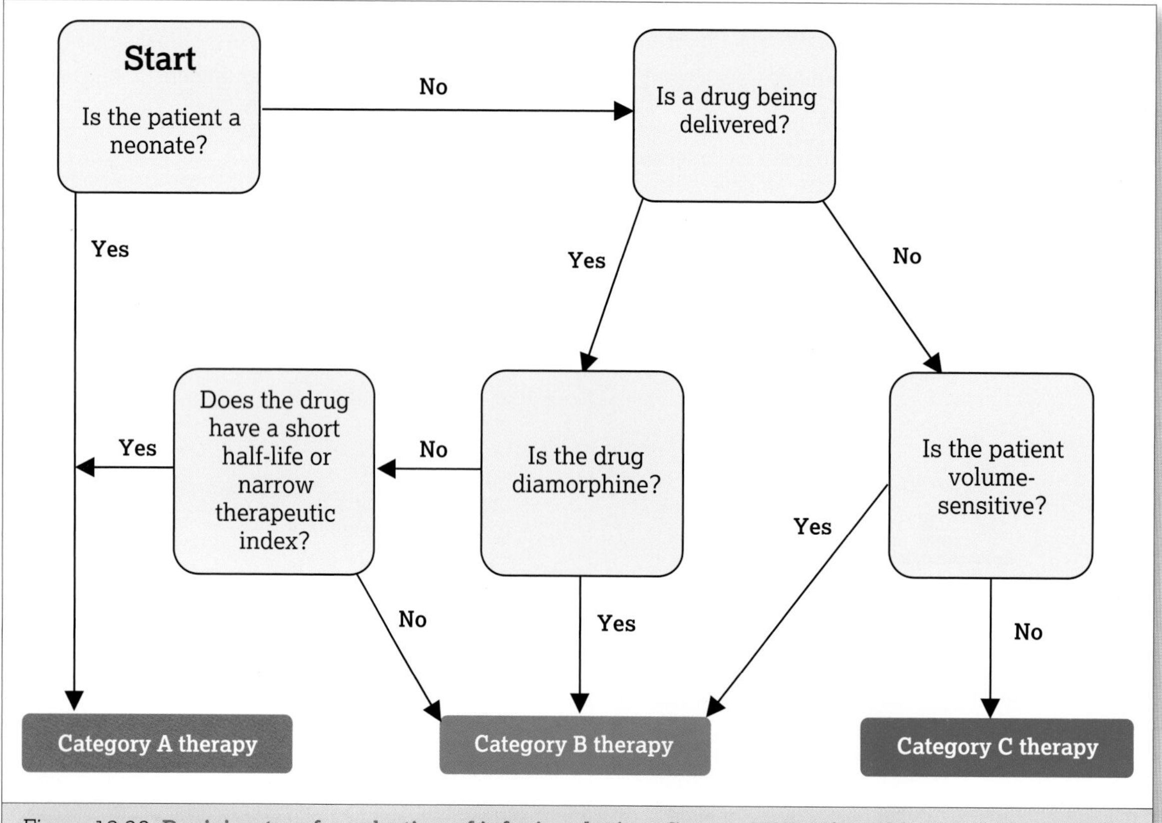

Figure 12.38 **Decision tree for selection of infusion device.** ***Source:*** **MHRA (2010b). © Crown copyright. Reproduced under the Open Government Licence v2.0.**

654

Paediatric considerations

The MHRA classifies infusion devices into categories of infusion risk. Neonatal infusions are the highest risk category; high-risk infusions are typically the infusion of fluids in children where accuracy of the flow rate is essential (MHRA 2014). Infusion therapy within the paediatric setting requires very specific skills (Frey and Pettit 2010). Competency in calculation of paediatric dosages, maintaining a stringent fluid balance, use of paediatric-specific devices and management of complications are paramount.

The MHRA has made recommendations on the safety and performance of infusion devices in order to enable users to make the appropriate choice of equipment to suit most applications (MHRA 2010b). The classification system is divided into three major categories according to the potential risks involved. These are shown in Table 12.11. A pump suited to the most risky category of therapy (A) can be safely used for the other categories (B and C). A pump suited to category B can be used for B and C, whereas a pump with the lowest specification (C) is suited only to category C therapies (MHRA 2010b) (Figure 12.38). Hospitals are required to label each infusion pump with its category and it is necessary to know the category of the proposed therapy and match it with a pump of the same or better category. A locally produced list of drugs/fluids by their categories will need to be provided to all device users (MHRA 2010b).

Procedure guideline 12.22 Medication: continuous infusion of intravenous drugs

This procedure may be carried out by the infusion of drugs from a bag, bottle or burette.

Essential equipment

- Clinically clean tray containing the prepared drug
- Patient's prescription chart
- Recording chart or book as required by law or hospital policy
- Non-sterile gloves
- Protective clothing as required by hospital policy for the administration of specific drugs
- Container of appropriate intravenous infusion fluid
- 2% chlorhexidine swab
- Drug additive label

Pre-procedure

Action	Rationale
1 Explain and discuss the procedure with the patient.	To ensure that the patient understands the procedure and gives their valid consent (Griffith and Jordan 2003, **E**; NMC 2013, **C**; NMC 2015, **C**).
2 Inspect the infusion in progress.	To check it is the correct infusion being administered at the correct rate and that the contents are due to be delivered on time in order for the next prepared infusion bag to be connected. To check whether the patient is experiencing any discomfort at the site of insertion, which might indicate the peripheral device needs to be resited (NPSA 2007d, **C**).
3 Before administering any prescribed drug, check that it is due and has not already been given.	To protect the patient from harm (NPSA 2007d, **C**).
4 Before administering any prescribed drug, look at the patient's prescription chart and check the following. (a) The correct patient (b) Drug (c) Dose (d) Date and time of administration (e) Route and method of administration (f) Diluent as appropriate (g) Validity of prescription (h) Signature of prescriber (i) The prescription is legible	To ensure that the correct patient is given the correct drug in the prescribed dose using the appropriate diluent and by the correct route (DH 2003b, **C**; NMC 2010a, **C**). To protect the patient from harm (DH 2003b, **C**; NMC 2010a, **C**).
If any of these pieces of information are missing, are unclear or illegible then the nurse should not proceed with administration and should consult with the prescriber.	To prevent any errors occurring. **E**
5 Wash hands with bactericidal soap and water or bactericidal alcohol handrub, and assemble the necessary equipment.	To minimize the risk of infection (DH 2007, **C**; Fraise and Bradley 2009, **E**).
6 Prepare the drug for injection as described in Procedure guidelines 12.12, 12.13, 12.14 and 12.15.	To ensure the drug is prepared (NPSA 2007d, **C**).
7 Check the name, strength and volume of intravenous fluid against the prescription chart.	To ensure that the correct type and quantity of fluid are administered (NMC 2010a, **C**; NPSA 2007d, **C**).
8 Check the expiry date of the fluid.	To prevent an ineffective or toxic compound being administered to the patient (NPSA 2007d, **C**).

(continued)

Procedure guideline 12.22 Medication: continuous infusion of intravenous drugs *(continued)*

Action	Rationale
9 Check that the packaging is intact and inspect the container and contents in a good light for cracks, punctures and air bubbles.	To check that no contamination of the infusion container has occurred (NPSA 2007d, **C**).
10 Inspect the fluid for discoloration, haziness and crystalline or particulate matter.	To prevent any toxic or foreign matter being infused into the patient (NPSA 2007d, **C**).
11 Check the identity and amount of drug to be added. Consider: (a) compatibility of fluid and additive (b) stability of mixture over the prescribed duration of the infusion (c) any special directions for dilution, for example pH, optimum concentration (d) sensitivity to external factors such as light (e) any anticipated allergic reaction. If any doubts exist about the listed points, consult the pharmacist or appropriate reference works.	To minimize any risk of error. To ensure safe and effective administration of the drug. To enable anticipation of toxicities and the nursing implications of these (NPSA 2007d, **C**).
12 Any additions must be made immediately before use.	To prevent any possible microbial growth or degradation (NPSA 2007d, **C**).
13 Wash hands thoroughly using bactericidal soap and water or bactericidal alcohol handrub.	To minimize the risk of cross-infection (DH 2007, **C**; Fraise and Bradley 2009, **E**).
14 Place infusion bag on flat surface.	To prevent puncturing the side of the infusion bag when making additions (NPSA 2007d, **C**).
15 Remove any seal present.	To expose the injection site on the container. **E**
Procedure	
16 Clean the site with the swab and allow it to dry.	To reduce the risk of contamination (NPSA 2007d, **C**).
17 Inject the drug using a new sterile needle into the bag, bottle or burette. A 23 or 25 G needle should be used. If the addition is made into a burette at the bedside: (a) avoid contamination of the needle and inlet port (b) check that the correct quantity of fluid is in the chamber (c) switch the infusion off briefly (d) add the drug.	To minimize the risk of contamination. To enable resealing of the latex or rubber injection site (NPSA 2007d, **C**). To minimize the risk of contamination (NPSA 2007d, **C**). To ensure the correct dilution (NPSA 2007d, **C**). To ensure a bolus injection is not given (NPSA 2007d, **C**).
18 Invert the container a number of times, especially if adding to a flexible infusion bag.	To ensure adequate mixing of the drug (NPSA 2007d, **C**).
19 Check again for haziness, discoloration and particles. This can occur even if the mixture is theoretically compatible, thus making vigilance essential.	To detect any incompatibility or degradation (NPSA 2007d, **C**).
20 Complete the drug additive label and fix it on the bag, bottle or burette.	To identify which drug has been added, when and by whom (NPSA 2007d, **C**).
21 Place the container in a clean receptacle. Wash hands and proceed to the patient.	To minimize the risk of contamination (DH 2007, **C**).
22 Check the identity of the patient against the prescription chart and infusion bag.	To minimize the risk of error and ensure the correct infusion is administered to the correct patient (NPSA 2007d, **C**).
23 Check that the contents of the previous container have been fully delivered.	To ensure that the preceding prescription has been administered (NPSA 2007d, **C**).
24 Switch off the infusion. Apply gloves. Place the new infusion bag on a flat surface and then disconnect empty infusion bag.	To ensure that the administration set spike will not puncture the side wall of the infusion bag (Finlay 2008, **E**; NPSA 2007d, **C**).
25 Push the spike in fully without touching it and hang the new infusion bag on the infusion stand. Insert tubing into an infusion pump where appropriate.	To reduce the risk of contamination (DH 2007, **C**). To ensure accuracy of delivery (Quinn 2008, **E**).
26 For gravity infusion, restart the infusion and adjust the rate of flow as prescribed. If via an infusion pump, start the pump and set rate.	To ensure that the infusion will be delivered at the correct rate over the correct period of time (NPSA 2007d, **C**).

Action	Rationale
27 If the addition is made into a burette, the infusion can be restarted immediately following mixing and recording and the infusion rate adjusted accordingly.	To ensure that the infusion will be delivered correctly (NPSA 2007d, **C**).
28 Ask the patient whether any abnormal sensations are experienced.	To ascertain whether there are any problems that may require nursing care and refer to medical staff where appropriate. **E**.

Post-procedure

Action	Rationale
29 Discard waste, making sure that it is placed in the correct containers, for example sharps into a designated receptacle.	To ensure safe disposal and avoid injury to staff. To prevent reuse of equipment (DH 2005, **C**; EU 2010, **C**; MHRA 2004, **C**).
30 Complete the patient's recording chart and other hospital and/or legally required documents.	To maintain accurate records. To provide a point of reference in the event of any queries. To prevent any duplication of treatment (NMC 2010a, **C**; NMC 2010b, **C**).

Procedure guideline 12.23 **Medication: intermittent infusion of intravenous drugs**

Essential equipment

- Patient's prescription chart
- Recording chart
- Protective clothing as required by hospital policy for the administration of specific drugs
- Container of appropriate intravenous infusion fluid
- Drug additive label
- Intravenous administration set
- Intravenous infusion stand
- Clean dressing trolley
- Clinically clean receiver or tray containing the prepared drug to be administered
- Sterile needles and syringes
- 10 mL for injection of a compatible flush solution, for example 0.9% sodium chloride or 5% dextrose
- Flushing solution to maintain patency plus sterile injection cap
- 2% chlorhexidine swab
- Non-sterile gloves
- Alcohol-based hand wash solution or rub
- Sterile dressing pack
- Hypoallergenic tape
- Sharps bin

Pre-procedure

Action	Rationale
1 Explain and discuss the procedure with the patient.	To ensure that the patient understands the procedure and gives their valid consent (Griffith and Jordan 2003, **E**; NMC 2013, **C**; NMC 2015, **C**).
2 Before administering any prescribed drug, check that it is due and has not been given already.	To protect the patient from harm (NMC 2010a, **C**; NPSA 2007d, **C**).
3 Before administering any prescribed drug, look at the patient's prescription chart and check the following. (a) The correct patient (b) Drug (c) Dose (d) Date and time of administration (e) Route and method of administration (f) Diluent as appropriate (g) Validity of prescription (h) Signature of prescriber (i) The prescription is legible	To ensure that the correct patient is given the correct drug in the prescribed dose using the appropriate diluent and by the correct route (DH 2003b, **C**; NMC 2010a, **C**). To protect the patient from harm (DH 2003b, **C**; NMC 2010a, **C**). To protect the patient from harm. To comply with NMC (2010a) *Standards for Medicines Management.*
If any of these pieces of information are missing, are unclear or illegible then the nurse should not proceed with administration and should consult with the prescriber.	To prevent any errors occurring. **E**
4 Wash hands with bactericidal soap and water or bactericidal alcohol handrub.	To prevent contamination of medication and equipment (DH 2007, **C**).
5 Prepare the intravenous infusion and additive as described in Procedure guidelines 12.12, 12.13, 12.14 and 12.15.	To ensure the drug is prepared correctly (NPSA 2007d, **C**).
6 Prime the intravenous administration set with infusion fluid mixture and hang it on the infusion stand.	To ensure removal of air from set and check that tubing is patent. To prepare for administration (NPSA 2007d, **C**).
7 Draw up 10 mL of compatible flush solution for injection using an aseptic technique.	To ensure sufficient flushing solution is available. **E**
8 Draw up solution (as advised by hospital policy) to be used for maintaining patency, for example 0.9% sodium chloride.	To prepare for administration. **E**

(continued)

Procedure guideline 12.23 Medication: intermittent infusion of intravenous drugs *(continued)*

Action	Rationale
9 Place the syringes in a clinically clean tray on the bottom shelf of the dressing trolley.	To ensure top shelf is used for sterile dressing pack in order to minimize the risk of contamination. **E**
10 Collect the other equipment and place it on the bottom shelf of the dressing trolley.	To ensure all equipment is available to commence procedure. **E**
11 Place a sterile dressing pack on top of the trolley.	To minimize risk of contamination. **E**
12 Check that all necessary equipment is present.	To prevent delays and interruption of the procedure. **E**
13 Wash hands thoroughly using bactericidal soap and water or bactericidal alcohol handrub before leaving the clinical room.	To minimize the risk of cross-infection (DH 2007, **C**; Fraise and Bradley 2009, **E**).
14 Proceed to the patient. Check patient's identity against prescription chart and prepared drugs.	To minimize the risk of error and ensure the correct drug is given to the correct patient (NMC 2010a, **C**; NPSA 2007d, **C**).
Procedure	
15 Open the sterile dressing pack.	To minimize the risk of cross-infection (DH 2007, **C**; Fraise and Bradley 2009, **E**).
16 Open the 2% chlorhexidine swab packet and empty it onto the pack.	To ensure the correct cleaning swab is available (DH 2007, **E**).
17 Wash hands with bactericidal soap and water or with a bactericidal alcohol handrub.	To minimize the risk of cross-infection. (DH 2007, **C**; Fraise and Bradley 2009, **E**).
18 If peripheral device is *in situ* remove the patient's bandage and dressing, where appropriate.	To observe the insertion site (Dougherty 2008, **E**).
19 Inspect the insertion site of the device.	To detect any signs of inflammation, infiltration, and so on. If present, take appropriate action (DH 2003c, **C**).
20 Wash and dry hands.	To minimize the risk of contamination (DH 2007, **C**).
21 Put on gloves.	To protect against contamination with hazardous substances, for example cytotoxic drugs (NPSA 2007d, **C**).
22 Place a sterile towel under the patient's arm.	To create a sterile area on which to work. **E**
23 Clean the needle-free cap with 2% chlorhexidine swab.	To minimize the risk of contamination and maintain a closed system (Loveday et al. 2014, **C**).
24 Gently inject 10 mL of 0.9% sodium chloride for injection.	To confirm the patency of the device. **E**
25 Check that no resistance is met, no pain or discomfort is felt by the patient, no swelling is evident, no leakage occurs around the device and there is a good backflow of blood on aspiration.	To ensure the device is patent (Dougherty 2008, **E**).
26 Connect the infusion to the device.	To commence treatment. **E**
27 Open the roller clamp and/or insert the tubing into an infusion pump and start pump.	To check the infusion is flowing freely. **E**
28 Check the insertion site and ask the patient if they are comfortable.	To confirm that the vein can accommodate the extra fluid flow and that the patient experiences no pain. **E**
29 Adjust the flow rate as prescribed.	To ensure that the correct speed of administration is established (NPSA 2007d, **C**).
30 Tape the administration set in a way that places no strain on the device, which could in turn damage the vein.	To reduce the risk of mechanical phlebitis or infiltration (Dougherty 2008, **E**).
31 If a peripheral device is *in situ*, cover it with a sterile topical swab and tape it in place.	To maintain asepsis (Dougherty 2008, **E**).
32 Remove gloves.	To ensure disposal. **E**
33 If the infusion is to be completed within 30 minutes, bandaging is unnecessary and the patient may be instructed to keep the arm resting on the sterile towel. Otherwise reapply bandage.	To reduce the risk of dislodging the device. **E**
34 The equipment must be cleared away and new equipment only prepared when required at the end of the infusion.	To ensure that the equipment used is sterile prior to use. **E**

Action	Rationale
35 Monitor flow rate and device site frequently.	To ensure the flow rate is correct and the patient is comfortable, and to check for signs of infiltration (NPSA 2007d, **C**).
36 When the infusion is complete, wash hands using bactericidal soap and water or bactericidal alcohol handrub, and recheck that all the equipment required is present.	To maintain asepsis and ensure that the procedure runs smoothly (DH 2007 **C**; Finlay 2008, **E**).
37 Stop the infusion when all the fluid has been delivered.	To ensure that all the prescribed mixture has been delivered and prevent air infusing into the patient (NPSA 2007d, **C**).
38 Put on non-sterile gloves.	To protect against contamination with hazardous substances. **E**
39 Disconnect the infusion set and flush the device with 10 mL of 0.9% sodium chloride or other compatible solution for injection. (A 'minibag' may be used to flush the drug through the tubing but the cost implications of this as well as the risk to patients on restricted intake should be considered before this is adopted routinely.)	To flush any remaining irritating solution away from the cannula. **E**
40 Attach a new sterile injection cap if necessary.	To maintain a closed system (Hart 2008, **E**).
41 Flushing must follow.	To maintain the patency of the device (Dougherty 2008, **E**).
42 Clean the injection site of the cap with 2% chlorhexidine swab.	To minimize the risk of contamination (Hart 2008, **E**).
43 Administer flushing solution using the push-pause technique and ending with positive pressure.	To maintain the patency of the device and if needle was used, to enable reseal of the injection site (Dougherty 2008, **E**).
44 If a peripheral device is *in situ*, cover the insertion site and cannula with a new sterile low-linting swab. Tape it in place. Apply a bandage.	To minimize the risk of contamination of the insertion site. To reduce the risk of dislodging the cannula. **E**
45 Remove gloves.	To ensure disposal. **E**
46 Assist the patient into a comfortable position.	To ensure the patient is comfortable. **E**
Post-procedure	
47 Discard waste, placing it in the correct containers, for example sharps into a designated container.	To ensure safe disposal and avoid injury to staff (DH 2005, **C**; EU 2010, **C**; MHRA 2004, **C**; NHS Employers 2007, **C**).
48 Record the administration on appropriate charts.	To maintain accurate records, provide a point of reference in the event of any queries and prevent any duplication of treatment (NMC 2010a, **C**; NMC 2010b, **C**).

Procedure guideline 12.24 Medication: injection (bolus or push) of intravenous drugs

Essential equipment

- Clinically clean tray containing the prepared drug(s) to be administered
- Patient's prescription chart
- Protective clothing as required by hospital policy for adminstering drugs
- Clean dressing trolley
- Sterile needles and syringes
- 0.9% sodium chloride, 20 mL for injection, or compatible solution
- Flushing solution, in accordance with hospital policy
- 2% chlorhexidine swab
- Sterile dressing pack
- Hypoallergenic tape
- Sharps container

Pre-procedure

Action	Rationale
1 Explain and discuss the procedure with the patient.	To ensure that the patient understands the procedure and gives their valid consent (Griffith and Jordan 2003, **E**; NMC 2013, **C**; NMC 2015, **C**).
2 Before administering any prescribed drug, check that it is due and has not been given already.	To protect the patient from harm (NMC 2010a, **C**).

(continued)

Procedure guideline 12.24 Medication: injection (bolus or push) of intravenous drugs *(continued)*

Action	Rationale
3 Before administering any prescribed drug, look at the patient's prescription chart and check the following. (a) The correct patient (b) Drug (c) Dose (d) Date and time of administration (e) Route and method of administration (f) Diluent as appropriate (g) Validity of prescription (h) Signature of prescriber (i) The prescription is legible	To ensure that the correct patient is given the correct drug in the prescribed dose using the appropriate diluent and by the correct route (DH 2003b, **C**; NMC 2010a, **C**). To protect the patient from harm (DH 2003b, **C**; NMC 2010a, **C**). To protect the patient from harm. To comply with NMC (2010a) *Standards for Medicines Management.*
If any of these pieces of information are missing, are unclear or illegible then the nurse should not proceed with administration and should consult with the prescriber.	To prevent any errors occurring. **E**
Procedure	
4 Select the required medication and check the expiry date.	Treatment with medication that is outside the expiry date is dangerous. Drugs deteriorate with storage. The expiry date indicates when a particular drug is no longer pharmacologically efficacious (NPSA 2007d, **C**).
5 Wash hands with bactericidal soap and water or bactericidal alcohol handrub, and assemble necessary equipment.	To minimize the risk of infection (DH 2007, **C**; Fraise and Bradley 2009, **E**).
6 Prepare the drug for injection as described in Procedure guidelines 12.12, 12.13, 12.14 and 12.15.	To prepare the drug correctly. **E**
7 Prepare a 20 mL syringe of 0.9% sodium chloride (or compatible solution) for injection, as described, using aseptic technique.	To use for flushing between each drug (NPSA 2007d, **C**).
8 Draw up the flushing solution, as indicated by local hospital policy.	To prepare for administration. **E**
9 Place syringes in a clinically clean receptacle on the bottom shelf of the dressing trolley, along with the receptacle containing any drug(s) to be administered.	To ensure top shelf is used for sterile dressing pack in order to minimize the risk of contamination. **E**
10 Collect the other equipment and place it on the bottom of the trolley.	To ensure all equipment is available to commence procedure. **E**
11 Place a sterile dressing pack on top of the trolley.	To minimize the risk of contamination. **E**
12 Check that all necessary equipment is present.	To prevent delays and interruption of the procedure. **E**
13 Wash hands thoroughly.	To minimize the risk of infection (DH 2007, **C**; Fraise and Bradley 2009, **E**).
14 Proceed to the patient and check their identity and the prepared drug against the prescription chart.	To minimize the risk of error and ensure the drug is given to the correct patient (NPSA 2007d, **C**).
15 Open the sterile dressing pack and 2% chlorhexidine swab and empty onto pack.	To gain access to equipment and to ensure there is a cleaning swab available (DH 2007, **C**).
16 Wash hands with bactericidal soap and water or with bactericidal alcohol handrub.	To reduce the risk of infection (DH 2007, **C**; Fraise and Bradley 2009, **E**).
17 If a peripheral device is *in situ*, remove the bandage and dressing (if appropriate).	To observe the insertion site. **E**
18 Inspect the insertion site of the device.	To detect any signs of inflammation, infiltration, and so on. If present, take appropriate action (see Problem-solving table 12.3) (DH 2003c, **C**).
19 Observe the infusion, if in progress.	To confirm that it is infusing as desired (NPSA 2007d, **C**).
20 Check whether the infusion fluid and the drugs are compatible. If not, change the infusion fluid to 0.9% sodium chloride to flush between the drugs if necessary.	To prevent drug interaction. Some manufacturers may recommend that the drug is given into the injection site of a rapidly running infusion (NPSA 2007d, **C**). A compatible fluid must be used to remove the medication and prevent precipitation or drug incompatibility if medications mix in the tubing (Whittington 2008, **E**).

21 Wash hands or clean them with an alcohol handrub.	To minimize the risk of infection (DH 2007, **C**; Fraise and Bradley 2009, **E**).
22 Place a sterile towel under the patient's arm.	To create a sterile field. **E**
23 Apply gloves and clean the injection site with a 2% chlorhexidine swab and allow to dry.	To reduce the number of pathogens introduced by the needle at the time of the insertion. To ensure complete disinfection has occurred (Loveday et al. 2014, **C**).
24 Switch off the infusion.	To prevent excessive pressure within the vein. To prevent contact with an incompatible infusion fluid. To allow the nurse to concentrate on the site of insertion and injection (NPSA 2007d, **C**).
25 If a peripheral device is *in situ*, gently inject 0.9% sodium chloride. This may not be necessary if the patient has a 0.9% sodium chloride infusion in progress.	To confirm patency of the vein. To prevent contact with an incompatible infusion solution (NPSA 2007d, **C**).
26 Open the roller clamp of the administration set fully. Inject the drug at a speed sufficient to slow but not stop the infusion and inject the drug smoothly in the direction of flow at the specified rate.	To prevent backflow of drug up the tubing. To prevent excessive pressure within the vein. To prevent speed shock (NPSA 2007d, **C**).
27 Ensure needles and syringes are disposed of immediately into appropriate sharps container (or are returned to tray). Do not leave any sharps on opened sterile pack.	To reduce the risk of needlestick injury and to prevent contamination of pack (RCN 2010, **C**).
28 Observe the insertion site of the device throughout.	To detect any complications at an early stage, for example extravasation or local allergic reaction (Dougherty 2008, **E**).
29 Blood return and/or 'flashback' must be checked frequently throughout the injection (that is, every 3–5 mL) but other signs and symptoms must be taken into consideration.	To confirm that the device is correctly placed and that the vein remains patent (Weinstein and Plumer 2007, **E**). Flashback alone is not an indicator that the vein is patent (Dougherty 2008, **E**).
30 Consult the patient during the injection about any discomfort, and so on.	To detect any complications at an early stage, and ensure patient comfort (Dougherty 2008, **E**).
31 If more than one drug is to be administered, flush with 0.9% sodium chloride between administrations by restarting the infusion or changing syringes.	To prevent drug interactions (NPSA 2007d, **C**).
32 At the end of the injection, flush with 0.9% sodium chloride by restarting the infusion or attaching a syringe containing 0.9% sodium chloride.	To flush any remaining irritant solution away from the device site (NPSA 2007d, **C**).
33 After the final flush of 0.9% sodium chloride, adjust the infusion rate as prescribed or open the fluid path of the tap/stopcock or administer the flushing solution using pulsatile flush and ending with positive pressure.	To continue delivery of therapy. To maintain the patency of the cannula (Finlay 2008, **E**).
34 If a peripheral device is *in situ*, cover the insertion site with new sterile low-linting swab and tape it in place.	To minimize the risk of contamination of the insertion site. **E**
35 Apply a bandage.	To reduce the risk of dislodging the cannula. **E**
36 Assist the patient into a comfortable position.	To ensure the patient is comfortable. **E**
Post-procedure	
38 Dispose of used syringes with the needle, unsheathed, directly into a sharps container during procedure or place back on to plastic tray and then dispose of in a sharps container as soon as possible. *Do not* disconnect needle from syringe prior to disposal. Other waste should be placed into the appropriate plastic bags.	To avoid needlestick injury (EU 2010, **C**; MHRA 2004, **C**; NHS Employers 2007, **C**).
37 Record the administration on appropriate charts.	To maintain accurate records, provide a point of reference in the event of any queries and prevent any duplication of treatment (NMC 2010a, **C**; NMC 2010b, **C**).

Problem-solving table 12.3 **Prevention and resolution (Procedure guidelines 12.22, 12.23 and 12.24)**

Problem	Cause	Prevention	Action
Infusion slows or stops (part 1).	Change in position of the following.		
	(a) Patient.	Check the height of the fluid container if the patient is active and receiving an infusion using gravity flow.	Adjust the height of the container accordingly. The infusion should not hang higher than 1 m above the patient as the increased height will result in increased pressure and possible rupture of the vessel/device (Quinn 2008).
	(b) Limb.	Prevent by avoiding inserting peripheral devices at joints of limbs.	Move the arm or hand until infusion starts again. Secure the device, then bandage or splint the limb again carefully in the desired position. Take care not to cause damage to the limb.
		Instruct the patient on the amount of movement permitted. Continued movement could result in mechanical phlebitis (Lamb and Dougherty 2008).	
	(c) Administration set.	Tape the administration set so that it cannot become kinked or occluded.	Check for kinks and/or compression if the patient is active or restless and correct accordingly.
	(d) Cannula.	Secure the cannula firmly to prevent movement. It may come into contact with the vein wall or a valve. Infusions sited in small veins are prone to this problem.	Remove the bandage and dressing and manoeuvre the peripheral device gently, without pulling it out of the vein, until the infusion starts again. Secure adequately.
Infusion slows or stops (part 2).	Technical problems.		
	(a) Negative pressure prevents flow of fluid.	Ensure that the container is vented using an air inlet.	Vent if necessary, using venting needle.
	(b) Empty container.	Check fluid levels regularly.	Replace the fluid container before it runs dry.
	(c) Venous spasm due to chemical irritation or cold fluids/drugs.	Dilute drugs as recommended. Remove solutions from the refrigerator a short time before use.	Apply a warm compress to soothe and dilate the vein, increase the blood flow and dilute the infusion mixture.
	(d) Injury to the vein.	Detect any injury early as it is likely to progress and cause more serious conditions.	Stop the infusion and resite the cannula.
	(e) Occlusion of the device due to fibrin formation.	Maintain a continuous, regular fluid flow or ensure that patency is maintained by flushing. Instruct the patient to keep arm below the level of the heart if ambulant and attached to a gravity flow infusion.	*If peripheral device:* remove extension set/ injection cap and attempt to flush the cannula gently using a 10 mL syringe of 0.9% sodium chloride. If resistance is met, stop and resite the peripheral device.
			If CVAD: remove injection cap and attempt to flush the cannula gently using a 10 mL syringe of 0.9% sodium chloride. If resistance is met, attempt to instil fibrinolytic agent such as urokinase.
	(f) The cannula has become displaced either completely or partially; that is, fluid or drug has leaked into the surrounding tissues (infiltration). If the drugs were vesicant in nature this would then be defined as extravasation.	Secure the cannula and tape the administration set to prevent pulling and dislodgement. Instruct the patient on the amount of movement permitted with the limb that has the device *in situ* (Fabian 2000).	Confirm that infiltration of drugs has/has not occurred by: (i) inspecting the site for leakage, swelling, and so on (ii) testing the temperature of the skin: it will be cooler if infiltration has occurred (iii) comparing the size of the limb with the opposite limb.

Problem	Cause	Prevention	Action
			Once infiltration has been confirmed, stop the infusion and request a resiting of the device. If the infusion is allowed to progress, discomfort and tissue damage will result. Apply cold or warm compresses to provide symptomatic relief, whichever provides the most comfort for the patient. Reassure the patient by explaining what is happening. Document in care plan and monitor site (Lamb and Dougherty 2008). If extravasation occurs, follow hospital policy and procedure.
Infusion pump alarming.			
(a) Air detected.	Air bubbles in administration set.	Ensure all air is removed from all equipment prior to use.	Remove all air from the administration set and restart the infusion.
(b) Tube misload.	Administration set has been incorrectly loaded.	Ensure set is loaded correctly.	Check that the set is loaded correctly and reload if necessary.
(c) Upstream occlusion.	Closed clamp, obstruction or kink in the administration set is preventing fluid flow.	Ensure the container/fluid bag has been adequately pierced by the administration spike.	Inspect the administration set and restart the infusion.
		Ensure that the tubing is taped to prevent kinking.	If tubing is kinked, reposition, tape and restart infusion.
		Ensure the regulating (roller) clamp is open.	Check the administration set and open the clamp; restart the infusion.
(d) Downstream occlusion.	Phlebitis/infiltration or extravasation.	Observe site regularly for signs of swelling, pain and erythema.	Remove peripheral device, provide symptomatic relief where appropriate. Initiate extravasation procedure. Resite as appropriate.
	Closed distal clamp.	Ensure clamps are open.	Locate distal occlusion, restart infusion.
(e) KVO alert (keep vein open).	The volume infused is complete and the device is infusing at the KVO rate.	Programme in a new volume as appropriate.	Do not turn the device off. Allow KVO mode to run to maintain patency of device. Prepare new infusion or discontinue as appropriate.
Infusion devices malfunctioning (electrical/ mechanical).	Not charging at mains.	Ensure that the device is kept plugged in where appropriate.	Change device and remove device from use until fully charged. Send to clinical engineering to check plug.
	Low battery.	Check lead is pushed in adequately.	
	Batteries keep requiring replacement.	Do not use small rechargeable batteries in ambulatory devices.	
	Technical fault.	Ensure all infusion devices are serviced regularly.	Remove infusion device from use and contact clinical engineering department or relevant personnel.
	Device soiled inside mechanism.	Maintain equipment and keep clean and free from contamination.	Remove administration set, wipe pump, reload. Do not use alcohol-based solutions on internal mechanisms.
Unstable infusion device.	Mounted on old, poorly maintained stands.	Ensure that stands are maintained and kept clean. Replace old stands.	Remove device from stand. Remove stand and send to clinical engineering for repair.
	Mounted on incorrect stands.	Ensure the correct stands are used.	Check the stand and change to appropriate stand.
	Equipment not balanced on stand.	Ensure that all equipment is balanced around the stand.	Remove devices and attach to two stands if necessary. Balance equipment.

POST-PROCEDURAL CONSIDERATIONS

Ongoing care

Monitoring of the infusion while in progress includes monitoring of the patient's condition and response to therapy, the VAD site, the rate and volume infused. It may also include the battery life and occlusion pressure. The frequency of monitoring is often based on the type of therapy and patient condition, for example checking the rate of infusion and the infusion site 15 minutes after setting up infusion, then at 1 hour and then 4 hourly (or more frequently depending on medication). This information must be documented on the patient's fluid balance chart or in their notes. The type and make of pump along with the serial number should also be documented (useful if any errors occur) (MHRA 2008).

COMPLICATIONS

Phlebitis

This is inflammation of the intima of the vein (Perucca 2010, Washington and Barrett 2012). It is characterized by pain and tenderness along the cannulated vein, erythema, warmth and streak formation with/without a palpable cord (Mermel et al. 2001).

There are three main types.

- *Mechanical* is related to irritation and damage to a vein by large-gauge cannulas, sited where there is movement, for example antecubital fossa, not secured adequately or increased dwell time.
- *Chemical* is related to chemical irritation from drugs such as antibiotics and chemotherapy.
- *Bacterial* is when the site becomes infected due to poor hand-washing or aseptic technique (Lamb and Dougherty 2008, Morris 2011).

Influencing factors that increase the risk of phlebitis include being female, dwell time, large-gauge cannulas, higher number of doses of irritating medications such as antibiotics,; factors that reduce risk include choice of vein (forearm), smaller gauge cannulas and use of IV teams (da Silva et al. 2010, Mestre et al. 2013, Wallis et al. 2014, Washington and Barrett 2012). Prevention is key and includes appropriate device and vein selection, dilution of drugs and pharmacological methods, for example application of glyceryl trinitrate (GTN) patches (Dougherty 2008). Treatment includes discontinuing the infusion at the first signs of phlebitis (grade 1). Warm or cold compresses can be applied to the affected site. The patient should be referred to the doctor if the phlebitis rating is over 3. If bacterial phlebitis is suspected then the insertion site should be cultured and the cannula tip sent to microbiology (Dougherty 2008, Morris 2011).

Haematoma

This is leakage of blood into the tissues indicated by rapid swelling which occurs during the insertion procedure or after removal (McCall and Tankersley 2012, Perucca 2010). It can be caused by:

- penetration of the posterior vein wall
- incorrect choice of needle to vein size
- fragile veins
- patients receiving anticoagulant therapy
- excessive or blind probing to locate the vein
- spontaneous rupture of the vessel on application of the tourniquet or cleaning of the skin
- inadequate pressure on venepuncture site following removal of the cannula (Dougherty 2008, McCall and Tankersley 2012, Moini 2013).

Prevention includes good vein and device selection and using a careful technique. The practitioner should always be aware of patients with fragile veins or those on anticoagulant therapy and inexperienced individuals should not attempt cannulation in these individuals (Perucca 2010). A tourniquet should not be applied to a limb where recent venepuncture has occurred and the tourniquet should not be left in place for any longer than necessary.

On removal of the cannula, adequate pressure should be applied to the site. Alcohol pads inhibit clotting and should not be used (Perucca 2010). In the event of a haematoma occurring, the needle should be removed immediately and pressure applied to the site for a few minutes (Garza and Becan McBride 2013, McCall and Tankersley 2013). Elevate the extremity if appropriate and reassure the patient and explain the reason for the bruise. Apply a pressure dressing if required and an ice pack if bruising is extensive (Moini 2013). Hirudoid or arnica ointment can help to reduce bruising and discomfort. Arnica is made of dried roots or flower of the arnica plant which stimulates activity of the white blood cells which process congested blood and reduce the bruise (http://emc.medicines.org.uk/medicine/19031/SPC). Hirudoid is a substance similar to heparin which acts by dissolving blood clots and improving blood supply to the skin (http://emc.medicines.org.uk/medicine/5001/SPC/Hirudoid+Cream/). They are both applied directly to the affected arm (BNF 2014). The incident should be documented and the patient given an information sheet with advice about when and who to contact if the haematoma gets worse or they develop any numbness in the limb (Dougherty 2008, Moini 2013, Morris 2011, Perucca 2010).

Infiltration

DEFINITION

Infiltration tends to refer to the leakage of non-vesicant solutions/medications into the surrounding tissues (INS 2011) and generally does not cause tissue necrosis but can result in long-term injury due to local inflammatory reactions or by compression of the surrounding tissues (if a large volume infiltrates) which is known as compartment syndrome (Doellman et al. 2009, RCN 2010, Schulmeister 2009).

Management of infiltration

Treatment is often dependent upon the severity of the infiltration. There should be ongoing observation and assessment of the infiltrated site. The presence and severity of the infiltration should be documented. Infiltration statistics should include frequency, severity and type of infusate. The infiltration rate should be calculated according to a standard formula (INS 2011, RCN 2010).

Allergic reaction

This is a complication associated with any medication administration but because it happens more rapidly when IV medication is administered, it is often considered as more of an issue.

An allergic reaction is a response to a medication or solution to which the patient is sensitive and may be immediate or delayed (Lamb and Dougherty 2008, Perucca 2010). Clinical features may start with chills and fever, with or without urticaria, erythema and itching. The patient could then go on to experience shortness of breath with or without wheezing, then angioneurotic oedema and in severe cases anaphylactic shock (Lamb and Dougherty 2008). Prevention is by assessment and recording of patient allergies (drug, food and products) and application of allergy identification wristbands (NPSA 2008a, Perucca 2010). In the event of an allergic reaction, the infusion should be stopped immediately, the tubing and container changed and the vein kept patent. The doctor should be notified and any interventions undertaken (Lamb and Dougherty 2008).

Circulatory overload (isotonic fluid expansion)

A critical and common complication of intravenous therapy is circulatory overload, which is *isotonic fluid expansion*. It is caused by infusion of fluids of the same tonicity as plasma into the vascular circulation, for example sodium chloride 0.9%. As isotonic solutions do not affect osmolarity, water does not flow from the extracellular to the intracellular compartment. The result is that the extracellular compartment expands in proportion to the fluid infused (Weinstein and Plumer 2007). Because of the electrolyte concentration, no extra water is available to enable the kidneys selectively to excrete and restore the balance. It can also occur due to:

- infusing excessive amounts of sodium chloride solutions
- large-volume infusions running over multiple days
- rapid fluid infusion into patients with compromised cardiac, liver or renal status (Lamb and Dougherty 2008, Macklin and Chernecky 2004).

Prevention includes thorough assessment of the patient before commencing IV therapy, close monitoring of patient, maintaining infusion rates as prescribed and use of infusion devices where required (Lamb and Dougherty 2008). If circulatory overload is detected early, sit the patient upright (Macklin and Chernecky 2004). Treatment consists of withholding all fluids until excess water and electrolytes have been eliminated by the body and/or administration of diuretics to promote rapid diuresis (Weinstein and Plumer 2007). However, careful monitoring should continue to prevent isotonic contraction occurring (where there is loss of fluid and electrolytes isotonic to the extracellular fluid such as blood and large volumes of fluid from diarrhoea and vomiting; Weinstein and Plumer 2007). If fluid administration is allowed to continue unchecked, it can result in left-sided heart failure, circulatory collapse and cardiac arrest (Dougherty 2002).

DEHYDRATION

Dehydration may be categorized as either hypertonic or hypotonic contraction and may be caused by underinfusion. Hypertonic contraction occurs when water is lost without corresponding loss of salts (Weinstein and Plumer 2007) and occurs in patients unable to take sufficient fluids (elderly, unconscious or incontinent patients) or who have excessive insensible water loss via skin and lungs or as a result of certain drugs in excess. Hypotonic contraction occurs when fluids containing more salt than water are lost and this results in a decrease in osmolarity of the extracellular compartment (Weinstein and Plumer 2007).

It is important that the nurse recognizes the symptoms of overinfusion or underinfusion and certain factors should be considered when monitoring patients (Weinstein and Plumer 2007) (Table 12.12).

Table 12.12 **Monitoring overinfusion and underinfusion**

Type of fluid/ electrolyte imbalance	Patients at risk	Signs and symptoms	Treatment
Circulatory overload (isotonic fluid expansion)	Early post-operative or post-trauma patients, older people, those with impaired renal and cardiac function and children	Weight gain A relative increase in fluid intake compared to output A high bounding pulse pressure, indicating a high cardiac output Raised central venous pressure measurements Peripheral hand vein emptying time longer than normal (peripheral veins will usually empty in 3–5 seconds when the hand is elevated and will fill in the same length of time when the hand is lowered to a dependent position) Peripheral oedema Hoarseness Dyspnoea, cyanosis and coughing due to pulmonary oedema and neck vein engorgement	If detected early: withholding all fluids until excess water and electrolytes have been eliminated by the body and/or administration of diuretics to promote rapid diuresis
Dehydration (hypertonic contraction or hypotonic contraction)	*Hypertonic:* elderly, unconscious or incontinent patients *Hypotonic*: infants are at greatest risk, especially if they have diarrhoea. Loss of salt from various sources: excess diuresis, fistula drainage, burns, vomiting or sweating	*Hyper/hypotonic contraction:* weight loss *Hypercontraction:* thirst (although this may be absent in the elderly) Irritability and restlessness and possible confusion Diminished skin turgor Dry mouth and furred tongue *Hypocontraction:* negative fluid balance Weak, thready, rapid pulse rate Increased 'hand filling time' Increased skin turgor	Replacement of fluids and electrolytes

SPEED SHOCK

Speed shock is a systemic reaction that occurs when a substance foreign to the body is rapidly introduced into the circulation (Perucca 2010, Weinstein and Plumer 2007). This complication can manifest following administration of intravenous bolus injections or when large volumes of fluid are given too rapidly (Perucca 2010). This should not be confused with pulmonary oedema, which relates to the volume of fluid infused into the patient. Rapid, uncontrolled administration of drugs will result in toxic concentrations reaching vital organs (Lamb and Dougherty 2008). Toxicity may be manifested by an exaggeration of the usual pharmacological actions of the drug or by signs and symptoms specific for that drug or class of drugs. The most extreme toxic response which can occur if a drug is given at a dose or rate exceeding that recommended is termed the lethal response.

Signs of speed shock may include:

- flushed face
- headache and dizziness
- congestion of the chest
- tachycardia and fall in blood pressure
- syncope
- shock
- cardiovascular collapse (Perucca 2010, Weinstein and Plumer 2007).

Prevention of speed shock involves the nurse having knowledge of the drug and the recommended rate of administration. When commencing an infusion using gravity flow, check that the solution is flowing freely before adjusting the rate and monitored regularly (Perucca 2010). Movement of the patient or the device within the vessel can cause the infusion to flow more or less freely after a few minutes of setting the rate (Weinstein and Plumer 2007). For high-risk medications an electronic flow control device is recommended (RCN 2010). Although most pumps have an anti-free flow mechanism, always close the roller clamp prior to removing the set from the pump (MHRA 2006a, Pickstone 1999).

If speed shock occurs, the infusion must be slowed down or discontinued. Medical staff should be notified immediately and the patient's condition treated as clinically indicated (Perucca 2010).

Learning Activity 12.8 **Case study: Complications of IV infusions**

Mrs Kyle is a 48-year-old woman who had abdominal surgery yesterday. She has a peripheral cannula *in situ* in her left forearm, through which she is having continuous intravenous fluids, as well as intravenous antibiotics, three times a day. Her observations are stable, but she is complaining of some discomfort around the cannula site.

1 What may be causing this discomfort?
2 In consultation with your supervising nurse, what actions would you suggest taking?

See the end of the chapter for the answers.

Learning for practice

After studying this chapter, list five key points you have learnt about medicines management that you will be able to apply to your clinical practice.

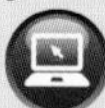
For further learning exercises visit **www.royalmarsdenmanual.com/student**.

Now Test Yourself

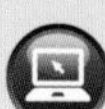
This section provides a range of exercises/activities to further test your learning. For additional exercises visit **www.royalmarsdenmanual.com/student**.

What have you learnt?

1 Pharmacokinetics can be described as:
  A The study of the effects of drugs on the function of living systems
  B The absorption, distribution, metabolism and excretion of drugs within the body: 'what the body does to the drug'
  C The study of the mechanisms of the action of drugs and other biochemical and physiological effects: 'what the drug does to the body'
  D All of the above

2 The Medicines and Healthcare Products Regulatory Agency (MHRA) is responsible for what?
  A Licensing medicinal products
  B Regulating the manufacture, distribution and importation of medicines
  C Regulating which medicines require a prescription and which can be available without a prescription and under what circumstances
  D All of the above

3 Give three examples of 'never events' related to medicines management.

4 Whose responsibility is it to update and document any identified allergies, hypersensitivities, anaphylaxis or drug intolerances?
  A Any members of the nursing team involved in the patient's care
  B Any members of the medical team involved in the patient's care
  C Any members of the pharmacy team involved in the patient's care
  D Any members of the healthcare team involved in the patient's care

5 Who has overall responsibility for the safe and appropriate management of controlled drugs within a clinical area?
A All registered nurses
B The nurse in charge
C The consultant in charge
D The pharmacist

6 Name three warning signs of opioid toxicity.

7 When administering pulmonary medication, how can you make it easier for a patient to use a metered dose inhaler?
A Practise their technique with them beforehand
B Adopt an upright position in the bed or chair
C Use a spacer device
D All of the above

8 When calculating medication doses, if 2 mL of diluent is added to a vial of 100 mg powder, how much volume of medication should you give if a patient requires a dose of 75 mg?
A 0.5 mL
B 1.0 mL
C 1.5 mL
D 2.0 mL

9 Winged infusion devices that are inserted for the administration of subcutaneous infusion of drugs should be inserted at an angle of 45°.
A True
B False

10 Which of the following IS NOT a type of phlebitis associated with peripheral cannulas?
A Mechanical
B Bacterial
C Infiltration
D Chemical

See the end of the chapter for the answers.

Key points

- All registered nurses have a professional responsibility with regard to procurement, prescription supply and disposal of medicines as defined in the NMC *Standards for Medicines Management* (2010a).
- All healthcare professionals involved in the patient's care have a responsibility to update and document any identified allergies, hypersensitivities, anaphylaxis reactions or drug intolerances in the patients' records.
- The nurse in charge of a clinical area is responsible for the safe and appropriate management of controlled drugs within the area.
- Before administering any prescribed drug, the patient's prescription chart should be reviewed and checked to ensure that the medication is being administered to the correct patient, that it is the right drug, dose, date and time of administration, route and method of administration and that the prescription is legible, signed and valid.
- Medications can be administered using a number of different routes. Oral administration is the most convenient route and may result in better compliance (Kelly and Wright 2009).
- Student nurses must never administer/supply medicinal products without direct supervision and both the student and registered nurse must sign the medication chart or document the administration in the notes (NMC 2010b).

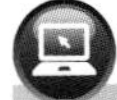

Websites

Institute for Healthcare Improvement
www.ihi.org/explore/adesmedicationreconciliation/Pages/default.aspx

MHRA – How we regulate medicines section
www.mhra.gov.uk
www.yellowcard.gov

REFERENCES

Absalom, A. & Struys, M. (2006) *An Overview of TCI & TIVA.* Ghent, Belgium: Academia Press.

Agius, C.R. (2012) Intelligent infusion technologies: integration of a smart system to enhance patient care. *Journal of Infusion Nursing*, 35(6), 364–368.

Aldridge, M. (2010) Miscellaneous routes of medication administration. In: Jevon, P., Payne, L., Higgins, D. & Endecott, R. (eds) *Medicines Management: A Guide for Nurses.* Hoboken, NJ: John Wiley & Sons, pp.239–261.

Alexander, M., Fawcett, J. & Runciman, P. (2007) *Nursing Practice: Hospital and Home*, 3rd edn. London: Churchill Livingstone.

Amoore, J. & Adamson, L. (2003) Infusion devices: characteristics, limitations and risk management. *Nursing Standard*, 17(28), 45–52.

Amoore, J., Dewar, D., Ingram, P. & Lowe, D. (2001) Syringe pumps and start-up time: ensuring safe practice. *Nursing Standard*, 15(17), 43–45.

Andrew, S. (2006) Pharmacology. In: Marsden, J. (ed.) *Ophthalmic Care.* Chichester: Whurr, pp.42–65.

Antipuesto, D.J. (2010) *Z Track Method.* Nursing Crib. Available at: www.nursingcrib.com

Appelbe, G.E. & Wingfield, J. (2005) *Dale and Appelbe's Pharmacy Law and Ethics*, 8th edn. London: Pharmaceutical Press.

Armitage, G. (2008) Double-checking medicines: defence against error or contributory factor? *Journal of Evaluation in Clinical Practice*, 14(4), 513–517.

Aronson, J.K. (ed.) (2006) *Meyler's Side Effects of Drugs: The International Encyclopedia of Adverse Drug Reactions and Interactions*, 15th edn. Philadelphia: Elsevier Science.

ASHP (1982) ASHP standard definition of a medication error. *American Journal of Hospital Pharmacy*, 3(2), 321.

Audit Commission (2001) *A Spoonful of Sugar: Medicines Management in NHS Hospitals.* London: Audit Commission.

Aulton, M.E. (ed.) (1988) *Pharmaceutics. The Science of Dosage Form Design.* Edinburgh: Churchill Livingstone.

Barker, P., Anderson, A.D. & MacFie, J. (2004) Randomised clinical trial of elective re-siting of intravenous cannulae. *Annals of the Royal College of Surgeons of England*, 86(4), 281–283.

Barton, A., Fuller, R. & Dudley, N. (2004) Using subcutaneous fluids to rehydrate older people: current practices and future challenges. *Quarterly Journal of Medicine*, 97(11), 765–768.

Barua, P. & Bhowmick, B. (2005) Hypodermoclysis: a victim of historical prejudice. *Age and Ageing*, 34(3), 215–217.

Bausone-Gazda, D., Lefaiver, C.A. & Walters, S.A. (2010) A randomized controlled trial to compare the complications of 2 peripheral intravenous catheter-stabilization systems. *Journal of Infusion Nursing*, 33(6), 371–384.

Baxter, K. (ed.) (2008) *Stockley's Drug Interactions*, 8th edn. London: Pharmaceutical Press.

Beijnen, J.H. & Schellens, J.H.M. (2004) Drug interactions in oncology. *Lancet Oncology*, 5, 489–496.

BNF (2014) *British National Formulary 67.* London: Pharmaceutical Press.

Bonsell, L. (2011) *8 Rights of Medication Administration.* Available at: www.nursingcenter.com/Blog/post/2011/05/27/8-rights-of-medication-administration.aspx

Brady, A.M., Malone, A.M. & Fleming, S. (2009) A literature review of the individual and systems factors that contribute to medication errors in nursing practice. *Journal of Nursing Management*, 17(6), 679–697.

Bregenzer, T., Conen, D., Sakmann, P., et al. (1998) Is routine replacement of peripheral intravenous catheters necessary? *Archives of Internal Medicine*, 158(2), 151–156.

Bridge, J., Hemingway, S. & Murphy, K. (2005) Implications of non-medical prescribing of controlled drugs. *Nursing Times*, 101(44), 32–33.

British Pharmacopoeia (2007) *British Pharmacopoeia.* London: Her Majesty's Stationery Office.

Brown, J., Moss, H. & Elliot, T. (1997) The potential for catheter microbial contamination from a needleless connector. *Journal of Hospital Infection*, 36(3), 181–189.

Catney, M.R., Hillis, S., Wakefield, B., et al. (2001) Relationship between peripheral intravenous catheter dwell time and the development of phlebitis and infiltration. *Journal of Infusion Nursing*, 24(5), 332–341.

Chan, H. (2001) Effects of injection duration on site-pain intensity and bruising associated with subcutaneous heparin. *Journal of Advanced Nursing*, 35(6), 882–892.

Chernecky, C., Butler, S.W., Graham, P. & Infortuna, H. (2002) *Drug Calculations and Drug Administration.* Philadelphia: W.B. Saunders.

Chumbley, G. & Mountford, L. (2010) Patient controlled analgesia infusion pumps for adults. *Nursing Standard*, 25(8), 35–40.

Chung, J.W., Ng, W.M. & Wong, T.K. (2002) An experimental study on the use of manual pressure to reduce pain in intramuscular injection. *Journal of Clinical Nursing*, 11, 457–461.

Constans, T., Dutertre, J. & Froge, E. (1991) Hypodermoclysis in dehydrated elderly patients – local effects with and without hyaluronidase. *Journal of Palliative Care*, 7(2), 10–12.

Dann, T.C. (1969) Routine skin preparation before injection: an unnecessary procedure. *Lancet*, ii, 96–97.

Da Silva, G.A., Priebe, S. & Dias, F.N. (2010) Benefits of establishing an intravenous team and the standardisation of peripheral intravenous catheters. *Journal of Infusion Nursing*, 33(3) 156–160.

Danzig, L.E., Short, L., Collins, K., et al. (1995) Bloodstream infections associated with a needleless intravenous infusion system in patients receiving home infusion therapy. *JAMA*, 273(23), 1862–1864.

Dawkins, L., Britton, D., Johnson, I., et al. (2000) A randomised trial of winged Vialon cannulae and metal butterfly needles. *International Journal of Palliative Nursing*, 6(3), 110–116.

Deeks, P. & Byatt, K. (2000) Are patients who self-administer their medicines in hospital more satisfied with their care? *Journal of Advanced Nursing*, 31(2), 395–400.

Dennison, R.D. (2007) A medication safety education program to reduce the risk of harm caused by medication errors. *Journal of Continuing Education in Nursing*, 38(4), 176–184.

Department of Health, Social Services and Public Safety (2006) *Controls Assurance Standards: Medical Devices and Equipment Management.* Available at: www.dhsspsni.gov.uk/medical_device_and_equipment_management_-_version_2008_-_pdf

DH (1989) *Report of the Advisory Group on Nurse Prescribing (Crown One).* London: Her Majesty's Stationery Office.

DH (1998) *Review of Prescribing, Supply and Administration of Medicines. A Report on the Supply and Administration of Medicines under Group Protocols (Crown Two).* London: Her Majesty's Stationery Office.

DH (1999) *Review of Prescribing, Supply and Administration of Medicines. Final Report (Crown Three).* London: Her Majesty's Stationery Office.

DH (2000a) *An Organization with a Memory.* London: Department of Health.

DH (2000b) *Patient Group Directions.* HSC 2000/026. London: Health and Safety Commission.

DH (2003a) *Supplementary Prescribing by Nurses and Pharmacists within the NHS in England: A Guide for Implementation.* London: National Health Service.

DH (2003b) *Building a Safer NHS for Patients: Improving Medication Safety.* London: Department of Health.

DH (2003c) *Winning Ways: Working Together to Reduce Healthcare-Associated Infection in England.* London: Department of Health.

DH (2004) *Extending Independent Nurse Prescribing within the NHS in England: A Guide to Implementation.* London: Department of Health.

DH (2007) *Safer Management of Controlled Drugs. A Guide to Good Practice in Secondary Care (England).* London: Department of Health.

DH (2009) *Changes to Medicines Legislation to Enable Mixing of Medicines Prior to Administration in Clinical Practice.* London: Department of Health. Available at: www.dh.gov.uk

DH (2010) *Clean Safe Care. High Impact Intervention. Central Venous Catheter Care Bundle and Peripheral IV Cannula Care Bundle.* London: Department of Health.

DH (2011) *High Impact Intervention – Central Venous Catheter Care Bundle.* London: Department of Health. Available at: http://webarchive.nationalarchives.gov.uk/20120118164404/hcai.dh.gov.uk/files/2011/03/2011-03-14-HII-Central-Venous-Catheter-Care-Bundle-FINAL.pdf

DH (2012) *The Never Events Policy Framework.* Available at: www.dh.gov.uk/publications

DHSS (1976) *Health Services Development, Addition of Drugs to Intravenous Fluids, HC(76)9 (Breckenridge Report).* London: Her Majesty's Stationery Office.

Dickerson, R.J. (1992) 10 tips for easing the pain of intramuscular injections. *Nursing*, 92, 55.

Dickman, A., Schneider, J. & Varga, J. (2007) *The Syringe Driver: Continuous Subcutaneous Infusions in Palliative Care*, 3rd edn. Oxford: Oxford University Press.

Doellman, D., Hadaway, L., Bowe-Geddes, L.A., et al. (2009) Infiltration and extravasation: update on prevention and management. *Journal of Infusion Nursing*, 32(4), 203–211.

Dougherty, L. (2002) Delivery of intravenous therapy. *Nursing Standard*, 16(16), 45–56.

Dougherty, L. (2008) Obtaining peripheral access. In: Dougherty, L. & Lamb, J. (eds) *Intravenous Therapy in Nursing Practice*, 2nd edn. Oxford: Blackwell Publishing.

Downie, G., MacKenzie, J. & Williams, A. (2003) Medicine management. In: Downie, G., MacKenzie, J. & Williams, A. (eds) *Pharmacology and Medicines Management for Nurses*, 3rd edn. London: Churchill Livingstone, pp.49–91.

Dychter, S.S., Gold, D.A. & Haller, M.F. (2012) Subcutaneous drug delivery: a route to increased safety, patient satisfaction, and reduced costs. *Journal of Infusion Nursing*, 35(3), 154–160.

Elkin, M.K., Perry, A.G. & Potter, P.A. (eds) (2007) *Nursing Interventions and Clinical Skills*, 4th edn. St Louis, MO: Mosby Elsevier.

Elliott, M. & Liu, Y. (2010) The nine rights of medication administration: an overview. *British Journal of Nursing*, 19(5), 300–305.

EU Directive (2010) *Directive 2010/32/EU – Prevention of Sharp Injuries in the Hospital and Healthcare Sector.* Available at: www.osha.europa.eu/en/legislation/directives/sector-specific-and-worker-related-provisions/osh-directives/council-directive-2010-32-eu-prevention-from-sharp-injuries-in-the-hospital-and-healthcare-sector

Fabian, B. (2000) IV complications: infiltration. *Journal of Intravenous Nursing*, 23(4), 229–231.

Fair, R. & Proctor, B. (2007) *Administering Medicines through Enteral Feeding Tubes*, 2nd edn. Belfast, NI: Royal Hospitals.

Federico, F. (2011) *The 5 Rights of Medication Administration.* Available at: www.ismp.org

Fields, M. & Peterson, J. (2005) Intravenous medication safety system averts high risk medication errors and provides actionable data. *Nursing Administration Quarterly*, 29(1) 78–87.

Finlay, T. (2008) Safe administration of IV therapy. In: Dougherty, L. & Lamb, J. (eds) *Intravenous Therapy in Nursing Practice*, 2nd edn. Oxford: Blackwell Publishing.

FIT (Forum for Injection Technique) (2011) *The First Injection Technique Recommendations*, 2nd edn. Available at: www.fit4diabetes.com/

Forrester, J., Dick, A.D., McMenamin, P.G. & Lee, W.R. (2002) *The Eye: Basic Science in Practice*, 2nd edn. Edinburgh: Saunders.

Fox, N. (2000) Armed and dangerous. *Nursing Times*, 96(44), 24–26.

Fraise, A.P. & Bradley, T. (eds) (2009) *Ayliffe's Control of Healthcare-Associated Infection: A Practical Handbook*, 5th edn. London: Hodder Arnold.

Frey, A.M. & Pettit, J. (2010) Infusion therapy in children. In: Alexander, M., Corrigan, A., Gorski, L., Hankins, J. & Perucca, R. (eds) *Infusion Nursing: An Evidence-Based Approach*, 3rd edn. St Louis, MO: Saunders Elsevier, pp.550–568.

Gabriel, J., Bravery, K., Dougherty, L., et al. (2005) Vascular access: indications and implications for patient care. *Nursing Standard*, 19(26), 45–52.

Garza, D. & Becan-McBride, K. (2013) *Phlebotomy Simplified*, 2nd edn. Upper Saddle River, NJ: Pearson Education.

Greenway, K. (2004) Using the ventrogluteal site for intramuscular injection. *Nursing Standard*, 18(25), 39–42.

Griffith, R. & Jordan, S. (2003) Administration of medicines part 1: the law and nursing. *Nursing Standard*, 18(2), 47–53.

Grissinger, M. (2008) Oops, sorry, wrong patient! Applying the Joint Commission's "two-identifier" rule goes beyond the patient's room. *Pharmacy & Therapeutics*, 33(11), 625, 651.

Groll, D., Davies, B., MacDonald, J., et al. (2010) Evaluation of the psychometric properties of the phlebitis and infiltration scales for the assessment of complications of peripheral vascular access devices. *Journal of Infusion Nursing*, 33(6), 385–390.

Gunningberg, L, Pöder, U., Donaldson, N. & Leo Swenne, C. (2014) Medication administration accuracy: using clinical observation and review of patient records to assess safety and guide performance improvement. *Journal of Evaluation in Clinical Practice*, 20(4), 411–416.

Hadaway, L.C. (2010) Anatomy and physiology related to infusion therapy. In: Alexander, M., Corrigan, A., Gorski, L., Hankins, J. & Perucca, R. (eds) *Infusion Nursing: An Evidence-Based Approach*, 3rd edn. St Louis, MO: Saunders Elsevier, pp.139–177.

Harding, A.D. (2011) Use of intravenous smart pumps for patient safety. *Journal of Emergency Nursing*, 37(1), 71–72.

Harding, A.D. (2012) Increasing the use of 'smart' pump drug libraries by nurses: a continuous quality improvement project. *American Journal of Nursing*, 112(1), 26–35.

Hardman, J.G., Limbird, L.E., Molinoff, P.B., et al. (eds) (1996) *Goodman and Gilman's The Pharmacological Basis of Therapeutics*, 9th edn. New York: McGraw-Hill.

Harkin, H. (2008) Guidance document in ear care. Available at: www.earcarecentre.com/HealthProfessionals/Protocols.aspx?id=8

Hart, S. (2008) Infection control in IV therapy. In: Dougherty, L. & Lamb, J. (eds) *Intravenous Therapy in Nursing Practice*, 2nd edn. Oxford: Blackwell Publishing.

Haw, C., Stubbs, J. & Dickens, G. (2007) An observational study of medication administration: errors in old age psychiatric inpatients. *International Journal of Quality in Health Care*, 19(4), 210–216.

Healthcare Commission (2007) *The Best Medicine – The Management of Medicines in Acute and Specialist Trusts*. London: Healthcare Commission.

Health Care Standards Unit (2007a) *First Domain – Safety (Info Bank) C4b*. Available at: www.hcsu.org.uk/index.php?option=com_content&task=view&id=197&Itemid=109

Health Care Standards Unit (2007b) *Updated Signpost C4b*. Available at: www.hcsu.org.uk/index.php?option=com_content&task=view&id=309&Itemid=111

Hertzel, C. & Sousa, V.D. (2009) The use of smart pumps for preventing medication errors. *Journal of Infusion Nursing*, 32(5), 257–267.

Hillery, A., Lloyd, A. & Swarbrick, J. (eds) (2001) *Drug Delivery and Targeting for Pharmacists and Pharmaceutical Scientists*. Boca Raton, FL: CRC Press.

Hilton, S. (1990) An audit of inhaler technique among patients of 34 general practitioners. *British Journal of General Practice*, 40(341), 505–506.

HMSO (1968) *Medicines Act*. London: Her Majesty's Stationery Office.

HMSO (1971) *Misuse of Drugs Act*. London: Her Majesty's Stationery Office.

Ho, C.Y., Dean, B.S. & Barber, N. (1997) When do medication administration errors happen to hospital in-patients? *International Journal of Pharmacy Practice*, 5, 91–96.

Homer, L.D. & Holmes, K.R. (1998) Risks associated with 72- and 96-hour peripheral intravenous catheter dwell times. *Journal of Intravenous Nursing*, 21(5), 301–305.

Huber, C. & Augustine, A. (2009) IV infusion alarms: don't wait for the beep. *American Journal of Nursing*, 109(4), 32–33.

Hunter, J. (2008) Intramuscular injection techniques. *Nursing Standard*, 22(24), 35–40.

Hyde, L. (2008) Legal and professional aspects of IV therapy. In: Dougherty, L. & Lamb, J. (eds) *Intravenous Therapy in Nursing Practice*, 2nd edn. Oxford: Blackwell Publishing.

Hypodermoclysis Working Group (1998) *Hypodermoclysis: Guidelines on the Technique*. Wrexham: CP Pharmaceuticals.

INS (2011) Infusion nursing standards of practice. *Journal of Infusion Nursing*, Supplement 34(15), S1–S110.

Jackson, A. (1998) Infection control – a battle in vein: infusion phlebitis. *Nursing Times*, 94(4), 68, 71.

Jarman, H., Jacobs, E. & Zielinski, V. (2002) Medication study supports registered nurses' competence for single checking. *International Journal of Nursing Practice*, 8, 330–335.

Jenkins, G.W. & Tortora, G.J. (2013) *Anatomy and Physiology: From Science to Life*, 3rd edn. Hoboken, NJ: John Wiley & Sons.

Jevon, P. (2008) Severe allergic reaction: management of anaphylaxis in hospital. *British Journal of Nursing*, 17(2), 104–108.

Jevon, P., Payne, L., Higgins, D. & Endecott, R. (eds) (2010) *Medicines Management: A Guide for Nurses*. Hoboken, NJ: John Wiley & Sons.

Jordan, S., Griffiths, H. & Griffith, R. (2003) Administration of medicines part 2: pharmacology. *Nursing Standard*, 18(3), 45–54.

Kelly, J. & Wright, D. (2009) Administering medication to adult patients with dysphagia. *Nursing Standard*, 23(29), 61–68.

Keohane, C.A., Hayes, J., Saniuk, C., et al. (2005) Intravenous medication safety and smart infusion systems. *Journal of Infusion Nursing*, 28(5), 321–328.

King, L. (2003) Subcutaneous insulin injection technique. *Nursing Standard*, 17(34), 45–52.

Kirkwood, B. (2006) The cornea. In: Marsden, J. (ed.) *Ophthalmic Care*. Chichester: Whurr, pp.339–369.

Koda-Kimble, M.A., Young, L.Y., Kradjan, W.A. & Guglielmo, B.J. (eds) (2005) *Applied Therapeutics: The Clinical Use of Drugs*, 8th edn. Philadelphia: Lippincott Williams & Wilkins.

Koivistov, V.A. & Felig, P. (1978) Is skin preparation necessary before insulin injection? *Lancet*, i, 1072–1073.

Lamb, J. & Dougherty, L. (2008) Local and systemic complications of intravenous therapy. In: Dougherty, L. & Lamb, J. (eds) *Intravenous Therapy in Nursing Practice*, 2nd edn. Oxford: Blackwell Publishing.

Lamblet, L.C.R., Meira, E.S.A., Torres, S., Ferreira, B.C. & Martucchi, S.D. (2011) Randomized clinical trial to assess pain and bruising in medicines administered by means of subcutaneous and intramuscular needle injection: is it necessary to have needles changed? *Revista Latino-Americana de Enfermagem*, 19(5), 1063–1071.

Lapham, R. & Agar, H. (2003) *Drug Calculations for Nurses: A Step-By-Step Approach*, 2nd edn. London: Arnold.

Larson, G.Y., Parker, H., Cash, J., et al. (2005) Standard drug concentrations and smart pump technology reduce continuous medication infusion errors in pediatric patients. *Pediatrics*, 116(1), 21–25.

Latter, S. (2008) Safety and quality in independent prescribing: an evidence review. *Nurse Prescribing*, 6(2), 59–65.

Latter, S., Maben, J., Myall, M., et al. (2005) *An Evaluation of Extended Formulary Independent Nurse Prescribing: Executive Summary of Final Report*. Southampton: University of Southampton.

Latter, S., Blenkinson, A., Smith, A., et al. (2010) *Evaluation of Nurse and Pharmacist Independent Prescribing*. Department of Health Policy Research Programme Project 016 0108. Southampton: University of Southampton.

Laverty, D., Mallett, J. & Mulholland, J. (1997) Protocols and guidelines for managing wounds. *Professional Nurse*, 13(2), 79–80.

Lee, W., Chen, H., Tsai, T., et al. (2009) Risk factors for peripheral intravenous catheter infection in hospitalized patients: a prospective study of 3165 patients. *American Journal of Infection Control*, 37(8), 683–686.

Lenz, C.L. (1983) Make your needle selection right to the point. *Nursing*, 13(2), 50–51.

Lilley, L.L., Collins, S.R. & Snyder, J.S. (2007) *Pharmacology and the Nursing Process*, 5th edn. St Louis, MO: Elsevier Health Sciences.

Longshore, L., Smith, T. & Weist, M. (2010) Successful implementation of intelligent infusion technology in a multihospital setting: nursing perspective. *Journal of Infusion Nursing*, 33(1), 38–47.

Loveday, H., Wilson, J., Pratt, R., et al. (2014) epic3: national evidence-based guidelines for preventing healthcare-associated infections in NHS hospitals in England. *Journal of Hospital Infection*, 86(suppl 1), S1–S70.

Luebke, M.A, Arduino, M., Duda, D., et al. (1998) Comparison of the microbial barrier properties of a needleless and conventional needle based intravenous access system. *American Journal of Infection Control*, 26, 437–441.

Luk, J., Chan, F. & Chu, L. (2008) Is hypodermoclysis suitable for frail Chinese elderly? *Asian Journal of Gerontology and Geriatrics*, 3(1), 49–50.

MacDonald, M. (2010) Patient safety: examining the adequacy of the 5 rights of medication administration. *Clinical Nurse Specialist*, 24(4), 196–201.

Macklin, D. & Chernecky, C.C. (2004) *IV Therapy*. St Louis, MO: Saunders.

Malkin, B. (2008) Are techniques used for intramuscular injection based on research evidence? *Nursing Times*, 104(50/51), 48–51.

Mallett, J., Faithfull, S., Guerrero, D., et al. (1997) Nurse prescribing by protocol. *Nursing Times*, 93(8), 50–52.

Marders, J. (2012) *Sounding the Alarm for IV Infiltration*. Medical Device Safety Communications. Available at: www.fda.gov/medical devices/safety/alertsandnotices/tipsandarticlesondevices

Marieb, E.N. & Hoehn, K. (2007) *Human Anatomy and Physiology*, 7th edn. San Francisco, CA: Pearson Benjamin Cummings.

Marriott, J.L. & Nation, R.L. (2002) Splitting tablets. *Australian Prescriber*, 25(6), 133–135.

McCall, R.E. & Tankersley, C.M. (2012) *Phlebotomy Essentials*, 5th edn. Philadelphia: Lippincott Williams & Wilkins..

McClelland, B. (2007) *Handbook of Transfusion Medicine*, 3rd edn. London: Her Majesty's Stationery Office.

McGoldrick, M. (2010) Infection prevention and control. In: Alexander, M., Corrigan, A., Gorski, L., Hankins, J. & Perucca, R. (eds) *Infusion Nursing: An Evidence-Based Approach*, 3rd edn. St Louis, MO: Saunders Elsevier, pp.204–228.

McHale, J. (2002) Extended prescribing: the legal implications. *Nursing Times*, 98(32), 36–38.

Medicines Partnership Programme (2007) *A Competency Framework For Shared Decision-Making With Patients: Achieving Concordance For Taking Medicines*. Keele: NPC Plus and Medicines Partnership Programme.

Mei, A. & Auerhahn, C. (2009) Hyperdermoclysis maintaining hydration in the frail older adult. *Annals of Long Term Care*, 17(5), 28–30.

Menahem, S. & Shvartzman, P. (2010) Continuous subcutaneous delivery of medications for home care palliative patients – using an infusion set or a pump? *Supportive Care in Cancer*, 18(9), 1165–1170.

Mendelson, M.H., Short, L., Schechter, C., et al. (1998) Study of a needleless intermittent intravenous access system for peripheral infusions: analysis of staff, patient and institutional outcomes. *Infection Control and Hospital Epidemiology*, 19(6), 401–406.

Merck (2014) *Merck Manual for Professionals 2014*, 19th edn. White House Station, NJ: Merck Sharp & Dohme.

Mermel, L.A., Farr, B.M., Sherertz, R.J., et al. (2001) Guidelines for the management of intravascular catheter-related infections. *Journal of Intravenous Nursing*, 24(3), 180–205.

Mestre, G., Berbel, C., Tortajada, P., et al. (2013) Successful multifaceted intervention aimed to reduce short peripheral venous catheter related adverse events. *American Journal of Infection Control*, 41(6), 520–526.

MHRA (2001) *Recommendations on the Control and Monitoring of Storage and Transportation of Medicinal Products*. London: Medicines and Healthcare Products Regulatory Agency.

MHRA (2004) *Reducing Needlestick and Sharps Injuries*. London: Medicines and Healthcare Products Regulatory Agency.

MHRA (2005) *Consultation on Options for the Future of Independent Prescribing by Extended Formulary Nurse Prescribers*. London: Medicines and Healthcare Products Regulatory Agency.

MHRA (2006a) *Free-flow Situations*. Available at: www.mhra.gov.uk/home/idcplg?IdcService=GET_FILE&dID=20057&noSaveAs=0&Rendition=WEB

MHRA (2006b) *Reporting Adverse Incidents and Disseminating Medical Device Alerts*. DB2006(01). Available at: www.mhra.gov.uk/Publications/Safetyguidance/DeviceBulletins/CON2030705

MHRA (2007) *Medical Device Alert /2007/089. Intravenous (IV) Infusion Lines All Brands*. London: Medicines and Healthcare Products Regulatory Agency.

MHRA (2008) *Devices in Practice: A Guide for Professionals in Health and Social Care*. London: Medicines and Healthcare Products Regulatory Agency.

MHRA (2009) *Drug Safety Update: Volume 2, Issue 9*. London: Medicines and Healthcare Products Regulatory Agency.

MHRA (2010a) *Good Pharmacovigilance Practice*. London: Medicines and Healthcare Products Regulatory Agency.

MHRA (2010b) *Device Bulletin Infusion Systems*. DB 2003 (02) v2.0 November. London: Medicines and Healthcare Products Regulatory Agency.

MHRA (2011) *Report on Devices Adverse Incidents in 2010*. DB2011(02). Available at: www.mhra.gov.uk/home/groups/dts-bs/documents/publication/con129234.pdf

MHRA (2014) *Devices in Practice: Checklist for Using Medical Devices*. London: Medicines and Healthcare Products Regulatory Agency.

Mirakian, R., Ewan, P.W., Durham, S.R., et al. (2009) BSACI guidelines for the management of drug allergy. *Clinical and Experimental Allergy*, 39, 43–61.

Mitten, T. (2001) Subcutaneous drug infusions: a review of problems and solutions. *International Journal of Palliative Nursing*, 7(2), 75–85.

Moini, J. (2013) *Phlebotomy: Principles and Practice*. Burlington, MA: Jones & Bartlett Learning.

Moriarty, D. & Hudson, E. (2001) Hypodermoclysis for rehydration in the community. *British Journal of Community Nursing*, 6(9), 437–443.

Morris, W. (2011) Complications. In: Phillips, S., Collins, M. & Dougherty, L. (eds) *Venepuncture and Cannulation*. Oxford: John Wiley & Sons, pp.175–222.

Moureau, N.L. & Iannucci, A.L. (2003) Catheter securement: trends in performance and complications associated with the use of either traditional methods or adhesive anchor devices. *Journal of Vascular Access Devices*, 8(1), 29–33.

Murray, W. & Glenister, H. (2001) How to use medical devices safely. *Nursing Times*, 97(43), 36–38.

NHSCLU (2009) Available at: www.corelearningunit.nhs.uk

NHS (2009) *Connecting for Health: Electronic Prescribing in Hospitals: Challenges and Lessons Learned*. Available at: www.connectingforhealth.nhs.uk/systemsandservices/eprescribing/challenges/Final_report.pdf

NHS Employers (2007) *The Management of Health, Safety and Welfare Issues for NHS Staff*. London: NHS Confederation (Employers).

NHS Litigation Authority (2013) *NHSLA Risk Management Standards for Acute Trusts*. Available at: www.nhsla.com/Safety/Documents/NHS LA Risk Management Standards 2013-14.doc

NICE (2003) *Technology Appraisal Guidance No 57. Guidance on the Use of Continuous Subcutaneous Insulin Infusion for Diabetes*. London: National Institute for Health and Clinical Excellence.

NICE (2009) *Medicines Adherence: Involving Patients in Decisions about Prescribed Medicines and Supporting Adherence*. Available at: www.nice.org.uk/guidance/CG76

NICE (2010) *Chronic Obstructive Pulmonary Disease: Management of Chronic Obstructive Pulmonary Disease in Adults in Primary and Secondary Care (Partial Update)*. CG101. Available at: www.nice.org.uk/guidance/CG101

NICE (2014a) *Competency Framework: For People Developing and/or Reviewing and Updating Patient Group Directions*. Manchester: National Institute for Health and Care Excellence.

NICE (2014b) *Drug allergy: diagnosis and management of drug allergy in adults, children and young people. CG 183*. London: National Institute for Health and Care Excellence.

NICE/NPSA (2007) *Patient Safety Guidance 001. Technical Patient Safety Solutions for Medicines Reconciliation on Admission of Adults to Hospital*. London: National Patient Safety Agency.

Nichols, C. & O'Brien, E. (2012) Ear irrigation. In: O'Brien, L. (ed.) *District Nursing Manual of Clinical Procedures*. Oxford: John Wiley & Sons, pp.84–92.

Nisbet, A. (2006) Intramuscular gluteal injections in the increasingly obese population: retrospective study. *BMJ*, 332, 637–638.

NMC (2001a) *UKCC Position Statement on the Covert Administration of Medicines – Disguising Medicine in Food and Drink*. London: Nursing and Midwifery Council.

NMC (2001b) *Circular 25/2002*. London: Nursing and Midwifery Council.

NMC (2006) *Standards of Proficiency for Nurse and Midwife Prescribers*. London: Nursing and Midwifery Council.

NMC (2010a) *Standards for Medicines Management*. London: Nursing and Midwifery Council.

NMC (2010b) *Record Keeping: Guidance for Nurses and Midwives*. London: Nursing and Midwifery Council.

NMC (2013) *Consent*. London: Nursing and Midwifery Council. Available at: www.nmc-uk.org/Nurses-and-midwives/Advice-by-topic/A/Advice/Consent/

NMC (2015) *The Code: Standards of Conduct, Performance and Ethics for Nurses and Midwives*. London: Nursing and Midwifery Council.

NPC (2001) *Maintaining Competency in Prescribing: An Outline Framework to Help Nurse Prescribers*. London: National Health Service.

NPC (2003a) *Supplementary Prescribing. A Resource to Help Healthcare Professionals to Understand the Framework and Opportunities*. London: National Health Service.

NPC (2003b) *Maintaining Competency in Prescribing: An Outline Framework to Help Nurse Supplementary Prescribers*. London: National Health Service.

NPC (2007a) *Self Administration of Medicines: 5-Minute Guide Series*. Keele: National Prescribing Centre. Available at: www.npc.nhs.uk/patients_medicines/self_admin/resources/5mg_sam.pdf

NPC (2007b) *Medicines Reconciliation: A Guide To Implentation*. Keele: National Prescribing Centre. Available at: www.npc.nhs.uk/improving_safety/medicines_reconciliation/resources/reconciliation_guide.pdf

NPC (2009) *Patient Group Directions: A Practical Guide and Framework of Competencies for All Professionals Using Patient Group Directions*.

London: National Prescribing Centre. Available at: http://www.npc.nhs.uk/non_medical/resources/patient_group_directions.pdf

NPSA (2003) *Risk Analysis of Infusion Devices.* London: National Patient Safety Agency.

NPSA (2004) *Safer Practice Notice 01: Infusion Devices.* London: National Patient Safety Agency. Available at: www.npsa.nhs.uk/Patientsafety/alerts-and-directives/notices/infusion-device

NPSA (2005) *Wristbands for Hospital Inpatients Improve Safety (Safer Practice Notice 11).* London: National Patient Safety Agency.

NPSA (2006) *Ensuring Safer Practice with High Dose Ampoules of Morphine and Diamorphine. Alert No. 2006/12.* London: National Patient Safety Agency.

NPSA (2007a) *Safety in Doses: Medication Safety Incidents in the NHS, PSO/4.* London: National Patient Safety Agency.

NPSA (2007b) *Standardising Wristbands Improves Patient Safety.* Safer Practice Notice 0507. London: National Patient Safety Agency.

NPSA (2007c) *Patient Safety Alert 19. Promoting Safer Measurement and Administration of Liquid Medicines via Oral and other Enteral Routes.* London: National Patient Safety Agency.

NPSA (2007d) *Promoting Safer Use of Injectable Medicines. Alert No. 2007/20.* London: National Patient Safety Agency. Available at: www.npsa.nhs.uk/Patientsafety/alerts-and-directives/alerts/injectable-medicines

NPSA (2008a) *Rapid Response Report 05: Reducing Dosing Errors with Opioid Medicines.* London: National Patient Safety Agency.

NPSA (2008b) *Rapid Response Report 11: Reducing Risk of Overdose with Midazolam Injection in Adults.* London: National Patient Safety Agency.

NPSA (2009) *Safety in Doses. Improving the Use of Medicines in the NHS.* London: National Patient Safety Agency.

NPSA (2010) *New Insulin Safety Guidance Issued to Reduce Wrong Dosages.* Available at: http://npsa.nhs.uk/corporate/news/the-national-patient-safety-agency-npsa-has-today-issued-guidance-for-all-nhs-organisations-across-england-and-wales-aimed-at-re/

Ostendorf, W. (2012) Preparation for safe medication administration. In: Perry, A.G., Potter, P.A. & Elkin, M.K. (eds) *Nursing Interventions & Clinical Skills*, 5th edn. St Louis, MO: Elsevier, pp.486–583.

Palese, A., Cassone, A., Kulla, A., et al. (2011) Factors influencing nurses' decision-making process on leaving in the peripheral intravascular catheter after 96 hours: a longitudinal study. *Journal of Infusion Nursing*, 34(5), 319–326.

Peragallo-Dittko, V. (1997) Rethinking subcutaneous injection technique. *American Journal of Nursing*, 97(5), 71–72.

Perry, A.G. (2007) Administration of injections. In: Elkin, M.K., Perry, A.G. & Potter, P.A. (eds) *Nursing Interventions and Clinical Skills*, 4th edn. St Louis, MO: Mosby Elsevier, pp.416–446.

Perucca, R. (2010) Peripheral venous access devices. In: Alexander, M., Corrigan, A., Gorski, L., Hankins, J. & Perucca, R. (eds) *Infusion Nursing: An Evidence-Based Approach*, 3rd edn. St Louis, MO: Saunders Elsevier, pp.456–479.

Pickstone, M. (1999) *A Pocketbook for Safer IV Therapy.* Medical Technology and Risk Series. Broadstairs, Kent: Scitech Educational Ltd.

Pickstone, M. (2000) Using the technology triangle to assess the safety of technology-controlled clinical procedures in critical care. *International Journal of Intensive Care*, 7(2), 90–96.

Polovich, M., Whitford, J.M. & Olsen, M. (eds) (2014) *Chemotherapy and Biotherapy Guidelines and Recommendations for Practice*, 4th edn. Pittsburgh, PA: Oncology Nursing Society.

Pope, B.B. (2002) How to administer subcutaneous and intramuscular injection. *Nursing*, 32(1), 50–51.

Potter, P.A. (2011) Administration of nonparenteral medications. In: Perry, A.G., Potter, P.A. & Elkin, M.K. (eds) *Nursing Interventions & Clinical Skills*, 5th edn. St Louis, MO: Elsevier, pp.501–540.

Quinn, C. (2000) Infusion devices: risks, functions and management. *Nursing Standard*, 14(26), 35–41.

Quinn, C. (2008) Intravenous flow control and infusion devices. In: Dougherty, L. & Lamb, J. (eds) *Intravenous Therapy in Nursing Practice*, 2nd edn. Oxford: Blackwell Publishing, pp.197–224.

Rang, H.P & Dale, M.M. (2012) *Pharmacology*, 7th edn. Edinburgh: Elsevier Churchill Livingstone.

Rawlins, M.D. & Thompson, J.W. (1977) Pathogenesis of adverse drug reactions. In: Davies, D.M. (ed.) *Textbook of Adverse Drug Reactions.* Oxford: Oxford University Press.

Ray-Barruel, G., Polit, D., Murfield, J. & Rickard, C. (2013) Infusion phlebitis assessment scales: a systematic review of their use and psychometric adequacy. *Journal of the Association for Vascular Access*, 18(4), 217.

RCN (2010) *Standards for Infusion Therapy*, 3rd edn. London: Royal College of Nursing.

Reckmann, M.H., Westbrook, J.I., Koh, Y., Lo, C. & Day, R.O. (2009) Does computerised provider order entry reduce prescribing errors for hospital inpatients? A systematic review. *JAMA*, 10, 1197.

Regnard, C. & Hockley, J. (2004) *A Guide to Symptom Relief in Palliative Care*, 5th edn. Oxford: Radcliffe Medical Press.

Reid, A. (2012) Changing practice for safe insulin administration. *Nursing Times*, 108(10), 22–26.

Relihan, E., O'Brien, V., O'Hara, S. & Silke, B. (2010) The impact of a set of interventions to reduce interruptions and distractions to nurses during medication administration. *Quality and Safety in Health Care*, 19, e52.

Riedl, M.A. & Casillas, A.M. (2003) Adverse drug reactions: types and treatment options. *American Family Physician*, 68, 1781–1790.

Rickard, C.M., Webster, J., Wallis, M.C., et al. (2012) Routine versus clinically indicated replacement of peripheral intravenous catheters: a randomised controlled equivalence trial. *Lancet*, 380(9847), 1066–1074.

Ripamonti, C. & Bruera, E. (1997) Current status of patient controlled analgesia in cancer patients. *Oncology*, 11(3), 373–380.

Rodger, M.A. & King, L. (2000) Drawing up and administering intramuscular injection: a review of the literature. *Journal of Advanced Nursing*, 31(3), 574–582.

Rosenthal, M.M. (2003) *Check the Wristband.* Available at: http://webmm.ahrq.gov/case.aspx?caseID=22

Rothschild, J.M., Keohane, C.A., Cook, E.F., et al. (2005) A controlled trial of smart infusion pumps to improve medication safety in critically ill patients. *Critical Care Medicine*, 33, 533–540.

RPSGB (2005) *The Safe and Secure Handling of Medicines. A Team Approach.* London: Royal Pharmaceutical Society of Great Britain.

RPSGB (2007a) *Developing and Implementing Standard Operating Procedures for Dispensing.* London: Royal Pharmaceutical Society of Great Britain.

RPSGB (2007b) *Legal and Advisory Service Fact Sheet Six. Monitored Dosage Systems and Compliance Aids.* London: Royal Pharmaceutical Society of Great Britain.

RPSGB (2012) *Medicines, Ethics and Practice. The Professional Guide for Pharmacists*, 36th edn. London: Royal Pharmaceutical Society of Great Britain.

Sasson, M. & Shvartzman, P. (2001) Hypodermoclysis: an alternative infusion technique. *American Family Physician*, 64(9), 1575–1578.

Savage, P. & Tripp, K. (2008) *A Study of Independent Double-Checking Processes for Chemotherapy Administration via an Ambulatory Infusion Pump.* 15th International Conference on Cancer Nursing, Singapore 17–21 August 2008. Abstract Q116.

Scales, K. (2008) Anatomy and physiology related to intravenous therapy. In: Dougherty, L. & Lamb, J. (eds) *Intravenous Therapy in Nursing Practice*, 2nd edn. Oxford: Blackwell Publishing, pp.23–48.

Scales, K. (2011) Use of hypodermoclysis to manage dehydration. *Nursing Older People*, 23(5), 16–22.

Schulmeister, L. (2008) Patient misidentification. *Clinical Journal of Oncology Nursing*, 12(3), 495–498.

Schulmeister, L. (2009) Antineoplastic therapy. In: Alexander, M. et al. (eds) *Infusion Nursing An Evidence Based Approach.* St Louis, MO: Saunders Elsevier, pp.351–371.

Shelton, B.K. & Shivnan, J. (2011) *Acute Hypersensitivity Reactions: What Nurses Need to Know.* Available at: http://magazine.nursing.jhu.edu/2011/04/acute-hypersensitivity-reactions-what-nurses-need-to-know/

Shepherd, M. (2002a) Medicines 2. Administration of medicines. *Nursing Times*, 98(16), 45–48.

Shepherd, M. (2002b) Medicines 3. Managing medicines. *Nursing Times*, 98(17), 43–46.

Shuttleworth, A. (2005) Are nurses ready to take on the BNF? *Nursing Times*, 101(48), 29–30.

Smyth, J. (ed.) (2006) *The NEWT Guidelines for Administration of Medication to Patients with Enteral Feeding Tubes and Swallowing Difficulties.* Wrexham: North East Wales NHS Trust.

Springhouse (2005) *Intravenous Therapy Made Incredibly Easy*, 3rd edn. Philadelphia: Lippincott, Williams & Wilkins.

Stanley, A. (2002) Managing complications of chemotherapy administration. In: Allwood, M., Stanley, A. & Wright, P. (eds) *The Cytotoxics Handbook*, 4th edn. Oxford: Radcliffe Medical Press, pp.119–192.

Stollery, R., Shaw, M. & Lee, A. (2005) *Ophthalmic Nursing*, 3rd edn. Oxford: Blackwell Publishing.

Take 5 (2006) *Z Track Injections.* Nursing 2006. Available at: http://www.nursingcenter.com/upload/static/592775/Take5_Ztrack.pdf

Taxis, K., Dean, B. & Barber, N. (1999) Hospital drug distribution systems in the UK and Germany: a study of medication errors. *Pharmacy World and Science*, 21(1), 25–31.

The Misuse of Drugs and Misuse of Drugs (Safe Custody) (Amendment) (England, Wales and Scotland) Regulations (2014). *Statutory Instrument No.1275.* London: Her Majesty's Stationery Office.

Thomas, J.R., Wallace, M., Yocum, R., et al. (2009) The INFUSE morphine study: use of recombinant human hyaluronidase (rHuPH20) to enhance the absorption of subcutaneously administered morphine in patients with advanced illness. *Journal of Pain and Symptom Management*, 38, 663–672.

Torrance, C. (1989) Intramuscular injection, part 1 and 2. *Surgical Nurse*, 2(5), 6–10; 2(6), 24–27.

Torre, M. (2002) Subcutaneous infusion: non-metal cannulae vs metal butterfly needles. *British Journal of Community Nursing*, 7(7), 365–369.

Tortora, G.J. & Derrickson, B. (2011) *Principles of Anatomy and Physiology*, 13th edn. Hoboken, NJ: John Wiley & Sons.

Treloar, A., Beats, B. & Philpot, M. (2000) A pill in the sandwich: covert medication in food and drink. *Journal of the Royal Society of Medicine*, 93, 408–411.

Trounce, J. & Gould, D. (2000) *Clinical Pharmacology for Nurses*, 16th edn. London: Churchill Livingstone.

Turner, M.S. & Hankins, J. (2010) Pharmacology. In: Alexander, M., Corrigan, A., Gorski, L., Hankins, J. & Perucca, R. (eds) *Infusion Nursing: An Evidence-Based Approach*, 3rd edn. St Louis, MO: Saunders Elsevier.

Twycross, R., Wilcock, A., Dean, M. and Kennedy, B. (2007) *Palliative Care Formulary*, 3rd edn. Available at: www.palliativedrugs.com

Van Donk, P., Rickard, C., McGrail, M. & Doolan, G. (2009) Routine replacement versus clinical monitoring of peripheral intravenous catheters in a regional hospital in the home program: a randomized controlled trial. *Infection Control and Hospital Epidemiology*, 30(9) 915–917.

Walker, R. & Edwards, C. (2003) *Clinical Pharmacy and Therapeutics*, 3rd edn. London: Churchill Livingstone.

Wallis, M., McGrail, M., Webster, J., et al. (2014) Risk factors for peripheral intravenous catheter failure: a multivariate analysis of data from a randomized controlled trial. *Infection Control and Hospital Epidemiology*, 35(1), 63–8.

Walsh, G. (2005) Hypodermoclysis: an alternate method for rehydration in long-term care. *Journal of Infusion Nursing*, 28(2), 123–129.

Washington, G.T. & Barrett, R. (2012) Peripheral phlebitis: a point-prevalence study. *Journal of Infusion Nursing*, 35(4), 252–258.

Watt, S. (2003) Safe administration of medicines to children: part 2. *Paediatric Nurse*, 15(5), 40–44.

Webster, J., Clarke, S., Paterson, D., et al. (2008) Routine care of peripheral intravenous catheters versus clinically indicated replacement: randomised controlled trial. *BMJ*, 337(7662), 157–160.

Weeks, K.W., Lyne, P. & Torrance, C. (2000) Written drug dosage errors made by students: the threat to clinical effectiveness and the need for a new approach. *Clinical Effectiveness in Nursing*, 4, 20–29.

Weeks, K.W., Lyne, P., Mosely, L. & Torrance, C. (2001) The strive for clinical effectiveness in medication dosage calculation problem solving skills: the role of constructivist learning theory in the design of a computer-based 'authentic world' learning environment. *Clinical Effectiveness in Nursing*, 5, 18–25.

Weinstein, S. & Plumer, A. (2007) *Plumer's Principles and Practices of Intravenous Therapy*, 8th edn. Philadelphia: Lippincott, Williams & Wilkins.

Westbrook, J., Woods, A., Rob, M., Dunsmuir, W. & Day, R. (2010) Association of interruptions with an increased risk of severity of medication administration errors. *Archives of Internal Medicine*, 170(8), 683–690.

Westbrook, J., Rob, M., Woods, A. & Parry, D. (2011) Errors in the administration of intravenous medications and the role of correct procedures and nurse experience. *BMJ Quality and Safety*, 20, 1027–1034.

Whittington, Z. (2008) Pharmacological aspects of IV therapy. In: Dougherty, L. & Lamb, J. (eds) *Intravenous Therapy in Nursing Practice*, 2nd edn. Oxford: Blackwell Publishing.

WHO (2004) *Immunization in Practice. Module 6: Holding an Immunization Session.* Geneva: World Health Organization.

WHO (2008) *Medicines: Safety of Medicines – Adverse Drug Reactions. Factsheet No.293.* Available at: www.medicines.org.uk/EMC/medicine/21309/SPC/Kentura+oxybutynin+transdermmal+patch

Wilkes, G. & Barton Burke, M. (2011) *Oncology Nursing Drug Handbook.* Sudbury, MA: Jones & Bartlett.

Wilson, K. & Sullivan, M. (2004) Preventing medication errors with smart infusion technology. *American Journal of Health System Pharmacists*, 61(2), 177–183.

Workman, B. (1999) Safe injection techniques. *Nursing Standard*, 13(39), 47–52.

Wright, K. (2010) Do calculation errors by nurses cause medication errors in clinical practice? A literature review. *Nurse Education Today*, 30(1), 85–97.

Answers

Learning Activity 12.1 Scenario: Verbal orders

You have been asked to ring the doctor on-call, as one of your patients, who has just been admitted to the ward, is complaining of pain and there is currently no analgesia prescribed on their medication chart. The doctor asks you if you can give the patient some paracetamol and he will come down shortly to prescribe it. What would you do? Discuss this scenario with your mentor/supervising nurse.

- The guidance from the NMC (2010a) (see the section on 'Verbal orders' earlier in this chapter) advises that a verbal order is not acceptable on its own, particularly where a medication has not been previously prescribed, as is the case in this scenario.

Learning Activity 12.3 Scenario: Allergy status

You have been looking after a female patient who has had an allergic reaction to her antibiotics, in the form of a raised, itchy, skin rash.

1 What actions should be taken to ensure that such a reaction is avoided in the future?
   - The medication that caused the allergy is removed from her medication prescription chart and the allergy information is recorded clearly in the patient's medical records, including paper and electronic records.
   - The patient is given information regarding what substance she should avoid.
   - While an inpatient, she should have her allergy indicated by wearing a red-coloured identity band (NPSA 2007b).
   - The allergic drug reaction should also be reported using the Yellow Card Scheme (Mirakian et al. 2009).
   - Prior to administering any medication, the nurse must confirm the patient's allergy status and where necessary document any changes.

Learning Activity 12.5 Scenario: Drug administration

You have been asked to give some oral medication to a patient you are looking after.

What should you check before administering the medication?

- Correct patient
- Correct drug, dose, date and time
- Correct route and method of administration
- Correct diluent (if appropriate)
- Validity and legibility of prescription
- Signature of prescriber

Learning Activity 12.7 Scenario: Calculating flow rate

One of the patients you are looking after has an intravenous infusion of fluids (sodium chloride 0.9%), which is being administered using a gravity solution set. Your supervising nurse has just put up a new 1 L bag of fluids which needs to infuse over 8 hours and you have been asked to calculate the flow rate based on the principle that crystalloid fluids administered via a solution set is delivered at the rate of 20 drops/mL.

1 What should the flow rate be?

$$\frac{1000 \times 20}{8 \times 60} = 42 \text{ drops/minute}$$

2 What else should you consider to help ensure the accuracy of the flow rate?

- Type of fluid
- Height of the infusion container
- Administration set/roller clamps
- Vascular access devices
- Advising the patient not to interfere with the infusion device

Learning Activity 12.8 Case study: Complications of IV infusions

Mrs Kyle is a 48-year-old woman who had abdominal surgery yesterday. She has a peripheral cannula *in situ* in her left forearm, through which she is having continuous intravenous fluids, as well as intravenous antibiotics, three times a day. Her observations are stable, but she is complaining of some discomfort around the cannula site.

1 What may be causing this discomfort?

- Phlebitis, infiltration

2 In consultation with your supervising nurse, what actions would you suggest taking?

- Ensure the fluid is being administered at the correct rate.
- Ongoing assessment of the site: document any swelling, pain, erythema, warmth around the site or up the length of the vein.
- Use of a scale, e.g. VIP.
- Ensure all fluid being administered is accurately documented on the fluid prescription and balance chart.

Now Test Yourself What have you learnt?

1 Pharmacokinetics can be described as:
A The study of the effects of drugs on the function of living systems
B The absorption, distribution, metabolism and excretion of drugs within the body: 'what the body does to the drug'
C The study of the mechanisms of the action of drugs and other biochemical and physiological effects: 'what the drug does to the body'
D All of the above

2 The Medicines and Healthcare Products Regulatory Agency (MHRA) is responsible for what?
A Licensing medicinal products
B Regulating the manufacture, distribution and importation of medicines
C Regulating which medicines require a prescription and which can be available without a prescription and under what circumstances
D All of the above

3 Give three examples of 'never events' related to medicines management.
Never events are largely preventable patient safety incidents that should not occur if the available preventative measures have been implemented by healthcare providers (DH 2011, p.4). Examples include: wrongly prepared high-risk injectable medications, maladministration of a potassium-containing solution, air embolism, misidentification of patients, maladministration of insulin.

4 Whose responsibility is it to update and document any identified allergies, hypersensitivities, anaphylaxis or drug intolerances?
A Any members of the nursing team involved in the patient's care
B Any members of the medical team involved in the patient's care
C Any members of the pharmacy team involved in the patient's care
D Any members of the healthcare team involved in the patient's care

5 Who has overall responsibility for the safe and appropriate management of controlled drugs within a clinical area?
A All registered nurses
B The nurse in charge
C The consultant in charge
D The pharmacist

6 Name three warning signs of opioid toxicity.
Warning signs may include: pin-point pupils, confusion, hallucinations, respiratory depression, myoclonus.

7 When administering pulmonary medication, how can you make it easier for a patient to use a metered dose inhaler?
A Practise their technique with them beforehand
B Adopt an upright position in the bed or chair
C Use a spacer device
D All of the above

8 When calculating medication doses, if 2 mL of diluent is added to a vial of 100 mg powder, how much volume of medication should you give if a patient requires a dose of 75 mg?
A 0.5 mL
B 1.0 mL
C 1.5 mL
D 2.0 mL

9 Winged infusion devices that are inserted for the administration of subcutaneous infusion of drugs should be inserted at an angle of 45°.
A True
B False

10 Which of the following IS NOT a type of phlebitis associated with peripheral cannulas?
A Mechanical
B Bacterial
C Infiltration
D Chemical

Perioperative care

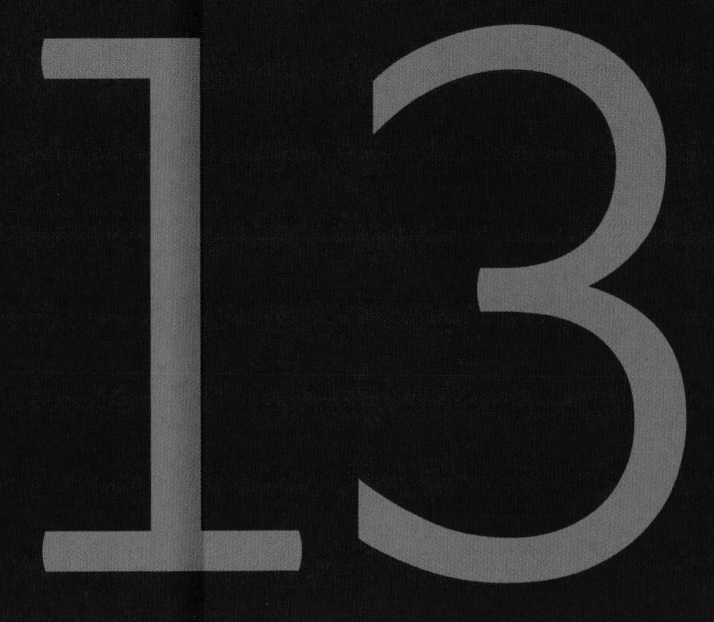

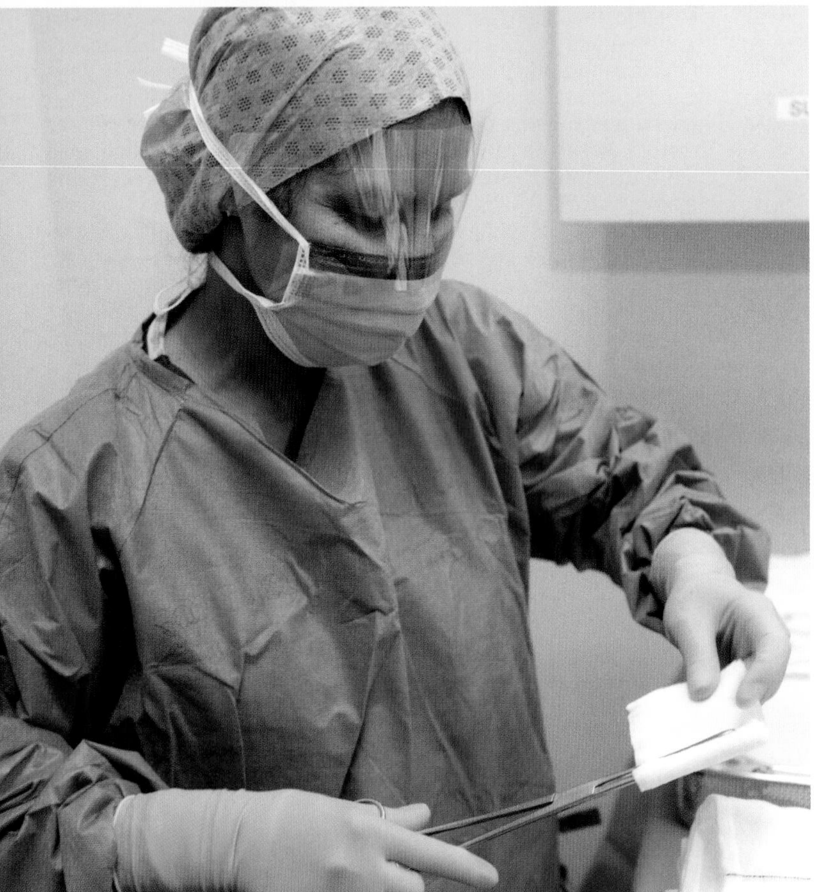

By reading this chapter and undertaking the learning activities within it, you should be able to:

1. Demonstrate an understanding of the pre-assessment phase in order to ensure patients are physically and mentally able to undergo a surgical procedure.
2. Identify the care required in the immediate pre-operative phase to ensure the patient is correctly prepared for their procedure.
3. Gain insight into the phases of intraoperative care, including induction of anaesthesia, surgery and recovery of the patient.
4. Demonstrate an understanding of the variety and complexity of post-operative care both before and after discharge from hospital.

Procedure guidelines

The Royal Marsden Manual of Clinical Nursing Procedures: Student Edition, Ninth Edition. Edited by Lisa Dougherty, Sara Lister and Alexandra West-Oram

Overview

Care of the patient undergoing any surgical procedure begins pre-operatively. The patient is pre-assessed and any appropriate investigations are undertaken to ensure they are physically able to undergo the surgery and be mentally prepared for the process. The care continues in the immediate pre-operative phase to ensure the patient is prepared adequately for the surgical procedure and to mitigate associated risks. Intraoperative care usually comprises three phases: induction of anaesthesia, surgery and recovery of the patient within the post-anaesthetic care unit (PACU). As care within surgery is delivered by a multidisciplinary team, a thorough handover of the patient is essential at every stage. The care continues beyond the intraoperative phase when the patient receives post-operative care both before and after discharge from hospital. The amount and complexity of post-operative care required will vary significantly according to the nature of the surgery (minor, major, laparoscopic, robotic, etc.) and the physical, mental and social status of the patient.

This chapter relates to the care provided to the patient in all three stages of surgery:

- pre-operative care
- intraoperative care
- post-operative care.

Pre-operative care

DEFINITION

Pre-operative care is the physical and psychosocial care provided to the patient to help them prepare to safely undergo surgery. Psychosocial preparation includes assessing and managing stress, patient education and informed consent, whilst physical preparation is concerned with the prevention of peri- and post-operative complications (Liddle 2012, Scott et al. 2007).

RELATED THEORY

Optimal pre-operative care is underpinned by thorough assessment and planning. The assessment aims to reduce cancellations on the day of surgery, rationalize the amount of investigations and tests required pre-operatively (so ensuring there are no unnecessary costs) and reduce patient anxiety whilst improving post-operative outcomes for patients (Pritchard 2012). This is ensured by properly managing and optimizing any co-morbidities pre-operatively that may affect the perioperative care of the patient. Because general anaesthesia is considered a risk to the patient, it is necessary to 'consider the patient's health and quality of life and to question whether the proposed benefits of surgery outweigh the attendant risks' (Avidan 2003).

Traditionally, patients were admitted to hospital 1–2 days pre-operatively to allow for the appropriate assessment, tests and investigations to be completed prior to their surgery. Once they were admitted, it was frequently found that patients were presenting with complicated, newly identified or inappropriately managed co-morbidities so surgery was often delayed or cancelled. It was also found that a large number of cancelled operations occurred because patients did not arrive for their scheduled operation fasted. Some did not arrive because the date provided was inconvenient (due to childcare or work-related concerns) or the surgery was no longer wanted or needed. Pre-operative assessment clinics were established to address these issues. It has been found that providing patients with a time and place to explore their concerns and gain the information they need has increased the attendance of patients and therefore made more effective use of operating theatre time and other associated resources (NHS Modernization Agency 2005).

Pre-operative assessment (POA) and planning carried out prior to treatment is an essential part of the planned surgical care pathway (NHSIP 2008). POA and planning should take into account the physiological, psychological and social needs of the patient undergoing surgery with the aim of optimizing patient safety at all times and minimizing intra-/post-operative complications. Depending on the complexity of the surgery, POA can be undertaken during face-to-face or telephone clinics, which are increasingly nurse led.

EVIDENCE-BASED APPROACHES

Principles of care

Pre-operative assessment should include a comprehensive history taking, physical examination and the ordering of appropriate investigations.

Pre-operative history taking includes the following.

Medical history

Medical history should start with the history of the presenting illness. For the pre-operative assessment, this starts with the reason why the patient is having the planned procedure. It is important to include how the patient first presented with the symptoms of the condition, and any treatments provided. Details of treatments such as previous chemotherapy or radiotherapy are important to obtain within the health history. A full history of current and previous medical problems should be taken. This would include any history of disorders such as diabetes mellitus, hypertension, asthma, epilepsy, strokes or cardiac symptoms such as chest pains or shortness of breath. It is valuable to obtain information such as dates of diagnosis, severity, ongoing treatments and any history of hospitalizations for the disorders. By obtaining a reliable and clear record of the patient's medical history, the foundations for creating a plan of care are laid. 'This ensures the patient's surgical journey is effective, reducing the risk of suboptimal management and increasing safety with the least possible distress for the patient and their significant others' (Walsgrove 2011).

Family history

Asking the patient about common familial illnesses, such as hypertension, coronary artery disease, stroke, diabetes and hypercholesterolaemia, will alert the anaesthetist to any potential medical problems.

Body system review

It is essential to assess each of the following body systems in more detail as this contributes to the information about the patient's overall health status.

CARDIOVASCULAR SYSTEM

- Cardiac function.
- History of cardiovascular disease such as ischaemia, anaemias and clotting disorders.
- Blood pressure.
- Patient's risk of thrombosis, excessive bleeding. If the patient has a history of thrombosis or is undergoing surgery where this presents a significant risk, they may require anticoagulation pre-operatively.

RESPIRATORY SYSTEM

- History of respiratory disease such as asthma, chronic obstructive airway disease.
- Respiratory infections.

GASTROINTESTINAL SYSTEM

- Digestive history.
- Nutritional and BMI status.
- Hepatic functioning.
- Renal function including urination patterns.

CENTRAL NERVOUS SYSTEM

- History of neurological disease such as epilepsy, transient ischaemic attacks.
- Pain profile.

ENDOCRINE SYSTEM

- Thyroid function.
- Blood glucose levels measured with HbA1c test.
- History of any other endocrine disorder.

MUSCULOSKELETAL SYSTEM

- This should include a review of the range of movement and any musculoskeletal disease that may either give the patient pain or restrict their movement.

Surgical and anaesthetic history

Assessors must gather history of previous surgery. History of previous major surgeries or recent anaesthetics gives the assessor a good idea of the fitness of the patient for the planned surgery. It is also important to find out about previous anaesthetic problems such as post-operative nausea and vomiting, as well as a history of malignant hyperthermia. Identifying these factors is important in assessing the potential risk in performing the designated procedure on the patient. The American Society of Anesthesiologists (ASA) developed a scale with which to classify patients on the basis of their existing co-morbidities (Table 13.1). The scale is a well-established scoring tool that is useful for calculating patient risk of anaesthetic complications in relation to existing conditions (Walsgrove 2011).

The anaesthetic assessment also includes any cardiovascular, hepatic or pulmonary impairment, bleeding disorders, significant history of reflux or a hiatus hernia, breathing difficulties such as sleep apnoea, paroxysmal nocturnal dyspnoea or orthopnoea.

Medications and allergies

A full list of the patient's current medications, including over-the-counter medications as well as vitamin and herbal supplements, is essential. Many medications interact with anaesthetic agents or will negatively affect the patient in the intra- or post-operative period. These include anticoagulants, diabetic medications, calcium channel antagonists, beta-blockers and some antidepressants. If a patient is taking steroids or opiates, these require careful titration intra- or post-operatively. Specific medications may need to be discontinued days or weeks prior to surgery (Figure 13.1).

The patient's allergy status should be determined and specific details of reactions recorded. Medication 'intolerance' should also be documented to avoid severe side-effects such as nausea and vomiting. History of previous anaphylactic reactions should be thoroughly documented to avoid potential incidents. Patients who are allergic to latex will need to be first on the theatre list, and theatre staff will need to be alerted to avoid complications (see Latex sensitivity and allergy).

Table 13.1 **Modified ASA Physical Status Classification System**

Class	Physical status	Example
I	A healthy patient	A fit patient with an inguinal hernia
II	A patient with mild systemic disease	Essential hypertension, mild diabetes without end organ damage
III	A patient with severe systemic disease that is a constant threat to life	Angina, moderate-to-severe chronic obstructive pulmonary disease (COPD)
IV	A patient with an incapacitating disease that is a constant threat to life	Advanced COPD, cardiac failure
V	A moribund patient who is not expected to live 24 hours with or without surgery	Ruptured aortic aneurysm, massive pulmonary embolism
E	Emergency case	

Source: Adapted from American Society of Anesthesiologists (2013).

Social history

Social history encompasses social situations such as home life and occupation. Within the social history, the assessor develops a general idea about the social practices of the patient that may affect their fitness for surgery but also influence their recovery.

It is important to know about the patient's past and current occupational picture. The patient's occupation will give the assessor a picture of not only the patient's home and financial situation, but also potential occupational disorders such as respiratory or musculoskeletal problems.

Understanding the patient's support systems such as family or wider community is important. This will allow the assessor to pick up on potential 'road blocks' for a timely discharge. If the patient is found to have little or no available support in the community, the assessor has the opportunity to initiate any discharge planning or Social Services referrals prior to admission. This allows the patient to avoid any potential delays in their discharge.

It is also necessary to explore smoking, drug and alcohol use. Long-term abuse of alcohol, tobacco products or drugs can lead to organ damage, related medical complications, and therefore a higher incidence of perioperative morbidity and mortality. Intra- and post-operative events such as delirium tremens (acute episode of delirium) are considered medical emergencies.

ALCOHOL

It is imperative to communicate to the patient the importance of honesty with regard to alcohol or drug intake. Many patients will often admit to usage, but may deny they have excessive intake or a problem. It is important to assess the amount consumed on a daily or weekly basis. The recommended maximum intake for males is 21 units per week, and for females 14 units per week.

SMOKING

It is important to assess smoking behaviour. The length of time an individual has smoked, the number smoked a week, the pattern of their smoking, i.e. times of day, smoking with specific activities such as waking up, going to sleep or managing stress. Pre-operative smoking cessation is important and help with this should be offered during the assessment. The extent of smoking-related effects is dependent upon the amount, and the length of time, of smoking. Smokers have hyper-reactive airways that lead them to become more susceptible to incidents of laryngospasm or bronchospasm. They have an increased chance of developing post-operative lung infections due to a compromised ability to clear secretions. Smoking also affects the liver, which may mean that the patient will require higher dosages of medications. Post-operative healing is also affected by smoking as nicotine is a vasoconstrictor. NICE (2013) recommends the implementation of a smoking cessation service for people having elective surgery where:

- patients who smoke are identified
- patients receive appropriate information, referral and intervention
- patients have a seamless pathway between secondary and primary care.

The Royal Marsden Foundation NHS Trust
Peri-operative Guidelines for Drug Therapy

- Medication to Omit
- Medication to Omit unless specifically asked to give by Doctor (see comments below)
- Medication to continue can be given up to 2 hours before surgery, with a sip of water

Gastro-intestinal System	**H_2 antagonists, e.g. ranitidine**	
	Proton pump inhibitors, e.g. lansoprazole	
Cardiovascular System	**Alpha antagonists, e.g. doxazosin**	
	Anti-arrythmics, e.g. digoxin, amiodarone	
	Beta-blockers, e.g. atenolol	Avoid stopping suddenly. Continue iv if prolonged NBM
	Calcium antagonists, e.g. amlodipine	
	Loop & thiazide diuretics, e.g. furosemide, bendroflumethiazide	
	Nitrates, e.g. isosorbide mononitrate	
	ACE inhibitors, e.g. lisinopril	Consult Anaesthetist. May cause hypotension on induction of anaesthesia
	Angiotensin receptor II antagonists, e.g. losartan	Consult Anaesthetist. May cause hypotension on induction of anaesthesia
	Aspirin	If to be withheld, stop 7-10 days pre-op
	Clopidogrel	Stop 7 days pre-op unless Cardiologist states continue
	Dipyridamole	If procedure high risk, omit on day of surgery
	Low molecular weight heparin, e.g. tinzaparin, enoxaparin	Omit 12 hrs pre-op
	Potassium sparing diuretics, e.g. spironolactone, amiloride	Omit on day of surgery. May contribute to hyperkalaemia post-op
	Warfarin	Stop 3 days pre-op. If appropriate admit 3 days pre-op and start a heparin infusion until 4 hrs before surgery. Aim for APPT ratio < 1.5
Respiratory System	**Aminophylline / Theophylline**	
	Inhalers, e.g. salbutamol, beclomethasone	
Central Nervous System	**Anti-epileptics, e.g. phenytoin**	
	Antipsychotics, e.g. haloperidol, risperidone	
	Benzodiazepines, e.g. diazepam	
	Opioid analgesics, e.g. morphine, methadone, codeine	Consult Anaesthetist to plan post-op analgesia
	Paracetamol	
	Parkinson's treatment, e.g. co-careldopa, co-beneldopa	
	Selective serotonin re-uptake inhibitors (SSRIs), e.g. paroxetine, fluoxetine	
	Anti-dementia drugs, e.g. donepezil, rivastigmine, galantamine (acetylcholinesterase inhibitors)	May prolong neuromuscular blockade and exaggerate muscle relaxation with succinylcholine-type muscle relaxants. Alert Anaesthetist to the potential for prolonged neuromuscular blockade. Omit rivastigmine and galantamine 24-48 hours prior to surgery It is recommended to stop donepezil 2-3 weeks prior to surgery; however these patients may not return to their baseline mental function, therefore may be unethical to stop
	Lithium	Check levels pre-op. Continue for minor surgery. Discuss with Anaesthetist plan for major surgery. Restart ASAP post-op
	Non-steroidal anti-inflammatory (NSAIDs), e.g. diclofenac, COX II inhibitors	Increased risk of bleeding. Can stop 1-3 days pre-op depending on half-life. Stop piroxicam 7 days pre-op
	Tricyclic antidepressants, e.g. amitriptyline	Increased risk of arrhythmias. Consult Anaesthetist
	Clozapine	Stop 12 hrs pre-op. Restart ASAP. Contact pharmacy for advice
	Monoamine-oxidase inhibitors (non-reversible), e.g. phenelzine	Stop 14 days pre-op (discuss with Psychiatrist). If not withdrawn inform Anaesthetist
	Reversible MAOIs, e.g. moclobemide	Omit on day of surgery
Infections	**Antibiotics**	
	Anti-virals, e.g. HIV antiretroviral drugs, aciclovir	

Figure 13.1 **Guide to pre-operative medication.** ***Source:*** **Reproduced with permission from Dr David Chisholm, Anaesthetist, The Royal Marsden Hospital NHS Foundation Trust, 2010.**

Endocrine System	**Corticosteroids, e.g. prednisolone (Current or stopped within last 3 months)**	May need additional hydrocortisone bolus intra/post operation: **Minor surgery**: 25mg hydrocortisone at induction (or usual oral dose) **Moderate surgery**: 25mg hydrocortisone at induction (or usual oral dose) then 25mg hydrocortisone TDS for 24 hours and then restart usual steroid dose **Major surgery**: 25mg hydrocortisone at induction (or usual oral dose) then 50mg TDS hydrocortisone for 48-72 hours and then restart usual steroid dose
	Desmopressin (DDAVP)	
	Hormone antagonists, e.g. tamoxifen, anastrozole	Thromboprophylaxis and TEDS
	Hormone replacement therapy (HRT)	Thromboprophylaxis and TEDS
	Levothyroxine	
	Progesterone only oral contraceptives	Thromboprophylaxis and TEDS
	Combined oral contraceptives (i.e. containing oestrogen)	Omit 4 weeks prior to major surgery, institute thromboprophylaxis and TEDS. Advise on alternative family planning
	Glibenclamide, glipizide, gliclazide, tolbutamide & glitazones (e.g. pioglitazone)	Refer to Anaesthetist. Omit all oral hypoglycaemics on morning of surgery
	Insulin	Continue until morning of surgery. Omit morning dose & breakfast. **Minor surgery**: Re-start s/c insulin post-op with first meal. **Major surgery**: Omit breakfast and S/C insulin and start intravenous sliding scale insulin
	Metformin	Refer to Anaesthetist. Omit 48-72 hrs pre-op in patients with renal impairment
Malignant Disease & Immunosuppression	**Drugs to prevent adverse effects, e.g. allopurinol**	Seek advice from Oncologist/Haematologists
	DMARDS, e.g. methotrexate for Rheumatoid Arthritis	Continue unless at risk of renal complications. Discuss with specialist
	Immunosuppressants, e.g. azathioprine, ciclosporin	Seek advice from Oncologist/Haematologists
	Cytotoxics, e.g. alkylating agents, antimetabolites	Seek advice from Oncologist/Haematologists
Complementary Alternative Medicines	**Echinacea** (activates cell-mediated immunity allergic reactions, poor wound healing, increased risk of infection, reduced action of immunosuppressive medicines).	Discontinue as far in advance as possible before surgery
	Ephedra (causes dose-dependent increases in blood pressure and heart rate. Risk of MI and stroke from tachycardia and hypertension. Long-term use depletes endogenous catecholamines & may cause intraoperative haemodynamic instability. Interacts with MAOIs).	Discontinue 24 hrs before surgery
	Garlic (inhibits platelet aggregation (may be irreversible) so may increase risk of bleeding, especially when combined with other platelet inhibitors).	Discontinue at least 7 days before surgery
	Ginkgo (inhibits platelet activating factor so may increase risk of bleeding, especially when combined with other platelet inhibitors).	Discontinue at least 36 hrs before surgery
	Ginseng (lowers blood glucose & inhibits platelet aggregation so can lead to hypoglycaemia risk of bleeding. Platelet inhibition may be irreversible and increased).	Discontinue at least 7 days before surgery
	Kava (sedates and reduces anxiety so could increase sedative effect of anaesthetics. Has potential for tolerance).	Sedates & reduces anxiety Discontinue at least 24 hrs before surgery
	St John's Wort (inhibits neurotransmitter serotonin, norepinephrine and dopamine reuptake by neurons. Induces cytochrome P450 therefore concentrations of alfentanil, midazolam, and lidocaine may be reduced. Also reduces concentrations of digoxin, warfarin and ciclosporin).	Discontinue at least 5 days before surgery
	Valerian (sedates via modulation of GABA transmission and receptor function so increases the sedative effect of anaesthetics, especially those via GABA receptor e.g. midazolam. Long-term use could increase amount of anaesthetic required).	Reduce dose gradually over several weeks before surgery: risk of benzodiazepine-like withdrawal. If a patient is dependent on valerian, can be taken up until day of sugery. Benzodiazepines can be used to treat withdrawal in the post-operative period
Nutrition & Blood	**Drugs for nutrition, e.g. iron, folic acid, calcium, magnesium**	Continue unless specifically asked not to

This information applies to all types of surgery (minor or major). Please contact local pharmacy for administration advice if the patient requires a prolonged NBM period.

Figure 13.1 ***(continued)***

Physical examination

Within the POA, baseline vital signs and a physical examination are essential and should be completed by a trained assessor. The physical examination should include specific attention to the respiratory and cardiac systems, as they are 'most obviously affected by anaesthetics and which themselves exert an influence on the course of anaesthesia and the post-operative period' (Cashman 2001, p.9). Examination of further organ systems, such as abdominal or neurological systems, should also be completed if indicated by the patient's history. For example, patients with known alcohol or drug abuse should be further examined for hepatic and neurological impairments.

Within the pre-operative assessment, it is vital to perform an airway assessment. This includes:

- range of motion of the neck and jaw
- mouth opening, including ability to protrude lower incisors in front of the upper incisors
- dentition – condition of teeth
- history of temporomandibular joint dysfunction and other airway abnormalities.

If there are any problems with the airway, the anaesthetist needs to be informed so that appropriate equipment can be ordered for the day of surgery. Alert the anaesthetist if the patient has previously experienced a difficult intubation; has disease, surgical or radiotherapy scarring of the head, neck or mediastinum; difficult or noisy breathing; morbid obesity; poor mouth opening; rigid or deformed neck; receding chin or an overbite (Ong and Pearce 2011). Further explanation on physical assessment can be found in Chapter 2: Assessment and discharge.

Pre-operative investigations

Another aspect of the pre-operative assessment is the ordering and interpreting of pre-operative investigations. Investigations are often ordered to establish baseline values, support or refute differential diagnoses, and support or monitor the management of existing disease processes. The results of the physical examination and history taking direct the practitioner to the types of pre-operative investigations necessary. Investigations are often ordered based on routine rather than on patient health indicators or for aiding in perioperative management. *Pre-operative Tests: The Use of Routine Pre-operative Tests for Elective Surgery* (NICE 2003) is an evidence-based guide for the ordering and use of routine pre-operative testing in elective surgeries. The investigations are based on ASA status (see Table 13.1), the age of the patient and their co-morbidities. Table 13.2 lists various laboratory tests.

Table 13.2 **Pre-operative laboratory tests**

Test	Rationale
Haematology	
Full blood count (FBC), including haemoglobin, haematocrit	Patients with a history of: • smoking • malignancy • respiratory disease • cardiac disease may be at increased risk for anaemia and polycythaemia
White blood cell count	Patients with a history of: • recent chemotherapy and/or radiotherapy • malignancy • recent infection may have either raised or lowered white blood cell count
Platelet count	Platelet count should be checked on patients with a history of: • bleeding tendencies • renal or hepatic disease • recent treatment with chemotherapy
Coagulation screening, including prothrombin and activated partial thromboplastin time	This is not recommended unless the patient: • is taking anticoagulants • has a history of bleeding disorders • has a history of post-surgical bleeding • has a bleeding history (such as liver disease or malignancy) (Chee et al. 2008)
Group and save or cross-match	Having the blood tested prior to the date of surgery gives the blood bank more time to find the appropriate blood required for the specific patient. Patients with unusual blood typing or rare antibodies may need to have special blood obtained from a national blood bank, and having the sample collected in advance will decrease the chance of errors and of the patient having their surgery postponed
Serum biochemistry	
Glycosylated haemoglobin (HbA1c) level	Patients presenting with a history of: • steroid use • obesity • cardiovascular disease • symptoms suggestive of diabetes. The HbA1c is a more accurate measurement of the patient's long-term glucose control and compliance

Test	Rationale
Baseline serum creatinine and blood urea nitrogen level	Patients with a history of: • renal dysfunction • diabetes • cardiovascular disease • obesity • medications such as steroids or diuretics
Liver function tests, such as albumin	Patients presenting with: • liver disease • malignancy • alcohol abuse • malnutrition • jaundice. The liver and kidneys aid the metabolism and elimination of many anaesthetics and medications. Therefore it is vital to ensure these are checked pre-operatively to ensure adequate organ function
Electrolyte levels	Electrolyte levels should be checked pre-operatively in patients with a history of: • renal dysfunction • diabetes • malignancy • malnutrition • vomiting or diarrhoea • medications such as diuretics or chemotherapy. These patients may require pre-operative prescribing of supplements such as potassium to optimize electrolyte levels prior to surgery. Electrolyte imbalances such as hypokalaemia or hyponatraemia can be potentially life-threatening in the perioperative period
Other tests	
Thyroid function testing	Patients with a history of hypo- or hyperthyroidism. Patients with untreated or severe thyroid disease are at increased risk of developing 'thyroid storm' (dangerously raised heart rate, blood pressure and temperature) relating to the stress of surgery or illness (Weinberg et al. 1983)
Urinalysis	Patients presenting with symptoms of a urinary tract infection or those presenting for procedures of the urinary tract, e.g. cystoscopy
Pregnancy testing	Pregnancy testing should be completed based on findings of the medical history, date of last menstrual cycle. This should ideally be done on the day of admission unless the patient suspects she might be pregnant during pre-assessment

ELECTROCARDIOGRAMS

A standard 12-lead electrocardiogram is frequently performed if indicated by the age of the patient, risk factors, co-morbidities and findings of the physical examination. The patient's ASA grading and the surgical grading of the planned surgery may also indicate an ECG. The proportion of patients with an abnormal ECG increases with age and the presence of co-morbidities. An ECG can also be completed to establish a baseline prior to surgery for post-operative comparison.

IMAGING: CHEST X-RAY (CXR)

A CXR can give the practitioner valuable information to support or refute potential diagnoses or further assess the severity of a specific disease. Patients presenting with history of cardiovascular or respiratory symptoms or disease processes should have a CXR completed pre-operatively. If the patient has had a CXR within the last 6 months, it does not need to be repeated unless new problems have arisen or the existing problems have worsened.

CARDIOPULMONARY EXERCISE TESTING

Older and Smith (1988) introduced the concept of cardiopulmonary exercise testing (CPET) (Figure 13.2). CPET is a dynamic, non-invasive test, involving the use of an exercise bicycle (cycle ergometer) where the work rate is gradually and imperceptibly increased in a stepped or ramped manner until the patient is unable to continue. This enables examination of the ability of the patient's cardiorespiratory system to adapt to a 'stress' situation of increased oxygen demand, in effect mimicking the conditions of surgery.

Cardiopulmonary exercise testing relies upon accurate breath-by-breath measurements of pulmonary gas exchange through a mouthpiece measuring respiratory gas exchange. In addition, electrocardiography, blood pressure, pulse oximetry and heart rate are monitored during exercise (American Thoracic Society and American College of Chest Physicians 2003, Wasserman 2012). From the CPET, two key indicators are derived: the body's maximum oxygen uptake (VO_{2max}) and the point at which anaerobic metabolism exceeds aerobic metabolism (anaerobic threshold, AT). Together these broadly indicate the ability of the cardiovascular system to deliver oxygen to the peripheral tissues and the ability of the tissues to utilize that oxygen. In addition, the AT has been shown to be a useful predictor of post-operative cardiac complications in abdominal surgery (Older et al. 1999).

Exercise testing is commonly used to reproduce common symptoms such as impaired exercise capacity, fatigue and exertional breathlessness. This enables accurate physiological measurements to be obtained, assisting with the overall assessment of suitability for surgery, and can predict post-operative mortality and morbidity (Cooper and Storer 2001). This assessment will reveal to both the healthcare professional and the patient what needs to be considered if optimum results are to be achieved from surgery.

Cardiopulmonary exercise testing is often referred to as 'the gold standard for measuring exercise tolerance'. It enables clinicians to triage patients to the appropriate level of care after surgery, allowing the efficient use of intensive care facilities (MacGregor et al. 2009). It also assists surgeons in assessing

Figure 13.2 **Cardiopulmonary exercise testing (CPET).**

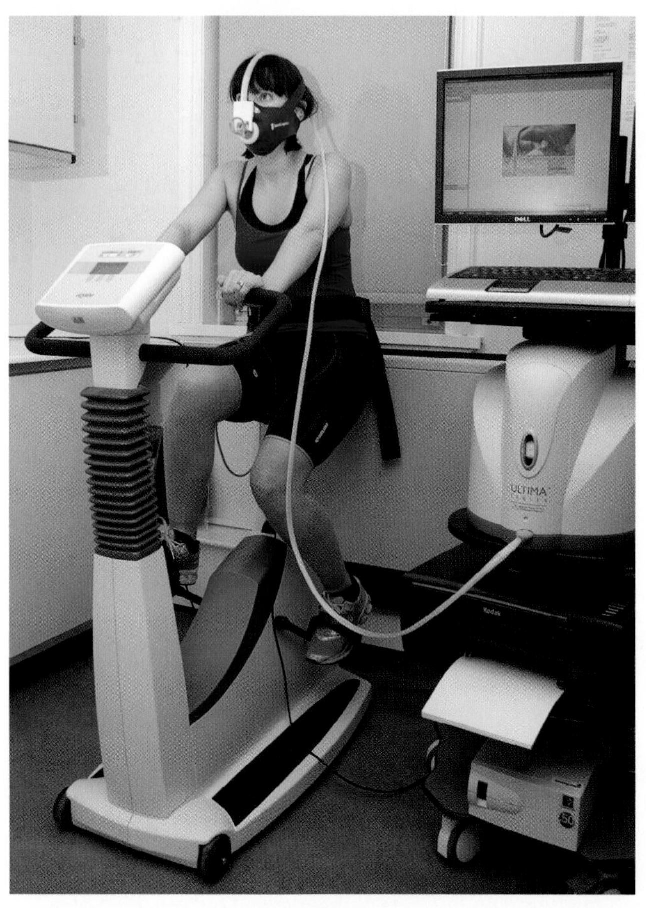

treatment options more easily (Older et al. 1993). The patient is then in a better position to evaluate their own risk/benefit ratio for surgery and thus make a more informed decision on consent for an operation (American Thoracic Society and American College of Chest Physicians 2003, Lee et al. 2006).

FURTHER REFERRALS

During the patient's pre-operative assessment, it is often deemed necessary to refer for further expert assessment or advice. This is helpful in providing valuable information regarding the patient's condition and creating an appropriate plan of action for the patient in the perioperative or post-operative period. Patients are seen by a specialist to further assess whether they are in the optimum condition for the desired surgery and/or if their health can be 'optimized' prior to surgery to improve their post-operative outcomes.

Learning Activity 13.1

Learning in practice: Pre-operative assessment

Ensuring that patients are seen as an outpatient for a pre-operative assessment, prior to their admission for surgery, is now a common and recommended practice.

- Speak to your colleagues within your clinical area to arrange a visit to the pre-operative assessment clinic.
- Identify which core assessments and investigations are carried out for all patients and for what reason.
- Identify which members of the multidisciplinary team are involved in the pre-operative assessment clinic.

Anticipated patient outcomes

Ensure patient safety at all times and minimize intra- and post-operative complications. According to the *National Good Practice Guidance on Pre-operative Assessment for Inpatient Surgery* (NHS Modernization Agency 2003), pre-operative assessment clinics were created with several objectives in mind.

- Provide the opportunity to further explain and discuss any information provided by the surgeon to the patient. This process should aid in minimizing any patient fears or anxieties, through ensuring that the patient understands the upcoming surgery, as well as what the recovery following the surgery will entail. This gives the patient time to prepare psychologically, reducing stress and thereby enhancing recovery.
- Assist in the assessment of the patient's fitness for the surgery, as well as anaesthesia and post-operative recovery. This will provide information for a comprehensive assessment of the risks and benefits of the required surgery and anaesthesia, allowing the patient to make an informed decision. This is achieved through a comprehensive medical history, physical examination and the ordering of appropriate investigations (NICE 2003).
- Identify any co-morbidities that may require intervention prior to admission and surgery likely to affect the intra- and post-operative care of the patient.This should allow enough time to take appropriate action before admission to make changes to the patient's treatment regimen, such as discontinuation of anticoagulants or implementation of antihypertensive medications.
- Assist in ensuring that the patient is in optimum health prior to surgery, through further referrals to secondary care specialists as necessary, for example cardiologists.
- Perform necessary investigations prior to surgery and ensure that the results of these investigations are actioned (for example, haematological investigations).
- Identify the need for and arrange supply of any specialist equipment and special requirements for the post-operative period (for example, critical care beds, bariatric equipment).
- Provide information to the patient about any specific pre-operative preparation that may be required (for example, fasting, bowel preparation). This may also include involving members of the multidisciplinary team such as clinical nurse specialists, physiotherapists or dieticians.
- Give the patient a point of contact for further questions or concerns, or if they want to postpone or cancel the surgery.
- Provide information to the patient on what they should anticipate in the post-operative period. This may include leaflets and videos to help the patient understand the planned procedure. This would also include discussion with the anaesthetist about pain control, intubation and potential critical care admission.
- Provide any assistance with health promotion activities such as smoking cessation, weight loss and alcohol use that will help to improve the outcome in the perioperative and post-operative periods. This may include further referrals to primary care services such as stop smoking services or dietetic advice.
- Identify any cultural, religious or communication needs for the patient.
- Individual admission and discharge planning, ensuring that the patient and carer(s) know what to expect, facilitating earlier discharge and enabling follow-up care to be undertaken in the primary care setting.
- Provide the appropriate pre-operative documentation for the multidisciplinary team. See Chapter 2: Assessment and discharge for further insight into POA processes (Liddle 2012, NICE 2003, Oakley and Bratchell 2010).

Thorough POA results in good clinical outcomes and enhanced patient experience as evidenced by the success of the Enhanced Recovery Partnership Programme, which has transformed elective

Box 13.1 Enhanced Recovery Partnership Programme

Enhanced Recovery, also known as fast track, rapid or accelerated surgery, is transforming elective surgical care pathways across the NHS and improving both patient experience and clinical outcomes (including reduced length of stay) (NHSIP 2008). Since 2009, Enhanced Recovery pathways have been established and become standard practice in the vast majority of NHS hospitals in England (DH 2011).

The underlying principle of the Enhanced Recovery Programme involves ensuring patients are in the optimal condition for surgery, have the best possible care during their operation and experience optimal post-operative rehabilitation (DH 2009a). Shared decision making is integral to the Enhanced Recovery pathway, incorporating elements of patient self-care through to highly specialist care (DH 2011). Shared decision making involves the patient as an active participant in their care, first clarifying the range of clinically acceptable treatment options for the patient and then working in partnership with the patient in determining the best treatment, management and support for them, which best meets their individual needs, values and preferences at the time (DH 2011).

The Enhanced Recovery Programme includes the following.

1 Pre-operative assessment, planning and preparation before admission – optimize health (including encouraging patients to exercise and eat well) and pre-existing medical conditions (e.g. diabetes); discharge planning and information giving.
2 Reducing the physical stress of the operation – using minimally invasive surgical techniques (e.g. laparoscopic); individualized goal-directed fluid therapy; use of quick-offset anaesthetic agents, allowing quick recovery; prevent hypothermia; effective opiate-sparing analgesia, to facilitate early mobilization, e.g. nerve blocks; minimize the risk of post-operative nausea and vomiting; minimize the use of drains and nasogastric tubes.
3 Post-operative rehabilitation – early nutrition; early mobilization; early removal of catheters; post-operative education and support, e.g. stoma care; follow-up advice and support.

Box 13.2 Role of the assessor in the POA clinic

- Work to guidelines and compentencies agreed by anaesthetists, surgeons and other allied health professionals to ensure a consistent approach.
- Take a targeted history and conduct a relevant physical examination of the patient, including airway assessment.
- Refer patients who fall outside the agreed criteria to the anaesthetist, who may then make further referrals.
- Arrange and perform investigations in accordance with NICE guidelines.
- Ensure that the results of tests are evaluated and refer abnormal investigation results to the available anaesthetist, surgeon and/or primary care, according to local guidelines.
- Refer a patient back to primary care or another healthcare professional to optimize the patient's medical condition, according to local guidelines.
- Take responsibility for following up referrals to ensure the patient remains in the pre-operative system.
- Liaise actively with the anaesthetic department.
- Arrange and co-ordinate any assessment and/or investigations needed near time of surgery. Take responsibility for all communication with the patient throughout their pre-operative journey.
- Commence necesssary planning for the perioperative stay and ensure a timely discharge.
- Identify factors that may influence the dates of surgery offered, for example school holidays.
- Collate all information prior to surgery and ensure that the multidisciplinary documentation is available for anaesthetists to see at least 48 hours prior to admission.
- Communicate approximate length of operation, any special requirements and essential resources to the waiting list office, bed management, operating theatre department and/or theatre scheduler.
- Contact all patients failing to attend pre-operative assessment to identify the reason. Act on the reason, following local protocols for the management of DNAs (did not attend) in pre-operative assessment.

surgical care pathways across the NHS since 2009 (DH 2011) (Box 13.1). It also minimizes length of hospital stay through:

- reduced cancellations due to patient ill health or DNAs (did not attend)
- increased number of same-day surgery admissions
- earlier discharge.

LEGAL AND PROFESSIONAL ISSUES

The POA should only be performed by assessors trained and deemed competent in the process. Assessors can include not only doctors or anaesthetists but also nurses or operating department practitioners (ODPs). The role of the assessor is broad (Box 13.2), but they should be competent in the following procedures:

- take a comprehensive health history
- perform a physical examination
- order appropriate investigations.

The Association of Anaesthetists of Great Britain and Ireland (AAGBI 2010) states that trained staff 'play an essential role when, by working to agreed protocols, they screen patients for fitness for anaesthesia and surgery' although they are not qualified to make the final decision about a patient's fitness for surgery, but play an important role in 'identifying problem patients'. Non-complicated patients often do not require further assessment by an anaesthetist until the day of admission. Patients considered complicated by the trained assessor are further reviewed by an anaesthetist. This is supported by Kenny (2011) who found that approximately 20% of patients assessed by pre-assessment nurses were referred to the anaesthetic clinic. Of these, 10% were due to the discovery of poorly controlled, undiagnosed or complex health problems and 10% due to the nature of surgery required.

While the POA can be performed by non-anaesthetic personnel such as nurses, it is vital that the anaesthetist in charge of the patient's case is aware of the patient's co-morbidities. Competency assessement is also carried out in pre-assessment in the form of a competency portfolio as advocated by Walsgrove (2011), which was designed in correlation with the NHS Modernization Agency's (2003) guidance for pre-operative assessment. This covers administrative function, physical assessment (medical and nursing history), psychological and social assessment, decision making, interventions (referral, pre-operative counselling, ordering and performing tests and investigations). To ensure quality, regular audits on the pre-assessment documentation should be carried out. Any incidents stemming from a pre-assessment, for example if a patient is cancelled on the day, must be reported immediately and investigated, so ensuring that the unit is continually improving its practice.

Patient information and education

RELATED THEORY

Patients undergoing surgery have information and supportive care needs before and after their surgery. Providing information to patients is considered a crucial issue and the central focus in patient educational activities. Patients require information that is meaningful for them as individuals. It is necessary to educate patients on the nature of the outcomes and the benefits and risks of procedures so they can be involved in the decision-making process and enabled to give fully informed consent. Accurate, reliable and complete information plays a pivotal role in helping patients make informed decisions.

EVIDENCE-BASED APPROACHES

Principles of care

The way in which information is delivered and understood will help determine whether a patient's actual post-operative experiences are congruent with expected ones; therefore it is essential that information is provided at the right time and in a variety of formats. Information materials must contain scientifically reliable information and be presented in a form that is acceptable and useful to patients, i.e. suitable for the patient's educational level. Patient education has been found to be extremely beneficial, reducing anxiety levels and promoting patient well-being (Bondy et al. 1999, Klopfenstein et al. 2000, Liddle 2012, Walker 2002).

Pre-operatively, pain and anaesthesia are amongst patients' greatest worries and need to be discussed so that anxiety can be reduced (Mitchell 2005), which may ultimately result in patients requiring less analgesia. Patients should also be provided with information about the equipment and intravenous access extension sets that they will be attached to post-operatively so that they know what to expect as this can be distressing to both the patient and their family/friends when they return from theatre. Patients should also be provided with information on the recovery period, including when they will be expected to mobilize, when they can eat and drink and the length of time they can expect to be in hospital.

There are currently three main forms of patient education: face to face; paper based and internet/web based (Table 13.3).

Patient education has been found to be extremely beneficial, reducing anxiety levels and promoting patient well-being (Jlala et al. 2010, Klopfenstein et al. 2000, Walker 2002). However, it is important that any form of patient education is tailored to individual patients to ensure that the needs of those patients requiring additional follow-up information, practical or psychosocial support are met. These can be identified through face-to-face education programmes or web-based consultations.

Any verbal information should be supported by paper or web-based written information, from reliable, evidence-based sources, which are tailored to the patient's educational level. Written patient information in particular can help patients to gain a greater understanding of surgery and what is expected of them and can:

- ensure patients arrive on time and are properly prepared for surgery, e.g. pre-operative fasting
- increase patient confidence, improving their overall experience
- refamiliarize patients with what they have already been told
- enhance patient and carer involvement in their treatment and condition (NHSIP 2008).

LEGAL AND PROFESSIONAL ISSUES

Competencies

One of the principal responsibilities of a nurse is to educate patients (Anderson and Klemm 2008); however, time and work-related constraints can interfere with the provision of patient education. Timing is crucial and can influence a patient's ability to retain information. Furthermore, it is essential to consider the educational level of the patient, to ensure that any patient education/information is appropriate and meaningful. Effective patient education also requires evaluation to ensure the patient has understood and retained the information they have been given.

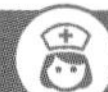
Learning Activity 13.2

Scenario: Pre-operative patient information

You are looking after a female patient who is due to have her surgery tomorrow morning.

1 Although you can see from her documentation that she has had information about her procedure given to her in the pre-operative assessment clinic, what key elements of information regarding perioperative care are most important to reiterate with her prior to surgery?
2 How would you ensure that she has understood the information you have given her?

See the end of the chapter for the answers.

Table 13.3 **Forms of patient education**

Patient education	Definition	Advantages	Disadvantages
Face to face	Includes any education delivered verbally by a healthcare provider to a single patient or group of patients. This remains the most common form of patient education	Can be tailored to individual patient needs	Time consuming Consistency problems Relies on patient's ability to absorb, understand and retain the verbal information
Paper based	Includes any written information – patient information leaflets	Develop comprehensive educational materials that are consistently presented Patients can refer back to material	Unable to tailor to individual patient needs
Web based	Includes any verbal and written patient information. Web-based seminars, patient groups, programmes of care; interactive websites; podcasts; video/YouTube	Wide-ranging and current information A variety of teaching formats; patient empowerment – patient control vs healthcare professional control Support 24 hours a day Develop comprehensive educational materials that are consistently presented Patients can refer back to material Accessed all over world	Potential for inaccurate information Lack of access Poor quality of online resources Security and privacy issues

Consent

DEFINITION

NHS Choices (2012) defines consent as: 'the principle that a person must give their permission before they receive any type of medical treatment'.

EVIDENCE-BASED APPROACHES

There are different types of consent in healthcare: written, verbal (explicit) and non-verbal (implied or implicit) (DH 2009b). The Department of Health (DH 2009b) and professional bodies including the Nursing and Midwifery Council (NMC) and General Medical Council (GMC) have produced comprehensive guidance about consent (GMC 2008, NMC 2013). The DH guidance (DH 2009b) includes information about what consent is, the different types of consent, when consent should be obtained, by whom and in what circumstances.

Principles of care

Unless it is an emergency, the gaining of consent should be treated as a process rather than a one-off event (DH 2009b). For major operations, it should be considered good practice to gain a person's consent to the proposed procedure well in advance, ideally prior to pre-assessment when there is time to respond to the person's questions and provide adequate information so that the person has time to develop an understanding to allow an informed decision to be made (Hughes 2011).

Whilst the validity of consent does not depend on the form in which it is given (DH 2009b), it is good practice to use forms for written consent where an intervention such as surgery is to be undertaken. Most hospitals' local consent policies will require written consent to be obtained in these circumstances and this practice is supported by the Department of Health (DH 2009b). However, written consent merely serves as evidence of consent and a signature on a form alone will not make the consent valid. For example, if a person's signature to confirm their consent is gained immediately before the surgical procedure is due to start, at a time when they may be feeling particularly vulnerable, this would raise concerns about its validity (DH 2009b). Furthermore, patients should not in any situation be given routine pre-operative medication before being asked for their consent to proceed with the treatment (NMC 2013).

LEGAL AND PROFESSIONAL ISSUES

It is accepted that when a patient gives valid consent, this is valid indefinitely unless withdrawn by the patient; therefore no specific time limit is designated from signature to procedure (Hughes 2011). However, it is good practice to confirm the patient's wishes if significant time has elapsed since the initial process. The patient is entitled to withdraw consent at any time (Hughes 2011).

For consent to be valid, it must encompass several factors.

- *Consent must be given willingly*: this is without pressure or undue influence to either undertake or not undertake treatment.
- *Consent must be informed*: the person must have an understanding of the procedure and the purpose behind it, and has been given relevant information about the benefits and risks of the procedure as well as potential alternatives. This information needs to be explained or presented in a way that is meaningful and easy to understand by the person in a variety of formats (both verbal and written) to enable them to make an informed decision.
- *The person must have the capacity to consent to the procedure in question*: that is, the ability to understand and retain the information provided, especially around the consequences of having or not having the procedure (NMC 2013). An assessment of a person's capacity must be based on their ability to make a specific decision at the time it needs to be made, and not their ability to make a decision in general (DH 2009b). Under the Mental Capacity Act 2005 (DCA 2007), which became fully effective in England and Wales in 2007, a person must be presumed to have capacity unless it is established that they lack capacity. If there is any doubt, then the healthcare professional should assess the capacity of the patient to take the decision in general (see Chapter 4: Communication).

Competencies

All healthcare professionals should be aware of the different types of consent and the importance of ensuring that the person understands what is going to happen to them and what is involved. Healthcare professionals should also be familiar with their local hospital consent policy and be aware of and understand what to do if people refuse care or treatment or when consent is not valid or is no longer valid.

Current guidance states that the person obtaining consent must either be capable of performing the procedure themselves or have received specialist training in advising patients about the procedure (DH 2009b, Oakley and Bratchell 2010). The person obtaining the patient's consent for surgery should ideally be the surgeon performing the procedure. The anaesthetist should also discuss the risks related to the chosen method of anaesthesia and obtain consent from the patient (Hughes 2011).

Physical pre-operative preparation

DEFINITION

Physical pre-operative preparation is concerned with reducing harm and complications in the peri- and post-operative period (NPSA 2007, Scott et al. 2007).

RELATED THEORY

Peri- and post-operative physical complications include wrong site surgery, infection (e.g. chest infection and wound infection), deep vein thrombosis, pain and allergies/anaphylaxis (Scott et al. 2007).

LEGAL AND PROFESSIONAL ISSUES

The National Patient Safety Agency (NPSA 2008a) received over 128,000 reports of patient safety incidents from surgical specialties from October 2006 to September 2007. The nature of these incidents varied widely from wrong site surgery to misplaced patient notes. Not all of these incidents were serious but some have led to patient harm or in some instances death. In 2008, this resulted in the World Health Organization (WHO) developing a Surgical Safety Checklist, which is a structured communication aid to enhance safety intraoperatively (www.who.int/patientsafety/safesurgery/ss_checklist/en/) (see 'Intraoperative' section and Box 13.11 for detailed information about the WHO surgical safety checklist). This checklist is currently mandated in many countries including the UK (NPSA 2008b).

Whilst the WHO Surgical Safety Checklist (2008) is used during the intraoperative period, several measures can be undertaken pre-operatively to help prevent peri- and post-operative complications from arising (Box 13.3).

Namebands

Namebands (otherwise known as identity bands or wristbands) are fundamental in the identification of patients. Patient misidentification contributes to errors and is a cause of patient

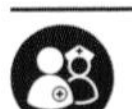

Box 13.3 **Pre-operative patient safety measures**

- Namebands.
- Antiembolic stockings and prophylactic anticoagulation.
- Pre-operative fasting.
- Skin preparation.
- Marking skin for surgery.
- Pre-operative pregnancy testing.
- Preventing toxic shock syndrome from tampons.
- Assessment for latex allergy.
- Comprehensive pre-operative checks.

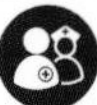

Box 13.4 **Information to be included on a nameband**

- Date of birth, in the format dd.mm.yyyy (e.g. 01-Mar-2013).
- Name (surname first in capitals followed by the first name with the first letter in capitals, e.g. MARSDEN, William).
- Patient's 10-digit NHS number.

safety incidents with potentially grave consequences. In 2007, the NPSA reported that incorrect namebands were the cause of more than 2900 incidents involving patients being mismatched to their planned care. In the most recent guidance by the NPSA (2007) and Information Standards Board for Health and Social Care (ISB 2009), it is suggested that standardizing the design of patient wristbands, the information on them and the processes used to produce and check them will improve patient safety. Since 1st July 2011, it has been mandatory for all hospitals to have electronically printed namebands (ISB 2009). Where possible, colour coding for individual risks should be avoided. If a healthcare organization believes colour coding is necessary to alert healthcare professionals to a known risk, e.g. patient allergy, then the NPSA (2007) recommends the use of only one colour, red. Box 13.4 sets out the recommended information to be included on the nameband (NPSA 2007).

Antiembolic stockings and prophylactic anticoagulation

DEFINITION

Antiembolic stockings (also known as graduated elastic compression stockings or thromboembolic deterrents [TEDs]) and prophylactic anticoagulation (e.g. low molecular weight heparin) are used as a preventive measure against the formation of venous thromboembolism (VTE – blood clots).

RELATED THEORY

Venous thromboembolism is a condition where a blood clot is formed inside a vein. This is normally due to stasis of blood within the vessel, trauma to the vessel or an increase in the ability of the blood to clot (Figure 13.3, Figure 13.4). This most frequently happens in the deep veins of the leg which is termed a deep vein thrombosis or DVT. If one of these clots dislodges from the leg and travels to the lung via the bloodstream, it is called a pulmonary embolus or PE (Figure 13.5). This is a potentially fatal event (NICE 2010). Potential clinical signs of DVT or PE are outlined in Box 13.5.

In January 2010 NICE guidance *Venous Thromboembolism: Reducing the Risk* was issued. This updated guidance specified that VTE 'at-risk' patients must be assessed on admission and again for risk of VTE and bleeding within 24 hours of admission and prophylaxis commenced where necessary (NICE 2010). Venous thrombus risk factors include the following.

- Surgical patients, including day surgery patients, where total anaesthetic and surgery time is over 90 minutes or 60 minutes if surgery involves the pelvis or lower limbs
- Immobility, for example prolonged bedrest
- Active cancer
- Severe cardiac failure or recent myocardial infarction
- Acute respiratory failure
- Elderly
- Previous history of DVT or PE
- Acute infection/inflammation
- Diabetes
- Smoker
- Obesity
- Gross varicose veins
- Paralysis of lower limbs
- Clotting disorders
- Hormone replacement therapy
- Oral contraceptives (House of Commons Health Committee 2005, NICE 2010, Rashid et al. 2005, Scottish Intercollegiate Guidelines Network 2002).

Figure 13.4 **Deep vein thrombosis. Source: Adapted from The Royal Marsden NHS Foundation Trust (2010).**

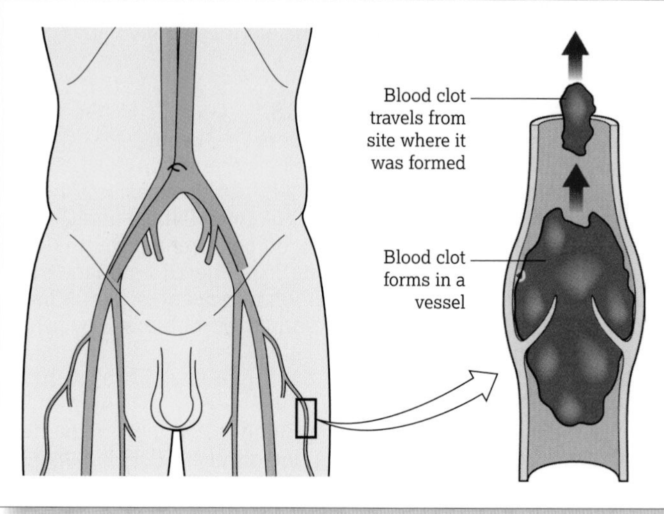

Figure 13.3 **Pulmonary embolism.** ***Source:*** **Adapted from The Royal Marsden NHS Foundation Trust (2010).**

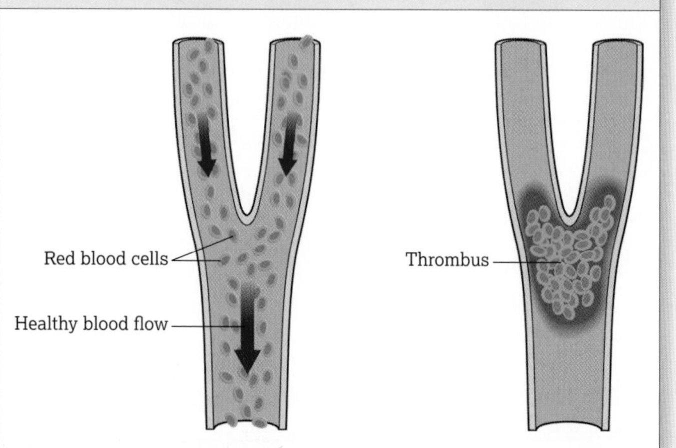

Figure 13.5 **Thrombus.** ***Source:*** **Adapted from The Royal Marsden NHS Foundation Trust (2010).**

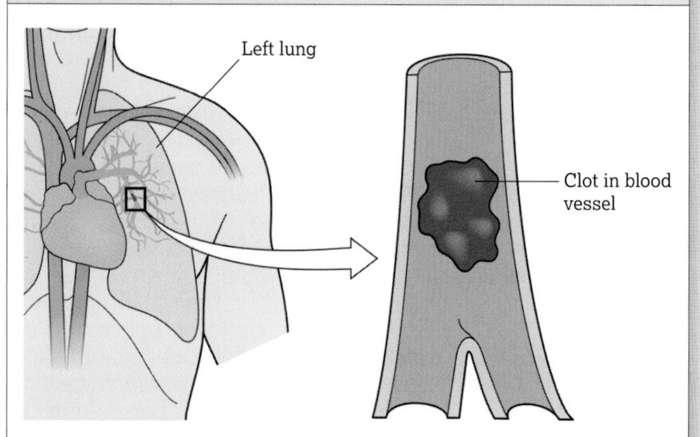

Box 13.5 **Signs of deep vein thrombosis/pulmonary embolism**

- Complaints of calf or thigh pain.
- Erythema, warmth, tenderness and abnormal swelling of the calf or thigh in the affected limb.
- Numbness or tingling of the feet.
- Dyspnoea, chest pain or signs of shock.
- Pain in the chest, back or ribs which gets worse when the patient breathes in deeply.
- Coughing up blood.

All patients requiring an inpatient stay for surgery should have prophylactic treatment to reduce the risk of DVT, which may include prophylactic anticoagulation (e.g. low molecular weight heparin) and mechanical compression methods. Antiembolic stockings are the most common form of mechanical compression method, but extremely high-risk patients may also use intermittent pneumatic compression devices (e.g. Flowtron boots) or venous foot pumps (NICE 2010, Roderick et al. 2005, Scottish Intercollegiate Guidelines Network., 2002) in the intraoperative and post-operative period (Figure 13.6, Figure 13.7). If antiembolic stockings are contraindicated (Box 13.6) then alternative forms of mechanical compression aids may need to be considered by the surgical team.

Figure 13.6 **Antiembolic stockings.**

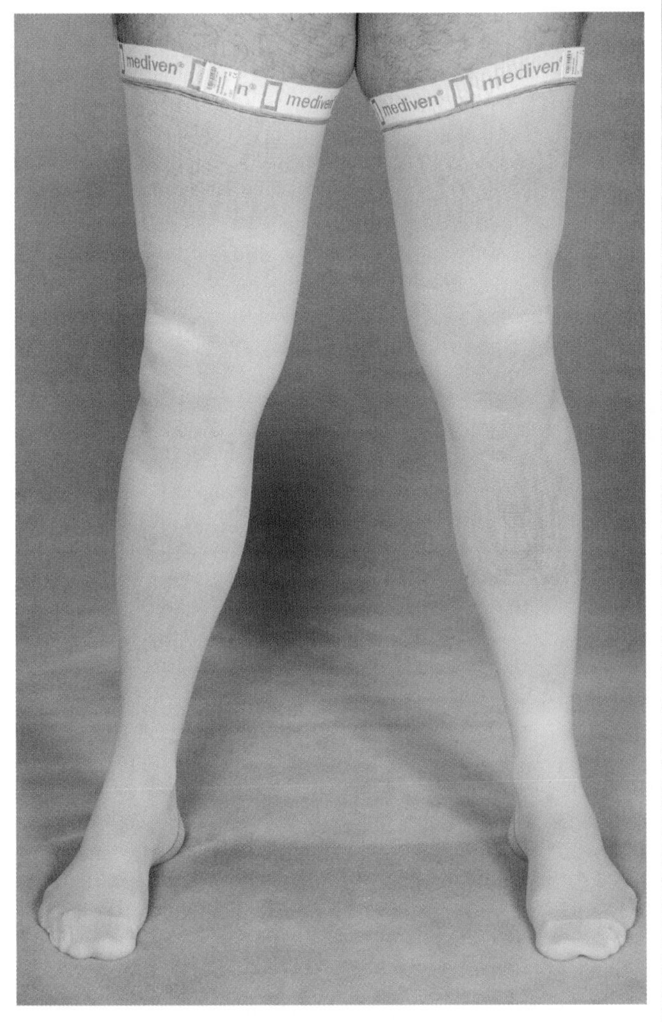

Figure 13.7 **Flowtron machine and boots.**

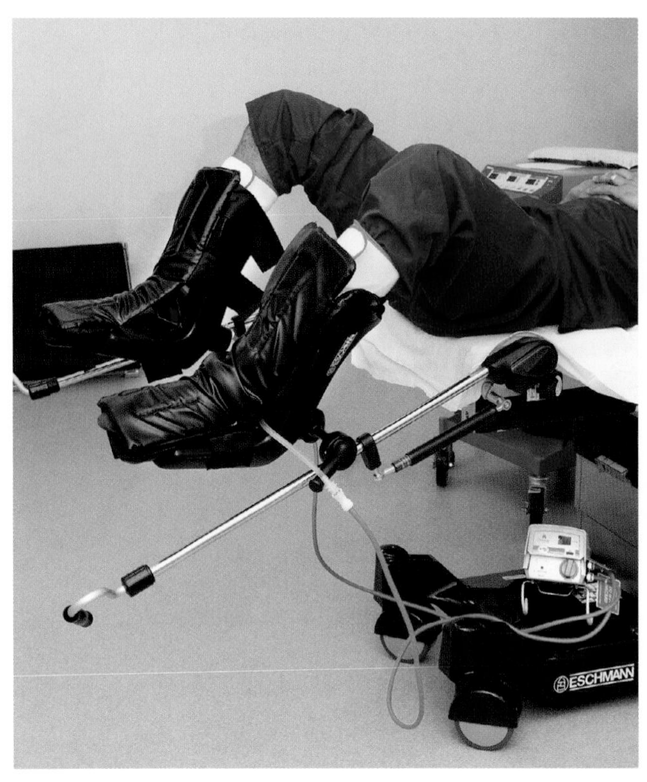

Patients should be given verbal and written information before surgery about the risks of VTE and the effectiveness of prophylaxis (NICE 2010) (see Figure 13.8 for an example of a patient information leaflet). It is estimated that 20% of patients undergoing major surgery will develop a DVT with the risk increasing to 40% of patients undergoing major orthopaedic surgery (Scottish Intercollegiate Guidelines Network 2002). Mechanical compression methods reduce the risk of DVT by about two-thirds when used as monotherapy and by about half when added to pharmacological methods (Roderick et al. 2005). Graduated compression (antiembolic) stockings promote venous flow and reduce venous stasis not only in the legs but also in the pelvic veins and inferior vena cava (Hayes et al. 2002, Rashid et al. 2005, Roderick et al. 2005).

Stockings should be applied according to manufacturer's instructions and must be removed daily to assess the condition of the skin and tissues. Information concerning the frequency of stocking removal, daily skin care and assessment is outlined in the section on immobility in the post-operative section.

Box 13.6 **Contraindications for antiembolism stockings**

- Suspected or proven peripheral arterial disease.
- Peripheral arterial bypass grafting.
- Peripheral neuropathy or other causes of sensory impairment.
- Local condition in which stockings may cause damage, such as fragile tissue paper skin.
- Pressure sores to heels. Pressure sores are a complication of antiembolic stockings and stockings should not be applied (NICE 2005b).
- Use caution and clinical judgement when applying antiembolism stockings over venous ulcers or wounds.

Source: Adapted from NICE (2005a), NICE (2010).

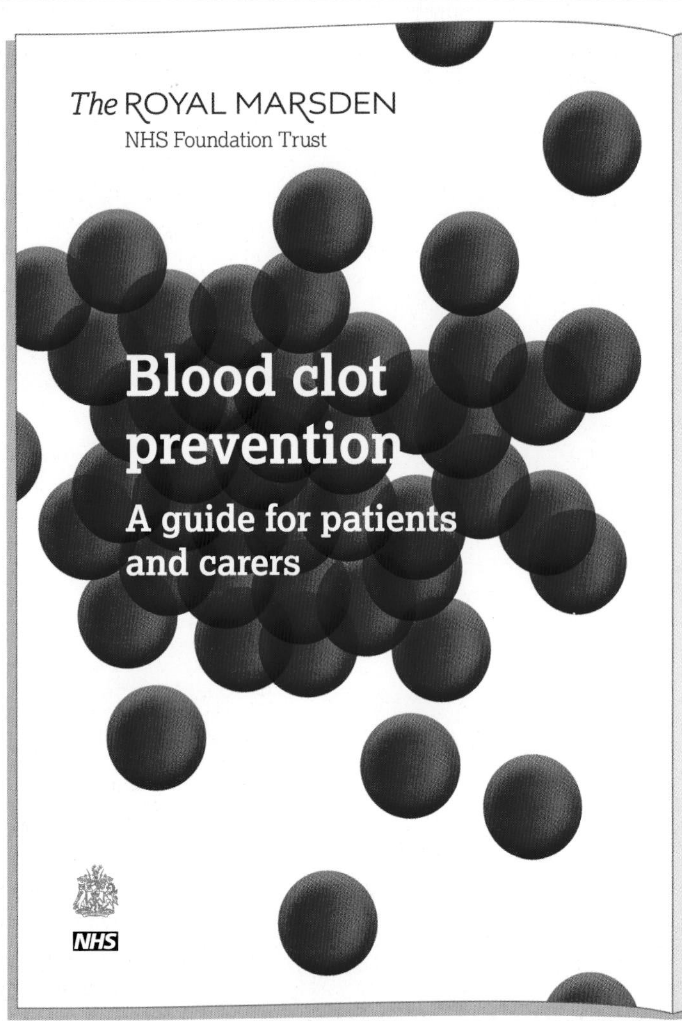

When I am in hospital what will be done to help prevent a VTE?

- **Stay hydrated** – if you are allowed to do so, drink plenty of fluid. However, if you are not allowed to do this, the doctors will give you fluids via a vein.
- **Move around** – keep mobile as much as you can. The physiotherapist will teach you some appropriate leg exercise.
- **Anti-embolic stockings** – If the doctor decides that you would be suitable for these, the nursing staff will fit you with a pair of stockings.
- **Intermittent calf pumps** – some surgical patients will have a special device which fits like a cuff around each calf (a bit like a blood pressure cuff). This will inflate and deflate alternately. These are designed to help prevent clot formation in the calf. They are not necessary for all surgical patients.
- **Medication (anticoagulants)** – your doctor might consider it necessary to prescribe you an anticoagulant (blood-thinning) drug to reduce your risk of developing a blood clot. Depending on the type of surgery you may be asked to continue this medication for 28 days following the operation.

Not all methods mentioned above are appropriate for all patients. Your doctor will assess which methods are most suitable for you as an individual.

If you are already taking blood-thinning medication such as warfarin please tell your doctor.

Figure 13.8 **Patient information sheet: DVT.** *Source:* Adapted from The Royal Marsden NHS Foundation Trust (2010).

Procedure guideline 13.1 Step-by-step guide to measuring and applying antiembolic stockings

Essential equipment

- Disposable tape measure (patient specific)
- Antiembolic stocking sizing chart
- Apron
- Patient records/documentation

Pre-procedure

Action	Rationale
1 Assess and record in the patient's documentation the patient's risk factors for VTE, that is, DVT and PE.	All patients admitted to hospital should undergo a risk assessment for venous thrombosis to determine the most appropriate preventive measures, that is thromboprophylaxis (House of Commons Health Committee 2005, **C**; NICE 2010, **C**; Roderick et al. 2005, **R1a**; Scottish Intercollegiate Guidelines Network 2002, **C**). The higher the number of risk factors, the greater the risk for VTE (NICE 2010, **C**; Scottish Intercollegiate Guidelines Network 2002, **C**).
2 Assess and record in the patient's documentation the patient's suitability for antiembolic stockings, identifying whether the patient has any contraindications to wearing antiembolic stockings (see Box 13.6).	To comply with national guidelines and hospital policy/ guidelines. To ensure that antiembolic stockings are used appropriately (All Wales Tissue Viability Nurse Forum 2009, **E**; House of Commons Health Committee 2005, **C**; NICE 2010, **C**; Rashid et al. 2005, **E**; Scottish Intercollegiate Guidelines Network 2002, **C**).
3 Explain and discuss the procedure with the patient.	To ensure that the patient understands the procedure and gives their valid consent (NMC 2010, **C**; NMC 2013, **C**).

Procedure	
4 Perform hand hygiene and put on apron prior to the procedure.	To prevent cross-infection (Loveday et al. 2014, **C**).
5 *Measurement* A Thigh length 1 Measure upper thigh circumference at widest part of thigh (Measurement #1) (**Action figure 5**). 2 Measure calf circumference at greatest dimension. NB: Please refer to individual manufacturer's instructions to ensure that no other measurements are necessary, e.g. length of leg. 3 Consult the product packaging to determine the appropriate size. (a) If right and left legs measure differently, order two different stocking sizes. (b) If thigh or calf circumference is greater than that stocked by manufacturer then refer to local trust guidelines to determine appropriate course of action. In some cases, knee length stocking may be appropriate. B Knee length 1 Measure calf circumference at greatest dimension. NB: Please refer to individual manufacturer's instructions to ensure that no other measurements are necessary, e.g. length of leg. 2 Consult the product packaging to determine the appropriate size. (a) If right and left legs measure differently, order two different stocking sizes. C Order two pairs of stockings.	To comply with the manufacturer's instructions. **C** Incorrect sizing causes swelling and bruising to ankles and can constrict blood supply, leading to long-term complications. **C** It has also been suggested that 15–20% of patients cannot effectively wear thigh-length antiembolic stockings because of unusual limb size or shape (Scottish Intercollegiate Guidelines Network 2002, **C**). To ensure that prophylaxis is uninterrupted during laundering care (if in accordance with local trust guidelines) or to send a pair home with the patient if appropriate. **C**
6 *Applying* (a) Insert hand into stocking as far as the heel pocket. (b) Grasp centre of heel pocket and turn stocking inside out to heel area. (c) Position stocking over foot and heel, ensuring patient's heel is centred in heel pocket (**Action figure 6a**). (d) Pull a few inches of the stocking up around the ankle and calf (**Action figure 6b**). (e) Continue pulling the stocking up the leg as described in manufacturer's instructions. When using thigh length, the top band rests in the gluteal furrow. (f) Smooth out wrinkles. (g) Align inspection window to fall under the toes (toes should not stick out).	To ensure correct size of stocking is fitted correctly. **C**. Thigh-length stockings are difficult to put on and can roll down, creating a tourniquet just above the knee which restricts blood supply, so patient monitoring and/or assistance should take place to ensure that stockings are fitted smoothly, are not rolled down or the top band folded down.
Post-procedure	
7 Document appropriate leg measurements and size of stockings applied in nursing documentation. Instruct patient and provide written information about the following: (a) reasons for wearing antiembolic stockings (b) how to fit and wear stockings (c) what to report to the nurse, for example any feelings of pain or numbness or skin problems (d) skin care, that is, wash and dry legs daily, applying emollient if clinically indicated (e) reasons for early mobilization and adequate hydration (f) reasons for not crossing legs or ankles – to prevent constriction of blood supply (g) length of time that the stockings should be worn, e.g. stockings should be removed for a maximum of 30 minutes daily and worn until the patient returns to their usual level of mobility.	To ensure that the patient understands how to fit and wear stockings, including self-care measures and what to report to the nurse so as to detect complications early, for example pressure sores, circulation difficulties of wearing antiembolic stockings (NICE 2010, **C**; Scottish Intercollegiate Guidelines Network 2002, **C**).

Procedure guideline 13.1 **Step-by-step guide to measuring and applying antiembolic stockings *(continued)***

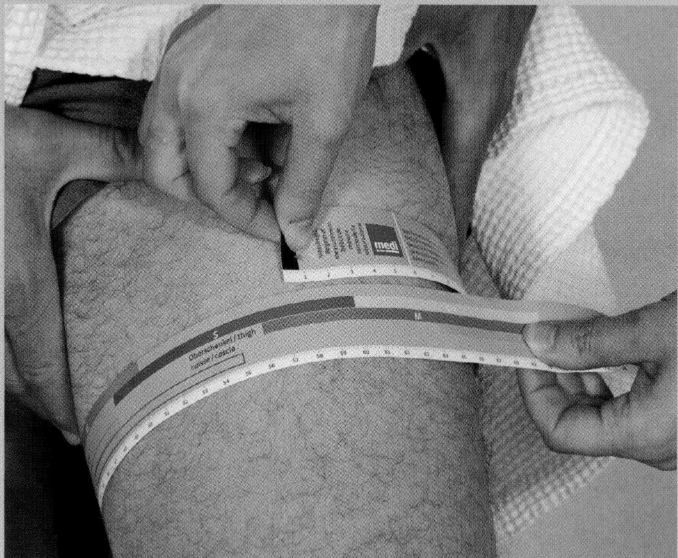

Action Figure 5 Measuring thigh diameter.

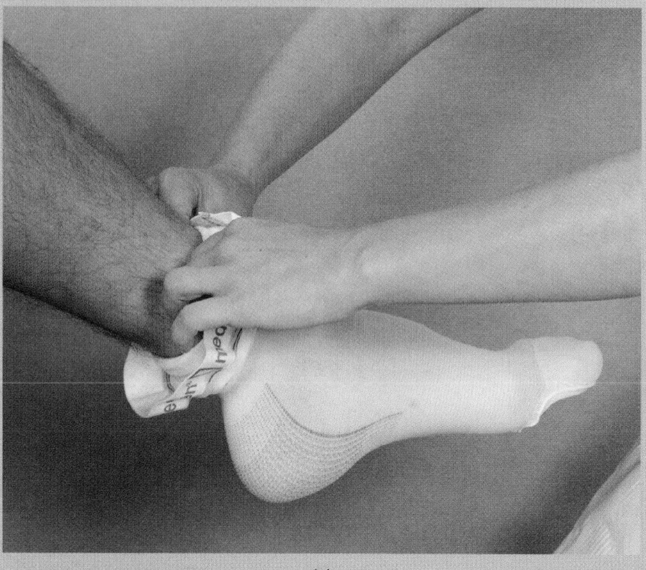

(a)

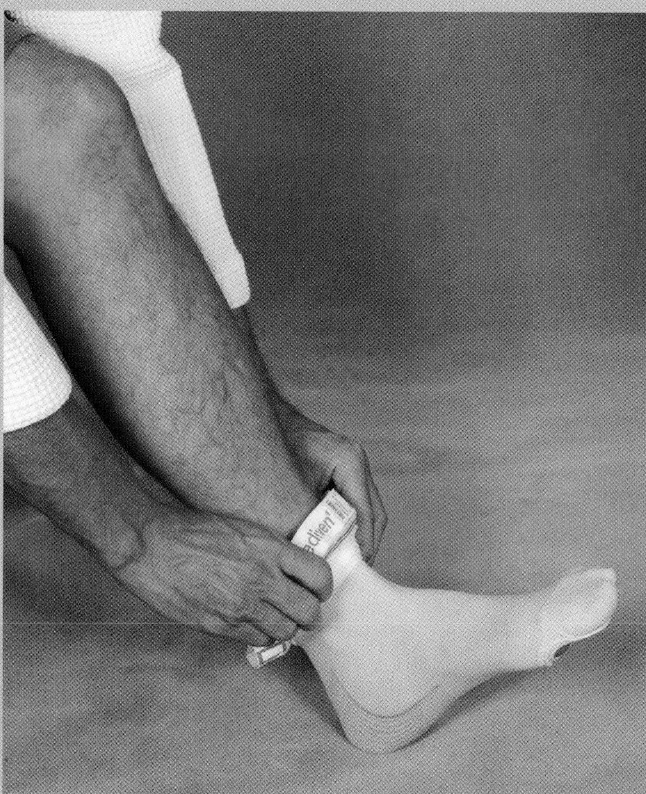

(b)

Action Figure 6 (a) Ensuring heel is centred in heel pocket. (b) Pull stocking up over the ankle.

Pre-operative fasting

DEFINITION

Pre-operative fasting is the practice of a patient abstaining from oral food and fluid intake for a determined period of time before an operation is performed.

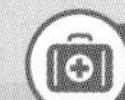

Learning Activity 13.3

Learning in practice: Pre-operative fasting

In your clinical area:

- Find out where the organization's policy on pre-operative fasting is located.
- Within the policy, check the guidance on times to stop taking solid food, fluids and clear fluids prior to surgery.

RELATED THEORY

General anaesthesia carries the risk of the patient inhaling gastric contents during induction, which could result in respiratory problems (including aspiration pneumonitis and aspiration pneumonia) or at worst acute respiratory failure and death (King 2010). This is due to the potential for airway reflexes (such as coughing or laryngospasm) or gastrointestinal motor responses (such as gagging or recurrent swallowing) occurring during surgery (AAGBI 2010). The lower oesophageal sphincter (LOS) is functionally distinct from the oesophagus, and acts as a valve preventing the reflux of gastric contents. Barrier pressure is the difference between LOS pressure (normally 20–30 mmHg) and intragastric pressure (normally 5–10 mmHg) (King 2010). LOS pressure is reduced by several factors, including various drugs used during anaesthesia, including propofol and opioids. This drop in barrier pressure increases the risk of aspiration which increases if the gastric volume exceeds 1000 mL (King 2010). Surgery itself can be a factor as manipulation of organs in the chest or abdominal cavities may force gastric contents up the oesophagus (AAGBI 2010).

Gastric volume is influenced by the rate of gastric secretions (approximately 0.6 mL/kg/h), swallowing of saliva (1 mL/kg/h), ingestion of solids/liquids and the rate of gastric emptying (King 2010). In order to reduce this risk, patients need to be fasted pre-operatively for long enough to allow the stomach to empty (AAGBI 2010, Benington and Severn 2007). Fasting before general anaesthesia aims to reduce the volume and acidity of stomach contents during surgery, thus reducing the risk of regurgitation/aspiration (Brady et al. 2003). Patients at greatest risk of aspiration are those undergoing unplanned surgery, obese patients, those with abdominal pathology but also inadequate level of anaesthesia (King 2010). Other examples are outlined in Box 13.7.

However, the psychological and physiological effects of hypoglycaemia and fluid deprivation can be very unpleasant, leading to severe thirst, hunger, irritability and an increased incidence of headache and can affect the incidence of post-operative nausea and vomiting (RCN 2005). Dehydration is a particular problem, resulting in an exaggerated hypotensive effect on induction of anaesthesia and making central vein location difficult (AAGBI 2010).

Ensuring that the patient understands the rationale for fasting is important in order to reduce anxiety. Historically, there has been much debate over an optimum pre-operative fasting time. Box 13.8 outlines current best practice pre-operative fasting guidelines for healthy adults undergoing elective surgery.

It is important to be aware that several factors can delay gastric emptying (O'Callaghan 2002). These include:

- reduced conscious level
- systemic opiate therapy
- recent history of difficulty in eating, swallowing, digesting food
- recent history of dyspepsia – heartburn, particularly on lying down or bending over
- upper gastrointestinal surgery
- anxiety
- pregnancy or labour
- abdominal pain
- renal failure
- diabetes.

Box 13.7 **Predisposing factors for aspiration under general anaesthesia**

Patient factors	Increased gastric content	Intestinal obstruction Non-fasted Drugs Delayed gastric emptying
	Lower oesophageal sphincter incompetence	Hiatus hernia Gastro-oesophageal reflux Pregnancy Morbid obesity Neuromuscular disease
	Decreased laryngeal reflexes	Head injury Bulbar palsy
	Gender	Male
	Age	Elderly
Operation factors	Procedure	Emergency Laparoscopic
	Position	Lithotomy
Anaesthetic factors	Airway	Difficult intubation Gas insufflation
	Maintenance	Inadequate depth

Source: Adapted from King (2010).

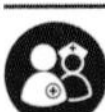

Box 13.8 **Pre-operative fasting guidelines**

- 6 hours fasting from solid food, provided this is a light meal (refer to local trust guidelines for examples of suitable light meal).
- Sweets, including lollipops, are solid food. A minimum pre-operative fasting time of 6 hours is recommended.
- Tea and coffee with milk are acceptable up to 6 hours before surgery.
- Clear fluids (those through which newsprint can be read) up to 2 hours prior to surgery (see Box 13.9).
- Patients being fed by nasogastric or gastrostomy tube should have their feed stopped 6 hours prior to surgery and water 2 hours prior to surgery.
- Chewing gum should be avoided on the day of surgery.
- Regular medication taken orally should be continued pre-operatively unless there is advice to the contrary. Patients can have up to 30 mL of water orally to help them take medication.

Source: Adapted from AAGBI (2010), RCN (2005).

Patients with hiatus hernia and suspected delayed gastric emptying are at high risk of aspirating. Advice on pre-operative fasting times should be given to these patients by the anaesthetist (AAGBI 2010, King 2010).

In patients with any suspicion of delayed gastric emptying, the anaesthetist responsible for performing the procedure will determine the period of pre-operative fasting. Patients undergoing emergency surgery should be treated as though they have a full stomach (RCN 2005) and the period of fasting will be prescribed by the anaesthetist responsible for the anaesthetic. It is important that all elderly patients, anyone who has undergone bowel preparation, sick patients and mothers who are breastfeeding should not spend long periods without hydration. In these groups intravenous fluids should be considered (AAGBI 2010).

It is recognized that fasting times may be prolonged due to alterations in the operating list. Some alterations are unavoidable, but patients should be kept informed of changes to the theatre list and those without disorders of gastric emptying allowed to continue drinking clear fluids up to 2 hours prior to rescheduled surgery (Box 13.9) (Powell-Tuck et al. 2011). Patients with disorders of gastric emptying or in cases where the theatre time is difficult to ascertain should be offered mouthwashes to keep their mouths moist and intravenous fluids considered if not contraindicated for the surgery being performed, e.g. liver surgery.

Skin preparation

DEFINITION

The purpose of pre-operative skin preparation is to remove visible contaminants and to reduce the levels of naturally occurring skin

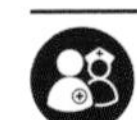

Box 13.9 **Examples of clear fluids**

- Water
- Tea/coffee *without* milk
- Fruit/herb tea
- Fruit squash
- Polycal diluted half and half with water
- Fortijuice
- Enlive

flora, particularly Staphylococcus aureus, to reduce the risk of surgical site infection (Wicker and O'Neill 2010).

RELATED THEORY

Normal bacterial flora live in the nose, groin, armpit, gut, skin and hair of everybody. Organisms may become pathogenic when they move out of their normal area on the body to an open wound (Wicker and O'Neill 2010). NICE (2008) guidelines advise patients to shower or have a bath using soap, either the day before or on the day of surgery. Whilst there is no evidence concerning patient theatre attire, NICE (2008) guidelines advise that patients are given a clean theatre gown to wear and asked to remove their own clothing (depending on the operation). Theatre gowns should maintain the patient's comfort and dignity whilst allowing easy access to the operative site (NICE 2008). Furthermore, theatre gowns avoid placing patients' own clothes at risk of contamination from blood, body and washout fluids (Pudner 2010).

A controversial aspect of skin preparation concerns the removal of body hair from the surgical site. Current NICE (2008) guidance advises against routine hair removal to reduce the risk of surgical site infection. If hair has to be removed in order to adequately view or access the operative site then the best practice as shown in Table 13.4 is advised.

Marking skin for surgery

DEFINITION

To identify unambiguously the intended site of surgical incision. The mark should be an arrow, drawn with an indelible, latex-free marker pen and should extend to, or near to, the exact incision site.

RELATED THEORY

The surgeon may need to mark an area of the body for surgery, e.g. a limb to be operated on or the position of an organ such as a specific kidney in a patient undergoing a nephrectomy. Marking the surgical site is essential for the planning of any surgical procedure and for the prevention of wrong-site surgery (Mears et al. 2009, NPSA 2005). The incidence of wrong-site surgery is low but any error can be devastating and in some cases fatal. In 2005 the NPSA published recommendations promoting correct-site surgery. These establish a consistent method of marking patients prior to surgery and provide a checklist of steps to be taken to avoid errors.

The marking should be undertaken by the surgeon performing the operation or competent deputy (i.e. an individual capable of performing the procedure themselves) who will be present at the surgery, to ensure the correct site is marked and this should be checked against the patient's consent form (Haynes et al. 2009). The mark should be an arrow, drawn with an indelible, latex-free marker pen and should extend to, or near to, the exact incision site. The majority of surgical site marking pens contain gentian violet ink, which has antifungal properties (Pennsylvania Patient Safety Authority 2008). Other types of marking pens include permanent ink markers, which despite their lack of antifungal properties have not been found to affect the sterility of the surgical field (Zhao et al. 2009). Marking must be undertaken before pre-medication or anaesthesia so that patients can be involved in ensuring the mark is in the right place. It needs to remain visible after the application of antiseptic (aqueous or alcohol-based) skin preparation (e.g. povidone-iodine or chlorhexidine) and ideally remain visible after the application of theatre drapes (Mears et al. 2009, NPSA 2005). The surgical site mark should not be easily removed with skin preparation but should not be so permanent as to last weeks or months after the surgical procedure.

Following surgery, once the wound has healed, residual traces of the marker pen can be gently removed using warm, soapy water. It is important not to rub too hard to prevent irritating the skin as well as sinking the ink deeper into skin tissues, making it harder to extract. This process may need to be repeated over a series of days.

There are circumstances where marking may not be appropriate.

- Emergency surgery.
- Surgery on teeth or mucous membranes.
- Bilateral procedures such as tonsillectomy and squint surgery.
- Situations where laterality of surgery will be confirmed during the procedure (NPSA 2005).

If a patient refuses pre-operative skin marking, local policy should be followed but include documentation in the patient's nursing and medical notes and on the Surgical Safety Checklist (WHO 2008), clearly stating that the patient refuses marking.

There are some situations in which a specialist nurse may mark the skin. For example, stoma therapists mark the position on the patient's skin which is the optimum place for the stoma to be placed (see Chapter 5: Elimination).

Table 13.4 Skin preparation

Principle	Rationale
Electric clippers with a single-use disposable head should be used	Clippers do not come into contact with the skin and therefore reduce the risk of cuts and abrasions (JBI 2008, NICE 2008, Pudner 2010). Single-use head prevents cross-infection (AORN 2008). Electric clippers with single-use disposable heads are the most cost-effective method of hair removal (NICE 2008)
If hair removal is required to facilitate access or view of surgical site then where possible, this should be undertaken on the day of surgery	Undertaken as close to the surgery as possible (NICE 2008, Wicker and O'Neill 2010)
Only hair interfering with the surgical procedure should be removed	To prevent unnecessary trauma or visible difference for the patient (Murkin 2009, Wicker and O'Neill 2010)

Pre-operative pregnancy testing

RELATED THEORY

There is an increased risk of spontaneously aborting the fetus when undergoing surgery during the first trimester of pregnancy (Allaert et al. 2007). It is possible that this is affected by surgical manipulation and the patient's underlying medical condition rather than exposure to anaesthesia (Allaert et al. 2007, Kuczkowski 2004).

Prior to consenting to surgery, all female patients who have commenced menstruation (menarche) need to be informed of the risks surgery may pose to a pregnancy (NICE 2003). The clinician performing the procedure or the appropriately delegated representative (i.e. an individual capable of performing the procedure themselves) is responsible for informing patients of the risks of surgery and is therefore responsible for ensuring that a female patient has had her pregnancy status assessed

(DH 2001, GMC 2008). Once informed of the risks, the patient will need to take responsibility for her own contraception (NICE 2003).

All female patients who have commenced menstruation (menarche) should be considered for pregnancy testing if they express a concern that they may be pregnant or are undergoing gynaecology surgery (NICE 2003). Any pregnancy testing requires informed consent and documentation in the patient's medical record, including test results or patient refusal and the responsible surgical team must be informed prior to the initiation of surgery (NICE 2003). If a previously unknown pregnancy is detected, the risks and benefits of the surgery can be discussed with the patient. Surgery may be postponed or, if the decision is to go ahead, the anaesthetic and surgical approaches can be modified if necessary (NPSA 2010). In emergency situations, confirmation of pregnancy should not delay treatment and should be judged within the clinical assessment of risk.

LEGAL AND PROFESSIONAL ISSUES

The practice of checking and documenting current pregnancy status in the immediate pre-operative period has been shown to be inconsistent (NPSA 2010). Pre-operative assessment may take place weeks in advance of a planned operation but pregnancy status may change in the intervening time, so pregnancy status must be rechecked by asking the patient in the immediate pre-operative period on the ward and documented in the perioperative documentation used by staff performing the final clinical and identity checks before the surgical intervention (NPSA 2010).

Prevention of toxic shock syndrome from tampon use

DEFINITION

Staphylococcal toxic shock syndrome (TSS) is a rare, life-threatening systemic bacterial infection, historically associated with the use of superabsorbent tampons. TSS is characterized by high fever, hypotension, rash and multiorgan dysfunction (Deresiewicz 2004).

RELATED THEORY

Toxic shock syndrome occurs when the bacteria *Staphylococcus aureus* and *Streptococcus pyrogenes*, which normally live harmlessly on the skin, enter the bloodstream and produce poisonous toxins. These toxins cause severe vasodilation which in turn causes a large drop in blood pressure (shock), resulting in dizziness and confusion. They also begin to damage tissue, including skin and organs, and can disturb many vital organ functions. If TSS is left untreated, the combination of shock and organ damage can result in death.

Whilst TSS can also affect men and children, the first reported cases of TSS involved women who were using tampons during menstruation (Eckert and Lentz 2012). Female patients of menstruating age therefore need to be made aware of the dangers of using tampons which can cause infection leading to TSS. At the time of admission, it is important to ask female patients if they are menstruating and to highlight the dangers of using tampons during surgery. If tampons are left *in situ* for longer than 6 hours, infection may develop. Nurses can offer a sanitary pad as an alternative.

Latex sensitivity and allergy

RELATED THEORY

Latex is a natural rubber composed of proteins and added chemicals. Its durable, flexible properties give it a high degree of protection from many micro-organisms, which makes it an ideal fibre to use for many healthcare products. It currently provides the best protection against infection and gives the sensitivity and control needed in the healthcare field. It is found in the following products (AORN 2010, HSE 2004).

- Gloves
- Airways
- Intravenous tubing
- Stethoscopes
- Catheters
- Wound drains
- Dressings and bandages

Some of the proteins in the natural rubber latex can cause sensitivity and allergic reactions and the incidence of latex hypersensitivity seems to be increasing (Rose 2005). Powdered gloves can create the greatest risk as proteins leak into the powder which can become airborne when gloves are removed and inhaling the powder may lead to respiratory sensitization. The amount of latex exposure needed to produce sensitization is unknown. Sensitivity can be described as the development of an immunological memory to specific latex proteins, which can be asymptomatic. A substance which causes sensitization is one which is capable of causing an allergic reaction in certain people. Allergy is the visible reaction of the sensitivity, for example hives, rhinitis, conjunctivitis, anaphylaxis, which can be serious or potentially life-threatening (Table 13.5) (AORN 2010, HSE 2012).

Once sensitization has taken place, further exposure will cause symptoms to recur and increasing exposure to latex proteins increases the risk of developing allergic symptoms (HSE 2012); therefore sensitivities and allergies should be treated in the same way (AORN 2010). Routes of exposure include:

- direct external contact (i.e. to gloves or other latex products)
- airborne exposure
- direct contact of the mucous membranes
- internal patient exposure from healthcare provider use of natural rubber latex gloves during surgical procedures
- internally placed devices (e.g. wound drains) (AORN 2010).

Latex allergies are classified as: irritant contact dermatitis; type I and type IV reactions.

LEGAL AND PROFESSIONAL ISSUES

Healthcare providers have an ethical responsibility to prevent latex sensitization and, because there is no cure, protection must be paramount. Employers should have a latex allergy policy and procedure which should provide information and instruction on measures to identify patients at risk, patient education, interventions to reduce undue latex exposure, recognizing symptoms of sensitization and the action to be taken if a sensitization is suspected (AORN 2010, HSE 2012).

Assessment and monitoring for symptoms of latex allergy in both the conscious and unconscious patient are required at all stages of perioperative care. The assessment should cover the following known risk factors for latex allergy.

- History of multiple surgeries beginning at an early age (e.g. spina bifida, urinary malformation).
- History of hayfever or asthma.
- History of an allergic reaction to latex. For example, a history suggestive of reactivity to latex may be gained by anecdotal accounts of swelling or itching of the lips when blowing up balloons, following dental examinations or swelling and itching of the hands when using household gloves.
- History of an allergic reaction during an operation.
- Past experience of itchy skin, skin rash or redness when in contact with rubber products.

Table 13.5 **Allergic reactions**

Reaction	Description	Symptoms
Irritation	Irritant contact dermatitis, a non-allergenic reaction caused by soaps, gloves, glove powder and hand creams	Dry, crusty, itchy skin Rashes and inflammation
Type I reaction: immediate hypersensitivity – occurs within minutes and can fade rapidly after removal of the latex	Immediate hypersensitivity, sometimes called immunoglobulin E response. Caused by exposure to proteins in latex on glove surface and/or bound to powder	Most severe reaction Wheal and flare response Irritant and allergic contact Dermatitis Facial swelling Rhinitis Urticaria Respiratory distress and asthma Rarely, anaphylactic shock
Type IV reaction: delayed hypersensitivity – usually occurring within 6–48 hours of contact	Sometimes known as allergic contact dermatitis, caused by exposure to chemicals used in latex manufacturing	Red, raised, palpable area with bumps, sores and cracks

Source: Adapted from AORN (2010), HSE (2004), Rose (2005).

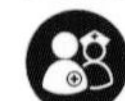

Box 13.10 **Pre-operative actions for patients with potential or confirmed latex allergy**

- Notify operating theatre of potential or confirmed latex allergy 24–48 hours (or as soon as possible) before scheduled procedure.
- Identify the patient's risk factors for latex allergy and communicate them to the healthcare team.
- Schedule the procedure as the first case of the day if the facility is not latex safe.
- Plan for a latex-safe environment of care.
- The theatre must be cleaned with latex-free gloves and equipment.
- All latex products must be removed or covered with plastics so that the rubber elements are not exposed.
- All healthcare staff in direct contact with the patient must wear vinyl gloves during procedures and in the vicinity of the patient.
- Secure latex-free products for all latex-containing items used by surgeons and anaesthetists.
- A latex-free contents box or trolley (this holds stock of all latex-free products that will be required during surgery and anaesthetic) should be ready in every theatre department and recovery room. There should be a list of all latex-free equipment with the manufacturers listed available in the box or trolley.
- Notify surgeon if no alternative product is available.
- Notify anaesthetist if latex-containing product to be used and develop plan of emergency care if necessary.
- Where a type I (immediate hypersensitivity reaction) allergy is suspected, suitable clinical management procedures must be ready for use in the event of the patient having a hypersensitivity reaction.

Source: Adapted from AORN (2004), AORN (2010).

- Past skin irritation from an examination by a doctor or dentist wearing rubber gloves.
- Past sneezing, wheezing or chest tightness when exposed to rubber (AORN 2010).

If a suspected or confirmed latex sensitivity or allergy is found, this information must be documented in the patient's medical notes and communicated to all members of the healthcare team and departments that the patient may visit, including theatre, recovery, pathology and radiology (AORN 2010, Rose 2005). Box 13.10 outlines the pre-operative actions for patients with potential or confirmed latex allergy. The anaesthetist will need to be informed so that decisions can be made regarding potential allergy prophylaxis pre-operatively. A latex-safe environment is recommended – one where every reasonable effort has been made to prevent high-allergen and airborne latex sources from coming into direct contact with affected individuals. Latex-free alternative items should be collected and stored in a quick-access location for ease of access and identification. At present, best practice dictates that patients with a suspected or confirmed latex allergy be scheduled first on the morning list because it is assumed that the inactivity in the room during the previous evening hours causes the content of latex-coated powder in the ambient air to be lowest in the morning (AORN 2010, Rose 2005). Further guidance may be sought online from the Association of Perioperative Registered Nurses (AORN: www.aorn.org).

There is also a voluntary scheme in place for reporting cases of latex sensitization, both of staff and patients, to the Medical Devices Agency (MDA), which is an executive agency of the Department of Health (HSE 2012).

Pre-operative theatre checklist

The pre-operative theatre checklist (see Procedure guideline 13.2: Pre-operative care: checking that the patient is fully prepared for surgery and Figure 13.9) is the final check between the ward and the operating theatre and should be completed as fully as possible to reduce the possibility of any complications during the period that the patient is put under anaesthetic or during surgery itself.

One item on the list is ensuring that blood results and X-rays or imaging accompany the patient. The blood results are important for assessing patient haemoglobin levels which will help in transporting oxygen and also the electrolytes to identify any imbalances such as low sodium or potassium as these can interfere with anaesthetic agents and can cause cardiovascular disturbances such as arrhythmias (Higgins and Higgins 2013) (Table 13.6, Table 13.7).

Prior to taking the patient to the operating theatre, the clinician performing the procedure should check that the patient still consents (see Consent section earlier in this chapter). Patients should not in any situation be given routine pre-operative medication before being asked for their consent to proceed with the treatment (NMC 2013).

Ward & Anaesthetic Room – Pre-operative Checklist

Each entry below must be ticked to indicate Yes, No, or N/A (not applicable) with the relevant details

1st Check by Ward/Unit Nurse before pre-medication if prescribed or prior to leaving the ward				2nd Check by Theatre Practitioner / Nurse in anaesthetic room / appropriate area		
SECTION A To be checked from nursing/medical notes/EPR	Yes	No	N/A	Yes	No	N/A
Consent to anaesthetic / operation form signed						
Patient has undergone pre-anaesthetic examination						
Medical case notes / Adult Peri-operative Care Plan to accompany patient						
Imaging / Blood Results / Electrocardiogram (ECG) accompany patient or available on PACS						
Confirm blood has been cross-matched and ordered						
Confirm Infection Status and swab results e.g. MRSA results and liaise with infection control, clinical team and theatres if appropriate						
SECTION B To be checked from nursing/medical notes/EPR	Yes	No	N/A	Yes	No	N/A
Confirm Pregnancy Status: Check and confirm pregnancy status on all women of childbearing age Date of last menstrual period:............................... Pregnancy Test Date:.................. Result:........................ If positive, has the surgeon been informed: Yes: 0 No 0 Comments:						

1st Check by Ward/Unit Nurse before pre-medication if prescribed or prior to leaving the ward				2nd Check by Theatre Practitioner / Nurse in anaesthetic room / appropriate area		
SECTION C To be checked by observing/asking patient	Yes	No	N/A	Yes	No	N/A
Two Identification Bands (e.g. wrist & ankle) present and correct						
Red Identification Bands (in case of allergy) present and correct						
Operation Site Marked if appropriate						
Time of Last Food (24 Hr Clock):............... Time of Last Drink (24 Hr Clock):............... Type of Drink:.......................................						
Time pre-medication given (24 Hr Clock):.....................						
Braces / Caps / Crowns / Bridge work / Loose Teeth (If Yes, specify)						
False Teeth / Dentures removed / with patient (Please circle) Supply denture pot with patient's details						

Figure 13.9 **Pre-operative ward–theatre checklist.**

Shower/Bath taken on day of surgery						
Valuables placed in hospital property						
Theatre gown						
Anti-embolic Stockings applied (please document why if removed)						
Cottonbased underwear worn or consent for removal of underwear						
Contact Lenses removed						
Glasses removed / worn / (Please circle) Supply patient's glasses case with patient's details Kept on Ward / Sent back to Ward / Kept in Operating Theatre						
Hearing Aid removed/to be removed by Anaesthetist (Please circle) Supply envelope with patient's details Kept on Ward / Sent back to Ward / Kept in Operating Theatre						
False Nails / Nail Varnish / Make Up removed (Please circle)						
Jewellery / Ring(s) / Metal Hair Clip(s) are removed or taped						
Body Piercing is removed or taped Area of piercing(s)..						
Prosthesis e.g. knee replacements, implants, pacemaker (specify):..						
Waterlow Score:.................................... Pressure Area Problems / Aids (If Yes, specify)						
Time of last micturition .... OR urinary catheter / nephrostomy tube (please circle)						

	Signature	Full Name (PRINT)	Date	Time
Ward/Unit Nurse				
Ward/Escort Nurse (i.e. transfers/handovers patient to theatre staff)				
Theatre Practitioner / Nurse				

Figure 13.9 *(continued)*

Table 13.6 **Haematology values**

Test	Reference range	Functions/additional information
Red blood cells (RBC)	Men: 4.5–6.5 × 10^{12}/L Women: 3.9–5.6 × 10^{12}/L	The main function of the RBC is the transport of oxygen and carbon dioxide
Haemoglobin	Men: 13.5–13.5 g/dL Women: 11.5–15.5 g/dL	Haemoglobin (Hb) is a protein pigment found within the RBC which carries the oxygen Anaemia (deficiency in the number of RBC or in the Hb content) may occur for many reasons. Changes to cell production, deficient dietary intake or blood loss may be relevant and need to be investigated further
White blood cells (WBC)	Men: 3.7–9.5 × 10^9/L Women: 3.9–11.1 × 10^9/L	The function of the WBC is defence against infection. There are different kinds of WBC: neutrophils, lymphocytes, monocytes, eosinophils and basophils. Leucopenia is a WBC count lower than 3.7 and is usually associated with the use of cytotoxic drugs. Leucocytosis (high levels of neutrophils and lymphocytes) occurs as the body's normal response to infection and after surgery. Leukaemia involves an increased WBC count caused by changes in cell production in the bone marrow. The leukaemic cells enter the blood in increased numbers in an immature state
Platelets	Men: 150–400 × 10^9/L Women: 150–400 × 10^9/L	Clot formation occurs when platelets and the blood protein fibrin combine. A patient may be thrombocytopenic (low platelet count) due to drugs/poor production or have a raised count (thrombocytosis) with infection or autoimmune disease
Coagulation/ international normalized ratio (INR)	INR range 2–3 (in some cases a range of 3–4.5 is acceptable)	Coagulation occurs to prevent excessive blood loss by the formation of a clot (thrombus). However, a clot that forms in an artery may block the vessel and cause an infarction or ischaemia which can be fatal. Aspirin, warfarin and heparin are three drugs used for the prevention and/or treatment of thrombosis. It is imperative that patients on warfarin therapy receive regular monitoring to ensure a balance of slowing the clot-forming process and maintaining the ability of the blood to clot

Table 13.7 **Biochemistry values**

Test	Reference range	Functions/additional information
Sodium	135–145 mmol/L	The main function of sodium is to maintain extracellular volume (water stored outside the cells), acid/base balance and the transmitting of nerve impulses. *Hypernatraemia* (serum sodium >145 mmol/L) may be an indication of dehydration due to fluid loss from diarrhoea, excessive sweating, increased urinary output or a poor oral intake of fluid. An increased salt intake may also cause an elevation. *Hyponatraemia* (serum sodium <135 mmol/L) may be indicated in fluid retention (oedema)
Potassium	3.5–5.2 mmol/L	Potassium plays a major role in nerve conduction, muscle function, acid/base balance and osmotic pressure. It has a direct effect on cardiac muscle, influencing cardiac output by helping to control the rate and force of each contraction. The most common cause of *hyperkalaemia* (serum potassium >5.2 mmol/L) is chronic renal failure. The kidneys are unable to excrete potassium. The level may be elevated due to an increased intake of potassium supplements during treatment. Tissue cell destruction caused by trauma/cytotoxic therapy may cause a release of potassium from the cells and an elevation in the potassium plasma level. It may also be observed in untreated diabetic ketoacidosis. Urgent treatment is required as hyperkalaemia may lead to changes in cardiac muscle contraction and cause subsequent cardiac arrest. The main cause of *hypokalaemia* (serum potassium <3.5 mmol/L) is the loss of potassium via the kidneys during treatment with thiazide diuretics. Excessive/chronic diarrhoea may also cause a decreased potassium level
Urea	2.5–6.5 mmol/L	Urea is a waste product of metabolism that is transported to the kidneys and excreted as urine. Elevated levels of urea may indicate poor kidney function
Creatinine	55–105 μmol/L	Creatinine is a waste product of metabolism that is transported to the kidneys and excreted as urine. Elevated levels of creatinine may indicate poor kidney function
Calcium	2.20–2.60 mmol/L	Most of the calcium in the body is stored in the bone but ionized calcium, which circulates in the blood plasma, plays an important role in the transmission of nerve impulses and for the functioning of cardiac and skeletal muscle. It is also vital for blood coagulation. High calcium levels (hypercalcaemia >2.6 mmol/L) can be due to hyperthyroidism, hyperparathyroidism or malignancy. Elevation in calcium levels may cause cardiac arrhythmia, potentially leading to cardiac arrest. Tumour cells can cause excessive production of a protein called parathormone-related polypeptide (PTHrP) which causes loss of calcium from the bone and an increase in blood calcium levels. This is a major reason for hypercalcaemia in cancer patients (Higgins and Higgins 2013). *Hypocalcaemia* (<2.20 mmol/L) is often associated with vitamin D deficiency due to inadequate intake or increased loss due to GI disease. Mild hypocalcaemia may be symptomless but severe disease may cause increased neuromuscular excitability and cardiac arrhythmias. It is also a common feature of chronic renal failure (Higgins and Higgins 2013)
C-reactive protein (CRP)	<10 mg/L	Elevation in the CRP level can be a useful indication of bacterial infection. CRP is monitored after surgery and for patients who have a high risk of infection. The CRP level can help monitor the severity of inflammation and assist in the diagnosis of conditions such as systemic lupus erythematosus (SLE), ulcerative colitis and Crohn's disease (Higgins and Higgins 2013)
Albumin	35–50 g/L	Albumin is a protein found in blood plasma which assists in the transport of water-soluble substances and the maintenance of blood plasma volume
Bilirubin	(total) <13 μmol/L	Bilirubin is produced from the breakdown of haemoglobin; it is transported to the liver for excretion in bile. Elevated levels of bilirubin may cause jaundice

Procedure guideline 13.2 Pre-operative care: checking that the patient is fully prepared for surgery

Essential equipment

- Two namebands
- Theatre gown
- Cotton-based underwear or disposable pants can be worn if this does not interfere with surgery
- Antiembolic stockings
- Labelled containers for dentures, glasses and/or hearing aid if necessary
- Hypoallergenic tape
- Patient records/documentation including medical records, consent form, drug chart, X-ray films, blood test results, anaesthetic assessment, record and pre-operative checklist

(continued)

Procedure guideline 13.2 Pre-operative care: checking that the patient is fully prepared for surgery *(continued)*

Procedure

Action	Rationale
1 Discuss with the patient: • if they know what surgery they are having and why • if they can tell you about the wound, any intravenous infusions or drains, etc. that they may expect after the surgery • if they have been told about levels of pain and how it will be controlled • how they can be involved in ensuring they recover as quickly as possible, etc.	To ensure that the patient understands the nature and outcome of the surgery, to reduce anxiety and possible post-operative complications (Walker 2002, **E**).
2 Check that the patient has undergone relevant investigative procedures and that the results are included with the patient's notes. Examples include X-ray, ECG, MRI, CT, ECHO, blood test, urinalysis.	To ensure all relevant information is available to the nurses, anaesthetists and surgeons (AORN 2000, **C**).
3 Confirm and document when the patient last had food or drink, ensuring that this complies with pre-operative instructions and document in pre-operative documentation.	To reduce the risk of regurgitation and inhalation of stomach contents on induction of anaesthesia. It can take 9 hours or more for a substantial meal to be emptied from the stomach (AAGBI 2010, **C**; King 2010, **C**; RCN 2005, **C**).
4 Confirm and document which medications the patient has taken and when. Ensure this complies with pre-operative instructions and document in pre-operative documentation.	To ensure the patient does not take and/or omit any medication which could adversely affect surgery e.g. continuation of high dose warfarin.
5 If the patient is female and of child-bearing age:	
(a) check her pregnancy status and document the result in the pre-operative documentation. If a pregnancy test is required (e.g. if the patient expresses a concern that she may be pregnant or she is undergoing gynaecology surgery) (NICE 2003), test results should be given to the patient and documented in the pre-operative documentation	To eliminate the possibility of unknown pregnancy prior to the planned surgical procedure (NPSA 2010, **E**).
(b) if appropriate, ask the patient if she is menstruating and ensure that she has a sanitary towel in place and not a tampon.	This is to prevent infection if the tampon is left in place for longer than 6 hours (www.tamponalert.org.uk, **C**).
6 In the presence of the patient, check the consent form is correctly completed, signed and dated.	To comply with legal requirements and hospital policy and to ensure that the patient has understood the surgical procedure (NMC 2013, **C**).
7 If applicable, check the operation site has been marked correctly with the patient and the consent form.	To ensure the patient undergoes the correct surgery for which they have consented (AORN 2000, **C**; Haynes et al. 2009, **C**).
8 Check that the patient has undergone pre-anaesthetic assessment by the anaesthetist.	To ensure that the patient can be given the most suitable anaesthetic and any special requirements for anaesthetic have been highlighted (AORN 2000, **C**).
9 Measure and record the patient's pulse, blood pressure, respirations, oxygen saturations, temperature, weight and blood sugar (if required) in pre-operative documentation.	To provide baseline data for comparison intra- and post-operatively. The weight is recorded so that the anaesthetist can calculate the correct dose of drugs to be administered (AORN 2000, **C**).
10 Ask the patient to remove all jewellery, cosmetics and nail varnish. Wedding rings may be left on fingers, but must be covered and secured with hypoallergenic tape. Patients requesting to wear other forms of metal jewellery (e.g. chains) for personal or religious reasons will need to discuss this with the operating team.	Metal jewellery may be accidentally lost or may cause harm to the patient, for example diathermy burns. Facial cosmetics make the patient's colour difficult to assess. Nail varnish makes the use of the pulse oximeter, used to monitor the patient's pulse and oxygen saturation levels, impossible and masks peripheral cyanosis (Vedovato et al. 2004, **C**).
11 If a patient has valuables, these must be recorded and stored away securely according to hospital policy.	To prevent loss of valuables. **E**

Action	Rationale
12 Ask the patient to shower or bath as close to the planned time of the operation as possible and before a pre-medication is administered (if this has been prescribed). If the patient has long hair, this needs to be tied back with a non-metallic tie.	To minimize risk of post-operative wound infection and prevent patient accidents when sedated (Loveday et al. 2014, **C**). For safety, to prevent hair getting caught in equipment and to reduce the risk of infection. **E**
13 Apply antiembolic stockings according to local trust procedure (see Procedure guideline 13.1: Step-by-step guide to measuring and applying antiembolic stockings).	To reduce the risk of post-operative deep vein thrombosis or pulmonary emboli (NICE 2010, **C**).
14 Ensure the patient is wearing two electronic namebands containing their full name, date of birth and NHS number. One should be placed on the patient's wrist and the other on the ankle. Prior to placing the namebands on the patient, the details should be verbally checked and confirmed as accurate by the patient and against the patient's medical notes. The namebands will be white unless local trust policy stipulates that colour coding is necessary to alert healthcare professionals to a risk, e.g. allergy, in which case the wristbands will be red (NPSA 2007).	To ensure correct identification and prevent possible patient misidentification (AORN 2000, **C**). To reduce allergic reactions to known causative agents and to alert all involved in the care of the patient in the operating theatre (AORN 2004, **C**).
15 Record whether the patient has dental caps, crowns, bridge work or loose teeth in the pre-operative checklist.	The anaesthetist needs to be informed to prevent accidental damage. Loose teeth or a dental prosthesis could be inhaled by the patient when an endotracheal tube is inserted. **E**
16 Document any patient prostheses in the pre-operative checklist and whether they are removable (e.g. artificial limb, dentures, hearing aid) or irremovable (e.g. pacemaker, knee replacement). Removable prostheses may be retained until the patient is in the anaesthetic room. Spectacles and hearing aids may be retained until the patient has been anaesthetized (these may be left in position if a local anaesthetic is used). Any prosthesis that is removed should be labelled clearly (ideally with a patient identifier) and retained in the recovery room.	To promote patient safety during surgery. For example, dentures may obstruct the airway, contact lenses can cause corneal abrasions. Internal non-removable prostheses may be affected by the electric current used in diathermy. To enable the patient to communicate fully, thus reducing anxiety and enabling the patient to understand any procedures carried out. **E** To enable patients with prosthetic limbs to mobilize independently to theatre.
17 Check whether the patient passed urine before pre-medication or anaesthetic.	To prevent urinary incontinence when sedated and/or unconscious and possible contamination of sterile area. **E**
18 Once the pre-operative checklist is fully completed, administer any pre-medication, if prescribed, in accordance with the anaesthetist's instructions. Patients who receive a sedative pre-medication should be advised to remain in bed and to use the nurse call system if assistance is needed.	Different drugs may be prescribed to complement the anaesthetic to be given, for example temazepam to reduce patient anxiety by inducing sleep and relaxation. E Questioning pre-medicated patients is not a reliable source of checking information as the patient may be drowsy and/or disorientated (AORN 2000, **C**). To reduce the risk of accidental patient injury as the pre-medication may make the patient drowsy and disorientated. **E**
19 Accompany the patient to theatre, taking their notes, medication chart, X-rays/scans, blood results, completed consent form and pre-operative checklist. The patient should be accompanied to the theatre by an appropriately trained healthcare professional. Mobile patients who have not received a sedative pre-medication will be able to walk to theatre wearing appropriately fitting footwear. Immobile patients or patients who have received a sedative pre-medication will need to be taken to theatre on a theatre trolley.	To prevent delays which can increase the patient's anxiety and to ensure that the anaesthetist and surgeon have all the information they require for safe treatment of the patient. **E** To reduce patient anxiety and ensure a safe environment during anaesthetic induction. **E** To reduce the risk of accidental patient injury. **E** To reduce the risk of accidental patient injury as the pre-medication may make the patient drowsy and disorientated. **E**
20 Give a full handover to the anaesthetic nurse or operating department practitioner on arrival in the anaesthetic room, using patient records and the pre-operative checklist. The escorting healthcare professional will stay with the patient until they have been fully checked in by the anaesthetic assistant/nurse.	To ensure the patient has the correct operation. To ensure continuity of care and to maintain the safety of the patient by exchanging all relevant information (AORN 2000, **C**).

Intraoperative care

Intraoperative care: anaesthesia

DEFINITION

Intraoperative care is the physical and psychological care given to the patient in the anaesthetic room and operating theatre until transfer to the post-operative area. In the anaesthetic room patients are admitted and checked into the operating suite. The patient is normally transferred already anaesthetized into the theatre on a trolley and moved across to the operating table. For emergency surgery (e.g. dissecting aortic aneurysm or ruptured ectopic pregnancy) and in the case of bariatric patients, it is safer to induce anaesthesia inside the operating theatre with the patient already positioned on the operating table (Leonard and Thompson 2008). A crucial role of the anaesthetic nurse is to support the patient who is often frightened or anxious due to the unfamiliar, often intimidating environment and apprehensive about both the anaesthesia and impending surgery (Lindwall et al. 2003, Mitchell 2010).

RELATED THEORY

The safe administration of anaesthesia has been evolving since the early 1840s. At this time surgery was often seen as a final attempt to save life and very few operations were performed. This was because surgery was very painful and patients were conscious during the procedure and could hear everything that was being said and done. In order to overcome these difficulties, surgeons would administer alcohol, morphine and other sedatives. This was usually ineffective and most patients were restrained either with straps or physically held down. Surgery (such as amputation of limbs) had to be performed speedily and often patients would either faint from pain or die from the bleeding.

Modern anaesthesia began in October 1846 when William Morton administered ether for the first time at Massachusetts General Hospital, Boston. This was shortly followed that year by James Robinson who administered the first ether anaesthetic in England. The following year James Simpson, Professor of Obstetrics, introduced chloroform anaesthesia in Edinburgh. Although chloroform had severe side-effects such as sudden death and delayed liver damage, it still became popular because it worked well and was easier to use than ether. John Snow, the first dedicated anaesthetist, administered chloroform to Queen Victoria during labour in 1853 (Simpson et al. 2002). Local anaesthetic (cocaine) was introduced in 1877 which progressed during the 1900s with newer, less toxic local anaesthetics which facilitated further developments such as infiltration anaesthesia, nerve blocks, spinal and epidural analgesia (Cobbold and Money 2010).

However, it was not until the turn of the 20th century that control of the airway, using tubes in the trachea to facilitate ventilation and prevent aspiration of stomach contents, and intravenous induction agents were introduced. This practice enabled patients to be anaesthetized more quickly and safely.

Modern general anaesthesia is usually described as a triad of components that include hypnosis (sleep), analgesia and muscle relaxation. The proportion of each component may vary according to the surgery. For example, modern muscle relaxants, which emerged from the 1940s, enable adequate relaxation of the abdomen (for example) without relying on very deep anaesthesia (from a single agent) to achieve the same effect (Simpson et al. 2002). Today anaesthesia is very safe and there are very few deaths – less than 1 in 250,000 directly related to anaesthesia (Royal College of Anaesthetists 2013).

EVIDENCE-BASED APPROACHES

Anticipated patient outcomes

- To ensure that the patient understands what will happen in the operating theatres at all times in order to minimize anxiety.
- To ensure that the patient has the correct surgery for which the consent form was signed.
- To ensure patient safety at all times and minimize post-operative complications by:
  - giving the required care for the unconscious patient
  - ensuring injury is not sustained from hazards associated with the use of swabs, needles, instruments, diathermy and power tools
  - minimizing post-operative problems associated with patient positioning, such as nerve or tissue damage
  - maintaining asepsis during surgical procedures to reduce the risk of post-operative wound infection in accordance with hospital policies on infection control.

LEGAL AND PROFESSIONAL ISSUES

The WHO Surgical Safety Checklist is a structured aid to enhance communication and improve safety within surgery (www.who.int/patientsafety/safesurgery/en/). It is mandated in many countries including the UK. The purpose of this checklist is to ensure that the correct procedure is performed on the correct patient, encourage team work and improve communication amongst the surgical team. The safety checklist comprises three parts: sign in, time out and sign out (Box 13.11). Sign in is completed in the anaesthetic room before the patient is induced. It has to be read out loud with the anaesthetist and the anaesthetic assistant present. The checklist may be modified to ensure relevance within different surgical specialties/settings (WHO 2008). However, local modifications that increase the complexity of the checklist may negatively impact on team compliance (Alnaib et al. 2012).

PRE-PROCEDURAL CONSIDERATIONS

Pharmacological support

Prior to commencing anaesthesia, the patient is usually assessed by the anaesthetist and/or the nursing pre-assessment team. The type of anaesthetic administered will depend on a number of factors including the age/risk of the patient, planned surgery and patient/clinician preference. However, the following components are usually included.

- *Analgesia*: this will be administered intravenously with the muscle relaxants and sleep-inducing drugs. Drugs used are dependent on anaesthetic preference and technique. Commonly used agents include fentanyl, remifentanil and morphine as well as non-steroidal anti-inflammatory drugs (NSAIDs) such as ketorolac. This is to ensure that the patient does not feel any pain at the time of skin incision, during the surgery and post-operatively.
- *Antiemetics* are given with analgesia. These medications, such as cyclizine, ondansetron and granisetron, moderate the side-effects of opioid analgesics and inhalational anaesthesia and reduce post-operative nausea and vomiting (PONV).
- *Induction agents* are drugs which help to induce unconsciousness. The mostly commonly used is propofol, a short-acting medication that can also be used to maintain anaesthesia as an intravenous infusion.
- *Inhalation agents*: after induction, the anaesthesia can be maintained by either inhalational agents or intravenous infusion (propofol). Examples of inhalation agents are sevoflurane and isoflurane. While these are very effective, they are associated with a higher incidence of PONV (Apfel et al. 2005). These are administered through vaporizers which are attached to the anaesthetic machines (Figure 13.10).
- *Muscle relaxants* are the last drugs to be administered during induction as they relax all muscles (except the cardiac muscle), leading to paralysis. This is done when patients are unconscious otherwise it would be a very frightening experience for them to be aware but unable to move. The most commonly used relaxants/paralysing agents are atracurium, vecuronium and rocuronium.

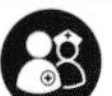

Box 13.11 **WHO Surgical Safety Checklist**

DATE:
THEATRE:

The ROYAL MARSDEN

PATIENT DETAILS

Last name ....
First name ....
DOB ....
Hospital number ....

SURGICAL SAFETY CHECKLIST
V3.1 *pilot*

CHECK IN

Has the patient confirmed their identity, procedure, site and consent?

Has the patient identity been confirmed with two staff members?

Is the site marked?

Does the patient have:
- A known allergy?
- A difficult airway?
- Aspiration risk?

What are the patient-specific concerns?
ASA grade
Are the required blood products available?
Have required antibiotic been given?
Is glycaemic control an issue?
Are warming devices prepared for use?
Has the VTE assessment been completed?
Are VTE prophylaxis devices in place for use?

SIGNATURE:
NAME:

TIME OUT

Are the regular team member names written on the board?

Have new team members been introduced?

Is the patient's name and planned procedure confirmed?

Is anticipated blood loss >500mL ?
Blood is/not in the fridge

Are there specific equipment or investigation requirements?

Are there any critical or unusual steps the team needs to know?

Has the sterility of the instruments been confirmed?

SIGNATURE:
NAME:

SIGN OUT

Has the name of the procedure been recorded?

Is the instrument and sharps count correct?

Have the specimens been labeled?

Were there any problems during this case?

Could they have been dealt with differently?

Is the operation note written?

Is the immediate post-op plan agreed?
LMWH/ABx/NGT/Feeding

SIGNATURE:
NAME:

Source: WHO (2008).

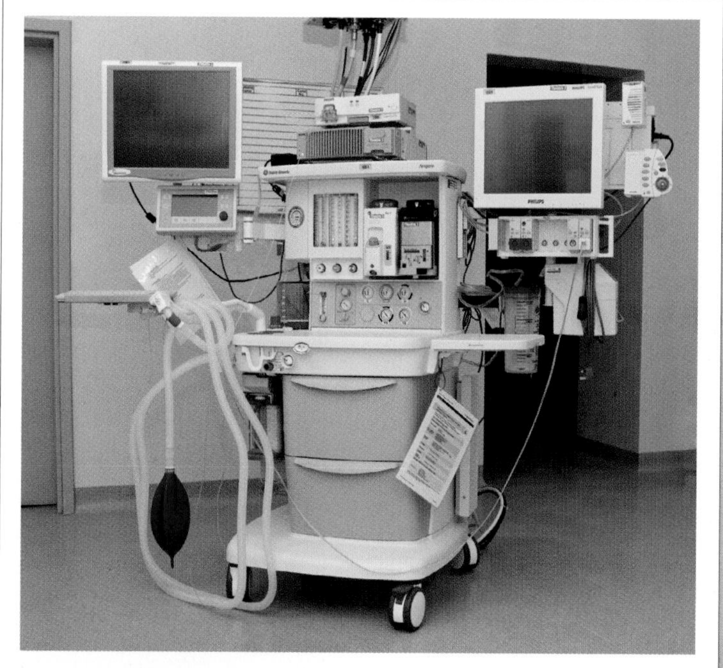

Figure 13.10 **Anaesthetic machine.**

Specific patient preparation

When the patient arrives in the anaesthetic room, it is important to check their details to ensure that the correct patient is being received. At this point, consent is verified with the patient in order to confirm the planned surgery and the patient's identity. This completes the final phase of the pre-operative checklist. As this is the final patient check prior to commencing anaesthesia and surgery, it is crucial to ensuring the patient's safety.

Procedure guideline 13.3 Caring for the patient in the anaesthetic room

Essential equipment

- Suction
- Anaesthetic machine
  - Airway equipment
- Medical gases (including back-up O_2 cylinders)
- Monitoring equipment
  - Emergency drugs

Action	Rationale
Pre-procedure	
1 Greet the patient by name. Confirm with the ward nurse that it is the correct patient for the scheduled operation.	To reduce patient anxiety. **P**
Procedure	
2 Identify the patient by checking the identification band (name and patient number) against the patient's notes and the operating list.	To safeguard against patient misidentification (AFPP 2011, **C**).
3 Check and confirm the correct completion of the pre-operative checklist.	To ensure that all the listed measures have been completed and that any additional information has been recorded. **E**
4 Check that the results of the investigative procedures, for example blood results, X-rays, and so on, are included with the patient's notes.	To ensure that all the required results are available for the theatre team's use. **E**
5 Maintain a calm, quiet environment and explain all the procedures to the patient, including the monitoring of blood pressure, pulse and oxygen saturation.	To reduce anxiety and enhance the smooth induction of anaesthesia (Mitchell 2010, **E**).
6 When the patient is anaesthetized, ensure that the eyes are closed and secured with hypoallergenic tape/padding.	To prevent corneal damage due to eyes drying out or accidental abrasion. For longer cases a sterile lubricant may also be applied to the surface of the eye (White and Crosse 1998, **E**).
Post-procedure	
7 When the patient has been anaesthetized, they are transferred into the operating theatre.	

Intraoperative care: theatre

RELATED THEORY

Before surgical intervention (skin incision)

The team in theatre normally consists of at least one surgeon (often more, including surgical trainees), an anaesthetist and the theatre staff which as well as Registered Nurses often also includes registered ODPs and healthcare assistants. Within this team there will be a scrub nurse (or ODP) who works in the sterile field, managing the instrumentation, swabs and sutures and assisting the surgeon. There will normally be at least one circulating person who remains outside the sterile field and provides items as required for the scrub nurse/ODP. There will also be a designated nurse/ODP who assists the anaesthetist (Figure 13.11).

Once the patient has been positioned on the operating table, before surgical intervention, the theatre team will complete the second section of the WHO safety checklist which is 'time out'. This ensures that the team is fully aware and readily equipped for

Figure 13.11 **Surgical team.**

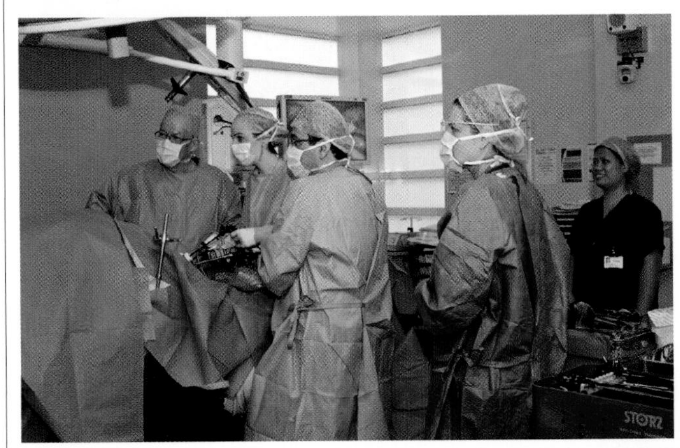

any eventuality that may arise during the procedure. The WHO checklist (part 2) 'time out' has to be read out loud for all team members to hear and respond to and has to be completed before the start of any surgical intervention such as the first skin incision (see Box 13.11).

Control of infection and asepsis in the operating theatre

As part of intraoperative care, the aim of operating theatres is to provide an environment that minimizes the presence of pathogens (both airborne and surface). The general principle is that the actual operating theatre is the cleanest area within the suite as this is the area where patients are at most risk of surgical site infection. Ventilation systems within theatres support this principle by using positive pressure ventilation to carry pathogens away from the surgical wound (Al-Benna 2012).

Large quantities of bacteria are present in the nose and mouth, on the skin, hair and the attire of personnel. The skin of staff becomes dispersed in the air and is a potential source of wound infection (Sivanandan et al. 2011). Therefore staff working in operating theatres wear clean scrub suits and lint-free surgical hats to eliminate the possibility of these bacteria, hair or dandruff being shed into the environment (AFPP 2011). Well-fitting shoes with impervious soles should be worn and regularly cleaned to remove splashes of blood and body fluids (Woodhead et al. 2002). Facemasks are worn to prevent droplets falling from the mouth into the operating field. The extent to which facemasks are capable of preventing droplet spread is disputed (Lipp and Edwards 2002). It is, however, accepted that masks offer protection to the wearer from blood splashes and for safety reasons should be worn by the scrub team. Instruments must be handled carefully and needle holders and forceps used to manipulate sutures to minimize the risk of needlestick or sharps injury.

Minimally invasive surgery (laparoscopic surgery) and robotically assisted laparoscopic surgery

Abdominal and pelvic surgeries are often performed using this technique. Laparoscopy is often referred to as keyhole surgery and involves the introduction of a number of small ports through the skin to allow access into the abdominal cavity. Specialized cameras, lights and instruments (Figure 13.12) are introduced through these ports in order to perform this minimally invasive surgery.

Minimally invasive surgery involves the insufflation of the abdomen with carbon dioxide (CO_2). This is necessary in order to expand the space in which the surgeon is operating to facilitate the surgery and is known as pneumoperitoneum (Figure 13.13). Carbon dioxide is used as, unlike air or oxygen, it does not

Figure 13.12 **Laparoscopic equipment.**

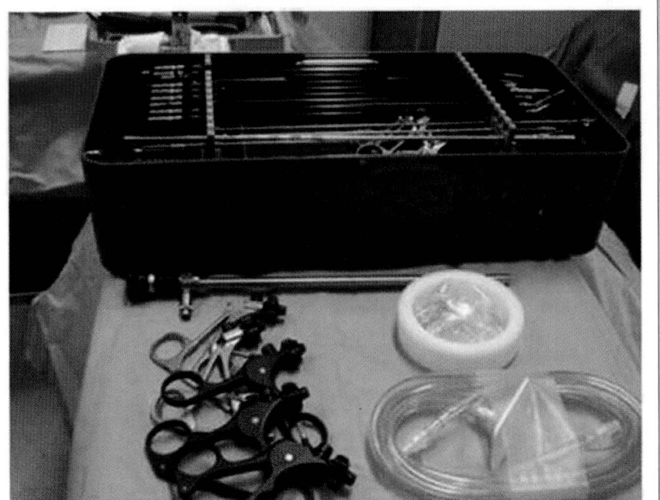

Figure 13.13 **Pnuemoperitoneum/port placement.**

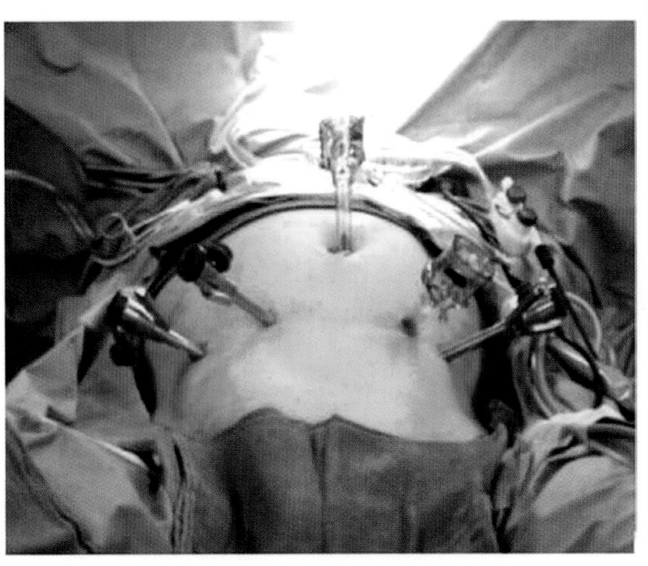

support combustion in the presence of electricity and is readily excreted by the patient via the respiratory system. Prolonged insufflation may cause hypothermia as, although the gas is equal to room temperature, the temperature in the abdomen decreases because of the high gas flow and the volume of gas used (Jacobs et al. 2000). Sharma et al. (1997) refer to the increased risk of hypercarbia and surgical emphysema during insufflation with CO_2. Careful monitoring and recording of the patient's vital signs, including oxygen saturation and expiratory gas levels, are therefore essential during laparoscopy.

Haemorrhage can occur during any surgical procedure and may be difficult to detect and control in laparoscopic procedures. Therefore the theatre staff should always have the equipment necessary to convert to an open procedure. Theatre staff must also ensure that equipment is used safely and according to the manufacturer's instructions.

Robotic surgery

Robotic surgery is a relatively recent development (the Da Vinci system was licensed in 2000). The robot is controlled remotely by the surgeon who sits at a console inside the theatre. The robot is able to manipulate instruments (introduced laparoscopically) through 360° which is something even the most talented and dextrous surgeon cannot do. This means that robotic surgery is of particular value in confined, hard-to-reach spaces such as the pelvis. Therefore it is most commonly used in urological and gynaecological surgery. In common with regular laparoscopic surgery, patients often spend a much shorter time in hospital compared to those having open surgery for the same procedure. The market is currently dominated by one single supplier, Integra, which manufactures the Da Vinci surgical robot (Figure 13.14).

Staff involved with robotic surgery have to receive special training in order to set up and assist with robotic procedures (Figure 13.15). The robot is a sophisticated and very expensive item of equipment and a dedicated team of staff are often assigned to this specialty (Figure 13.16).

EVIDENCE-BASED APPROACHES

Positioning of the patient on the table

The position of the patient on the operating table must be such as to facilitate access to the operative site(s) by the surgeon, and the patient's airway for the anaesthetist. It will also be dependent upon the type of surgery being performed, position of

Figure 13.14 Da Vinci surgical robot.

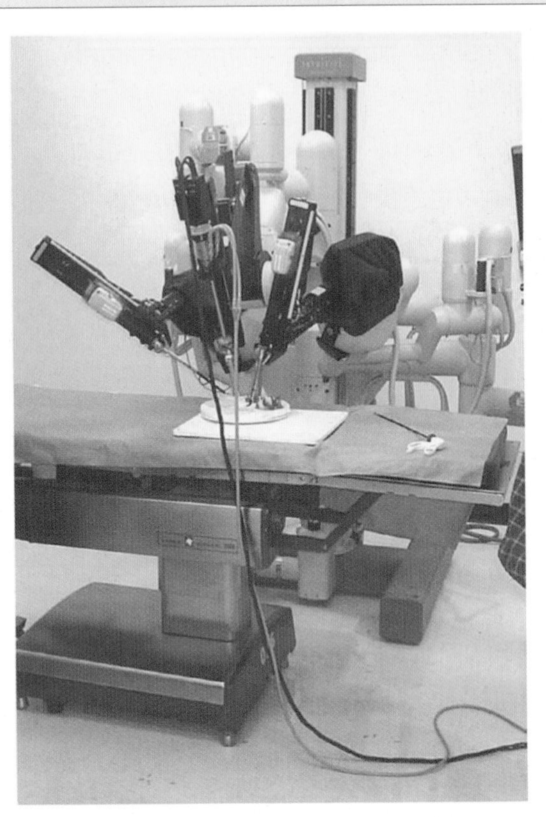

Figure 13.15 Specialist staff using the robotic equipment.

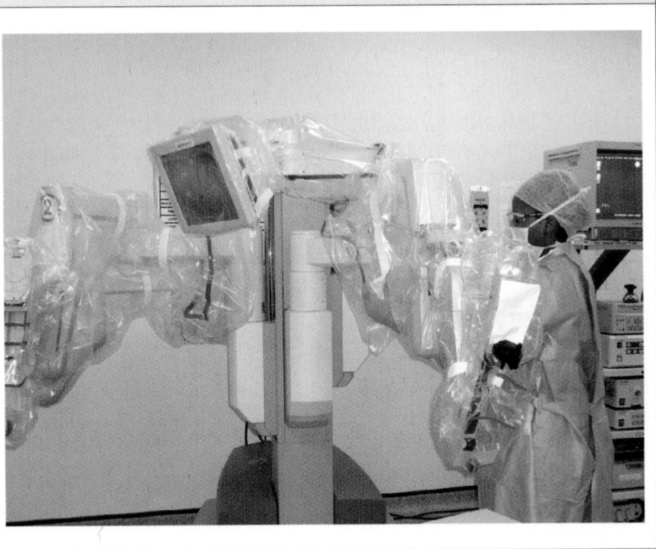

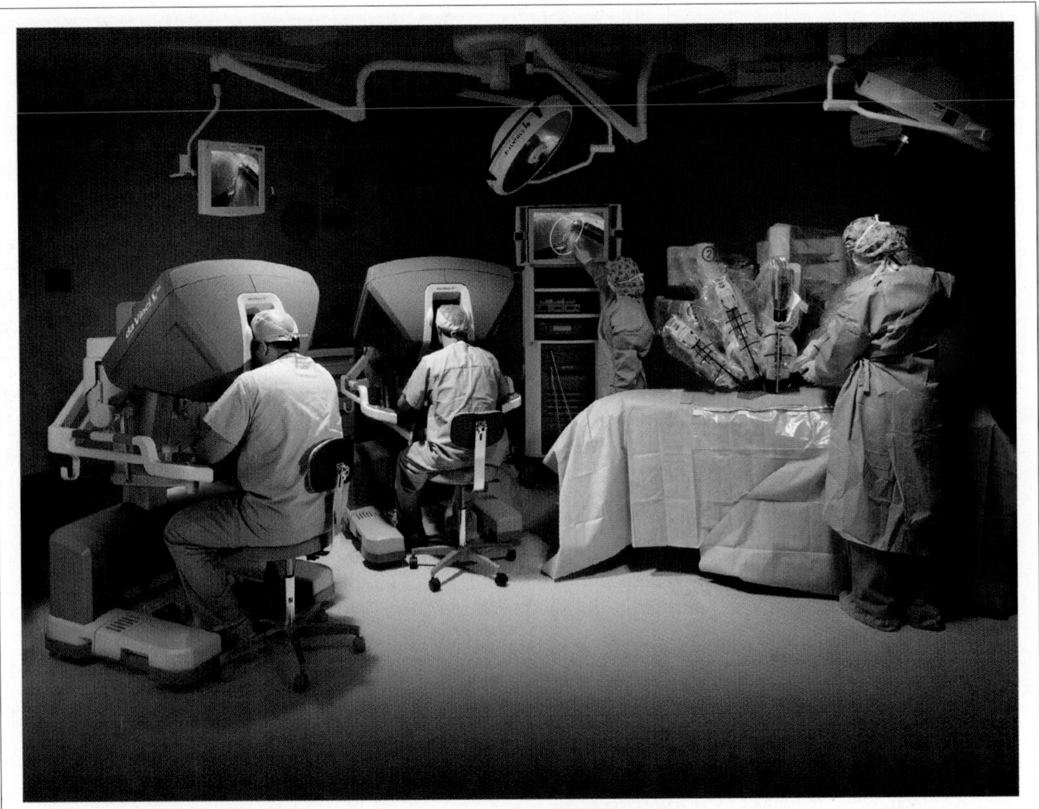

Figure 13.16 Robotic surgical team. *Source:* Reproduced with permission from Intuitive Medical, Inc. © 2014 Intuitive Surgical, Inc.

Figure 13.17 Lithotomy position.

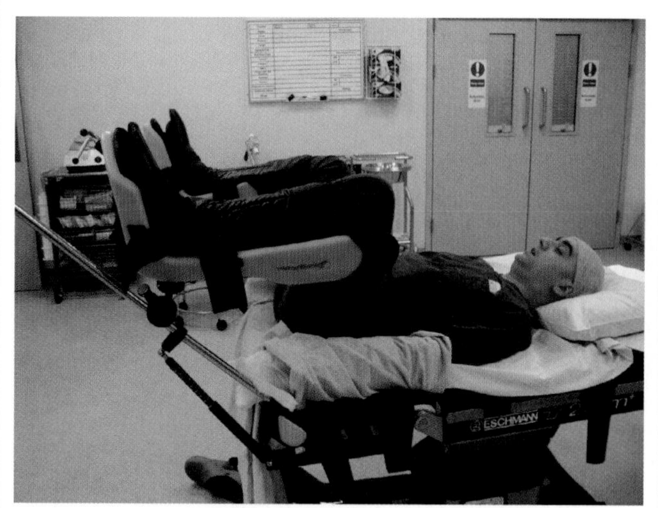

Figure 13.18 Armboard.

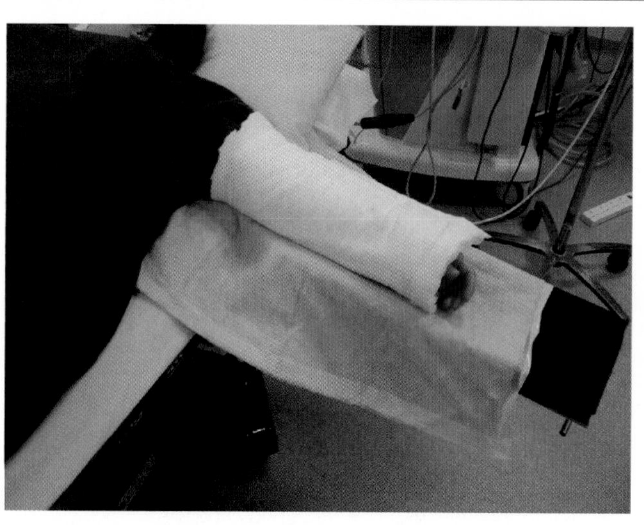

monitoring equipment and intravenous devices *in situ*. It should not compromise the patient's circulation or respiratory system or cause damage to the skin or nerves.

Pre-operative assessment will identify patients who may need extra precautions during positioning because of their weight, nutritional state, age, skin condition or pre-existing disease. The increased numbers of obese patients requiring surgery present specific challenges and staff must be familiar with the weight limits of patient trolleys and operating tables. Many departments now have specialist bariatric equipment for the safe positioning of obese patients (Bale and Berrecloth 2010).

Pre-existing conditions such as backache or sciatica can be exacerbated, particularly if the patient is in the lithotomy position (Figure 13.17), as the sciatic nerve can be compressed against the poles (AFPP 2011). Most post-operative palsies are due to incorrect positioning of the patient on the operating table (Beckett 2010). Consideration by and co-operation of all theatre personnel can help prevent many of the post-operative complications related to intraoperative positioning and this remains a team responsibility (AFPP 2011, Beckett 2010).

All movements of the limbs of the unconscious patient should take into account the anatomy and natural planes of movement of that limb to avoid stretching and pressure on the related nerve planes (AFPP 2011). Hyperabduction of the arm when placed on a board, for example, could stretch the brachial plexus, causing some post-operative loss of sensation and reduced movement of the forearm, wrist and fingers. To prevent this, the board should be angled at 45° and not 90° with hands facing more towards the feet rather than the head (Figure 13.18). The ulnar and radial nerves may be affected by direct pressure as a result of insufficient padding on arm supports.

Compartment syndrome is a life-threatening complication of the Lloyd Davies position (Figure 13.19) and occurs when perfusion falls below tissue pressure in a closed anatomical space or compartment such as hand, forearm, buttocks, legs, upper arms and feet. It develops through a combination of prolonged ischaemia and reperfusion of muscle within a tight osseofascial compartment (Raza et al. 2004). Untreated, it can lead to necrosis, functional impairment, possible renal failure and death (Callum and Bradbury 2000, Paula 2002).

If patients are placed in Lloyd Davies position and Trendelenburg tilt for longer than 4 hours, the legs should be removed from the support every 2 hours, or as close to 2 hours as possible, for a short period of time to prevent reperfusion injury (Raza et al. 2004). The use of compression stockings and intermittent compression devices in the Lloyd Davies position should be approached with caution as these devices may contribute to compartment syndrome (Malik et al. 2009). The use of these devices will depend on the clinical judgement of the surgeon and anaesthetist and the physical status of the patient.

Methods of infection prevention

It is imperative that during surgical procedures, infection control and prevention are maintained at all times. The area immediately around the patient and the instrument trolley is known as the sterile field. Only those staff who have donned sterile gloves and gowns after washing and decontaminating their hands and

Figure 13.19 Lloyd Davies position.

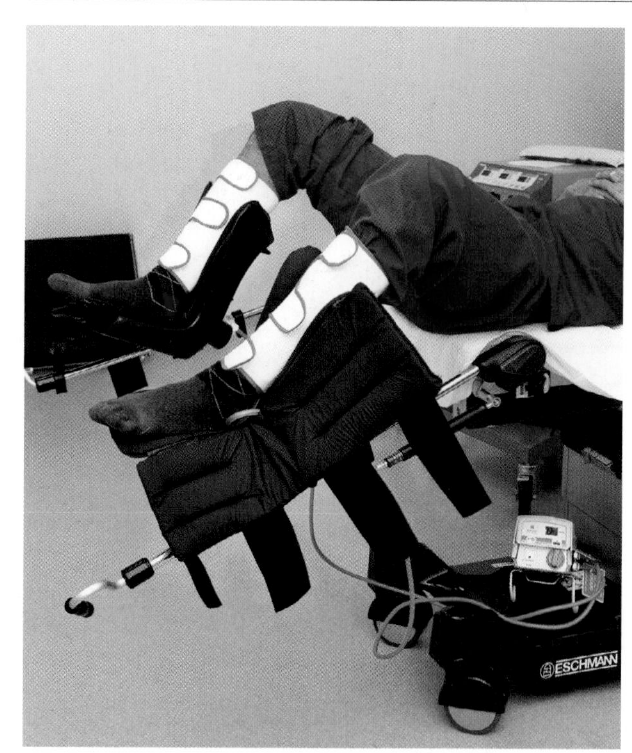

forearms (scrubbing-up) can enter the sterile field. Pre-surgical hand washing or scrubbing up (Figure 13.20) is an essential step in the prevention of infection during surgery.

The aim of surgical hand antisepsis is to remove dirt and transient micro-organisms and also to reduce to a minimum resident micro-organisms on the hands, nails and forearms (AORN 2013). For minor surgical procedures, current research supports a 1-minute hand wash with a non-antiseptic soap followed by hand rubbing with liquid aqueous alcoholic solution prior to the first procedure of the day and before any subsequent procedures (Tanner et al. 2007). This has been shown to be as effective as traditional hand scrubbing with an antiseptic soap containing 4 % chlorhexidine gluconate or 7.5% povidone-iodine in preventing surgical site infection (Parienti et al. 2002). However, for more major cases it is usual to perform surgical hand antisepsis using either a solution containing chlorhexidine or iodine. The duration of the wash is usually 2–5 minutes (AFPP 2011). The six steps of hand washing should be followed and also the arms up to the elbow should be washed (Loveday et al. 2014).

Surgeons and staff who are working within the sterile field wear sterile surgical gowns. These gowns are designed to function as both a sterile barrier between the wearer's body and the surgical field and as protection for the wearer against exposure to blood, body fluids and tissue. The gown should be resistant to microbial and liquid penetration and minimize the release of particles (AFPP 2011).

Surgical gloves have a dual role, acting as a barrier for personal protection from the patient's blood and other exudates and preventing bacterial transfer from the surgeon's hand to the operating site. Surgical gloves must conform to international standards and different types are used for various procedures. It is essential that the glove is the correct size, not only for reasons of comfort but also for dexterity and sensitivity. It is common practice for many surgeons and theatre staff to double glove. Evidence suggests that double gloving significantly reduces the number of perforations to the innermost glove, thus reducing infection rates during surgical procedures (Tanner and Parkinson 2006).

Figure 13.20 **Surgical scrub.**

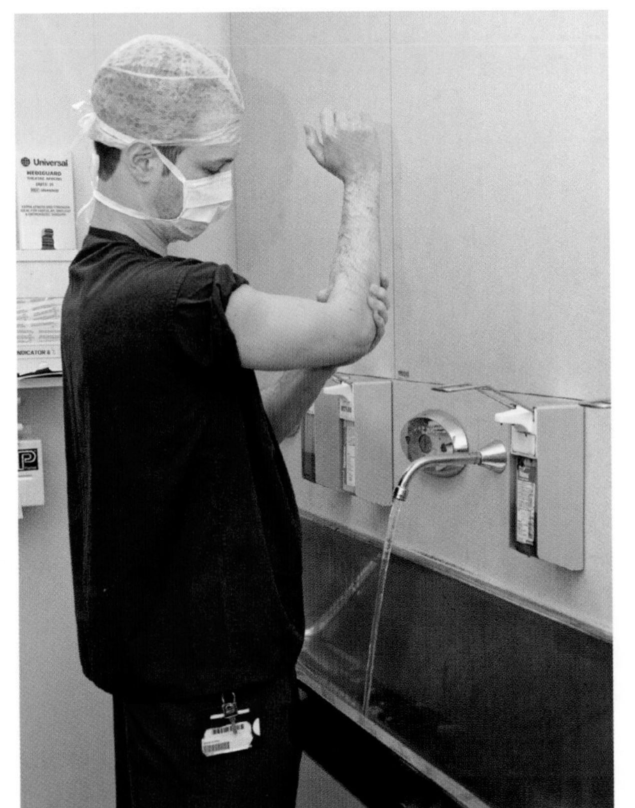

Prior to skin incision, the skin of the patient is cleaned with an antiseptic solution. The purpose of this is to reduce the amount of both transient and resident skin bacteria. Most surgical wound infections are caused by bacteria living on the patient's own skin. Several types of skin preparation are used but commonly include povidone-iodine or chlorhexidine gluconate. These agents are included in either aqueous or alcoholic solutions. Which is used depends on both the condition of the patient's skin and whether they are allergic to either of the agents (AFPP 2011).

LEGAL AND PROFESSIONAL ISSUES

Transferring and positioning

When a patient is transferred between the trolley or bed and operating table, adequate personnel should be present to ensure patient and staff safety (AFPP 2011). It is recommended that an approved sliding device is used to transfer patients from trolley to operating table, in compliance with national legislation on manual handling and local hospital policy/guidelines.

Safe manual handling and the safety of the patient depend on the participation of the correct number of staff in the specified handling manoeuvre. There should be a minimum of four staff: one at either end of the patient to support the head and the feet and one on either side. Additional staff and/or specialist transfer devices may be required if the patient weighs over 90 kg (Figure 13.21).

Once the patient has been positioned safely, the intermittent compression device is attached. Figure 13.22 shows the Flowtron machine used in prevention of deep vein thrombosis in conjunction with venous compression garments.

PRE-PROCEDURAL CONSIDERATIONS

Equipment

In the operating room, the staff should ensure that all equipment is ready and checked before the first patient is sent for.

Anaesthetic machine and patient monitoring (Figure 13.23)

This allows the anaesthetists to administer the correct proportions of oxygen, air and inhalational agents. Cardiovascular and respiratory monitoring is essential throughout the anaesthetic and surgery and includes ECG, blood pressure, respiratory rate/volume, oxygen saturation and expired CO_2 monitoring. To ensure adequate depth of anaesthesia, either the expired anaesthetic agent or brain electrical activity is monitored by the anaesthetist (depending on the anaesthetic technique).

Suction unit (Figure 13.24)

This is attached to the anaesthetic machine and is used in the event of obstruction (to clear secretions) or to remove regurgitated stomach contents.

Vaporizer

This is also attached to the anaesthetic machine and is used to administer inhalational anaesthetic agents.

Scavenging system

This removes the inhalational agents that the patient exhales so it is important to ensure that this is operational. Contamination of the atmosphere with these agents can be harmful to staff.

Operating table (Figure 13.25)

As part of the equipment check, the operating table is assessed to ensure it is fully operational and performs all the required functions to enable correct positioning of the patient. The height of the operating table is adjusted in relation to the height of the surgeon and team to prevent any unnecessary strain on the back and neck.

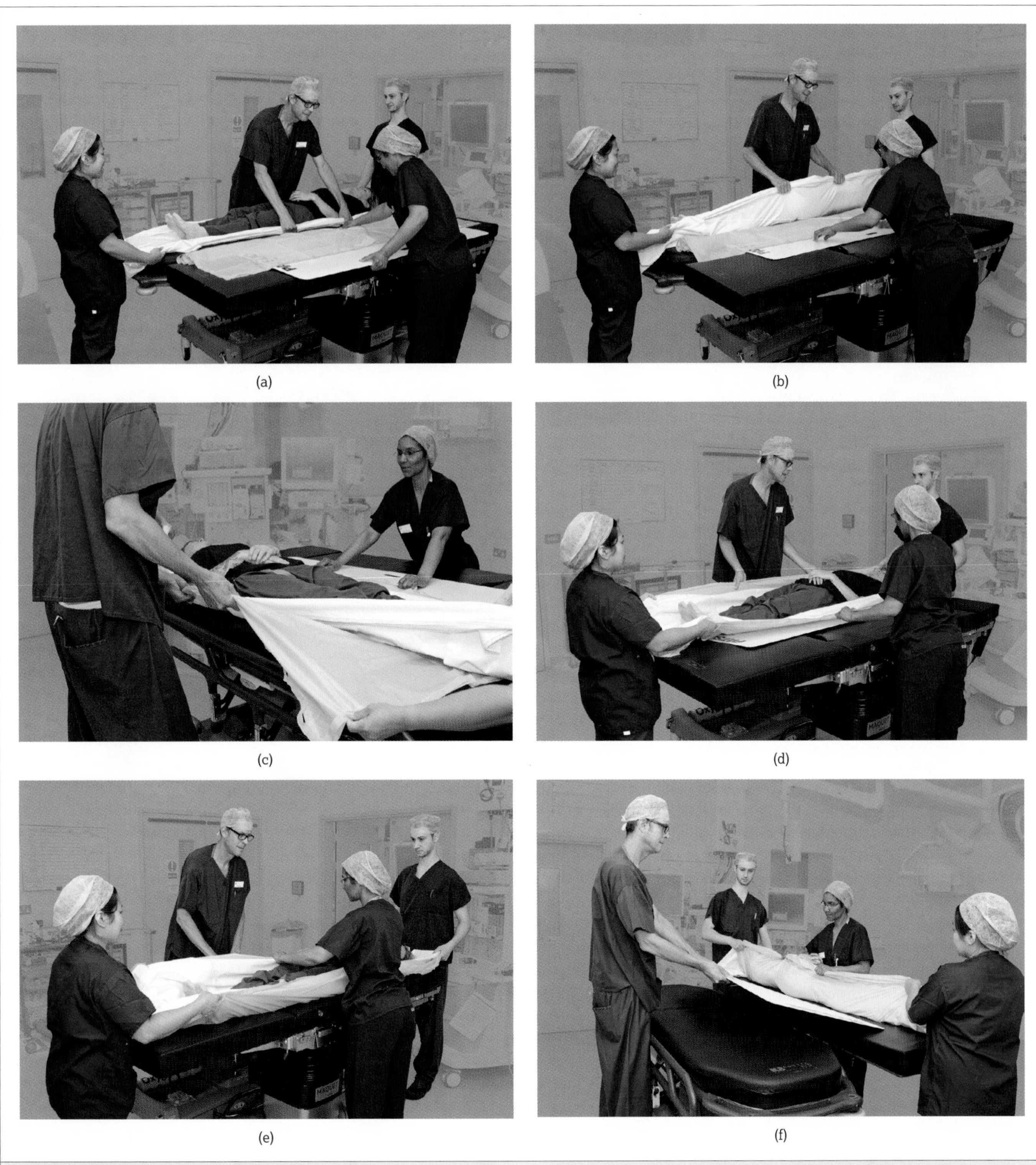

Figure 13.21 **Lateral transfer.**

Modern operating tables are powered by a battery that needs to be charged when not in use. Therefore it is essential that the table is plugged into the main power supply at the end of the operating list.

Diathermy machine (Figure 13.26)

Diathermy (or electrosurgery) is used routinely during surgery to cut tissue and control haemorrhage by sealing bleeding vessels. It uses heat from electricity and this is achieved by passing a normal electrical current through the diathermy machine which converts it into a high-frequency alternating current. There are two types of diathermy.

- *Monopolar*: this works by producing current from an active electrode such as the diathermy forceps, which is then returned back to the machine through the patient's body via another electrode, such as a patient diathermy plate/pad, which creates a complete circuit. It is the most commonly used type of electrosurgery as a wider range of effects can be achieved

Figure 13.22 **Flowtron boots and heel pads.**

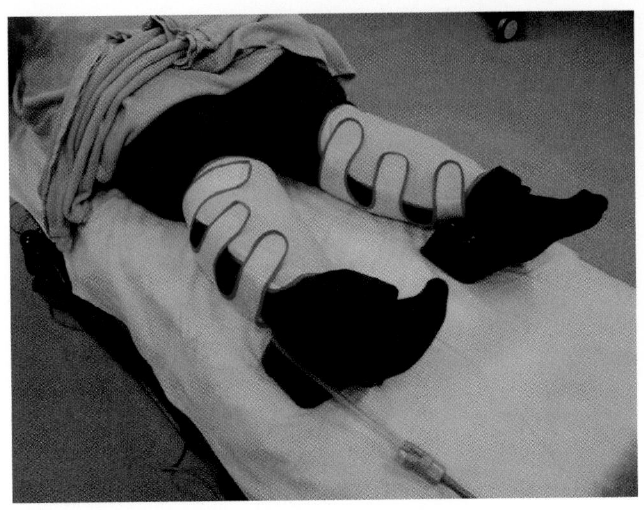

(cutting, coagulating, fulgurating). The current is delivered by the surgeon operating a hand switch or foot pedal.

- *Bipolar*: this does not require a patient diathermy plate/pad to complete the circuit. The current produced by the machine passes down one side of the forceps prong, through the tissue and back to the machine via the other side of the forceps prong (rather than through the patient's body and returning to the machine via the plate/pad). Again the surgeon operates the device by a hand switch or foot pedal. Biopolar diathermy is often used in laparoscopic surgery and in hand/foot surgery (AFPP 2011).

Diathermy is potentially hazardous to the patient if used incorrectly. The main risk when using diathermy is of thermoelectrical burns. The most common cause is incorrect application of the patient plate or a break in the connecting lead (Vedovato et al. 2004); burns can also be caused if the patient comes into contact with metal which allows the current to earth through the patient's skin. The machine automatically switches off or alarms if the neutral electrodes come loose from the patient. However, if the patient is in contact with metal, this is harder to identify. Care must therefore be taken during positioning that no part of the patient's body is in contact with metal and that the return electrode (plate/pad), if used, is placed close to the operative site (AFPP 2011).

It is important that theatre staff know how to test and use diathermy equipment to prevent patient injury (Molyneux 2001, Wicker and O'Neill 2010). This involves checking that the cables and plugs are not damaged and indicator lights are all in working order. It is also important that the theatre staff check the equipment before every operating list to ensure that the alarms

Figure 13.23 **Anaesthetic machine and patient monitoring.**

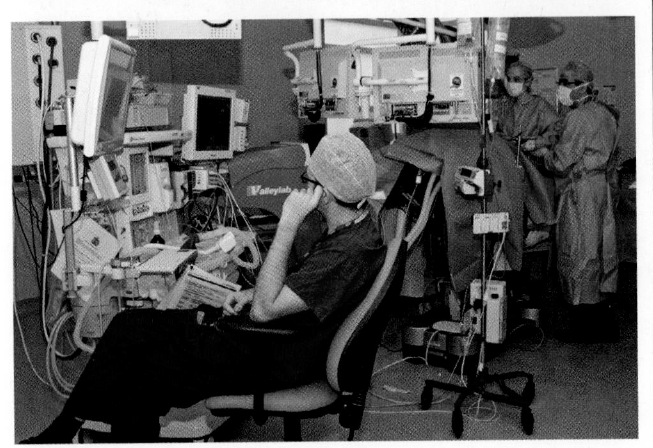

Figure 13.24 **High vacuum suction unit.**

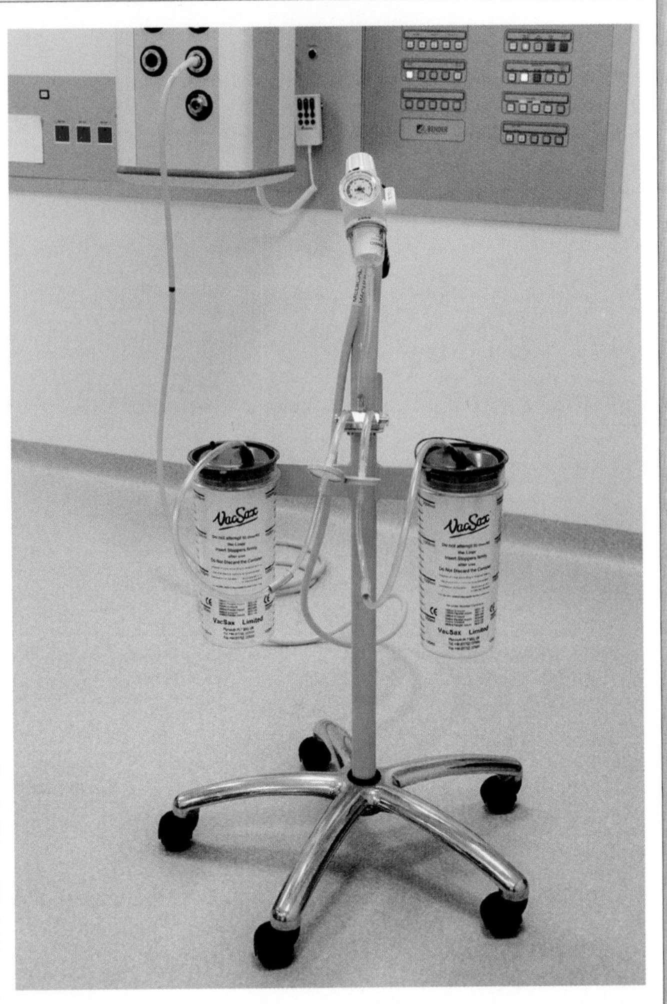

Figure 13.25 **Operating table.**

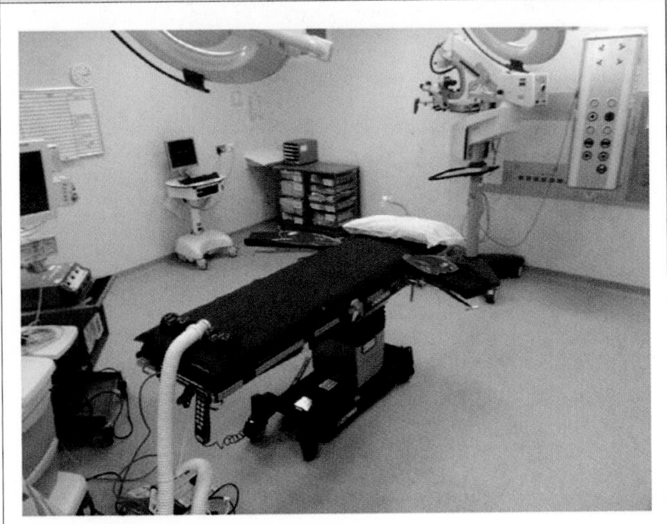

Figure 13.26 **Diathermy equipment.**

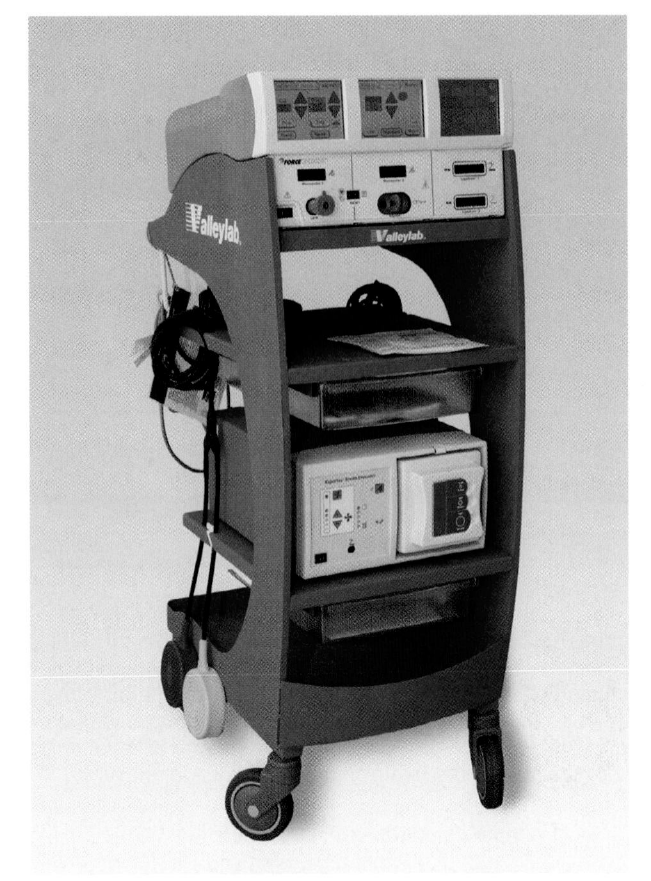

Figure 13.27 **Operating lights.**

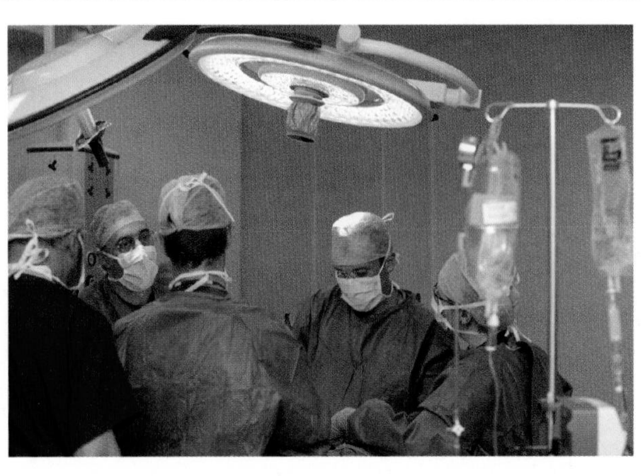

are operational (these should alert the surgical team if the circuit is broken, e.g. the plate/pad detaches from the patient) (AFPP 2011). If the patient's position is changed during the operation, the diathermy patient plate should be rechecked to ensure that it is still in contact and that the connecting clamp or lead is not causing pressure to the skin. Use of diathermy and the plate position should be noted on the nursing care plan and the patient's skin condition (plate site, pressure areas and other areas where exposure to metal could have occurred) should be assessed before the patient is transferred from theatre.

Other causes of burns include alcohol-based skin preparations or other liquids pooling around the plate site. When using alcohol-based skin preparations, the skin should be dried or the alcohol allowed to evaporate before diathermy is used to avoid the risk of ignition (AFPP 2011, Fong et al. 2000).

The use of diathermy during surgical procedures results in a smoke by-product from the coagulation or cutting of the tissue. This smoke plume can be harmful to the perioperative team as it may contain:

- toxic gases and vapours such as benzene, hydrogen cyanide and formaldehyde
- bio-aerosols
- dead and live cellular material, including blood fragments
- viruses (Allen 2004).

To reduce the risk to staff and patients, an efficient filtered evacuation system should be used, such as a smoke evacuation machine; piped hospital suction must not be used (Scott et al. 2004). The patient suction unit is also checked to ensure that it is patent and the suction power is adequate to withdraw excessive bodily fluids from the operating site.

Operating lights (Figure 13.27)

The lights must be bright enough to ensure that the procedure is fully illuminated but not generate excess heat which would dry the exposed tissue. These are checked prior to every operation to ensure they are bright and all the lamps are in working order.

Equipment for laparoscopy procedure

- Camera system (consisting of light source, camera, insufflator, DVD recorder and monitors × 2) (Figure 13.28).

Figure 13.28 **Laparoscopic stack system.**

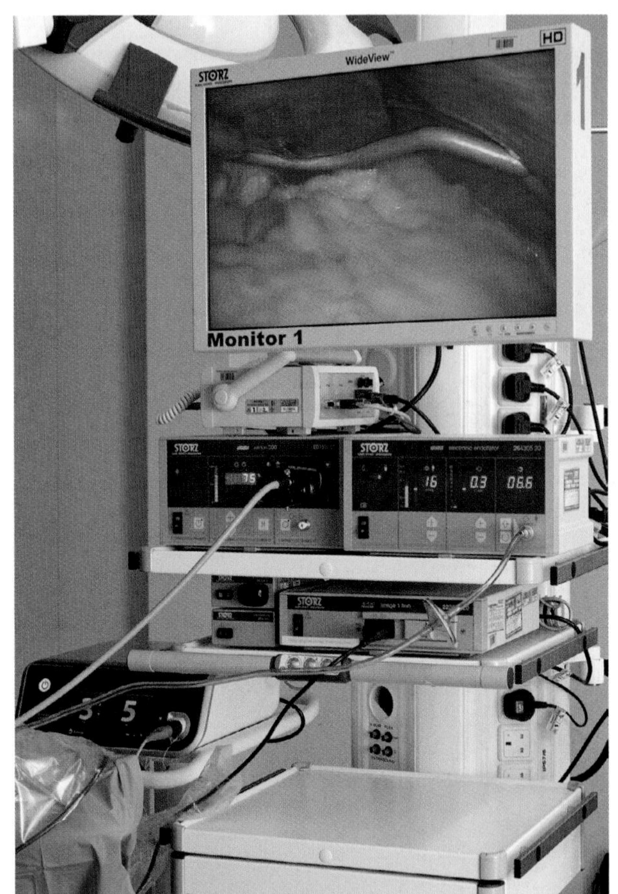

Figure 13.29 **Laparoscope.**

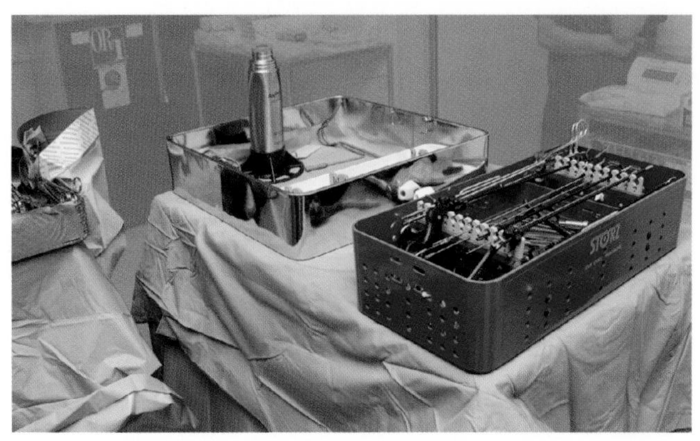

Figure 13.30 **Laparoscopic equipment.**

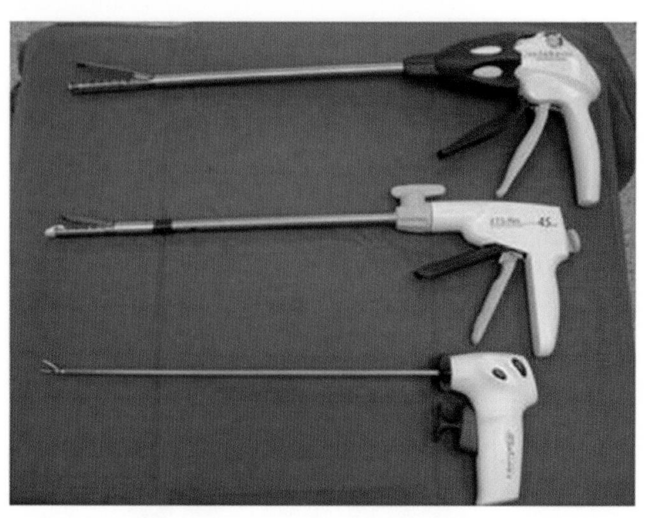

- Laparoscope (Figure 13.29).
- Laparoscopy-specific instruments (scissors, biopsy forceps, grabbers, dissectors, ports, retrieval pouches, insufflating tube, light lead) (Figure 13.30).

The equipment used for laparoscopic surgery is very specialized. The AORN recommends that all equipment is regularly and competently maintained and a maintenance record kept in a log (AORN 2000, Wicker and O'Neill 2010). Policies should be developed for the checking procedure, and all staff thoroughly instructed in the operation of laparoscopic equipment. The staff must be able to properly check the equipment prior to use to ensure the clarity of colour and picture and set the pressure and flow rate of the insufflator for inflating the abdomen with carbon dioxide. The surgeon will determine the level to achieve and this will be activated at the beginning of the procedure.

Procedure guideline 13.4 **Operating theatre procedure: maintaining the safety of a patient while undergoing surgery**

Pre-procedure

Action	Rationale
1 Prior to transferring the patient from the trolley to the operating table, check with the anaesthetist that the patient's airway is protected, patent and safe.	To prevent complications with airway/breathing. **E**
2 There mut be adequate staff (a minimum of 4 is recommended) to transfer the patient onto the operating table. The team must ensure that the brakes on the trolley and operating table have been applied. Ensure the patient's head and limbs are supported when transferring to the operating table. When transferring anaesthetized patients, the anaesthetist takes charge of the patient's head and airway and co-ordinates the transfer. See Figure 13.21.	To prevent patient injury during the transfer between trolley and operating table (AORN 2001, **C**).
3 When positioning the patient, the theatre staff ensure that limbs are supported and secure on the table and that bony prominences are padded/cushioned.	If the patient is unconscious and unable to maintain a safe environment, support is necessary to prevent injury. Nerve damage due to compression or stretching must be prevented.
4 The patient's position will be dictated by the nature of the surgery and can include lateral (**Action figure 4a**) and prone positions (**Action figure 4b**) and the theatre staff will verify the position with the surgeon and anaesthetist and prepare any required positioning equipment/devices.	The patient is at risk from skin/nerve damage during surgery, especially if it is prolonged. Measures must be taken to preserve the integrity of the skin (e.g. use of pressure-relieving mattress/pads). Positioning must take into account the natural movement of the back, neck and limbs to safeguard against injury (AFPP 2011, **C**).
5 Cover the patient with a gown or blanket. The patient must remain covered until immediately before surgery.	To maintain the patient's dignity. To help prevent a reduction in body temperature or accidental hypothermia. **E**

Action	Rationale
6 Use a warming mattress and/or blanket on the operating table (**Action figure 6**). Both intravenous and irrigation fluids should be warmed prior to administration. The theatre staff must ensure that patient and fluid warming devices are available for every operating list.	To help maintain the patient's body temperature, prevent inadvertent perioperative hypothermia and reduce post-operative complications due to hypothermia (NICE 2008, **E**).
7 Ensure the diathermy patient plate is attached securely in accordance with the manufacturer's instructions and sited correctly as close to the operative site as possible (**Action figure 7**).	To ensure that no injury is sustained from the use of diathermy during surgery.
8 Before, during and at the end of surgery, theatre staff perform thorough counts of surgical instruments, swabs, sutures, needles and blades (**Action figure 8**). If an item is not accounted for prior to closure of the surgical wound, the surgeon is notified.	To ensure that all items used in surgery are accounted for at the end of the operation in order to guard against items being retained inside the patient's body following surgery (AFPP 2011, **C**).
9 The scrub nurse/ODP is responsible for ensuring the wound is covered with an appropriate surgical dressing (**Action figure 9**).	The dressing facilitates healing by preventing the wound from drying out and also acting as barrier against external contaminants which can cause wound infection (Wicker and O'Neill 2010). To reduce the risk of injury to the patient and staff (Loveday et al. 2014, **C**).
10 After the surgery has concluded, the theatre staff follow hospital policy regarding the disposal of sharps and clinical waste that are no longer required.	
11 The scrub nurse/ODP is responsible for ensuring that any tissue samples, organs or swabs taken from the patient during the surgery are correctly labelled with the patient details and the exact nature of the specimen before being sent for histological/microbiological examination as specified by the operating surgeon.	The examination of specimens within the laboratory will decide any subsequent treatment for the patient. It is essential that labelling and documentation accompanying the specimen are accurate and that it arrives in the laboratory within the specified time frame (AFPP 2011, **C**).
12 The scrub nurse/ODP together with the anaesthetist and the other theatre staff take responsibility for the safety and well-being and dignity of the patient during the phase between the surgery finishing and the transfer/handover to the post-operative care team. During this period, when patients who have undergone general anaesthesia are usually emerging from the anaesthetic, the theatre staff prepare to hand over the patient and ensure that the relevant documentation has been completed. This is also when the time-out phase of the WHO Surgical Safety Checklist is completed by the whole theatre team (see Box 13.11). The patient will require reassurance and safe transfer from the operating table to a trolley/bed.	

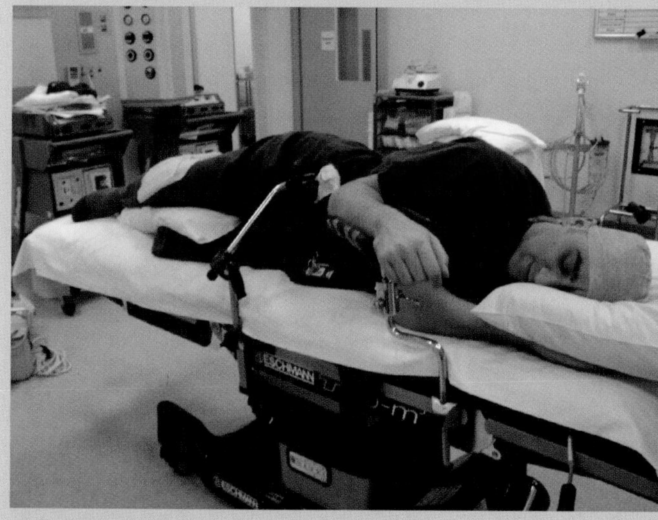
(a)

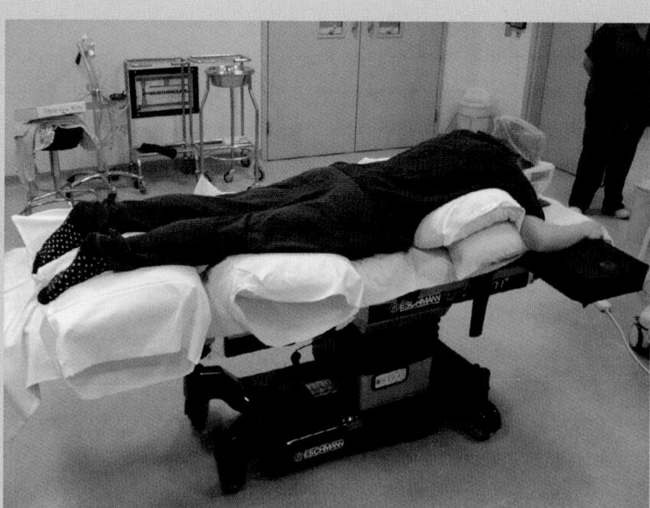
(b)

Action Figure 4 (a) Lateral position. (b) Prone position.

(continued)

Procedure guideline 13.4 **Operating theatre procedure: maintaining the safety of a patient while undergoing surgery *(continued)***

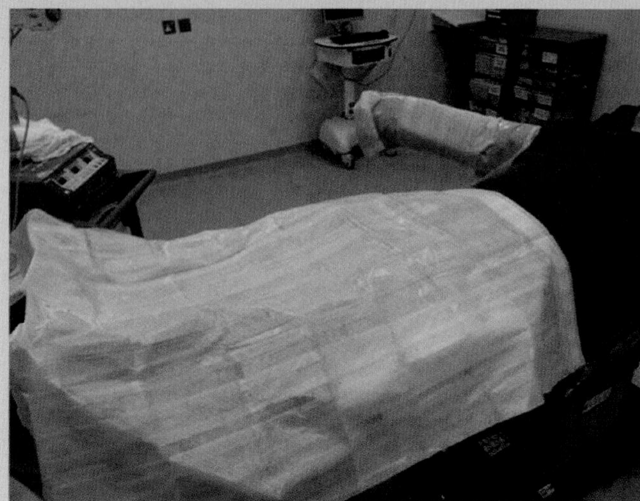

Action Figure 6 Warming blanket.

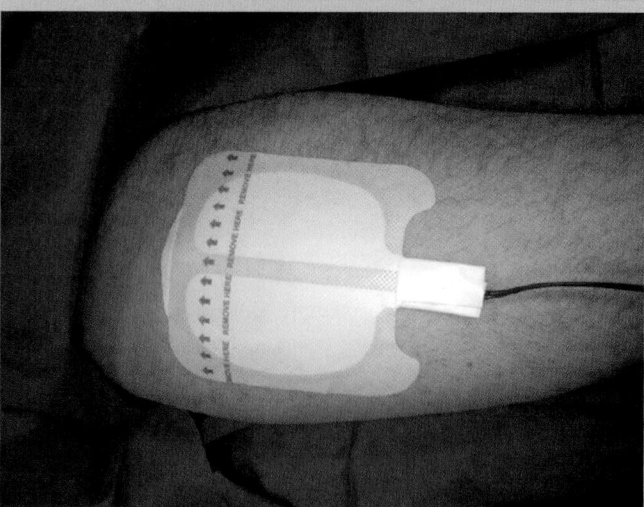

Action Figure 7 Diathermy plate in position.

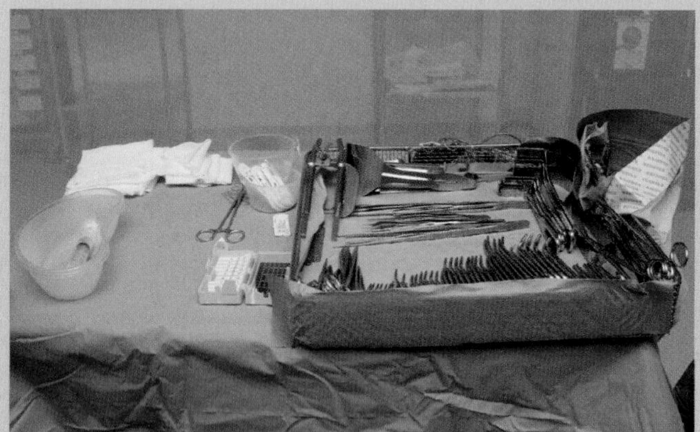

Action Figure 8 Surgical equipment in sterile field.

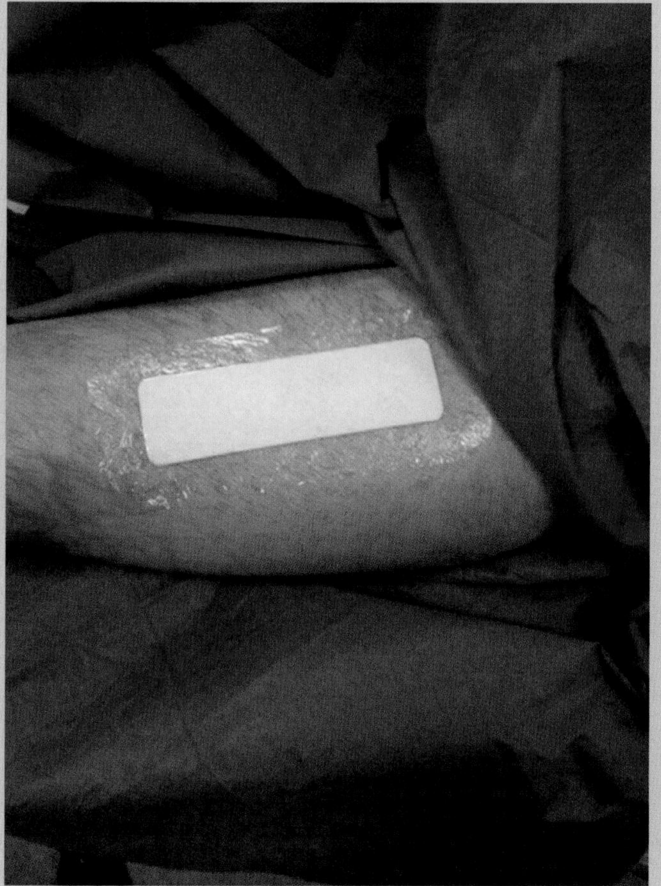

Action Figure 9 Surgical dressing *in situ.*

Intraoperative care: post-anaesthetic care unit (PACU)

DEFINITION

Post-anaesthetic recovery involves the short- to medium-term care required by patients (following general, epidural or spinal anaesthesia) during the immediate post-operative period until they are stable, conscious, orientated and safe to transfer back to the ward, day unit or higher dependency area. The post-anaesthetic recovery room is an area within the operating department specifically designed, equipped and staffed for the support, monitoring and assessment of patients immediately following anaesthesia and surgery.

Transfer of patient from operating theatre to post-anaesthetic care unit

The patient is transferred from the operating theatre to the PACU by the anaesthetist and/or anaesthetic nurse/ODP and/or the scrub nurse/ODP. It is the anaesthetist's responsibility to ensure the safe transfer of the patient. The patient should be assessed as stable prior to leaving the operating theatre and the anaesthetist will decide on the level of monitoring required which will depend on the distance of the transfer, the patient's level of consciousness and both their cardiovascular and respiratory status.

Oxygen is usually administered to the patient during the transfer unless they did not receive supplemental oxygen during the procedure. It is vital that the anaesthetist flush the patient's IV lines to ensure that there are no residual anaesthetic drugs remaining (AAGBI et al. 2013).

EVIDENCE-BASED APPROACHES

Post-anaesthetic care

Post-anaesthetic care can best be described and understood as a series of nursing procedures performed sequentially and simultaneously on patients immediately post anaesthesia/surgery. These patients will display varying degrees of responsiveness and physical and emotional states.

The recovery period is potentially hazardous. Therefore, when the patient arrives in the PACU, individual nursing care is required until the nurse is satisfied that the patient can maintain their own airway and is sufficiently oxygenated (AAGBI et al. 2013, AFPP 2011).

Procedure guideline 13.5 **Handover in post-anaesthetic care unit: scrub nurse/ODP to recovery practitioner**

Procedure

Action	Rationale
1 Accompany the patient with the anaesthetist to the recovery area. Hand over the following:	To ensure continuity and effective communication of care for the patient. To ensure that the recovery practitioner has all the information required to assess the patient's recovery needs. **C**
• the surgical procedure performed	The actual procedure performed may be different from the proposed procedure. **E**
• information including allergies or pre-existing medical conditions, for example diabetes mellitus	To highlight specific potential post-operative complications to be assessed and monitored. **E**
• the patient's cardiovascular state and type of anaesthesia administered	To safely maintain the patient's cardiovascular system and airway immediately post-operatively. **E**
• the presence, position and nature of any drains, infusions or intravenous or arterial devices	To ensure care and management of these drains are continued and the positioning of the patient is assessed to prevent any occlusion of drains or infusions. **E**
• information about any anxieties of the patient expressed before surgery, such as a fear of not waking after anaesthesia or fear about coping with pain	To ensure that the recovery practitioner can respond appropriately as the patient regains consciousness and to enable assessment of the efficacy of subsequent nursing interventions. **E**
• specific instructions from the surgeon/anaesthetist for post-operative care.	To facilitate effective communication of the patient's care and treatment and to ensure that the appropriate post-operative clinical care is delivered. **E**
Post-procedure	
2 Record all information in the perioperative nursing care plan.	

PRE-PROCEDURAL CONSIDERATIONS

Equipment required in the PACU

Whereas in the past, post-anaesthetic care meant a relatively brief period of observation in an area close to theatres, it has now evolved into a distinct critical care area where patients of varying dependency receive specialist clinical care from trained staff using a variety of drugs, monitoring and equipment (AAGBI et al. 2013). The following items are the minimum required in each bed space (Figure 13.31). The equipment should be compatible between the operating theatres and the PACU. It must be arranged for ease of access and always be clean and in full working order.

- *Patient monitoring*: pulse oximetry, non-invasive blood pressure monitoring, ECG, invasive pressure monitoring, temperature monitoring and capnography.
- *Basic equipment for airway maintenance*: wall-mounted piped oxygen with tubing and facemask (with both fixed and variable settings), a Mapleson C breathing circuit and a self-inflating resuscitator bag, for example Ambu-bag with facemask, a full range of oral and nasopharyngeal airways. These allow for maintenance of the airway, delivery of oxygen and artificial ventilation of the patient should it be necessary. Spare oxygen cylinders with flowmeters should also be available in case of piped oxygen failure.
- *Suction*: regulator with tubing and a range of oral and endotracheal suction catheters. An electric-powered portable suction machine should also be available in case of pipeline vacuum failure.
- *Sphygmomanometer and stethoscope*: in case of failure of the electronic patient monitor, manual blood pressure monitoring equipment must always be available.

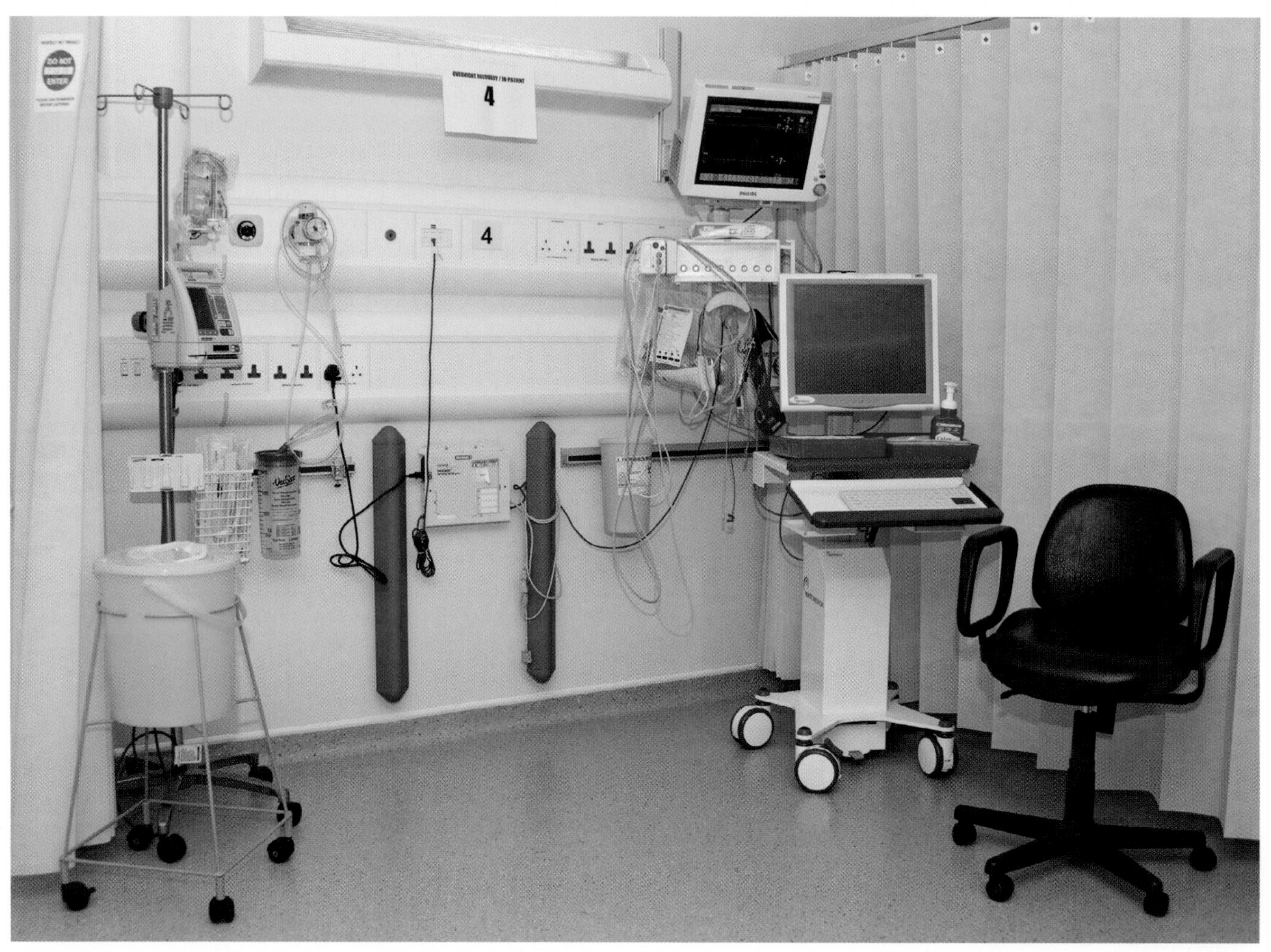

Figure 13.31 **Recovery bay.**

- Electrical sockets and individual lamps.
- *Miscellaneous items*: receivers, tissues, disposable gloves, sharps container and waste receptacle (AAGBI et al. 2013, AFPP 2011).

Other equipment should be available centrally for respiratory and cardiovascular support.

- *Intubation and difficult airway equipment:* fibreoptic laryngoscopes with spare batteries and a range of blades (including McCoy tip), range of endotracheal tubes, bougies, Magill forceps, syringe and catheter mount. This is to ensure that the patient can be intubated quickly during an emergency.
- *Ventilator:* to ensure that the patient can be mechanically ventilated if extubated too early, not fully reversed from the anaesthetic.
- *Range of tracheostomy tubes and tracheal dilator*: in case an emergency tracheostomy needs to be performed.
- *Intravenous infusion sets, cannula, central venous catheters and a range of intravenous fluids.*
- *Defibrillator*: required during a cardiac arrest to restart the heart.
- *Nerve stimulators* should be available to monitor level of neuromuscular blockade.
- *Patient and fluid warming devices* to maintain normothermia and correct inadvertent perioperative hypothermia.

The relevant resuscitation equipment, drugs, fluids and algorithms should be immediately available for the management of both surgical and anaesthetic complications. Ideally these items are contained in dedicated trolleys (AAGBI et al. 2013, AFPP 2011).

PACU staff

No less than two staff (at least one must be a registered practitioner) should be present when there is a patient in the PACU who does not fulfil the discharge criteria. The staffing level should allow one-to-one observation of every patient by an anaesthetist or registered PACU practitioner until the patient has regained control of their airway, is haemodynamically and respiratory stable and able to communicate. One member of staff present should be a certified Acute Life Support (ALS) provider. Life-threatening complications can occur during the immediate post-operative/anaesthesia phase. Any failure to provide adequate care could have devastating consequences for patients, their families and staff. Patients must be kept under clinical observation at all times. The frequency of the observations is dependent upon the procedure performed, the physical status of the patient and the stage of recovery. Box 13.12 outlines the minimum information that should be routinely monitored/recorded for patients in PACU.

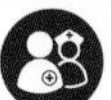

Box 13.12 **Minimum information to be recorded for patients in the post-anaesthesia care unit**

- Level of consciousness.
- Patency of the airway.
- Respiratory rate and adequacy.
- Oxygen saturation.
- Oxygen administration.
- Blood pressure.
- Heart rate and rhythm.
- Pain intensity on an agreed scale.
- Nausea and vomiting.
- Intravenous infusions.
- Drugs administered.
- Core temperature.
- Other parameters depending on circumstances, e.g. urinary output, central
- venous pressure, expired CO_2, surgical drainage volume.

Source: AAGBI et al. (2013). Reproduced with permission from John Wiley & Sons.

COMPLICATIONS

Pain

Pain is the most common adverse effect of surgery for the majority of patients (McMain 2010). Pain is a subjective experience and patients in the PACU should receive both effective and empathetic care to relieve their pain (AFPP 2011). A patient should not be discharged from the PACU until satisfactory pain control has been achieved. PACU staff must be trained and competent in the use of intravenous analgesia, patient-controlled analgesia, management of epidurals, spinals and peripheral nerve blocks (AAGBI et al. 2013). It is important to recognize that pain may not only be due to the surgery. Other reasons include pre-existing medical conditions, poor positioning during surgery, headache as a result of anaesthetic drugs and muscle aches from the use of depolarizing muscle relaxants (suxamethonium) (Wicker and O'Neill 2010).

Nausea and vomiting

Post-operative nausea and vomiting (PONV) may arise from many causes. These include hypotension, swallowing of blood (for example in oral surgery), abdominal surgery, anxiety, but most commonly, as a side-effect of opioid administration. Nausea, vomiting and retching may exist independently and therefore require individual assessment (AFPP 2011). No patient should be discharged from the PACU unless their PONV is controlled and suitable medication prescribed (AAGBI et al. 2013).

Hypothermia

Inadvertent perioperative hypothermia (which is defined as below 36.0°C) is a common but preventable complication of surgery and is associated with poor outcomes for patients. Adult surgical patients may develop hypothermia at any stage of the perioperative journey though the elderly, malnourished and those who have undergone long surgery or where large amounts of blood or fluid replacement therapy have been used are especially at risk (Nunney 2008).

During the first 30–40 minutes of anaesthesia, a patient's temperature can fall to below 35.0°C. Reasons for this include:

- loss of the behavioural response to cold
- impairment of thermoregulatory heat-preserving mechanisms (due to general or regional anaesthesia)
- anaesthesia-induced peripheral vasodilation (with associated heat loss)
- the patient becoming cold while waiting for surgery in the pre-operative area (NICE 2008).

On admission to the PACU, the patient's temperature should be measured and documented. If it is below 36.0°C, active warming should be commenced until the patient is warm/discharged from the recovery room. They should not be discharged until the temperature is 36.0°C or above. Hypothermia produces symptoms which mimic those of other post-operative complications, which may result in inappropriate treatment. Hypothermia interferes with the effective reversal of muscle relaxants, so monitor patients who are shivering, restless, confused or with respiratory depression. Shivering puts an increased demand on cardiopulmonary systems as oxygen consumption is increased (Feldmann 1988, Frank et al. 1993). Other complications such as arrhythmias or myocardial infarct can result and the longer the duration of the post-operative hypothermia, the greater the patient mortality (Crayne and Miner 1988).

Other complications

When emerging from the final stage of anaesthesia, some patients can behave in an emotional and disinhibited fashion, at variance with their normal behaviour (Eckenhoff et al. 1961, Radtke et al. 2008). Therefore it is important to establish a rapport with each individual to gain the patient's confidence and co-operation and to aid assessment. These displays are always transient and fortunately patients seldom have any recollection of them. All actions must be accompanied by commentary and explanation regardless of the patient's apparent responsiveness, as the sense of hearing returns before the patient's ability to respond (Levinson 1965, Starritt 1999).

Procedure guideline 13.6 **Safe management of the patient in the PACU**

The following recommended actions are not necessarily listed in order of priority. Many will be carried out simultaneously and will depend on the patient's condition, type of surgery and level of consciousness.

Procedure

Action	Rationale
1 Assess the patency of the airway by feeling for movement of expired air.	To determine the presence of any respiratory depression or neuromuscular blockade. Observe chest and abdominal movement, respiratory rate, depth and pattern (Drummond 1991, **C**).
2 Listen for inspiration and expiration. Observe any use of accessory muscles of respiration and check for tracheal tug which might indicate airway obstruction.	To ensure airway is clear and laryngeal spasm is not present. **E**
3 If indicated, support the chin with the neck extended.	In the unconscious patient the tongue is liable to fall back and obstruct the airway, and protective reflexes are absent. **E**

(continued)

Procedure guideline 13.6 Safe management of the patient in the PACU *(continued)*

Action	Rationale
4 Suction of the upper airway is indicated if: • gurgling sounds are present on respiration • blood secretions or vomitus are evident or suspected • the patient is unable to swallow • the patient is unable to cough adequately or at all. Suction must be applied with care to avoid damage to mucosal surfaces and further irritation or initiation of a gag reflex or laryngeal spasm.	Foreign matter can obstruct the airway or cause laryngeal spasm in light planes (induction and emergence) of anaesthesia. Foreign matter can also be inhaled when protective laryngeal reflexes are absent (Dhara 1997, **C**).
5 (a) Apply a facemask and administer oxygen at the rate prescribed by the anaesthetist. (b) If an endotracheal tube or laryngeal mask is in position, check whether the cuff or mask is inflated and administer oxygen by means of a T-piece system.	To maintain adequate oxygenation. Oxygen should be administered to all patients in the recovery room (Nimmo et al. 1994, **C**).
6 Check the colour of lips and conjunctiva, then peripheral colour and perfusion (skin temperature and peripheral pulse).	Central cyanosis indicates impaired gaseous exchange between the alveoli and pulmonary capillaries. Peripheral cyanosis indicates low cardiac output (Nimmo et al. 1994, **C**).
7 Record blood pressure, pulse and respiratory rate measurements on admission to the PACU and at a minimum of 5-minute intervals unless the patient's condition dictates otherwise.	To enable any fluctuations or gross abnormalities in cardiovascular and respiratory functions to be detected immediately (Peskett 1999, **C**). To assess cardiovascular function and establish a post-operative baseline for future comparisons (Peskett 1999, **C**).
8 Obtain full handover from the surgical/anaesthetic team.	To ensure effective communication of the patient's care and treatment and to aid the planning of subsequent care. **E**
9 Check the temperature of the patient.	Peri- and post-operative hypothermia is common and preventable.
10 Check and observe wound site(s), dressings and drains on admission to the PACU and at regular intervals. Note and record leakage/drainage on the post-operative chart and also on the drain bottle/bag.	To assess and monitor for signs of haemorrhage (Eltringham et al. 1989, **C**).
11 Check that intravenous infusions are running at the correct prescribed rate in accordance with local policy and the site of the venous access device is assessed as patent in accordance with local protocol.	Care of venous devices/sites prevents complications and ensures that fluid replacement and balance are achieved safely. **E**
12 Check the prescription chart for medications to be administered during the immediate post-operative period, for example analgesia and antiemetics.	To treat and prevent symptoms such as pain and nausea swiftly and appropriately and further monitor their effectiveness. **E**
13 Orientate the patient to time and place as frequently as is necessary.	To alleviate anxiety, provide reassurance and gain the patient's confidence and co-operation. Pre-medication and anaesthesia can induce a degree of amnesia and disorientation. **C**
14 Give mouth care including moistened mouth swabs, sips of water and petroleum jelly for the lips.	Pre-operative fasting, drying gases and manipulation of lips, and so on, leave mucosa vulnerable, sore and foul tasting. **E**
15 After regional and/or spinal anaesthesia, assess the return of sensation and mobility of limbs. Check that the limbs are anatomically aligned.	To prevent inadvertent injury following sensory loss (AAGBI 2002, **C**).

Problem-solving table 13.1 Prevention and resolution (Procedure guideline 13.6)

Problem	Cause	Prevention	Suggested action
Airway obstruction.	Tongue occluding the airway.	Do not remove the laryngeal mask or the Guedel airway until the patient starts responding to commands.	Support chin forward from the angle of the jaw. If necessary, insert a Guedel airway. Use a nasopharyngeal airway if the teeth are clenched or crowned.

Problem	Cause	Prevention	Suggested action
	Foreign material, blood, secretions, vomitus.	Use suction to remove secretions when removing airway.	Apply suction. Always check for the presence of a throat pack.
	Laryngeal spasm.	Do not remove airway until patient responds to commands and ensure oxygen flow is high (5–10 litres) on arrival in PACU.	Increase the rate of oxygen. Assist ventilation with an ambu-bag and facemask. If there is no improvement, inform anaesthetist and have intubation equipment ready. Offer the patient reassurance by talking to them and telling them what you are doing.
Hypoventilation.	Respiratory depression from medications, for example opiates, inhalations, barbiturates.	Monitor depth and rate of respiration before administering analgesia.	Inform the anaesthetist, keeping oxygen on, and administer antagonist on instruction, for example naloxone (opiate antagonist), doxapram (respiratory stimulant). Note: if naloxone is given it can reverse the analgesic effects of opiates and has a duration of action of only 20–30 minutes. The patient must be observed for signs of returning hyperventilation (Nimmo et al. 1994).
	Decreased respiratory drive from a low partial pressure of carbon dioxide ($PaCO_2$), loss of hypoxic drive in patients with chronic pulmonary disease.	Ensure that Venturi masks are available and close to hand in the recovery bay.	Administer oxygen using a Venturi mask with graded low concentrations (Atkinson et al. 1982).
	Residual neuromuscular blockade from continued action of non-depolarizing muscle relaxants, potentiation of relaxants caused by electrolyte imbalance, impaired excretion with renal or liver disease. Signs include: difficulty breathing/speaking, generalized weakness, visual disturbances, patient distress.		Inform the anaesthetist, have available neostigmine and glycopyrrolate, or atropine, potassium chloride and 10% calcium chloride. Often the blockade is mild and will wear off in minutes without treatment, but it is extremely frightening and patients will need continuous reassurance that their condition is not unnoticed and is resolving and that they will not be left alone.
Hypotension.	Hypovolaemia.	Increase the rate of fluids and ensure more fluids are prescribed.	Take manual reading of the blood pressure. Take central venous pressure (CVP) readings if catheter is in place. Give oxygen. Lower the head of the trolley unless contraindicated, for example hiatus hernia, gross obesity. Check the record of anaesthetic agents used which might cause hypotension, for example enflurane, beta-blockers, nitroprusside, opiates, droperidol, sympathetic blockade following spinal anaesthesia. Check the peripheral perfusion. If the CVP is low, increase intravenous infusion unless contraindicated, for example congestive cardiac failure. Check drains and dressings for visible bleeding and haematoma. Inform the anaesthetist or surgeon.
Hypertension.	Pain.	Ensure pain is assessed as soon as patient is responding to commands and scores are recorded.	Treat pain with prescribed analgesia and provide a quiet environment to enable the patient to rest/sleep. Pain from certain operation sites can also be alleviated by changing the patient's position.
	Fluid overload.	Slow the intravenous rate.	Check fluid balance sheet and the rate of intravenous infusion.
	Distended bladder.	Check if the bladder is distended and catheter is patent.	Offer a bedpan or urinal and if necessary catheterize the patient.

(continued)

Problem-solving table 13.1 **Prevention and resolution (Procedure guideline 8.12)** ***(continued)***

Problem	Cause	Prevention	Suggested action
	Some anaesthetic drugs given during reversal of anaesthetic.	Ensure the anaesthetist monitors patient when reversing effects of anaesthetic drugs.	Check the prescription chart for those patients on regular antihypertensive therapy. If the situation is not resolved, inform the anaesthetist. Also check patient's past medical history.
Bradycardia.	Very fit patient, opiates, reversal agents, beta-blockers, pain, vagal stimulation, hypoxaemia from respiratory depression.	Ensure oxygen is administered and anaesthetist identifies any adverse episodes of bradycardia during surgery.	Connect the patient to the ECG monitor to exclude heart block and monitor cardiac activity. Ascertain pre-operative cardiac function. Check the prescription chart and anaesthetic sheet for medication administered that may cause bradycardia. Inform and liaise with the anaesthetist.
Tachycardia.	Pain, hypovolaemia, some anaesthetic drugs, for example ephedrine, septicaemia, fear, fluid overload.	Ensure pain is managed and intravenous fluids are adminstered.	Assess patient's pain and provide analgesia. Check the anaesthetic chart to ascertain which anaesthetic drugs were used. Connect the patient to the ECG monitor to exclude ventricular tachycardia. Provide reassurance for the patient. Assess fluid balance.
Pain.	Surgical trauma, worsened by fear, anxiety and restlessness.	Adminster analgesia after assessing patient's pain.	Provide prescribed analgesia and assess its efficacy. Reassure and orientate the patient. Try positional changes where feasible; for example, after breast surgery raise the back support by 20–40°; abdominal or gynaecological surgery patients may be more comfortable lying on their side. Elevate limbs to reduce swelling where appropriate. If significant relief is not obtained, inform the anaesthetist and the pain control specialist nurse.
Nausea and vomiting.	Anaesthetic agents, opiates, hypotension, abdominal surgery, pain; high-risk patients who have a history of post-operative nausea and vomiting.	Administer antiemetics with the analgesia and ensure intravenous fluids are administered as prescribed.	Administer intravenous antiemetics and monitor effectiveness. Encourage slow, regular breathing. If the patient is unconscious, turn onto the side, tip the head down and suck out pharynx; give oxygen.
Hypothermia.	Depression of the heat-regulating centre, vasodilation, following abdominal surgery, large infusions of unwarmed blood and fluids.	Measure and record the patient's temperature upon arrival in the PACU and maintain temperature using a Bair Hugger.	Use extra blankets or a Bair Hugger (Kumar et al. 2005). Monitor the patient's temperature. Administer warm intravenous fluids. Bladder irrigation may also be warmed to normal body temperature.
Shivering.	Some inhalational anaesthetics, hypothermia.	Measure and record the patient's temperature on arrival in the PACU and maintain temperature using a Bair Hugger. Measure temperature every 30–60 mins.	Give oxygen, reassure the patient and take their temperature. Provide a Bair Hugger and warm blankets.
Hyperthermia.	Infection, blood transfusion reaction.	Measure and record temperature at least every 30–60 mins.	Give oxygen, use a fan or tepid sponging if this is warranted. Medical assessment of antibiotic therapy and obtaining blood cultures. Administer intravenous paracetamol if prescribed.
	Malignant hyperpyrexia (above 40°).	This may be identified during the anaesthetic. All anaesthetic and theatre personnel must know the location of the emergency drug (dantrolene) which is kept in every operating theatre suite.	Malignant hyperpyrexia is a medical emergency. Dantrolene is used to treat this life-threatening condition.

Problem	Cause	Prevention	Suggested action
Oliguria.	Mechanical obstruction of catheter, for example clots, kinking.	Check patency and drainage upon arrival in the PACU and every 30–60 mins.	Check the patency of the catheter. Consider bladder irrigation. If clots present, inform surgeon.
	Inadequate renal perfusion, for example hypotension, systolic pressures under 60 mmHg, hypovolaemia, dehydration.		Take blood pressure and CVP if available. Increase intravenous fluids. Inform the anaesthetist.
	Renal damage, for example from blood transfusion, infection, drugs, surgical damage to the ureters.		Inform the anaesthetist or surgeon.

POST-PROCEDURAL CONSIDERATIONS

Discharge from PACU

Discharge from the PACU is ultimately the responsibility of the anaesthetist but is usually delegated to the PACU practitioner who uses discharge criteria to assess whether the patient has achieved the optimum recovery, enabling them to return to the ward safely. In the event of complications or deterioration, the anaesthetist must be informed and should assess the patient before their return to the ward (AAGBI et al. 2013, AFPP 2011).

The PACU must specify minimum criteria that patients must meet prior to their discharge to the general ward or other clinical areas (Box 13.13).

Learning Activity 13.4 Case study: Safe discharge from the post-anaesthetic care unit

Jane Ward, 38 years old, is being discharged back to the ward from the post-anaesthetic care unit (PACU). She has had laparoscopic gynaecological surgery and, so far, is recovering well. She has oxygen via a face mask and her respiration rate is 14 breaths/minute, oxygen saturations 99%. Her pulse is 76, blood pressure 110/60 and her temperature is 36.2°C. 30 minutes ago she was feeling rather sick so was given some more antiemetic and is now managing to take a few sips of water. She still has a bag of IV fluids that is running through a peripheral cannula, no drains or catheter *in situ*. Her stomach is feeling a little painful but she hasn't mentioned this to the nurse yet.

You have been asked by the ward to go and collect Jane from PACU. When you arrive you find she is awake and alert and the nurse hands over the information provided above. You ask Jane how she is feeling and she says she is ok but her stomach isn't feeling great.

1 Using the criteria for discharging patients from PACU (see Box 13.13) and the information from handover, what else would you want to check before accepting Jane and returning her to the ward?
2 You find that Jane has a pain score of 7/10; her wound dressings are all clean and intact. What would you do next?

See the end of the chapter for the answers.

Post-operative care

DEFINITION

Post-operative care is the physical and psychological care given to the patient immediately after transfer from the recovery room to the ward. Post-operative care continues until the patient is discharged from hospital, and in some cases continues on as ambulatory care as an outpatient.

EVIDENCE-BASED APPROACHES

Principles of care

Although different surgical procedures require specific and specialist nursing care, the principles of post-operative care

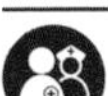

Box 13.13 Minimum criteria for discharge of patients from the post-anaesthesia care unit

- The patient is fully conscious, able to maintain a clear airway and has protective airway reflexes.
- Breathing and oxygenation are satisfactory.
- The cardiovascular system is stable, with no unexplained cardiac irregularity or persistent bleeding. The specific values of pulse and blood pressure should approximate to normal pre-operative values or be at an acceptable level, ideally within parameters set by the anaesthetist, and peripheral perfusion should be adequate.
- Pain and post-operative nausea and vomiting should be adequately controlled, and suitable analgesic and antiemetic regimens prescribed.
- Temperature should be within acceptable limits. Patients should not be returned to the ward if significantly hypothermic.
- Oxygen therapy should be prescribed if appropriate.
- Intravenous cannulae should be patent, flushed if necessary to ensure removal of any residual anaesthetic drugs and intravenous fluids should be prescribed if appropriate.
- All surgical drains and catheters should be checked.
- All health records should be complete and medical notes present.

Source: AAGBI et al. (2013). Reproduced with permission from John Wiley & Sons.

remain the same, underpinned by the application of evidence-based care. Optimal management of patients throughout the post-operative phase requires appropriate clinical assessment, monitoring and timely and accurate documentation. The nursing care given during the post-operative period is directed towards the prevention of those potential complications resulting from surgery and anaesthesia. Potential complications are outlined in Figure 13.32.

Anticipated patient outcomes

Safety of the patient at all times and the minimizing of post-operative complications by:

- delivering the required nursing care for the post-operative patient. This includes fully informing the patient of the post-operative care requirements so that they can enhance their recovery, facilitating earlier discharge home
- optimizing the patient's post-operative physical and psychological condition to minimize the risk of potential post-operative complications occurring. This is achieved through comprehensive nursing assessment and planning to ensure early identification and management of any post-operative complications.

Figure 13.32 **Post-operative complications.**

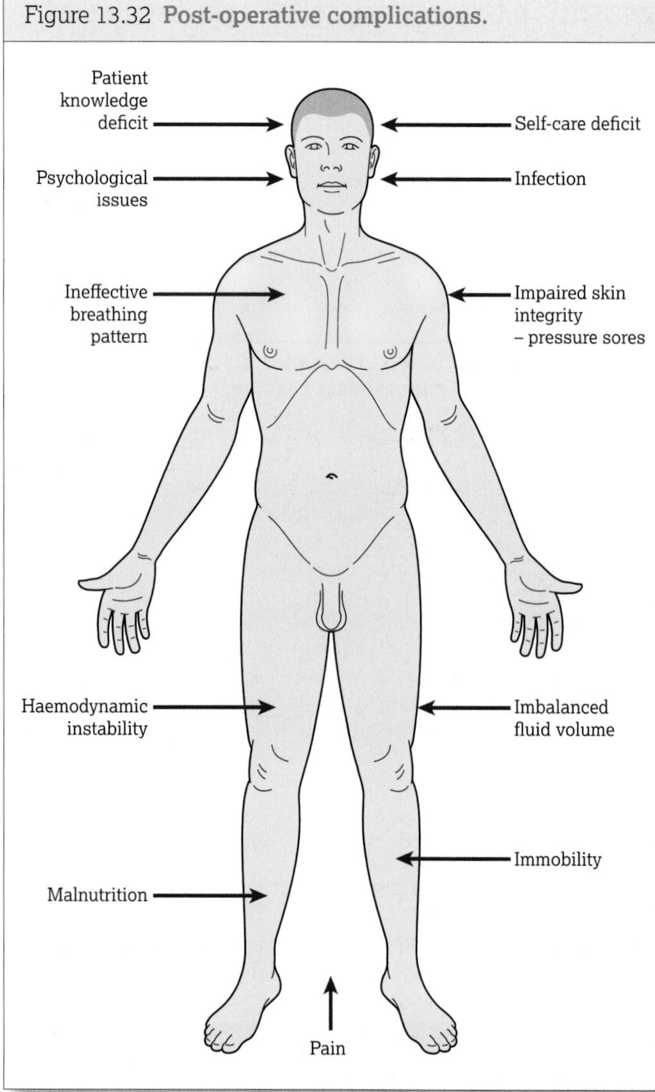

Post-operative observations

EVIDENCE-BASED APPROACHES

Principles of care

Regular monitoring and accurate reporting of the patient's clinical observations in the post-operative period are an essential part of the planned surgical care pathway, which can identify potential complications. Post-operative observations are outlined in Table 13.8. A clear physiological monitoring plan should be made for each patient, detailing frequency of observations and parameters (NCEPOD 2011). All nurses should be aware of the parameters for these observations and what is normal for the patient under observation. Post-operative observations should be compared with baseline observations taken pre-operatively, during surgery and in the recovery area (Liddle 2013). The regularity of post-operative observations should be determined in accordance with local policies or guidelines and will be affected by the type of surgery performed as well as the method of pain control (e.g. epidural) and as indicated by the patient's clinical condition. All vital signs and assessments should be recorded in accordance with guidelines for record keeping (NMC 2010).

Critical care outreach and acute care teams have long encouraged the use of early warning scoring (EWS) systems to enable a more timely response to, and assessment of, acutely ill patients (Royal College of Physicians 2012). EWS is a simple physiological scoring system, based on the observations previously outlined, that identifies patients at risk of deterioration who may require increased levels of care (DH 2000, NICE 2007) (see Chapter 11: Observations).

LEGAL AND PROFESSIONAL ISSUES

The National Confidential Enquiry into Patient Outcome and Death (NCEPOD 2011) report established that patients whose clinical condition was deteriorating post-operatively were not always identified and referred for a higher level of care. When assessing the post-operative patient, it is vital that the patient is observed for signs of haemorrhage, shock, sepsis and the effects of analgesia and anaesthetic (Liddle 2013). It is therefore imperative that nurses are able to interpret the results of

Table 13.8 **Post-operative observations**

Routine post-operative observations include:	Normal range:
• Blood pressure	• <101–149 mmHg systolic
• Pulse (rate, rhythm and amplitude)	• 51–100 beats per minute
• Respiration rate (rate, depth, effort and pattern)	• Respirations: 9–14 per minute
• Peripheral oxygen saturation	• >95% on room air
• Temperature	• 36.1–37.9°C
• Accurate fluid balance (to include input and output)	• Desired balance guided by surgeons and surgery performed
• Pain score	• Verbal numeric pain scale: 0–1/10 at rest; 3/10 on movement/coughing
• Sedation score	• Sedation score: 0/4 (see Chapter 11: Observations)
Additional observations if clinically indicated:	
• Blood glucose	• 4–7 mmol/L
• Central venous pressure	• 5–10 cm H_2O
• Neurological response	• Glasgow Coma Scale: 14–15/15 or AVPU: AV

Source: Adapted from Bickley et al. (2009), DH (2000), Liddle (2013).

post-operative observations and, if reliant on appropriately trained care assistants to take the observations, that nurses themselves interpret the results, thereby ensuring that patients who require a higher level of care are given immediate priority.

If obtaining blood pressure measurements using an electronic sphygmomanometer, the trained health professional should be aware that errors in measurement can occur. For example, a weak, thready or irregular pulse may not be identified by the monitor and/or produce an inaccurate blood pressure reading. Best practice indicates that prior to using an electronic sphygmomanometer, the patient's pulse should be palpated for rate, rhythm, volume and character. If an irregular, weak or thready pulse is identified, then the patient's blood pressure should be measured with a manual sphygmomanometer to ensure accuracy of the reading. This information should be clearly documented to alert other health professionals. It is therefore essential that trained health professionals develop the skill and dexterity to monitor patients' vital signs with traditional manual equipment (see Chapter 11: Observations).

It has also been reported that pulse oximeters can be open to misinterpretation and therefore should not replace a respiratory assessment, which is an early and sensitive indicator of deterioration (NCEPOD 2011) (see 'Ineffective breathing pattern').

An abnormal pulse oximeter recording may be due to shivering, peripheral vasoconstriction or dried blood on the finger probe. Prior to taking a recording, appropriately trained healthcare professionals should ensure that the finger probe is clean, residual nail varnish (if applicable) is removed and the position of the probe is changed regularly to prevent fingers becoming sore.

Haemodynamic instability

RELATED THEORY

Haemodynamic instability is most commonly associated with an abnormal or unstable blood pressure, especially hypotension (Anderson 2003). A reduction in systolic blood pressure following surgery can indicate hypovolaemic shock, a condition in which the blood vessels do not contain sufficient blood (Hatfield and Tronson 2009). Bleeding is the most common cause but other causes can occur when tissue fluid is lost from the circulation, for example bowel obstruction and nausea and vomiting (Hughes 2004). Hatfield and Tronson (2009, p.348) outline three stages of hypovolaemic shock.

- *Compensated shock:* blood flow to the brain and heart is preserved at the expense of the kidneys, gastrointestinal system, skin and muscles.
- *Decompensated shock:* the body's compensatory mechanisms begin to fail and organ perfusion is severely reduced.
- *Irreversible shock:* tissues become so deprived of oxygen that multiorgan failure occurs.

EVIDENCE-BASED APPROACHES

Principles of care

During compensated shock, some patients can lose up to 30% of their circulatory volume before the effects of hypovolaemia are reflected in the systolic blood pressure measurements or heart rate (Hughes 2004). Therefore, when assessing post-operative patients it is also useful to consider the early signs of reduced tissue perfusion in detecting signs of hypovolaemic shock, which include:

- restlessness, anxiety or confusion (as a result of cerebral hypoperfusion or hypoxia)
- increased respiratory rate, becoming shallow (frequently occurring before signs of tachycardia and hypotension)
- rising pulse rate (tachycardia as the heart attempts to compensate for the low circulatory blood volume)
- low urine output of <0.5 mL/kg/h (as the kidneys experience a reduction in perfusion and pressure, which activates the renin-angiotensin system in an attempt to conserve fluid and increase circulatory blood volume)
- pallor (pale, cyanotic skin) and later sweating
- cool peripheries (pale, cyanotic lips and nailbed), resulting in a poor signal on the pulse oximeter
- visible bleeding and haematoma from drains and wounds.

In most cases, if impending hypovolaemic shock is recognized and treated promptly, its progression through the aforementioned stages of shock can be circumvented (Hatfield and Tronson 2009).

Irrespective of the cause of hypovolaemic shock, the aim of treatment is to restore adequate tissue perfusion (Hughes 2004). Excessive blood loss might require blood transfusion and occasionally surgical intervention. However, if signs are in the compensatory phase, fluid resuscitation with crystalloid or colloid and increased oxygenation to maintain saturation above 95% are sufficient to promote recovery for many patients.

Ineffective breathing pattern

RELATED THEORY

Respiratory function post-operatively can be influenced by a number of factors:

- increased bronchial secretions from inhalation anaesthesia
- decreased respiratory effort from opiate medication
- pain or anticipated pain from surgical wounds
- surgical trauma to the phrenic nerve
- pneumothorax as a result of surgical or anaesthetic procedures
- co-morbidity, for example asthma, chronic obstructive airways disease (COAD).

All factors affecting adequate expansion of the lung and the ejection of bronchial secretions will encourage the development of atelectasis and consolidation of the affected lung tissue (AAGBI 2002). To prevent this, deep breathing exercises (DBE), coughing exercises and early mobilization may be undertaken post-operatively. DBE help remove mucus which can form and remain in the lungs due to the effects of general anaesthetic and analgesics (which depress action of cilia of the mucous membranes lining the respiratory tract and the respiratory centre in the brain). DBE prevent pneumonia by increasing lung expansion and preventing the accumulation of secretions. DBE also initiate the coughing reflex; voluntary coughing in conjunction with DBE facilitates the expectoration of respiratory tract secretions. A physiotherapist will often provide pre-/post-operative advice and/or assessment for DBE. Note that the patient will require adequate analgesia and support for the wound to enable DBE and mobilization.

EVIDENCE-BASED APPROACHES

Principles of care

Respiratory rate and function is often the first vital sign to be affected if there is a change in cardiac or neurological state. It is therefore imperative that this observation is performed accurately; however, studies show it is often omitted or poorly assessed (NPSA 2007). Routine post-operative respiratory observations will include:

- airway
- respiratory rate (regular and effortless), rhythm and depth (chest movements symmetrical)
- *respiratory depression*: indicated by hypoventilation or bradypnoea, and whether opiate-induced or due to anaesthetic gases
- listening for audible signs of stridor, wheeze or secretions
- observing any changes in the patient's colour for signs of peripheral/central cyanosis
- *pulse oximetry*: should be above 95% on air, unless the patient has lung disease, and maintained above 95% if oxygen therapy is prescribed to prevent hypoxia or hypoxaemia

- *use of oxygen therapy*: flow and method of delivery
- observing any chest drains (if applicable).

Oxygen is administered to enable the anaesthetic gases to be transported out of the body, and is prescribed when patients have an epidural, patient-controlled analgesia or morphine infusion. Nurses should ensure and record the following.

- Oxygen therapy is prescribed.
- Oxygen is administered at the correct rate.
- Continuous oxygen therapy is humidified to prevent mucous membranes from drying out.
- The skin above the ears is protected from elastic on the mask/nasal prongs.

Fluid balance

DEFINITION

The balance of the input and output of fluids in the body to allow metabolic processes to function correctly (Welch 2010).

EVIDENCE-BASED APPROACHES

Principles of care

Iatrogenic factors potentially contributing to fluid imbalance (circulating and tissue fluid volumes) in the post-operative patient are outlined in Box 13.14. Some patients may require fluid replacement in the post-operative period to ensure an adequate fluid balance, avoiding dehydration and the resulting concentration of the blood that, along with venous stasis, is conducive to thrombus formation (Hughes 2004, NICE 2010).

Post-operative fluid replacements should be based on the following considerations:

- maintenance requirements
- extra needs resulting from systemic factors (e.g. pyrexia, losses from surgical drains)
- requirements resulting from third space losses, for example oedema and ileus (Doherty and Way 2006, NICE 2013, Powell-Tuck et al. 2011).

Daily maintenance fluids for sensible losses (i.e. measurable losses, e.g. urine output) and insensible losses (i.e. not measurable, e.g. sweating) will be dependent upon age, gender, weight and body surface area and will increase with pyrexia, hyperventilation and conditions that increase the catabolic rate.

Deciding on the optimal amount and composition of intravenous fluids to be administered and the best rate at which to give them can be a difficult and complex task, and decisions must be based on careful assessment of the patient's individual needs (NICE 2013). Where possible and clinically indicated, euvolaemic and haemodynamically stable patients should return to oral fluids as soon as possible (Powell-Tuck et al. 2011). If intravenous fluids are required, the most commonly used replacement fluids are crystalloids and colloids, which have different effects on a range of important physiological parameters (Perel et al. 2013). All patients continuing to receive intravenous fluids need regular monitoring. This should initially include at least daily reassessments of clinical fluid status, laboratory values (urea, creatinine and electrolytes) and fluid balance charts, along with weight measurement twice weekly (NICE 2013).

In December 2013, NICE published guidance outlining recommendations and algorithms for the general principles for managing intravenous fluids for adults in hospital. Refer to the guidance (www.nice.org.uk/nicemedia/live/14330/66015/66015.pdf) for information/algorithms on the following: patient assessment; fluid resuscitation; routine maintenance fluids; replacement and redistribution.

Box 13.14 Iatrogenic factors with potential to contribute to fluid imbalance

- Pre-operative bowel preparation.
- Pre-operative fasting times.
- Potential fluid volume excess.
- Fluid loss perioperatively.
- Inappropriate fluid prescription.
- Reduced intake post-operatively.
- Ongoing losses from bleeding.
- Paralytic ileus and/or vomiting.

Source: Adapted from Anderson (2003), Hatfield and Tronson (2009).

LEGAL AND PROFESSIONAL ISSUES

The NCEPOD (2011) found there was insufficient recording of post-operative fluid balance in 30% of patient data reviewed. Post-operatively, it is essential that accurate fluid balance charts are maintained, outlining all fluid input (intravenous and oral) and output (e.g. urine, vomiting, wound exudate, drains, nasogastric drainage, stoma). This will facilitate the early identification of fluid loss or excess, which should be raised with a surgical colleague for appropriate management. If intravenous fluids are required, details of the fluids administered must be clearly recorded and easily accessible (Powell-Tuck et al. 2011). Fluid requirements should be frequently re-evaluated with intravenous prescriptions being rewritten every 12–24 hours or more often if clinically indicated.

Surgical drains

DEFINITION

A device, such as a tube, inserted intraoperatively into a body cavity (e.g. bladder, chest wall) or opening of a surgical wound to facilitate discharge of fluid or air.

RELATED THEORY

Surgical drains are used in many different types of surgery with the aim of decompressing, draining or diverting either fluid (blood, pus, gastric fluids, lymph or urine) or air from the site of surgery (Hatfield and Tronson 2009).

Drains can be open or closed and are made from latex, silicone or PVC (Table 13.9; Figure 13.33). All drains induce some degree of tissue reaction (inflammation, fibrosis) as they are foreign bodies; however, the softer the drain, the less likely it is to cause tissue erosion. The type of drain used will be determined by the substance being drained (e.g. viscous versus thin fluid), the reason for the drain, drain location and volume of drainage (Ngo et al. 2004, Walker 2007).

EVIDENCE-BASED APPROACHES

Principles of care

While drains serve an important function, they are also associated with complications such as haemorrhage, tissue inflammation, retrograde bacterial migration and drain entrapment (Walker 2007). It is therefore essential that nurses are familiar with the monitoring and management of surgical drains, but also the process involved in their removal.

The management of a surgical drain is determined by its type, purpose and location (refer to your trust's local procedural guidelines). If a patient has more than one drain, each one should be numbered to prevent confusion. Drains should be firmly secured at the exit site (e.g. with a suture) and if attached to a drainage bag or bottle, they should also be secured at one other point (e.g. with adhesive tape).

To minimize the risk of cross-infection, the drainage bag or bottle should not be placed directly on the floor but should be placed below the level of the wound to facilitate drainage.

Table 13.9 **Open and closed drains**

Type of drain	Example
Open drains are 'open' to the air with the exudate 'passively' collecting onto a sterile dressing, e.g. gauze (if only minimal) or a drainage bag (if copious) from the surgical wound bed. These drains are cheap, simple and versatile and can be used in any part of the body in both clean and infected wounds. They can be brought out through the end of a wound or more commonly through a separate stab incision. It is important to suture open drains to the skin to prevent them from falling out. As these drains are 'open', there is an associated risk of infection; however, the development of deep infection from retrograde tracking of micro-organisms is rare owing to the continuous outward flow of exudate	*Penrose drains*: thin-walled soft rubber latex tubes which collapse to resemble a flat ribbon. Being very soft, they are considered safe to lay adjacent to bowel or other internal organs. *Yates drains:* quite flat but composed of multiple small tubules stuck side by side and are much stiffer. The tubules can be peeled off longitudinally to create any width of drain required. *Corrugated drain:* wavy strips of PVC, still relatively stiff. They usually have a radiopaque strip down the middle (see Figure 13.33a)
Closed drains are 'closed' to the air with the fluid collecting into a sealed collection system (bags or bottles); thus the drain contents remain clean. Closed drains can be divided broadly into those that employ suction (active drains, e.g. Redivac, chest) and those that do not (passive drains).	
– Closed non-suction drains (passive) work by pressure gradient, gravity effect, capillary action or a combination of these (Hatfield and Tronson 2009, Ngo et al. 2004). They are commonly used after abdominal/pelvic surgery. They are characterized by a collapsible plastic bag on the end of the drainage tubing.	Examples include urinary catheter (Foley), nasogastric tube (Ryle), Robinson's, Bonanno catheter (see Figure 13.33b)
– Closed suction drains (active) combine gravity drainage with active suction created by the drainage system, which also acts as a reservoir for drained fluid. They are commonly used in the subcutaneous tissues after abdominal, breast, plastic or orthopaedic surgery to obliterate dead spaces and prevent blood or serous fluid collections. They typically comprise a fine-bore tube with an end hole and multiple side perforations/drainage holes. These are either attached to a pre-vacuumed hard plastic bottle, e.g. Redivac (see Figure 13.33c), or to a soft concertina-style bottle (designed to be squeezed before connection to generate negative pressure) (see Figure 13.33d). For suction to be effective, all drainage holes must be located inside the drainage cavity (i.e. inside the skin)	

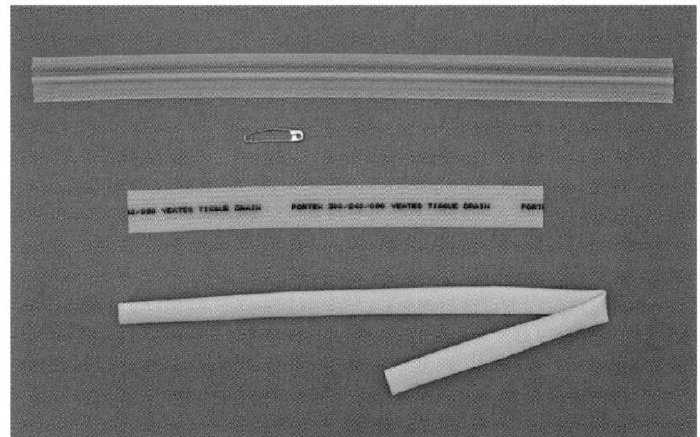

(a)

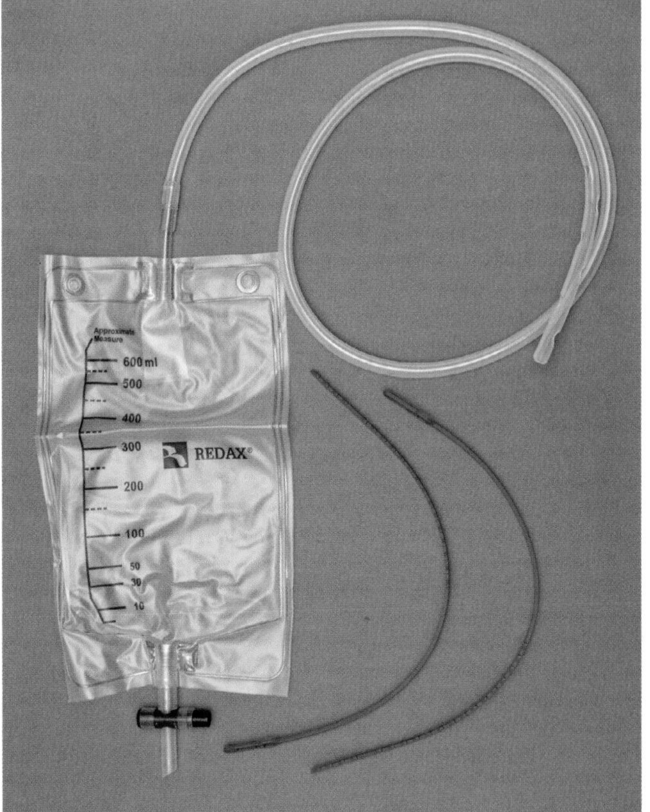

(b)

Figure 13.33 **(a) Corrugate, Yates and Penrose drains. (b) Robinson's drain attached to sterile closed drainage bag. (c) Redivac drain. (d) Concertina drain.**

(continued)

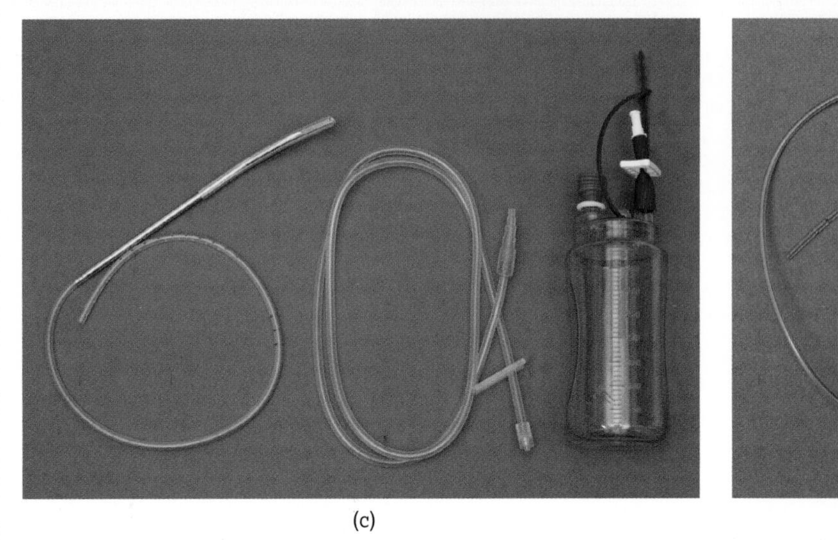

(c)

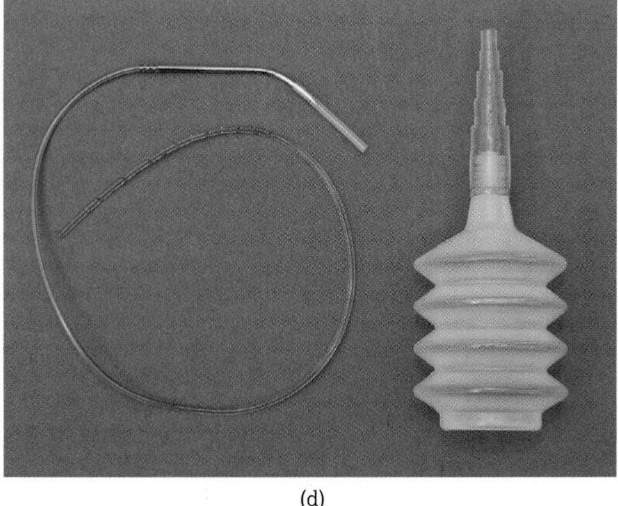

(d)

Figure 13.33 *(continued)*

Drainage output should be measured and recorded on the fluid balance chart as accurate 24-hour totals are necessary for making decisions about drain management. This should be undertaken as clinically indicated (e.g. each time clinical observations are recorded). In particular, nurses should monitor changes in the character (colour, viscosity, odour) or volume of drainage fluid. Unexpected drainage volume (too high or low) or type (unexpected fluids, e.g. blood in urinary catheter) should always prompt further investigation by the clinical team and could indicate that something is wrong (see Problem-solving table 13.2). The length of the drainage tubing (from drain exit point) should also be documented on nursing/surgery documentation and regularly observed for signs of dislodgement (withdrawal or retraction). Furthermore, drain tubing and connections should be regularly inspected for signs of disconnection (e.g. suction pressure source), damage, blockages (viscous fluid, e.g. blood clots, pus, gastric contents) or kinks. For wound drains, it is also important that nurses observe the skin surrounding the drain site for signs of swelling, infection or haematoma. Swabs of wound/drain sites should only be taken if infection is suspected, e.g. inflammation of wound margins, pain, oedema, pyrexia and/or purulent exudates.

Drains should be emptied frequently using clean technique/standard precautions to reduce the strain on the suture line and ensure maximum drainage (Lippincott Williams & Wilkins 2012). However, the dangers of introducing infection should be weighed against the need to empty the drain. Vacuum bottles (e.g. Redivac bottles) and underwater sealed drains (e.g. chest drains) are not emptied but renewed when full (see Procedure guideline 13.8: Closed drainage systems: changing a vacuum bottle).

With the exception of urinary catheters and Ryle's tubes, surgical drains are usually removed once the drainage has stopped or become less than approximately 25–50 mL/day. In some instances drains are 'shortened' by withdrawing them gradually (typically 2 cm/day) before they are completely removed or fall out, to promote gradual closure of the tract. The drain may also be 'cut and bagged' to facilitate easier mobilization. In each of these circumstances, the decision is taken by the surgical team. See Procedure guideline 13.9 for instructions concerning surgical wound drain removal.

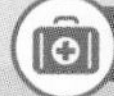 Learning Activity 13.5

Learning in practice: Drains

Within your clinical area:

- Find out what sort of drains are used for patients undergoing different procedures (note the variety of different drains outlined in Figure 13.33).
- Where feasible, ask to be involved in the care of a patient with a drain. Find out for what purpose the drain was inserted. Is it a closed or open drain? Is it a suction or non-suction drain?
- If appropriate, talk to the patient about how the drain feels, and whether a particular position makes it more or less comfortable for them.

Procedure guideline 13.7 Drainage systems: changing the dressing around the drain site for both open and closed drains

Essential equipment

- Dressing trolley or other suitable surface (cleaned according to local trust guidelines) and detergent wipe
- Apron
- Sterile fluids for cleaning and/or irrigation, e.g. sodium chloride 0.9%
- Appropriate absorbent dry dressing. Special features of a dressing should be referred to in the patient's nursing care plan
- Dressing pack, including sterile towel, gauze and gallipot, disposable bag
- Gloves: one disposable pair, one sterile pair

- Alcohol handrub or hand-washing facilities (see local trust guidelines)
- Hypoallergenic tape

Optional equipment

- Any extra equipment that may be needed during procedure, for example sterile scissors, forceps, microbiological swab

Pre-procedure

Action	Rationale
1 Check the medical notes to identify which drain is to be removed. Explain and discuss the procedure with the patient and gain their consent and co-operation.	To ensure that the patient understands the procedure and gives their valid consent and participates in care (NMC 2013, **C**; Walker 2007, **C**).
2 Check patient comfort, for example position and pain level. Offer the patient analgesia as described on their chart or encourage self-administration via a PCA pump (if applicable) and allow appropriate time for medication to take effect.	To promote comfort (NMC 2015, **C**).
3 Clean trolley/tray (see local trust guidelines) and gather equipment, checking the sterility and expiry date of equipment and solutions, and place on the bottom of the trolley.	To minimize the risk of infection (Fraise and Bradley 2009, **E**).
4 Take the trolley/tray to the bed and adjust the bed to the correct height to avoid stooping.	To promote good manual handling. **E**
5 Wash and dry hands thoroughly and put on apron.	To minimize the risk of infection (Fraise and Bradley 2009, **E**).

Procedure

Action	Rationale
6 Remove dressing pack from the outer pack and place on top of the clean dressing trolley/tray. Using aseptic technique, open packaging for other equipment required during procedure (e.g. sterile gloves, dressing, etc.) and place on the sterile field.	To minimize the risk of infection (Fraise and Bradley 2009, **E**).
7 Expose drain site, adjusting the patient's clothes to expose the wound, taking care to maintain their dignity.	To minimize the amount of skin exposed; to maintain dignity. **E**
8 Wearing disposable gloves, remove the dressing covering the drain site and place in a soiled dressing bag away from the sterile field. (a) Closed drains may have a small sterile gauze dressing surrounding the exit site. (b) Open drains will be covered with either a wound drainage bag (if copious exudate) or a small, absorbent, non-adhesive sterile gauze dressing (if only minimal exudate). Once the drainage bag/dressing has been removed from an open drain, the volume and character of exudate should be measured and recorded. If requested by surgical team, gauze dressings can be weighed once saturated to ascertain volume of drainage.	To minimize the risk of infection (Fraise and Bradley 2009, **E**).
9 Observe the drain to ensure the skin suture holding the drain in position is intact.	To ensure drain is well secured and not withdrawn/retracted. Dislodgement can increase the risk of infection, erosion into adjacent structures (e.g. blood vessels/organs) and irritation to surrounding skin. **E**
10 Observe skin surrounding drain site for signs of excoriation, fluid collection, infection (inflammation of wound margins, pain, oedema, purulent exudate, pyrexia). NB: Swabs of wound/drain sites should only be taken if infection is suspected.	Recognize and treat suspected complications (Fraise and Bradley 2009, **E**; Walker 2007, **E**).
11 Using aseptic technique, clean the surrounding skin with an appropriate sterile solution such as 0.9% sodium chloride.	To minimize the risk of infection (Fraise and Bradley 2009, **E**).

(continued)

Procedure guideline 13.7 Drainage systems: changing the dressing around the drain site for both open and closed drains *(continued)*

Action	Rationale
12 If appropriate, cover the drain site as follows. (a) Closed drains should only be covered with a non-adherent, absorbent dressing if there is exudate or to promote patient comfort. (b) Open drains should be covered with a wound drainage bag (if exudate copious) or a small, absorbent, non-adhesive sterile gauze dressing (if only minimal exudate).	To allow effluent to drain, prevent excoriation of the skin, promote patient comfort and contain any odour. **E**
Post-procedure	
13 If applicable, tape dressing securely. If the drain is attached to a drainage bag or bottle, it should also be secured at one other point (e.g. with adhesive tape).	To prevent drain coming loose. **E**
14 If the drain is attached to a drainage bag or bottle, this should not be placed on the floor but placed below the level of the wound to allow drainage. If the drain is attached to a suction drain, ensure this is working correctly.	To ensure continuity of drainage. Ineffective drainage can result in oedema/haematoma (Hess 2005, **E**). To minimize the risk of cross-infection.
15 Check dressing/bag is secure and comfortable for the patient.	For patient comfort. **E**
16 Dispose of all clinical equipment in clinical waste bag or sharps bin according to local trust guidelines.	To ensure safe disposal. **E**
17 Document in patient's notes that the dressing has been changed, reporting any unusual signs or complications to surgical colleagues (Fraise and Bradley 2009; NMC 2010). If the volume of exudate on the dressing has been measured, this should be documented on the fluid balance chart.	To ensure effective communication and instructions for ongoing care. For accurate documentation of drainage (NMC 2010, **C**).

Procedure guideline 13.8 Closed drainage systems: changing a vacuum bottle

(NB: this guideline is not for underwater sealed drains, e.g. chest drain)

Essential equipment

- Dressing trolley or other suitable surface (cleaned according to local trust guidelines) and detergent wipe
- Apron
- Sterile fluids for cleaning and/or irrigation, e.g. sodium chloride 0.9%
- Vacuum drainage bottle, e.g. Redivac
- Dressing pack, including sterile towel, gauze and gallipot, disposable bag
- Gloves: one disposable pair, one sterile pair
- Alcohol handrub or hand-washing facilities

Optional equipment

- Any extra equipment that may be needed during procedure, for example a clamp (although this is usually part of the drainage system in place) or hypoallergenic tape (to place on side of vacuum bottle to facilitate measurement of drain exudate)

Pre-procedure

Action	Rationale
1 Explain and discuss the procedure with the patient and gain their consent and co-operation.	To ensure that the patient understands the procedure and gives their valid consent and participates in care (NMC 2013, **C**; Walker 2007, **C**).
2 Clean trolley/tray and gather equipment, checking the sterility and expiry date of equipment and solutions, and place on the bottom of the trolley.	To minimize the risk of infection (Fraise and Bradley 2009, **E**).

Action	Rationale
3 Take the trolley/tray to the bed and adjust the bed to the correct height to avoid stooping.	To promote good manual handling. **E**
4 Wash and dry hands thoroughly and put on apron and disposable gloves.	To minimize the risk of infection (Fraise and Bradley 2009, **E**).
Procedure	
5 Remove dressing pack from the outer pack and place on the top of the clean dressing trolley/tray. Using aseptic technique, open packaging for other equipment required during procedure (e.g. sterile gloves, vacuum bottle, etc.) and place on the sterile field.	To minimize the risk of infection (Fraise and Bradley 2009, **E**).
6 Clean hands with alcohol gel. Seal off the bottle by closing both sliding clamps on the drainage tubing leading from the patient and the bottle connector.	To prevent air and contamination entering the wound via the drain. **E**
7 Put on sterile gloves and, using non-touch technique, place sterile field/towel under drain tubing at connection point between the vacuum bottle and drain tubing.	To minimize the risk of infection (Fraise and Bradley 2009, **E**).
8 Disconnect the bottle by unscrewing the Luer-Lok, clean the end of the tube with a sterile solution (sterile water or 0.9% NaCl) and securely screw new sterile bottle into the connecting tube at the Luer-Lok.	To maintain sterility. **E**
9 Unclamp both tubing clamps. Suction is established if the concertina bung remains compressed.	To re-establish the drainage system. **E**
10 Check the drainage tubing is secured with adhesive tape dressing at one point (other than at entry site).	To prevent drain coming loose. **E**
11 Vacuum bottle should not be placed on the floor but placed below the level of the wound to allow drainage.	To ensure continuity of drainage. Ineffective drainage can result in oedema/haematoma (Hess 2005, **E**). To minimize the risk of cross-infection.
Post-procedure	
12 Measure the contents of the used drainage system and document any additional drainage in the appropriate documents.	To maintain an accurate record of drainage from the wound (NMC 2010, **E**).
13 Place used vacuum drainage system into the clinical waste bag and dispose of according to local trust policy.	To safely dispose of used system. **E**
14 Document in patient's notes that the vacuum bottle has been changed (Fraise and Bradley 2009; NMC 2010).	To ensure effective communication and instructions for ongoing care and accurate documentation of drainage (NMC 2010, **C**).

Procedure guideline 13.9 **Wound drain removal: closed drainage system**

Essential equipment

- Dressing trolley or other suitable surface (cleaned according to local trust guidelines) and detergent wipe
- Apron
- Stitch cutter
- Sterile fluids for cleaning and/or irrigation, e.g. sodium chloride 0.9%
- Appropriate absorbent dry dressing. Special features of a dressing should be referred to in the patient's nursing care plan
- Dressing pack, including sterile towel, gauze and gallipot, disposable bag
- Gloves: one disposable pair, one sterile pair
- Sterile dressing
- Alcohol handrub or hand-washing facilities
- Hypoallergenic tape

Optional equipment

- Any extra equipment that may be needed during procedure, for example microbiological swab, sterile specimen pot

(continued)

Procedure guideline 13.9 Wound drain removal: closed drainage system *(continued)*

Action	Rationale
Pre-procedure	
1 Explain and discuss the procedure with the patient and gain their consent and co-operation.	To ensure that the patient understands the procedure and gives their valid consent and participates in care (NMC 2013, **C**; Walker 2007, **C**).
2 Check patient comfort, for example position and pain level. Offer the patient analgesia according to chart or encourage self-administration via a PCA pump (if applicable) and allow appropriate time for medication to take effect. Another member of staff may be needed to reassure the patient during the procedure.	To promote comfort (NMC 2015, **C**).
3 If applicable, release vacuum on the drainage bottle by clamping the tubing coming from the patient; keep clamp on green connection open. Loosen the Luer-Lok to allow air into the bottle. Reattach the Luer-Lok and release clamp coming from the patient. Leave for 2–3 minutes. Note amount of drainage in the bottle.	This releases the vacuum and prevents suction during the removal of the drain which may cause tissue damage or pain (Walker 2007, **C**).
4 Clean trolley/tray and gather equipment, checking the sterility and expiry date of equipment and solutions, and place on the bottom of the trolley.	To minimize the risk of infection (Fraise and Bradley 2009, **E**).
5 Take the trolley/tray to the bed and adjust the bed to the correct height to avoid stooping.	To promote good manual handling. **E**
6 Wash and dry hands thoroughly and put on apron.	To minimize the risk of infection (Fraise and Bradley 2009, **E**).
Procedure	
7 Remove dressing pack from the outer pack and place on the top of the clean dressing trolley/tray. Using aseptic technique, open packaging for other equipment required during procedure (e.g. sterile gloves, dressing, etc.) and place on the sterile field.	To minimize the risk of infection (Fraise and Bradley 2009, **E**).
8 Expose drain site, adjusting patient's clothes to expose wound, taking care to maintain their dignity.	To minimize the amount of skin exposed; to maintain dignity. **E**
9 Wearing disposable gloves, remove the dressing covering the drain site and place in a soiled dressing bag away from the sterile field.	To minimize the risk of cross-infection (Fraise and Bradley 2009, **E**).
10 Wash and dry hands thoroughly and put on apron and sterile gloves using aseptic technique.	To minimize the risk of infection. Use of aseptic technique is essential when caring for and removing drains because micro-organisms may pass through the drain to tissue and body cavities, which may result in infection and surgical complications (Fraise and Bradley 2009, **E**; Walker 2007, **C**).
11 Observe skin surrounding drain site for signs of excoriation, fluid collection, infection (inflammation of wound margins, pain, oedema, purulent exudate, pyrexia). If the drain site appears inflamed or purulent, a swab should be obtained and sent for microbiology and sensitivity analysis.	To recognize and treat suspected complications (Fraise and Bradley 2009, **E**; Walker 2007, **C**).
12 The skin surrounding the drain site should only be cleansed (with 0.9% sodium chloride) if necessary, that is, the drain site is purulent or to ensure the suture is visible and accessible.	To reduce the risk of infection (Fraise and Bradley 2009, **E**; Walker 2007, **C**).

Action	Rationale
13 Using non-touch technique, place sterile field under drain tubing and gently lift up the knot of the suture with sterile forceps. Use the stitch cutter to cut the shortest end of the suture as close to the skin as possible and remove the suture with the forceps.	To allow space for the scissors or stitch cutter to be placed underneath. To minimize cross-infection by allowing the suture to be liberated from the drain without drawing the exposed part through tissue (Pudner 2010, **E**).
14 Warn the patient of the pulling sensation they will experience and reassure throughout.	To promote comfort and co-operation (Walker 2007, **C**).
15 Fold up a sterile gauze swab several times to create an absorbent pad (Ngo et al. 2004). Loosening up of the drain should be done if possible, especially for a drain that has been in for some time. For round drains, this can be done by gently rotating the drain to 'break' it free. For flat ones, gentle movement from side to side can achieve this.	To minimize pain and reduce trauma. **E** Drains that have been left in for an extended period will sometimes be more difficult due to tissue growing around the tubing (Walker 2007, **C**).
16 With gloved hand, place one finger on each side of the drain exit site, first stabilizing the skin around the drain with firm pressure. With the other hand, the drain should be firmly grasped as close to the skin as possible and gently removed. Steady gentle traction should be used to remove the drain rather than sudden jerky movements. If there is resistance, place free gloved hand against the tissue to oppose the removal from the wound. Maintain gentle pressure for a few seconds until the drainage/bleeding has stopped or is minimal.	Firm grasp of shortest length should be done to minimize patient discomfort. This is especially important for supple drains such as those made from silicone or rubber which can stretch for some distance then suddenly break free (Walker 2007, **C**).
17 The edge of the drain should be clean cut and not jagged. The drain should be inspected to ensure that it is intact. If there is any doubt that the drain is not intact, the surgeons should be contacted to inspect the drain before disposal.	This clean appearance ensures that the whole drain has been removed. **E**
18 Cover the drain site securely with a sterile dressing and tape. A wound management bag may be placed over a mature exit site if fluid discharge remains high after drain removal.	To prevent infection entering the drain site. **E** To prevent fluid collection/haematoma.
19 If the site is inflamed or there is a request for the tip to be sent to microbiology, cut it cleanly with sterile scissors and place in a sterile specimen container, maintaining asepsis.	To recognize and treat suspected infection (Fraise and Bradley 2009, **E**; Walker 2007, **C**).
20 Check dressing/bag is secure and comfortable for the patient.	To promote patient comfort. **E**
Post-procedure	
21 Measure and record the contents of the drainage bottle in the appropriate documents.	To maintain an accurate record of drainage from the wound and enable evaluation of state of wound (NMC 2010, **C**).
22 Dispose of all clinical equipment in clinical waste bag or sharps bin according to local trust guidelines.	To safely dispose of used equipment. **E**
23 Document in patient's notes that the drain has been removed, reporting complications to surgical colleagues (Fraise and Bradley 2009, NMC 2010).	To ensure effective communication and instructions for ongoing care. To ensure accurate documentation of drainage.
24 Observe drain site dressing for signs of excess fluid discharge (soaked dressing). On routine dressing change, observe site for signs of infection (inflammation, oedema, purulent exudate, pyrexia) and obtain a wound swab if appropriate. Report any unusual signs or complications and record in appropriate documentation (see Procedure guideline 13.7: Drainage systems: changing the dressing around the drain site for both open and closed drains).	To recognize and treat potential complications (Fraise and Bradley 2009, **E**; Walker 2007, **C**). To ensure accurate documentation of any unusual signs or complications (NMC 2010, **C**).

Problem-solving table 13.2 **Prevention and resolution (Procedure guidelines 13.7, 13.8, 13.9)**

This refers to open and closed drainage systems only (not chest drains). The surgical team must be contacted in the event of any of the following problems occurring.

Problem	Cause	Prevention	Action
1 Blocked drain. Blockage should be suspected when there is a sudden drop in drainage output, lower output than expected, or no output at all. **ALERT:** Unexpected fall in drain output may result from drain dislodgement rather than blockage. Advice should be obtained from the surgical team prior to any intervention.	Overly tight sutures, kinking. Ingrowth or collapse of surrounding tissues. Debris accumulation and blood clots in the lumen. Commonly a drain is blocked due to lumenal debris which may not be visible from external inspection.	Drain tubing and connections should be regularly inspected for blockages or kinks.	**Surgical team should be informed prior to any action being taken.** *(a) 'Milk'* Manual 'milking' of debris out through the drain can help to dislodge the obstruction or break it up into smaller debris. This can be done by gently squeezing the tube between your thumb and index finger while moving your fingers along the tubing towards the suction bottle. *(b) Aspirate* After ruling out external compression, a drain can usually be unblocked by aspirating the drain according to local trust guidelines. **ALERT: This should not be undertaken without instruction from surgical team.** *(c) Flush* Failing aspiration and milking, one may attempt to flush the drain with sterile saline using aseptic technique according to local trust guidelines. This can push back in any debris too large to be aspirated through the drain. Flushing also helps to re-establish drainage where tissue collapse or adhesion around the drain interferes with its function. **ALERT: No attempts should be made to flush a drain without instruction and guidance from the surgical team who inserted the drain.**
2 Leaking drain.	Determined by site of leakage. Leakage occurring around the exit site of a suction drain is usually due to a blocked drain rather than a perforation in the drain. The drainage fluid may find its way out along the external surface of the drain when the lumen is blocked. Leakage around the tubing or connections is due to damaged tubing or connections. Skin incision too big for the drain.	Drain tubing and connections should be regularly inspected for blockages, kinks or damaged tubing/ connectors. Ensure the drainage bag is lower than the drain site.	Blocked drain – unblock drain using methods outlined in point 1: Blocked drain. Connections – using aseptic technique, replace the tubing according to manufacturer's instructions and tighten connections as appropriate. Reduce size of skin incision – if skin incision is too big, report to surgical team for guidance. They may either consider an additional suture or may cut and bag the drain to collect the leaking exudate.
3 Loose drain.	Causes may include drain-securing suture cutting through the skin, loose knot tying or traction on the drain.	The majority of drains need to be well secured, preferably at two points. Regular observation of drain to check it is firmly secured at its exit site (e.g. with a suture) and one other point (e.g. with adhesive tape). Awareness of length of drain from exit site at skin to drainage bag (if applicable) – documented in nursing/medical notes.	**Surgical team should be informed prior to any action being taken.** Loose drains must be resecured appropriately and promptly. If the suture around the drain appears loose, the surgical team should be contacted immediately, who may consider placing a stitch through the skin next to the drain exit site under local anaesthetic, then tying the suture securely around the drain. Extra security can be provided by taping the drain/tubing to the skin. Open drains should be prevented from falling into the drainage cavity, e.g. by passing a large sterile safety pin through the drain.

Problem	Cause	Prevention	Action
4 Drain retraction.	Drain retraction is due to a loose drain being pushed inwards, e.g. during dressing change or from patient movement.	Virtually all drains need to be well secured, preferably at two points. Regular observation of drain to check it is firmly secured at its exit site (e.g. with a suture) and one other point (e.g. with adhesive tape). Awareness of length of drain from exit site at skin to drainage bag (if applicable) – documented in nursing/medical notes.	**Surgical team should be informed prior to any action being taken for guidance.** *(a) Resecure* This should be dealt with as a loose drain (see point 3: Loose drain). **ALERT**: Drains suspected to have partially retracted inside a wound should be left in place and properly resecured by a member of the surgical team and a safety pin placed through the tubing to prevent further retraction. **ALERT:** Attempts to pull the drain back out **should be avoided** unless the distance of retraction is known, e.g. drain retraction witnessed or length at skin surface marked. Otherwise any attempt to pull the drain back out may lead to it being dislodged altogether. *(b) Reposition* Drains that have clearly retracted inwards should be pulled out by a member of the surgical team to a length that allows removal at a later date before being resecured. **ALERT**: A drain that is 'cut and bagged' must always be secured with a large, sterile safety pin placed through the external tubing close to the skin to prevent retraction.
5 Drain appears to be falling/fallen out.	This is due to: – failure of the sutures to secure the drain – tethering of the drain or drainage bottle/bag – breakage of the drain – tugging of the drain by the patient/staff – retraction of the drain.	All drains need to be well secured, preferably at two points. Regular observation of drain to check it is firmly secured at its exit site (e.g. with a suture) and one other point (e.g. with adhesive tape). Awareness of length of drain from exit site to drainage bag (if applicable) – documented in nursing/medical notes.	**In this event a member of the surgical team should be contacted immediately for guidance.** *(a) Resecure* A drain that has only partially migrated out should be resecured and the surgical team informed. It **should not be pushed back in** as the externalized part is now contaminated. *(b) Examine* If a drain has fallen out completely, the tube must be inspected to ensure that the drain is intact and saved for inspection by the surgeon. Also ensure that no part of the drain is left inside. If there is any doubt, an X-ray should be performed to ensure no part of the drain remains inside the body. The surgeon will decide if the drain requires replacement and make the necessary arrangements. A wound management bag may be placed over the exit site to catch any ongoing drainage from a mature tract.
6 Broken drain/ tubing/retained drain.	This is usually from repetitive physical trauma with potential contributing factors including: – manufacturing defects – drain weakness as a result of prolonged use – contact with digestive enzymes in body fluids – accidental tethering of the tube/ bag.	All drains need to be well secured, preferably at two points. Regular observation of drain to check it is firmly secured at its exit site (e.g. with a suture) and one other point (e.g. with adhesive tape).	**In this event a member of the surgical team should be contacted immediately for guidance.** *(a) Replacement* If breakage occurs to the external part of the drain or tubing, then the drain might still be able to function. It may be reconnected to a new reservoir or have tubing replaced as appropriate. A safety pin should be placed through the tubing to prevent retraction.

(continued)

Problem-solving table 13.2 **Prevention and resolution (Procedure guidelines 13.7, 13.8, 13.9)** ***(continued)***

Problem	Cause	Prevention	Action
	A high-risk factor is a drain that is 'cut and bagged' without use of a safety pin.		*(b) Removal* If the break is flush with the skin exit site, the surgeon should be contacted immediately and then it should be VERY CAREFULLY removed by the surgeon so as not to push it further inside the wound. The surgeon will perform this using aseptic technique taking care to avoid pushing the broken part further inside or creating tissue bleeding which may further obscure vision. If the surgeon is unable to remove the drain, intraoperative removal under X-ray guidance or an open procedure may be necessary.
7 Inflamed drain exit site	Minimal redness can often be seen around drain exit sites due to local irritation. Cellulitis at the drain exit site may appear as a more pronounced zone of redness, warmth and tenderness. Fever and/or tachycardia may also be present as part of systemic inflammatory response. Purulent discharge at the drain exit site may persist around drains which have been in place beyond the acute post-operative phase. However, the discharge must be examined by the surgical team to distinguish between purulent drainage fluid coming up around the outside of the drain and local abscess collection (unusual).	Well-secured drain to prevent local irritation to skin at drain exit site. All drains need to be well secured, preferably at two points. Regular observation of drain to check it is firmly secured at the exit site (e.g. with a suture) and one other point (e.g. with adhesive tape). Cleanliness of site.	*Irritation:* if local irritation is suspected, no treatment is required other than good wound care according to local trust guidelines to keep drain exit site clean and dry and regularly monitoring drain to ensure it is firmly secured at the exit site (e.g. with a suture) and one other point (e.g. with adhesive tape). *Cellulitis:* surgical team should be informed if cellulitis is suspected as this can indicate inadequate drainage. Antibiotics are NOT indicated unless there is significant associated cellulitis or systemic immunosuppression. *Purulent discharge:* if an abscess has been excluded, then local care for a small wound should be given according to local trust guidelines. Where there is an abscess collection, the treatment in some cases is drainage by a member of the surgical team using appropriate aseptic technique. This can usually be done by a simple incision after infiltration with local anaesthetic. Antibiotics are NOT indicated unless there is significant associated cellulitis or systemic immunosuppression.
8 Atypical drainage fluids.	Unexpected fluids coming up from around a drain or in the drain lumen may be due to: – anastomotic leaks – drain erosion into adjacent structures, e.g. bowel, bladder or blood vessels. The likelihood of tissue erosion is increased by fragility of the local tissues (e.g. in the presence of local inflammation, infection or necrosis), the use of large or rigid drains, and the use of continuous high-pressure suction which sucks surrounding tissues into the drain holes. *Blood* Bleeding can be deep or superficial, early or delayed.	Well-secured drain to minimize risk of tissue erosion into adjacent structures.	**In this event a member of the surgical team should be contacted immediately for guidance.** *(a) Bleeding* The team registrar or consultant must be notified of any significant bleeding. Superficial bleeding will usually settle with local pressure but on occasion may require additional suturing by a member of the surgical team. Deep bleeding may need angiography or surgery.

Problem	Cause	Prevention	Action
	Early bleeding: usually results from a vessel being accidentally pierced by the trocar during insertion or by the drain stitch. *Delayed bleeding:* may indicate erosion of a vessel by the drain anywhere along the drain tract. Erosion into blood vessels may appear as an initial 'herald bleed' consisting of a brief and brisk fresh bleed which may be followed by a more catastrophic haemorrhage at a later stage.		*(b) Anastomotic leak or tissue erosion* There are several approaches including observation only, reducing or stopping suction (if applicable), partial withdrawal of the drain, removal of the drain or intraoperative repair. The approach taken will be determined by the surgical team. Anastomotic leaks may be verified by testing for appropriate biochemical markers, e.g. amylase for suspect pancreatic anastomotic leak or creatinine for urinary tract anastomotic leak. If the concentration of the particular biochemical marker in the drainage fluid is significantly higher than the serum concentration then leakage should be suspected.
9 High drainage output.	Unless it is suspected that the drain is blocked, sudden increase in drain output usually signifies a complication, e.g. anastomotic leak or erosion into adjacent organs (see point 8).	n/a	**In this event a member of the surgical team should be contacted immediately for guidance.** Management steps appropriate to the cause should be undertaken.
10 Vacuum failure for suction drains. When the vacuum suction reservoir fills with air, loss of vacuum has occurred.	This may be the result of: – an air leak in the actual drain or the connecting tubing – a problem with the actual reservoir, e.g. failure to close a cap or presence of a puncture in the reservoir – less commonly, this may be due to the development of a communication between the drainage cavity and the external environment (e.g. wound dehiscence) or an adjacent hollow viscus (e.g. fistula development).	Drain tubing and connections should be regularly inspected to ensure the maintenance of the vacuum within the bottle (according to manufacturer's instructions).	If the vacuum of the drainage system is continually being lost, check all connections for evidence of an air leak and for any wound drain perforations exposed above skin level. Any drain hole outside the skin should be covered with occlusive dressing/bandaging using aseptic technique to stop the air leak. Air leaks elsewhere in the system should be stopped preferably by tightening of connections and/or replacement of any defective component. Otherwise occlusive tape may also be used to seal such defects. If no air leak or suction reservoir defect is found, an opened wound edge or some abnormal communication from the drainage cavity ought to be suspected. The surgical team must be notified.
11 Drain appears stuck and will not come out on attempted removal.	Potential causes include: – stitches remain *in situ* – the drain may just have been in for so long that tissue has grown into it, or perhaps tissue has been sucked into the side holes.	Check operation notes to determine number and types of sutures *in situ* prior to attempting drain removal.	Recheck operation notes to ensure all non-absorbable stitches have been removed. Loosening up of the drain should be done if possible, especially for a drain that has been in for some time. For round drains, this can be done by gently rotating the drain to release it. For flat drains, gentle movement from side to side can achieve this. NB: Removal using excess force should not be attempted. Assistance from the surgical team should be sought if the drain does not come easily.

Source: Adapted from Ngo et al. (2004) and Nottingham University Hospital/Rushcliffe PCT Nursing Practice Guidelines (2006).

Surgical wounds

DEFINITION

A surgical wound is an incision through the skin made by a cutting instrument (e.g. scalpel) to allow the surgeon to gain access to the deeper tissues or organs. Surgical wounds are made in a sterile environment, where many variables can be controlled such as bacteria, size, location and the nature of the wound itself (Toon et al. 2013).

RELATED THEORY

Surgical wounds are usually closed fully at the end of the procedure (primary closure), using one of four devices depending on the type of surgery and determined by surgeon preference: sutures (absorbable and non-absorbable), adhesive skin closure strips (e.g. Steri-Strips), tissue adhesive and staples. Non-absorbable sutures, Steri-Strips and staples will need to be removed but only on the advice of the surgical team, usually 7–10 days post-operatively.

Dressings for surgical wounds

RELATED THEORY

The location of the wound and the method of wound closure usually determine whether the wound is dressed or not. In a closed surgical wound (i.e. one closed by sutures or clips), the main functions of a wound dressing are to:

- promote healing by providing a moist environment without causing maceration (softening and deterioration) of the surrounding skin
- protect the wound from potentially harmful agents (e.g. bacterial contamination) or injury
- allow appropriate assessment of the wound post-operatively
- absorb exudates, e.g. blood or haemoserous fluids
- ease discomfort (preventing the wound rubbing on clothing) (NICE 2008).

NICE (2008) describes three categories of wound dressing used post-operatively.

- *Passive*: designed solely to cover the wound, neither promoting nor intentionally hindering the wound-healing process, e.g. 'gauze-like' materials.
- *Interactive*: designed to promote the wound-healing process through the creation and maintenance of a warm, moist environment underneath the chosen dressing, e.g. alginates, foams, hydrocolloids, semi-permeable film.
- *Active*: designed to manipulate or alter the wound-healing environment to either restimulate or further promote the healing process, e.g. collagen, negative pressure therapy (see Chapter 14: Wound management).

Current guidance recommends that surgical incisions should be covered with an appropriate interactive dressing at the end of an operation (NICE 2008). However, a systematic review published by the Cochrane Library in 2011 (Dumville et al. 2011), evaluating the clinical effectiveness of wound dressings for preventing surgical site infection (SSI), concluded that there is no evidence to suggest that applying a wound dressing to a surgical wound healing by primary intention reduces the risk of surgical site infection. Whether or not a dressing is applied in theatre will be determined by the type of surgery performed and surgical advice.

When dressings are applied in theatre, it is recommended that they are not removed unless exudate, commonly termed 'strike-through', is evident or clinical signs of local or systemic infection (e.g. malodour, fever) occur. Unless contraindicated, dressings changes required within 48 hours of surgery should be undertaken using aseptic non-touch technique and sterile normal saline (see Chapter 3: Infection prevention and control). Whilst some dressings allow early bathing or showering of the rest of the patient after 48 hours, this should be confirmed with the surgeon performing the procedure (NICE 2008).

Studies have demonstrated that it is unnecessary to dress surgical wounds after 72 hours as a surgical wound which has good apposition is sealed against pathogenic invasion by epithelialization in approximately 48–72 hours (Dumville et al. 2011, Toon et al. 2013); however, the application of wound dressings and their removal and subsequent renewal will depend upon local trust protocols. If a dressing is required, it should be changed using aseptic non-touch technique, to prevent micro-organisms being introduced into the wound (NICE 2008).

The choice of dressing will depend on which qualities are required (i.e. absorbtive or supportive) and according to surgical recommendation (Dumville et al. 2011). Gauze-based dressings should not be used to dress surgical wounds as these can completely adhere to the wound and become part of the healing tissue, causing excessive pain and wound damage (Vermeulen et al. 2005). Patient education and psychological support will be required prior to exposing a wound as it may cause patient distress.

On discharge, the patient should be referred to a community nurse and/or be educated about how to care for the surgical wound. Verbal and written information should be given to the patient and include observing for signs of infection and swelling/seroma formation and information on how to seek support/advice if such an event arises (Figure 13.34).

Figure 13.34 **Surgical wound dressings.**

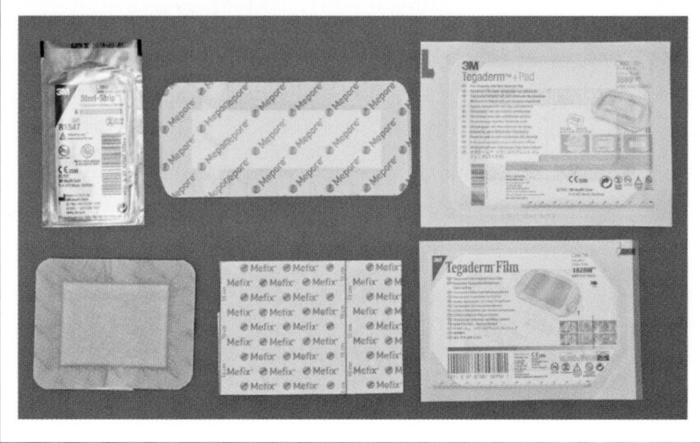

Surgical wound complications

Surgical wound complications are important causes of early and late post-operative morbidity (Mizell 2012). Surgical wounds in normal, healthy individuals heal through an orderly sequnce of physiological events that include inflammation, epithelialization, fibroplasia and maturation. Failure of wound healing following surgery can lead to various complications including dehiscence, surgical site infection, seroma and haematoma.

> **Learning Activity 13.6**
>
> **Scenario: Surgical wound complications**
>
> You have been asked to redress a surgical wound for a male patient who had abdominal surgery three days ago. On assessing the wound you notice that one end of the wound is red, inflamed and tender to touch, with a small amount of oozing from one end. You have only just done his observations and his temperature was 36.7°C.
>
> What actions would you take?
>
> See the end of the chapter for the answers.

Problem-solving table 13.3 Surgical wound complications: prevention and resolution

The surgical team must be contacted in the event of any of the following problems occurring.

Problem	Potential causes/risk factors	Prevention	Action
Dehiscence: partial or total disruption of any or all layers of the surgical wound.	• Systemic factors such as diabetes mellitus, cancer, immunosuppression. • Local factors: – inadequate closure of surgical wound site – tight suturing can tear the skin and affect vascularity of the wound edges, and may result in necrosis and wound breakdown – increased intra-abdominal pressure (ileus) – suboptimal wound care – impaired wound healing caused by infection, seroma, haematoma, drains – impaired wound healing caused by poor perfusion of wound bed due to risk factors including: smoking, male gender, obesity, rheumatoid arthritis, malnutrition.	Reduction in risk factors (refer to cause) identified through comprehensive pre-assessment. Adequate closure of surgical wound intraoperatively.	Action is dependent upon level of dehiscence, which can range from a sudden discharge of fluid or cellulitis along the suture line to the splitting open of the skin layers to complete dehiscence of the muscle and fascia, exposing internal organs, and occasionally incisional hernia with outer layers intact. NB: If dehiscence is suspected then a member of the surgical team should be contacted immediately for guidance. *Minor dehiscence:* local care for a small wound should be given according to local trust guidelines. Wound manager bags are occasionally indicated to drain the excessive exudate from a partially dehisced wound, particularly if skin integrity is compromised. *Partial (deep) or full dehiscence:* in this event, a member of the surgical team should be contacted **immediately** for guidance. Management steps appropriate to the cause should be undertaken.
Surgical site infection (SSI): when pathogenic organisms multiply in a wound, giving rise to local and systemic signs and symptoms. SSI can occur at the incision site or in subcutaneous dead space. Symptoms include localized erythema, purulent exudates, tenderness, wound odour at the incision site. In more serious cases, systemic signs of infection including temperature and raised white cell count may be present. Infection in the surgical wound may prevent healing taking place so that the wound edges separate or it may cause an abscess to form in the deeper tissues.	• Systemic factors such as diabetes mellitus, cancer, immunosuppression. • Local factors: – inadequate closure of surgical wound site – suboptimal wound care – impaired wound healing caused by poor perfusion of wound bed due to risk factors including: smoking, male gender, rheumatoid arthritis, malnutrition. • Obesity – causes increased subcutaneous dead space, rendering the patient more susceptible to incidence of infection. • Drains and sutures. • Poor hand hygiene contaminating surgical site.	Reduction in risk factors (refer to cause) identified through comprehensive pre-assessment. Adequate closure of surgical wound intraoperatively. Optimal wound care.	Some signs of SSI including erythema and tenderness are also seen in the normal post-operative inflammatory response, lasting up to 48 hours. Persistent inflammation beyond this period or the presence of pus or purulent discharge, or pyrexia of the patient may indicate infection. NB: If infection is suspected then a member of the surgical team should be contacted immediately for guidance. A swab, pus sample and blood cultures (if systemic signs of infection, e.g. pyrexia, are present) should be taken to identify the causative micro-organism and appropriate treatment commenced to eradicate it. Antibiotics will usually only be given if adjacent tissue is inflamed or there are systemic signs of infection. In more serious cases, infected wounds may need to be opened and explored or debrided.
Haematoma: collection of blood. The blood seeps from blood vessels that are cut during the operation to remove tissue.	• Inadequate haemostasis. • Use of coagulants. • Obesity – causes increased subcutaneous dead space, rendering the patient more susceptible to haematoma formation.	Adequate haemostasis. Reduction in risk factors (refer to cause) identified through comprehensive pre-assessment.	Action is dependent upon manifestation. Haematomas can be asymptomatic or manifest as swelling with pain. They can cause the incision to separate and predispose to wound infection since bacteria can gain access to deeper layers and multiply uninhibited in the stagnant blood. *Small haematomas:* can be managed expectantly and may resolve with no intervention as, once the small vessels heal, no further blood collects and the haematoma will gradually be absorbed by the body. *Large haematomas:* may require drainage under sterile conditions by needle aspiration. This will be undertaken by a member of the surgical team.

(continued)

Problem-solving table 13.3 **Surgical wound complications: prevention and resolution *(continued)***

Problem	Potential causes/risk factors	Prevention	Action
Seroma: collection of serous fluid. The fluid seeps from small blood and lymph vessels that are cut during the operation to remove the tissue or lymph nodes. Most frequently seen under split-thickness skin grafts and in areas with large dead spaces (e.g. axilla, groin, neck or pelvis).	• Challenging dissection. • Obesity – causes increased subcutaneous dead space, rendering the patient more susceptible to seroma formation.	Reduction in risk factors (refer to cause) identified through comprehensive pre-assessment.	Action is dependent upon manifestation. Seromas can be asymptomatic or manifest as swelling with pain. Seromas can cause the incision to separate and predispose to wound infection since bacteria can gain access to deeper layers and multiply uninhibited in the stagnant fluid. *Small seromas:* can be managed expectantly and may resolve with no intervention as, once the small vessels heal, no further fluid collects and the seroma will gradually be absorbed by the body, usually over 1 month. *Large seromas*: may require drainage under sterile conditions by needle aspiration. This will be undertaken by a member of the surgical team.
Allergic reaction: local rash, redness, itching at site of surgical wound.	• Allergic reaction to surgical dressing or topical ointment applied intraoperatively.	Identification of allergies identified through comprehensive pre-assessment.	Removal of allergen (dressing or ointment). If a severe allergic reaction then give antihistamine. Documentation of allergy according to local policy, e.g. updating patient records to alert other healthcare professionals; informing patient.

Source: Adapted from Escobar and Knight (2012), Mizell (2012), NICE (2008), Sorensen et al. (2005).

Urinary output and catheters

RELATED THEORY

It is important that patients pass urine within 6–8 hours of surgery or pass more than 0.5 mL/kg/h (i.e. half the patient's bodyweight, for example 60 kg = 30 mL) if a urinary catheter is in situ (Liddle 2013). Urinary catheters are used to relieve or prevent urinary retention and bladder distension, or to monitor urine output. Most urinary catheters are inserted urethrally but, where this is contraindicated, suprapubic catheters can be used (see Chapter 5: Elimination).

EVIDENCE-BASED APPROACHES

Principles of care

Urine output should be measured and accurately recorded on the fluid balance chart. This should be undertaken as clinically indicated (e.g. hourly in the immediate post-operative period). Nurses should also monitor and report changes in the character (colour, viscosity, odour) or volume of urine output, e.g. oliguria (urine output of less than 0.5 mL/kg/h for two consecutive hours in the catheterized patient) could indicate the patient is hypovolaemic and should be reported to surgical staff immediately (once catheter tubing has been checked to confirm it is not kinked or blocked). If a patient does not have a catheter *in situ*, it is important that the patient is asked to pass urine into a jug/commode so that the volume of urine can be measured and recorded.

The inability to pass urine post-operatively is usually caused by a condition called neurogenic bladder, a type of bladder dysfunction that interferes with the nerve impulses from the brain to the bladder, preventing it from emptying. For patients with no history of difficulty urinating prior to surgery, the problem is often attributed to a combination of risk factors that include abdominal surgery, general anaesthesia and pain medications and fluids given perioperatively. Signs that a patient is in urinary retention include the patient reporting discomfort or pain or a full bladder and inability to urinate, despite feeling the urge. A bladder scan can be used to determine the residual volume of urine in the bladder and if encouraging the patient to urinate on several occasions is unsuccessful then an in/out urinary catheter can be inserted to drain the bladder. No attempts should be made to catheterize the patient without seeking confirmation from the surgical team that this is the appropriate course of action to take.

Bowel function

RELATED THEORY

Gastrointestinal (GI) peristalsis usually returns within 24 hours after most operations that do not involve the abdominal cavity and within 48 hours after laparotomy (Crainic et al. 2009). Patients undergoing abdominal surgery experience reduced GI peristalsis due to surgical manipulation of the bowel and post-operative opioid medication (Litkouhi 2013). The motility of the small intestine is affected to a lesser degree, except in patients who have had small bowel resection or who were operated on to relieve small bowel obstruction (Crainic et al. 2009). Prolonged inhibition of GI peristalsis (more than 3 days post surgery) is referred to as paralytic ileus (Litkouhi 2013). The duration of post-operative ileus correlates with the degree of surgical trauma, occurring less frequently following laparoscopic than open surgery (Baig and Wexner 2004). Traditional interventions to prevent post-operative ileus or stimulate bowel function after surgery include:

- decompression of the stomach until return of bowel function with a nasogastric tube
- reduction in opioid use
- early mobilization of the patient to stimulate bowel function
- early post-operative feeding (Crainic et al. 2009, Nelson et al. 2005).

Post-operative ileus usually leads to slight abdominal distension and absent bowel sounds. Return of peristalsis is often noted by the patient as mild cramps, passage of flatus and return of appetite. Unless clinically indicated, food or enteral feeds should be withheld until there is evidence of return of normal GI motility.

EVIDENCE-BASED APPROACHES

Principles of care

Post-operatively, nurses should monitor and document when patients pass flatus, when bowels first open and ongoing bowel movements to facilitate early identification of return to GI motility or if complications are arising (e.g. prolonged ileus or infection). Bowel motions should be documented according to the Bristol Stool Chart and any abnormalities, e.g. blood or pale stools, should be escalated to the surgical team. If the patient has undergone abdominal surgery or if clinically appropriate, the surgical team should also be made aware of any evidence of return to GI motility so that food or enteral feeds can be recommenced if clinically indicated (see Chapter 5: Elimination).

Nutrition

RELATED THEORY

For normally nourished patients, the primary objective of post-operative care is restoration of normal GI function to allow adequate food and fluid intake and rapid recovery. Prolonged delays in oral feeding may compromise post-operative nutrition, which can lead to poor wound healing, susceptibility to infection and the need for nutritional support (Litkouhi 2013, SIGN 2012). Post-operatively, energy and protein requirements depend on body composition, clinical status and mobility. Surgery places the body under extraordinary stressors (hypo/hypervolaemia, bacteraemia, medications) and wound healing requires the intake of appropriate vitamins (A, C, zinc) and adequate calories from protein (see Chapter 7: Nutrition, fluid balance and blood transfusion).

EVIDENCE-BASED APPROACHES

Principles of care

Surgery may exert a detrimental effect on appetite and the ability to maintain adequate nutritional intake post-operatively. Causative factors include the surgery itself; post-operative nausea and vomiting; anorexia; altered bowel movements (constipation, ileus, diarrhoea); medication; oral candida; sore mouth; dysphagia and/or early satiety.

Unless contraindicated by the surgery performed (e.g. major abdominal or head and neck surgery) or the patient's current clinical status (e.g. risk of pulmonary aspiration, vomiting and/or ileus), the majority of patients will be able to meet their nutritional requirements orally in the post-operative period. If clinically indicated, any food or drink taken by the patient should be accurately recorded (volume and type of food) on a food chart and fluid balance chart. It is essential that appropriately trained healthcare professionals undertake ongoing oral and nutritional screening assessments in accordance with local trust policy, put preventive measures in place (e.g. good oral hygiene, offering appetising food and drink, provide assistance with eating and drinking) and alert the dietician/surgeon when there is cause for concern (see Chapter 7: Nutrition, fluid balance and blood transfusion). Any patient unable to meet their nutritional requirements orally will require referral to a dietician who will assess the patient's nutritional requirements and tailor any nutritional replacement (oral, e.g. nutritional supplements, enteral or parenteral) to their needs.

Post-operative nutritional support has potentially serious complications (NICE 2006). Enteral nutrition uses the physiological route of nutrient intake, is cheaper and is generally safer, and should be the preferred method of nutritional support, in the presence of a functioning gastrointestinal tract (SIGN 2012). Types of enteral feed tubes include nasogastric, nasoduodenal, nasojejunal, gastrostomy or jejunostomy (see Chapter 7: Nutrition, fluid balance and blood transfusion). Whilst enteral feeding is the preferred route of nutritional support (NCCAC and NICE 2006), parenteral nutrition may be indicated for some post-operative patients who have undergone major abdominal surgery or those with prolonged ileus, uncontrolled vomiting or diarrhoea, short bowel syndrome or gastrointestinal obstruction.

LEGAL AND PROFESSIONAL ISSUES

In the fourth Nutrition Screening Week survey (spring 2011), undertaken by the British Association for Parenteral and Enteral Nutrition (BAPEN 2012), malnutrition was found to affect one in four adults on admission to hospitals. The survey found that nutritional screening policies and practice vary between and within healthcare settings, and so malnutrition continues to be under-recognized and undertreated (BAPEN 2012). It is therefore essential that screening and ongoing assessment of nutritional screening are undertaken by healthcare professionals with the appropriate skills and training.

The Francis Report (Francis 2013) highlights that nutrition and hydration are still not being recognized as an essential part of an individual's recovery from illness in hospital. In line with the Francis Report, it is essential that the environment is conducive to enabling patients to eat. This encompasses the implementation of protected mealtimes, assistance to eat and drink (including provision of eating aids), provision of regular snacks and maintenance of oral hygiene (Box 13.15).

Post-operative pain

Effective management of pain following surgery requires that information about the patient's goals for pain relief, previous history with analgesics, and type of surgical procedure is used to guide decisions about analgesic regimens (Bell and Duffy 2009, Layzell 2008). It is imperative that the patient's pain is managed well, initially by the anaesthetist and then the ward staff and pain team to ensure that the patient has adequate analgesia but is alert enough to be able to communicate and co-operate with staff (Liddle 2013). Analgesics are selected based on the location of surgery, degree of anticipated pain and patient characteristics, such as co-morbidities, and routes of administration and dosing schedules are determined to maximize the effectiveness and safety of analgesia while minimizing the potential for adverse events (Layzell 2008).

Pain management can be delivered using the following routes: oral, rectal, epidural, intravenous, including patient-controlled analgesia (PCA) and opioid continuous infusion (Liddle 2013). A pain tool, e.g. verbal numeric rating score, should be used to assess the effectiveness of prescribed analgesia and action taken if the patient's pain is not controlled. See Chapter 8: Patient comfort and end-of-life care for further information concerning effective management of pain following surgery, including assessment tools.

Immobility

RELATED THEORY

Post-operatively, patients are at increased risk of developing deep vein thrombosis (DVT) as a result of muscular inactivity, post-operative respiratory and circulatory depression, abdominal and pelvic surgery, prolonged pressure on calves (e.g. from lithotomy poles), increased production of thromboplastin as a result of surgical trauma and pre-existing coronary artery disease (Rashid et al. 2005). To prevent this complication, many patients undergoing surgery will be treated with anticoagulants, for example low molecular weight heparin subcutaneous injections or a continuous heparin infusion if the patient was previously anticoagulated (NICE 2010) (see Pre-operative

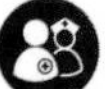

Box 13.15 **Francis Report recommendations for nutrition**

- Food and drink that are, as far as possible, palatable to patients must be made available and delivered to them at a time and in a form they are able to consume.
- Food and drink should, where possible, be delivered to patients in containers and with utensils which enable them to feed themselves, taking account of any physical incapacity.
- Systems, such as specially marked trays or jugs or other prompts, should be employed to remind staff of those patients who need assistance with eating and drinking.
- It is essential that appropriate assistance is made available to patients needing it as and when necessary to consume food or drink.
- No meal or drink should ever be left out of reach of patients able to feed themselves.
- Where patients have not eaten or drunk what is provided at mealtimes this must be noted and the reasons established. Steps should also be taken to remedy the deficit in nutrition and hydration.
- Proper records should be kept of the food and drink supplied to and consumed by elderly patients or as clinically indicated.
- Time for meals should be protected in the daily schedule, but if it is necessary for therapeutic reasons to interrupt mealtimes for a patient, alternatives should be made available.
- For patients capable of eating out of bed, where possible, facilities should be made available on the ward for them to eat at tables.
- Mealtimes should be considered as an opportunity for non-intrusive forms of observation and interaction where this is desirable and appropriate.
- Patients' supporters should not be prevented from joining them at mealtimes provided that this does not interfere with the preservation of appropriate levels of nutrition and hydration or with other patients on the ward, and should be encouraged to help with feeding where this is needed and they wish to provide such help.
- Feedback should be regularly obtained (preferably in real time) from patients, supporters and volunteer helpers on the quality of food and drink and about any necessary adjustments required for individual patients.

Source: Francis (2013).

section: Antiembolic stockings and prophylactic anticoagulation for information relating to DVTs and their prevention). Unless contraindicated, patients will also be wearing antiembolic stockings. Stockings should only be removed for up to 30 minutes daily; however, they can be removed more frequently if clinically indicated, e.g. patient complains of pain or discomfort. Patients should be supported to provide daily skin hygiene by careful washing and application of an emollient cream if the skin is dry. Appropriately trained healthcare professionals should also undertake a daily assessment of the following:

- the fit of the stocking – checking for any change in leg circumference
- consideration of abnormalities or complications of antiembolic stockings, e.g. any discoloration, numbness or tingling, swelling or coldness of the toes/feet; pressure sores; circulation difficulties (e.g. arterial occlusion, thrombosis, gangrene), which can be linked to the tourniquet effect of bunched-up stockings combined with swelling of the leg (House of Commons Health Committee 2005, SIGN 2012).

If the stocking no longer fits, i.e. painful/uncomfortable, loose or tight, there are circulation difficulties or skin damage, remeasure and replace with the correct size of stockings if appropriate, ensuring that they fit smoothly with no wrinkles (see Procedure guideline 13.1: Step-by-step guide to measuring and applying antiembolic stockings).

Post-operative instructions should describe any special positioning of the patient. Where a patient's condition allows, early mobilization (wearing non-slip slippers or shoes to prevent falls) is encouraged to reduce venous stasis unless otherwise contraindicated. For patients on bedrest, a physiotherapist should provide the patient with verbal and written information about deep breathing and leg exercises (flexion/extension and rotation of the ankles). Furthermore, patients on bedrest should be encouraged to change position hourly to minimize atelectasis and circumvent the development of pressure sores. Patients on bedrest may also have intermittent pneumatic compression or foot impulse devices in addition to graduated compression/antiembolic stockings whilst in hospital (NICE 2010).

Ongoing care on discharge

RELATED THEORY

All patients, whether day case, short or long stay, those with few needs or those with complex needs, should receive comprehensive discharge planning. Post-operatively, discharge planning needs to be tailored to the individual needs of the patient, particularly in relation to advice and information on recovery and self-management (DH 2004) (see Chapter 2: Assessment and discharge).

The increase in same-day surgical admissions combined with shorter hospital stays means that more post-operative recovery, including wound healing, takes place at home. This means that where appropriate, patients need to have assimilated the knowledge of usual post-operative outcomes and management with the ability to recognize when professional intervention and/or advice are required.

Surgery can be physically and psychologically stressful, resulting in patients forgetting pre-operative information/teaching (Mitchell 2005). Nurses therefore need to reinforce pre-operative education post-operatively, ensuring that information and discussions are tailored to the patient's individual needs, taking into account their level of anxiety and distress (Mitchell 2005). Ongoing assessment of the patient's understanding of the information given should be carried out and documented. Nurses should teach the patient and carers any necessary skills (including how to use equipment), allowing sufficient time to practise before discharge. This will enable the patient to be as independent as possible post-operatively and promote an understanding of any self-care initiatives required on discharge. This should be supported with centralized evidence-based written information concerning post-discharge care at home.

Learning for practice

After studying this chapter, list five key points you have learnt about perioperative care that you will be able to apply to your clinical practice.

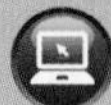

For further learning exercises visit **www.royalmarsdenmanual.com/student**.

Now Test Yourself

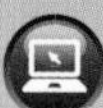

This section provides a range of exercises/activities to further test your learning. For additional exercises visit **www.royalmarsdenmanual.com/student**.

What have you learnt?

1 What is often referred to as the gold standard for measuring exercise tolerance?
A Pre-operative assessment
B Cardiopulmonary exercise testing
C A brisk 10 minute walk with pre- and post-vital signs monitoring
D 12-lead electrocardiogram

2 How many hours before surgery should a patient stop taking clear fluids and be nil-by-mouth?
A 2 hours
B 3 hours
C 4 hours
D 6 hours

3 What are the last anaesthetic agents to be administered during induction prior to surgery?
A Induction agents
B Inhalation agents
C Muscle relaxants
D Antiemetics

4 Which gas is used to inflate the abdomen during laparoscopic surgery?
A Oxygen
B Carbon dioxide
C Air
D Any of the above

5 What is the most common adverse effect of surgery, experienced by the majority of patients immediately post-anaesthetic?
A Pain
B Nausea and vomiting
C Hypothermia
D Behaviour changes

6 Which three interventions can help to maximize respiratory function and prevent complications post-operatively?

7 There are a range of different drainage systems that are used for different purposes. Which of the following is an example of an active, closed suction drain?
A Robinson's drain
B Chest drain
C Nasogastric (Ryle's) tube
D Urinary catheter

8 NICE (2008) describe three categories of wound dressing that can be used post-operatively. Which of the following is an example of an interactive wound dressing that is designed to promote healing by creating a warm, moist environment?
A Gauze dressing
B Semi-permeable film
C Negative pressure therapy
D All of the above

9 How long after surgery does evidence suggest that dressings are no longer required in a wound with good apposition?
A 48 hours
B 72 hours
C 4 days
D 5 days

10 Post-operatively, what are the key nursing interventions to assess GI function and identify any complications?

See the end of the chapter for the answers.

Key points

- Optimal pre-operative care is underpinned by thorough assessment and planning. The aim of the assessment is to reduce cancellations on the day of surgery, rationalize the number of investigations required pre-operatively, and reduce patient anxiety whilst improving post-operative outcomes.
- Immediately prior to surgery it is the nurses' responsibility to ensure that the patient is adequately prepared both physically and psychologically for their procedure and that all appropriate documentation accompanies the patient to the operating department.
- Nurses have an important role to play intraoperatively to support the patient, ensuring that the appropriate equipment is available for the procedure and that all necessary precautions are taken by the multidisciplinary team to avoid peri- and post-operative complications.
- Post-anaesthetic care can best be described and understood as a series of nursing procedures performed sequentially and simultaneously on patients immediately post-anaesthesia/surgery. The post-anaesthetic care unit (PACU) must specify minimum criteria that patients must meet prior to their discharge to the general ward or other clinical areas.
- Optimal management of patients throughout the post-operative phase requires appropriate clinical assessment, monitoring and timely and accurate documentation. The nursing care given during the post-operative period is directed towards the prevention of those potential complications resulting from surgery and anaesthesia.

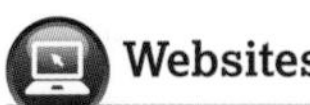

Websites

www.nhs.uk/Conditions/Toxic-shock-syndrome/Pages/Introduction.aspx

www.nhs.uk/conditions/toxic-shock-syndrome/pages/prevention.aspx

http://www.who.int/patientsafety/safesurgery/ss_checklist/en/)

http://www.nice.org.uk/nicemedia/live/14330/66015/66015.pdf

REFERENCES

AAGBI (2002) *Immediate Postanaesthetic Recovery.* London: Association of Anaesthetists of Great Britain and Ireland. Available at: www.aagbi.org/sites/default/files/postanaes02.pdf

AAGBI (2010) *Pre-Operative Assessment and Patient Preparation: The Role of the Anaesthetist: AAGBI Guideline 2.* London: Association of Anaesthetists of Great Britain and Ireland. Available at: www.aagbi.org/publications/guidelines/docs/preop2010.pdf

AAGBI, Membership of the Working Party, Whitaker, D.K., Chair, et al. (2013) Immediate post-anaesthesia recovery 2013: Association of Anaesthetists of Great Britain and Ireland. *Anaesthesia*, 68(3), 288–297.

AFPP (2011) *Standards and Recommendations for Safe Perioperative Practice.* Harrogate: Association for Perioperative Practice.

Al-Benna, S. (2012) Infection control in operating theatres. *Journal of Perioperative Practice*, 22(10), 318–322.

All Wales Tissue Viability Nurse Forum (2009) Guidelines for best nursing: the nursing care of patients wear anti-embolic stockings. *British Journal of Nursing* (supplement). Available at: http://tinyurl.com/kjkanqk

Allaert, S.E., Carlier, S.P., Weyne, L.P., Vertommen, D.J., Dutre, P.E. & Desmet, M.B. (2007) First trimester anesthesia exposure and fetal outcome: a review. *Acta Anaesthesiologica Belgica*, 58(2), 119–123.

Allen, G. (2004) Smoke plume evacuation; antibiotic prophylaxis; alcohol's effect on infection; misuse of prophylactic techniques. *AORN Journal*, 79(4), 866–870.

Alnaib, M., Al Samaraee, A. & Bhattacharya, V. (2012) The WHO surgical safety checklist. *Journal of Perioperative Practice*, 22(9), 289–292.

American Society of Anesthesiologists (2013) *ASA Physical Status Classification System.* Available at: www.asahq.org/clinical/physicalstatus.htm

American Thoracic Society & American College of Chest Physicians (2003) ATS/ACCP Statement on cardiopulmonary exercise testing. *American Journal of Respiratory and Critical Care Medicine*, 167(2), 211–277.

Anderson, A.S. & Klemm, P. (2008) The Internet: friend or foe when providing patient education? *Clinical Journal of Oncology Nursing*, 12(1), 55–63.

Anderson, I.D. (2003) *Care of the Critically Ill Surgical Patient*, 2nd edn. London: Arnold.

AORN (2000) Recommended practices for safety through identification of potential hazards in the perioperative environment. *AORN Journal*, 72(4), 690–692, 695–698.

AORN (2001) Recommended practices for positioning the patient in the perioperative practice setting. *AORN Journal*, 73(1), 231–235, 237–238.

AORN (2004) AORN latex guideline. *AORN Journal*, 79(3), 653–672.

AORN (2008) *Perioperative Standards and Recommended Practices.* Denver, CO: Association of Perioperative Registered Nurses.

AORN (2010) *AORN Latex Guideline.* Denver, CO: Association of Perioperative Registered Nurses. Available at: http://isgweb.aorn.org/ISGWeb/downloads/CIA11008-4061.pdf

AORN (2013) *Hand Antisepsis.* Denver, CO: Association of Perioperative Registered Nurses. Available at: www.aorn.org/secondary.aspx?id=20976

Apfel, C.C., Stoecklein, K. & Lipfert, P. (2005) PONV: a problem of inhalational anaesthesia? *Best Practice & Research Clinical Anaesthesiology*, 19(3), 485–500.

Atkinson, R.S., Rushman, G.B. & Lee, J.A. (1982) *A Synopsis of Anaesthesia*, 9th edn. Bristol: Wright-PSG.

Avidan, M. (2003) *Perioperative Care, Anaesthesia, Pain Management, and Intensive Care: An Illustrated Colour Text.* Edinburgh: Churchill Livingstone.

Baig, M.K. & Wexner, S.D. (2004) Postoperative ileus: a review. *Diseases of the Colon and Rectum*, 47(4), 516–526.

Bale, E. & Berrecloth, R. (2010) The obese patient. Anaesthetic issues: airway and positioning. *Journal of Perioperative Practice*, 20(8), 294–299.

BAPEN (2012) *Nutritional Screening Survey in the UK and Republic of Ireland in 2011.* London: British Association of Parenteral and Enteral Nutrition. Available at: www.bapen.org.uk/pdfs/nsw/nsw-2011-report.pdf

Beckett, A.E. (2010) Are we doing enough to prevent patient injury caused by positioning for surgery? *Journal of Perioperative Practice*, 20(1), 26–29.

Bell, L. & Duffy, A. (2009) Pain assessment and management in surgical nursing: a literature review. *British Journal of Nursing*, 18(3), 153–156.

Benington, S. & Severn, A. (2007) Preventing aspiration and regurgitation. *Anaesthesia and Intensive Care Medicine*, 8(9), 368–372.

Bickley, L.S., Bates, B. & Szilagyi, P.G. (2009) *Bates' Pocket Guide to Physical Examination and History Taking*, 6th edn. Philadelphia: Lippincott Williams & Wilkins.

Bondy, L.R., Sims, N., Schroeder, D.R., Offord, K.P. & Narr, B.J. (1999) The effect of anesthetic patient education on preoperative patient anxiety. *Regional Anesthesia and Pain Medicine*, 24(2), 158–164.

Brady M.C., Kinn, S., Stuart, P. & Ness, V. (2003) Preoperative fasting for adults to prevent perioperative complications. *Cochrane Database of Systematic Reviews*, 4, CD004423. Available at: http://onlinelibrary.wiley.com/doi/10.1002/14651858.CD004423/pdf

Callum, K. & Bradbury, A. (2000) ABC of arterial and venous disease: acute limb ischaemia. *BMJ (Clinical Research Edition)*, 320(7237), 764–767.

Cashman, J.N. (2001) The preoperative visit. In: *Preoperative Assessment.* London: BMJ Books, pp.3–20.

Chee, Y., Crawford, J., Watson, H. & Greaves, M. (2008) Guidelines on the assessment of bleeding risk prior to surgery or invasive procedures. British Committee for Standards in Haematology. *British Journal of Haematology*, 140, 496–504.

Cobbold, A. & Money, T. (2010) Regional anaesthesia: back to basics. *Journal of Perioperative Practice*, 20(8), 288–293.

Cooper, C.B. & Storer, T.W. (2001) *Exercise Testing and Interpretation: A Practical Guide.* Cambridge: Cambridge University Press.

Crainic, C., Erickson, K., Gardner, J., et al. (2009) Comparison of methods to facilitate postoperative bowel function. *Medsurg Nursing*, 18(4), 235–238.

Crayne, H.L. & Miner, D.G. (1988) Thermo-resuscitation for postoperative hypothermia. Using reflective blankets. *AORN Journal*, 47(1), 222–233, 226–227.

DCA (2007) *Mental Capacity Act: Code of Practice.* London: The Stationery Office. Available at: www.direct.gov.uk/prod_consum_dg/groups/dg_digitalassets/@dg/@en/@disabled/documents/digitalasset/dg_186484.pdf

Deresiewicz, R.L. (2004) *Toxic Shock Removal Syndrome Information Service.* Guildford: Toxic Shock Syndrome Information Service. Available at: www.toxicshock.com/healthprofessionalsinfo/

DH (2000) *Comprehensive Critical Care: A Review of Adult Critical Care Services.* London: Department of Health. Available at: http://webarchive.nationalarchives.gov.uk/20130107105354/http://www.dh.gov.uk/prod_consum_dh/groups/dh_digitalassets/@dh/@en/documents/digitalasset/dh_4082872.pdf

DH (2001) *Good Practice in Consent. Implementation Guide: Consent to Examination or Treatment.* London: Department of Health. Available at: http://webarchive.nationalarchives.gov.uk/20130107105354/http://www.dh.gov.uk/prod_consum_dh/groups/dh_digitalassets/@dh/@en/documents/digitalasset/dh_4019061.pdf

DH (2004) *Achieving Timely "Simple" Discharge from Hospital: A Toolkit for the Multi-Disciplinary Team.* London: Department of Health. Available at: http://webarchive.nationalarchives.gov.uk/+/www.dh.gov.uk/en/Publicationsandstatistics/Publications/PublicationsPolicyAndGuidance/DH_4088366

DH (2009a) *Enhanced Recovery for Elective Surgery.* London: Department of Health.

DH (2009b) *Reference Guide to Consent for Examination or Treatment.* London: Department of Health. Available at: http://webarchive.nationalarchives.gov.uk/20130107105354/http://www.dh.gov.uk/prod_consum_dh/groups/dh_digitalassets/documents/digitalasset/dh_103653.pdf

DH (2011) *Enhanced Recovery Partnership Project Report.* Available at: www.gov.uk/government/uploads/system/uploads/attachment_data/file/215511/dh_128707.pdf

Dhara, S.S. (1997) Complications in the recovery room. *Singapore Medical Journal*, 38(5), 190–191.

Doherty, G.M. & Way, L.W. (2006) Current surgical diagnosis and treatment. In: Levinson, W.E. (ed.) *Lange Medical Book*, 12th edn. London: Lange Medical Books/McGraw-Hill.

Drummond, G.B. (1991) "Keep a clear airway". *British Journal of Anaesthesia*, 66(2), 153–156.

Dumville J.C., Walter, J., Sharp, A. & Page, T. (2011) Dressings for the prevention of surgical site infection. *Cochrane Database of Systematic Reviews*, 7, CD004423. Available at: http://onlinelibrary.wiley.com/doi/10.1002/14651858.CD004423/pdf

Eckenhoff, J.E., Kneale, D.H. & Dripps, R.D. (1961) The incidence and etiology of postanesthetic excitement. A clinical survey. *Anesthesiology*, 22, 667–673.

Eckert, L.O. & Lentz, G.M. (2012) Infections of the lower genital tract: vulva, cervix, toxic shock syndrome, endometritis, and salpingitis. In: Lentz, G.M., Lobo, R.A., Gershenson, D.M. & Katz, V.L. (eds) *Comprehensive Gynecology*, 6th edn. Philadelphia: Elsevier Mosby, pp.519–560.

Eltringham, R., Durkin, M., Andrewes, S. & Casey, W. (1989) *Post-Anaesthetic Recovery: A Practical Approach*, 2nd edn. London: Springer-Verlag.

Escobar, P. & Knight, J. (2012) *Surgical Wounds: Strategies for Minimizing Complications*. Available at: http://contemporaryobgyn.modernmedicine.com/contemporary-obgyn/news/modernmedicine/modern-medicine-now/surgical-wounds-strategies-minimizing-com?id=&pageID=1&sk=&date=

Feldmann, M.E. (1988) Inadvertent hypothermia: a threat to homeostasis in the postanesthetic patient. *Journal of Post Anesthesia Nursing*, 3(2), 82–87.

Fong, E.P., Tan, W.T. & Chye, L.T. (2000) Diathermy and alcohol skin preparations – a potential disastrous mix. *Burns*, 26(7), 673–675.

Fraise, A.P. & Bradley, C. (2009) *Ayliffe's Control of Healthcare-Associated Infection: A Practical Handbook*, 5th edn. London: Hodder Arnold.

Francis, R. (2013) *Report of the Mid Staffordshire NHS Foundation Trust Public Inquiry*, London: The Stationery Office. Available at: www.midstaffspublicinquiry.com/report

Frank, S. M., Beattie, C., Christopherson, R., et al. (1993) Unintentional hypothermia is associated with postoperative myocardial ischemia. The Perioperative Ischemia Randomized Anesthesia Trial Study Group. *Anesthesiology*, 78(3), 468–476.

GMC (2008) *Consent Guidance: Patients and Doctors Making Decisions Together*. London: General Medical Council. Available at: www.gmc-uk.org/guidance/ethical_guidance/consent_guidance_index.asp

Hatfield, A. & Tronson, M. (2009) *The Complete Recovery Room Book*, 4th edn. Oxford: Oxford University Press.

Hayes, J.M., Lehman, C.A. & Castonguay, P. (2002) Graduated compression stockings: updating practice, improving compliance. *Medsurg Nursing*, 11(4), 163–166.

Haynes, A.B., Weiser, T.G., Berry, W.R., et al. (2009) A surgical safety checklist to reduce morbidity and mortality in a global population. *New England Journal of Medicine*, 360(5), 491–499.

Hess, C.T. (2005) *Wound Care*, 5th edn. Philadelphia: Lippincott, Williams & Wilkins.

Higgins, C. & Higgins, C. (2013) *Understanding Laboratory Investigations: A Guide for Nurses, Midwives and Healthcare Professionals*, 3rd edn. Oxford: John Wiley & Sons.

House of Commons Health Committee (2005) *The Prevention of Venous Thromboembolism in Hospitalised Patients*. London: The Stationery Office. Available at: www.publications.parliament.uk/pa/cm200405/cmselect/cmhealth/99/99.pdf

HSE (2004) *Latex and You*. Sudbury: Health and Safety Executive. Available at: www.hse.gov.uk/pubns/indg320.pdf

HSE (2012) *Latex Allergies in Health and Social Care*. Sudbury: Health and Safety Executive. Available at: www.hse.gov.uk/healthservices/latex/

Hughes, C. (2011) Consent and the perioperative patient. In: Radford, M., Williamson, A. & Evans, C. (eds) *Preoperative Assessment and Perioperative Management*. Keswick: M & K Update, pp.303–318.

Hughes, E. (2004) Principles of post-operative patient care. *Nursing Standard*, 19(5), 43–51.

ISB (2009) *Data Set Change Notice*. Birmingham: NHS Executive. Available at: www.isb.nhs.uk/documents/dscn/dscn2009/dataset/042009v2.pdf

Jacobs, V.R., Morrison, J.E. Jr., Mundhenke, C., Golombeck, K. & Jonat, W. (2000) Intraoperative evaluation of laparoscopic insufflation technique for quality control in the OR. *Journal of the Society of Laparoendoscopic Surgeons*, 4(3), 189–195.

JBI (2008) Pre-operative hair removal to reduce surgical site infection. *Australian Nursing Journal*, 15(7), 27–30.

Jlala, H.A., French, J.L., Foxall, G.L., Hardman, J.G. & Bedforth, N.M. (2010) Effect of preoperative multimedia information on perioperative anxiety in patients undergoing procedures under regional anaesthesia. *British Journal of Anaesthesia*, 104(3), 369–374.

Kenny, L. (2011) The evolving role of the preoperative assessment team. In: Radford, M., Williamson, A. & Evans, C. (eds) *Preoperative Assessment and Perioperative Management*. Keswick: M & K Update, pp.1–13.

King, W. (2010) *Pulmonary Aspiration of Gastric Contents*. Available at: www.frca.co.uk/Documents/192%20Pulmonary%20aspiration%20of%20gastric%20contents.pdf

Klopfenstein, C.E., Forster, A. & van Gessel, E. (2000) Anesthetic assessment in an outpatient consultation clinic reduces preoperative anxiety. *Canadian Journal of Anaesthesia*, 47(6), 511–515.

Kuczkowski, K.M. (2004) Nonobstetric surgery during pregnancy: what are the risks of anesthesia? *Obstetrical & Gynecological Survey*, 59(1), 52–56.

Kumar, S., Wong, P.F., Melling, A.C. & Leaper, D.J. (2005) Effects of perioperative hypothermia and warming in surgical practice. *International Wound Journal*, 2(3), 193–204.

Layzell, M. (2008) Current interventions and approaches to postoperative pain management. *British Journal of Nursing*, 17(7), 414–419.

Lee, J.T., Chaloner, E.J. & Hollingsworth, S.J. (2006) The role of cardiopulmonary fitness and its genetic influences on surgical outcomes. *British Journal of Surgery*, 93(2), 147–157.

Leonard, A. & Thompson, J. (2008) Anaesthesia for ruptured abdominal aortic aneurysm. *Continuing Education in Anaesthesia, Critical Care & Pain*, 8(1), 11–15.

Levinson, B.W. (1965) States of awareness during general anaesthesia. Preliminary communication. *British Journal of Anaesthesia*, 37(7), 544–546.

Liddle, C. (2012) Preparing patients to undergo surgery. *Nursing Times*, 108(48), 12–13.

Liddle, C. (2013) Principles of monitoring postoperative patients. *Nursing Times*, 109(22), 24–26.

Lindwall, L., von Post, I. & Bergbom, I. (2003) Patients' and nurses' experiences of perioperative dialogues. *Journal of Advanced Nursing*, 43(3), 246–253.

Lipp, A. & Edwards, P. (2002) Disposable surgical face masks for preventing surgical wound infection in clean surgery. *Cochrane Database of Systematic Reviews*, 1, CD002929.

Lippincott Williams & Wilkins (2012) *Lippincott's Nursing Procedures*, 6th edn. Philadelphia: Lippincott Williams & Wilkins.

Litkouhi, B. (2013) *UpToDate: Postoperative Ileus*. Netherlands: Wolters Kluwer. Available at: www.uptodate.com/contents/postoperative-ileus?source=search_result&search=postoperative&selectedTitle=3%7E150

Loveday, H., Wilson, J., Pratt, R., et al. (2014) epic3: national evidence-based guidelines for preventing healthcare-associated infections in NHS hospitals in England. *Journal of Hospital Infection*, 86(suppl 1), S1–S70.

MacGregor, T., Patel, N., Blick, C., Arya, M. & Muneer, A. (2009) Is there a role for cardiopulmonary exercise testing before major urological surgery? *BJU International*, 104(5), 579–580.

Malik, A.A., Khan, W.S., Chaudhry, A., Ihsan, M. & Cullen, N.P. (2009) Acute compartment syndrome – a life and limb threatening surgical emergency. *Journal of Perioperative Practice*, 19(5), 137–142.

McMain, L. (2010) Pain management in recovery. *Journal of Perioperative Practice*, 20(2), 59–65.

Mears, S.C., Davani, A.B. & Belkoff, S.M. (2009) Does the type of skin marker prevent marking erasure of surgical-site markings? *Eplasty*, 9, 342–346. Available at: www.ncbi.nlm.nih.gov/pmc/articles/PMC2743516/pdf/eplasty09e36.pdf

Mitchell, M. (2010) General anaesthesia and day-case patient anxiety. *Journal of Advanced Nursing*, 66(5), 1059–1071.

Mitchell, M.B. (2005) *Anxiety Management in Adult Day Surgery: A Nursing Perspective*. London: Whurr.

Mizell, J.S. (2012) *Complications of Abdominal Surgical Incisions*. UpToDate. Available at: www.uptodate.com/contents/complications-of-abdominal-surgical-incisions

Molyneux, C. (2001) Open forum. Electrosurgery policy... 'Electrosurgery in perioperative practice' (Wicker P 2000). *British Journal of Perioperative Nursing*, 11(10), 424–425.

Murkin, C.E. (2009) Pre-operative antiseptic skin preparation. *British Journal of Nursing*, 18(11), 665–669.

NCCAC & NICE (2006) *Nutrition Support for Adults. Oral Nutrition Support, Enteral Tube Feeding, and Parenteral Nutrition*. London: National Collaborating Centre for Acute Care. Available at: http://nice.org.uk/nicemedia/pdf/cg032fullguideline.pdf

NCEPOD (2011) *Knowing the Risk: A Review of the Peri-Operative Care of Surgical Patients*. London: National Confidential Enquiry into Patient Outcome and Death. Available at: www.ncepod.org.uk/2011report2/downloads/POC_fullreport.pdf

Nelson, R., Tse, B. & Edwards, S. (2005) Systematic review of prophylactic nasogastric decompression after abdominal operations. *British Journal of Surgery*, 92(6), 673–680.

Ngo, Q., Lam, V. & Deane, S. (2004) *Drowning in Drainage*. New South Wales, Australia: Liverpool Hospital. Available at: www.surgicaldrains.com/includes/DID.pdf

NHS Choices (2012) *Consent to Treatment*. Available at: www.nhs.uk/conditions/consent-to-treatment/pages/introduction.aspx

NHSIP (2008) *Preoperative Assessment & Planning*. London: NHS Institute for Innovation and Improvement. Available at: www.institute.nhs.uk/quality_and_service_improvement_tools/quality_and_service_improvement_tools/pre-operative_assessment_and_planning.html

NHS Modernization Agency (2005) Definition of preoperative assessment. In: *National Good Practice Guideline on Preoperative Assessment for Inpatient Surgery*. London: NHS Modernization Agency, pp.2–3.

NICE (2003) *Preoperative Tests: The Use of Routine Preoperative Tests for Elective Surgery: Evidence, Methods & Guidance*. London: National Institute for Clinical Excellence. Available at: www.nice.org.uk/nicemedia/live/10920/29094/29094.pdf

NICE (2005a) *The Prevention and Treatment of Pressure Ulcers*. London: National Institute for Clinical Excellence. Available at: www.nice.org.uk/nicemedia/pdf/CG29QuickRefGuide.pdf

NICE (2005b) *The Prevention and Treatment of Pressure Ulcers*. London: National Institute for Clinical Excellence. Available at: www.nice.org.uk/nicemedia/live/10972/29887/29887.pdf

NICE (2006) *Nutrition Support in Adults: Oral Nutrition Support, Enteral Tube Feeding and Parenteral Nutrition*. London: National Institute for Health and Clinical Excellence. Available at: www.nice.org.uk/page.aspx?o=cg032quickrefguide

NICE (2007) *Acutely Ill Patients in Hospital: Recognition of and Response to Acute Illness in Adults in Hospital*. London: National Institute for Health and Clinical Excellence. Available at: www.nice.org.uk/nicemedia/pdf/CG50FullGuidance.pdf

NICE (2008) *Surgical Site Infection: Prevention and Treatment of Surgical Site Infection*. London: RCOG Press. Available at: www.nice.org.uk/nicemedia/pdf/CG74NICEGuideline.pdf

NICE (2010) *Venous Thromboembolism: Reducing the Risk: Reducing the Risk of Venous Thromboembolism (Deep Vein Thrombosis and Pulmonary Embolism) in Patients Admitted to Hospital*. London: National Institute for Health and Clinical Excellence. Available at: www.nice.org.uk/guidance/cg92

NICE (2013) *Intravenous Fluid Therapy in Adults in Hospital*. London: National Institute for Health and Care Excellence. Available at: www.nice.org.uk/nicemedia/live/14330/66015/66015.pdf

Nimmo, W.S., Rowbotham, D.J. & Smith, G. (1994) *Anaesthesia*, 2nd edn. Oxford: Blackwell Scientific.

NMC (2010) *Record Keeping: Guidance for Nurses and Midwives*. London: Nursing and Midwifery Council. Available at: www.nmc-uk.org/Documents/NMC-Publications/NMC-Record-Keeping-Guidance.pdf

NMC (2013) *Consent*. London: Nursing and Midwifery Council. Available at: www.nmc-uk.org/Nurses-and-midwives/Regulation-in-practice/Regulation-in-practice-Topics/consent/

NMC (2015) *The Code*. London: Nursing and Midwifery Council. Available at: www.nmc-uk.org/Documents/Standards/The-code-A4-20100406.pdf

NPSA (2005) *Patient Safety Alert 06: Correct Site Surgery*. Number 0169DEC04. London: NPSA/Royal College of Surgeons.

NPSA (2007) *Fifth Report from the Patient Safety Observatory. Safer Care for the Acutely-ill Patient: Learning from Serious Incidents*. London: National Patient Safety Agency. Available at: www.nrls.npsa.nhs.uk/resources/?entryid45=59828

NPSA (2008a) *Patient Safety First*. London: National Patient Safety Agency. Available at: www.patientsafetyfirst.nhs.uk/content.aspx?path=/

NPSA (2008b) *UK Organisations Sign Up to World Health Organization Challenge: Safe Surgery Saves Lives*. London: National Patient Safety Agency. Available at: www.npsa.nhs.uk/corporate/news/surgical-safety-checklist-saves-lives/

NPSA (2010) *Checking Pregnancy Before Surgery: Rapid Response Report: NSPA/2010RRR011*. London: National Patient Safety Agency. Available at: www.nrls.npsa.nhs.uk/resources/?EntryId45=73838

Nunney, R. (2008) Inadvertent hypothermia: a literature review. *Journal of Perioperative Practice*, 18(4), 148, 150–152, 154.

Oakley, M. & Bratchell, J. (2010) Preoperative assessment. In: Pudner, R. (ed.) *Nursing the Surgical Patient*, 3rd edn. Edinburgh: Baillière Tindall/Elsevier, pp.3–16.

O'Callaghan, N. (2002) Pre-operative fasting. *Nursing Standard*, 16(36), 33–37.

Older, P. & Smith, R. (1988) Experience with the preoperative invasive measurement of haemodynamic, respiratory and renal function in 100 elderly patients scheduled for major abdominal surgery. *Anaesthesia and Intensive Care*, 16, 389–395.

Older, P., Hall, A. & Hader, R. (1999) Cardiopulmonary exercise testing as a screening test for perioperative management of major surgery in the elderly. *Chest*, 116(2), 355–362.

Older, P., Smith, R., Courtney, P. & Hone, R. (1993) Preoperative evaluation of cardiac failure and ischemia in elderly patients by cardiopulmonary exercise testing. *Chest*, 104(3), 701–704.

Ong, C. & Pearce, A. (2011) Assessment of the airway. In: Radford, M., Williamson, A. & Evans, C. (eds) *Preoperative Assessment and Perioperative Management*. Keswick: M & K Update.

Parienti, J.J., Thibon, P., Heller, R., et al. (2002) Hand-rubbing with an aqueous alcoholic solution vs traditional surgical hand-scrubbing and 30-day surgical site infection rates: a randomized equivalence study. *JAMA*, 288(6), 722–727.

Paula, R. (2002) *Compartment Syndrome Extremity*. Available at: http://emedicine.medscape.com/article/828456-overview

Pennsylvania Patient Safety Authority (2008) *Surgical Site Markers. Putting Your Mark on Patient Safety*. Harrisburg, PA: Pennsylvania Patient Safety Authority. Available at: http://patientsafetyauthority.org/ADVISORIES/AdvisoryLibrary/2008/Dec5(4)/Pages/130.aspx

Perel, P., Roberts, I. & Ker, K. (2013) Colloids versus crystalloids for fluid resuscitation in critically ill patients. *Cochrane Database of Systematic Reviews*, 2, CD000567. Available at: http://onlinelibrary.wiley.com/doi/10.1002/14651858.CD000567.pub6/abstract

Peskett, M.J. (1999) Clinical indicators and other complications in the recovery room or postanaesthetic care unit. *Anaesthesia*, 54(12), 1143–1149.

Powell-Tuck, J., Gosling, P., Lobol, D., et al. (2011) *British Consensus Guidelines on Intravenous Fluid Therapy for Adult Surgical Patients*. Redditch: British Association for Parenteral and Enteral Nutrition. Available at: www.bapen.org.uk/pdfs/bapen_pubs/giftasup.pdf

Pritchard, M.J. (2012) Pre-operative assessment of elective surgical patients. *Nursing Standard*, 26(30), 51–56; quiz 58.

Pudner, R. (2010) *Nursing the Surgical Patient*, 3rd edn. Edinburgh: Baillière Tindall.

Radtke, F.M., Franck, M., Schneider, M., et al. (2008) Comparison of three scores to screen for delirium in the recovery room. *British Journal of Anaesthesia*, 101(3), 338–343.

Rashid, S.T., Thursz, M.R., Razvi, N.A., et al. (2005) Venous thromboprophylaxis in UK medical inpatients. *Journal of the Royal Society of Medicine*, 98(11), 507–512.

Raza, A., Byrne, D. & Townell, N. (2004) Lower limb (well leg) compartment syndrome after urological pelvic surgery. *Journal of Urology*, 171(1), 5–11.

RCN (2005) *Perioperative Fasting in Adults and Children: An RCN Guideline for the Multidisciplinary Team*. London: Royal College of Nursing. Available at: www.rcn.org.uk/__data/assets/pdf_file/0009/78678/002800.pdf

RCP (2012) *National Early Warning Scores (NEWS). Standardising the Assessment of Acute-Illness Severity in the NHS*. London: Royal College of Physicians. Available at: www.rcplondon.ac.uk/sites/default/files/documents/national-early-warning-score-standardising-assessment-acute-illness-severity-nhs.pdf

Roderick, P., Ferris, G., Wilson, K., et al. (2005) Towards evidence-based guidelines for the prevention of venous thromboembolism: systematic reviews of mechanical methods, oral anticoagulation, dextran and regional anaesthesia as thromboprophylaxis. *Health Technology Assessment*, 9(49), 1–78.

Rose, D. (2005) Latex sensitivity awareness in preoperative assessment. *British Journal of Perioperative Nursing*, 15(1), 27–33.

Royal College of Anaesthetists (2013) *Risks Associated With Your Anaesthetic*. Section 14: Death or brain damage. London: Royal College of Anaesthetists. Available at: www.rcoa.ac.uk/system/files/PI-Risk14_2.pdf

Royal Marsden NHS Foundation Trust (2010) *Blood clot prevention. A guide for patients and carers*. London: The Royal Marsden NHS Foundation Trust.

Scott, C., McArthur-Rouse, D. & Prosser, S. (2007) Pre-operative assessment and preparation. In: McArthur-Rouse, F.J. & Prosser, S. (eds) *Assessing and Managing the Acutely Ill Adult Surgical Patient*. Oxford: Blackwell, pp.3–16.

Scott, E., Beswick, A. & Wakefield, K. (2004) The hazards of diathermy plume. Part 2. Producing quantified data. *British Journal of Perioperative Practice*, 14(10), 452, 454–456.

Scottish Intercollegiate Guidelines Network (2002) *Prophylaxis of Venous Thromboembolism: A National Clinical Guideline*. Edinburgh: Scottish Intercollegiate Guidelines Network.

Sharma, K.C., Kabinoff, G., Ducheine, Y., Tierney, J. & Brandstetter, R.D. (1997) Laparoscopic surgery and its potential for medical complications. *Heart & Lung: The Journal of Critical Care*, 26(1), 52–64.

SIGN (2012) *Audit Tool for SIGN Guideline 77: Postoperative Management in Adults*. Edinburgh: Scottish Intercollegiate Guidelines Network. Available at: www.sign.ac.uk/pdf/audit77_postop_audit_plus_instructions.pdf

Simpson, P.J., Popat, M.T. & Carrie, L.E. (2002) *Understanding Anaesthesia*, 4th edn. Oxford: Butterworth-Heinemann.

Sivanandan, I., Bowker, K.E., Bannister, G.C. & Soar, J. (2011) Reducing the risk of surgical site infection: a case controlled study of contamination of theatre clothing. *Journal of Perioperative Practice*, 21(2), 69–72.

Sorensen, L.T., Hemmingsen, U., Kallehave, F., et al. (2005) Risk factors for tissue and wound complications in gastrointestinal surgery. *Annals of Surgery*, 241(4), 654–658.

Starritt, T. (1999) Patient assessment in recovery. *British Journal of Theatre Nursing*, 9(12), 593–595.

Tanner, J. & Parkinson, H. (2006) Double gloving to reduce surgical cross-infection. *Cochrane Database of Systematic Reviews*, 3, CD003087. Available at: http://onlinelibrary.wiley.com/doi/10.1002/14651858.CD003087.pub2/abstract

Tanner, J., Blunsden, C. & Fakis, A. (2007) National survey of hand antisepsis practices. *Journal of Perioperative Practice*, 17(1), 27–37.

Toon, C.D., Ramamoorthy, R., Davidson, B.R. & Gurusamy, K.S. (2013) Early versus delayed dressing removal after primary closure of clean and clean-contaminated surgical wounds. *Cochrane Database of Systematic Reviews*, 9, CD010259. Available at: http://onlinelibrary.wiley.com/doi/10.1002/14651858.CD010259.pub2/abstract

Vedovato, J.W., Polvora, V.P. & Leonardi, D.F. (2004) Burns as a complication of the use of diathermy. *Journal of Burn Care & Rehabilitation*, 25(1), 120–123, discussion 119.

Vermeulen, H., Ubbink, D.T., Goossens, A., de Vos, R. & Legemate, D.A. (2005) Systematic review of dressings and topical agents for surgical wounds healing by secondary intention. *British Journal of Surgery*, 92(6), 665–672.

Walker, J. (2007) Patient preparation for safe removal of surgical drains. *Nursing Standard*, 21(49), 39–41.

Walker, J.A. (2002) Emotional and psychological preoperative preparation in adults. *British Journal of Nursing*, 11(8), 567–575.

Walsgrove, H. (2011) History taking. In: Radford, M., Williamson, A. & Evans, C. (eds) *Preoperative Assessment and Perioperative Management*. Keswick: M & K Update, pp.33–53.

Wasserman, K. (2012) *Principles of Exercise Testing and Interpretation: Including Pathophysiology and Clinical Applications*, 5th edn. Philadelphia: Lippincott Williams & Wilkins.

Weinberg, A.D., Brennan, M.D., Gorman, C.A., Marsh, H.M. & O'Fallon, W.M. (1983) Outcome of anesthesia and surgery in hypothyroid patients. *Archives of Internal Medicine*, 143(5), 893–897.

Welch, K. (2010) Fluid balance. *Learning Disability Practice*, 13(6), 33–38.

White, E. & Crosse, M.M. (1998) The aetiology and prevention of peri-operative corneal abrasions. *Anaesthesia*, 53(2), 157–161.

WHO (2008) *WHO Surgical Safety Checklist*. Geneva: World Health Organization. Available at: www.who.int/patientsafety/safesurgery/tools_resources/SSSL_Checklist_finalJun08.pdf?ua=1

Wicker, P. & O'Neill, J. (2010) *Caring for the Perioperative Patient*, 2nd edn. Oxford: John Wiley & Sons.

Woodhead, K., Taylor, E.W., Bannister, G., et al. (2002) Behaviours and rituals in the operating theatre. A report from the Hospital Infection Society Working Party on Infection Control in Operating Theatres. *Journal of Hospital Infection*, 51(4), 241–255.

Zhao, X., Chen, J., Fang, X.Q. & Fan, S.W. (2009) Surgical site marking will not affect sterility of the surgical field. *Medical Hypotheses*, 73(3), 319–320.

Answers

Learning Activity 13.2 **Scenario: Pre-operative patient information**

You are looking after a female patient who is due to have her surgery tomorrow morning.

1 Although you can see from her documentation that she has had information about her procedure given to her in the pre-operative assessment clinic, what key elements of information regarding perioperative care are most important to reiterate with her prior to surgery?
- The pathway of care through surgery.
- Anaesthetic and pain management.
- Equipment and intravenous access that may be in place following her return from theatre.
- Any additional tubes, for example, urinary catheter or wound drains.
- Any questions she may have.

2 How would you ensure that she has understood the information you have given her?
- Provide any written supporting material regarding the surgical procedure and what to expect afterwards.
- Clarify her understanding by asking her to repeat back what she has understood.

Learning Activity 13.4 **Case study: Safe discharge from the post-anaesthetic care unit**

Jane Ward, 38 years old, is being discharged back to the ward from the post-anaesthetic care unit (PACU). She has had laparoscopic gynaecological surgery and, so far, is recovering well. She has oxygen via a face mask and her respiration rate is 14 breaths/minute, oxygen saturations 99%. Her pulse is 76, blood pressure 110/60 and her temperature is 36.2°C. 30 minutes ago she was feeling rather sick so was given some more antiemetic and is now managing to take a few sips of water. She still has a bag of IV fluids that is running through a peripheral cannula, no drains or catheter *in situ*. Her stomach is feeling a little painful but she hasn't mentioned this to the nurse yet.

You have been asked by the ward to go and collect Jane from PACU. When you arrive you find she is awake and alert and the nurse hands over the information provided above. You ask Jane how she is feeling and she says she is ok but her stomach isn't feeling great.

1 Using the criteria for discharging patients from PACU (see Box 13.13), and the information from handover, what else would you want to check before accepting Jane and returning her to the ward?
- Explore her abdominal pain, using a pain score. She may require further analgesia prior to discharge from PACU.
- Check her abdominal wound dressings for any signs of oozing from the laparoscopy sites.
- Review her vital signs with the nurse in PACU to ensure they are within normal limits.
- Check that her documentation is completed.

2 You find that Jane has a pain score of 7/10; her wound dressings are all clean and intact. What would you do next?
- Ask the nurse if she can give Jane some analgesia prior to transferring her back to the ward. You should wait to ensure this has had sufficient effect prior to transfer.
- Reassess Jane to ensure that she still meets the minimum discharge criteria outlined in Box 13.13 prior to signing that you agree to return her to the ward.

Learning Activity 13.6 **Scenario: Surgical wound complications**

You have been asked to redress a surgical wound for a male patient who had abdominal surgery three days ago. On assessing the wound you notice that one end of the wound is red, inflamed and tender to touch, with a small amount of oozing from one end. You have only just done his observations and his temperature was 36.7°C.

What actions would you take?

- Wound swab. Note any sign of wound dehiscence.
- Inform the nurse in charge who may want to review the wound.
- Redress the wound ensuring the dressing has sufficient absorbency for the amount of exudate.
- Document in the wound care plan and inform the medical team.

Now Test Yourself **What have you learnt?**

1 What is often referred to as the gold standard for measuring exercise tolerance?
A Pre-operative assessment
B Cardiopulmonary exercise testing
C A brisk 10 minute walk with pre- and post-vital signs monitoring
D 12-lead electrocardiogram

2 How many hours before surgery should a patient stop taking clear fluids and be nil-by-mouth?
A 2 hours
B 3 hours
C 4 hours
D 6 hours

3 What are the last anaesthetic agents to be administered during induction prior to surgery?
A Induction agents
B Inhalation agents
C Muscle relaxants
D Antiemetics

4 Which gas is used to inflate the abdomen during laparoscopic surgery?
A Oxygen
B Carbon dioxide
C Air
D Any of the above

5 What is the most common adverse effect of surgery, experienced by the majority of patients immediately post-anaesthetic?
A Pain
B Nausea and vomiting
C Hypothermia
D Behaviour changes

6 Which three interventions can help to maximize respiratory function and prevent complications post-operatively?
- Deep breathing exercises
- Coughing exercises
- Early mobilization

7 There are a range of different drainage systems that are used for different purposes. Which of the following is an example of an active, closed suction drain?
A Robinson's drain
B Chest drain
C Nasogastric (Ryle's) tube
D Urinary catheter

8 NICE (2008) describe three categories of wound dressing that can be used post-operatively. Which of the following is an example of an interactive wound dressing that is designed to promote healing by creating a warm, moist environment?
A Gauze dressing
B Semi-permeable film
C Negative pressure therapy
D All of the above

9 How long after surgery does evidence suggest that dressings are no longer required in a wound with good apposition?
A 48 hours
B 72 hours
C 4 days
D 5 days

10 Post-operatively, what are the key nursing interventions to assess GI function and identify any complications?
- Monitor when patients pass flatus
- Note when bowels open
- Monitor nature of bowel movements (using the Bristol stool chart)
- Note abnormalities such as pale, bloody stool

Wound management

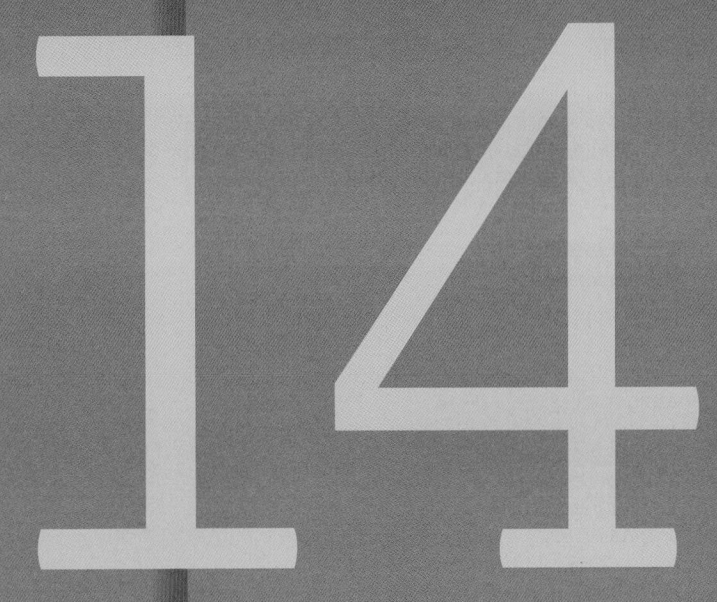

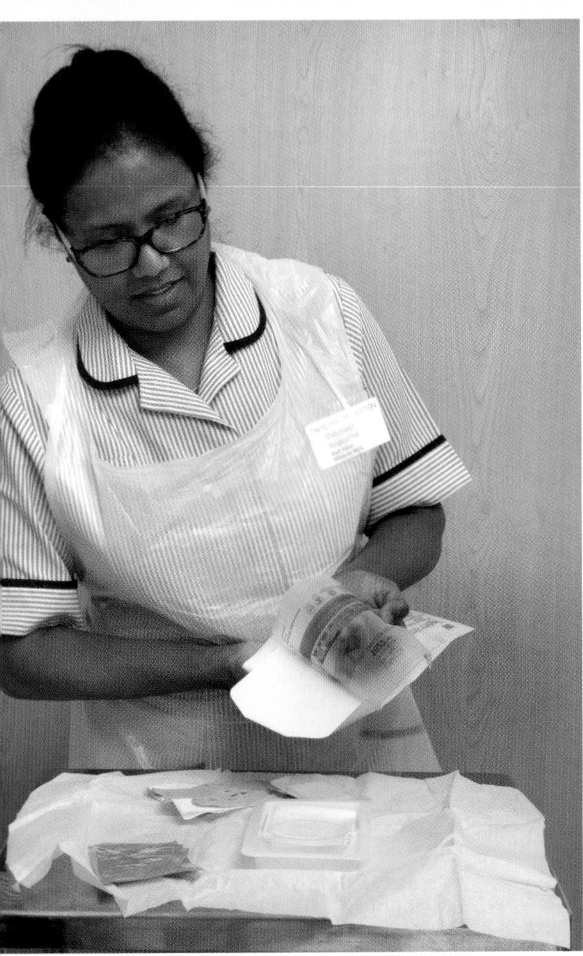

By reading this chapter and undertaking the learning activities within it, you should be able to:

1 Demonstrate an understanding of the principles of wound care.
2 Describe the different phases of wound healing.
3 Demonstrate an understanding of the need for a comprehensive wound assessment and identify appropriate tools.
4 Identify a range of dressings and their suitability for different types of wounds.

Procedure guidelines

The Royal Marsden Manual of Clinical Nursing Procedures: Student Edition, Ninth Edition. Edited by Lisa Dougherty, Sara Lister and Alexandra West-Oram

Overview

The aim of this chapter is to provide an overview of wound care principles and current practice.

Wounds

DEFINITION

A wound can be defined as an injury to living tissue, breaking its continuity (Martin 2010). Wounds can be divided into six basic categories:

1 contusion (bruise)
2 abrasion (graze)
3 laceration (tear)
4 incision (cut)
5 puncture (stab)
6 burn.

Both external and internal factors can contribute to the formation of a wound and a holistic approach is essential for accurate assessment and planning care (Eagle 2009).

- *External*: mechanical (friction, surgery), chemical, electrical, temperature extremes, radiation, micro-organisms, environment.
- *Internal*: circulatory system failure (venous, arterial, lymphatic), endocrine (diabetes), neuropathy, haematological (porphyria cutanea tarda, mycosis fungoides), nutritional status (smoking and alcohol history), malignancy, infection and age (Eagle 2009).

ANATOMY AND PHYSIOLOGY

The skin is the largest organ in the body and makes up about 10% of the adult total bodyweight (Hess 2005). The skin is important as it functions as an outer boundary for the body and helps preserve the balance within (Tortora and Derrickson 2011). The skin needs to remain intact to perform vital functions (Timmons 2006) and without it, humans would not survive insults from bacterial invasion or heat and water loss (Marieb and Hoehn 2010).

The skin varies in thickness from 1.5 to 4 mm depending upon which part of the body it is covering (Marieb and Hoehn 2010). The skin is made up of two main layers, the dermis and epidermis, which have six main functions: protection, sensation, thermoregulation, metabolism, excretion and non-verbal communication (Hess 2005, Timmons 2006).

The *epidermis* is the outermost layer and is avascular and thin. It regenerates every 4–6 weeks and functions as a protective barrier, preventing environmental damage and micro-organism invasion (Hess 2005). The thickness of the epidermis varies and it is thicker over the palms of the hands and soles of the feet (Marieb and Hoehn 2010).

The *dermis* provides support and transports nutrients to the epidermis. It contains blood and lymphatic vessels, sweat and oil glands and hair follicles. The dermis is made up of collagen and fibroblasts, elastins and other extracellular proteins which bind it together and keep it strong (Hess 2005). Its extracellular matrix (ECM) contains fibroblasts, macrophages and some mast cells and white blood cells (Marieb and Hoehn 2010). The connective tissue within the dermis is highly elastic and provides strength to maintain the skin's integrity and combat everyday stretching and wear and tear (Tortora and Derrickson 2011).

The subcutaneous layer just below the dermis is the deepest extension and binds the skin to underlying tissues (Tortora and Derrickson 2011). This layer is known as the *hypodermis* or superficial fascia and stores fat. It also assists the body as a protective layer and allows movement (Marieb and Hoehn 2010).

RELATED THEORY

Classification of wounds

An acute wound is traumatic or surgical and moves through the stages of the healing process in a predictable time frame. A chronic wound does not progress through the stages of healing and is not resolved over an expected period of time regardless of the cause (Broderick 2009).

EVIDENCE-BASED APPROACHES

Methods of wound healing

Wound healing is the process by which damaged tissue is restored to normal function. Healing may occur by primary, second or tertiary intention.

Healing by *primary intention* involves the union of the edges of a wound under aseptic conditions, for example, a laceration or incision that is closed with sutures or skin adhesive (Dealey 2005).

Healing by *secondary intention* occurs when the wound's edges cannot be brought together. The wound is left open and allowed to heal by contraction and epithelialization. Epithelialization encourages restoration of the skin's integrity (Giele and Cassell 2008). Wounds that heal by secondary intention include surgical or traumatic wounds where a large amount of tissue has been lost, heavily infected wounds, chronic wounds or, in some cases, where a better cosmetic or functional result will be achieved (Benbow 2005, Dealey 2005).

Healing by *tertiary intention*, or delayed primary closure, occurs when a wound has been left open and is then closed primarily after a few days' delay, usually once swelling, infection or bleeding has decreased (Giele and Cassell 2008).

> **Learning Activity 14.1**
>
> **Learning in practice: Wound healing**
>
> In your own clinical experience, think about the different types of wounds that you have been involved in the care of.
>
> - Jot down an example of each of the following:
>   - a wound that healed by primary intention.
>   - a wound that healed by secondary intention.
>   - a wound that healed by tertiary intention.
> - Note what sort of dressing was used to aid healing for each wound.

Phases of wound healing

Wound healing is a cellular and biochemical process which relies essentially on an inflammatory process (Hampton and Collins 2004). These processes are dynamic, depend upon each other and overlap (Dealey 2005, Timmons 2006). It is important to support a wound-healing environment that encourages progression from one phase to the next without bacterial contamination, as this increases slough and necrosis (Hampton and Collins 2004).

The generally accepted phases of healing are:

1 haemostasis
2 inflammatory phase
3 proliferation or reconstructive phase
4 maturation or remodelling phase (Dealey 2005).

Haemostasis (minutes)

Vasoconstriction occurs within a few seconds of tissue injury and damaged blood vessels constrict to stem the blood flow. When platelets come into contact with exposed collagen from damaged

Figure 14.1 **Haemostasis in a wound. *Source:* Reproduced with permission from Wayne Naylor.**

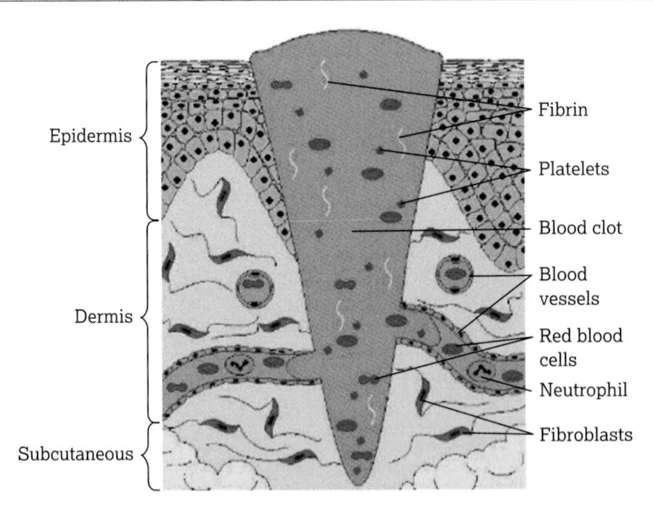

Figure 14.3 **The proliferative phase of wound healing. *Source:* Reproduced with permission from Wayne Naylor.**

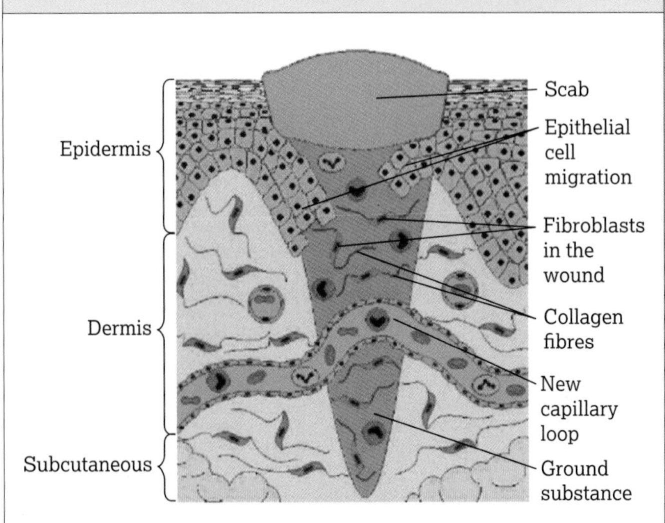

blood vessels, they release chemical messengers that stimulate a 'clotting cascade' (Hampton and Collins 2004, Timmons 2006). Platelets adhere to vessel walls and are stabilized by fibrin networks to form a clot. Bleeding ceases when the blood vessels thrombose, usually within 5–10 minutes of injury (Hampton and Collins 2004) (Figure 14.1).

Inflammatory phase (1–5 days)

With the activation of clotting factors comes the release of histamine and vasodilation begins (Dowsett 2002). The liberation of histamine also increases the permeability of the capillary walls and plasma proteins, leucocytes, antibodies and electrolytes exude into the surrounding tissues. The wound becomes red, swollen and hot. These signs are accompanied by pain and tenderness at the wound site, last for 1–3 days and can be mistaken for wound infection (Hampton 2013) (Figure 14.2).

Polymorphonuclear leucocytes and macrophages migrate to the wound within hours and these phagocytose debris and bacteria and begin the process of repair (Hart 2002). If the number and function of macrophages are reduced, as may occur in disease, for example diabetes (Springett 2002), healing processes are affected. Nutrients and oxygen are required to produce the cellular activity and therefore malnourished patients and hypoxic wounds are more susceptible to infection (Dealey 2005, Timmons 2006). The breakdown of debris causes an increased osmolarity within the area, resulting in further swelling. A chronic wound can get stuck in this phase of wound healing (Dealey 2005, Hampton and Collins 2004) with prolonged healing, tendency to infection and high levels of exudate (Timmons 2006). The phases that follow start the process of repair (Tortora and Derrickson 2011).

Figure 14.2 **The inflammatory phase of wound healing. *Source:* Reproduced with permission from Wayne Naylor.**

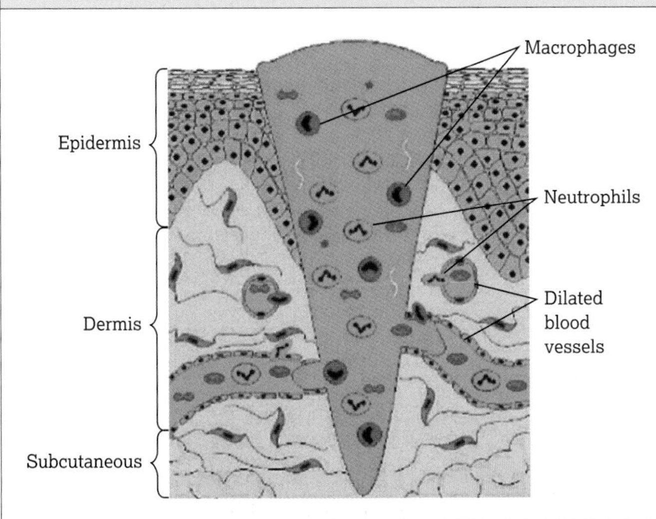

Proliferative phase (3–24 days)

Acute wounds will start to granulate within 3 days, but the inflammatory and proliferative phases can overlap, with both granulation and sloughy tissue present (Timmons 2006) (Figure 14.3).

The fibroblasts are activated to divide and produce collagen by processes initiated by the macrophages (Timmons 2006). Newly synthesized collagen creates a 'healing ridge' below an intact suture line, thus giving an indication of how primary wound healing is progressing. This mechanism is dependent on the presence of iron, vitamin C and oxygen. Vitamin C (ascorbic acid) and lactate are stimulants for fibroblast activity (Hampton and Collins 2004). Fibroblasts are also dependent on the local oxygen supply (Dealey 2005). The wound surface and the oxygen tension within encourage the macrophages to instigate the process of angiogenesis, forming new blood cell vessels. These vessels branch and join other vessels, forming loops. The fragile capillary loops are held within a framework of collagen. This complex is known as granulation tissue (Gray et al. 2010).

Endothelial buds grow and the fibroblasts continue the process of repair by laying down fibrous tissue (Hampton and Collins 2004). Epithelial cells will burrow under contaminated debris and unwanted material while also secreting an enzyme that separates the scab from underlying tissue. Through a mechanism called contact inhibition, epithelial cells will cease migrating when they come into contact with other epithelial cells (Tortora and Derrickson 2011).

Epithelialization (migration, mitosis and differentiation) occurs at an increased rate in a moist wound environment, as do the synthesis of collagen and formation of new capillaries. Wound contraction is a function of myofibroblasts, which are

Figure 14.4 **The maturation phase of wound healing.** *Source:* **Reproduced with permission from Wayne Naylor.**

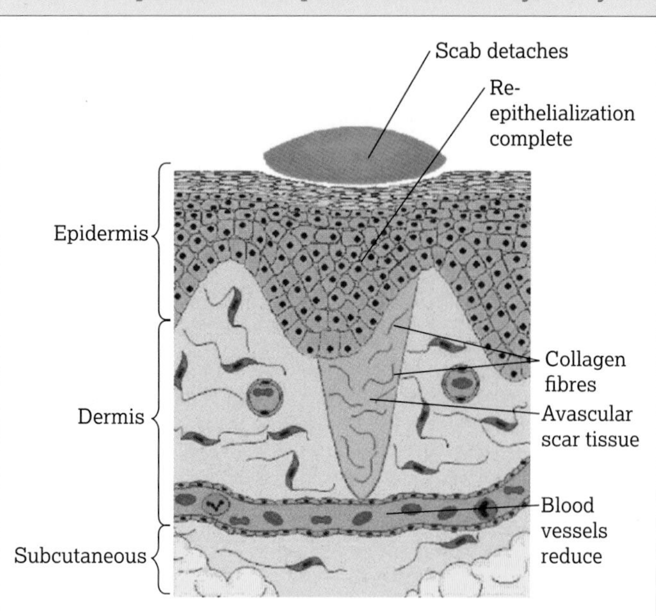

prominent in granulating tissue. The extent of wound contraction is dependent on the number of myofibroblasts present and it is maintained by collagen deposition and cross-linking (Giele and Cassell 2008).

Maturation phase (21 days onward)

Maturation or remodelling of the healed wound begins at around 21 days following the initial injury and may last for more than a year (Figure 14.4). Re-epithelialization occurs at this stage and covers the wound (Benbow 2005). Collagen is reorganized, the fibres becoming enlarged and orientated along the lines of tension in the wound (at right angles to the wound margin) (Silver 1994). This occurs via a process of lysis and resynthesis. Intermolecular cross-linking aids the tensile strength of the wound. During this reorganization, fibroblasts may constrict the neighbouring collagen fibres surrounding them, causing contraction of the tissue and reduction of blood vessels within the scar (Cho and Hunt 2001). At the end of the maturation phase, the delicate granulation tissue of the wound will have been replaced by stronger avascular scar tissue. Rationalization of the blood vessels also results in thinning and fading of the scar, although it is not fully known why this varies amongst people (Dealey 2005).

Methods of wound assessment

In order to provide a method of wound assessment and a simple way of selecting appropriate dressings, an international group of wound care experts developed a concept using 'TIME' (tissue, infection/inflammation, moisture balance and edge advancement) as an acronym to identify the key barriers to healing (Dowsett and Ayello 2004, Werdin et al. 2008) (Table 14.1).

Wound bed preparation

Wound bed preparation (WBP) focuses on controlling and optimizing the wound environment for healing chronic wounds (Falanga 2004). It provides a means of bringing together a cohesive plan of both patient and wound care and is a holistic dynamic process (Moffatt 2004).

Table 14.1 **TIME principles for wound bed preparation**

Clinical observations		Proposed pathophysiology	Wound bed preparation Clinical actions	Effect on wound bed preparation actions	Clinical outcomes
Tissue non-viable or deficient	T	Defective matrix and cell debris impair healing	Debridement (episodic or continuous) • Autolytic, sharp debridement, mechanical or biological (tissue viability nurse only) • Biological agents	Restoration of wound base and functional extracellular matrix proteins	Viable wound base
Infection or inflammation	I	High bacterial counts or prolonged inflammation ↑ Inflammatory cytokines ↑ Protease activity ↓ Growth factor activity	Remove infected foci Topical/systemic • Antimicrobials • Anti-inflammatories • Protease inhibition	Low bacterial counts or controlled inflammation ↓ Inflammatory cytokines ↓ Protease activity ↑ Growth factor activity	Bacterial balance and reduced inflammation
Moisture imbalance	M	Desiccation slows epithelial cell migration Excessive fluid causes maceration of wound margin	Apply moisture-balancing dressings Compression, negative pressure or other methods of removing fluids (tissue viability nurse only)	Restored epithelial cell migration Desiccation avoided Oedema, excessive fluid controlled Maceration avoided	Moisture balance
Edge of wound non-advancing or undermined	E	Non-migrating keratinocytes Non-responsive wound cells and abnormalities in extracellular matrix or abnormal protease activity	Reassess cause or consider corrective therapies • Debridement • Skin grafts • Biological agents • Adjunctive therapies	Migrating keratocytes and responsive wound cells Restoration of appropriate protease profile	Advancing edge of wound

Source: The Royal Marsden NHS Foundation Trust (2013).

Table 14.2 **Factors that may delay wound healing**

Extrinsic factor	Action	Intrinsic factor	Action
Cold	Any drop in temperature delays healing by up to 4 hours	Age	The elderly have a thinning of the dermis and underlying structural support for the wound (i.e. less moisture and subcutaneous fat). The metabolic process and circulation also slow with age
Excessive heat	Temperature over 30°C reduces tensile strength and causes vasoconstriction	Medical and general health conditions	Diabetes, cardiopulmonary disease, hypovolaemic shock, rheumatoid arthritis, anaemia, obesity
Chronic excessive exudate	Wounds should not be too wet or too dry (see moisture balance section in Table 14.1)	Malnutrition or protein–energy malnutrition	Poor healing, decreased tensile strength and higher risk of wound dehiscence and infection. Low serum albumin causes oedema
Poor dressing application and techniques	Gaping of dressing material or multiple layers Tape/adhesive not fastened securely and allowing slipping of wound exudates/dressing rnaterials and/or bandaging too tight/loose	Psychosocial factors	Alcohol and smoking (carbon monoxide affects the blood vessels and circulation of oxygen), poor mobility, stress, isolation, anxiety and altered body image
Poor surgical technique	Prolonged operating time, inappropriate use of diathermy and drains can lead to haematomas and infection	Drugs	Steroids and non-steroidal anti-inflammatories, anti-inflammatories, immunosuppressives, cytotoxic chemotherapy

Source: Adapted from Bale and Jones (2006), ConvaTec (2004), Hampton and Collins 2004.

Tissue factors affecting wound healing

The rate of wound healing varies depending on the general health, age and mobility of the individual, the location of the wound, the degree of damage and the treatment applied. It is necessary when treating a wound to appraise all potential detrimental factors and minimize them, where possible, in order to provide the optimum systemic, local and external conditions for healing.

Factors that may delay healing include disease, poor nutritional state and infection. Other influences involve the local microenvironment of the wound, including temperature, pH, humidity, air gas composition, oxygen tension, blood supply and inflammation (Storch and Rice 2005). Whether this influence is positive or negative may depend on the stage of wound healing that has been reached. Other important considerations are external variables such as continuing trauma or the presence of foreign bodies (Table 14.2).

Achieving a well-vascularized wound bed

Improving the blood flow to the wound bed will increase the availability of nutrients, oxygen, active cells and growth factors within the wound environment (Collier 2002). This may be achieved through the use of compression therapy, topical negative pressure therapy or wound management products that exert an osmotic pull on the wound bed, increasing capillary growth (Collier 2002).

Debridement of devitalized tissue

Surgical debridement is the most effective method of removing necrotic tissue (Woolcott et al. 2009). It is performed by a surgeon and usually involves excision of extensive or deep areas of necrosis, usually to the point of bleeding viable tissue to 'kickstart' healing (Hampton and Collins 2004). While this option is very effective, it carries the risks associated with general anaesthesia. An alternative method of rapid debridement is 'sharp' debridement, which may be utilized for the removal of loose, devitalized, superficial tissue only. Sharp debridement can be performed at the patient's bedside by an experienced healthcare professional with relevant training (Stephen-Hayes 2007). However, this can be a dangerous practice in inexperienced hands and is controversial (Fairbairn et al. 2002). Potentially, ligaments may be severed as they can have the appearance of sloughy tissue or vascular damage could occur (Hampton and Collins 2004). It is also acknowledged that informed patient consent is required as this is an invasive procedure with potential risks and complications (Fairbairn et al. 2002).

Autolytic debridement is recommended as a less invasive technique which utilizes the body's natural debriding mechanism. This effect is enhanced in a moist wound environment, which can be achieved through the use of hydrogel dressings or semi-occlusive dressings that maintain moisture at the wound surface. Many dressings are designed for this purpose and break down necrotic tissue naturally (Hampton and Collins 2004, Hess 2005) (Table 14.3).

Inflammation and infection (or bacterial burden)

It is generally agreed that all chronic wounds harbour a variety of bacteria to some degree and this can range from contamination through colonization to infection. There is also a stage between colonization and infection called 'critical colonization' where the bacterial load has reached a level just below clinical infection (Collier 2002). The virulence of the infection involves a complex interaction between the individual and condition of the wound (Butcher 2012). When a wound becomes infected, it will display the characteristic signs of heat, redness, swelling, pain, heavy exudate and malodour. The patient may also develop generalized pyrexia. An

Table 14.3 **Dressing groups. Please refer to manufacturer's recommendations with regard to individual products**

Dressings	Description	Advantages	Disadvantages
Activated charcoal	Contains a layer of activated charcoal that traps and reduces odour-causing molecules	Easy to apply as either primary or secondary dressing; can be combined with another dressing with absorbency	Need to obtain a good seal to prevent leakage of odour; some dressings lose effectiveness when wet*
Adhesive island	Consists of a low adherent absorbent pad located centrally on an adhesive backing	Quick and easy to apply; protects the suture line from contamination and absorbs exudate/blood	Only suitable for light exudate; some can cause skin damage (excoriation, blistering) if applied incorrectly
Alginates	A textile fibre dressing made from seaweed; the soft woven fibres gel as they absorb exudate and promote autolytic debridement. Available as a sheet, ribbon or packing	Are suitable for moderate to heavy exudate; can be used on infected wounds; useful for sinus and fistula drainage; have haemostatic properties; can be irrigated out of wound with warm saline	Cannot be used on dry wounds or wound with hard necrotic tissue (eschar); sometimes a mild burning or 'drawing' sensation is reported on application*
Antimicrobials	These topical dressings can be used as primary or secondary dressings and are available as a primary layer and impregnated in other dressings or as a cream	Suitable for chronic wounds with heavy exudate that need protection from bacterial contamination by providing a broad range of antimicrobial activity; can reduce or prevent infection	Sometimes sensitivity occurs with the use of silver and some skin staining can occur; instructions vary with products and dressings are expensive Evidence base for use is controversial and needs monitoring*
Capillary wound dressings	Composed of 100% polyester filament outer layers and a 65% polyester and 35% cotton woven inner layer; outer layer draws exudate, interstitial fluid and necrotic tissue into the inner layer via a capillary action	Suitable for light to heavy exudate; debride necrotic tissue; protect and insulate the wound; maintain a moist environment and prevent maceration; encourage development of granulation tissue; can be cut to any shape and are available in large rolls; can be used as a wick to drain sinus and cavity wounds	Can be hard to cut and are quite stiff to fit into wounds; cannot be used where there is the risk of bleeding due to the 'drawing' action and resultant increase in blood flow to the wound bed Expensive and should be used on a named patient basis
Collagen	This protein is fibrous and insoluble and produced by fibroblasts. Collagen encourages collagen fibres into the granulation tissue. It is available in sheets/gels	Conforms well to wound surface, maintains a moist environment, suitable for most wounds to accelerate healing. Supports ECM	Not recommended for necrotic wounds*
Foams	Produced in a variety of forms, most being constructed of polyurethane foam, and may have one or more layers; foam cavity dressings are also available	Suitable for use with open, exuding wounds; highly absorbent, non-adherent and maintain a moist wound bed Available for low-high exudates and/or bordered to simplify dressing choice	May be difficult to use in wounds with deep tracts and need a combined approach with an alginate
Honey – most widely used is Manuka honey	Available as tubes of liquid honey or impregnated dressings	Suitable for acute and chronic infected, necrotic or sloughy wounds; provides a moist wound environment; non-adherent; antibacterial; assists with wound debridement; eliminates wound malodour; has an anti-inflammatory effect	Can be messy to use and causes leakage if excess exudate is present* May have a burning/drawing effect when first applied
Hydrocolloid	Usually consists of a base material containing gelatin, pectin and carboxymethylcellulose combined with adhesives and polymers; base material may be bonded to either a semi-permeable film or a film plus polyurethane foam; some have a border	Suitable for acute and chronic wounds with low to no exudate; provides a moist wound environment; promotes wound debridement; provides thermal insulation; waterproof and barrier to micro-organisms; easy to use	May release degradation products into the wound; strong odour produced as dressing interacts with exudate; some hydrocolloids cannot be used on infected wounds

Dressings	Description	Advantages	Disadvantages
Hydrofibre	Same consistency as hydrocolloid but in a soft woven sheet (also available with silver)	Forms a soft, hydrophilic, gas-permeable gel on contact with the wound and manages exudate whilst preventing maceration of wound edge. Easy to remove without trauma to wound bed	Does not have haemostatic property of alginates*
Hydrogels	Contain 17.5–90% water depending on the product, plus various other components to form a gel or solid sheet	Suitable for light exudate wounds; absorb small amounts of exudate; donate fluid to dry necrotic tissue; reduce pain and are cooling; low trauma at dressing changes; can be used as carrier for drugs	Cool the wound surface; use with caution in infected wounds; can cause skin maceration due to leakage if too much gel is applied or the wound has moderate to heavy exudate* Moderate care of sheets so they do not dry out
Semi-permeable films	Polyurethane film with a hypoallergenic acrylic adhesive; have a variety of application methods often consisting of a plastic or cardboard carrier	Only suitable for shallow superficial wounds; prophylactic use against friction damage; useful as retention dressing; allow passage of water vapour; allow monitoring of the wound	Possibility of adhesive trauma if removed incorrectly; do not contain exudate and can macerate, slip or leak
Skin barrier film	Alcohol-free liquid polymer that forms a protective film on the skin	Non-cytotoxic; does not sting if applied to raw areas of skin; high wash-off resistance; protects the skin from body fluids, friction and shear and the effects of adhesive products	Requires good manual dexterity to apply; may cause skin warming on application

*Requires a secondary dressing.
Source: Adapted from Dealey (2005), Hess (2005).

essential role within wound management is therefore reducing bacterial burden and many dressings are impregnated with antimicrobial compounds, e.g. silver, iodine, honey (Butcher 2012). There is supporting evidence for the use of silver and other antimicrobials in reducing colonization and increasing healing rates (Leaper 2011).

However, immunosuppressed patients, diabetic patients or those on systemic steroid therapy may not present with the classic signs of infection. Instead, they may experience delayed healing, breakdown of the wound, presence of friable granulation tissue that bleeds easily, formation of an epithelial tissue bridge over the wound, increased production of exudate and malodour and increased pain.

Defining wound infection in all wounds is still debatable (Cutting 2011). The clinical presentation of a wound should lead to the diagnosis of an infection. A wound swab should only be taken if the clinical picture advocates it as the swab will only identify the type of bacteria present. The technique for swabbing a wound should be specified in local protocols and should include the cleaning of a wound prior to swabbing to remove surface contaminants and dressing residue (Young 2012). For further advice see Chapter 10: Interpreting diagnostic tests. Topical antibiotics are contraindicated as they may increase bacterial resistance and the use of antimicrobials prophylactically is controversial (Butcher 2012, Cutting 2011).

Moisture balance

Wound exudate usually performs a useful function by aiding autolytic debridement and providing nutrients to the healing wound bed. It is required in the process of epithelialization, to allow the movement of cells across the surface of the wound (Jones 2013). However, in the presence of excess exudate, the process of wound healing can be adversely affected. This is especially so in chronic wounds where there is an increased proteolytic activity, leading to damage in the wound bed. Matrix metalloproteases (MMPs) are found in exudate and, when present in chronic exudate, their beneficial properties, such as the provision of essential nutrients for cell metabolism, are hindered. This can be a significant factor in delayed healing (Hampton 2013).

The control of oedema or elevating the affected limb, e.g. in a lower leg wound, will undoubtedly help in the reduction of wound exudate. However, if the methods for achieving these goals are unsuccessful or contraindicated then exudate must be managed through the use of wound management products. These include such products as absorbent wound dressings (e.g. alginates, hydrofibre, foams), non-adherent wound contact layers with a secondary absorbent pad, wound manager bags and negative pressure wound therapy (NPWT). NPWT is highly effective in controlling excessive exudate (Probst and Huljev 2013). It is also vital to protect the skin surrounding the wound from maceration by excess exudate and excoriation from corrosive exudate. Useful products for skin protection include ointments/pastes, alcohol-free skin barrier films and thin hydrocolloid sheets used to 'frame' the wound (Flett et al. 2002).

Edge non-advancement

The clearest sign that the wound is failing to heal is when the epidermal edge is not advancing over time (Dowsett and Ayello 2004). In this case a thorough assessment should commence using the TIME principles and interventions.

Principles of wound cleansing

The aim of wound cleansing is to help create the optimum local conditions for wound healing.

If the wound is clean with little exudate and particularly with granulation tissue present, repeated cleaning may be detrimental to the healing process, damaging new tissue and decreasing the temperature of the wound unnecessarily (Watret and Armitage 2002). A fall in the temperature of the wound of 12°C is possible if the procedure is prolonged or the lotions are cold. It can take 3 hours or longer for the wound to return to normal temperature, during which time the cellular activity is reduced and therefore the healing process slowed (McKirdy 2001).

Sodium chloride (0.9%) is a physiologically balanced solution that has a similar osmotic pressure to that already present in living cells and is therefore compatible with human tissue. Although sodium chloride has no antiseptic properties, it dilutes bacteria and is non-toxic to tissue (Thomas 2009). There is an increasing use of tap water for irrigating chronic wounds; no significant difference has been shown in the healing and infection rates in wounds irrigated with tap water or 0.9% sodium chloride (Hall 2007). Evidence shows that although swabbing wounds may be effective in removing foreign bodies from the surface of a wound, irrigation is far less harmful to wound tissue (Hall 2007).

Principles of dressing a wound

With the exception of wounds where the main aim is to ameliorate symptoms such as malignant wounds, an ideal wound dressing must be capable of fulfilling the following functions.

- Allows gaseous exchange.
- Maintains optimum temperature and pH in the wound.
- Forms an effective barrier to bacteria (contains cellular debris or exudate to prevent the transmission of micro-organisms into and out of the wound).
- Allows removal of the dressing without pain or skin stripping.
- Is acceptable to the patient.
- Is highly absorbent (for heavily exuding wounds).
- Is cost-effective.
- Requires minimal replacement or disturbance.
- Appropriate to the wound; debridement activity, haemostatic properties, odour absorbing (Thomas 2009).

PRE-PROCEDURAL CONSIDERATIONS

Equipment

Dressings are named and categorized to make choices more clear (see Table 14.3 for details of groups of dressings). The dressing that is applied directly over the wound bed is the *primary* dressing. Dry dressings (such as gauze) do not fulfil most of the criteria for an ideal dressing and should not be used as a primary contact layer as they are likely to adhere and disturb healing (Dealey 2005). Silicone can be beneficial in protecting delicate wound beds and the peri-wound area due to its protective and atraumatic properties (Yarwood-Ross 2013). However, this also depends on the definition of 'dry' dressing as some dressings appear dry but 'gel' on contact with the wound, which maintains a moist environment, and are non-adhesive, thus becoming 'wet' (examples include hydrofibres, alginates and hydrocolloids). The wound itself has the ability to produce moisture. Wet dressings, such as hydrogels, can make a wound too wet and be responsible for maceration if used inappropriately (Hampton and Collins 2004).

Occlusive dressings achieve many of the criteria for an ideal dressing. They affect the wound and healing in several ways. They have the ability to maintain hydration and prevent the formation of an eschar. As they are designed for moderate exudates, chronic wounds and pressure sores are often dressed with occlusive dressings that are bordered with adhesive. They have a combined primary and secondary layer. If patients have sensitive skin and adhesive borders are traumatic, dressings should be held in place with netting (Netelast) or bandages (see Table 14.3). NB: A dressing used to hold another in place in this way would be a *secondary dressing*.

Dressings should be changed when leakage occurs or the dressing no longer absorbs exudates, around every 2–7 days or as instructed (Hess 2005).

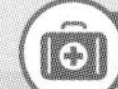 Learning Activity 14.2

Learning in practice: Dressing selection

In your clinical area, ask permission to access the dressing supplies.

- Take a selection of different dressings and, using Table 14.3, identify which group each dressing belongs to and for what type of wound each would be appropriate.
- Consider which dressing groups are not stocked on your unit and why this might be the case. You may want to discuss this with your mentor/supervising nurse.

Assessment and recording tools

The wound should be evaluated each time a dressing is applied or if it gives cause for concern. The aim of evaluating the wound is to assess healing and to establish which treatment will best provide the ideal environment for healing. The surface area or volume of the wound should be measured and recorded. Photography also provides a useful record in wound assessment, but patient consent should always be gained (Bianco and Williams 2002).

Figure 14.5 is an example of a wound assessment chart and Table 14.4 illustrates the types of wound and guidance on choice of dressing following assessment. The underlying cause of the wound should also be assessed, with the primary focus on details such as size and depth as well as the stage of healing (Teare and Barrett 2002). Links can then be made between the wound dressing and the optimal healing environment. The use of this type of documentation to assist in the assessment process is recommended to:

- facilitate continuity of care by providing a central reference point for wound progression
- facilitate appropriate evaluation of all relevant parameters
- fulfil legal and professional requirements (Teare and Barrett 2002).

Figure 14.5 **Wound assessment chart.** ***Source:*** **The Royal Marsden Hospital NHS Foundation Trust.**

THE ROYAL MARSDEN WOUND ASSESSMENT CHART
Complete one chart for each wound

Patient name:						
Hospital number:						
Date of assessment (weekly)						
	Wound dimensions					
Max length (cm)						
Max width (cm)						
Max depth (cm)						
	Wound bed – approximate % cover (enter %)					
Necrotic (BLACK)						
Slough (YELLOW)						
Granulating (RED)						
Epithelializing (PINK)						
	Skin around wound					
Intact						
Healthy						
Fragile						
Dry						
Scaly						
Erythema						
Maceration						
Oedema						
Eczema						
Skin nodules						
Skin stripping						
Dressing allergy						
Tape allergy						
Other (please state)						
	Exudate level					
None						
Low						
Moderate						
High						
Amount increasing						
Amount decreasing						
	Odour (see over for rating scale)					
None						
Slight						
Moderate						
Strong						
	Bleeding					
None						
Slight						
Moderate						
Heavy						
At dressing change						
	Pain from wound (see over for rating scale)					
Level (0–10)						
Continuous						
At specific times (specify)						
	Wound infection suspected					
Swab taken (Y/N)						
Swab result						
Treatment						
Assessment review date						
Initials of Assessor						

(continued)

Figure 14.5 ***(continued)***

Location (mark diagram):	**Visual Analogue Scale (VAS) for Patient's Rating of Pain.**
Right Left Left Right	0 1 2 3 4 5 6 7 8 9 10 No pain ... Worst pain imaginable

Rating Scale for Odour

Score	**Assessment**
None	No odour evident, even when at the patient's bedside with the dressing removed.
Slight	Wound odour is evident at close proximity to the patient when the dressing is removed.
Moderate	Wound odour is evident upon entering the room (1.5 to 3 metres from patient) with the dressing removed.
Strong	Wound odour is evident upon entering the room (1.5 to 3 metres from patient) with the dressing intact.

Diagram of wound if appropriate (or attach tracing/photograph):

Date: ______________	**Date:** ______________
Date: ______________	**Date:** ______________
Date: ______________	**Date:** ______________

Notes on use
Use one chart per wound.
Complete a wound assessment at least once a week.
Measure the wound at its widest points using a clean ruler, use a sterile wound swab or blunt probe to measure wound depth.
For the 'skin around wound' assessment more than one box may be ticked.
Odour and pain should be assessed using the scales at the top of page 2.
Following the assessment a wound management care plan should be written and updated if necessary after each reassessment.

Table 14.4 **Wound classification chart**

Wound picture	Type of wound	Primary dressings	Secondary dressings	Action	Examples of dressings available
	Necrotic Black/brown tissue Hard eschar	Hydrogel Honey-based dressing	Hydrocolloid foam Absorbent dressing Carbon-based dressing if odour present	Debride eschar Rehydrate Encourage a clean wound bed	Aquaform Novogel Intrasite gel Activon Honey Duoderm Allevyn Mepilex Border Carboflex Clinisorb Mepore
	Sloughy Green/yellow pus dying tissue +/– infection	Alginate Hydrofibre Honey-based dressing	Absorbent dressing Foam	Debrides Treats and prevents local wound infection	Sorbsan Aquacel Activon Allevyn Mepilex Border Granuflex Mepore
	Granulating Wound is moist, red or dark pink in appearance May appear bumpy Soft to touch	Hydrocolloid foam Adhesive/ non-adhesive		Protection	Duoderm Allevyn Granuflex Non-adhesive dressing
	Epithelializing Cells are migrating Wound is getting smaller and is healing	Hydrocolloid semi-permeable film Silicon-based product		Protects Reduces potential for infection	Duoderm Mepilex Border Mepilex
	Infected Odour Exudate Inflammation Pus Pain	Iodine/silver/ alginate/honey-based dressing	Low adherence dressing Absorbent carbon dressing	Treats local infection/ absorbs exudate	Aquacel AG Activon Alginate Mepilex Carboflex Allevyn Inadine

Source: Photographs courtesy of Smith and Nephew, Advancis Medical and Pauline Doran Williams.

Procedure guideline 14.1 **Dressing a wound**

Essential equipment

- Sterile dressing pack containing gallipots or an indented plastic tray, low-linting swabs and/or medical foam, disposable forceps, gloves, sterile field, disposable bag and disposable plastic apron
- Fluids for cleaning and/or irrigation
- Hypoallergenic tape
- Appropriate dressing
- Appropriate hand hygiene preparation
- Any other material will be determined by the nature of the dressing; special features of a dressing should be referred to in the patient's nursing care plan
- Detergent wipe
- Total traceability system for surgical instruments and patient record form

Optional equipment

- Sterile scissors

(continued)

Procedure guideline 14.1 Dressing a wound *(continued)*

Action	Rationale
Pre-procedure	
1 Explain and discuss the procedure with the patient and check analgesia requirements.	To ensure that the patient understands the procedure and gives his or her valid consent, and to reduce anxiety (NMC 2013, **E**).
2 Wash hands with soap and water, put on a disposable plastic apron.	Hands must be cleaned before and after every patient contact and before commencing the preparations for aseptic technique, to prevent cross-infection (Fraise and Bradley 2009, **E**).
3 Clean trolley with detergent wipe.	To provide a clean working surface (Fraise and Bradley 2009, **E**).
4 Place all the equipment required for the procedure on the bottom shelf of the clean dressing trolley. Check integrity and use-by dates of all equipment (i.e. packs are undamaged, intact and dry).	To maintain the top shelf as a clean working surface. To ensure sterility of equipment prior to use. **E**
5 Screen the bed area and provide privacy. Position the patient comfortably so that the area to be dealt with is easily accessible without exposing the patient unduly.	To allow any airborne organisms to settle before the sterile field (and in the case of a dressing, the wound) is exposed (Fraise and Bradley 2009, **E**). Maintain the patient's dignity and comfort. **E**
6 Take the trolley to the treatment room or patient's bedside, disturbing the screens as little as possible.	To minimize airborne contamination (Fraise and Bradley 2009, **E**).
Procedure	
7 Clean hands with a bactericidal alcohol handrub.	To reduce the risk of wound infection and cross-contamination (Fraise and Bradley 2009, **E**).
8 Open the outer cover of the sterile dressing pack and slide the contents onto the top shelf of the trolley.	To ensure that only sterile products are used (Fraise and Bradley 2009, **E**).
9 Open the sterile field using only the corners of the paper.	So that areas of potential contamination are kept to a minimum. **E**
10 Loosen the dressing tape (if necessary). If contamination on outer dressings, gloves should be worn.	To make it easier to remove the dressing. **E** For personal protection (Kingsley 2008, **E**).
11 Clean hands with a bactericidal alcohol handrub.	Hands may become contaminated by handling outer packets, dressing, and so on (Fraise and Bradley 2009, **E**).
12 Using the plastic bag in the pack, arrange the sterile field. Pour cleaning solution into gallipots or an indented plastic tray.	The time the wound is exposed should be kept to a minimum to reduce the risk of contamination. To prevent contamination of the environment. To minimize risk of contamination of cleaning solution. **E**
13 Remove dressing by placing a hand in the plastic bag, lifting the dressing off and inverting the plastic bag so that the dressing is now inside the bag. Thereafter use this as the 'dirty' bag. Use gloves if there is difficulty removing dressing.	To reduce the risk of cross-infection. To prevent contamination of the environment (Fraise and Bradley 2009, **E**).
14 Attach the bag with the dressing to the side of the trolley below the top shelf on the side next to the patient.	To avoid taking soiled dressings across the sterile area. Contaminated material should be disposed of below the level of the sterile field. **E**
15 Assess wound healing with reference to Table 14.1.	To evaluate wound care (Dealey 2005, **E**; Hampton and Collins 2004, **E**; Hess 2005, **E**).
16 Clean hands and put on sterile gloves.	To reduce the risk of infection to the wound and contamination of the nurse. Gloves provide greater sensitivity than forceps and are less likely to traumatize the wound or the patient's skin. **E**
17 If necessary, gently irrigate the wound with 0.9% sodium chloride, unless another solution is indicated.	To reduce the possibility of physical and chemical trauma to granulation and epithelial tissue (Hess 2005, **E**).
18 Apply the dressing that is most suitable for the wound using the criteria for dressings (see Table 14.2).	To promote healing and/or reduce symptoms. **E**
19 Make sure the patient is comfortable and the dressing is secure.	A dressing may slip or feel uncomfortable as the patient changes position. **E**

Post-procedure	
20 Dispose of waste in orange plastic clinical waste bags and sharps into a sharps bin. Remove gloves and wash hands.	To prevent environmental contamination and sharps injury. Orange is the recognized colour for clinical waste (DH 2005, **C**).
21 Ensure the patient is comfortable and draw back the curtains.	To promote well-being and maintain dignity and comfort. **E**
22 Clean hands with bactericidal alcohol rub. Wipe trolley with detergent wipe and return to storage.	To prevent the risk of cross-contamination from previous episode of care (Fraise and Bradley 2009, **E**).
23 Record assessment in relevant documentation at the end of the procedure.	To maintain an accurate record of wound-healing progress (NMC 2010, **C**).

POST-PROCEDURAL CONSIDERATIONS

Ongoing care

Dressings need to be changed when 'strike-through' occurs; that is, the dressing becomes soiled and damp at the surface or edge or leakage of wound exudate occurs (see individual dressing packs for instructions to guide practice). The medical team may take the dressing down to view the wound and the nurse should be present to monitor this and reapply an appropriate dressing. Record any changes and/or instructions in the patient's notes or wound care plan (NMC 2010). Included in the notes should be the amount of exudate, any signs of inflammation or odour and appearance of the tissue (Lippincott Williams & Wilkins 2008).

Pressure ulcers

DEFINITION

Pressure ulcers are areas of localized tissue damage caused by excess pressure, shearing or friction forces (NPUAP/EPUAP/PPPIA 2014). The extent of this damage can range from persistent erythema to necrotic ulceration involving muscle, tendon and bone (RCN 2005).

ANATOMY AND PHYSIOLOGY

A pressure ulcer usually results from compromised circulation secondary to pressure over time and is a local site of cell death (Hess 2005). Pressure ulcers are classified in four stages, according to depth. The first is superficial damage which is characterized by local inflammation and may present as a persistent area of redness with no breach of the epidermis. The second stage is partial loss of the epidermis or dermis, often with a blistering or abrasion. The third stage involves damage to the dermis and subcutaneous layers of tissue and clinically appears as an ulcer but does not involve the underlying fascia. The fourth stage involves tissue necrosis and full-thickness skin loss, often with tunnelling sinus tracts (Hess 2005, NPUAP/EPUAP/PPPIA 2014) as illustrated in Figure 14.6.

EVIDENCE-BASED APPROACHES

Pressure ulcers are a major healthcare issue and are associated with pain, infection, prolonged hospital stay, and in extreme cases can be a causative factor in a patient's death (Bennett et al. 2004, RCN 2005). It is important to use a structured approach that involves skin assessment and identification of risks (NPUAP/EPUAP/PPPIA 2014). The risk assessment should be carried out by a Registered Nurse or healthcare professional who has undergone appropriate training to recognize the risk factors that contribute to the development of pressure ulcers and how to initiate and maintain correct and suitable prevention measures (Waterlow 2007) (Figures 14.7, 14.8, 14.9). The use of assessment tools should be undertaken in conjunction with clinical judgement (RCN 2005, Waterlow 2007).

The three major extrinsic factors that are identified as being significant contributory factors in the development of pressure ulcers are pressure, shearing and friction. These factors should be removed or diminished to reduce injury (RCN 2005).

An individual's potential for developing pressure ulcers may be influenced by the following intrinsic factors.

- Reduced mobility or immobility
- Acute illness
- Level of consciousness
- Extremes of age
- Vascular disease
- Severe, chronic or terminal illness
- Previous history of pressure damage
- Malnutrition and dehydration
- Neurologically compromised
- Obesity
- Poor posture
- Use of equipment such as seating or beds which do not provide appropriate pressure relief (NPUAP/EPUAP/PPPIA 2014, RCN 2005, Royal Marsden NHS Foundation Trust 2013)

The potential of an individual to develop pressure ulcers may be exacerbated by the following factors, which therefore should be considered when performing a risk assessment.

- Sedatives and hypnotics may make the patient excessively sleepy and thus reduce mobility.
- Analgesics may reduce normal stimulus to relieve pressure.
- Inotropes cause peripheral vasoconstriction and tissue hypoxia.
- Non-steroidal anti-inflammatory drugs (NSAIDs) impair inflammatory responses to pressure injury.
- Cytotoxics and high-dose steroids may induce immunosuppression which impairs inflammatory responses to pressure injury and may lead to an increased risk of wound infection.
- Moisture to the skin (e.g. from incontinence, perspiration or wound exudate) (NPUAP/EPUAP/PPPIA 2014).

Skin inspection

Systematic skin inspection should occur regularly, with the frequency determined in response to changes in the individual's condition in relation to either deterioration or recovery. Individuals at risk should have their skin inspected at least once a day if an inpatient or at every visit in the community setting.

Skin inspection should be based on an assessment of the most vulnerable areas of risk for each patient, inclusive of daily removal of antiembolic stockings. Areas for observation include heels, sacrum, ischial tuberosities, elbows, temporal region of skull, shoulders, back of head and toes, femoral trochanters, parts of the body where pressure, friction and shear are exerted in the course of daily living activities, parts of the body where external forces are exerted by equipment and clothing. Other areas should be inspected as necessitated by the patient's condition.

Figure 14.6 **Pressure ulcer category system and decision making tool.** *Source:* **The Royal Marsden NHS Foundation Trust (2013).**

The ROYAL MARSDEN
NHS Foundation Trust

Pressure Ulcer Category System and Decision Making Tool

Category 1: Intact skin with non blanching*[1] Redness

The area may be: painful, firm or soft, warmer or cooler than adjacent tissue. It may be difficult to detect in people with darker skin tones.

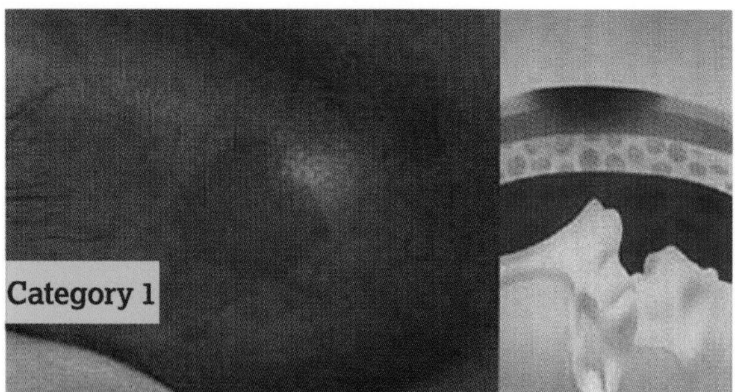

- Pressure area care*[2]
- Film spray
- Hydrocolloid dressing
- Skin barrier product

Category 2: Partial thickness

Loss of dermis presenting as a shallow ulcer with a pink wound bed without slough. May present as a shiny ulcer without slough or bruising.

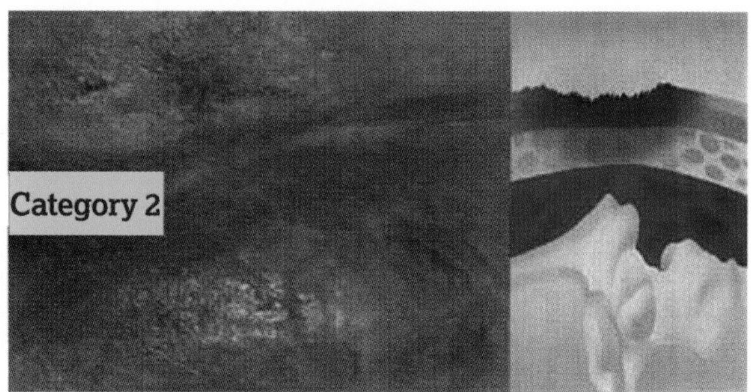

- Pressure area care*[2]
- Hydrocolloid dressing
- Skin barrier product
- Non-adhesive dressing
- Rapid capillary dressing
- Foam dressing

NHS

Figure 14.6 *(continued)*

Category 3: Full thickness tissue loss.

Subcutaneous fat may be visible, slough and undermining*[3] may be present.

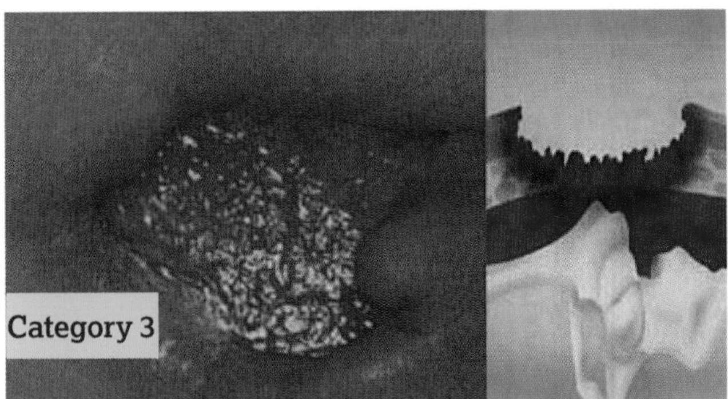

- Pressure area care*[2]
- Skin barrier product
- Rapid capillary dressing
- Negative pressure dressing
- Non-adhesive dressing
- Honey based dressing
- Alginate dressing
- Foam absorbent dressing

Category 4: Full thickness tissue loss with exposed bone, muscle and/or tendon.

Often includes wound undermining. This must be reported as a Serious Incident (SI). Slough may be obvious in the wound.

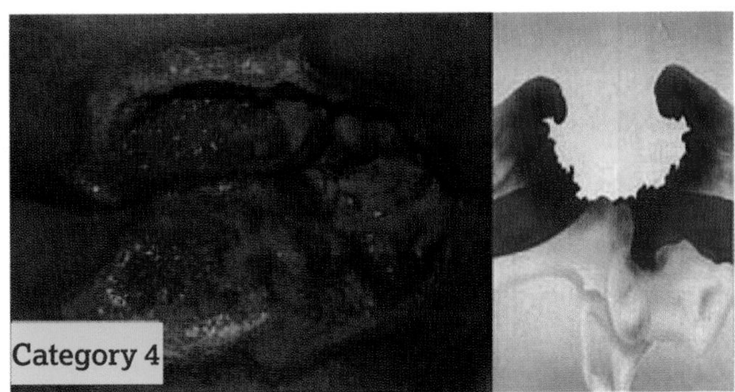

- Pressure area care*[2]
- Skin barrier product
- Negative pressure dressing
- Alginate dressing
- Rapid capillary dressing

*[1] Non-blanching, means that the area does not turn white when pressed.
*[2] Pressure area care includes assessing patient's skin regularly, moisturising the skin regularly with a suitable emollient, and turning the patient as condition allows, following hospital guideline. See pressure ulcer prevention protocol.
*[3] Undermining may present as tissue destruction in the periwound area under the intact skin.

Definitions and illustrations from European Pressure Ulcer Panel 2009
Pauline Doran Williams & Peta Hicks 2012 version 3

Printed March 2012

Figure 14.7 **Risk assessment flow diagram.** ***Source:*** **The Royal Marsden NHS Foundation Trust (2013).**

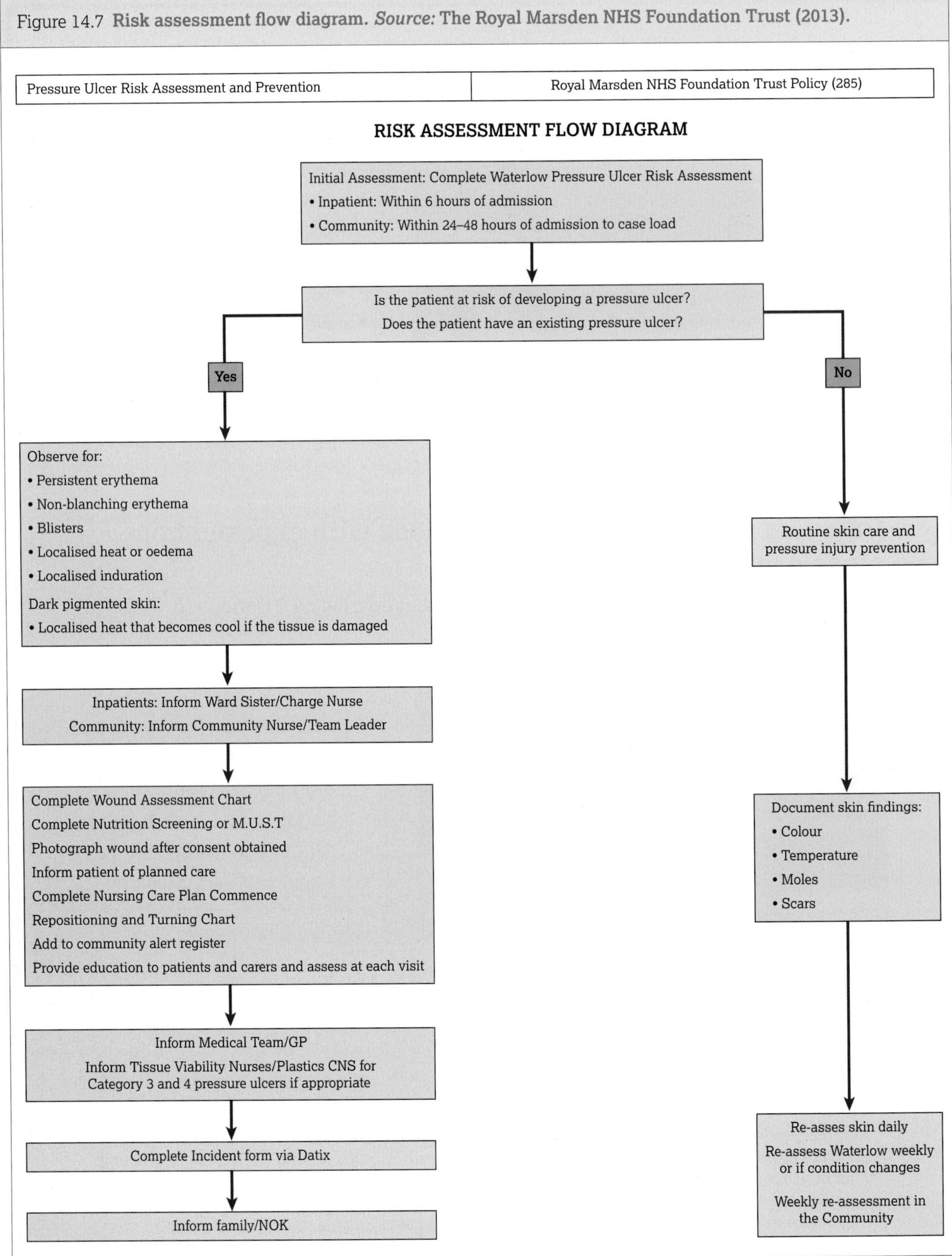

Pressure Ulcer Risk Assessment and Prevention
Royal Marsden NHS Foundation Trust Policy (285)
RISK ASSESSMENT FLOW DIAGRAM
Initial Assessment: Complete Waterlow Pressure Ulcer Risk Assessment
• Inpatient: Within 6 hours of admission
• Community: Within 24–48 hours of admission to case load
Is the patient at risk of developing a pressure ulcer?
Does the patient have an existing pressure ulcer?
Yes
No
Observe for:
• Persistent erythema
• Non-blanching erythema
• Blisters
• Localised heat or oedema
• Localised induration
Dark pigmented skin:
• Localised heat that becomes cool if the tissue is damaged
Inpatients: Inform Ward Sister/Charge Nurse
Community: Inform Community Nurse/Team Leader
Complete Wound Assessment Chart
Complete Nutrition Screening or M.U.S.T
Photograph wound after consent obtained
Inform patient of planned care
Complete Nursing Care Plan Commence
Repositioning and Turning Chart
Add to community alert register
Provide education to patients and carers and assess at each visit
Inform Medical Team/GP
Inform Tissue Viability Nurses/Plastics CNS for Category 3 and 4 pressure ulcers if appropriate
Complete Incident form via Datix
Inform family/NOK
Routine skin care and pressure injury prevention
Document skin findings:
• Colour
• Temperature
• Moles
• Scars
Re-asses skin daily
Re-assess Waterlow weekly or if condition changes
Weekly re-assessment in the Community

Figure 14.8 **Waterlow Pressure Ulcer Risk Assessment Tool.** ***Source:*** **The Royal Marsden NHS Foundation Trust (2013).**

Pressure Ulcer Risk Assessment and Prevention	Royal Marsden NHS Foundation Trust Policy (285)

WATERLOW PRESSURE ULCER RISK ASSESSMENT

THE ROYAL MARSDEN

Name: ____________________ **Hospital / RiO No:** ____________________

Instructions for Use:

1. Score on admission and update weekly or if significant change in patient's condition
2. Add scores together and insert total score
3. Document actions taken in the evaluation section
4. If total score is 10+ initiate core care plan At Risk of Pressure Damage/Pressure Ulcer Formation

10+ AT RISK
15+ HIGH RISK
20+ VERY HIGH RISK

		Date (day/month/year)								
		Time								
GENDER	Male	1								
	Female	2								
AGE	14 – 49	1								
	50 – 64	2								
	65 –74	3								
	75 – 80	4								
	81+	5								
BUILD	Average	0								
	Above average	1								
	Obese	2								
	Below average	3								
APPETITE (select one option ONLY)	Average	0								
	Poor	1								
	NG tube/fluids only	2								
	NBM/anorexic	3								
VISUAL ASSESSMENT OF AT RISK SKIN AREA (may select one or more options)	Healthy	0								
	Thin and fragile	1								
	Dry	1								
	Oedematous	1								
	Clammy (temp↑)	1								
	Previous pressure sore or scarring	2								
	Discoloured	2								
	Broken	3								
MOBILITY (select one option ONLY)	Fully	0								
	Restless/Fidgety	1								
	Apathetic	2								
	Restricted	3								
	Inert (due to ↓consciousness/traction	4								
	Chairbound	5								
CONTINENCE (select one option ONLY)	Continent/Catheterised	0								
	Occasional incontinence	1								
	Incontinent of urine	2								
	Incontinent of faeces	2								
	Doubly incontinent	3								
TISSUE MALNUTRITION (may select one or more options)	Smoking	2								
	Anaemia	2								
	Peripheral vascular disease	5								
	Cardiac failure	5								
	Cachexia	8								
NEUROLOGICAL DEFICIT (score depends on severity)	Diabetes, CVA, MS, Motor/sensory paraplegia, Epidural	4–6								
MAJOR SURGERY TRAUMA (up to 48 hours post surgery)	Above waist	2								
	Orthopaedic, Below waist, Spinal > 2 hours on theatre table	5								
MEDICATION	Cytotoxics, High dose steroids, Anti-inflammatory	4								
		TOTAL SCORE								
		NURSE SIGNATURE								

Figure 14.9 **Managing risk factors.** ***Source:*** **The Royal Marsden NHS Foundation Trust (2013).**

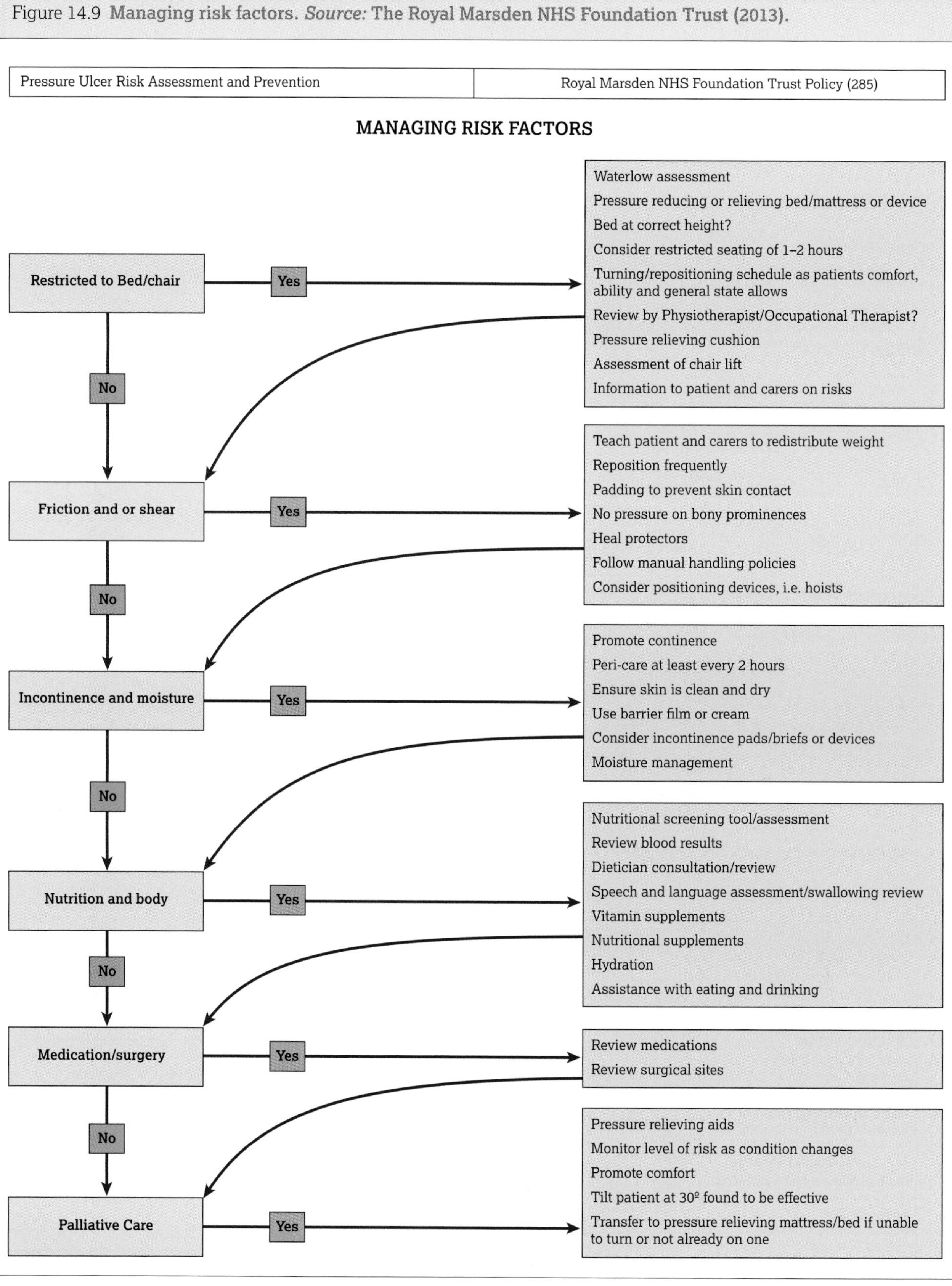
Pressure Ulcer Risk Assessment and Prevention
Royal Marsden NHS Foundation Trust Policy (285)
MANAGING RISK FACTORS
Restricted to Bed/chair
Yes
Waterlow assessment
Pressure reducing or relieving bed/mattress or device
Bed at correct height?
Consider restricted seating of 1–2 hours
Turning/repositioning schedule as patients comfort, ability and general state allows
Review by Physiotherapist/Occupational Therapist?
Pressure relieving cushion
Assessment of chair lift
Information to patient and carers on risks
No
Friction and or shear
Yes
Teach patient and carers to redistribute weight
Reposition frequently
Padding to prevent skin contact
No pressure on bony prominences
Heal protectors
Follow manual handling policies
Consider positioning devices, i.e. hoists
No
Incontinence and moisture
Yes
Promote continence
Peri-care at least every 2 hours
Ensure skin is clean and dry
Use barrier film or cream
Consider incontinence pads/briefs or devices
Moisture management
No
Nutrition and body
Yes
Nutritional screening tool/assessment
Review blood results
Dietician consultation/review
Speech and language assessment/swallowing review
Vitamin supplements
Nutritional supplements
Hydration
Assistance with eating and drinking
No
Medication/surgery
Yes
Review medications
Review surgical sites
No
Palliative Care
Yes
Pressure relieving aids
Monitor level of risk as condition changes
Promote comfort
Tilt patient at 30º found to be effective
Transfer to pressure relieving mattress/bed if unable to turn or not already on one

Individuals who are willing and able should be encouraged, following education, to inspect their own skin. Individuals who are wheelchair users should use a mirror to inspect the areas that they cannot see easily or get others to inspect them.

Healthcare professionals should be aware of the following signs that may indicate incipient pressure ulcer development: persistent erythema, non-blanching hyperaemia (previously identified as non-blanching erythema), blisters, discoloration, localized heat, localized oedema and localized induration. In those with darkly pigmented skin, the signs are purplish/bluish localized areas of skin, localized heat which, if tissue becomes damaged, is replaced by coolness, localized oedema and localized induration.

Skin changes should be documented/recorded immediately using the European Pressure Ulcer Advisory Panel Pressure Ulcer Grading (NPUAP/EPUAP/PPPIA 2014) to classify the ulcer stage and extent of tissue damage.

Maintaining skin integrity

Avoid excessive rubbing over bony prominences, as this does not prevent pressure damage and may actually cause additional damage.

Find the source of excess moisture due to incontinence, perspiration or wound drainage and eliminate this, where possible. When moisture cannot be controlled, interventions that can assist in preventing skin damage should be used.

Skin injury due to friction and shear forces should be minimized through correct positioning, transferring and repositioning techniques (see 'Positioning').

As the patient's condition improves, the potential for improving mobility and activity status exists. Rehabilitation efforts may be instituted if consistent with the overall goals of therapy and referral to a physiotherapist should be considered. Maintaining activity level, mobility and range of movement is an appropriate goal for most individuals.

All interventions and outcomes should be monitored and documented/recorded.

Equipment

The data currently available to evaluate the clinical effectiveness of pressure-relieving devices are variable (RCN 2005). A systematic review of support surfaces for the prevention of pressure ulcers reported that alternative foam mattresses show improvement over standard foam whilst the benefits of alternating pressure (AP) and continuous low pressure (CLP) mattresses are unclear (McInnes et al. 2011). The AP mattresses mould themselves around the person's shape, thereby redistributing the pressure, whilst CLP mattresses alter the pressure surface (RCN 2005). The cost of these systems is also a consideration in planning prevention (McInnes et al. 2011).

The following recommendations are supported.

- Patients with pressure ulcers should have access to pressure-relieving support surfaces and strategies, for example mattresses and cushions, 24 hours a day and this applies to all support surfaces.
- All individuals assessed as having a grade 1–2 pressure ulcer should, as a minimum provision, be placed on a high-specification foam mattress or cushion with pressure-reducing properties. Observation of skin changes, documentation of positioning and repositioning scheme must be combined in the patient's care.
- If there is any potential or actual deterioration of affected areas or further pressure ulcer development, an AP (replacement or overlay) or sophisticated CLP system (e.g. low air loss, air fluidized, air flotation, viscous fluid) should be used.
- Depending on the location of ulcer, individuals assessed as having grade 3–4 pressure ulcers (including intact eschar where depth, and therefore grade, cannot be assessed) should be, as a minimum provision, placed on an AP mattress or sophisticated CLP system.
- If AP equipment is required, the first choice should be an overlay system. However, circumstances such as patient weight or patient safety may indicate the need for a replacement system (RCN 2005).

Positioning

- Individuals who are 'at risk' of pressure ulcer development should be repositioned and the frequency of repositioning determined by the results of skin inspection and individual needs, not by a ritualistic schedule.
- Repositioning should take into consideration other relevant matters, including the patient's medical condition, their comfort, the overall plan of care and the support surface.
- A patient positioning chart should be used to document the patient's position each hour. In the community this should be at each nursing visit. This will give clear documented evidence of repositioning and injury resultant from prolonged periods in a certain position (Figure 14.10).
- Individuals who are considered to be acutely at risk of developing pressure ulcers should restrict chair sitting to less than 2 hours at a time until their general condition improves. Caution should also be exercised once their condition has improved.
- Positioning of patients should ensure that prolonged pressure on bony prominences is minimized, that bony prominences are kept from direct contact with one another, and friction and shear damage are prevented.
- A repositioning schedule, agreed with the individual, should be recorded and established for each person 'at risk'.
- Correct positioning of devices such as pillows or foam wedges should be used to keep bony prominences (for example, knees, heels or ankles) from direct contact with one another in accordance with a written plan. Care should be taken to ensure that these do not interfere with the action of any other pressure-relieving support surfaces in use.
- Individuals who are willing and able should be taught how to redistribute weight every 15 minutes. Carers should be taught how to assist in patient weight distribution.
- Manual handling devices should be used correctly in order to minimize shear and friction damage. After manoeuvring, slings, sleeves or other parts of the handling equipment should be removed from underneath individuals.
- In the community setting, patients and carers (both formal and informal) should be informed of the importance of repositioning (Royal Marsden NHS Foundation Trust 2013).

PRE-PROCEDURAL CONSIDERATIONS

Nurses must consistently question whether they are employing measures for preventing pressure ulcers and whether the patient and caregivers are following the care plan. Nutritional status and the patient's ability to self-care and mobilize should also be evaluated and documented (NPUAP/EPUAP/PPPIA 2014).

Patients who are able and willing should be informed and educated about risk assessment and resulting prevention strategies. This strategy should, where appropriate, include carers.

Patient/carer education leaflets are available and should include information on the following.

- The risk factors associated with them developing pressure ulcers.
- The sites that are at the greatest risk of pressure damage.
- How to inspect skin and recognize skin changes.
- How to care for skin; methods for pressure relief/reduction.
- Where they can seek further advice and assistance should they need it.
- Emphasize the need for immediate visits to a healthcare professional should signs of damage be noticed (Royal Marsden NHS Foundation Trust 2013).

Figure 14.10 **Patient positioning chart.** ***Source:*** **The Royal Marsden NHS Foundation Trust (2013).**

Pressure Ulcer Risk Assessment and Prevention		Royal Marsden NHS Foundation Trust Policy **(285)**

THE ROYAL MARSDEN

Repositioning and Turning Chart

Repositioning and Turning Chart

Name: ______________________ Hospital / RiO No: _____ _______ Need No: ______________

DOB: ____________ Date: ______________

Community Services:
GP Name: ______________________ Pressure Ulcer Form Sent: Yes ☐ No ☐
Base Practice: ______________________

Plan	
Patients position to be changed every……………….hours Patient can sit on a chair for………………………..hours	Document reason for not turning / repositioning………………… ……………………………………………… Reassess 12 hourly

Time	Date	Left Side	Right Side	Supine	30° Tilt	In Chair	Observed Skin Integrity	Comments	Print Name

Administration of analgesia as prescribed and the setting of a time frame with the patient's agreement are recommended to improve the experience for the patient (NPUAP/EPUAP/PPPIA 2014). If the patient refuses care, this should be documented, and/or evaluation of whether the patient improves or deteriorates should be recorded to keep the care plan up to date (Royal Marsden NHS Foundation Trust 2013). Nurses should consult additional guidance if unfamiliar with the patient or regimen (NMC 2015, NPUAP/EPUAP/PPPIA 2014).

Assessment

The use of a pressure ulcer classification system to estimate tissue loss and assess skin by colour, temperature and consistency (i.e. firm/turgid or soft/boggy) is recommended (NPUAP/EPUAP/PPPIA 2014).

- *Stages 1–2 with light exudates*: for reddened areas, barrier cream and relief of pressure are recommended, whilst superficial ulcers require dressing with transparent films as they effectively retain moisture and prevent friction (Bluestein and Javaheri 2008).
- *Stage 3 ulcers* should be dressed with synthetic dressings rather than gauze as these cause less pain and require less frequent changes (Bluestein and Javaheri 2008, NPUAP/EPUAP/PPPIA 2014). These dressings include alginates, hydrocolloids and foams and are often available in site-specific shapes to ease application and removal and minimize leakage. See previous guidance on 'Wound bed preparation' (see Table 14.1).

Learning Activity 14.3 Case study: Pressure ulcer

Mr Toomey is an 83-year-old gentleman who has had a previous above-knee amputation for peripheral vascular disease. He has very limited mobility and recently has become increasingly confused, in that he has been forgetting to eat and drink. He now spends the majority of his days sitting in his armchair and has had some episodes of urinary incontinence. He was seen at home by his GP who identified that he has a pressure sore on his right buttock and also diagnosed that he has a severe urinary tract infection. He has been admitted to the ward for intravenous antibiotics and also assessment of his pressure ulcer.

1. What factors contributed to the pressure ulcer occurring? Were any of these avoidable?

You have been asked to assess his skin integrity including the pressure ulcer on his right buttock.

2. What should you be observing for?
3. What tool(s) would help you to carry out a comprehensive assessment?

His pressure ulcer has been assessed as grade 2.

4. What measures should be put in place to manage the pressure ulcer and avoid any further skin deterioration?

See the end of the chapter for the answers.

Surgical wounds

EVIDENCE-BASED APPROACHES

Methods of wound closure

There are four main methods of wound closure:

- sutures
- adhesive skin closure strips
- tissue adhesive
- clips.

See Table 14.5 for advantages and disadvantages of each method.

Wounds may vary and therefore careful assessment is required before the method of closure is selected. The following guiding principles can assist with decision making (Richardson 2007).

- *What is the aim of the wound closure?* For example, eliminating dead space where a haematoma can develop, realigning tissue correctly or holding aligned tissues until healing has occurred.
- *What is the history of the wound?* This informs the practitioner about the depth of the wound and likelihood of infection.
- *What is the wound site pattern?* This and biomechanical properties may rule out some methods of closure.

Suturing

EVIDENCE-BASED APPROACHES

Rationale

Suturing as a method of wound closure is appropriate in managing deep, large wounds. As there is a direct relationship between the time of wound closure and infection risk, suturing is usually best suited for primary closure in recently acquired, non-infected wounds (Jain 2013).

Indications

This method is used to promote primary healing, realign tissue layers and hold the skin edges together until enough healing occurs to withstand stress without mechanical support (Wicker and O'Neill 2010). There are a number of common suturing errors as listed in Table 14.6.

Contraindications

Experts are usually required to manage wounds of a certain depth or in complex areas such as the face or hand. This is to minimize scarring and not restrict movement by poor technique. Therefore local policy will probably prevent nurses from suturing these wounds (Reynolds and Cole 2006).

LEGAL AND PROFESSIONAL ISSUES

Competencies

Nurses should decline to carry out procedures that they have not been prepared for (NMC 2015). Suturing wounds requires skill and should be performed by practitioners who have undergone appropriate training.

PRE-PROCEDURAL CONSIDERATIONS

The environment should be warm, quiet, relaxed and private prior to suturing in order to promote patient comfort and maintain dignity (Hughes and Mardell 2009). It is advisable to lie the patient down to relieve anxiety and prevent further injury that could occur if the patient faints (Reynolds and Cole 2006).

Before closing the wound by any method, the wound must be thoroughly cleansed to minimize the risk of wound infection and ensure that any dirt or foreign bodies are removed (Reynolds and Cole 2006). Dirty wounds should be thoroughly cleansed with irrigation of sterile 0.9% sodium chloride using a large syringe until cleared of visible debris (Giddings 2013).

The wound area needs to be prepared by administering local anaesthetic and as a result suturing is more painful and takes longer than other methods of wound closure (Reynolds and Cole 2006). Prophylactic antibiotics are not indicated after a simple laceration repair but should be given in cases of probable contamination, i.e. dirty wounds (Jain 2013).

Table 14.5 **Advantages and disadvantages of methods of wound closure**

Method	Advantages	Disadvantages
Suturing	Provides secure closure. Allows accurate approximation of tissue layers. Necessity of local anaesthesia use provides good conditions for thorough wound cleansing	Suturing must be performed by an experienced practitioner. Incorrect technique can lead to delayed healing, tissue necrosis and/or dehiscence. More time consuming than other methods. Requires local anaesthetic. Suture material is a foreign body and thus increases infection risk
Interrupted sutures are separate sutures each with its own knot	This is the simplest suture to appose two wound edges. Wound support is not reliant on any individual suture, therefore if there is a weakness or breakage in one, the others should continue to provide support.	Relatively time consuming to perform as each suture requires its own knot. Time consuming to remove if non-absorbable material used
Continuous sutures consist of a continuous over-and-over suture that forms a spiral within the tissues	Quick to perform with knots placed only at the beginning and end of the suture line. Easy to remove	The whole suture line may unravel if there is weakness or breakage anywhere along it. Difficult to drain localized subcutaneous collections by opening part of a wound, therefore interrupted sutures are preferable for wounds particularly at risk of infection
Subcuticular sutures are continuous or interrupted sutures placed in the dermis, with each bite placed horizontally in the dermal layer	This technique avoids suture marks on the skin so can be very neat and thus is popular in skin closure. Easy to remove	If continuous, the same disadvantages apply as above. If the sutures are not placed at the correct depth on each side of the wound, a 'step' can occur, resulting in poor cosmesis and delayed healing
Adhesive skin closure strips	No local anaesthetic required and tissue damage is minimal	Only suitable for clean wounds as lack of local anaesthesia may reduce ability to thoroughly cleanse wound and remove all foreign bodies
	Strips are cheap and simple to apply and remove	Shear forces may cause blistering of the skin Oedema at the site may cause taped wound edges to invert, causing delayed healing
Tissue adhesive	No local anaesthetic required and tissue damage is minimal	Only suitable for clean wounds as lack of local anaesthesia may reduce ability to thoroughly cleanse wound and remove all foreign bodies
	Rapidly produces a strong flexible bond	Requires a second person to assist in getting skin edges accurately aligned
	Sloughs off as skin re-epithelializes, producing good cosmetic results	Not suitable over joints, areas of excessive tension or wounds on the eyes, mouth or scalp
	Less painful than suturing	Care must be taken to avoid any contact with the open wound as adhesive in the wound will create a barrier to healing
	No statistically significant difference from suturing for infection and patient satisfaction (Coulthard et al. 2004)	Sutured wounds were less likely to dehisce (Coulthard et al. 2004)
Skin clips	Can be used on many types of surgical incisions	Clips are more expensive than sutures
	Reduce operating time and tissue trauma	Must be inserted by an experienced practitioner
	Produce excellent cosmetic results when correctly applied	Failure to align tissue edges may cause scar deformity
	Produce uniform tension along the suture line and less distortion from the stress of individual suture points	An extractor is required for clip removal

Source: Adapted from Kirk (2010), Tulloh and Lee (2007).

Table 14.6 **Common suturing errors**

Error	Resulting problems
Sutures too loose	Fails to bring wound edges together, leading to gaping, poor healing and poor cosmetic outcomes Sutures may fall out
Sutures too tight	Tissues tend to swell with oedema fluid in the first few hours after suturing. Does not allow for normal wound swelling. This may cause the tissues bound up within the suture line to strangulate and necrose with subsequent wound breakdown. Care must be taken to allow for this by gently apposing the tissues, ensuring sutures are neither too loose nor too tight May induce vascular compromise of the wound edges leading to necrosis. May lead to the stitch breaking, delayed healing, poor cosmetic results
Uneven tension on interrupted sutures	The tightest suture is exposed to excess tension and may give way
Sutures spaced too widely apart	Gaping between adjacent sutures leading to poor healing
Wound edge overlapping	The resultant 'step' caused by the overlap is likely to delay healing and produce a more obvious scar
Sutures too near the wound edge	These are likely to pull out
Traumatic tissue handling	Tissue handling (e.g. with forceps) should be gentle to preserve tissue integrity and blood supply, thereby promoting healing

Source: Adapted from Kirk (2010), Tulloh and Lee (2007).

Procedure guideline 14.2 Suturing a simple wound

Essential equipment

- Plastic apron
- Sterile gloves
- Electric clippers with disposable head
- Suture pack (containing needle holder, tissue forceps, dressing forceps, scissors, low-linting swabs, solution pot)
- Sutures in varying gauges and materials
- 10 mL syringe and needles (21 and 25 G)
- Dressing
- Traceability form

Medicinal products

- Local anaesthetic (1% lidocaine hydrochloride)
- Sterile 0.9% sodium chloride solution

Pre-procedure

Action	Rationale
1 Explain and discuss the procedure with the patient.	To ensure that the patient understands the procedure and gives their valid consent (NMC 2013, **C**).
2 Follow the procedure for aseptic technique, i.e. use of a trolley, clean hands, apply apron and gloves.	To reduce the risk of contamination (Fraise and Bradley 2009, **E**).

Procedure

Action	Rationale
3 Using a bright light, assess the wound, clean if necessary and decide the type of material and gauge of needle to use.	To ensure that the wound is closed using most appropriate material to promote healing (Reynolds and Cole 2006, **E**).
4 The skin surrounding the wound may require clipping to remove hair. This should be performed using electric clippers with disposable head immediately prior to the procedure.	To prevent hairs from becoming trapped in the closed wound. Clipping has been demonstrated to cause significantly fewer surgical site infections than shaving and is the only method of perioperative hair removal recommended (Tanner et al. 2006, **E**).
5 Draw up the local anaesthetic and first administer an intracutaneous bleb, using a fine needle. Wait for this to take effect then inject the remainder through the anaesthetized area, infiltrating deeper using a longer, larger needle. Keep the point moving as you inject to ensure the needle is not in a vessel.	To reduce pain during the procedure. Inadvertent injection of local anaesthetic into a blood vessel can result in local anaesthetic toxicity. Signs and symptoms are dose related and can include metallic taste, tinnitus and circumoral numbness, progressing to seizures and cardiac arrest (Rothrock 2011, **E**).

(continued)

Procedure guideline 14.2 Suturing a simple wound *(continued)*

Action	Rationale
6 Wait a minimum of 4–5 minutes and test the area gently with a needle tip or instrument prior to beginning. Do not begin the procedure until the anaesthetic has had time to act.	Beginning the procedure before the wound is fully anaesthetized will cause pain and undermine the confidence and trust of the patient (Kirk 2010, **E**).
7 Select approriate tissue forceps, needle and needle holder.	In readiness to perform the procedure. **E**
8 The needle should be grasped in the needle holder on its flattened area about a third of the way along from the suture material **(Action figure 8)**.	To prepare the suture material for use. Holding it where the needle is flat in cross-section will prevent it from rotating in the jaws of the needle holder and enable good control (Tulloh and Lee 2007, **E**).
9 The needle holder should be held in the dominant hand and support the wound edge with the closed tips of tissue forceps.	To facilitate control of the equipment and to promote accurate tissue apposition. Tissue approximation should err on the side of slight eversion (an outward turning) and avoid inversion (an inward turning) or overlapping (Tulloh and Lee 2007, **E**).
10 If a linear wound, suturing should begin at the centre.	To evenly distribute the tissue and promote accurate apposition (Kirk 2010, **E**).
11 The needle should be inserted at a 90° angle to the skin and traverse the full thickness of the wound. The distance of the needle puncture from the edge of the wound should be equal to the depth of the layer of tissue being sutured **(Action figure 11)**. NB: This does not apply to deep wounds where layered closure is required.	To create secure tension-free apposition of the wound edges (Giddings 2013, **E**; Jain 2013, **E**). To ensure that the correct tension of the sutures as this can affect healing and cosmetic appearance (Hampton and Collins 2004) with inflammation occurring when they are too tight (leading to devitalized tissue (Reynolds and Cole 2006)). If too loose, the scar will not align and hold the wound edges in apposition (Clark 2004, Reynolds and Cole 2006). See Table 14.6 for common suturing errors.
12 Bring the needle up in between the wound edges **(Action figure 12)**.	To allow visualization of the depth of bite and enable matching of this on each side of the wound (Tulloh and Lee 2007, **E**).
13 Pull the suture through the tissue until a short tail of approximately 2 cm remains at the initial skin entry site.	To ensure there is enough suture to use for knot tying (Giddings 2013, **E**).
14 Reinsert the needle at a 90° angle from the base of the wound on the other side and push the suture through the tissue, following the curve of the needle, so as to emerge perpendicular to the skin **(Action figure 14)**.	To bring the wound edges together and promote accurate apposition. If the tissues are not pierced perpendicular to the upper and lower surfaces of the wound, an inverted or everted effect will result (Kirk 2010, **E**).
15 Hold the needle parallel to the skin and, grasping the needle end of the suture, make two clockwise loops around the needle holder to produce a surgeon's knot **(Action figure 15)**.	To begin to create a knot (Giddings 2013, **E**).
16 Grasp the tail of the suture with the needle holder. The wrapped suture will slide off the holder to encircle the tail **(Action figure 16)**.	To 'set a throw' (Giddings 2013, **E**).
17 Pull the tail end of the suture toward you and the long suture strand away from you, making sure the suture lies flat.	To 'tighten the throw' (Giddings 2013, **E**).
18 Follow this by a single anticlockwise loop around the needle holder and move the needle to the opposite side of the wound **(Action figure 18)**.	To square the knot (Giddings 2013, **E**).
19 Then create a third throw of one loop. Do not tie it too tightly, just sufficient to secure the knot, thus approximating wound edges without constriction **(Action figure 19)**.	Sutures tied too tightly may cause tissue necrosis, delayed healing and increased scarring (Jain 2013, **E**).
20 The suture can then be cut free from the knot, leaving tails of about 5 mm **(Action figure 20)**.	If the tails are left too long they may entangle with the next suture. If they are too short there is a risk of knot slippage and they will also be difficult to remove (Jain 2013, **E**).
21 Insert each suture in the same way until the wound is entirely closed. The distance between adjacent sutures should be about the same as the depth and width of each one.	To close the wound securely with even spacing and no gaping between adjacent sutures (Tulloh and Lee 2007, **E**).
22 Once completed, discard needle in sharps bin.	To prevent potential sharps injury (Hughes and Mardell 2009, **E**).

Post-procedure	
23 Clean any blood from the surrounding area using aseptic technique and sterile saline solution of 0.9% sodium chloride.	To prevent any possible wound infection (Fraise and Bradley 2009, **E**).
24 Apply a suitable dressing.	To protect the wound from further trauma or contamination and ensure optimum healing (Fraise and Bradley 2009, **E**).
25 Record the date, time and name of the practitioner, amount of local anaesthetic used and size and type of suture material and number of sutures on the appropriate charts.	To maintain accurate records and provide a point of reference in the event of any queries (NMC 2010,**C**; Reynolds and Cole 2006, **E**).

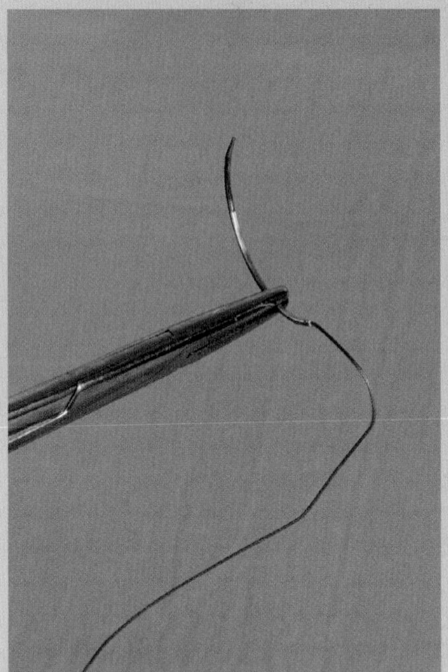
Action Figure 8 Grasp the needle.

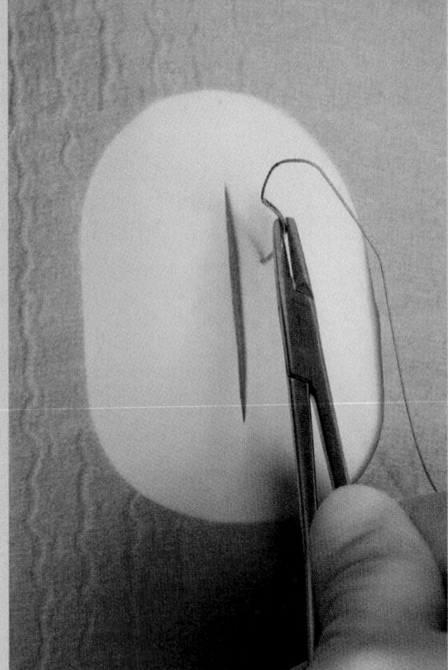
Action Figure 11 Insert the needle at a 90° angle.

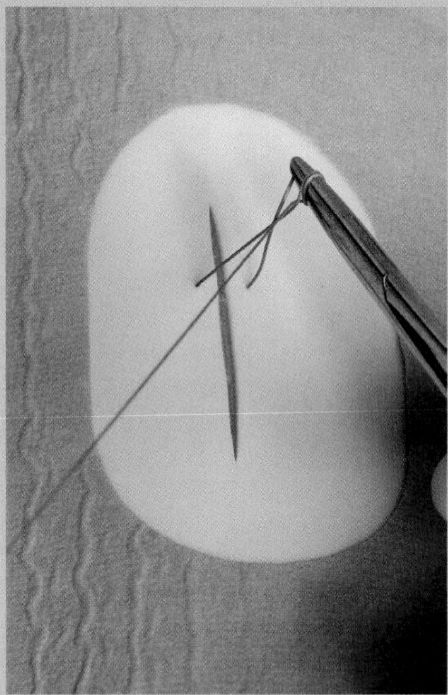
Action Figure 12 Bring the needle up between the wound edges.

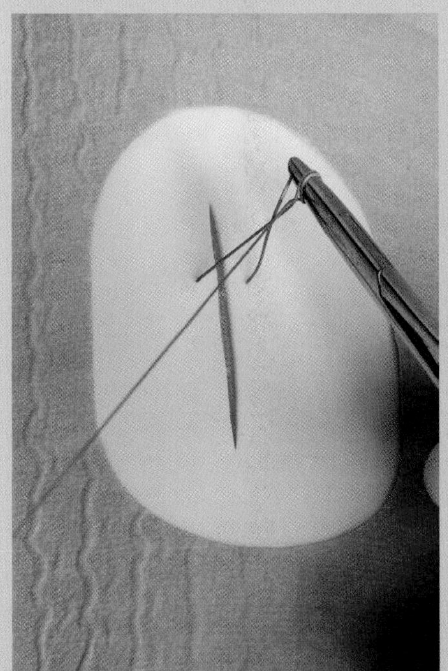
Action Figure 14 Reinsert the needle on the other side.

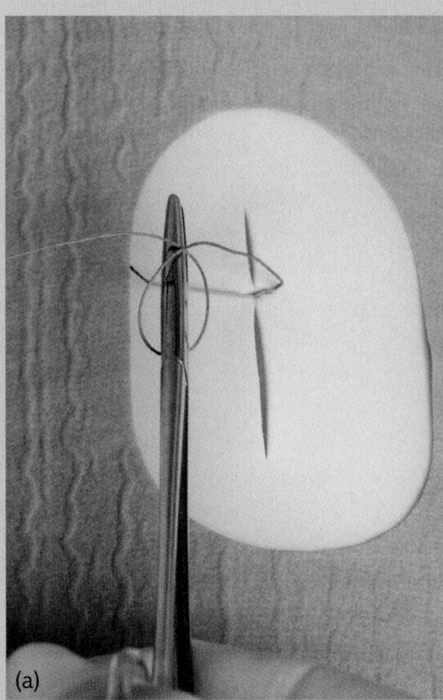

Action Figure 15 Make two clockwise loops.

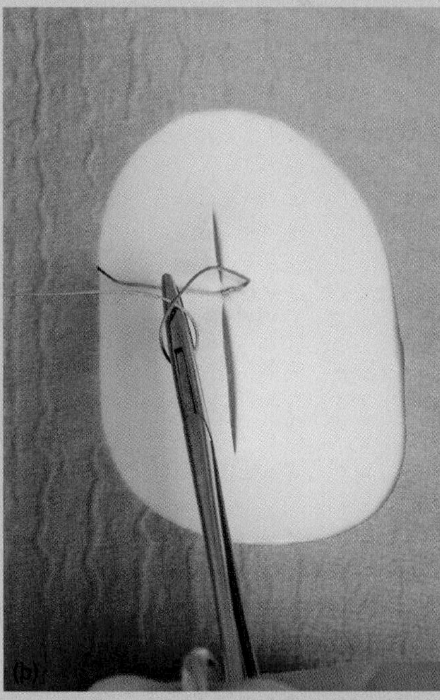

Action Figure 16 Grasp the tail of the suture with the needle holder.

(continued)

Procedure guideline 14.2 Suturing a simple wound *(continued)*

Action	Rationale
26 Provide the patient with written and verbal advice regarding wound care and when the sutures should be removed.	To ensure optimum care for the wound and correct removal time. Premature suture removal may lead to wound dehiscence and sutures kept in too long cause excessive scarring (Weinzweig 2010, **E**).

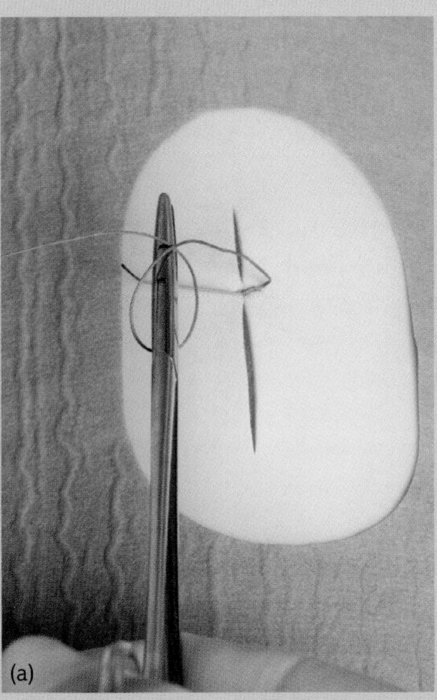

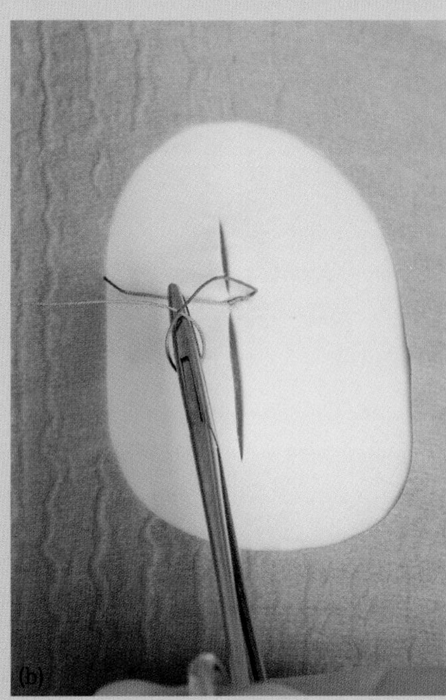

Action Figure 18 (a) Loop the suture around the needle holder. (b) Move the needle to the opposite side of the wound.

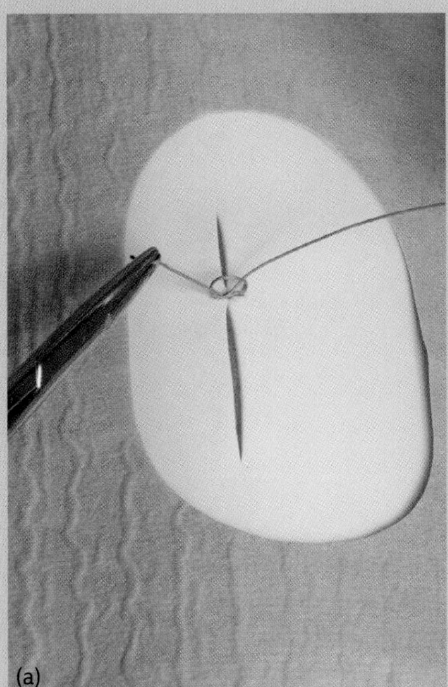

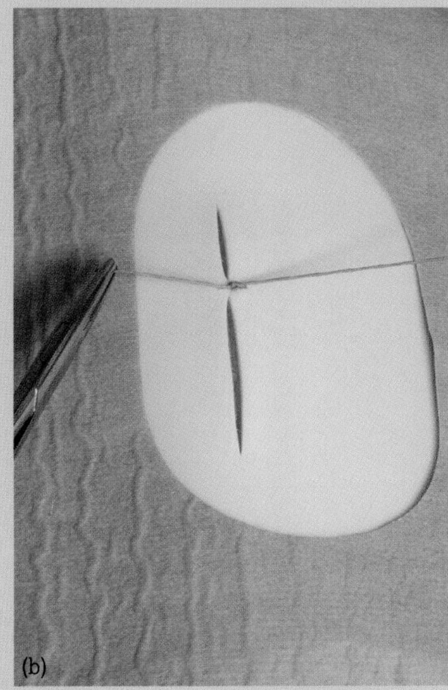

Action Figure 19 (a) Tying the knot to approximate the edges of the wound. (b) Tying the knot to approximate the edges of the wound.

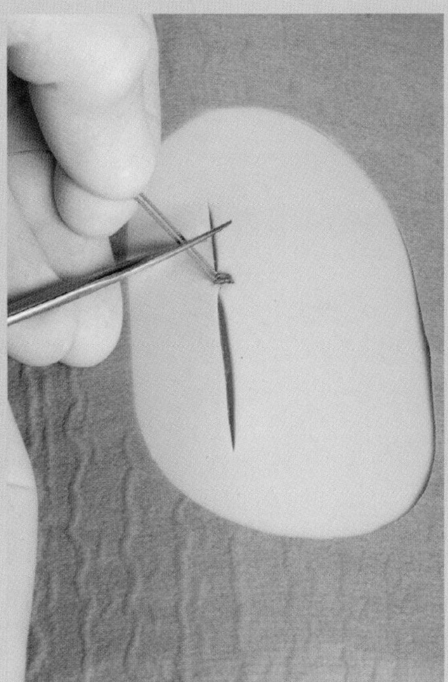

Action Figure 20 The suture can be freed from the knot.

POST-PROCEDURAL CONSIDERATIONS

On completion of suturing, a dressing should be applied. The nurse should then document the following: how many sutures were inserted, type of material, and when they should be removed (NMC 2010).

Removal of sutures or clips

EVIDENCE-BASED APPROACHES

Rationale

Removal of sutures is usually performed between 7 and 10 days post insertion, but this is dependent on where the wound is and whether it has healed. Routinely, every other suture or clip is removed first, with the rest removed if the incision remains securely closed. If any sign of suture line separation is evident during the removal process, the remaining sutures should be left in place and reported to the medical team (Pudner 2005).

PRE-PROCEDURAL CONSIDERATIONS

Assess the wound, as the time period for removal of sutures depends upon the patient's underlying pathology, condition of their skin and the wound position (Pudner 2005). Surgical notes and instructions should also be taken into account along with the skills of the practitioner (NMC 2010). Analgesia may be offered depending on the patient and wound site.

Procedure guideline 14.3 **Suture removal**

Essential equipment

- Sterile dressing pack containing gallipots or an indented plastic tray, low-linting swabs and/or medical foam, disposable forceps, gloves, sterile field, disposable bag
- Apron
- Fluids for cleaning and/or irrigation
- Hypoallergenic tape
- Appropriate dressing
- Appropriate hand hygiene preparation
- Any other material will be determined by the nature of the dressing; special features of a dressing should be referred to in the patient's nursing care plan
- Detergent wipe for cleaning trolley
- Total traceability system for surgical instruments and patient record form

Optional equipment

- Any extra equipment that may be needed during procedure, for example sterile scissors, stitch cutter, staple remover, sterile adhesive sutures

Action	Rationale
Pre-procedure	
1 Explain and discuss the procedure with the patient.	To ensure that the patient understands the procedure and gives their valid consent (NMC 2013, **C**).
2 Perform procedure using aseptic technique, i.e. use of a trolley, clean hands, apply apron and gloves.	To prevent infection (Fraise and Bradley 2009, **E**).
Procedure	
3 Clean the wound with an appropriate sterile solution such as 0.9% sodium chloride.	To prevent infection (Fraise and Bradley 2009, **E**).
4 Lift knot of suture with metal forceps.	Plastic forceps tend to slip against nylon sutures. **E**
5 Using stitch cutter or scissors, snip stitch close to the skin. Pull suture out gently towards the side that has been cut. For intermittent sutures, alternate sutures should be removed first before remaining sutures are removed.	To prevent infection by drawing exposed suture through the tissue (Pudner 2005, **E**). To ensure wound closure and predict dehiscence (Pudner 2005, **E**).
6 Use tips of scissors slightly open or the side of the stitch cutter to gently press the skin when the suture is being drawn out. Continue until all the sutures are removed as required.	To minimize pain by counteracting the adhesion between the suture and surrounding tissue. **E**
7 Apply a suitable dressing.	To protect the wound from further trauma or contamination and ensure optimum healing (Fraise and Bradley 2009, **E**).
Post-procedure	
8 Dispose of waste in orange plastic clinical waste bags and sharps into a sharps bin. Remove gloves and wash hands.	To prevent environmental contamination and sharps injury. Orange is the recognized colour for clinical waste (DH 2005, **C**).
9 Record condition of suture line and surrounding skin (amount of exudate, pus, inflammation, pain, and so on).	To document care and enable evaluation of the wound (Bale and Jones 2006, **E**; Dealey 2005, **E**; NMC 2010, **C**) .

Procedure guideline 14.4 Clip removal

Essential equipment

- Sterile dressing pack containing gallipots or an indented plastic tray, low-linting swabs and/or medical foam, disposable forceps, gloves, sterile field, disposable bag
- Fluids for cleaning and/or irrigation
- Hypoallergenic tape
- Appropriate dressing
- Appropriate hand hygiene preparation
- Any other material will be determined by the nature of the dressing; special features of a dressing should be referred to in the patient's nursing care plan
- Detergent wipe for cleaning trolley
- Total traceability system for surgical instruments and patient record form

Optional equipment

- Any extra equipment that may be needed during procedure, for example sterile scissors, stitch cutter, clip remover, sterile adhesive sutures

Action	Rationale
Pre-procedure	
1 Explain and discuss the procedure with the patient and gain their consent.	To ensure that the patient understands the procedure and gives their valid consent (NMC 2013, **C**).
2 Perform procedure using aseptic technique, i.e. use of a trolley, clean hands, apply apron and gloves.	To prevent infection (Fraise and Bradley 2009, **E**).
Procedure	
3 Clean the wound with an appropriate sterile solution such as 0.9% sodium chloride.	To prevent infection (Fraise and Bradley 2009, **E**).
4 If the suture line is under tension, use free hand to gently guide the skin either side of the surgical incision line.	To reduce tension of skin around suture line and lessen pain on removal of clip. **E**
5 Slide the lower bar of the clip remover with the V-shaped groove under the clip at an angle of 90°. Squeeze the handles of the clip removers together to open the clip.	To release the clip atraumatically from the wound. If the angle of the clip remover is not correct, the clip will not come out freely (Pudner 2005, **E**).
6 Continue till all clips are removed.	Clips should all be removed at the earliest possible point to avoid marks from the clips along the suture line (Widgerow 2013, **E**).
7 Apply a suitable dressing.	To protect the wound from further trauma or contamination and ensure optimum healing (Fraise and Bradley 2009, **E**).
Post-procedure	
8 Dispose of waste in orange plastic clinical waste bags and sharps into a sharps bin. Remove gloves and wash hands.	To prevent environmental contamination and sharps injury. Orange is the recognized colour for clinical waste (DH 2005, **C**).
9 Record condition of suture line and surrounding skin (amount of exudate, pus, inflammation, pain, etc.).	To document care and enable evaluation of the wound (Bale and Jones 2006, **E**; Dealey 2005, **E**; NMC 2010, **C**).

Plastic surgery

DEFINITION

Plastic surgery is the process of reconstructing or repairing parts of the body by the transfer of tissue, to restore normal functional ability and aesthetic form. This may be following trauma, disease or congenital malformations (Storch and Rice 2005). This is achieved by using flaps and skin grafts for reconstruction purposes, in addition to using the natural elasticity and mobility of the skin. Surgical reconstruction is often required following extensive surgery for cancer, trauma or congenital abnormalities.

There are several reconstructive options available, ranging in complexity from split-skin graft, full-thickness skin graft, local tissue transfer, distant tissue transfer to free flap-based reconstruction. This initial philosophy of reconstruction was of a 'reconstructive ladder' whereby the simplest procedure was performed first, and where this was not possible, to proceed up the ladder in a step-wise approach to the next most complex. This philosophy has now given way to a reconstructive menu or toolbox approach where the optimal procedure for the individual patient is selected, and a more complex procedure may be the first choice if this is likely to produce a better overall outcome (Giele and Cassell 2008).

RELATED THEORY

A surgical flap is a strip of tissue, usually consisting of skin, underlying fat, fascia, muscle and/or bone, which is transferred from one part of the body (known as the donor site) to another (known as the recipient site) (Storch and Rice 2005).

A skin graft is living but devascularized (separated from its blood supply) tissue consisting of all or some of the layers of the skin which is removed from one area of the body and applied to a wound on another area of the body. The common methods of skin grafting are full-thickness skin grafts (FTSG), in which the entire epidermis and dermis is removed, and split-thickness or split-skin graft (SSG), which consists of the epidermis and the upper part of the dermis only (Giele and Cassell 2008).

EVIDENCE-BASED APPROACHES

Principles of care

Each patient will require individually planned, and therefore unique, surgery. Reconstructive surgery of this type often results in altered anatomy, in both appearance and function, which may affect the psychological and physical well-being of the patient. Pre-operative patient assessment must be as detailed as possible; this should include information on past and present medical conditions that may delay wound healing.

The complexity of the surgery will often require intensive nursing care. Post-operative observation of the wound sites, flap, dressings and drains is crucial as deterioration of a wound can occur suddenly, necessitating the need for prompt nursing action and/or surgical intervention. The main aim following flap reconstruction is to ensure easy access for observation so that monitoring can be carried out effectively and efficiently during the crucial first 72 hours. Figure 14.11 shows a flap observation chart. These should adhere to medical notes and instructions as per patient. The principles are clarified in the procedure guidelines (e.g. change of wound dressing, removal of drains).

Negative pressure wound therapy

DEFINITION

Negative pressure wound therapy (NPWT), previously known as topical negative pressure (TNP), is the application of a controlled negative pressure across the wound bed to promote healing (Ubbink et al. 2008). The benefits of NPWT include the management of exudate, reduction of wound odour and an increase in local blood flow in the periwound area, a reduction in the number of dressing changes required and an improvement in quality of life (Milne 2013, Ubbink et al. 2008).

EVIDENCE-BASED APPROACHES

Rationale

Negative pressure wound therapy optimizes wound healing by stimulating granulation in an enhanced well-vascularized wound bed. It creates a moist wound environment and removes

Figure 14.11 **Flap observation chart.**

Name: .... Hospital No: .... Ward:.................................... THE ROYAL MARSDEN

Flap Observation Chart

Instructions	Criteria for Assessment	Normal	Arterial Insufficiency	Venous Congestion
1. **Confirm with the surgeon the frequency of flap observations (see medical notes / nursing care plan)** Suggested immediate post-op assessment frequency: • every 15 minutes for first 4 hours, • every 30 minutes for the next 4 hours, • hourly for 24–36 hours, • then 2–4 hourly thereafter	**Colour** • If it is an external flap then check with the donor site for original colour • If it is an internal flap then monitor for extremes of colour	Usual skin tone	Paler than usual skin tone	Blue / Purple / Mottled
	Temperature • An external or internal flap should always feel warm to touch • If the flap feels cool or has increased warmth, ***seek medical assessment immediately*** • A warmer flap may be due to an abnormal inflammatory response, e.g. infection	Warm	Cold	Increased warmth
	Turgidity (Texture) • The flap should usually feel soft (spongy), not hard or flaccid • Hard or swollen flap indicates possible oedema or haematoma	Soft	Flaccid	Turgid (hard)
2. **If signs of venous or arterial occlusion seek immediate help**	**Capillary Refill** (Blanching) • If possible this should be timed (in seconds) • If timing not possible and an alteration in perfusion is suspected, ***seek medical assessment immediately***	2–3 seconds	Absent / Sluggish > 6 seconds	Brisk < 3 seconds
3. **At each handover, confirm flap status/observations at the bedside**	**Specific Monitoring Instructions** (*e.g. Monitor the tension on the flap and check for kinking*)			

Type & Location of Flap: .... **Donor Area (if appropriate):** ....

Timing		**Colour** (*tick one*)			**Temperature** (*tick one*)			**Turgidity** (Texture) (*tick one*)			**Capillary Refill** (Blanching) (*tick one*)			**Specific Instructions (specify):**	**Signature and Print Name**
Date	Time	Usual skin tone	Paler than usual skin tone	Blue / purple / mottled	Warm	Cold	Increased warmth	Soft	Flaccid	Turgid (hard)	2–3 seconds	Absent / sluggish > 6 seconds	Brisk < 3 seconds		

exudate from the wound (KCI 2007) whilst protecting from outside contaminants and potentially reducing wound bioburden (Smith and Nephew 2011). The interstitial fluid that mechanically compromises healing is gently removed whilst the capillary circulation is increased (Ubbink et al. 2008). Pressures are set dependent on the wound aetiology and patient tolerance (Henderson et al. 2010). The suction can be set on continuous or intermittent according to the therapy required (Benbow 2005). Continuous therapy can be used for high-volume wounds, and is recommended for use over unstable structures to minimize movement and help to stabilize the wound bed, when used on flaps and grafts and for patients with a high risk of bleeding (Smith and Nephew 2011). Intermittent therapy stimulates more granulation tissue and improves the rate of healing, and can be used on any wounds other than those with high exudate (Milne 2013). It has proven to be cost-efficient, safe and effective as a treatment modality for wound care (KCI 2007).

The benefits to chronic wound healing of using NPWT versus other treatments have been shown in a number of clinical trials, but further research is needed with fewer methodological flaws and clearer reporting of infection rates and length of hospital stay (NICE 2009, Ubbink et al. 2008).

Indications

Negative pressure wound therapy is indicated for:

- chronic wounds, e.g. venous insufficiency and pressure ulcers
- diabetic and neuropathic ulcers
- post-operative and dehisced surgical wounds
- partial-thickness burns
- skin flaps and grafts
- traumatic wounds
- explored fistulae (Milne 2013, Smith and Nephew 2011).

Contraindications

Negative pressure wound therapy is contraindicated in:

- grossly contaminated wounds
- malignant wounds due to the potential to stimulate proliferation of malignant cells (with the exception of palliative care to improve quality of life)
- untreated osteomyelitis
- non-enteric and unexplored fistulae (KCI 2007)
- the force of the negative pressure can damage or rupture vessels if used over anastomotic sites or organs, exposed vasculature or nerves (Benbow 2005, Henderson et al. 2010)
- wounds with necrotic tissue with eschar present or thick slough will require debridement prior to the application of NPWT (Henderson et al. 2010). (See individual company precautions for use of NPWT systems.)

Precautions should be exercised when there is active bleeding in the wound, difficult haemostasis or when the patient is taking anticoagulants (Benbow 2005), on spinal cord injury, vascular anastomoses and wounds with sharp edges such as bone fragments (Henderson et al. 2010). The wound site must be carefully assessed to ensure that NPWT is indeed the appropriate treatment modality. If signs of infection or complications develop, the therapy should be discontinued (KCI 2007). There is currently not enough evidence to recommend NPWT for open abdominal wounds (NICE 2009). See Figure 14.12 and Figure 14.13 for examples of NPWT.

PRE-PROCEDURAL CONSIDERATIONS

Consulting the appropriate company representative for training is essential as application and approaches are individually determined and companies have their own comprehensive clinical guidelines. There are specific types of foams and gauze dressings which should be used in undermined wounds, tunnels or sinus tracts. See the list of websites at the end of the chapter for contact details. If the patient is discharged into the community with

Figure 14.12 **Negative pressure wound therapy: dressing.**

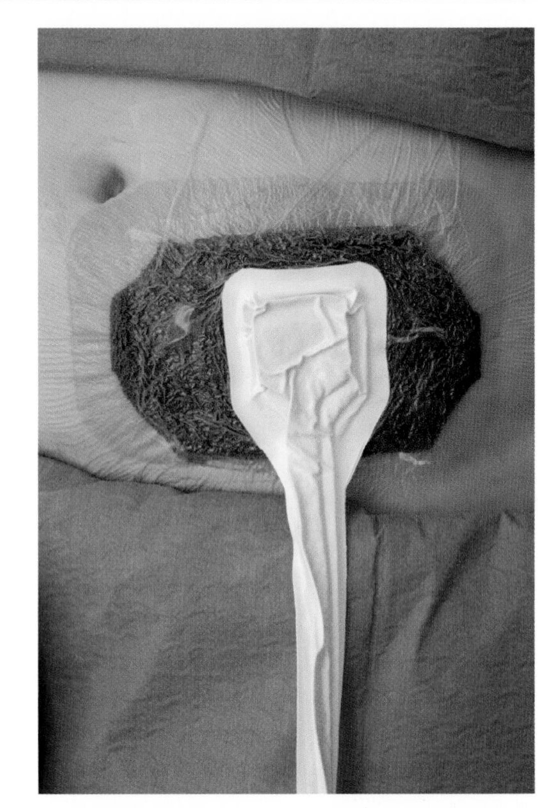

Figure 14.13 **Negative pressure wound therapy: pump.**

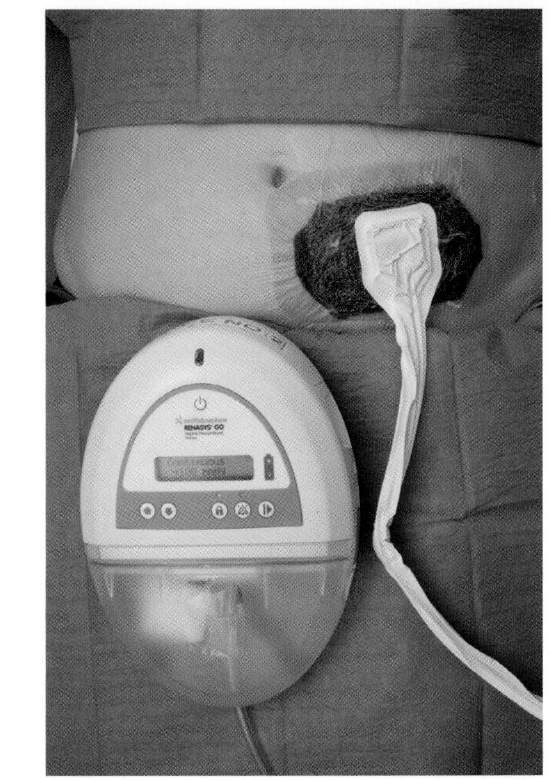

NPWT, consideration should be given to the managment of the dressings, the patient's mobility, risk of falls and psychological capability to cope with the therapy (Milne 2013).

Equipment

All equipment used should be the manufacturer's recommended materials for the relevant system (KCI 2007).

Procedure guideline 14.5 Negative pressure wound therapy

Essential equipment

- NPWT unit
- NPWT dressing pack; foam or gauze
- NPWT canister and tubing
- Forceps
- Sterile scissors
- Sterile gloves
- Apron
- Dressing procedure pack
- Sterile 0.9% sodium chloride for irrigation (warmed to approx. 37°C in a jug of warm water)

Optional equipment

- Extra semi-permeable film dressings to seal any leaks
- Non-adherent wound contact layer to prevent foam adhering to wound bed
- Alcohol-free skin barrier film to protect any fragile or macerated skin around the wound or thin hydrocolloid to protect peri-wound area

Pre-procedure

Action	Rationale
1 Explain and discuss the procedure with the patient and gain thier consent.	To ensure the patient understands the procedure and other options available and gives their valid consent (NMC 2013, **C**).
2 Provide routine analgesia prior to dressing procedure.	To prevent unnecessary procedural pain. **E**
3 Ensure there is adequate lighting and the patient is comfortable and in a position where the wound can be accessed and viewed easily. Assemble all necessary equipment.	To allow access to area for dressing change. Dressing application can be complicated and prolonged so the patient should be in a comfortable position for the procedure. **E**

Procedure

Action	Rationale
4 Use aseptic technique and sterile equipment (as listed above). See Figure 14.12 and Figure 14.13.	To prevent infection (Fraise and Bradley 2009, **E**; Pudner 2005, **E**).
5 To remove the NPWT dressing, put on a pair of non-sterile gloves.	To reduce the risk of cross-infection (Pudner 2005, **E**).
6 Clamp the dressing tubing and disconnect it from the canister tubing. Allow any fluid in the canister tubing to be sucked into the canister. Switch off the pump and clamp the canister tubing.	To prevent spillage of body fluid waste from the tubing or canister. **E**
7 Remove and discard the canister (if full or at least weekly).	To prevent pump alarming and for infection control. **E**
8 Carefully remove the occlusive film drape by gently lifting one edge and then stretching the drape horizontally and slowly remove from the skin.	To prevent damage to the periwound skin. **E**
9 Carefully remove the wound filler.	To prevent damage to newly formed tissue within the wound bed and prevent pain. **E**
10 Irrigate with sterile 0.9% sodium chloride if indicated.	To prevent infection and remove surface debris/necrotic tissue (Dealey 2005, **E**).
11 Debride the wound if applicable.	To remove loose necrotic tissue that may be a focus for infection (Vowden and Vowden 2002, **E**).
12 To apply the dressing, cut the NPWT foam to fit the size and shape of the wound. Appropriate foam or gauze should be used if tunnelling and undermined areas are present.	The foam should fit the wound exactly to ensure full benefit of the negative pressure therapy. **E**
13 Avoid cutting the foam over the wound bed.	To prevent loose particles of foam falling into the wound. **E**
14 Place the foam into the wound cavity.	The whole wound bed must be covered with foam. If the foam is touching, it will transfer the negative pressure to the next piece. **E**

(continued)

Procedure guideline 14.5 Negative pressure wound therapy *(continued)*

Action	Rationale
15 If the wound bed is friable/granulating and likely to bleed, a non-adherent contact layer may be used under the foam to protect the extracellular matrix (ECM).	The ECM requires a trauma-free dressing removal and, once the exudate subsides, the wound bed may become less moist (Flett et al. 2002, **E**).
16 Cut the occlusive film drape to size and apply over the top of the foam. The film should extend 5 cm from the wound margin and not be stretched or applied under pressure. (NB: Do not compress the foam into the wound.)	To obtain a good seal around the wound edges. **E**
17 Choose a location on the sealed occlusive film drape to apply the tubing where the tubing will not rub or cause pressure. Cut a hole through the film (size dependent on system being used), leaving the foam intact.	To reduce the risk of pressure injury to skin. **E**
18 Align the opening of the port over the hole in the film. Apply gentle pressure to anchor the port to the film.	To ensure correct position and seal of the pad (Smith and Nephew 2011, **C**).
19 To commence the NPWT, insert the canister into the pump until it clicks into place. (Do not clamp any part of the canister tubing.)	Indicates the canister is positioned correctly and is secure. **E** The pump will alarm if the tubing is clamped or not connected. **E**
20 Connect the dressing tubing to the canister tubing.	To complete the circuit set-up. **E**
21 Press POWER button and follow the on-screen instructions to set the level and type of pressure required according to instructions from the patient's medical/surgical team.	To ensure the therapy is set to the individual requirements of the patient. **E**
22 When therapy is commenced the foam should collapse into the wound, be firm to touch and have a wrinkled appearance (Smith and Nephew 2011).	Any small air leak will prevent the foam dressing from contracting and reassessment is required. **E**
Post-procedure	
23 Document the dressings and settings, frequency of changes, wound description and exudate in the patient's notes.	To provide a record of care in the patient's care plan (NMC 2010, **C**).

POST-PROCEDURAL CONSIDERATIONS

Ongoing care

Careful monitoring of the periwound area for signs of infection, skin breakdown or oedema and checking the equipment whilst *in situ* are imperative to ensure patient safety. The dressings should be changed every 48–72 hours. The NPWT unit should not be switched off for more than 2 hours without the dressing being replaced (KCI 2007).

Learning for practice

After studying this chapter, list five key points you have learnt about wound management that you will be able to apply to your clinical practice.

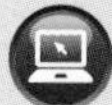

For further learning exercises visit **www.royalmarsdenmanual.com/student**.

Now Test Yourself

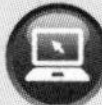

This section provides a range of exercises/activities to further test your learning. For additional exercises visit **www.royalmarsdenmanual.com/student**.

What have you learnt?

1 The skin is the largest organ in the body. What percentage of adult total bodyweight does it represent?
A 1%
B 5%
C 10%
D 20%

2 A chronic wound moves through the stages of the healing process in a predictable time frame.
A True
B False

3 How long is the inflammatory phase of wound healing?
- A A few minutes
- B Up to 5 days
- C Up to 24 days
- D 21 days and beyond

4 What are the three major extrinsic factors that are significant in the development of pressure ulcers?

5 What are the benefits of negative pressure wound therapy?
- A Creates a moist wound environment
- B Stimulates granulation
- C Protects the wound from contamination
- D All of the above

See the end of the chapter for the answers.

Key points

- Both external and internal factors can contribute to the formation of a wound so a holistic approach is essential for accurate assessment and planning care.
- Wound healing is the process by which damaged tissue is restored to normal function. Healing may occur by primary, secondary or tertiary intention.
- The four phases of wound healing are haemostasis, inflammatory phase, proliferation or reconstructive phase and maturation phase.
- The wound should be evaluated each time a dressing is applied or if the wound gives cause for concern. The aim of evaluating the wound is to assess healing and to establish which treatment will best provide the ideal environment for healing.
- Healthcare professionals should be aware of signs that may indicate incipient pressure ulcer development including persistent erythema, non-blanching hyperaemia, blisters, discoloration, localized heat, localized oedema and localized induration.

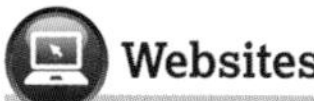

Websites

Aspen Medical: www.aspenmedicaleurope.com
Coloplast: www.coloplast.co.uk
Convatec: www.convatec.co.uk
European Pressure Ulcer Advisory Panel (EUAP): www.epuap.org
Insight Medical: www.insightmedical.net
KCI: www.kci-medical.com
Molnlycke Health Care: www.molnlycke.com
Smith and Nephew: www.wound.smith-nephew.com/uk
World Wide Wounds: Dressings Datacards: www.worldwidewounds.com
World Wide Wounds: Product Reviews: www.wounds-uk.com

REFERENCES

Bale, S. & Jones, V. (2006) *Wound Care Nursing: A Patient-Centred Approach.* Edinburgh: Mosby Elsevier.

Benbow, M. (2005) *Evidence-Based Wound Management.* London: Whurr Publishers.

Bennett, G., Dealey, C. & Posnett, J. (2004) The cost of pressure ulcers in the UK. *Age and Aging*, 33(3), 230–235.

Bianco, M. & Williams, C. (2002) Using photography in wound assessment. *Practice Nursing*, 13(11), 505–508.

Bluestein, D. & Javaheri, A. (2008) Pressure ulcers: prevention, evaluation, and management. *American Family Physician*, 78(10), 1186–1194.

Broderick, N. (2009) Understanding chronic wound healing. *Nurse Practitioner*, 34(10), 16–22.

Butcher, M. (2012) PHMB: an effective antimicrobial in wound bioburden management. *British Journal of Nursing (Tissue Viability Supplement)*, 21(12), S16–19.

Cho, M. & Hunt, T.K. (2001) The overall approach to wounds. In: Falanga, V. (ed.) *Cutaneous Wound Healing.* London: Martin Dunitz.

Clark, A. (2004) Understanding the principles of suturing minor skin lesions. *Nursing Times*, 100(29), 32–34.

Collier, M. (2002) Wound-bed preparation. *Nursing Times*, 98(2), 55–57.

Coulthard, P., Worthington, H., Esposito, M., et al. (2004) Tissue adhesives for closure of surgical incisions. *Cochrane Database of Systematic Reviews*, 2, CD004287.

ConvaTec (2004) *ConvaTec Wound Care Reference Guide.* Uxbridge: ConvaTec.

Cutting, K. (2011) Why use topical antiseptics? *Journal of Wound Care*, Supplement: The Silver Debate, 4–7.

Dealey, C. (2005) *The Care of Wounds: A Guide for Nurses.* Oxford: Blackwell Science.

DH (2005) *Saving Lives: A Delivery Programme to Reduce Health Associated Infection Including MRSA.* London: Department of Health.

Dowsett, C. (2002) The role of the nurse in wound bed preparation. *Nursing Standard*, 16(44), 69–72, 74, 76.

Dowsett, C. & Ayello, E. (2004) TIME principles of chronic wound bed preparation and treatment. *British Journal of Nursing*, 13(15), S16–23.

Eagle, M. (2009) Wound assessment: the patient and the wound. *Wound Essentials*, 4, 14–24.

Fairbairn, K., Grier, J., Hunter, C. & Preece, J. (2002) A sharp debridement procedure devised by specialist nurses. *Journal of Wound Care*, 11(10), 371–375.

Falanga, V. (2004) *Position Document: Wound Bed Preparation: Science Applied to Practice.* London: European Wound Management Association, pp.2–5.

Flett, A., Russell, F., Stringfellow, S., Cooper, P. & Gray, D. (2002) Modern wound management: an update of common products. *Nursing and Residential Care*, 4(7), 328–342.

Fraise, A.P. & Bradley, T. (eds) (2009) *Ayliffe's Control of Healthcare-Associated Infection: A Practical Handbook*, 5th edn. London: Hodder Arnold.

Giddings, F. (2013) *Surgical Knots and Suturing Techniques*, 4th edn. Fort Collins, CO: Giddings Studio Publishing.

Giele, H. & Cassell, O. (2008) *Plastic and Reconstructive Surgery.* Oxford: Oxford University Press.

Gray, D., White, R., Cooper, P. & Kingsley, A. (2010) Applied wound management and using the wound healing continuum in practice. *Wound Essentials*, 5, 131–139.

Hall, S. (2007) A review of the effect of tap water versus normal saline on infection rates in acute traumatic wounds. *Journal of Wound Care*, 16(1), 38–41.

Hampton, S. (2013) Exudate management. *Exudate Management*, 4–7.

Hampton, S. & Collins, F. (2004) *Tissue Viability: The Prevention, Treatment, and Management of Wounds.* London: Whurr Publishers.

Hart, J. (2002) Inflammation. 1: Its role in the healing of acute wounds. *Journal of Wound Care*, 11(6), 205–209.
Henderson, V., Timmins, J., Hurd, T., et al. (2010) NPWT in everyday practice made easy. *Wounds International*, 1(5).
Hess, C. (2005) *Wound Care*. Philadelphia: Lippincott Williams & Wilkins.
Hughes, S. & Mardell, A. (2009) *Oxford Handbook of Perioperative Practice*. Oxford: Oxford University Press.
Jain, S. (2013) *Basic Surgical Skills and Techniques*, 2nd edn. London: Jaypee Brothers Medical Publishers Ltd.
Jones, J. (2013) Exploring the link between the clinical challenges of wound exudate and infection. *Exudate Management*, 8–12.
KCI (2007) *V.A.C. Therapy Clinical Guidelines: A Reference Source for Clinicians*. Available at: www.kci1.com/KCI1/vacfaq.
Kingsley, A. (2008) Aseptic technique: a review of the literature. *Wound Essentials*, 3, 134–141.
Kirk, R. (2010) *Basic Surgical Techniques*, 6th edn. London: Churchill Livingstone.
Leaper, D. (2011) An overview of the evidence on the efficacy of silver dressings. *Journal of Wound Care, Supplement: The Silver Debate*, 8–13.
Lippincott Williams & Wilkins (2008) *Wound Care Made Incredibly Visual!* Philadelphia: Wolters Kluwer Health/Lippincott Williams & Wilkins.
Marieb, E.N. & Hoehn, K. (2010) *Human Anatomy & Physiology*. San Francisco: Benjamin Cummings.
Martin, E.A. (2010) *Concise Colour Medical Dictionary*. Oxford: Oxford University Press.
McInnes, E., Jammali-Blasi, A., Bell-Syer, S., et al. (2011) Support surfaces for pressure ulcer prevention. *Cochrane Database of Systematic Reviews*, 4, CD001735.
McKirdy, L.W. (2001) Burn wound cleansing. *Journal of Community Nursing*, 15(5), 24–29.
Milne, J. (2013) Effective use of negative pressure wound therapy. *Practice Nursing*, 24(1), 14–19.
Moffatt, C. (2004) Wound bed preparation in practice. EWMA Position Document. Medical Education Partnership Ltd. Available at: www.woundsinternational.com
NICE (2009) *Negative Pressure Wound Therapy for the Open Abdomen*. Available at: www.nice.org.uk/nicemedia/pdf/IPG322Guidance.pdf.
NMC (2010) *Record Keeping: Guidance for Nurses and Midwives*. Available at: www.nmc-uk.org/Documents/NMC-Publications/NMC-Record-Keeping-Guidance.pdf.
NMC (2013) *Consent*. London: Nursing and Midwifery Council. www.nmc-uk.org/Nurses-and-midwives/Regulation-in-practice/Regulation-in-Practice-Topics/consent/
NMC (2015) *The Code: Standards of Conduct, Performance and Ethics for Nurses and Midwives*. Available at: www.nmc-uk.org/Publications/Standards/The-code/Introduction/.
NPUAP/EPUAP/PPPIA (2014) *Prevention and treatment of pressure ulcers: Quick reference guide*. Available at: www.epuap.org/wp-content/uploads/2010/10/NPUAP-EPUAP-PPPIA-quick-reference-guide-2014-digital.pdf
Probst, S. & Huljev, D. (2013) The effective management of wounds with high levels of exudate. *British Journal of Nursing (Tissue Viability Supplement)*, 22(6), S34.
Pudner, R. (2005) *Wound Healing in the Surgical Patient*. Edinburgh: Churchill Livingstone Elsevier.
RCN (2005) *The Management of Pressure Ulcers in Primary and Secondary Care: A Clinical Practice Guideline*. London: Royal College of Nursing.
Reynolds, T. & Cole, E. (2006) Techniques for acute wound closure. *Nursing Standard*, 20(21), 55–64.
Richardson, M. (2007) Exploring various methods for closing traumatic wounds. *Nursing Times*, 103(5), 30–31.
Rothrock, J. (2011) *Alexander's Care of the Patient in Surgery*, 14th edn. St Louis, MO: Mosby Elsevier.
Royal Marsden NHS Foundation Trust (2013) *Pressure Ulcer Risk Assessment and Prevention*. Royal Marsden Hospital Intranet, 1–39.
Silver, I. (1994) The physiology of wound healing. *Journal of Wound Care*, 3(2), 106–109.
Smith and Nephew (2011) *NPWT Clinical Guidelines*. Hull: Smith & Nephew.
Springett, K. (2002) The impact of diabetes on wound management. *Nursing Standard*, 16(30), 72–74, 76, 78–80.
Stephen-Hayes, J. (2007) The different methods of wound debridement. *British Journal of Community Nursing*, 12(6 Supplement), 6–16.
Storch, J.E. & Rice, J. (2005) *Reconstructive Plastic Surgical Nursing: Clinical Management and Wound Care*. Oxford: Blackwell Publishing.
Tanner, J., Woodings, D. & Moncaster, K. (2006) Preoperative hair removal to reduce surgical site infection. *Cochrane Database of Systematic Reviews*, 3, CD004122.
Teare, J. & Barrett, C. (2002) Using quality of life assessment in wound care. *Nursing Standard*, 17(6), 59–60, 64, 67–58.
Thomas, S. (2009) *Formulary of Wound Management Products*. Liphook: Euromed Communications.
Timmons, J. (2006) Skin function and wound healing physiology. *Wound Essentials*, 8–17.
Tortora, G.J. & Derrickson, B. (2011) *Principles of Anatomy and Physiology*, 13th edn. Hoboken, NJ: John Wiley & Sons.
Tulloh, B. & Lee, D. (2007) *Foundations of Operative Surgery: An Introduction to Surgical Techniques*. Oxford: Oxford University Press.
Ubbink, D., Westerbos, S., Evans, D., et al. (2008) Topical negative pressure for treating chronic wounds. *Cochrane Database of Systematic Reviews*, 3, CD001898.
Vowden, K. & Vowden, P. (2002) *Wound Bed Preparation*. World Wide Wounds. Available at: www.worldwidewounds.com/2002/april/Vowden/Wound-Bed-Preparation.html
Waterlow, J. (2007) *The Waterlow Assessment Tool*. Available at: www.judy–waterlow.co.uk/waterlow_score.htm.
Watret, L. & Armitage, M. (2002) Making sense of wound cleansing. *Journal of Community Nursing*, 16(4), 27–34.
Weinzweig, J. (2010) *Plastic Surgery Secrets Plus*, 2nd edn. Philadelphia: Mosby Elsevier.
Werdin, F., Tenenhaus, M. & Rennekampff, H. (2008) Chronic wound care. *Lancet*, 372(9653), 1860–1862.
Wicker, P. & O'Neill, J. (2010) *Caring for the Perioperative Patient*, 2nd edn. Chichester: Wiley–Blackwell.
Widgerow, A. (2013) *Surgical Wounds*. Oxford: John Wiley & Sons.
Woolcott, R., Kennedy, J. & Dowd, S. (2009) Regular debridement is the main tool for maintaining a healthy wound in most chronic wounds. *Journal of Wound Care*, 18(2), 54–56.
Yarwood-Ross, L. (2013) Silicone dressings are a good fit in the wound care jigsaw. *British Journal of Nursing (Tissue Viability Supplement)*, 22(6), S22.
Young, T. (2012) Managing wound infection. *Independent Nurse*, 2(4).

Answers

Learning Activity 14.3 Case study: Pressure ulcer

Mr Toomey is an 83-year-old gentleman who has had a previous above-knee amputation for peripheral vascular disease. He has very limited mobility and recently has become increasingly confused, in that he has been forgetting to eat and drink. He now spends the majority of his days sitting in his armchair and has had some episodes of urinary incontinence. He was seen at home by his GP who identified that he has a pressure sore on his right buttock and also diagnosed that he has a severe urinary tract infection. He has been admitted to the ward for intravenous antibiotics and also assessment of his pressure ulcer.

1 What factors contributed to the pressure ulcer occurring? Were any of these avoidable?
- Contributory factors include: immobility, impaired nutrition, peripheral vascular disease, incontinence, confusion and infection. The impaired nutritional intake and the limited mobility could have been reduced with appropriate care. The incontinence could have been assessed earlier and steps taken to manage it appropriately and to treat the urinary tract infection.

You have been asked to assess his skin integrity including the pressure ulcer on his right buttock.

2 What should you be observing for?
- Assess all his pressure areas for erythema.
- Any broken areas of skin.

3 What tool(s) would help you to carry out a comprehensive assessment?
- Use of the Waterlow pressure ulcer risk assessment would assess his overall risk of developing further pressure ulcers.
- Use of a pressure ulcer classification system would identify the stage of his pressure sore.
- A wound assessment chart would accurately document his existing pressure ulcer and intended management.

His pressure ulcer has been assessed as grade 2.

4 What measures should be put in place to manage the pressure ulcer and avoid any further skin deterioration?
- Repositioning equipment
- Correct use of manual handling devices
- Patient information and orientation aids/prompts to boost, and then maintain, his nutritional status and hydration
- Transparent film dressing (retains moisture, prevents friction)

Now Test Yourself **What have you learnt?**

1 The skin is the largest organ in the body. What percentage of adult total bodyweight does it represent?
A 1%
B 5%
C 10%
D 20%

2 A chronic wound moves through the stages of the healing process in a predictable time frame.
A True
B False – an acute wound does; a chronic wound does not heal over a set period of time regardless of the cause

3 How long is the inflammatory phase of wound healing?
A A few minutes
B Up to 5 days
C Up to 24 days
D 21 days and beyond

4 What are the three major extrinsic factors that are significant in the development of pressure ulcers?
- Pressure
- Shearing
- Friction

5 What are the benefits of negative pressure wound therapy?
A Creates a moist wound environment
B Stimulates granulation
C Protects the wound from contamination
D All of the above

Appendix: The Code

The Royal Marsden Manual of Clinical Nursing Procedures: Student Edition, Ninth Edition. Edited by Lisa Dougherty, Sara Lister and Alexandra West-Oram

The Code

Professional standards of practice and behaviour for nurses and midwives

Introduction

The Code contains the professional standards that registered nurses and midwives must uphold. UK nurses and midwives must act in line with the Code, whether they are providing direct care to individuals, groups or communities or bringing their professional knowledge to bear on nursing and midwifery practice in other roles, such as leadership, education or research. While you can interpret the values and principles set out in the Code in a range of different practice settings, they are not negotiable or discretionary.

Our role is to set the standards in the Code, but these are not just our standards. They are the standards that patients and members of the public tell us they expect from healthcare professionals. They are the standards shown every day by good nurses and midwives across the UK.

When joining our register, and then renewing their registration, nurses and midwives commit to upholding these standards. This commitment to professional standards is fundamental to being part of a profession. We can take action if registered nurses or midwives fail to uphold the Code. In serious cases, this can include removing them from the register.

The Code should be useful for everyone who cares about good nursing and midwifery:

- patients and service users, and those who care for them, can use it to provide feedback to nurses and midwives about the care they receive
- nurses and midwives can use it to promote safe and effective practice in their place of work
- employer organizations should support their staff in upholding the standards in their professional Code as part of providing the quality and safety expected by service users and regulators
- educators can use the Code to help students understand what it means to be a registered professional and how keeping to the Code helps to achieve that.

For the many committed and expert practitioners on our register, this Code should be seen as a way of reinforcing their professionalism. Through revalidation, you will provide fuller, richer evidence of your continued ability to practise safely and effectively when you renew your registration. The Code will be central in the revalidation process as a focus for professional reflection. This will give the Code significance in your professional life, and raise its status and importance for employers.

The Code contains a series of statements that taken together signify what good nursing and midwifery practice looks like. It puts the interests of patients and service users first, is safe and effective, and promotes trust through professionalism.

Prioritize people

You put the interests of people using or needing nursing or midwifery services first. You make their care and safety your main concern and make sure that their dignity is preserved and their needs are recognized, assessed and responded to. You make sure that those receiving care are treated with respect, that their rights are upheld and that any discriminatory attitudes and behaviours towards those receiving care are challenged.

1 Treat people as individuals and uphold their dignity

To achieve this, you must:

1.1 treat people with kindness, respect and compassion
1.2 make sure you deliver the fundamentals of care effectively
1.3 avoid making assumptions and recognize diversity and individual choice
1.4 make sure that any treatment, assistance or care for which you are responsible is delivered without undue delay, and
1.5 respect and uphold people's human rights.

(The fundamentals of care include, but are not limited to, nutrition, hydration, bladder and bowel care, physical handling and making sure that those receiving care are kept in clean and hygienic conditions. It includes making sure that those receiving care have adequate access to nutrition and hydration, and making sure that you provide help to those who are not able to feed themselves or drink fluid unaided.)

2 Listen to people and respond to their preferences and concerns

To achieve this, you must:

2.1 work in partnership with people to make sure you deliver care effectively
2.2 recognize and respect the contribution that people can make to their own health and wellbeing
2.3 encourage and empower people to share decisions about their treatment and care
2.4 respect the level to which people receiving care want to be involved in decisions about their own health, wellbeing and care
2.5 respect, support and document a person's right to accept or refuse care and treatment, and
2.6 recognize when people are anxious or in distress and respond compassionately and politely.

3 Make sure that people's physical, social and psychological needs are assessed and responded to

To achieve this, you must:

3.1 pay special attention to promoting wellbeing, preventing ill health and meeting the changing health and care needs of people during all life stages

3.2 recognize and respond compassionately to the needs of those who are in the last few days and hours of life

3.3 act in partnership with those receiving care, helping them to access relevant health and social care, information and support when they need it, and

3.4 act as an advocate for the vulnerable, challenging poor practice and discriminatory attitudes and behaviour relating to their care.

4 Act in the best interests of people at all times

To achieve this, you must:

4.1 balance the need to act in the best interests of people at all times with the requirement to respect a person's right to accept or refuse treatment

4.2 make sure that you get properly informed consent and document it before carrying out any action

4.3 keep to all relevant laws about mental capacity that apply in the country in which you are practising, and make sure that the rights and best interests of those who lack capacity are still at the centre of the decision-making process, and

4.4 tell colleagues, your manager and the person receiving care if you have a conscientious objection to a particular procedure and arrange for a suitably qualified colleague to take over responsibility for that person's care.

(You can only make a 'conscientious objection' in limited circumstances. For more information, please visit our website at www.nmc-uk.org/standards.)

5 Respect people's right to privacy and confidentiality

As a nurse or midwife, you owe a duty of confidentiality to all those who are receiving care. This includes making sure that they are informed about their care and that information about them is shared appropriately.

To achieve this, you must:

5.1 respect a person's right to privacy in all aspects of their care

5.2 make sure that people are informed about how and why information is used and shared by those who will be providing care

5.3 respect that a person's right to privacy and confidentiality continues after they have died

5.4 share necessary information with other healthcare professionals and agencies only when the interests of patient safety and public protection override the need for confidentiality, and

5.5 share with people, their families and their carers, as far as the law allows, the information they want or need to know about their health, care and ongoing treatment sensitively and in a way they can understand.

Practise effectively

]You assess need and deliver or advise on treatment, or give help (including preventative or rehabilitative care) without too much delay and to the best of your abilities, on the basis of the best evidence available and best practice. You communicate effectively, keeping clear and accurate records and sharing skills, knowledge and experience where appropriate. You reflect and act on any feedback you receive to improve your practice.

6 Always practise in line with the best available evidence

To achieve this, you must:

6.1 make sure that any information or advice given is evidence-based, including information relating to using any healthcare products or services, and

6.2 maintain the knowledge and skills you need for safe and effective practice.

7 Communicate clearly

To achieve this, you must:

7.1 use terms that people in your care, colleagues and the public can understand

7.2 take reasonable steps to meet people's language and communication needs, providing, wherever possible, assistance to those who need help to communicate their own or other people's needs

7.3 use a range of verbal and non-verbal communication methods, and consider cultural sensitivities, to better understand and respond to people's personal and health needs

7.4 check people's understanding from time to time to keep misunderstanding or mistakes to a minimum, and

7.5 be able to communicate clearly and effectively in English.

8 Work cooperatively

To achieve this, you must:

8.1 respect the skills, expertise and contributions of your colleagues, referring matters to them when appropriate

8.2 maintain effective communication with colleagues

8.3 keep colleagues informed when you are sharing the care of individuals with other healthcare professionals and staff

8.4 work with colleagues to evaluate the quality of your work and that of the team

8.5 work with colleagues to preserve the safety of those receiving care

8.6 share information to identify and reduce risk, and

8.7 be supportive of colleagues who are encountering health or performance problems. However, this support must never compromise or be at the expense of patient or public safety.

9 Share your skills, knowledge and experience for the benefit of people receiving care and your colleagues

To achieve this, you must:

9.1 provide honest, accurate and constructive feedback to colleagues

9.2 gather and reflect on feedback from a variety of sources, using it to improve your practice and performance

9.3 deal with differences of professional opinion with colleagues by discussion and informed debate, respecting their views and opinions and behaving in a professional way at all times, and

9.4 support students' and colleagues' learning to help them develop their professional competence and confidence.

10 Keep clear and accurate records relevant to your practice

This includes but is not limited to patient records. It includes all records that are relevant to your scope of practice.

To achieve this, you must:

10.1 complete all records at the time or as soon as possible after an event, recording if the notes are written some time after the event
10.2 identify any risks or problems that have arisen and the steps taken to deal with them, so that colleagues who use the records have all the information they need
10.3 complete all records accurately and without any falsification, taking immediate and appropriate action if you become aware that someone has not kept to these requirements
10.4 attribute any entries you make in any paper or electronic records to yourself, making sure they are clearly written, dated and timed, and do not include unnecessary abbreviations, jargon or speculation
10.5 take all steps to make sure that all records are kept securely, and
10.6 collect, treat and store all data and research findings appropriately.

11 Be accountable for your decisions to delegate tasks and duties to other people

To achieve this, you must:

11.1 only delegate tasks and duties that are within the other person's scope of competence, making sure that they fully understand your instructions
11.2 make sure that everyone you delegate tasks to is adequately supervised and supported so they can provide safe and compassionate care, and
11.3 confirm that the outcome of any task you have delegated to someone else meets the required standard.

12 Have in place an indemnity arrangement which provides appropriate cover for any practice you take on as a nurse or midwife in the United Kingdom

To achieve this, you must:

12.1 make sure that you have an appropriate indemnity arrangement in place relevant to your scope of practice.

For more information, please visit: www.nmc-uk.org/indemnity.

Preserve safety

You make sure that patient and public safety is protected. You work within the limits of your competence, exercising your professional 'duty of candour' and raising concerns immediately whenever you come across situations that put patients or public safety at risk. You take necessary action to deal with any concerns where appropriate.

13 Recognize and work within the limits of your competence

To achieve this, you must:

13.1 accurately assess signs of normal or worsening physical and mental health in the person receiving care
13.2 make a timely and appropriate referral to another practitioner when it is in the best interests of the individual needing any action, care or treatment
13.3 ask for help from a suitably qualified and experienced healthcare professional to carry out any action or procedure that is beyond the limits of your competence
13.4 take account of your own personal safety as well as the safety of people in your care, and
13.5 complete the necessary training before carrying out a new role.

14 Be open and candid with all service users about all aspects of care and treatment, including when any mistakes or harm have taken place

To achieve this, you must:

14.1 act immediately to put right the situation if someone has suffered actual harm for any reason or an incident has happened which had the potential for harm
14.2 explain fully and promptly what has happened, including the likely effects, and apologize to the person affected and, where appropriate, their advocate, family or carers, and
14.3 document all these events formally and take further action (escalate) if appropriate so they can be dealt with quickly.

(The professional duty of candour is about openness and honesty when things go wrong. 'Every healthcare professional must be open and honest with patients when something goes wrong with their treatment or care which causes, or has the potential to cause, harm or distress.' Joint statement from the Chief Executives of statutory regulators of healthcare professionals.)

15 Always offer help if an emergency arises in your practice setting or anywhere else

To achieve this, you must:

15.1 only act in an emergency within the limits of your knowledge and competence
15.2 arrange, wherever possible, for emergency care to be accessed and provided promptly, and
15.3 take account of your own safety, the safety of others and the availability of other options for providing care.

16 Act without delay if you believe that there is a risk to patient safety or public protection

To achieve this, you must:

16.1 raise and, if necessary, escalate any concerns you may have about patient or public safety, or the level of care people are receiving in your workplace or any other healthcare setting and use the channels available to you in line with our guidance and your local working practices
16.2 raise your concerns immediately if you are being asked to practise beyond your role, experience and training
16.3 tell someone in authority at the first reasonable opportunity if you experience problems that may prevent you working within the Code or other national standards, taking prompt action to tackle the causes of concern if you can
16.4 acknowledge and act on all concerns raised to you, investigating, escalating or dealing with those concerns where it is appropriate for you to do so
16.5 not obstruct, intimidate, victimize or in any way hinder a colleague, member of staff, person you care for or member of the public who wants to raise a concern, and
16.6 protect anyone you have management responsibility for from any harm, detriment, victimization or unwarranted treatment after a concern is raised.

For more information, please visit: www.nmc-uk.org/raisingconcerns.

17 Raise concerns immediately if you believe a person is vulnerable or at risk and needs extra support and protection

To achieve this, you must:

17.1 take all reasonable steps to protect people who are vulnerable or at risk from harm, neglect or abuse
17.2 share information if you believe someone may be at risk of harm, in line with the laws relating to the disclosure of information, and
17.3 have knowledge of and keep to the relevant laws and policies about protecting and caring for vulnerable people.

18 Advise on, prescribe, supply, dispense or administer medicines within the limits of your training and competence, the law, our guidance and other relevant policies, guidance and regulations

To achieve this, you must:

18.1 prescribe, advise on, or provide medicines or treatment, including repeat prescriptions (only if you are suitably qualified) if you have enough knowledge of that person's health and are satisfied that the medicines or treatment serve that person's health needs
18.2 keep to appropriate guidelines when giving advice on using controlled drugs and recording the prescribing, supply, dispensing or administration of controlled drugs
18.3 make sure that the care or treatment you advise on, prescribe, supply, dispense or administer for each person is compatible with any other care or treatment they are receiving, including (where possible) over-the-counter medicines
18.4 take all steps to keep medicines stored securely, and
18.5 wherever possible, avoid prescribing for yourself or for anyone with whom you have a close personal relationship.

For more information, please visit: www.nmc-uk.org/standards.

19 Be aware of, and reduce as far as possible, any potential for harm associated with your practice

To achieve this, you must:

19.1 take measures to reduce as far as possible, the likelihood of mistakes, near misses, harm and the effect of harm if it takes place
19.2 take account of current evidence, knowledge and developments in reducing mistakes and the effect of them and the impact of human factors and system failures (see the note below)
19.3 keep to and promote recommended practice in relation to controlling and preventing infection, and
19.4 take all reasonable personal precautions necessary to avoid any potential health risks to colleagues, people receiving care and the public.

('Human factors refer to environmental, organisational and job factors, and human and individual characteristics, which influence behaviour at work in a way which can affect health and safety' Health and Safety Executive. You can find more information at www.hse.gov.uk.)

Promote professionalism and trust

You uphold the reputation of your profession at all times. You should display a personal commitment to the standards of practice and behaviour set out in the Code. You should be a model of integrity and leadership for others to aspire to. This should lead to trust and confidence in the profession from patients, people receiving care, other healthcare professionals and the public.

20 Uphold the reputation of your profession at all times

To achieve this, you must:

20.1 keep to and uphold the standards and values set out in the Code
20.2 act with honesty and integrity at all times, treating people fairly and without discrimination, bullying or harassment
20.3 be aware at all times of how your behaviour can affect and influence the behaviour of other people
20.4 keep to the laws of the country in which you are practising
20.5 treat people in a way that does not take advantage of their vulnerability or cause them upset or distress
20.6 stay objective and have clear professional boundaries at all times with people in your care (including those who have been in your care in the past), their families and carers
20.7 make sure you do not express your personal beliefs (including political, religious or moral beliefs) to people in an inappropriate way
20.8 act as a role model of professional behaviour for students and newly qualified nurses and midwives to aspire to
20.9 maintain the level of health you need to carry out your professional role, and
20.10 use all forms of spoken, written and digital communication (including social media and networking sites) responsibly, respecting the right to privacy of others at all times.

For more guidance on using social media and networking sites, please visit: www.nmc-uk.org/guidance.

21 Uphold your position as a registered nurse or midwife

To achieve this, you must:

21.1 refuse all but the most trivial gifts, favours or hospitality as accepting them could be interpreted as an attempt to gain preferential treatment
21.2 never ask for or accept loans from anyone in your care or anyone close to them
21.3 act with honesty and integrity in any financial dealings you have with everyone you have a professional relationship with, including people in your care
21.4 make sure that any advertisements, publications or published material you produce or have produced for your professional services are accurate, responsible, ethical, do not mislead or exploit vulnerabilities and accurately reflect your relevant skills, experience and qualifications
21.5 never use your professional status to promote causes that are not related to health, and
21.6 cooperate with the media only when it is appropriate to do so, and then always protecting the confidentiality and dignity of people receiving treatment or care.

22 Fulfil all registration requirements

To achieve this, you must:

22.1 meet any reasonable requests so we can oversee the registration process
22.2 keep to our prescribed hours of practice and carry out continuing professional development activities, and
22.3 keep your knowledge and skills up to date, taking part in appropriate and regular learning and professional development activities that aim to maintain and develop your competence and improve your performance.

For more information, please visit: www.nmc-uk.org/standards.

23 Cooperate with all investigations and audits

This includes investigations or audits either against you or relating to others, whether individuals or organizations. It also includes cooperating with requests to act as a witness in any hearing that forms part of an investigation, even after you have left the register.

To achieve this, you must:

23.1 cooperate with any audits of training records, registration records or other relevant audits that we may want to carry out to make sure you are still fit to practise

23.2 tell both us and any employers as soon as you can about any caution or charge against you, or if you have received a conditional discharge in relation to, or have been found guilty of, a criminal offence (other than a protected caution or conviction)

23.3 tell any employers you work for if you have had your practice restricted or had any other conditions imposed on you by us or any other relevant body.

23.4 tell us and your employers at the first reasonable opportunity if you are or have been disciplined by any regulatory or licensing organization, including those who operate outside of the professional healthcare environment, and

23.5 give your NMC Pin when any reasonable request for it is made.

(When telling your employers, this includes telling (i) any person, body or organization you are employed by, or intend to be employed by, as a nurse or midwife; and (ii) any person, body or organization with whom you have an arrangement to provide services as a nurse or midwife.)

For more information, please visit: www.nmc-uk.org.

24 Respond to any complaints made against you professionally

To achieve this, you must:

24.1 never allow someone's complaint to affect the care that is provided to them, and

24.2 use all complaints as a form of feedback and an opportunity for reflection and learning to improve practice.

25 Provide leadership to make sure people's wellbeing is protected and to improve their experiences of the healthcare system

To achieve this, you must:

25.1 identify priorities, manage time, staff and resources effectively and deal with risk to make sure that the quality of care or service you deliver is maintained and improved, putting the needs of those receiving care or services first, and

25.2 support any staff you may be responsible for to follow the Code at all times. They must have the knowledge, skills and competence for safe practice; and understand how to raise any concerns linked to any circumstances where the Code has, or could be, broken.

About us

The Nursing and Midwifery Council exists to protect the public. We do this by making sure that only those who meet our requirements are allowed to practise as a nurse or midwife in the UK. We take action if concerns are raised about whether a nurse or midwife is fit to practise.

It is illegal to practise as a nurse or midwife in the UK if you are not on our register.

For more information about the Code, please visit: www.nmc-uk.org/code.

Published 29 January 2015
Effective from 31 March 2015

Index

Page numbers in *italics* refer to figures, and those in **bold** to tables and boxes.

The Royal Marsden Manual of Clinical Nursing Procedures: Student Edition, Ninth Edition. Edited by Lisa Dougherty, Sara Lister and Alexandra West-Oram